a LANGE medical book

Smith & Tanagho's General Urology

EIGHTEENTH EDITION

Edited by

Jack W. McAninch, MD, FACS, FRCS(E)(Hon)
Professor of Urology
University of California School of Medicine
Chief, Department of Urology
San Francisco General Hospital
San Francisco, California

Tom F. Lue, MD, FACS, ScD (Hon)
Professor of Urology
Department of Urology
University of California School of Medicine
San Francisco, California

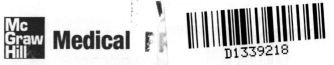

Mc Graw Hill **Medical**

New York   Chicago   San Francisco   Lisbon   London
Milan   New Delhi   San Juan   Seoul   Singapore   Sydney   Toronto

Smith & Tanagho's General Urology, Eighteenth Edition

Copyright © 2013 by The McGraw-Hill Companies, Inc. All rights reserved. Printed in the United States of America. Except as permitted under the United States Copyright Act of 1976, no part of this publication may be reproduced or distributed in any form or by any means, or stored in a data base or retrieval system, without the prior written permission of the publisher.

Previous editions copyright © 2008, 2004, 2001, 2000 by The McGraw-Hill Companies, Inc.

1 2 3 4 5 6 7 8 9 0   DOC/DOC   17 16 15 14 13 12

ISBN 978-0-07-162497-8
MHID 0-07-162497-X
ISSN 0892-1245

Notice

Medicine is an ever-changing science. As new research and clinical experience broaden our knowledge, changes in treatment and drug therapy are required. The authors and the publisher of this work have checked with sources believed to be reliable in their efforts to provide information that is complete and generally in accord with the standards accepted at the time of publication. However, in view of the possibility of human error or changes in medical sciences, neither the authors nor the publisher nor any other party who has been involved in the preparation or publication of this work warrants that the information contained herein is in every respect accurate or complete, and they disclaim all responsibility for any errors or omissions or for the results obtained from use of the information contained in this work. Readers are encouraged to confirm the information contained herein with other sources. For example and in particular, readers are advised to check the product information sheet included in the package of each drug they plan to administer to be certain that the information contained in this work is accurate and that changes have not been made in the recommended dose or in the contraindications for administration. This recommendation is of particular importance in connection with new or infrequently used drugs.

This book was set in Times Roman by Aptara, Inc.
The editors were Brian Belval and Regina Brown.
The production supervisor was Sherri Souffrance.
Project management provided by Indu Jawwad, Aptara, Inc.
The designer was Alan Barnett.
Cover image: X-ray of prostatic adenoma (VEM/Photo Researchers, Inc.)
RR Donnelley was printer and binder.

This book is printed on acid-free paper.

McGraw-Hill books are available at special quantity discounts to use as premiums and sales promotions, or for use in corporate training programs. To contact a representative, please e-mail us at bulksales@mcgraw-hill.com.

International Edition ISBN 978-0-07-174279-5; MHID 0-07-174279-4

Copyright © 2013. Exclusive rights by The McGraw-Hill Companies, Inc., for manufacture and export. This book cannot be reexported from the country to which it is consigned by McGraw-Hill. The International Edition is not available in North America.

Dedication

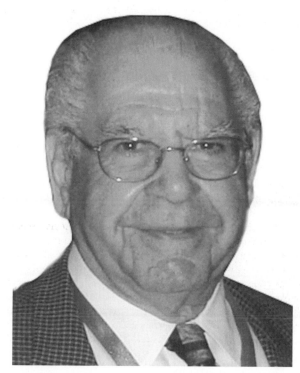

Emil A. Tanagho, MD

Contents

Contributors

Sherif R. Aboseif, MD
Director, West Coast Center for Urinary
  Incontinence and Reconstructive Urology
St. John Medical Center
Oxnard, California

Karl-Erik Andersson, MD, PhD
Institute for Regenerative Medicine
Wake Forest University School of Medicine
Winston Salem, North Carolina

Susan Barbour, RN, MS, WOCN
Clinical Nurse Specialist
University of California Medical Center
San Francisco, California

Laurence S. Baskin, MD
Chief of Pediatric Urology
Department of Urology
University of California Children's Medical Center
San Francisco, California
Attending Urologist
Children's Hospital Oakland
Oakland, California

Peter R. Carroll, MD, MPH
Professor
Ken and Donna Derr-Chevron Endowed Chair in Prostate
  Cancer
Department of Urology
University of California School of Medicine
San Francisco, California

Matthew R. Cooperberg, MD, MPH
Assistant Professor
Department of Urology
UCSF Helen Diller Family Comprehensive Cancer Center
San Francisco, California

Donna Y. Deng, MD, MS
Ken and Donna Derr-Chevron Endowed Chair in Prostate
  Cancer
Department of Urology
University of California School of Medicine
San Francisco, California

Stuart M. Flechner, MD, FACS
Ken and Donna Derr-Chevron Endowed Chair in Prostate
  Cancer
Department of Urology
Cleveland Clinic Foundation
Cleveland, Ohio

Scott Gerst, MD
Associate Attending
Radiology
Memorial Hospital, Memorial Sloan-Kettering Cancer
  Center
New York, New York

Rolf Gillitzer, MD
Associate Professor
Department of Urology
Johannes Gutenberg University
Mainz, Germany

Roy L. Gordon, MD
Professor of Radiology
Department of Radiology
University of California
San Francisco, California

Alexander R. Gottschalk, MD, PhD
Associate Professor
Director of Cyberknife
Department of Radiation Oncology
University of California, San Francisco
San Francisco, California

Kirsten L. Greene, MD, MS
Department of Urology
University of California, San Francisco
San Francisco, California

Hedvig Hricak, MD, PhD
Chairman
Department of Radiology
Memorial Sloan-Kettering Cancer Center
Professor of Radiology
Cornell University
New York, New York

Christopher J. Kane, MD, FACS
Associate Professor of Urology
University of California School of Medicine
Chief
Department of Urology
Veterans Affairs Medical Center
San Francisco, California

Barry A. Kogan, MD
Professor, Surgery and Pediatrics
Falk Chair in Urology
Albany Medical College
Albany, New York

Badrinath R. Konety, MD, MBA
Assistant Professor of Urology and Epidemiology
Department of Urology
University of Iowa
Iowa City, Iowa

John N. Krieger, MD
Professor of Urology
University of Washington
School of Medicine
Seattle, Washington

Brian K. Lee, MD
Assistant Clinical Professor
The Connie Frank Kidney Transplant Center
UCSF Medical Center
San Francisco, California

Tom F. Lue, MD, FACS, ScD (Hon)
Professor of Urology
Department of Urology
University of California School of Medicine
San Francisco, California

Jack W. McAninch, MD, FACS, FRCS(E)(Hon)
Professor of Urology
University of California School of Medicine
Chief
Department of Urology
San Francisco General Hospital
San Francisco, California

Maxwell V. Meng, MD, MPH
Associate Professor
Department of Urology
University of California School of Medicine
San Francisco, California

Hiep T. Nguyen, MD
Associate Professor
Surgery and Urology
Harvard Medical School and Children's Hospital
Boston, Massachussets

Sima P. Porten, MD, MPH
Urology Resident
Department of Urology
University of San Francisco
San Francisco, California

Joseph C. Presti, Jr., MD
Associate Professor of Urology
Director, Genitourinary Oncology Program
Department of Urology
Stanford University School of Medicine
Stanford, California

Mack Roach III, MD
Professor of Radiation Oncology and Urology
Department of Urology
University of California School of Medicine, San Francisco
    Comprehensive Cancer Center
San Francisco, California

Alan W. Shindel, MD
Assistant Professor
Department of Urology
University of California, Davis
Sacramento, California

Katsuto Shinohara, MD
Professor
Helen Diller Family Chair in Clinical Urology
Department of Urology
University of California, San Francisco
San Francisco, California

Eric J. Small, MD
Professor of Medicine and Urology
Urologic Oncology Program
University of California School of Medicine
Program Member
UCSF Comprehensive Cancer Center
San Francisco, California

James F. Smith, MD, MS
Assistant Professor-in-Residence
Director, Male Reproductive Health
Departments of Urology, Obstetrics, Gynecology, and
    Reproductive Sciences
University of California, San Francisco
San Francisco, California

Joycelyn L. Speight, MD, PhD
Clinical Instructor of Radiation Oncology
University of California School of Medicine
Member
UCSF Comprehensive Cancer Center
San Francisco, California

Marshall L. Stoller, MD
Professor of Urology
Department of Urology
University of California School of Medicine
San Francisco, California

Emil A. Tanagho, MD
Professor of Urology
Department of Urology
University of California School of Medicine
San Francisco, California

Joachim W. Thüroff, MD
Professor
Department of Urology
University Medical Center
Mainz, Germany

Flavio G. Vincenti, MD
Clinical Professor
The Connie Frank Kidney Transplant Center
UCSF Medical Center
San Francisco, California

Daniel A. Vaena, MD
Associate Professor
Hematology, Oncology & BMT Service
Departments of Internal Medicine and Urology
University of Iowa
Iowa City, Iowa

Thomas J. Walsh, MD, MS
Assistant Professor
Department of Urology
University of Washington School of Medicine
Seattle, Washington

Richard D. Williams, MD
Professor and Head
Rubin H. Flocks Chair
Department of Urology
University of Iowa
Iowa City, Iowa

J. Stuart Wolf, Jr., MD, FACS
The David A Bloom Professor of Urology
University of Michigan
Ann Arbor, Michigan

Preface

Smith & Tanagho's General Urology, Eighteenth Edition, provides in a concise, well-organized format the information necessary for the understanding, diagnosis, and treatment of diseases managed by urologic surgeons. The book is current, to the point, and readable.

Medical students will find this book useful because of its concise, easy to follow format and organization and its breadth of information on common diseases urologists see and manage. Residents, as well as practicing physicians in urology, family practice, or general medicine will find it an efficient and current reference, particularly because of its emphasis on diagnosis and treatment.

The eighteenth edition has been completely updated with clinical information and current references. The reader will find this edition is written in an uncomplicated, straightforward manner that provides relevant clinical information and guidelines for diagnosis and management of urologic conditions. Chapters on chemotherapy of urologic tumors, neoplasms of the prostate, and vascular interventional radiology have all undergone extensive revision. For this edition, we have added a chapter on the timely topic of robotic surgery in urology.

Many illustrations and figures have been modernized and improved with color being added. The classic fine anatomic drawings demonstrate well the important clinical findings.

This edition is dedicated to Professor Emil A. Tanagho, who served as the principal editor of this text since the eleventh edition. His untiring efforts have made this book one of the leading sources of information for students, trainees, and urologists around the world. In addition to English, the book has been published in Chinese, French, Greek, Italian, Japanese, Korean, Portuguese, Russian, Spanish, and Turkish.

We greatly appreciate the patience and efforts of our McGraw-Hill staff, the expertise of our contributors, and the support of our readers.

Jack W. McAninch, MD, FACS, FRCS(E)(Hon)
Tom F. Lue, MD, FACS, ScD (Hon)
San Francisco, California
August 2012

Anatomy of the Genitourinary Tract

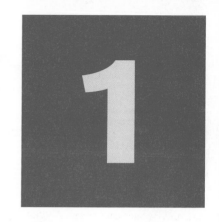

Emil A. Tanagho, MD, & Tom F. Lue, MD, FACS, ScD (Hon)

Urology deals with diseases and disorders of the male genitourinary tract, the female urinary tract, and the adrenal gland. These systems are illustrated in Figures 1–1 and 1–2.

ADRENALS

▶ Gross Appearance

A. Anatomy

Each kidney is capped by an adrenal gland, and both organs are enclosed within Gerota's (perirenal) fascia. Each adrenal weighs about 5 g. The right adrenal is triangular in shape; the left is more rounded and crescentic. Each gland is composed of a cortex, chiefly influenced by the pituitary gland, and a medulla derived from chromaffin tissue (Avisse et al, 2000; O'Donoghue et al, 2010).

B. Relations

Figure 1–2 shows the relation of the adrenals to other organs. The right adrenal lies between the liver and the vena cava. The left adrenal lies close to the aorta and is covered on its lower surface by the pancreas. The spleen lies superior and lateral to it.

▶ Histology

The adrenal cortex, which makes up 90% of the mass, is composed of three distinct layers: the outer zona glomerulosa, the middle zona fasciculata, and the inner zona reticularis. The medulla lies centrally and is made up of polyhedral cells containing eosinophilic granular cytoplasm. These chromaffin cells are accompanied by ganglion and small round cells.

▶ Blood Supply

A. Arterial

Each adrenal receives three arteries: one from the inferior phrenic artery, one from the aorta, and one from the renal artery.

B. Venous

Blood from the right adrenal is drained by a very short vein into the vena cava; the left adrenal vein terminates in the left renal vein.

▶ Lymphatics

The lymphatic vessels accompany the suprarenal vein and drain into the lumbar lymph nodes.

KIDNEYS

▶ Gross Appearance

A. Anatomy

The kidneys lie along the borders of the psoas muscles and are therefore obliquely placed. The position of the liver causes the right kidney to be lower than the left (Figures 1–2 and 1–3). The adult kidney weighs about 150 g each.

The kidneys are supported by the perirenal fat (which is enclosed in the perirenal fascia), the renal vascular pedicle, abdominal muscle tone, and the general bulk of the abdominal viscera (Rusinek et al, 2004). Variations in these factors permit variations in the degree of renal mobility. The average descent on inspiration or on assuming the upright position is 4–5 cm. Lack of mobility suggests abnormal fixation (eg, perinephritis), but extreme mobility is not necessarily pathologic.

On longitudinal section (Figure 1–4), the kidney is seen to be made up of an outer cortex, a central medulla, and the internal calices and pelvis. The cortex is homogeneous in appearance. Portions of it project toward the pelvis between the papillae and fornices and are called the columns of Bertin. The medulla consists of numerous pyramids formed by the converging collecting renal tubules, which drain into the minor calices at the tip of the papillae.

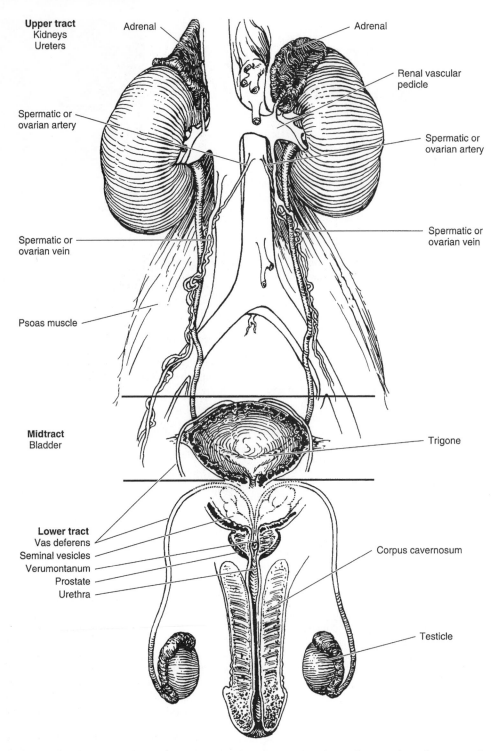

Upper tract
Kidneys
Ureters

Adrenal

Adrenal

Spermatic or
ovarian artery

Renal vascular
pedicle

Spermatic or
ovarian artery

Spermatic or
ovarian vein

Spermatic or
ovarian vein

Psoas muscle

Midtract
Bladder

Trigone

Lower tract
Vas deferens
Seminal vesicles
Verumontanum
Prostate
Urethra

Corpus cavernosum

Testicle

▲ **Figure 1–1.** Anatomy of the male genitourinary tract. The upper and midtracts have urologic function only. The lower tract has both genital and urinary functions.

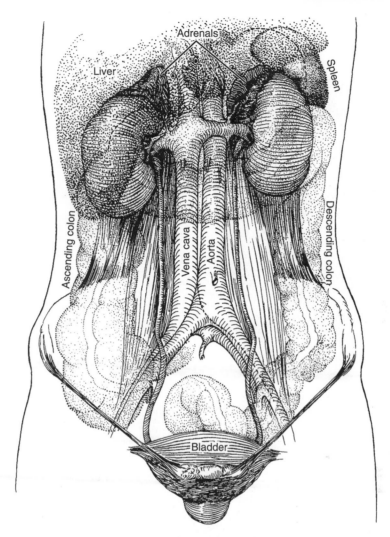

▲ **Figure 1–2.** Relations of kidney, ureters, and bladder (anterior aspect).

B. Relations

Figures 1–2 and 1–3 show the relations of the kidneys to adjacent organs and structures. Their intimacy with intraperitoneal organs and the autonomic innervation they share with these organs explain, in part, some of the gastrointestinal symptoms that accompany genitourinary disease (Glassberg, 2002).

▶ Histology

A. Nephron

The functioning unit of the kidney is the nephron, which is composed of a tubule that has both secretory and excretory functions (Figure 1–4). The secretory portion is contained largely within the cortex and consists of a renal corpuscle and the secretory part of the renal tubule. The excretory portion of this duct lies in the medulla. The renal corpuscle is composed of the vascular glomerulus, which projects into Bowman's capsule, which, in turn, is continuous with the epithelium of the proximal convoluted tubule. The secretory portion of the renal tubule is made up of the proximal convoluted tubule, the loop of Henle, and the distal convoluted tubule.

The excretory portion of the nephron is the collecting tubule, which is continuous with the distal end of the ascending limb of the convoluted tubule. It empties its contents through the tip (papilla) of a pyramid into a minor calyx.

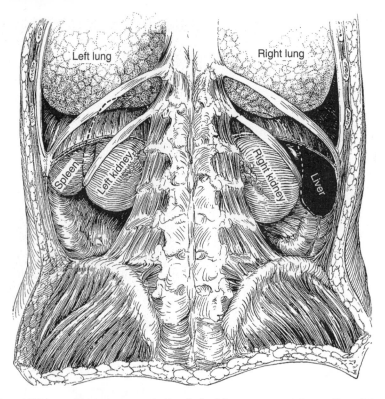

▲ **Figure 1–3.** Relations of kidneys (posterior aspect). The dashed lines represent the outline of the kidneys where they are obscured by overlying structures.

B. Supporting Tissue

The renal stroma is composed of loose connective tissue and contains blood vessels, capillaries, nerves, and lymphatics.

▶ Blood Supply (Figures 1–2, 1–4, and 1–5)

A. Arterial

Usually there is one renal artery, a branch of the aorta that enters the hilum of the kidney between the pelvis, which normally lies posteriorly, and the renal vein. It may branch before it reaches the kidney, and two or more separate arteries may be noted (Budhiraja et al, 2010). In duplication of the pelvis and ureter, it is common for each renal segment to have its own arterial supply.

The renal artery divides into anterior and posterior branches. The posterior branch supplies the midsegment of the posterior surface. The anterior branch supplies both upper and lower poles as well as the entire anterior surface. The renal arteries are all end arteries.

The renal artery further divides into interlobar arteries, which travel in the columns of Bertin (between the pyramids) and then arch along the base of the pyramids (arcuate arteries). These arteries then divide as interlobular arteries. From these vessels, smaller (afferent) branches pass to the glomeruli. From the glomerular tuft, efferent arterioles pass to the tubules in the stroma.

B. Venous

The renal veins are paired with the arteries, but any of them will drain the entire kidney if the others are tied off.

Although the renal artery and vein are usually the sole blood vessels of the kidney, accessory renal vessels are common and may be of clinical importance if they are so placed to compress the ureter, in which case hydronephrosis may result.

▶ Nerve Supply

The renal nerves derived from the renal plexus accompany the renal vessels throughout the renal parenchyma.

▶ Lymphatics

The lymphatics of the kidney drain into the lumbar lymph nodes.

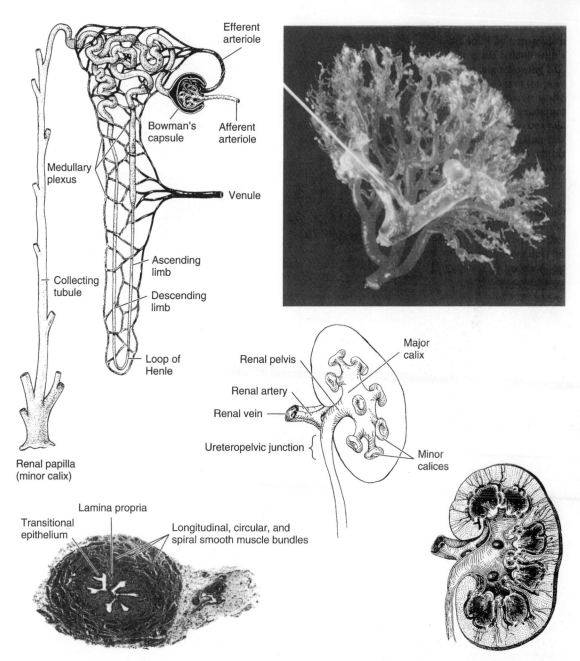

▲ **Figure 1–4.** Anatomy and histology of the kidney and ureter. ***Upper left:*** Diagram of the nephron and its blood supply. (Courtesy of Merck, Sharp, Dohme: Seminar. 1947;9[3].) ***Upper right:*** Cast of the pelvic caliceal system and the arterial supply of the kidney. ***Middle:*** Renal calices, pelvis, and ureter (posterior aspect). ***Lower left:*** Histology of the ureter. The smooth-muscle bundles are arranged in both a spiral and a longitudinal manner. ***Lower right:*** Longitudinal section of kidney showing calices, pelvis, ureter, and renal blood supply (posterior aspect).

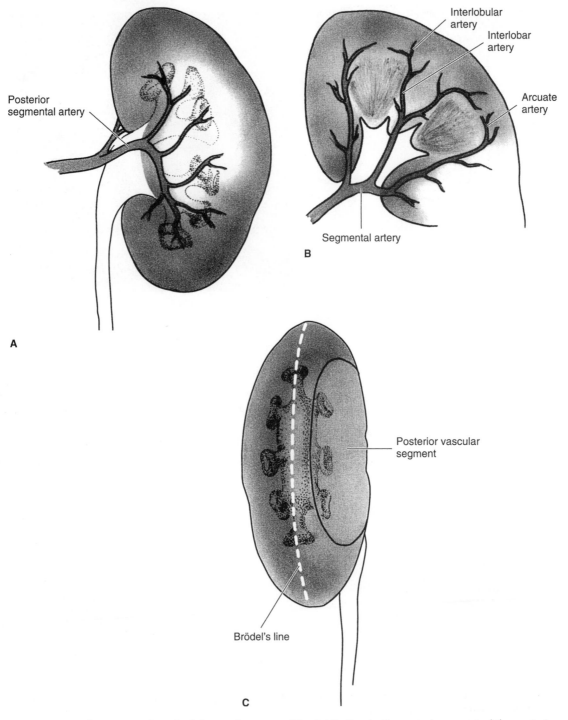

▲ **Figure 1–5.** **A:** The posterior branch of the renal artery and its distribution to the central segment of the posterior surface of the kidney. **B:** Branches of the anterior division of the renal artery supplying the entire anterior surface of the kidney as well as the upper and lower poles at both surfaces. The segmental branches lead to interlobar, arcuate, and interlobular arteries. **C:** The lateral convex margin of the kidney. Brödel's line, which is 1 cm from the convex margin, is the bloodless plane demarcated by the distribution of the posterior branch of the renal artery.

CALICES, RENAL PELVIS, AND URETER

▶ Gross Appearance

A. Anatomy

1. Calices—The tips of the minor calices (8–12 in number) are indented by the projecting pyramids (Figure 1–4). These calices unite to form two or three major calices that join to form the renal pelvis (Sozen et al, 2008).

2. Renal pelvis—The pelvis may be entirely intrarenal or partly intrarenal and partly extrarenal. Inferomedially, it tapers to join the ureter.

3. Ureter—The adult ureter is about 30 cm long, varying in direct relation to the height of the individual. It follows a rather smooth S curve. Areas that stones are often impacted are (1) at the ureteropelvic junction, (2) where the ureter crosses over the iliac vessels, and (3) where it courses through the bladder wall.

B. Relations

1. Calices—The calices are intrarenal and are intimately related to the renal parenchyma.

2. Renal pelvis—If the pelvis is partly extrarenal, it lies along the lateral border of the psoas muscle and on the quadratus lumborum muscle; the renal vascular pedicle is just anterior to it. The left renal pelvis lies at the level of the first or second lumbar vertebra; the right pelvis is a little lower.

3. Ureter—On their course downward, the ureters lie on the psoas muscles, pass medially to the sacroiliac joints, and then swing laterally near the ischial spines before passing medially to penetrate the base of the bladder (Figure 1–2). In females, the uterine arteries are closely related to the juxtavesical portion of the ureters. The ureters are covered by the posterior peritoneum; their lowermost portions are closely attached to it, while the juxtavesical portions are embedded in vascular retroperitoneal fat (Koff, 2008).

The vasa deferentia, as they leave the internal inguinal rings, sweep over the lateral pelvic walls anterior to the ureters (Figure 1–6). They lie medial to the latter before joining the seminal vesicle and penetrating the base of the prostate to become the ejaculatory ducts.

▶ Histology (Figure 1–4)

The walls of the calices, pelvis, and ureters are composed of transitional cell epithelium under which lies loose connective tissue (lamina propria). External to these are a mixture of helical and longitudinal smooth muscle fibers. They are not arranged in definite layers. The outermost adventitial coat is composed of fibrous connective tissue.

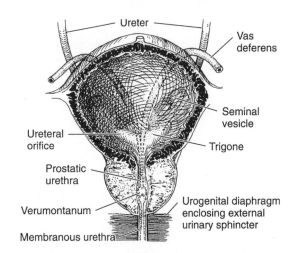

▲ **Figure 1–6.** Anatomy and relations of the ureters, bladder, prostate, seminal vesicles, and vasa deferentia (anterior view).

▶ Blood Supply

A. Arterial

The renal calices, pelvis, and upper ureters derive their blood supply from the renal arteries; the midureter is fed by the internal spermatic (or ovarian) arteries. The lowermost portion of the ureter is served by branches from the common iliac, internal iliac (hypogastric), and vesical arteries.

B. Venous

The veins of the renal calices, pelvis, and ureters are paired with the arteries.

▶ Lymphatics

The lymphatics of the upper portions of the ureters as well as those from the pelvis and calices enter the lumbar lymph nodes. The lymphatics of the midureter pass to the internal iliac (hypogastric) and common iliac lymph nodes; the lower ureteral lymphatics empty into the vesical and hypogastric lymph nodes.

BLADDER

▶ Gross Appearance

The bladder is a hollow muscular organ that serves as a reservoir for urine. In women, its posterior wall and dome are invaginated by the uterus. The adult bladder normally has a capacity of 400–500 mL.

A. Anatomy

When empty, the adult bladder lies behind the pubic symphysis and is largely a pelvic organ. In infants and children, it is situated higher (Berrocal et al, 2002). When it is full, it rises well above the symphysis and can readily be palpated or percussed. When overdistended, as in acute or chronic urinary retention, it may cause the lower abdomen to bulge visibly.

Extending from the dome of the bladder to the umbilicus is a fibrous cord, the median umbilical ligament, which represents the obliterated urachus. The ureters enter the bladder posteroinferiorly in an oblique manner and at these points are about 5 cm apart (Figure 1–6). The orifices, situated at the extremities of the crescent-shaped interureteric ridge that forms the proximal border of the trigone, are about 2.5 cm apart. The trigone occupies the area between the ridge and the bladder neck.

The internal sphincter, or bladder neck, is not a true circular sphincter but a thickening formed by interlaced and converging muscle fibers of the detrusor as they pass distally to become the smooth musculature of the urethra.

B. Relations

In males, the bladder is related posteriorly to the seminal vesicles, vasa deferentia, ureters, and rectum (Figures 1–7 and 1–8). In females, the uterus and vagina are interposed between the bladder and rectum (Figure 1–9). The dome and posterior surfaces are covered by peritoneum; hence, in this area, the bladder is closely related to the small intestine and sigmoid colon. In both males and females, the bladder is related to the posterior surface of the pubic symphysis, and, when distended, it is in contact with the lower abdominal wall.

▶ Histology (Figure 1–10)

The mucosa of the bladder is composed of transitional epithelium. Beneath it is a well-developed submucosal layer formed largely of connective and elastic tissues. External to the submucosa is the detrusor muscle that is made up of a mixture of smooth muscle fibers arranged at random in a longitudinal, circular, and spiral manner without any layer formation or specific orientation except close to the internal meatus, where the detrusor muscle assumes three definite layers: inner longitudinal, middle circular, and outer longitudinal (John et al, 2001).

▶ Blood Supply

A. Arterial

The bladder is supplied by the superior, middle, and inferior vesical arteries, which arise from the anterior trunk of the internal iliac (hypogastric) artery, and by smaller branches from the obturator and inferior gluteal arteries. In females, the uterine and vaginal arteries also send branches to the bladder.

B. Venous

Surrounding the bladder is a rich plexus of veins that ultimately empties into the internal iliac (hypogastric) veins.

▶ Nerve Supply

The bladder receives innervation from sympathetic and parasympathetic nervous systems. The sensory afferent of the bladder originates from both subepithelial nerve endings and nerve fibers between detrusor muscle bundles (Andersson, 2010; Birder et al, 2010; McCloskey, 2010).

▶ Lymphatics

The lymphatics of the bladder drain into the vesical, external iliac, internal iliac (hypogastric), and common iliac lymph nodes.

PROSTATE GLAND

▶ Gross Appearance

A. Anatomy

The prostate is a fibromuscular and glandular organ lying just inferior to the bladder (Figures 1–6 and 1–7). The normal prostate weighs about 20 g and contains the posterior urethra, which is about 2.5 cm in length. It is supported anteriorly by the puboprostatic ligaments and inferiorly by the urogenital diaphragm (Figure 1–6). The prostate is perforated posteriorly by the ejaculatory ducts, which pass obliquely to empty through the verumontanum on the floor of the prostatic urethra just proximal to the striated external urinary sphincter (Figure 1–11).

According to the classification of Lowsley, the prostate consists of five lobes: anterior, posterior, median, right lateral, and left lateral. This classification is often used in cystourethroscopic examinations. After a comprehensive analysis of 500 prostates, McNeal (1981) divides the prostate into four zones: peripheral zone, central zone (surrounds the ejaculatory ducts), transitional zone (surrounds the urethra), and anterior fibromuscular zone (Myers et al, 2010) (Figure 1–12). The segment of urethra that traverses the prostate gland is the prostatic urethra. It is lined by an inner longitudinal layer of muscle (continuous with a similar layer of the vesical wall). Incorporated within the prostate gland is an abundant amount of smooth musculature derived primarily from the external longitudinal bladder musculature. This musculature represents the true smooth involuntary sphincter of the posterior urethra in males.

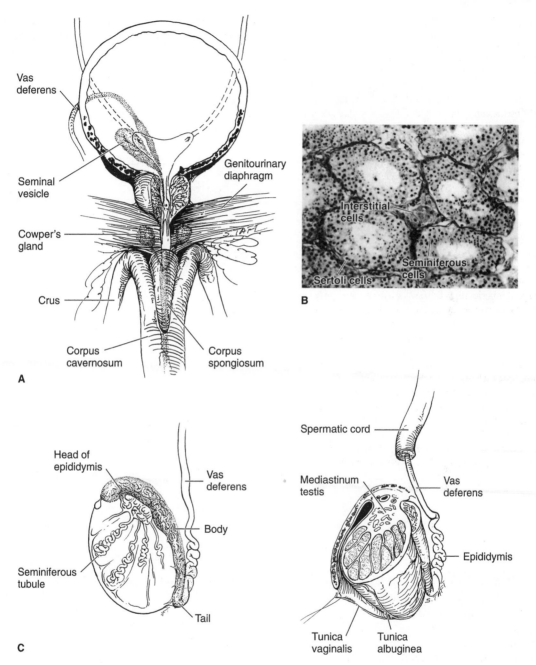

▲ **Figure 1–7.** **A:** Anatomic relationship of the bladder, prostate, prostatomembranous urethra, and root of the penis. **B:** Histology of the testis. Seminiferous tubules lined by supporting basement membrane for the Sertoli and spermatogenic cells. The latter are in various stages of development. **C:** Cross sections of the testis and epididymis. (A and C are reproduced, with permission, from Tanagho EA: Anatomy of the lower urinary tract. In: Walsh PC et al [eds] Campbell's Urology, 6th edn., Vol. 1. Saunders, Philadelphia, PA, 1992.)

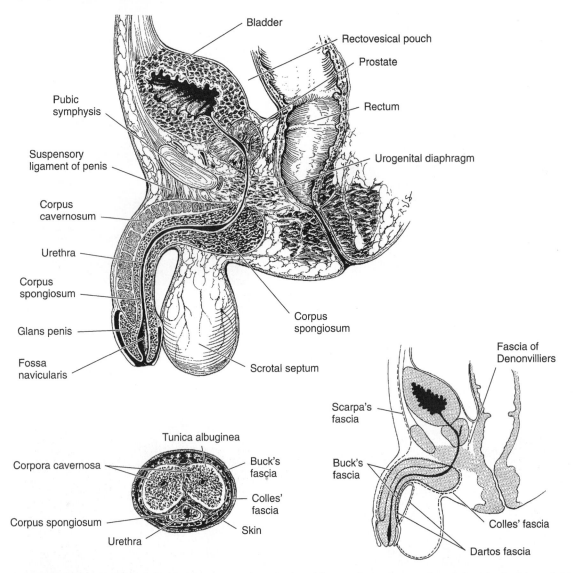

▲ **Figure 1–8.** ***Top:*** Relations of the bladder, prostate, seminal vesicles, penis, urethra, and scrotal contents. ***Lower left:*** Transverse section through the penis. The paired upper structures are the corpora cavernosa. The single lower body surrounding the urethra is the corpus spongiosum. ***Lower right:*** Fascial planes of the lower genitourinary tract. (After Wesson.) (Tanagho EA: Anatomy of the lower urinary tract. In: Walch PC et al [eds] Campbell's Urology. 6th edn., Vol. 1. Saunders, Philadelphia, PA, 1992.)

B. Relations

The prostate gland lies behind the pubic symphysis. Located closely to the posterosuperior surface are the vasa deferentia and seminal vesicles (Figure 1–7). Posteriorly, the prostate is separated from the rectum by the two layers of Denonvilliers' fascia, serosal rudiments of the pouch of Douglas, which once extended to the urogenital diaphragm (Raychaudhuri and Cahill, 2008) (Figure 1–8).

▶ Histology (Figure 1–10)

The prostate consists of a thin fibrous capsule under which are circularly oriented smooth muscle fibers and collagenous tissue that surrounds the urethra (involuntary sphincter). Deep in this layer lies the prostatic stroma, composed of connective tissues and smooth muscle fibers in which are embedded the epithelial glands. These glands drain into the major excretory ducts (about 25 in number), which open chiefly on

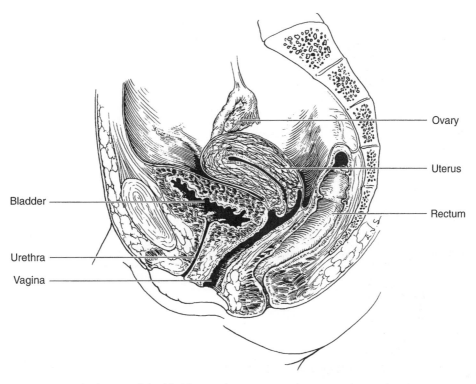

▲ **Figure 1–9.** Anatomy and relations of the bladder, urethra, uterus and ovary, vagina, and rectum.

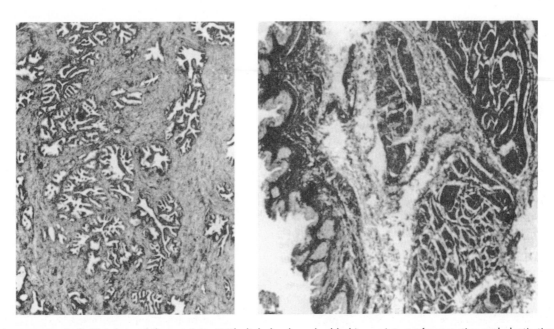

▲ **Figure 1–10.** *Left:* Histology of the prostate. Epithelial glands embedded in a mixture of connective and elastic tissue and smooth muscle. *Right:* Histology of the bladder. The mucosa is transitional cell in type and lies on a well-developed submucosal layer of connective tissue. The detrusor muscle is composed of interlacing longitudinal, circular, and spiral smooth-muscle bundles.

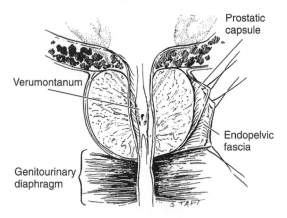

▲ **Figure 1–11.** Section of the prostate gland shows the prostatic urethra, verumontanum, and crista urethralis, in addition to the opening of the prostatic utricle and the two ejaculatory ducts in the midline. Note that the prostate is surrounded by the prostatic capsule, which is covered by another prostatic sheath derived from the endopelvic fascia. The prostate is resting on the genitourinary diaphragm. (Reproduced, with permission, from Tanagho EA: Anatomy of the lower urinary tract. In: Walsh PC et al [eds] Campbell's Urology, 6th edn., Vol. 1. Saunders, Philadelphia, PA, 1992.)

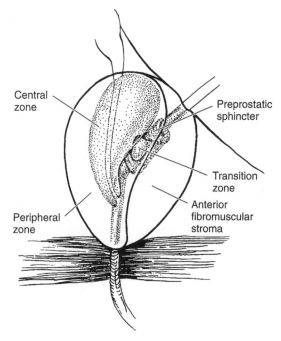

▲ **Figure 1–12.** Anatomy of the prostate gland (adapted from McNeal JE: The zonal anatomy of the prostate. Prostate 1981;2:35–49). (Reproduced, with permission, from Tanagho EA: Anatomy of the lower urinary tract. In: Walsh PC et al [eds] Campbell's Urology, 6th edn., Vol. 1. Saunders, Philadelphia, PA, 1992.) **Prostatic adenoma develops from the periurethral glands at the site of the median or lateral lobes. The posterior lobe, however, is prone to cancerous degeneration.**

the floor of the urethra between the verumontanum and the vesical neck. Just beneath the transitional epithelium of the prostatic urethra lie the periurethral glands.

▶ Blood Supply

A. Arterial

The arterial supply to the prostate is derived from the inferior vesical, internal pudendal, and middle rectal (hemorrhoidal) arteries.

B. Venous

The veins from the prostate drain into the periprostatic plexus, which has connections with the deep dorsal vein of the penis and the internal iliac (hypogastric) veins.

▶ Nerve Supply

The prostate gland receives a rich innervation from the sympathetic and parasympathetic nerves of the inferior hypogastric plexus.

▶ Lymphatics

The lymphatics from the prostate drain into the internal iliac (hypogastric), sacral, vesical, and external iliac lymph nodes (Saokar et al, 2010).

SEMINAL VESICLES

▶ Gross Appearance

The seminal vesicles lie just cephalic to the prostate under the base of the bladder (Figures 1–6 and 1–7). They are about 6 cm long and quite soft. Each vesicle joins its corresponding vas deferens to form the ejaculatory duct (Kim et al, 2009). The ureters lie medial to each, and the rectum is contiguous with their posterior surfaces.

▶ Histology

The mucous membrane is pseudostratified. The submucosa consists of dense connective tissue covered by a thin layer of muscle that in turn is encapsulated by connective tissue.

▶ Blood Supply

The blood supply is similar to that of the prostate gland.

Nerve Supply

The nerve supply is mainly from the sympathetic nerve plexus.

Lymphatics

The lymphatics of the seminal vesicles are those that serve the prostate.

SPERMATIC CORD

Gross Appearance

The two spermatic cords extend from the internal inguinal rings through the inguinal canals to the testicles (Figure 1–7). Each cord contains the vas deferens, the internal and external spermatic arteries, the artery of the vas, the venous pampiniform plexus (which forms the spermatic vein superiorly), lymph vessels, and nerves (Jen et al, 1999). All of the preceding are enclosed in investing layers of thin fascia. A few fibers of the cremaster muscle insert on the cords in the inguinal canal (Bhosale et al, 2008; Kim et al, 2009).

Histology

The fascia covering the cord is formed of loose connective tissue that supports arteries, veins, nerve, and lymphatics. The vas deferens is a small, thick-walled tube consisting of an internal mucosa and submucosa surrounded by three well-defined layers of smooth muscle encased in a covering of fibrous tissue. Above the testes, this tube is straight. Its proximal 4 cm tends to be convoluted.

Blood Supply

A. Arterial

The external spermatic artery, a branch of the inferior epigastric, supplies the fascial coverings of the cord. The internal spermatic artery passes through the cord on its way to the testis. The deferential artery is close to the vas.

B. Venous

The veins from the testis and the coverings of the spermatic cord form the pampiniform plexus, which, at the internal inguinal ring, unites to form the spermatic vein.

Lymphatics

The lymphatics from the spermatic cord empty into the external iliac lymph nodes.

EPIDIDYMIS

Gross Appearance

A. Anatomy

The upper portion of the epididymis (globus major) is connected to the testis by numerous efferent ducts from the testis

(Figure 1–7). The epididymis consists of a markedly coiled duct that, at its lower pole (globus minor), is continuous with the vas deferens. An appendix of the epididymis is often seen on its upper pole; this is a cystic body that in some cases is pedunculated, but in others, it is sessile.

B. Relations

The epididymis lies posterolateral to the testis and is nearest to the testis at its upper pole. Its lower pole is connected to the testis by fibrous tissue. The vas lies posteromedial to the epididymis.

Histology

The epididymis is covered by serosa. The ductus epididymidis is lined by pseudostratified columnar epithelium throughout its length.

Blood Supply

A. Arterial

The arterial supply to the epididymis comes from the internal spermatic artery and the artery of the vas (deferential artery).

B. Venous

The venous blood drains into the pampiniform plexus, which becomes the spermatic vein.

Lymphatics

The lymphatics drain into the external iliac and internal iliac (hypogastric) lymph nodes.

TESTIS

Gross Appearance

A. Anatomy

The average testicle measures about $4 \times 3 \times 2.5$ cm (Figure 1–7). It has a dense fascial covering called the tunica albuginea testis, which, posteriorly, is invaginated somewhat into the body of the testis to form the mediastinum testis. This fibrous mediastinum sends fibrous septa into the testis, thus separating it into about 250 lobules.

The testis is covered anteriorly and laterally by the visceral layer of the serous tunica vaginalis, which is continuous with the parietal layer that separates the testis from the scrotal wall (Bidarkar and Hutson, 2005). Small amount of fluid normally exists within the tunica vaginalis sac. At the upper pole of the testis is the appendix testis, a small pedunculated or sessile body similar in appearance to the appendix of the epididymis.

B. Relations

The testis is closely attached posterolaterally to the epididymis, particularly at its upper and lower poles (Klonisch et al, 2004).

Histology(Figure 1–7)

Each lobule contains one to four markedly convoluted seminiferous tubules, each of which is about 60 cm long. These ducts converge at the mediastinum testis, where they connect with the efferent ducts that drain into the epididymis.

The seminiferous tubule has a basement membrane containing connective and elastic tissue. This supports the seminiferous cells that are of two types: (1) Sertoli (supporting) cells and (2) spermatogenic cells. The stroma between the seminiferous tubules contains connective tissue in which the interstitial Leydig cells are located.

Blood Supply

The blood supply to the testes is closely associated with that to the kidneys because of the common embryologic origin of the two organs.

A. Arterial

The arteries to the testes (internal spermatics) arise from the aorta just below the renal arteries and course through the spermatic cords to the testes, where they anastomose with the arteries of the vasa deferentia that branch off from the internal iliac (hypogastric) artery.

B. Venous

The blood from the testis returns in the pampiniform plexus of the spermatic cord. At the internal inguinal ring, the pampiniform plexus forms the spermatic vein.

The right spermatic vein enters the vena cava just below the right renal vein; the left spermatic vein empties into the left renal vein.

Lymphatics

The lymphatic vessels from the testes pass to the lumbar lymph nodes, which in turn are connected to the mediastinal nodes.

SCROTUM

Gross Appearance

Beneath the corrugated skin of the scrotum lies the dartos muscle. Deep to this are the three fascial layers derived from the abdominal wall at the time of testicular descent. Beneath these is the parietal layer of the tunica vaginalis (Kim et al, 2007).

The scrotum is divided into two sacs by a septum of connective tissue. The scrotum not only supports the testes but also, by relaxation or contraction of its muscular layer, helps to regulate their temperature.

Histology

The dartos muscle, under the skin of the scrotum, is unstriated. The deeper layer is made up of connective tissue.

Blood Supply

A. Arterial

The arteries to the scrotum arise from the femoral, internal pudendal, and inferior epigastric arteries.

B. Venous

The veins are paired with the arteries.

Lymphatics

The lymphatics drain into the superficial inguinal and subinguinal lymph nodes.

PENIS AND MALE URETHRA

Gross Appearance

The penis is composed of two corpora cavernosa and the corpus spongiosum, which contains the urethra. The corpus spongiosum enlarges distally and caps the glans penis. Each corpus is enclosed in a fascial sheath (tunica albuginea), and all are surrounded by a thick fibrous envelope known as Buck's fascia. A covering of skin, devoid of fat, is loosely applied about these bodies. The prepuce forms a hood over the glans.

Beneath the skin of the penis (and scrotum) and extending from the base of the glans to the urogenital diaphragm is Colles' fascia, which is continuous with Scarpa's fascia of the lower abdominal wall (Figure 1–8).

The proximal ends of the corpora cavernosa are attached to the pelvic bones just anterior to the ischial tuberosities. The ischiocavernosus muscles insert to the lateral surface of the tunica albuginea at the proximal corpora cavernosa. Occupying a depression of their ventral surface in the midline is the corpus spongiosum, which is connected proximally to the undersurface of the urogenital diaphragm, through which emerges the membranous urethra. This portion of the corpus spongiosum is surrounded by the bulbospongiosus muscle.

The suspensory ligament of the penis arises from the linea alba and pubic symphysis and inserts into the fascial covering of the corpora cavernosa.

Histology

A. Corpora and Glans Penis

The corpora cavernosa, the corpus spongiosum, and the glans penis are composed of smooth muscles, intracavernosal struts (corpus cavernosum only), and endothelium-lined sinusoids. The sympathetic and parasympathetic (continuing neuronal nitric oxide synthase) nerve terminals are often seen around the vessels and near the smooth muscles.

B. Urethra

The urethral mucosa that traverses the glans penis is formed of squamous epithelium. Proximal to this, the mucosa is transitional in type. Underneath the mucosa is the submucosa that contains connective and elastic tissue and smooth muscle. In the submucosa are the numerous glands of Littre, whose ducts connect with the urethral lumen. The urethra is surrounded by the vascular corpus spongiosum and the glans penis.

▶ Blood Supply

A. Arterial

The penis and urethra are supplied by the internal pudendal arteries. Each artery divides into a cavernous artery of the penis (which supplies the corpora cavernosa), a dorsal artery of the penis, and the bulbourethral artery. These branches supply the corpus spongiosum, the glans penis, and the urethra. Accessory pudendal arteries originate from inferior vesical, obturator, or other arteries may also supply the penis.

B. Venous

The superficial dorsal vein lies external to Buck's fascia and drains to the saphenous vein. The deep dorsal vein is placed beneath Buck's fascia and lies between the dorsal arteries. The cavernous veins drain the crura of the penis. These veins connect with the pudendal plexus that drains into the internal pudendal vein and periprostatic plexus.

▶ Lymphatics

Lymphatic drainage from the skin of the penis is to the superficial inguinal and subinguinal lymph nodes. The lymphatics from the glans penis pass to the subinguinal and external iliac nodes. The lymphatics from the proximal urethra drain into the internal iliac (hypogastric) and common iliac lymph nodes (Wood and Angermeier, 2010).

FEMALE URETHRA

▶ Gross Appearance

The adult female urethra is about 4 cm long and 8 mm in diameter. It is slightly curved and lies beneath the pubic symphysis just anterior to the vagina.

▶ Histology

The epithelial lining of the female urethra is squamous in its distal portion and pseudostratified or transitional in the remainder. The submucosa is made up of connective and elastic tissues and spongy venous spaces. Embedded in it are many periurethral glands, which are most numerous distally; the largest of these are the periurethral glands of Skene that open on the floor of the urethra just inside the meatus.

External to the submucosa is a longitudinal layer of smooth muscle continuous with the inner longitudinal layer of the bladder wall. Surrounding this is a heavy layer of circular smooth muscle fibers extending from the external vesical muscular layer. This constitutes the involuntary ure-

thral sphincter. External to this is the circular striated (voluntary) sphincter surrounding the middle third of the urethra. The smooth and striated muscles within the midurethra constitute the external urethral sphincter (Ashton-Miller and Delancey, 2009; Thor and de Groat, 2010).

▶ Blood Supply

The arterial supply to the female urethra is derived from the inferior vesical, vaginal, and internal pudendal arteries. Blood from the urethra drains into the internal pudendal veins.

▶ Lymphatics

Lymphatic drainage from the external portion of the urethra is to the inguinal and subinguinal lymph nodes. Drainage from the deep urethra is into the internal iliac (hypogastric) lymph nodes.

BIBLIOGRAPHY

Adrenals

Avisse C et al: Surgical anatomy and embryology of the adrenal glands. Surg Clin North Am 2000;80:403–415.

O'Donoghue PM et al: Genitourinary imaging: Current and emerging applications. J Postgrad Med 2010;56:131–139.

Kidneys

Budhiraja V et al: Renal artery variations: Embryological basis and surgical correlation. Rom J Morphol Embryol 2010;51:533–536.

Glassberg KI: Normal and abnormal development of the kidney: A clinician's interpretation of current knowledge. J Urol 2002; 167:2339.

Rusinek H et al: Renal magnetic resonance imaging. Curr Opin Nephrol Hypertens 2004;13:667–673.

Calices, Renal Pelvis, and Ureter

Koff SA: Requirements for accurately diagnosing chronic partial upper urinary tract obstruction in children with hydronephrosis. Pediatr Radiol 2008;38(Suppl 1):S41–S48.

Sozen S et al: Significance of lower-pole pelvicaliceal anatomy on stone clearance after shockwave lithotripsy in nonobstructive isolated renal pelvic stones. J Endourol 2008;22(5):877–881.

Bladder

Andersson KE: Detrusor myocyte activity and afferent signaling. Neurourol Urodyn 2010;29(1):97–106.

Berrocal T et al: Anomalies of the distal ureter, bladder, and urethra in children: Embryologic, radiologic, and pathologic features. Radiographics 2002;22:1139.

Birder L et al: Neural control of the lower urinary tract: Peripheral and spinal mechanisms. Neurourol Urodyn 2010;29(1):128–139.

John H et al: Ultrastructure of the trigone and its functional implications. Urol Int 2001;67(4):264–271.

McCloskey KD: Interstitial cells in the urinary bladder—localization and function. Neurourol Urodyn 2010;29(1):82–87.

Prostate Gland

McNeal JE: The zonal anatomy of the prostate. Prostate 1981;2:35–49.

Myers RP et al: Making anatomic terminology of the prostate and contiguous structures clinically useful: Historical review and suggestions for revision in the 21st century. Clin Anat 2010;23:18–29.

Raychaudhuri B, Cahill D: Pelvic fasciae in urology. Ann R Coll Surg Engl 2008;90:633–637.

Saokar A et al: Detection of lymph nodes in pelvic malignancies with computed tomography and magnetic resonance imaging. Clin Imaging 2010;34:361–366.

Spermatic Cord and Seminal Vesicles

Bhosale PR et al: The inguinal canal: Anatomy and imaging features of common and uncommon masses. Radiographics 2008; 28(3):819–835.

Jen PY et al: Colocalisation of neuropeptides, nitric oxide synthase and immunomarkers for catecholamines in nerve fibres of the adult human vas deferens. J Anat 1999;195(Pt 4):481–489.

Kim B et al: Imaging of the seminal vesicle and vas deferens. Radiographics 2009;29(4):1105–1121.

Testis, Scrotum, and Penis

Bidarkar SS, Hutson JM: Evaluation and management of the abnormal gonad. Semin Pediatr Surg 2005;14:118.

Kim W et al: US MR imaging correlation in pathologic conditions of the scrotum. Radiographics 2007;27(5):1239–1253.

Klonisch T et al: Molecular and genetic regulation of testis descent and external genitalia development. Dev Biol 2004;270:1.

Wood HM, Angermeier KW. Anatomic considerations of the penis, lymphatic drainage, and biopsy of the sentinel node. Urol Clin North Am 2010;37(3):327–334.

Female Urethra

Ashton-Miller JA, Delancey JO: On the biomechanics of vaginal birth and common sequelae. Annu Rev Biomed Eng 2009;11: 163–176.

Delancey JO: Why do women have stress urinary incontinence? Neurourol Urodyn 2010;29(Suppl 1):S13–S17.

Thor KB, de Groat WC: Neural control of the female urethral and anal rhabdosphincters and pelvic floor muscles. Am J Physiol Regul Integr Comp Physiol 2010;299:R416–R438.

Embryology of the Genitourinary System

2

Emil A. Tanagho, MD, & Hiep T. Nguyen, MD

At birth, the genital and urinary systems are related only in the sense that they share certain common passages. Embryologically, however, they are intimately related. Because of the complex interrelationships of the embryonic phases of the two systems, they are discussed here as five subdivisions: the nephric system, the vesicourethral unit, the gonads, the genital duct system, and the external genitalia.

NEPHRIC SYSTEM

The nephric system develops progressively as three distinct entities: pronephros, mesonephros, and metanephros.

▶ Pronephros

The pronephros is the earliest nephric stage in humans, and it corresponds to the mature structure of the most primitive vertebrate. It extends from the 4th to the 14th somites and consists of six to ten pairs of tubules. These open into a pair of primary ducts that are formed at the same level, extend caudally, and eventually reach and open into the cloaca. The pronephros is a vestigial structure that disappears completely by the 4th week of embryonic life (Figure 2–1).

▶ Mesonephros

The mature excretory organ of the larger fish and amphibians corresponds to the embryonic mesonephros. It is the principal excretory organ during early embryonic life (4–8 weeks). It too gradually degenerates, although parts of its duct system become associated with the male reproductive organs. The mesonephric tubules develop from the intermediate mesoderm caudal to the pronephros shortly before pronephric degeneration. The mesonephric tubules differ from those of the pronephros in that they develop a cuplike outgrowth into which a knot of capillaries is pushed. This is called Bowman's capsule, and the tuft of capillaries is called a glomerulus. In their growth, the mesonephric tubules extend toward and establish a connection with the nearby primary nephric duct as it grows caudally to join the cloaca (Figure 2–1). This primary nephric duct is now called the mesonephric duct. After establishing their connection with the nephric duct, the primordial tubules elongate and become S-shaped. As the tubules elongate, a series of secondary branchings increase their surface exposure, thereby enhancing their capacity for interchanging material with the blood in adjacent capillaries. Leaving the glomerulus, the blood is carried by one or more efferent vessels that soon break up into a rich capillary plexus closely related to the mesonephric tubules. The mesonephros, which forms early in the 4th week, reaches its maximum size by the end of the 2nd month.

▶ Metanephros

The metanephros, the final phase of development of the nephric system, originates from both the intermediate mesoderm and the mesonephric duct. Development begins in the 5- to 6-mm embryo with a budlike outgrowth from the mesonephric duct as it bends to join the cloaca. This ureteral bud grows cephalad and collects mesoderm from the nephrogenic cord of the intermediate mesoderm around its tip. This mesoderm with the meta-nephric cap moves, with the growing ureteral bud, more and more cephalad from its point of origin. During this cephalic migration, the metanephric cap becomes progressively larger, and rapid internal differentiation takes place. Meanwhile, the cephalic end of the ureteral bud expands within the growing mass of metanephrogenic tissue to form the renal pelvis (Figure 2–1). Numerous outgrowths from the renal pelvic dilatation push radially into this growing mass and form hollow ducts that branch and rebranch as they push toward the periphery. These form the primary collecting ducts of the kidney. Mesodermal cells become arranged in small vesicular masses that lie close to the blind end of the collecting ducts. Each of these vesicular masses will form a uriniferous tubule draining into the duct nearest to its point of origin.

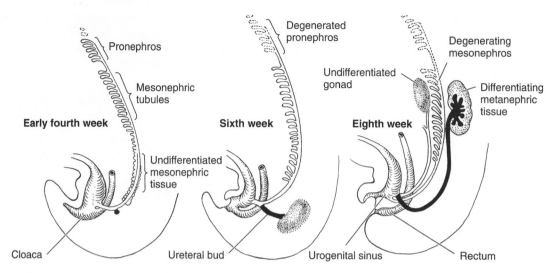

▲ **Figure 2–1.** Schematic representation of the development of the nephric system. Only a few of the tubules of the pronephros are seen early in the 4th week, while the mesonephric tissue differentiates into mesonephric tubules that progressively join the mesonephric duct. The first sign of the ureteral bud from the mesonephric duct is seen. At 6 weeks, the pronephros has completely degenerated and the mesonephric tubules start to do so. The ureteral bud grows dorsocranially and has met the metanephrogenic cap. At the 8th week, there is cranial migration of the differentiating metanephros. The cranial end of the ureteric bud expands and starts to show multiple successive outgrowths. (Adapted from several sources.)

As the kidney grows, increasing numbers of tubules are formed in its peripheral zone. These vesicular masses develop a central cavity and become S-shaped. One end of the S coalesces with the terminal portion of the collecting tubules, resulting in a continuous canal. The proximal portion of the S develops into the distal and proximal convoluted tubules and into Henle's loop; the distal end becomes the glomerulus and Bowman's capsule. At this stage, the undifferentiated mesoderm and the immature glomeruli are readily visible on microscopic examination (Figure 2–2). The glomeruli are fully developed by the 36th week or when the fetus weighs 2500 g (Osathanondh and Potter, 1964a and 1964b). The metanephros arises opposite the 28th somite (fourth lumbar segment). At term, it has ascended to the level of the first lumbar or even the twelfth thoracic vertebra. This ascent of the kidney is due not only to actual cephalic migration but also to differential growth in the caudal part of the body. During the early period of ascent (7th to 9th weeks), the kidney slides above the arterial bifurcation and rotates 90°. Its convex border is now directed laterally, not dorsally. Ascent proceeds more slowly until the kidney reaches its final position.

Certain features of these three phases of development must be emphasized: (1) The three successive units of the system develop from the intermediate mesoderm. (2) The tubules at all levels appear as independent primordia and only secondarily unite with the duct system. (3) The nephric duct is laid down as the duct of the pronephros and develops from the union of the ends of the anterior pronephric tubules. (4) This pronephric duct serves subsequently as the mesonephric duct and as such gives rise to the ureter. (5) The nephric duct reaches the cloaca by independent caudal growth. (6) The embryonic ureter is an outgrowth of the nephric duct, yet the kidney tubules differentiate from adjacent metanephric blastema.

▶ Molecular Mechanisms of Renal and Ureteral Development

The kidney and the collecting system originate from the interaction between the mesonephric duct (Wolffian duct) and the metanephric mesenchyme (MM). The uretic bud (UB) forms as an epithelial outpouching from the mesonephric duct and invades the surrounding MM. Reciprocal induction between the UB and MM results in branching and elongation of the UB from the collecting system and in condensation and epithelial differentiation of MM around the branched tips of the UB. Branching of the UB occurs approximately 15 times during human renal development, generating approximately 300,000 and 1 million nephrons per kidney (Nyengaard and Bendtsen, 1992).

This process of reciprocal induction is dependent on the expression of specific factors. Glial cell–derived neurotrophic

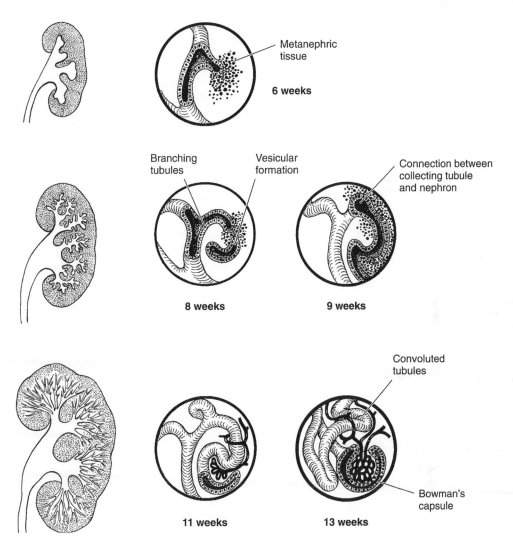

▲ **Figure 2–2.** Progressive stages in the differentiation of the nephrons and their linkage with the branching collecting tubules. A small lump of metanephric tissue is associated with each terminal collecting tubule. These are then arranged in vesicular masses that later differentiate into a uriniferous tubule draining into the duct near which it arises. At one end, Bowman's capsule and the glomerulus differentiate; the other end establishes communication with the nearby collecting tubules.

factor (GDNF) is the primary inducer of ureteric budding (Costantini and Shakya, 2006). GDNF interacts with several different proteins from the MM (eg, *Wt-1, Pax2, Eyal, Six1, Sall 1*) and from the UB itself (*Pax2, Lim1, Ret*) resulting in outgrowth of the UB (reviewed by Shah et al, 2004). Proper activation of the *Ret*/GDNF signaling pathway in the tip of UB epithelium appears to be essential in the progression of branching morphogenesis (reviewed by Michos, 2009). B-catenin and Gata-3 are important regulators of *Ret* expression, and correct activity of *Ret* is regulated by positive (Wnt-11 from MM) and negative (Sprouty1 from the UB)

feedback signaling. Additional specific factors are required for (1) early branching (eg, *Wnt-4 and 11, fgf 7–10*); (2) late branching and maturation (*bmp2*, activin); and (3) branching termination and tubule maintenance (hepatocyte growth factor, transforming growth factor-alpha, epidermal growth factor receptor) (reviewed by Shah et al, 2004). BMP-7, SHH, and Wnt-11 produced from the branching ureteric bud induce the MM to differentiate. These factors induce the activation of Pax2, alpha-8-integrin, and Wnt-4 in the renal mesenchymal cells, resulting in condensation of the MM and the formation of pretubular aggregate and primitive renal vesicle (reviewed by Burrow, 2000). With the continued induction from the UB and the autocrine activity of Wnt-4, the pretubular aggregates differentiate into comma-shaped bodies. Platelet derived growth factor alpha-beta and vascular endothelial growth factor expression are required for initiating the migration of endothelial cells into the cleft of the comma-shaped bodies to form rudimentary glomerular capillary tufts (reviewed by Burrow, 2000). Wt-1 and *Pod*-1 may have important functions in the regulation of gene transcription necessary for the differentiation of podocytes (Ballermann, 2005).

ANOMALIES OF THE NEPHRIC SYSTEM

Failure of the metanephros to ascend leads to an **ectopic kidney**. An ectopic kidney may be on the proper side but low (simple ectopy) or on the opposite side (crossed ectopy) with or without fusion. Failure to rotate during ascent causes a **malrotated kidney**.

Fusion of the paired metanephric masses leads to various anomalies—most commonly a **horseshoe kidney**.

The ureteral bud from the mesonephric duct may bifurcate, causing a **bifid ureter** at various levels depending on the time of the bud's subdivision. An accessory ureteral bud may develop from the mesonephric duct, thereby forming a **duplicated ureter**, usually meeting the same metanephric mass. Rarely, each bud has a separate metanephric mass, resulting in **supernumerary kidneys**.

If the double ureteral buds are close together on the mesonephric duct, they open near each other in the bladder. In this case, the main ureteral bud, which is the first to appear and the most caudal on the mesonephric ducts, reaches the bladder first. It then starts to move upward and laterally and is followed later by the second accessory bud as it reaches the urogenital sinus. The main ureteral bud (now more cranial on the urogenital sinus) drains the lower portion of the kidney. The two ureteral buds reverse their relationship as they move from the mesonephric duct to the urogenital sinus. This is why double ureters always cross (Weigert-Meyer law). If the two ureteral buds are widely separated on the mesonephric duct, the accessory bud appears more proximal and ends in the bladder with an ectopic orifice lower than the normal one. This ectopic orifice could still be in the bladder close to its outlet, in the urethra, or even in the genital duct system (Figure 2–3). A single ureteral bud that arises higher than normal on the mesonephric duct can also end in a similar ectopic location.

Lack of development of a ureteral bud results in a **solitary kidney** and a hemitrigone.

VESICOURETHRAL UNIT

The blind end of the hindgut caudal to the point of origin of the allantois expands to form the cloaca, which is separated from the outside by a thin plate of tissue (the cloacal membrane) lying in an ectodermal depression (the proctodeum) under the root of the tail. At the 4-mm stage, starting at the cephalic portion of the cloaca where the allantois and gut meet, the cloaca progressively divides into two compartments by the caudal growth of a crescentic fold, the urorectal fold. The two limbs of the fold bulge into the lumen of the cloaca from either side, eventually meeting and fusing. The division of the cloaca into a ventral portion (urogenital sinus) and a dorsal portion (rectum) is completed during the 7th week. During the development of the urorectal septum, the cloacal membrane undergoes a reverse rotation, so that the ectodermal surface is no longer directed toward the developing anterior abdominal wall but gradually is turned to face caudally and slightly posteriorly. This change facilitates the subdivision of the cloaca and is brought about mainly by development of the infraumbilical portion of the anterior abdominal wall and regression of the tail. The mesoderm that passes around the cloacal membrane to the caudal attachment of the umbilical cord proliferates and grows, forming a surface elevation, the genital tubercle. Further growth of the infraumbilical part of the abdominal wall progressively separates the umbilical cord from the genital tubercle. The division of the cloaca is completed before the cloacal membrane ruptures, and its two parts therefore have separate openings. The ventral part is the primitive urogenital sinus, which has the shape of an elongated cylinder and is continuous cranially with the allantois; its external opening is the urogenital ostium. The dorsal part is the rectum, and its external opening is the anus.

Traditionally, it is believed that the urogenital sinus receives the mesonephric ducts. The caudal end of the mesonephric duct distal to the ureteral bud (the common excretory duct) is progressively absorbed into the urogenital sinus. By the 7th week, the mesonephric duct and the ureteral bud have independent opening sites. This introduces an island of mesodermal tissue amid the surrounding endoderm of the urogenital sinus. As development progresses, the opening of the mesonephric duct (which will become the ejaculatory duct) migrates downward and medially. The opening of the ureteral bud (which will become the ureteral orifice) migrates upward and laterally. The absorbed mesoderm of the mesonephric duct expands with this migration to occupy the area limited by the final position of these tubes (Figure 2–3). This will later be differentiated as the trigonal structure, which is the only mesodermal inclusion in the endodermal vesicourethral unit.

Recent studies suggest an alternative path of development (reviewed by McInnes and Michaud, 2009). The right and left common excretory duct appears to undergo gradual programmed cell death; the elimination of the common excretory ducts brings the distal ureters in immediate contact with the urogenital sinus epithelium. Concurrently, the ureters undergo a 180° rotation around the axis of the mesonephric duct (also known as the Wolffian duct). The distal segment of the ureters then also undergoes apoptosis. As a

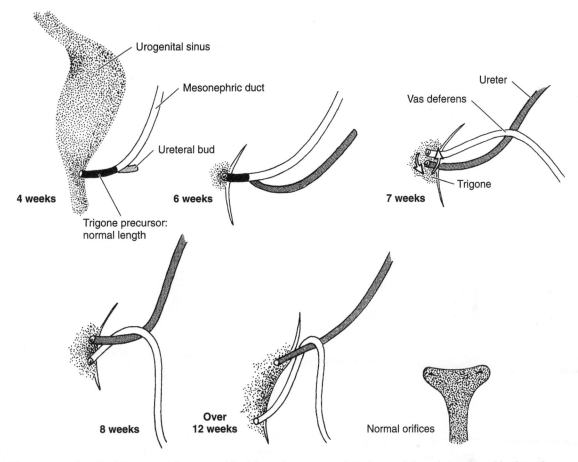

▲ **Figure 2–3.** The development of the ureteral bud from the mesonephric duct and the relationship of both to the urogenital sinus. The ureteral bud appears at the 4th week. The mesonephric duct distal to this ureteral bud is gradually absorbed into the urogenital sinus, resulting in separate endings for the ureter and the mesonephric duct. The mesonephric tissue that is incorporated into the urogenital sinus expands and forms the trigonal tissue.

result, this process generates a new ureteral connection point in the urogenital sinus region that will give rise to the bladder, while the Wolffian duct remains in the region giving rise to the urethra. Further growth of the bladder and urethra moves the ureteral orifices cranially, while those to the Wolffian ducts move caudally. This pattern of development is supported by recent studies that suggest the trigone is formed mostly from bladder smooth muscle and less so from the ureters. Condensation of myoblasts in the region between the openings of the ureters and Wolffian ducts at 12 weeks of gestation gives rise to the trigone, as a single circular muscular layer and the muscles from the distal ureters cross midline to form the interureteral fold (Oswald et al, 2006).

The urogenital sinus can be divided into two main segments. The dividing line, the junction of the combined Müllerian ducts with the dorsal wall of the urogenital sinus, is an elevation called Müller's tubercle, which is the most fixed reference point in the whole structure and which is discussed in a subsequent section. The segments are as follows:

1. The ventral and pelvic portion forms the bladder, part of the urethra in males, and the whole urethra in females. This portion receives the ureter.

2. The urethral, or phallic, portion receives the mesonephric and the fused Müllerian ducts. This will be part of the urethra in males and forms the lower fifth of the vagina and the vaginal vestibule in females.

During the 3rd month, the ventral part of the urogenital sinus starts to expand and forms an epithelial sac whose apex tapers into an elongated, narrowed urachus. The

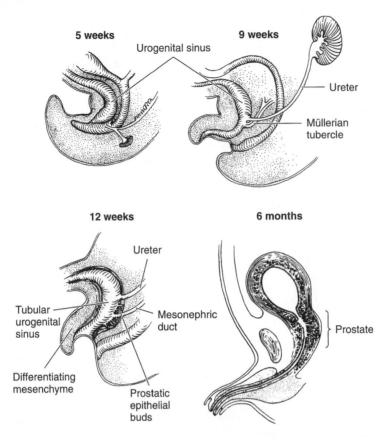

5 weeks   **9 weeks**

Urogenital sinus

Ureter

Müllerian
tubercle

12 weeks   **6 months**

Ureter

Tubular
urogenital   Mesonephric
sinus   duct   Prostate

Differentiating
mesenchyme   Prostatic
                    epithelial
                    buds

▲ **Figure 2–4.** Differentiation of the urogenital sinus in males. At the 5th week, the progressively growing urorectal septum separates the urogenital sinus from the rectum. The former receives the mesonephric duct and the ureteral bud. It retains its tubular structure until the 12th week, when the surrounding mesenchyme starts to differentiate into the muscle fibers around the whole structure. The prostate gland develops as multiple epithelial outgrowths just above and below the mesonephric duct. During the 3rd month, the ventral part of the urogenital sinus expands to form the bladder proper; the pelvic part remains narrow and tubular, forming part of the urethra. (Reproduced, with permission, from Tanagho EA, Smith DR: Mechanisms of urinary continence. 1. Embryologic, anatomic, and pathologic considerations. J Urol 1969;100:640.)

pelvic portion remains narrow and tubular; it forms the whole urethra in females and the supramontanal portion of the prostatic urethra in males. The splanchnic mesoderm surrounding the ventral and pelvic portion of the urogenital sinus begins to differentiate into interlacing bands of smooth muscle fibers and an outer fibrous connective tissue coat. By the 12th week, the layers characteristic of the adult urethra and bladder are recognizable (Figure 2–4).

The part of the urogenital sinus caudal to the opening of the Müllerian duct forms the vaginal vestibule and contributes to the lower fifth of the vagina in females (Figure 2–5). In males, it forms the inframontanal part of the prostatic urethra and the membranous urethra. The penile

urethra is formed by the fusion of the urethral folds on the ventral surface of the genital tubercle. In females, the urethral folds remain separate and form the labia minora. The glandular urethra in males is formed by canalization of the urethral plate. The bladder originally extends up to the umbilicus, where it is connected to the allantois that extends into the umbilical cord. The allantois usually is obliterated at the level of the umbilicus by the 15th week. The bladder then starts to descend by the 18th week. As it descends, its apex becomes stretched and narrowed, and it pulls on the already obliterated allantois, now called the urachus. By the 20th week, the bladder is well separated from the umbilicus, and the stretched urachus becomes the middle umbilical ligament.

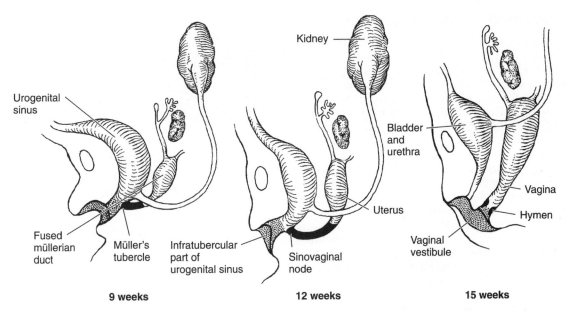

▲ **Figure 2–5.** Differentiation of the urogenital sinus and the Müllerian ducts in the female embryo. At 9 weeks, the urogenital sinus receives the fused Müllerian ducts at Müller's tubercle (sinovaginal node), which is solidly packed with cells. As the urogenital sinus distal to Müller's tubercle becomes wider and shallower (15 weeks), the urethra and fused Müllerian duct will have separate openings. The distal part of the urogenital sinus forms the vaginal vestibule and the lower fifth of the vagina (shaded area), and that part above Müller's tubercle forms the urinary bladder and the entire female urethra. The fused Müllerian ducts form the uterus and the upper four-fifths of the vagina. The hymen is formed at the junction of the sinovaginal node and the urogenital sinus.

PROSTATE

The prostate develops as multiple solid outgrowths of the urethral epithelium both above and below the entrance of the mesonephric duct. These simple tubular outgrowths begin to develop in five distinct groups at the end of the 11th week and are complete by the 16th week (112-mm stage). They branch and rebranch, ending in a complex duct system that encounters the differentiating mesenchymal cells around this segment of the urogenital sinus. These mesenchymal cells start to develop around the tubules by the 16th week and become denser at the periphery to form the prostatic capsule. By the 22nd week, the muscular stroma is considerably developed, and it continues to increase progressively until birth.

From the five groups of epithelial buds, five lobes are eventually formed: anterior, posterior, median, and two lateral lobes. Initially, these lobes are widely separated, but later they meet, with no definite septa dividing them. Tubules of each lobe do not intermingle with each other but simply lie side by side.

The anterior lobe tubules begin to develop simultaneously with those of the other lobes. Although in the early stages, the anterior lobe tubules are large and show multiple branches; gradually, they contract and lose most of the branches. They continue to shrink so that at birth, they show no lumen and appear as small, solid embryonic epithelial outgrowths. In contrast, the tubules of the posterior lobe are fewer in number yet larger, with extensive branching. These tubules, as they grow, extend posterior to the developing median and lateral lobes and form the posterior aspect of the gland, which may be felt rectally.

Prostate development results from complex interaction between urogenital sinus epithelium and mesenchyme in the presence of androgens (reviewed by Cunha et al, 2004, and Thomson, 2008). Early in development, the androgen receptors are solely expressed in the urogenital sinus mesenchyme. Under the influence of androgen, the mesenchyme induces epithelial bud formation, regulates the growth and branching of epithelial bud, promotes differentiation of a secretory epithelium, and specifies differential expression of prostatic secretory proteins. Several members of the fibroblast growth factor (eg, FGF7 and FGF10) play essential role in prostate development, though they do not appear to be directly regulated by androgens. Other factors involved in prostatic duct branching and patterning include *Hoxa*10, *Fut*1, and *Shh/Ptc*. In contrast, other factors such as Activin A serve to inhibit ductal branching in order to maintain tissue homeostasis and regulated growth in the prostate.

ANOMALIES OF THE VESICOURETHRAL UNIT

Failure of the cloaca to subdivide is rare and results in a **persistent cloaca**. Incomplete subdivision is more frequent, ending with **rectovesical**, **rectourethral**, or **rectovestibular fistulas** (usually with **imperforate anus** or **anal atresia**).

Failure of descent or incomplete descent of the bladder leads to a **urinary umbilical fistula (urachal fistula)**, **urachal cyst**, or **urachal diverticulum** depending on the stage and degree of maldescent.

Development of the genital primordia in an area more caudal than normal can result in formation of the corpora cavernosa just caudal to the urogenital sinus outlet, with the urethral groove on its dorsal surface. This defect results in complete or incomplete **epispadias** depending on its degree. A more extensive defect results in **vesical exstrophy**. Failure of fusion of urethral folds leads to various grades of **hypospadias**. This defect, because of its mechanism, never extends proximal to the bulbous urethra. This is in contrast to epispadias, which usually involves the entire urethra up to the internal meatus.

GONADS

Most of the structures that make up the embryonic genital system have been taken over from other systems, and their readaptation to genital function is a secondary and relatively late phase in their development. The early differentiation of such structures is therefore independent of sexuality. Furthermore, each embryo is at first morphologically bisexual, possessing all the necessary structures for either sex. The development of one set of sex primordia and the gradual involution of the other are determined by the sex of the gonad.

The sexually undifferentiated gonad is a composite structure. Male and female potentials are represented by specific histologic elements (medulla and cortex) that have alternative roles in gonadogenesis. Normal differentiation involves the gradual predominance of one component.

The primitive sex glands make their appearance during the 5th and 6th weeks within a localized region of the thickening known as the urogenital ridge (this contains both the nephric and the genital primordia). At the 6th week, the gonad consists of a superficial germinal epithelium and an internal blastema. The blastemal mass is derived mainly from proliferative ingrowth from the superficial epithelium, which comes loose from its basement membrane.

During the 7th week, the gonad begins to assume the characteristics of a testis or ovary. Differentiation of the ovary usually occurs somewhat later than differentiation of the testis.

If the gonad develops into a testis, the gland increases in size and shortens into a more compact organ while achieving a more caudal location. Its broad attachment to the mesonephros is converted into a gonadal mesentery known as the mesorchium. The cells of the germinal epithelium grow into the underlying mesenchyme and form cordlike masses. These are radially arranged and converge toward the mesorchium, where a dense portion of the blastemal mass is also emerging as the primordium of the rete testis. A network of strands soon forms that is continuous with the testis cords. The latter also split into three to four daughter cords. These eventually become differentiated into the seminiferous tubules by which the spermatozoa are produced. The rete testis unites with the mesonephric components that will form the male genital ducts, as discussed in a subsequent section (Figure 2–6).

If the gonad develops into an ovary, it (like the testis) gains a mesentery (mesovarium) and settles in a more caudal position. The internal blastema differentiates in the 9th week into a primary cortex beneath the germinal epithelium and a loose primary medulla. A compact cellular mass bulges from the medulla into the mesovarium and establishes the primitive rete ovarii. At 3–4 months of age, the internal cell mass becomes young ova. A new definitive cortex is formed from the germinal epithelium as well as from the blastema in the form of distinct cellular cords (Pflüger's tubes), and a permanent medulla is formed. The cortex differentiates into ovarian follicles containing ova.

The molecular mechanism that regulates testis and ovary differentiation remains to be fully defined. In the presence of a Y chromosome, SRY (as known as testis determining factor [TDF]) induces the upregulation of *Sox9* in the undifferentiated gonad (reviewed by Sekido, 2010). This in turn upregulates the expression of FGF9 and increases PGD2 synthesis, both helping to maintain *Sox9* expression. *Sox9* directs the differentiation of cells into Sertoli cell by activating several downstream genes such as *Amh*, *Cbln4*, FGF9, and *Ptgds*. In the absence of a Y chromosome and SRY, *Rspo1* is upregulated in the undifferentiated gonads (reviewed by Nef and Vassalli, 2009). *Rspo1* is required for Wnt-4 expression and together they activate β-catenin, which, in turn, suppresses the formation of the testis cords by inhibiting *Sox9* and FGF9. A second pathway involving the upregulation of *Foxl2* also serves to inhibit *Sox9* and FGF9 activity, contributing to the development of the ovary.

▶ Descent of the Gonads

A. Testis

In addition to its early caudal migration, the testis later leaves the abdominal cavity and descends into the scrotum. By the 3rd month of fetal life, the testis is located retroperitoneally in the false pelvis. A fibromuscular band (the gubernaculum) extends from the lower pole of the testis through the developing muscular layers of the anterior abdominal wall to terminate in the subcutaneous tissue of the scrotal swelling. The gubernaculum also has several other subsidiary strands that extend to adjacent regions. Just below the lower pole of the testis, the peritoneum herniates as a diverticulum along the anterior aspect of the gubernaculum, eventually reaching the scrotal sac through the anterior abdominal muscles (the processus vaginalis). The testis remains at the abdominal end of the inguinal canal until the 7th month. It then passes through the inguinal canal behind (but invaginating) the processus vaginalis. Normally, it reaches the scrotal sac by the end of the 8th month.

B. Ovary

In addition to undergoing an early internal descent, the ovary becomes attached through the gubernaculum to the tissues of the genital fold and then attaches itself to the developing uterovaginal canal at its junction with the uterine (fallopian) tubes. This part of the gubernaculum between the ovary and uterus becomes the ovarian ligament; the part between the uterus and the labia majora becomes the round ligament of the uterus. These ligaments prevent extra-abdominal descent, and the ovary enters the true pelvis. It eventually lies posterior to the uterine tubes on the superior surface of the urogenital mesentery, which has descended with the ovary and now forms the broad ligament. A small processus vaginalis forms and passes toward the labial swelling, but it is usually obliterated at full term.

GONADAL ANOMALIES

Lack of development of the gonads is called **gonadal agenesis**. Incomplete development with arrest at a certain phase is called **hypogenesis**. **Supernumerary gonads** are rare. The commonest anomaly involves descent of the gonads, especially the testis. Retention of the testis in the abdomen or arrest of its descent at any point along its natural pathway is called **cryptorchidism**, which may be either unilateral or bilateral. If the testis does not follow the main gubernacular structure but follows one of its subsidiary strands, it will end in an abnormal position, resulting in an **ectopic testis**.

Failure of union between the rete testis and mesonephros results in a testis separate from the male genital ducts (the epididymis) and azoospermia.

GENITAL DUCT SYSTEM

Alongside the indifferent gonads, there are, early in embryonic life, two different yet closely related ducts. One is primarily a nephric duct (Wolffian duct), yet it also serves as a genital duct if the embryo develops into a male. The other (Müllerian duct) is primarily a genital structure from the start.

Both ducts grow caudally to join the primitive urogenital sinus. The Wolffian duct (known as the pronephric duct at the 4-mm stage) joins the ventral part of the cloaca, which will be the urogenital sinus. This duct gives rise to the ureteral bud close to its caudal end. The ureteral bud grows cranially and meets metanephrogenic tissue. The part of each

mesonephric duct caudal to the origin of the ureteric bud becomes absorbed into the wall of the primitive urogenital sinus so that the mesonephric duct and ureter open independently. This is achieved at the 15-mm stage (7th week). During this period, starting at the 10-mm stage, the Müllerian ducts start to develop. They reach the urogenital sinus relatively late—at the 30-mm stage (9th week); their partially fused blind ends producing the elevation called Müller's tubercle. Müller's tubercle is the most constant and reliable point of reference in the whole system.

If the gonad starts to develop into a testis (17-mm stage, 7th week), the Wolffian duct will start to differentiate into the male duct system, forming the epididymis, vas deferens, seminal vesicles, and ejaculatory ducts. At this time, the Müllerian duct proceeds toward its junction with the urogenital sinus and immediately starts to degenerate. Only its upper and lower ends persist, the former as the appendix testis and the latter as part of the prostatic utricle.

If the gonad starts to differentiate into an ovary (22-mm stage, 8th week), the Müllerian duct system forms the uterine (fallopian) tubes, uterus, and most of the vagina. The Wolffian ducts, aside from their contribution to the urogenital sinus, remain rudimentary.

MALE DUCT SYSTEM

▶ Epididymis

Because of the proximity of the differentiating gonads and the nephric duct, some of the mesonephric tubules are retained as the efferent ductules, and their lumens become continuous with those of the rete testis. These tubules, together with the part of the mesonephric duct into which they empty, will form the epididymis. Each coiled ductule makes a conical mass known as the lobule of the epididymis. The cranial end of the mesonephric duct becomes highly convoluted, completing the formation of the epididymis. This is an example of direct inclusion of a nephric structure into the genital system. Additional mesonephric tubules, both cephalad and caudal to those that were included in the formation of the epididymis, remain as rudimentary structures, that is, the appendix of the epididymis and the paradidymis.

▶ Vas Deferens, Seminal Vesicles, and Ejaculatory Ducts

The mesonephric duct caudal to the portion forming the epididymis forms the vas deferens. Shortly before this duct joins the urethra (urogenital sinus), a localized dilatation (ampulla) develops, and the saccular convoluted structure that will form the seminal vesicle is evaginated from its wall. The mesonephric duct between the origin of the seminal vesicle and the urethra forms the ejaculatory duct. The whole mesonephric duct now achieves its characteristic thick investment of smooth muscle, with a narrow lumen along most of its length.

Both above and below the point of entrance of the mesonephric duct into the urethra, multiple outgrowths of urethral epithelium mark the beginning of the development of the prostate. As these epithelial buds grow, they meet the developing muscular fibers around the urogenital sinus, and some of these fibers become entangled in the branching tubules of the growing prostate and become incorporated into it, forming its muscular stroma (Figure 2–4).

FEMALE DUCT SYSTEM

The Müllerian ducts, which are a paired system, are seen alongside the mesonephric duct. It is not known whether they arise directly from the mesonephric ducts or separately as an invagination of the celomic epithelium into the parenchyma lateral to the cranial extremity of the mesonephric duct, but the latter theory is favored. The Müllerian duct develops and runs lateral to the mesonephric duct. Its opening into the celomic cavity persists as the peritoneal ostium of the uterine tube (later it develops fimbriae). The other end grows caudally as a solid tip and then crosses in front of the mesonephric duct at the caudal extremity of the mesonephros. It continues its growth in a caudomedial direction until it meets and fuses with the Müllerian duct of the opposite side. The fusion is partial at first, so there is a temporary septum between the two lumens. This later disappears, leaving one cavity that will form the uterovaginal canal. The potential lumen of the vaginal canal is completely packed with cells. The solid tip of this cord pushes the epithelium of the urogenital sinus outward, where it becomes Müller's tubercle (33-mm stage, 9th week). The Müllerian ducts actually fuse at the 63-mm stage (13th week), forming the sinovaginal node, which receives a limited contribution from the urogenital sinus. (This contribution forms the lower fifth of the vagina.)

The urogenital sinus distal to Müller's tubercle, originally narrow and deep, shortens, widens, and opens to form the floor of the pudendal or vulval cleft. This results in separate openings for the vagina and urethra and also brings the vaginal orifice to its final position nearer the surface. At the same time, the vaginal segment increases appreciably in length. The vaginal vestibule is derived from the infratubercular segment of the urogenital sinus (in males, the same segment will form the inframontanal part of the prostatic urethra and the membranous urethra). The labia minora are formed from the urethral folds (in males they form the pendulous urethra). The hymen is the remnant of the Müllerian tubercle. The lower fifth of the vagina is derived from the portion of the urogenital sinus that combines with the sinovaginal node. The remainder of the vagina and the uterus are formed from the lower (fused) third of the Müllerian ducts. The uterine tubes (fallopian tubes, oviducts) are the cephalic two-thirds of the Müllerian ducts (Figure 2–6).

ANOMALIES OF THE GONADAL DUCT SYSTEM

Nonunion of the rete testis and the efferent ductules can occur and, if bilateral, causes **azoospermia** and **sterility**. Failure of the Müllerian ducts to approximate or to fuse completely can lead to various degrees of **duplication** in the genital ducts. **Congenital absence** of one or both uterine tubes or of the uterus or vagina occurs rarely.

Arrested development of the infratubercular segment of the urogenital sinus leads to its persistence, with the urethra and vagina having a common duct to the outside (**urogenital sinus**).

EXTERNAL GENITALIA

During the 8th week, external sexual differentiation begins to occur. Not until 3 months, however, do the progressively developing external genitalia attain characteristics that can be recognized as distinctively male or female. During the indifferent stage of sexual development, three small protuberances appear on the external aspect of the cloacal membrane. In front is the genital tubercle, and on either side of the membrane are the genital swellings.

With the breakdown of the urogenital membrane (17-mm stage, 7th week), the primitive urogenital sinus achieves a separate opening on the undersurface of the genital tubercle.

MALE EXTERNAL GENITALIA

The urogenital sinus opening extends on the ventral aspect of the genital tubercle as the urethral groove. The primitive urogenital orifice and the urethral groove are bounded on either side by the urethral folds. The genital tubercle becomes elongated to form the phallus. The corpora cavernosa are indicated in the 7th week as paired mesenchymal columns within the shaft of the penis. By the 10th week, the urethral folds start to fuse from the urogenital sinus orifice toward the tip of the phallus. At the 14th week, the fusion is complete and results in the formation of the penile urethra. The corpus spongiosum results from the differentiation of the mesenchymal masses around the formed penile urethra.

The glans penis becomes defined by the development of a circular coronary sulcus around the distal part of the phallus. The urethral groove and the fusing folds do not extend beyond the coronary sulcus. The glandular urethra develops as a result of canalization of an ectodermal epithelial cord that has grown through the glans. This canalization reaches and communicates with the distal end of the previously formed penile urethra. During the 3rd month, a fold of skin at the base of the glans begins growing distally and, 2 months later, surrounds the glans. This forms the prepuce. Meanwhile, the genital swellings shift caudally and are recognizable as scrotal swellings. They meet and fuse, resulting in the formation of the scrotum, with two compartments partially separated by a median septum and a median raphe, indicating their line of fusion.

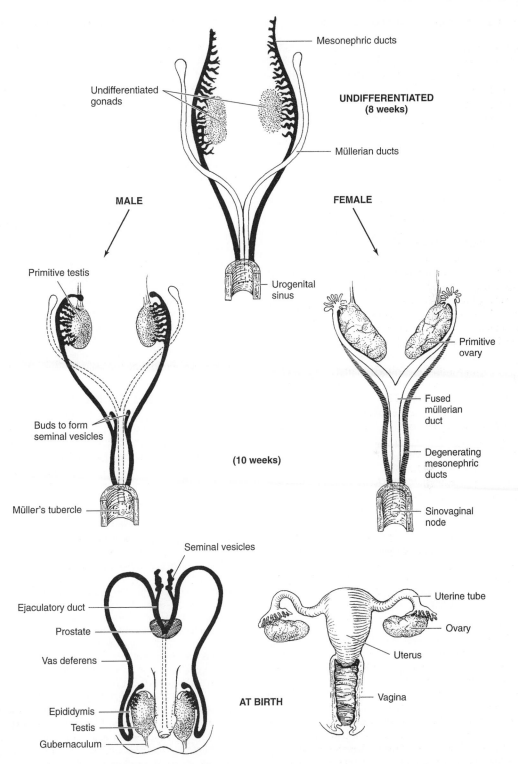

▲ Figure 2–6. Transformation of the undifferentiated genital system into the definitive male and female systems.

FEMALE EXTERNAL GENITALIA

Until the 8th week, the appearance of the female external genitalia closely resembles that of the male genitalia except that the urethral groove is shorter. The genital tubercle, which becomes bent caudally and lags in development, becomes the clitoris. As in males (though on a minor scale), mesenchymal columns differentiate into corpora cavernosa, and a coronary sulcus identifies the glans clitoridis. The most caudal part of the urogenital sinus shortens and widens, forming the vaginal vestibule. The urethral folds do not fuse but remain separate as the labia minora. The genital swellings meet in front of the anus, forming the posterior commissure, while the swellings as a whole enlarge and remain separated on either side of the vestibule and form the labia majora.

ANOMALIES OF THE EXTERNAL GENITALIA

Absence or duplication of the penis or clitoris is very rare. More commonly, the penis remains rudimentary or the clitoris shows hypertrophy. These anomalies may be seen alone or, more frequently, in association with pseudohermaphroditism. Concealed penis and transposition of penis and scrotum are relatively rare anomalies.

Failure or incomplete fusion of the urethral folds results in **hypospadias** (see preceding discussion). Penile development is also anomalous in cases of **epispadias** and **exstrophy** (see preceding discussion).

BIBLIOGRAPHY

General

Arey LB: Developmental Anatomy: A Textbook and Laboratory Manual of Embryology. 7th ed. Saunders, Philadelphia, 1974.

Ballermann BJ: Glomerular endothelial cell differentiation. Kidney Int 2005;67(5):1668–1671.

Burrow CR: Regulatory molecules in kidney development. Pediatr Nephrol 2000;131(7):240–253.

Carlson BM: Patten's Foundations of Embryology. 6th ed. McGraw-Hill, New York, 1996.

Costantini F, Shakya R: GDNF/Ret signaling and the development of the kidney. Bioessays 2006;28(2):117–127.

Cunha GR et al: Hormonal, cellular, and molecular regulation of normal and neoplastic prostatic development. J Steroid Biochem Mol Biol 2004;92(4):221–236.

Fine RN: Diagnosis and treatment of fetal urinary tract abnormalities. J Pediatr 1992;121:333.

FitzGerald MJT: Human Embryology: A Regional Approach. Harper & Row, London, 1978.

Gilbert SG: Pictorial Human Embryology. University of Washington Press, Seattle, 1989.

Marshall FF: Embryology of the lower genitourinary tract. Urol Clin North Am 1978;5:3.

Michos O: Kidney development: From ureteric bud formation to branching morphogenesis. Curr Opin Genet Dev 2009;19: 484–490.

Mcinnes RR, Michaud JL: Plumbing in the embryo: Development defects of the urinary tracts. Clin Genet 2009;75:307–317.

Nef S, Vassalli JD: Complementary pathways in mammalian female sex determination. J Biol 2009;8:74.

Nyengaard JR, Bendtsen TF: Glomerular number and size in relation to age, kidney weight, and body surface in normal man. Anat Rec 1992;232(2):194–201.

Oswald J et al: Reevaluation of the fetal muscle development of the vesical trigone. J Urol 2006;176(3):1166–1170.

Reddy PP, Mandell J: Prenatal diagnosis: Therapeutic implications. Urol Clin North Am 1998;25:171.

Sekido R: SRY: A transcriptional activator of mammalian testis determination. Int J Biochem Cell Biol 2010;42(3):417–420.

Shah MM et al: Branching morphogenesis and kidney disease. Development 2004;131(7):1449–1462.

Stephens FD: Embryopathy of malformations. J Urol 1982;127:13.

Stephens FD: Congenital Malformations of the Urinary Tract. Praeger, New York, 1983.

Tanagho EA: Embryologic development of the urinary tract. In: Ball TP (ed) AUA Update Series. American Urological Association, Philadelphia, 1982.

Tanagho EA: Developmental anatomy and urogenital abnormalities. In: Raz S (ed) Female Urology. 2nd ed. Saunders, Philadelphia, 1986.

Thomson AA: Mesenchymal mechanisms in prostate organogenesis. Differentiation 2008;76(6):587–598.

Vaughan ED Jr, Middleton GW: Pertinent genitourinary embryology: Review for practicing urologist. Urology 1975;6:139.

Anomalies of the Nephric System

Avni EF et al: Multicystic dysplastic kidney: Natural history from in utero diagnosis and postnatal followup. J Urol 1987;138:1420.

Bomalaski MD et al: Vesicoureteral reflux and ureteropelvic junction obstruction: Association, treatment options and outcome. J Urol 1997;157:969.

Chevalier RL: Effects of ureteral obstruction on renal growth. Pediatr Nephrol 1995;9:594.

Churchill BM et al: Ureteral duplication, ectopy and ureteroceles. Pediatr Clin North Am 1987;34:1273.

Corrales JG, Elder JS: Segmental multicystic kidney and ipsilateral duplication anomalies. J Urol 1996;155:1398.

Cox R et al: Twenty-year follow-up of primary megaureter. Eur Urol 1990;17:43.

Decter RM: Renal duplication and fusion anomalies. Pediatr Clin North Am 1997;44:1323.

El-Galley RE, Keane TE: Embryology, anatomy, and surgical applications of the kidney and ureter. Surg Clin North Am 2000;80:381.

Glassberg KI: Normal and abnormal development of the kidney: A clinician's interpretation of current knowledge. J Urol 2002; 167:2339.

Keating MA et al: Changing concepts in management of primary obstructive megaureter. J Urol 1989;142:636.

MacDermot KD et al: Prenatal diagnosis of autosomal dominant polycystic kidney disease (PKD1) presenting in utero and prognosis for very early onset disease. J Med Genet 1998;35:13.

Magee MC: Ureteroceles and duplicated systems: Embryologic hypothesis. J Urol 1980;123:605.

Maher ER, Kaelin WG Jr: Von Hippel-Lindau disease. Medicine (Baltimore) 1997;76:381.

Mesrobian HG et al: Unilateral renal agenesis may result from in utero regression of multicystic renal dysplasia. J Urol 1993; 150:793.

Murcia NS et al: New insights into the molecular pathophysiology of polycystic kidney disease. Kidney Int 1999;55:1187.

Nguyen HT, Kogan BA: Upper urinary tract obstruction: Experimental and clinical aspects. Br J Urol 1998;81(Suppl 2):13.

Osathanondh V, Potter EL: Pathogenesis of polycystic kidneys: Survey of results of microdissection. Arch Pathol 1964a;77:510.

Osathanondh V, Potter EL: Pathogenesis of polycystic kidneys: Type 4 due to urethral obstruction. Arch Pathol 1964b;77:502.

Pope JC IV et al: How they begin and how they end: Classic and new theories for the development and deterioration of congenital anomalies of the kidney and urinary tract, CAKUT. J Am Soc Nephrol 1999;10:2018.

Prasad PV, Priatna A: Functional imaging of the kidneys with fast MRI techniques. Eur J Radiol 1999;29:133.

Robson WL et al: Unilateral renal agenesis. Adv Pediatr 1995;42:575.

Ross JH, Kay R: Ureteropelvic junction obstruction in anomalous kidneys. Urol Clin North Am 1998;25:219.

Scherz HC et al: Ectopic ureteroceles: Surgical management with preservation of continence. Review of 60 cases. J Urol 1989;142:538.

Soderdahl DW et al: Bilateral ureteral quadruplication. J Urol 1976;116:255.

Somlo S, Markowitz GS: The pathogenesis of autosomal dominant polycystic kidney disease: An update. Curr Opin Nephrol Hypertens 2000;9:385.

Tanagho EA: Ureteroceles: Embryogenesis, pathogenesis and management. J Cont Educ Urol (Feb) 1979;18:13.

Tanagho EA: Development of the ureter. In: Bergman H (ed) The Ureter. 2nd ed. Springer-Verlag, New York, 1981.

Thomsen HS et al: Renal cystic diseases. Eur Radiol 1997;7:1267.

Tokunaka S et al: Morphological study of ureterocele: Possible clue to its embryogenesis as evidenced by locally arrested myogenesis. J Urol 1981;126:726.

Zerres K et al: Autosomal recessive polycystic kidney disease. Contrib Nephrol 1997;122:10.

Anomalies of the Vesicourethral Unit

Asopa HS: Newer concepts in the management of hypospadias and its complications. Ann R Coll Surg Engl 1998;80:161.

Austin PF et al: The prenatal diagnosis of cloacal exstrophy. J Urol 1998;160(3, Pt 2):1179.

Baskin LS: Hypospadias and urethral development. J Urol 2000; 163:951.

Begg RC: The urachus, its anatomy, histology and development. J Anat 1930;64:170.

Belman AB: Hypospadias update. Urology 1997;49:166.

Burbige KA et al: Prune belly syndrome: 35 years of experience. J Urol 1987;137:86.

Churchill BM et al: Emergency treatment and long-term follow-up of posterior urethral valves. Urol Clin North Am 1990;17:343.

Chwalle R: The process of formation of cystic dilatations of the vesicle end of the ureter and of diverticula at the ureteral ostium. Urol Cutan Rev 1927;31:499.

Connor JP et al: Long-term follow-up of 207 patients with bladder exstrophy: An evolution in treatment. J Urol 1989;142:793.

Dinneen MD, Duffy PG: Posterior urethral valves. Br J Urol 1996;78:275.

Duckett JW: The current hype in hypospadiology. Br J Urol 1995;76(Suppl 3):1.

Eagle JR Jr, Barrett GS: Congenital deficiency of abdominal musculature with associated genitourinary abnormalities: A syndrome. Report of nine cases. Pediatrics 1950;6:721.

Elmassalme FN et al: Duplication of urethra—case report and review of literature. Eur J Pediatr Surg 1997;7:313.

Escham W, Holt HA: Complete duplication of bladder and urethra. J Urol 1980;123:773.

Goh DW et al: Bladder, urethral, and vaginal duplication. J Pediatr Surg 1995;30:125.

Greskovich FJ III, Nyberg LM Jr: The prune belly syndrome: A review of its etiology, defects, treatment and prognosis. J Urol 1988; 140:707.

Hinman F Jr: Surgical disorders of the bladder and umbilicus of urachal origin. Surg Gynecol Obstet 1961;113:605.

Jaramillo D et al: The cloacal malformation: Radiologic findings and imaging recommendations. Radiology 1990;177:441.

Jeffs RD: Exstrophy, epispadias, and cloacal and urogenital sinus abnormalities. Pediatr Clin North Am 1987;34:1233.

Landes RR et al: Vesical exstrophy with epispadias: Twenty-year follow-up. Urology 1977;9:53.

Mackie GG: Abnormalities of the ureteral bud. Urol Clin North Am 1978;5:161.

Manzoni GA et al: Cloacal exstrophy and cloacal exstrophy variants: A proposed system of classification. J Urol 1987;138:1065.

Massad CA et al: Morphology and histochemistry of infant testes in the prune belly syndrome. J Urol 1991;146:1598.

Mesrobian HG et al: Long-term followup of 103 patients with bladder exstrophy. J Urol 1988;139:719.

Mouriquand PD et al: Hypospadias repair: Current principles and procedures. Br J Urol 1995;76(Suppl 3):9.

Nguyen HT, Kogan BA: Fetal bladder physiology. Adv Exp Med Biol 1999;462:121.

Orvis BR et al: Testicular histology in fetuses with the prune belly syndrome and posterior urethral valves. J Urol 1988;139:335.

Randall A, Campbell EW: Anomalous relationship of the right ureter to the vena cava. J Urol 1935;34:565.

Rosenfeld B et al: Type III posterior urethral valves: Presentation and management. J Pediatr Surg 1994;29:81.

Shapiro E: Embryologic development of the prostate: Insights into the etiology and treatment of benign prostatic hyperplasia. Urol Clin North Am 1990;17:487.

Silver RI: What is the etiology of hypospadias? A review of recent research. Del Med J 2000;72:343.

Stein R, Thuroff JW: Hypospadias and bladder exstrophy. Curr Opin Urol 2002;12:195.

Stephens FD: The female anus, perineum and vestibule: Embryogenesis and deformities. J Obstet Gynaecol Br Commonw 1968; 8:55.

Tanagho EA: Embryologic basis for lower ureteral anomalies: A hypothesis. Urology 1976;7:451.

Uehling DT: Posterior urethral valves: Functional classification. Urology 1980;15:27.

Van Savage JG et al: An algorithm for the management of anterior urethral valves. J Urol 1997;158(3, Pt 2):1030.

Wakhlu AK et al: Congenital megalourethra. J Pediatr Surg 1996; 31:441.

Workman SJ, Kogan BA: Fetal bladder histology in posterior urethral valves and the prune belly syndrome. J Urol 1990;144:337.

Gonadal Anomalies

Barteczko KJ, Jacob MI: The testicular descent in humans: Origin, development and fate of the gubernaculum Hunteri, processus vaginalis peritonei, and gonadal ligaments. Adv Anat Embryol Cell Biol 2000;156:III–X, 1.

Belville C et al: Persistence of Müllerian derivatives in males. Am J Med Genet 1999;89:218.

Ben-Chaim J, Gearhart JP: Current management of bladder exstrophy. Scand J Urol Nephrol 1997;31:103.

Borzi PA, Thomas DF: Cantwell-Ransley epispadias repair in male epispadias and bladder exstrophy. J Urol 1994;151:457.

Crankson SJ, Ahmed S: Female bladder exstrophy. Int Urogynecol J Pelvic Floor Dysfunct 1997;8:98.

de Palma L et al: Epididymal and vas deferens immaturity in cryptorchidism. J Urol 1988;140:1166.

Diez Garcia R et al: Peno-scrotal transposition. Eur J Pediatr Surg 1995;5:222.

Elder JS et al: Androgenic sensitivity of gubernaculum testis: Evidence for hormonal/mechanical interactions in testicular descent. J Urol 1982;127:170.

Gad YZ et al: 5 alpha-reductase deficiency in patients with micropenis. J Inherit Metab Dis 1997;20:95.

Hadziselimovic F et al: The significance of postnatal gonadotropin surge for testicular development in normal and cryptorchid testes. J Urol 1986;136:274.

Honoré LH: Unilateral anorchism: Report of 11 cases with discussion of etiology and pathogenesis. Urology 1978;11:251.

Johnson P et al: Inferior vesical fissure. J Urol 1995;154:1478.

Mollard P et al: Female epispadias. J Urol 1997;158:1543.

Nef S, Parada LF: Hormones in male sexual development. Genes Dev 2000;14:3075.

Newman K et al: The surgical management of infants and children with ambiguous genitalia: Lessons learned from 25 years. Ann Surg 1992;215:644.

Pagon RA: Diagnostic approach to the newborn with ambiguous genitalia. Pediatr Clin North Am 1987;34:1019.

Parker KL et al: Gene interactions in gonadal development. Annu Rev Physiol 1999;61:417.

Rajfer J, Walsh PC: Testicular descent: Normal and abnormal. Urol Clin North Am 1978;5:223.

Toppari J, Kaleva M: Maldescendus testis. Horm Res 1999;51:261.

Zaontz MR, Packer MG: Abnormalities of the external genitalia. Pediatr Clin North Am 1997;44:1267.

Symptoms of Disorders of the Genitourinary Tract

3

Jack W. McAninch, MD, FACS, FRCS(E)(Hon)

In the workup of any patient, the history is of paramount importance; this is particularly true in urology. It is necessary to discuss here only those urologic symptoms that are apt to be brought to the physician's attention by the patient. It is important to know not only whether the disease is acute or chronic but also whether it is recurrent, since recurring symptoms may represent acute exacerbations of chronic disease.

Obtaining the history is an art that depends on the skill and methods used to elicit information. The history is only as accurate as the patient's ability to describe the symptoms. This subjective information is important in establishing an accurate diagnosis.

SYSTEMIC MANIFESTATIONS

Symptoms of fever and weight loss should be sought. The presence of fever associated with other symptoms of urinary tract infection may be helpful in evaluating the site of the infection. Simple acute cystitis is essentially an afebrile disease. Acute pyelonephritis or prostatitis is apt to cause high temperatures (up to 40°C [104°F]), often accompanied by violent chills. Infants and children who have acute pyelonephritis may have high temperatures without other localizing symptoms or signs. Such a clinical picture, therefore, *invariably* requires bacteriologic study of the urine.

A history of unexplained attacks of fever occurring even years before may otherwise represent asymptomatic pyelonephritis. Renal carcinoma sometimes causes fever that may reach 39°C (102.2°F) or more. The absence of fever does not by any means rule out renal infection, for it is the rule that chronic pyelonephritis does not cause fever.

Weight loss is to be expected in the advanced stages of cancer, but it may also be noticed when renal insufficiency due to obstruction or infection supervenes. In children who have "failure to thrive" (low weight and less than average height for their age), chronic obstruction, urinary tract infection, or both should be suspected.

General malaise may be noted with tumors, chronic pyelonephritis, or renal failure. The presence of many of these symptoms may be compatible with human immunodeficiency virus (HIV; see Chapter 15).

LOCAL AND REFERRED PAIN

Two types of pain have their origins in the genitourinary organs: local and referred. The latter is especially common.

Local pain is felt in or near the involved organ. Thus, the pain from a diseased kidney (T10–12, L1) is felt in the costovertebral angle and in the flank in the region of and below the 12th rib. Pain from an inflamed testicle is felt in the gonad itself.

Referred pain originates in a diseased organ but is felt at some distance from that organ. The ureteral colic (Figure 3–1) caused by a stone in the upper ureter may be associated with severe pain in the ipsilateral testicle; this is explained by the common innervation of these two structures (T11–12). A stone in the lower ureter may cause pain referred to the scrotal wall; in this instance, the testis itself is not hyperesthetic. The burning pain with voiding that accompanies acute cystitis is felt in the distal urethra in females and in the glandular urethra in males (S2–3).

Abnormalities of a urologic organ can also cause pain in any other organ (eg, gastrointestinal, gynecologic) that has a sensory nerve supply common to both (Figures 3–2 and 3–3).

▶ Kidney Pain (Figure 3–1)

Typical renal pain is felt as a dull and constant ache in the costovertebral angle just lateral to the sacrospinalis muscle and just below the 12th rib. This pain often spreads along the subcostal area toward the umbilicus or lower abdominal quadrant. It may be expected in the renal diseases that cause sudden distention of the renal capsule. Acute pyelonephritis (with its sudden edema) and acute ureteral obstruction (with its sudden renal back pressure) both cause this typical

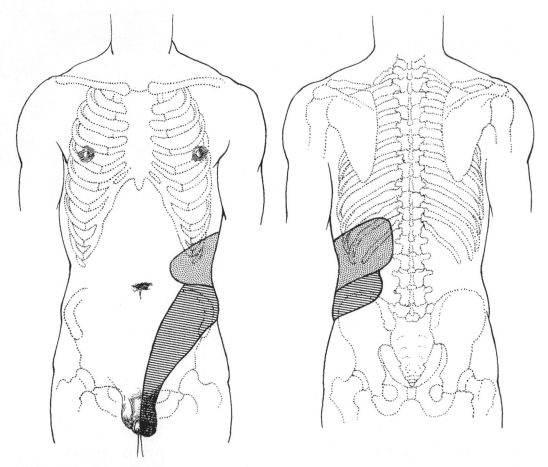

▲ **Figure 3–1.** Referred pain from kidney (dotted areas) and ureter (shaded areas).

pain. It should be pointed out, however, that many urologic renal diseases are painless because their progression is so slow that sudden capsular distention does not occur. Such diseases include cancer, chronic pyelonephritis, staghorn calculus, tuberculosis, polycystic kidney, and hydronephrosis due to chronic ureteral obstruction.

▶ Ureteral Pain (Figure 3–1)

Ureteral pain is typically stimulated by acute obstruction (passage of a stone or a blood clot). In this instance, there is back pain from renal capsular distention combined with severe colicky pain (due to renal pelvic and ureteral muscle spasm) that radiates from the costovertebral angle down toward the lower anterior abdominal quadrant, along the course of the ureter. In men, it may also be felt in the bladder, scrotum, or testicle. In women, it may radiate into the vulva. The severity and colicky nature of this pain are caused by the

hyperperistalsis and spasm of this smooth muscle organ as it attempts to rid itself of a foreign body or to overcome obstruction.

The physician may be able to judge the position of a ureteral stone by the history of pain and the site of referral. If the stone is lodged in the upper ureter, the pain radiates to the testicle, since the nerve supply of this organ is similar to that of the kidney and upper ureter (T11–12). With stones in the midportion of the ureter on the right side, the pain is referred to McBurney's point and may therefore simulate appendicitis; on the left side, it may resemble diverticulitis or other diseases of the descending or sigmoid colon (T12, L1). As the stone approaches the bladder, inflammation and edema of the ureteral orifice ensue, and symptoms of vesical irritability such as urinary frequency and urgency may occur. It is important to realize, however, that in mild ureteral obstruction, as seen in the congenital stenoses, there is usually no pain, either renal or ureteral.

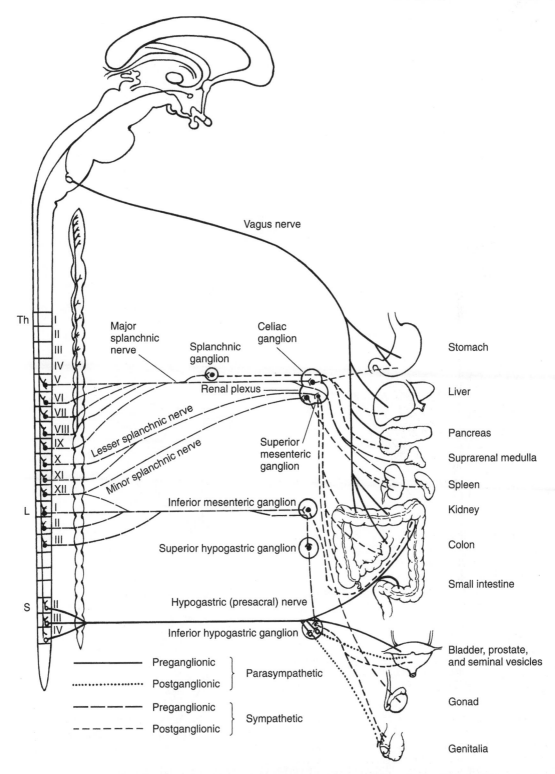

▲ **Figure 3–2.** Diagrammatic representation of autonomic nerve supply to gastrointestinal and genitourinary tracts.

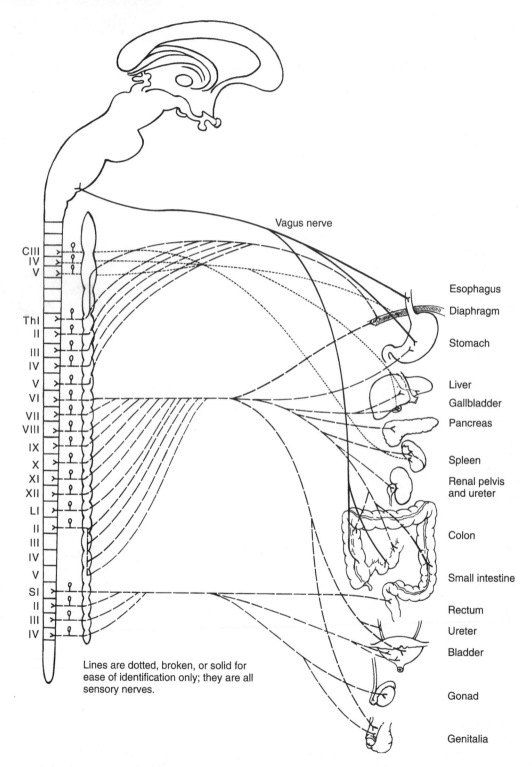

▲ **Figure 3–3.** Diagrammatic representation of sensory nerves of gastrointestinal and genitourinary tracts.

Vesical Pain

The overdistended bladder of the patient in acute urinary retention causes agonizing pain in the suprapubic area. Other than this, however, constant suprapubic pain not related to the act of urination is usually not of urologic origin.

The patient in chronic urinary retention due to bladder neck obstruction or neurogenic bladder may experience little or no suprapubic discomfort even though the bladder reaches the level of the umbilicus.

The most common cause of bladder pain is infection; the pain is usually not felt over the bladder but is referred to the distal urethra and is related to the act of urination. Terminal dysuria may be a major complaint in severe cystitis.

Prostatic Pain

Direct pain from the prostate gland is not common. Occasionally, when the prostate is acutely inflamed, the patient may feel a vague discomfort or fullness in the perineal or rectal area (S2–4). Lumbosacral backache is occasionally experienced as referred pain from the prostate, but is not a common symptom of prostatitis. Inflammation of the gland may cause dysuria, frequency, and urgency.

Testicular Pain

Testicular pain due to trauma, infection, or torsion of the spermatic cord is very severe and is felt locally, although there may be some radiation of the discomfort along the spermatic cord into the lower abdomen. Uninfected hydrocele, spermatocele, and tumor of the testis do not commonly cause pain. A varicocele may cause a dull ache in the testicle that is increased after heavy exercise. At times, the first symptom of an early indirect inguinal hernia may be testicular pain (referred). Pain from a stone in the upper ureter may be referred to the testicle.

Epididymal Pain

Acute infection of the epididymis is the only painful disease of this organ and is quite common. The pain begins in the scrotum, and some degree of neighborhood inflammatory reaction involves the adjacent testis as well, further aggravating the discomfort. In the early stages of epididymitis, pain may first be felt in the groin or lower abdominal quadrant. (If on the right side, it may simulate appendicitis.) This may be a referred type of pain but can be secondary to associated inflammation of the vas deferens.

GASTROINTESTINAL SYMPTOMS OF UROLOGIC DISEASES

Whether renal or ureteral disease is painful or not, gastrointestinal symptoms are often present. The patient with acute pyelonephritis not only has localized back pain, symptoms of vesical irritability, chills, and fever but also generalized abdominal pain and distention. A patient who is passing a stone down the ureter has typical renal and ureteral colic and, usually, hematuria and may experience severe nausea and vomiting as well as abdominal distention. However, the urinary symptoms so far overshadow the gastrointestinal symptoms that the latter are usually ignored. Inadvertent overdistention of the renal pelvis (eg, with opaque material in order to obtain adequate retrograde urograms) may cause the patient to become nauseated, to vomit, and to complain of cramplike pain in the abdomen. This clinical experiment demonstrates the renointestinal reflex, which may lead to confusing symptoms. In the very common "silent" urologic diseases, some degree of gastrointestinal symptomatology may be present, which could mislead the clinician into seeking the diagnosis in the intraperitoneal zone.

Cause of the Mimicry

A. Renointestinal Reflexes

Renointestinal reflexes account for most of the confusion. They arise because of the common autonomic and sensory innervations of the two systems (Figures 3–2 and 3–3). Afferent stimuli from the renal capsule or musculature of the pelvis may, by reflex action, cause pylorospasm (symptoms of peptic ulcer) or other changes in tone of the smooth muscles of the enteric tract and its adnexa.

B. Organ Relationships

The right kidney is closely related to the hepatic flexure of the colon, the duodenum, the head of the pancreas, the common bile duct, the liver, and the gallbladder (Figure 1–3). The left kidney lies just behind the splenic flexure of the colon and is closely related to the stomach, pancreas, and spleen. Inflammations or tumors in the retroperitoneum thus may extend into or displace intraperitoneal organs, causing them to produce symptoms.

C. Peritoneal Irritation

The anterior surfaces of the kidneys are covered by peritoneum. Renal inflammation, therefore, causes peritoneal irritation, which can lead to muscle rigidity and rebound tenderness.

The symptoms arising from chronic renal disease (eg, noninfected hydronephrosis, staghorn calculus, cancer, chronic pyelonephritis) may be entirely gastrointestinal and may simulate in every way the syndromes of peptic ulcer, gallbladder disease, or appendicitis, or other, less specific gastrointestinal complaints. If a thorough survey of the gastrointestinal tract fails to demonstrate suspected disease processes, the physician should give every consideration to study of the urinary tract.

SYMPTOMS RELATED TO THE ACT OF URINATION

Many conditions cause symptoms of "cystitis." These include infections of the bladder, vesical inflammation due to chemical or x-radiation reactions, interstitial cystitis, prostatitis, psychoneurosis, torsion or rupture of an ovarian cyst, and foreign bodies in the bladder. Often, however, the patient with chronic cystitis notices no symptoms of vesical irritability. Irritating chemicals or soap on the urethral meatus may cause cystitis-like symptoms of dysuria, frequency, and urgency. This has been specifically noted in young girls taking frequent bubble baths.

▶ Frequency, Nocturia, and Urgency

The normal capacity of the bladder is about 400 mL. Frequency may be caused by residual urine, which decreases the functional capacity of the organ. When the mucosa, submucosa, and even the muscularis become inflamed (eg, infection, foreign body, stones, tumor), the capacity of the bladder decreases sharply. This decrease is due to two factors: the pain resulting from even mild stretching of the bladder and the loss of bladder compliance resulting from inflammatory edema. When the bladder is normal, urination can be delayed if circumstances require it, but this is not so in acute cystitis. Once the diminished bladder capacity is reached, any further distention may be agonizing, and the patient may urinate involuntarily if voiding does not occur immediately. During very severe acute infections, the desire to urinate may be constant, and each voiding may produce only a few milliliters of urine. Day frequency without nocturia and acute or chronic frequency lasting only a few hours suggest nervous tension.

Diseases that cause fibrosis of the bladder are accompanied by frequency of urination. Examples of such diseases are tuberculosis, radiation cystitis, interstitial cystitis, and schistosomiasis. The presence of stones or foreign bodies causes vesical irritability, but secondary infection is almost always present.

Nocturia may be a symptom of renal disease related to a decrease in the functioning renal parenchyma with loss of concentrating power. Nocturia can occur in the absence of disease in persons who drink excessive amounts of fluid in the late evening. Coffee and alcoholic beverages, because of their specific diuretic effect, often produce nocturia if consumed just before bedtime. In older people who are ambulatory, some fluid retention may develop secondary to mild heart failure or varicose veins. With recumbency at night, this fluid is mobilized, leading to nocturia in these patients.

A very low or very high urine pH can irritate the bladder and cause frequency of urination.

▶ Dysuria

Painful urination is usually related to acute inflammation of the bladder, urethra, or prostate. At times, the pain is described as "burning" on urination and is usually located in the distal urethra in men. Women usually localize the pain to the urethra. The pain is present only with voiding and disappears soon after micturition is completed. More severe pain sometimes occurs in the bladder just at the end of voiding, suggesting that inflammation of the bladder is the likely cause. Pain also may be more marked at the beginning of or throughout the act of urination. Dysuria often is the first symptom suggesting urinary infection and is often associated with urinary frequency and urgency.

▶ Enuresis

Strictly speaking, enuresis means bedwetting at night. It is physiologic during the first 2 or 3 years of life but becomes troublesome, particularly to parents, after that age. It may be functional or secondary to delayed neuromuscular maturation of the urethrovesical component, but it may present as a symptom of organic disease (eg, infection, distal urethral stenosis in girls, posterior urethral valves in boys, neurogenic bladder). If wetting occurs also during the daytime, however, or if there are other urinary symptoms, urologic investigation is essential. In adult life, enuresis may be replaced by nocturia for which no organic basis can be found.

▶ Symptoms of Bladder Outlet Obstruction

A. Hesitancy

Hesitancy in initiating the urinary stream is one of the early symptoms of bladder outlet obstruction. As the degree of obstruction increases, hesitancy is prolonged and the patient often strains to force urine through the obstruction. Prostate obstruction and urethral stricture are common causes of this symptom.

B. Loss of Force and Decrease of Caliber of the Stream

Progressive loss of force and caliber of the urinary stream is noted as urethral resistance increases despite the generation of increased intravesical pressure. This can be evaluated by measuring urinary flow rates; in normal circumstances with a full bladder, a maximal flow of 20 mL/s should be achieved.

C. Terminal Dribbling

Terminal dribbling becomes more and more noticeable as obstruction progresses and is a most distressing symptom.

D. Urgency

A strong, sudden desire to urinate is caused by hyperactivity and irritability of the bladder, resulting from obstruction, inflammation, or neuropathic bladder disease. In most circumstances, the patient is able to control temporarily the sudden need to void, but loss of small amounts of urine may occur (urgency incontinence).

E. Acute Urinary Retention

Sudden inability to urinate may supervene. The patient experiences increasingly agonizing suprapubic pain associated with severe urgency and may dribble only small amounts of urine.

F. Chronic Urinary Retention

Chronic urinary retention may cause little discomfort to the patient even though there is great hesitancy in starting the stream and marked reduction of its force and caliber. Constant dribbling of urine (paradoxic incontinence) may be experienced; it may be likened to water pouring over a dam.

G. Interruption of the Urinary Stream

Interruption may be abrupt and accompanied by severe pain radiating down the urethra. This type of reaction strongly suggests the complication of vesical calculus.

H. Sense of Residual Urine

The patient often feels that urine is still in the bladder even after urination has been completed.

I. Cystitis

Recurring episodes of acute cystitis suggest the presence of residual urine.

▶ Incontinence (See also Chapter 27)

There are many reasons for incontinence. The history often gives a clue to its cause.

A. True Incontinence

The patient may lose urine without warning; this may be a constant or periodic symptom. The more obvious causes include previous radical prostatectomy, exstrophy of the bladder, epispadias, vesicovaginal fistula, and ectopic ureteral orifice. Injury to the urethral smooth muscle sphincters may occur during prostatectomy or childbirth. Congenital or acquired neurogenic diseases may lead to dysfunction of the bladder and incontinence.

B. Stress Incontinence

When slight weakness of the sphincteric mechanisms is present, urine may be lost in association with physical strain (eg, coughing, laughing, rising from a chair). This is common in multiparous women who have weakened muscle support of the bladder neck and urethra and in men who have undergone radical prostatectomy. Occasionally, neuropathic bladder dysfunction can cause stress incontinence. The patient stays dry while lying in bed.

C. Urge Incontinence

Urgency may be so precipitate and severe that there is involuntary loss of urine. Urge incontinence does not infrequently occur with acute cystitis, particularly in women, since women seem to have relatively poor anatomic sphincters. Urge incontinence is a common symptom of an upper motor neuron lesion.

D. Overflow Incontinence

Paradoxic incontinence is loss of urine due to chronic urinary retention or secondary to a flaccid bladder. The intravesical pressure finally equals the urethral resistance; urine then constantly dribbles forth.

▶ Oliguria and Anuria

Oliguria and anuria may be caused by acute renal failure (due to shock or dehydration), fluid-ion imbalance, or bilateral ureteral obstruction.

▶ Pneumaturia

The passage of gas in the urine strongly suggests a fistula between the urinary tract and the bowel. This occurs most commonly in the bladder or urethra but may be seen also in the ureter or renal pelvis. Carcinoma of the sigmoid colon, diverticulitis with abscess formation, regional enteritis, and trauma cause most vesical fistulas. Congenital anomalies account for most urethroenteric fistulas. Certain bacteria, by the process of fermentation, may liberate gas on rare occasions.

▶ Cloudy Urine

Patients often complain of cloudy urine, but it is most often cloudy merely because it is alkaline; this causes precipitation of phosphate. Infection can also cause urine to be cloudy and malodorous. A properly performed urinalysis will reveal the cause of cloudiness.

▶ Chyluria

The passage of lymphatic fluid or chyle is noted by the patient as passage of milky white urine. This represents a lymphatic–urinary system fistula. Most often, the cause is obstruction of the renal lymphatics, which results in forniceal rupture and leakage. Filariasis, trauma, tuberculosis, and retroperitoneal tumors have caused the problem.

▶ Bloody Urine

Hematuria is a danger signal that cannot be ignored. Carcinoma of the kidney or bladder, calculi, and infection are a few of the conditions in which hematuria is typically demonstrable at the time of presentation. It is important to know whether urination is painful or not, whether the hematuria is associated with symptoms of vesical irritability, and whether blood is seen in all or only a portion of the urinary stream. The hemoglobinuria that occurs as a feature of the hemolytic syndromes may also cause the urine to be red.

A. Bloody Urine in Relation to Symptoms and Diseases

Hematuria associated with renal colic suggests a ureteral stone, although a clot from a bleeding renal tumor can cause the same type of pain.

Hematuria is not uncommonly associated with nonspecific, tuberculous, or schistosomal infection of the bladder. The bleeding is often terminal (bladder neck or prostate), although it may be present throughout urination (vesical or upper tract). Stone in the bladder often causes hematuria, but infection is usually present, and there are symptoms of bladder neck obstruction, neurogenic bladder, or cystocele.

Dilated veins may develop at the bladder neck secondary to enlargement of the prostate. These may rupture when the patient strains to urinate, resulting in gross or microscopic hematuria.

Hematuria without other symptoms (silent hematuria) must be regarded as a symptom of tumor of the bladder or kidney until proved otherwise. It is usually intermittent; bleeding may not recur for months. Because the bleeding stops spontaneously, complacency must be condemned. Less common causes of silent hematuria are staghorn calculus, polycystic kidneys, benign prostatic hyperplasia, solitary renal cyst, sickle cell disease, and hydronephrosis. Painless bleeding is common with acute glomerulonephritis. Recurrent bleeding is occasionally seen in children suffering from focal glomerulitis. Joggers and people who engage in participatory sports frequently develop transient proteinuria and gross or microscopic hematuria.

B. Time of Hematuria

Learning whether the hematuria is partial (initial, terminal) or total (present throughout urination) is often of help in identifying the site of bleeding. Initial hematuria suggests an anterior urethral lesion (eg, urethritis, stricture, meatal stenosis in young boys). Terminal hematuria usually arises from the posterior urethra, bladder neck, or trigone. Among the common causes are posterior urethritis and polyps and tumors of the vesical neck. Total hematuria has its source at or above the level of the bladder (eg, stone, tumor, tuberculosis, nephritis).

OTHER OBJECTIVE MANIFESTATIONS

▶ Urethral Discharge

Urethral discharge in men is one of the most common urologic complaints. The causative organism is usually *Neisseria gonorrhoeae* or *Chlamydia trachomatis*. The discharge is often accompanied by local burning on urination or an itching sensation in the urethra (see Chapter 15).

▶ Skin Lesions of the External Genitalia (See Chapters 15 and 40)

An ulceration of the glans penis or its shaft may represent syphilitic chancre, chancroid, herpes simplex, or squamous cell carcinoma. Venereal warts of the penis are common.

▶ Visible or Palpable Masses

The patient may notice a visible or palpable mass in the upper abdomen that may represent renal tumor, hydronephrosis, or polycystic kidney. Enlarged lymph nodes in the neck may contain metastatic tumor from the prostate or testis. Lumps in the groin may represent spread of tumor of the penis or lymphadenitis from chancroid, syphilis, or lymphogranuloma venereum. Painless masses in the scrotal contents are common and include hydrocele, varicocele, spermatocele, chronic epididymitis, hernia, and testicular tumor.

▶ Edema

Edema of the legs may result from compression of the iliac veins by lymphatic metastases from prostatic cancer. Edema of the genitalia suggests filariasis, chronic ascites, or lymphatic blockage from radiotherapy for pelvic malignancies.

▶ Bloody Ejaculation

Inflammation of the prostate or seminal vesicles can cause hematospermia.

▶ Gynecomastia

Often idiopathic, gynecomastia is common in elderly men, particularly those taking estrogens for control of prostatic cancer. It is also seen in association with choriocarcinoma and interstitial cell and Sertoli cell tumors of the testis. Certain endocrinologic diseases, for example, Klinefelter syndrome, may also cause gynecomastia.

COMPLAINTS RELATED TO SEXUAL PROBLEMS

Many people have genitourinary complaints on a purely psychological or emotional basis. In others, organic symptoms may be increased in severity because of tension states. It is important, therefore, to seek clues that might give evidence of emotional stress.

In women, the relationship of the menses to ureteral pain or vesical complaints should be determined, although menstruation may exacerbate both organic and functional vesical and renal difficulties.

Many patients recognize that the state of their "nerves" has a direct effect on their symptoms. They often realize that their "cystitis" develops after a tension-producing or anxiety-producing episode in their personal or occupational environment.

▶ Sexual Difficulties in Men

Men may complain directly of sexual difficulty. However, they are often so ashamed of loss of sexual power that they cannot admit it even to a physician. In such cases, they may ask for "prostate treatment" and hope that the physician will understand that they have sexual complaints and that they will be treated accordingly. The main sexual symptoms include impaired quality of erection, premature loss of erection, absence of ejaculate with orgasm, premature ejaculation, and even loss of desire.

▶ Sexual Difficulties in Women

Women who have the psychosomatic cystitis syndrome almost always admit to have an unhappy sex life. They notice that frequency or vaginal–urethral pain often occurs on the day following the incomplete sexual act. Many of them recognize the inadequacy of their sexual experiences as one of the underlying causes of urologic complaints; too frequently, however, the physician either does not ask them pertinent questions or, if patients volunteer this information, ignores it.

BIBLIOGRAPHY

Abul F et al: The acute scrotum: A review of 40 cases. Med Princ Pract 2005;14(3):177.

Ahmed M et al: Ureteric bupivicaine infusion for loin pain haematuria syndrome. Ann R Coll Surg Engl 2010;92(2):139–141.

Ahn JH et al: Workup and management of traumatic hematuria. Emerg Med Clin North Am 1998;16:145.

Andreoli SP: Renal manifestations of systemic diseases. Semin Nephrol 1998;18:270.

Beni-Israel T et al: Clinical predictors for testicular torsion as seen in the pediatric ED. Am J Emerg Med 2010;28(7):786–789.

Blood in the urine: What does it mean for your health? Harv Mens Health Watch 2010;15(3):5–8.

Breyer BN, McAninch JW: Management of recalcitrant bladder neck contracture after radical prostatectomy for prostate cancer. Endoscopic and open surgery. J Urol 2011;185(2):390–391.

Catalano O et al: Real-time, contrast-enhanced sonographic imaging in emergency radiology. Radiol Med (Torino) 2004;108(5–6):454.

Chhor V et al: Misleading abdominal pain following extracorporeal renal lithotripsy. Urol Int 2009;83(2):246–248.

Ciftci AO et al: Clinical predictors for differential diagnosis of acute scrotum. Eur J Pediatr Surg 2004;14:333.

Crawford ED: Management of lower urinary tract symptoms suggestive of benign prostatic hyperplasia: The central role of the patient risk profile. BJU Int 2005;95(Suppl 4):1.

Eisner BH et al: Ureteral stone location at emergency room presentation with colic. J Urol 2009;182(1):165–168.

Elstad EA et al: Beyond incontinence: The stigma of other urinary symptoms. J Adv Nurs 2010;66(11):2460–2470.

Glassberg KI: Normal and abnormal development of the kidney: A clinician's interpretation of current knowledge. J Urol 2002;167:2339.

Green E, Ali Z: Flank pain and haematuria. BMJ 2009;339:b5443.

Heinberg LJ et al: Psychological factors in pelvic/urogenital pain: The influence of site of pain versus sex. Pain 2004;108(1–2):88.

Ho CH et al: Predictive factors for ureteral double-J-stent-related symptoms: A prospective, multivariate analysis. J Formos Med Assoc 2010;109(11):848–856.

Hollenbeck BK et al: Delays in diagnosis and bladder cancer mortality. Cancer 2010;116(22):5235–5242.

Hori S et al: Long-term outcome of epididymectomy for the management of chronic epididymal pain. J Urol 2009;182(4):1407–1412.

Kanematsu A et al: Objective patterning of uroflowmetry curves in children with daytime and nighttime wetting. J Urol 2010;184(4 Suppl):1674–1679.

Kaye JD, Palmer LS: Characterization and management of voiding dysfunction in children with attention deficit hyperactivity disorder. Urology 2010;76(1):220–224.

Kershen RT et al: Blood flow, pressure and compliance in the male human bladder. J Urol 2002;168:121.

Khadra MH et al: A prospective analysis of 1930 patients with hematuria to evaluate current diagnostic practice. J Urol 2000; 163:524.

Kumar P et al: Clinical management of chronic testicular pain. Urol Int 2010;84(2):125–131.

Kumar A et al: A prospective randomized comparison between early (<48 hours of onset of colicky pain) versus delayed shockwave lithotripsy for symptomatic upper ureteral calculi: A single center experience. J Endourol 2010;24(12):2059–2066.

Kurowski K: The women with dysuria. Am Fam Physician 1998;57(9):2155.

Lee YS et al: Most bothersome symptom and symptom specific goal achievement in patients with benign prostatic obstruction: A prospective open label study. J Urol 2011;185(3):1003–1009.

Lutz MC et al: Cross-sectional associations of urogenital pain and sexual function in a community based cohort of older men: Olmsted County, Minnesota. J Urol 2005;174:624.

Manger JP et al: Use of renal ultrasound to detect hydronephrosis after ureteroscopy. J Endourol 2009;23(9):1399–1402.

Mevcha A et al: Diagnosing urological disorders in ageing men. Practitioner 2010;254(1726):2–3, 25–26, 28–29.

Navanimitkul N, Lojanapiwat B: Efficacy of tamsulosin 0.4 mg/day in relieving double-J stent-related symptoms: A randomized controlled study. J Int Med Res 2010;38(4):1436–1441.

Nickel JC et al: Predictors of patient response to antibiotic therapy for the chronic prostatitis/chronic pelvic pain syndrome: A prospective multicenter clinical trial. J Urol 2001;165:1539.

Nickel JC et al: The patient with chronic epididymitis: Characterization of an enigmatic syndrome. J Urol 2002;167:1701.

Nitti VW et al: Lower urinary tract symptoms in young men: Videourodynamic findings and correlation with noninvasive measures. J Urol 2002;168:135.

Pabon-Ramos W et al: Excretory urography: Trends in clinical use and diagnostic yield. Abdom Imaging 2010;35(5):607–611.

Paryavi E et al: Acute exertional lumbar paraspinal compartment syndrome. Spine (Phila Pa 1976) 2010;35(25):E1529–E1533.

Payne C: Urodynamics for the evaluation of painful bladder syndrome/interstitial cystitis. J Urol 2010;184(1):15–16.

Persaud AC et al: Pediatric urolithiasis: Clinical predictors in the emergency department. Pediatrics 2009;124(3):888–894.

Quddus MB, Mahmud SM: Testicular torsion: A diagnosis not to be missed. J Pak Med Assoc 2011;61(4):391–392.

Roehrborn CG: Male lower urinary tract symptoms (LUTS) and benign prostatic hyperplasia (BPH). Med Clin North Am 2011;95(1):87–100.

Sea J et al: Review of exercise and the risk of benign prostatic hyperplasia. Phys Sportsmed 2009;37(4):75–83.

Swithinbank LV et al: The natural history of daytime urinary incontinence in children: A large British cohort. Acta Paediatr 2010;99(7):1031–1036.

Steinberg PL et al: A standardized pain management protocol improves timeliness of analgesia among emergency department patients with renal colic. Qual Manag Health Care 2011;20(1):30–36.

Sunela KL et al: Changes in symptoms of renal cell carcinoma over four decades. BJU Int 2010;106(5):649–653.

Swinn MJ et al: The cause and natural history of isolated urinary retention in young women. J Urol 2002;167:151.

Wampler SM, Llanes M.: Common scrotal and testicular problems. Prim Care 2010;37(3):613–626, x.

Weiss JP, Blaivas JG: Nocturia. J Urol 2000;163:5.

Wik L et al: Exertional paraspinal muscle rhabdomyolysis and compartment syndrome: A cause of back pain not to be missed. Clin Rheumatol 2010;29(7):803–805.

Wong LM et al: Creation and validation of a visual macroscopic hematuria scale for optimal communication and an objective hematuria index. J Urol 2010;184(1):231–236.

Wu JN et al: Palliative care in urology. Surg Clin North Am 2011;91(2):429–444, x.

Physical Examination of the Genitourinary Tract

Maxwell V. Meng, MD, MPH, & Emil A. Tanagho, MD

A careful history and assessment of symptoms will suggest whether a complete or limited examination is indicated, and also help direct the appropriate selection of subsequent diagnostic studies.

EXAMINATION OF THE KIDNEYS

▶ Inspection

A mass that is visible in the upper abdominal area may be difficult to palpate if soft, as with hydronephrosis. Fullness in the costovertebral angle may be consistent with cancer or perinephric infection. The presence and persistence of indentations in the skin from lying on wrinkled sheets suggest edema of the skin secondary to perinephric abscess.

▶ Palpation

The kidneys lie rather high under the diaphragm and lower ribs and are therefore well protected from injury. Because of the position of the liver, the right kidney is lower than the left. The kidneys are difficult to palpate in men because of (1) resistance from abdominal muscle tone and (2) more fixed position than in women, moving only slightly with change of posture or respiration. The lower part of the right kidney can sometimes be felt, particularly in thin patients, but the left kidney usually cannot be felt unless it is enlarged or displaced.

The most successful method of renal palpation is carried out with the patient lying in the supine position on a hard surface (Figure 4–1). The kidney is lifted by one hand in the costovertebral angle (CVA). On deep inspiration, the kidney moves downward; the other hand is pushed firmly and deeply beneath the costal margin in an effort to trap the kidney. When successful, the anterior hand can palpate the size, shape, and consistency of the organ as it slips back into its normal position.

Alternatively, the kidney may be palpated with the examiner standing behind the seated patient. At other times, if the patient is lying on one side, the uppermost kidney drops downward and medially, making it more accessible to palpation. Perlman and Williams (1976) described an effective method of identifying renal anomalies in newborns. The fingers are placed in the costovertebral angle, with the thumb anterior and performing the palpation.

An enlarged renal mass suggests compensatory hypertrophy (if the other kidney is absent or atrophic), hydronephrosis, tumor, cyst, or polycystic disease. However, a mass in this area may also represent a retroperitoneal tumor, spleen, lesion of the bowel (eg, tumor, abscess), lesion of the gallbladder, or pancreatic cyst. Tumors may have the consistency of normal tissue or be nodular, while hydronephrosis may be either firm or soft. Polycystic kidneys are usually nodular and firm.

An acutely infected kidney is tender, but the presence of marked muscle spasm may make this difficult to elicit. In addition, this sign may not always be helpful since the normal kidney is also often tender.

Although renal pain may be diffusely felt in the back, tenderness is usually well localized, just lateral to the sacrospinalis muscle and below the 12th rib (ie, CVA). Symptoms may be elicited by palpation or sharp percussion over the CVA.

▶ Percussion

At times, an enlarged kidney cannot be felt, particularly if it is soft as in some cases of hydronephrosis. However, such masses may be outlined by both anterior and posterior percussion and this part of the examination should not be omitted.

Percussion is of particular value in outlining an enlarging mass (progressive hemorrhage) in the flank following renal trauma, when tenderness and muscle spasm prevent palpation.

▶ Transillumination

Transillumination may prove helpful in children younger than 1 year who present with a suprapubic or flank mass. A dark room is required along with a flashlight with an opaque flange protruding beyond the lens. The flashlight is applied at right angles to the abdomen. The fiberoptic light cord, used

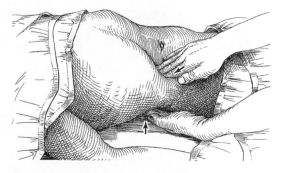

▲ **Figure 4–1.** Method of palpation of the kidney. The posterior hand lifts the kidney upward. The anterior hand feels for the kidney. The patient then takes a deep breath; this causes the kidney to descend. As the patient inhales, the fingers of the anterior hand are plunged inward at the costal margin. If the kidney is mobile or enlarged, it can be felt between the two hands.

to illuminate various optical instruments, is an excellent source of cold light. A distended bladder or cystic mass will transilluminate; a solid mass will not. Flank masses may be assessed by applying the light posteriorly.

▶ Differentiation of Renal and Radicular Pain

Radicular pain is commonly felt in the costovertebral and subcostal areas. It may also spread along the course of the ureter and is the most common cause of so-called "kidney pain." Every patient who complains of flank pain should be examined for evidence of nerve root irritation. Frequent causes are poor posture (scoliosis, kyphosis), arthritic changes in the costovertebral or costotransverse joints, impingement of a rib spur on a subcostal nerve, hypertrophy of costovertebral ligaments pressing on a nerve, and intervertebral disk disease (Smith and Raney, 1976). Radicular pain may be noted as an aftermath of a flank incision where a rib is dislocated, causing impingement of costal nerve on the edge of a ligament. Pain experienced during the preeruptive phase of herpes zoster involving any of the segments between T11 and L2 may simulate pain of renal origin.

Radiculitis usually causes hyperesthesia of the area of skin served by the irritated peripheral nerve. This hypersensitivity can be elicited by means of the pinwheel or grasping and pinching both skin and fat of the abdomen and flanks. Pressure exerted by the thumb over the costovertebral joints reveals local tenderness at the point of emergence of the involved nerve.

▶ Auscultation

Auscultation of the costovertebral areas and upper abdominal quadrants may reveal a systolic bruit, often associated with stenosis or aneurysm of the renal artery. Bruits over the femoral arteries may be found in association with Leriche syndrome, which may be a cause of impotence.

EXAMINATION OF THE BLADDER

The bladder cannot be felt unless it is moderately distended. In adults, it contains at least 150 mL of urine if it can be percussed. In acute or chronic urinary retention, the bladder may reach or even rise above the umbilicus, when its outline may be seen and usually felt. In chronic retention, the bladder may be difficult to palpate due to the flabby bladder wall, in which case percussion is of value.

In male infants or young boys, palpation of a hard mass deep in the center of the pelvis is compatible with a thickened, hypertrophied bladder secondary to obstruction caused by posterior urethral valves.

A sliding inguinal hernia containing some bladder wall can be diagnosed by compression of the scrotal mass when the bladder is full, leading to additional distension.

A few instances have been reported where marked edema of the legs has developed secondary to compression of the iliac vessels by a distended bladder. Bimanual (abdominorectal or abdominovaginal) palpation may reveal the extent of a vesical tumor; to be successful, it should be done under anesthesia.

EXAMINATION OF THE EXTERNAL MALE GENITALIA

▶ Penis

A. Inspection

If the patient has not been circumcised, the foreskin should be retracted. This may reveal tumor or balanitis as the cause of foul discharge. If retraction is not possible due to phimosis, surgical correction (dorsal slit or circumcision) is indicated.

The observation of a poor urinary stream is significant: in newborns, neurogenic bladder or the presence of posterior urethral valves should be considered, whereas in men such a finding suggests urethral stricture or prostatic obstruction.

The scars of healed syphilis may be an important clue. An active ulcer requires bacteriologic or pathologic study (eg, syphilitic chancre, epithelioma). Superficial ulcers or vesicles are compatible with herpes simplex and often interpreted by the patient as a serious sexually transmitted disease (eg, syphilis). Venereal warts may be observed.

Meatal stenosis is a common cause of bloody spotting in male infants. On occasion, it may be of such degree as to cause advanced bilateral hydronephrosis.

The position of the meatus should be noted. It may be located proximal to the tip of the glans on either the dorsal (epispadias) or the ventral surface (hypospadias). In either instance, there is apt to be abnormal curvature (chordee) of the penis in the direction of the displaced meatus.

Micropenis or macropenis may be noted during examination of the penis. In the neonate, the presence of hypospadias and bilateral undescended testes should raise the possibility of an intersex condition.

B. Palpation

Palpation of the dorsal surface of the shaft may reveal a fibrous plaque involving the tunica albuginea covering of the corpora cavernosa, typical of Peyronie's disease. Tender areas of induration felt along the urethra may signify periurethritis secondary to urethral stricture.

C. Urethral Discharge

Urethral discharge is the most common complaint referable to the male sex organ. Gonococcal pus is usually profuse, thick, and yellow or gray–brown. Nongonorrheal discharges may be similar in appearance but are often thin, mucoid, and scant. Although gonorrhea must be ruled out as the cause of urethral discharge, a significant percentage of cases is found to be caused by chlamydiae. Patients with urethral discharge should also be examined for other sexually transmitted diseases since multiple infection is not uncommon.

Bloody discharge suggests the possibility of a foreign body in the urethra, urethral stricture, or tumor.

Urethral discharge must always be sought before the patient is asked to void.

▶ Scrotum

Angioneurotic edema and infections and inflammation of the skin of the scrotum are not common. Small sebaceous cysts are occasionally seen while malignant tumors are rare. The scrotum is bifid when midscrotal or perineal hypospadias is present.

Elephantiasis of the scrotum is caused by obstruction to lymphatic drainage and endemic in the tropics due to filariasis. Genital lymphedema may also result from radical resection of the lymph nodes of the inguinal and femoral areas, in which case the skin of the penis is involved. Small hemangiomas of the skin are common and may bleed spontaneously.

Scrotal ultrasound is a helpful adjunct in evaluating the scrotal contents.

▶ Testis

The testes should be carefully palpated with the fingers of both hands. A hard area in the testis proper must be regarded as a malignant tumor until proven otherwise. Transillumination of scrotal masses should be done routinely. With the patient in a dark room, a flashlight or fiberoptic light is placed against the scrotal sac posteriorly. A hydrocele will cause the intrascrotal mass to glow red; conversely light is not transmitted through a solid tumor. Tumors are often smooth but may be nodular and the testes may seem abnormally heavy. A testis replaced by tumor or damaged by gumma is

insensitive to pressure, and the usual sickening sensation is absent. About 10% of tumors are associated with a secondary hydrocele that may require aspiration before definitive palpation can be performed.

The testis may be absent from the scrotum, and this may be transient (physiologic retractile testis) or true cryptorchidism. Palpation of the groins may reveal the presence of the organ.

The atrophic testis (postoperative orchiopexy, mumps orchitis, or torsion of the spermatic cord) may be flabby and at times hypersensitive but is usually firm and hyposensitive. Although spermatogenesis may be absent, androgen function is occasionally maintained.

▶ Epididymis

The epididymis is sometimes rather closely attached to the posterior surface of the testis, and at other times, it is quite free of it. The epididymis should be carefully palpated for size and induration, which implies infection since primary tumors are exceedingly rare.

In the acute stage of epididymitis, the testis and epididymis are indistinguishable by palpation; the testicle and epididymis may be adherent to the scrotum, which is usually red and exquisitely tender. With few exceptions, the infecting organism is *Neisseria gonorrhoeae*, *Chlamydia trachomatis*, or *Escherichia coli*.

Chronic painless induration suggests tuberculosis or schistosomiasis, although nonspecific chronic epididymitis is also possible. Other signs of genitourinary tuberculosis include sterile pyuria, thickened seminal vesicle, nodular prostate, and "beading" of the vas deferens.

▶ Spermatic Cord and Vas Deferens

A swelling in the spermatic cord may be cystic (eg, hydrocele or hernia) or solid (eg, connective tissue tumor) although the latter is rare. Lipoma in the investing fascia of the cord may simulate a hernia. Diffuse swelling and induration of the cord are seen with filarial funiculitis.

Careful palpation of the vas deferens may reveal thickening (eg, chronic infection), fusiform enlargements ("beading" caused by tuberculosis), or even absence of the vas. The latter finding is of importance in infertile males and may be associated with cystic fibrosis or ipsilateral Wolffian duct abnormality (eg, renal agenesis).

When a male patient stands, a mass of dilated veins (varicocele) may be noted behind and above the testis. The degree of dilatation decreases with recumbency and can be increased by the Valsalva maneuver. The major potential sequela of varicocele is infertility (see Chapter 42).

▶ Testicular Tunics and Adnexa

Hydroceles are usually cystic but on occasion so tense that they simulate solid tumors; transillumination confirms the diagnosis. The fluid may accumulate secondary to nonspecific acute or tuberculous epididymitis, trauma, or tumor of the testis. The latter is a distinct possibility if the hydrocele appears spontaneously between the ages of 18 and 35. It should be aspirated to permit careful palpation of underlying structures or further characterized with ultrasonography.

Hydroceles usually surround the testis completely. Cystic masses that are separate from but in the region of the upper pole of the testis are typically spermatoceles. Aspiration reveals the typical thin, milky fluid, which contains sperm.

EXAMINATION OF THE FEMALE GENITALIA

▶ Vaginal Examination

Diseases of the female genital tract may secondarily involve the urinary organs, making a thorough gynecologic examination essential, which should be performed by the male physician in the presence of a female nurse or health professional. Commonly associated conditions include urethrocystitis secondary to urethral diverticulitis or cervicitis, pyelonephritis during pregnancy, and ureteral obstruction from metastatic nodes or direct extension from cervical cancer.

A. Inspection

In newborns and children, the vaginal vestibule should be inspected for a single opening (common urogenital sinus), labial fusion, split clitoris and lack of fusion of the anterior fourchette (epispadias), or hypertrophied clitoris and scrotalization of the labia majora (adrenogenital syndrome).

The urinary meatus may reveal a reddened, tender, friable lesion (urethral caruncle) or a reddened, everted posterior lip often seen with senile urethritis and vaginitis. Biopsy is indicated if a malignant tumor cannot be ruled out. The diagnosis of senile vaginitis and urethritis is established by staining a smear of the vaginal epithelium with Lugol's solution. Cells lacking glycogen (hypoestrogenism) do not take up the stain, whereas normal cells do.

Multiple painful small ulcers or blister-like lesions may be noted, usually representing herpes virus type 2 infection, which may have serious sequelae.

Smears and cultures of urethral or vaginal discharge should be made. Gonococci are relatively easy to identify; culture of chlamydiae requires techniques seldom available to the physician.

The presence of skenitis and bartholinitis may reveal the source of persistent urethritis or cystitis. The condition of the vaginal wall should be observed. Urethrocele and cystocele, often found with stress incontinence, may be associated with residual urine and lead to persistent infection of the bladder. A bulge in the anterior vaginal wall may represent a urethral diverticulum. The cervix should be inspected for cancer or infection. Taking biopsy specimens or making Papanicolaou smears may be indicated.

B. Palpation

At times, the urethra, base of the bladder, and lower ureters may be tender on palpation, but little can be deduced from this finding. Induration of the urethra or trigonal area, or a mass involving either, may be a clue to an existing tumor. A soft mass could be a urethral diverticulum, and pressure may cause pus to extrude from the urethra. A stone in the lower ureter may be palpable. Evidence of enlargement of the uterus (eg, pregnancy, myoma) or diseases or inflammations of the colon or adnexa may afford a clue to the cause of urinary symptoms (eg, compression of ureter by ovarian tumor, endometriosis, or diverticulitis of the sigmoid colon adherent to the bladder).

Carcinoma of the cervix may invade the base of the bladder, causing vesical irritability or hematuria; metastases to iliac lymph nodes may compress the ureters.

Rectal examination may provide further information and is the obvious route of examination in children and virgins.

RECTAL EXAMINATION IN MALES

▶ Sphincter and Lower Rectum

The estimation of sphincter tone is of importance. Laxity of the muscle suggests similar changes in the urinary sphincter and detrusor and the possibility of neurogenic disease; the same is true for a spastic anal sphincter. In addition to the digital prostatic examination, the examiner should palpate the entire lower rectum to rule out stenosis, internal hemorrhoids, cryptitis, rectal fistulae, mucosal polyps, and rectal cancer. Testing perianal sensation is mandatory.

▶ Prostate

A specimen of urine for routine analysis should be collected before the rectal examination. This is of importance, since prostatic massage or even palpation at times forces prostatic secretion into the posterior urethra. If this secretion contains pus, a specimen of voided urine after the rectal examination will be contaminated.

A. Size

The average prostate is about 4 cm in both length and width. As the gland enlarges, the lateral sulci become relatively deeper and the median furrow becomes obliterated. The clinical importance of prostatic hyperplasia is measured by the severity of symptoms and the amount of residual urine rather than by the size of the gland on palpation. The prostate may be of normal size and consistency on examination in a patient with acute urinary retention or severe obstructive urinary complaints.

B. Consistency

Normally, the consistency of the gland is similar to that of the contracted thenar eminence of the thumb (with the thumb

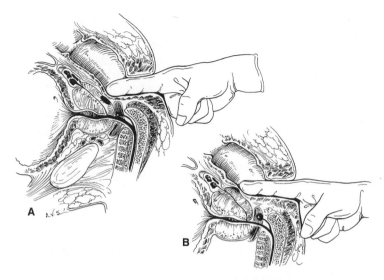

▲ **Figure 4–2.** Differential diagnosis of prostatic nodules. **A:** Inflammatory area is raised above the surface of the gland; induration decreases gradually at its periphery. **B:** Cancerous nodules is not raised; there is an abrupt change in consistency at its edges.

completely opposed to the little finger) and is rather rubbery. It may be mushy if congested (due to lack of intercourse or chronic infection with impaired drainage), indurated (due to chronic infection with or without calculi), or stony hard (due to advanced carcinoma).

The difficulty lies in differentiating firm areas in the prostate: fibrosis from nonspecific infection, granulomatous prostatitis, nodularity from tuberculosis, or firm areas due to prostatic calculi or early cancer. Generally, nodules caused by infection are raised above the surface of the gland. At their edges, the induration gradually fades to the normal softness of surrounding tissue. Conversely, the suspicious lesion in cases of prostate cancer is usually not raised; rather, it is hard and has a sharp edge (ie, there is an abrupt change in consistency on the same plane). It tends to arise in the lateral sulcus (Figure 4–2).

Even the most experienced clinician can have trouble differentiating cancer from other conditions. The serum prostate-specific antigen (PSA) level can be helpful if elevated and is currently the most common method of diagnosing prostate cancer (clinical stage T1c). Transrectal ultrasound-guided biopsy of the prostate can be diagnostic. Recent evidence suggests that rectal examination after radical prostatectomy is unnecessary when PSA is undetectable, since no case of locally recurrent cancer was identified in the absence of an elevated PSA.

C. Mobility

The mobility of the gland varies. Occasionally, it has great mobility while at other times, very little. With advanced carcinoma, it is fixed because of local extension through the capsule. In adults, the prostate should be routinely massaged and its secretion examined microscopically. However, prostatic massage should be avoided in the presence of an acute urethral discharge, acute prostatitis, or acute prostatocystitis; in men near the stage of complete urinary retention (because it may precipitate complete retention); or in men suffering from obvious cancer of the gland.

D. Massage and Prostatic Smear

Copious amounts of secretion may be obtained from some prostate glands and little or none from others. The amount obtained depends to some extent on the vigor with which the massage is carried out. If no secretion is obtained, the patient should be asked to void even a few drops of urine, as these will contain adequate secretion for examination. Microscopic examination of the secretion is done under low-power magnification. Normal secretion contains numerous lecithin bodies, which are refractile like red blood cells but much smaller. Only an occasional white cell is present. A few epithelial cells and, rarely, corpora amylacea are seen. Sperm may be present, but its absence is of no significance.

The presence of large numbers or clumps of leukocytes suggests prostatitis. Stained smears are usually impractical because it is difficult to fix the material on the slide; even when fixation and staining are successful, pyogenic bacteria are usually not found. Acid-fast organisms can often be found by appropriate staining methods.

On occasion, it may be necessary to obtain cultures of prostatic secretion in order to demonstrate nonspecific organisms, tubercle bacilli, gonococci, or chlamydiae. After thorough cleansing of the glans and emptying of the bladder to mechanically cleanse the urethra, the prostate is massaged. Drops of secretion are collected in a sterile tube of appropriate culture medium.

▶ Seminal Vesicles

Palpation of the seminal vesicles should be attempted. The vesicles are situated under the base of the bladder and diverge from below upward (Figure 1–8). Normal seminal vesicles are usually impalpable, but may feel cystic when overdistended. In the presence of chronic infection (particularly tuberculosis or schistosomiasis) or in association with advanced carcinoma of the prostate, they may be indurated. Stripping of the seminal vesicles should be done in association with prostatic massage, for the vesicles are usually infected when prostatitis is present. Primary tumors of the vesicles are very rare. A cystic mass may rarely be felt over the prostate or just above it. This probably represents a cyst of the Müllerian duct or the utricle; the latter is occasionally associated with severe hypospadias.

▶ Lymph Nodes

It should be remembered that generalized lymphadenopathy usually occurs early in human immunodeficiency syndrome (see Chapter 15).

A. Inguinal and Subinguinal Lymph Nodes

With inflammatory lesions of the skin of the penis and scrotum or vulva, the inguinal and subinguinal lymph nodes may be involved. Such diseases include chancroid, syphilitic chancre, lymphogranuloma venereum, and on occasion, gonorrhea.

Malignant tumors (squamous cell carcinoma) involving the penis, glans, scrotal skin, or distal urethra in women metastasize to the inguinal and subinguinal nodes. Testicular tumors do not spread to these nodes unless they have invaded the scrotal skin or the patient has previously undergone orchidopexy.

B. Other Lymph Nodes

Tumors of the testis and prostate may involve the left supraclavicular nodes (Virchow's or Troisier's node). Tumors of the bladder and prostate typically metastasize to the internal iliac, external iliac, and preaortic nodes, although rarely are they so large as to be palpable. Upper abdominal masses near the midline in a young man should suggest metastases from cancer of the testis; the primary growth may be minute and hidden in the substance of what appears to be a normal testicle.

NEUROLOGIC EXAMINATION

A careful neurologic survey may uncover sensory or motor impairment that account for residual urine or incontinence. Since the bladder and sphincter are innervated by the second to the fourth sacral segments, information can be gained by testing anal sphincter tone, evaluating sensation of the perianal skin, and testing Achilles tendon and bulbocavernosus reflexes. The bulbocavernosus reflex is elicited by placing a finger in the rectum and squeezing the glans penis or clitoris, or by jerking on an indwelling Foley catheter. The normal reflex involves contraction of the anal sphincter and bulbocavernosus muscles in response to these maneuvers.

It is wise, particularly in children, to seek a dimple over the lumbosacral area. One should palpate the sacrum to ensure it is present and normally formed. Sacral agenesis or partial development is compatible with deficits of S2–4. If findings seem abnormal, x-ray examination is indicated.

BIBLIOGRAPHY

Examination of the Kidneys

Lowe LH et al: Pediatric renal masses: Wilms tumor and beyond. Radiographics 2000;20:1585. [PMID: 11112813]

Mofenson HC, Greensher J: Transillumination of the abdomen in infants. Am J Dis Child 1968;115:428. [PMID: 5642347]

Perlman M, Williams J: Detection of renal anomalies by abdominal palpation in newborn infants. Br Med J 1976;3:347. [PMID: 947418]

Smith DR, Raney FL Jr: Radiculitis distress as a mimic of renal pain. J Urol 1976;116:269. [PMID: 957487]

External Genitalia in Males

Bemelmans BL et al: Penile sensory disorders in erectile dysfunction: Results of a comprehensive neuro-urophysiological diagnostic evaluation in 123 patients. J Urol 1991;146:777. [PMID: 1875492]

Galejs LE: Diagnosis and treatment of the acute scrotum. Am Fam Physician 1999;59:817. [PMID: 10068706]

Hanson P et al: Sacral reflex latencies in tethered cord syndrome. Am J Phys Med Rehabil 1993;72:39. [PMID: 8431266]

Horstman WG: Scrotal imaging. Urol Clin North Am 1997;24:653. [PMID: 9275983]

Lavoipierre AM: Ultrasound of the prostate and testicles. World J Surg 2000;24:198. [PMID: 10633147]

Kolettis PN et al: Clinical and genetic features of patients with congenital unilateral absence of the vas deferens. Urology 2002; 60:1073. [PMID: 12475673]

Lavoisier P et al: Bulbocavernosus reflex: Its validity as a diagnostic test of neurogenic impotence. J Urol 1989;141:311. [PMID: 2913351]

Leissner J et al: The undescended testis: Considerations and impact on fertility. BJU Int 1999;83:885. [PMID: 10368225]

Marcozzi D, Suner S: The nontraumatic, acute scrotum. Emerg Med Clin North Am 2001;19:547. [PMID: 11554275]

Sherrard J, Barlow D: Gonorrhoea in men: Clinical and diagnostic aspects. Genitourin Med 1996;72:422. [PMID: 9038638]

Wolf CK et al: The undescended testicle. Compr Ther 2001;27:11. [PMID: 11280851]

External Genitalia in Females

Edmonds DK: Congenital malformations of the genital tract. Obstet Gynecol Clin North Am 2000;27:49. [PMID: 10693182]

Redman JF: Techniques of genital examination and bladder catheterization in female children. Urol Clin North Am 1990;17:1. [PMID: 2305501]

Prostate

Carroll P et al: Prostate-specific antigen best practice policy—part II: Prostate cancer staging and post-treatment follow-up. Urology 2001;57:225. [PMID: 11182325]

Grossfeld GD, Coakley FV: Benign prostatic hyperplasia: Clinical overview and value of diagnostic imaging. Radiol Clin North Am 2000;38:31. [PMID: 10664665]

Lummus WE, Thompson I: Prostatitis. Emerg Med Clin North Am 2001;19:691. [PMID: 11554282]

Nickel JC: The Pre and Post Massage Test (PPMT): A simple screen for prostatitis. Tech Urol 1997;3:38. [PMID: 9170224]

Obek C et al: Comparison of digital rectal examination and biopsy results with the radical prostatectomy specimen. J Urol 1999; 161:494. [PMID: 9915434]

Pound CR et al: Digital rectal examination and imaging studies are unnecessary in men with undetectable prostate specific antigen following radical prostatectomy. J Urol 1999;162:1337. [PMID: 10492192]

Neurologic Examination

Cardenas DD et al: Lower urinary changes over time in suprasacral spinal cord injury. Paraplegia 1995;33:326. [PMID: 7644258]

Vodusek DB: Electromyogram, evoked sensory and motor potentials in neurourology. Neurophysiol Clin 1997;27:204. [PMID: 9260161]

Urologic Laboratory Examination

Sima P. Porten, MD, MPH, & Kirsten L. Greene, MD, MS*

Examination of specimens of urine, blood, and genitourinary secretions or exudates commonly directs the subsequent urologic workup and frequently establishes a diagnosis. Since approximately 20% of patients who visit a primary physician's office have a urologic problem, it is important for the physician to have a broad knowledge of the laboratory methods available to test appropriate specimens. Judicious use of such tests permits rapid, accurate, and cost-effective determination of the probable diagnosis and directs the management of patients with urologic disease.

EXAMINATION OF URINE

Urinalysis is one of the most important and useful urologic tests available, yet all too often, the necessary details are neglected and significant information is overlooked or misinterpreted. Reasons for inadequate urinalyses include (1) improper collection, (2) failure to examine the specimen immediately, (3) incomplete examination (eg, most laboratories do not perform a microscopic analysis unless it is specifically requested by the provider), (4) inexperience of the examiner, and (5) inadequate appreciation of the significance of the findings.

The necessity of routine urinalysis as a screen in asymptomatic individuals, those admitted to hospitals, or those undergoing elective surgery continues to be debated. Numerous studies indicate that in these situations, urinalysis is not routinely necessary (Godbole and Johnstone, 2004). However, patients presenting with urinary tract symptoms or signs should undergo urinalysis. Studies also indicate that, if macroscopic urinalysis (dip-strip) is normal, microscopic analysis is not necessary. If the patient has signs or symptoms suggestive of urologic disease, or the dip-strip is positive for protein, heme, leukocyte esterase, or nitrite, a complete urinalysis, including microscopic

examination of the sediment, should be carried out (Simerville et al, 2005).

▶ Urine Collection

A. Timing of Collection

It is best to examine urine that has been properly obtained in the office. First-voided morning specimens are helpful for qualitative protein testing in patients with possible orthostatic proteinuria and for specific-gravity assessment as a presumptive test of renal function in patients with minimal renal disease due to diabetes mellitus or sickle cell anemia or in those with suspected diabetes insipidus. Evaluation of sequential morning specimens may be required to obviate the variability often encountered. Urine specimens that are obtained immediately after the patient has eaten or that have been left standing for a few hours become alkaline and thus may contain lysed red cells, disintegrated casts, or rapidly multiplying bacteria; therefore, a freshly voided specimen obtained a few hours after the patient has eaten and examined within 1 hour of voiding is most reliable. The patient's state of hydration may alter the concentration of urinary constituents. Timed urine collections may be required for definitive assessment of renal function or proteinuria.

B. Method of Collection

Proper collection of the specimen is particularly important when patients have hematuria or proteinuria or are being evaluated for urinary tract infection. Examination of a urine specimen collected sequentially during voiding in several containers may help to identify the site of origin of hematuria or urinary tract infection. To gather consistent and meaningful urinalysis data, urine must be collected by a uniform method in the physician's office or laboratory. The specimen should be obtained before a genital or rectal examination in order to prevent contamination from the introitus or expressed prostatic secretions. Urine obtained from a

*Originally written by Karl J. Kreder Jr, MD, & Richard D. Williams, MD.

condom, chronic catheter, or intestinal conduit drainage bag is *not* a proper specimen for urinalysis.

1. Men—It is usually simple to collect a clean-voided midstream urine sample from men. Routine instructions may be printed on a sheet given to the patient or placed on the lavatory wall. The procedure should include (1) retraction of the foreskin (a common source of contamination of the specimen) and cleansing of the meatus with benzalkonium chloride or hexachlorophene, (2) passing the first part of the stream (15–30 mL) without collection, and (3) collecting the next or midstream portion (approximately 50–100 mL) in a sterile specimen container, which is capped immediately afterward. A portion of the specimen is prepared immediately for both macroscopic and microscopic examination, and the rest is saved in the sterile container for subsequent culture if this proves necessary.

With this midstream clean-catch method, the likelihood that the specimen will be contaminated by meatal or urethral secretions is markedly decreased, although not completely eliminated. In adult males, it is rarely necessary to collect urine by catheterization unless urinary retention is present.

2. Women—The best method for collecting a clean-voided midstream specimen from a woman is as follows: (1) the patient is placed on the examining table in the lithotomy position; (2) the vulva and urethral meatus are cleansed with benzalkonium chloride or hexachlorophene; (3) the labia are separated; and (4) the patient is instructed to initiate voiding into a container held close to the vulva. After she has passed the first 10–20 mL of urine, the next 50–100 mL is collected in a sterile container that is immediately capped. Because this technique requires considerable effort, it is acceptable to have the patient provide an initial specimen in a nonsterile container in the office lavatory. If results of urinalysis are normal, no further study is indicated; if abnormal, a urine specimen must be obtained by the more exacting technique. In either case, the specimen should be prepared for immediate examination.

If a satisfactory specimen cannot be obtained by the method described earlier, one should not hesitate to obtain a specimen by catheterization to eliminate nonvaginal sources of abnormal urinary constituents.

3. Children—Urine for analysis, other than bacterial cultures, can be obtained from males or females by covering the cleansed urethral meatus with a plastic bag; a urine specimen for culture may require catheterization or suprapubic needle aspiration. In girls, catheterization with a small catheter attached to a centrifuge tube is appropriate, but boys should *not* be routinely catheterized. It is often preferable in either sex to proceed with suprapubic needle aspiration. This is easier if the patient has been previously hydrated, so that the bladder is full. Suprapubic needle aspiration is performed as follows. (1) Cleanse the suprapubic area by

sponging with alcohol. (2) With a small amount of local anesthetic, raise an intradermal wheal on the midline 1–2 cm above the pubis (the bladder lies just above the pubis in young children). (3) Attach a 10-mL syringe to a 22-gauge needle. Insert the needle perpendicularly through the abdominal wheal into the bladder wall, maintaining gentle suction with the syringe so that urine will be aspirated as soon as the bladder is entered.

▶ Macroscopic Examination

Macroscopic examination of urine often provides a clue when diagnosis is difficult.

A. Color and Appearance

Urine is often colored owing to drugs: phenazopyridine (Pyridium) will turn the urine orange; rifampin will turn it yellow-orange; nitrofurantoin will turn it brown; and L-dopa, α-methyldopa, and metronidazole will turn it reddish-brown. Red urine does not always signify hematuria. A red discoloration unassociated with intact erythrocytes in the urine can result from betacyanin excretion after beet ingestion, phenolphthalein in laxatives, ingestion of vegetable dyes, concentrated urate excretion, myoglobinuria due to significant muscle trauma, or hemoglobinuria following hemolysis. In addition, *Serratia marcescens* bacteria can cause the "red diaper" syndrome. However, whenever red urine is seen, hematuria must be ruled out by microscopic analysis. Cloudy urine is commonly thought to represent pyuria, but more often the cloudiness is due to large amounts of amorphous phosphates, which disappear with the addition of acid, or urates, which dissolve with the use of alkali. The odor of urine is rarely clinically significant.

B. Specific Gravity

The specific gravity of urine (normal, 1.003–1.030) is often important for diagnostic purposes: that of patients with significant intracranial trauma may be low owing to a lack of antidiuretic hormone (vasopressin); that of patients with primary diabetes insipidus is <1.010 even after overnight dehydration; that of patients with extensive acute renal tubular damage is consistently 1.010 (similar to the specific gravity of plasma); and a low specific gravity can be an early sign of renal damage from conditions such as sickle cell anemia. Urine specific gravity is the simplest time-honored test for evaluating hydration in postoperative patients. The specific gravity of urine may affect the results of other urine tests: in dilute urine, a pregnancy test may be falsely negative; in concentrated urine, protein may be falsely positive on dip-strips yet unconfirmed on quantitative tests. The specific gravity of urine may be falsely elevated by the presence of glucose, protein, artificial plasma expanders, or intravenous contrast agents.

Studies of specific-gravity reagent strips (method based on ionic alteration of a polyelectrolyte solution) have shown the method to be rapid, reliable, and unaffected by elevated amounts of glucose or contrast medium; however, alkaline pH may falsely lower the result (0.005 per pH unit >7.0). In the routine office setting, these strips are as reliable as either the hydrometer or refractometer methods.

C. Chemical Tests

Chemically impregnated reagent strips are accurate and have simplified routine urinalysis greatly. However, they must be monitored routinely by appropriate standardized quality-control reagents. The dip-strips are reliable only when not outdated and when used with *room temperature* urine.

1. pH—The pH of urine is important in a few specific clinical situations. Patients with uric acid stones rarely have a urinary pH >6.5 (uric acid is soluble in alkaline urine). Patients with calcium stones, nephrocalcinosis, or both may have renal tubular acidosis and will be unable to acidify urine pH <6.0. With urinary tract infections caused by urea-splitting organisms (most commonly *Proteus* species), the urinary pH tends to be >7.0. It should be reemphasized that urine obtained within 2 hours of a large meal or left standing at room temperature for several hours tends to be alkaline. The indicator paper in most dip-strips is quite accurate; however, confirmation by a pH meter is occasionally required.

2. Protein—Dip-strips containing bromphenol blue can be used to determine the presence of >10 mg/dL protein in urine, but persistent proteinuria detected in this manner requires quantitative protein testing for confirmation. The dip-strip measures primarily albumin and is not sensitive to Bence-Jones proteins (immunoglobulins). Concentrated urine may give a false-positive result, as will urine containing numerous white blood cells (leukocytes) or vaginal secretions replete with epithelial cells. Orthostatic proteinuria can be demonstrated by detecting elevated protein levels in a urine specimen obtained after the patient has been in the upright position for several hours, whereas normal levels are found before ambulation. Prolonged fever and excessive physical exertion are also common causes of transient proteinuria.

Persistently elevated protein levels in the urine (>150 mg/24 h) may indicate significant disease. Therefore, specific quantitative protein tests, electrophoretic studies of the urine, or both may be required to determine the specific type of protein that is present.

3. Glucose—The glucose oxidase–peroxidase tests used in dip-strips are quite accurate and specific for urinary glucose. False-positive results may be obtained when patients have ingested large doses of aspirin, ascorbic acid, or cephalosporins. An occasional patient has a blood glucose level below 180 mg/dL and yet has significant glucosuria; this indicates a low renal threshold of glucose excretion. However, most patients with a positive reading have diabetes mellitus.

4. Hemoglobin—The dip-strip test for hemoglobin is not specific for erythrocytes and should be used only to *screen* for hematuria, with microscopic analysis of the urinary sediment used for confirmation. Free hemoglobin or myoglobin in the urine may give a positive reading; ascorbic acid in the urine can inhibit the dip-strip reaction and give a false-negative result. Note that dilute urine (<1.008) will lyse erythrocytes and thus provide a positive dip-strip reading for hemoglobin but no visible erythrocytes on microscopic analysis.

5. Bacteria and leukocytes—Test strips to determine the number of bacteria (nitrite) or leukocytes (leukocyte esterase) as predictors of bacteriuria are as accurate as microscopic sediment analysis in studies using quantitative urine cultures as the standard. The nitrite reductase test depends on the conversion of nitrate to nitrite. Many of the bacteria responsible for urinary tract infections, particularly enterobacteria, are capable of reducing nitrate to nitrite and, therefore, detectable by this test. When the nitrite test is positive, it suggests the presence of >100,000 organisms per milliliter; however, several factors can lead to false-negative results. The nitrite test is positive only for coagulase-splitting bacteria, and thus, when used alone it is only 40–60% accurate. Urine must be in the bladder for a sufficient time before sampling for the reduction of nitrate to occur (>4 hours); therefore, this test is most likely to be positive when first-voided morning urine is tested. A false-negative test will also result if the bacteria present do not contain nitrate reductase or if dietary nitrate is absent. A false-negative nitrite study may occur in a patient taking vitamin C. The leukocyte esterase test is a widely used chemical test that depends on the presence of esterase in granulocytic leukocytes. The leukocyte esterase test is an indication of pyuria and will remain positive even after the leukocytes have degenerated. The test accurately identifies patients with 10–12 leukocytes per high-power field in a centrifuged specimen. Although this test is a good indicator of pyuria, it does not detect bacteriuria. Therefore, it is often combined with the nitrite test to detect both bacteriuria and inflammation to maximize the chances of predicting urinary tract infection. Used together, the two tests are as predictive as the microscopic analysis but not as accurate as a urine culture. A false-negative leukocyte esterase study can be caused by glucosuria, or by phenazopyridine hydrochloride (Pyridium), nitrofurantoin, vitamin C, or rifampin in the urine.

▶ Microscopic Examination

To be most accurate, the microscopic sediment examination should be done personally by an experienced physician or technician. Early-morning urine is the best specimen if it can be examined within a few minutes of collection. In most cases, the sediment can be prepared as follows: (1) centrifuge a 10-mL specimen at 2000 rpm for 5 minutes; (2) decant the

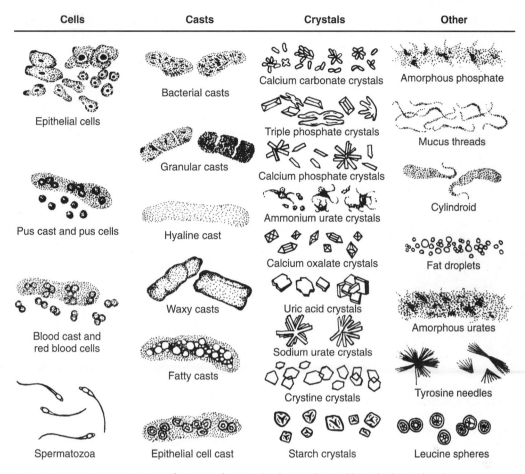

Cells	Casts	Crystals	Other

▲ **Figure 5–1.** Microscopic examination of urine sediment. (Redrawn after Todd–Sanford–Davidson.)

supernatant; (3) resuspend the sediment in the remaining 1 mL of urine by tapping the tube gently against a countertop; and (4) place one drop of the mixture on a microscope slide, cover with a coverslip, and examine first under a low-power (10×) lens and then under a high-power (40×) lens. For maximal contrast of the elements in the sediment, the microscope diaphragm should be nearly closed to prevent overillumination. Significant elements (particularly bacteria) are more easily seen if the slide is stained with methylene blue, but staining is not essential. Figure 5–1 shows typical findings in the urinary sediment.

A. Interpretation

1. Bacteria—The significance of bacteria in the urinary sediment is discussed in Section "Bacteriuria."

2. Leukocytes—Just as the presence of bacteria in the sediment is not an absolute indication of infection, neither is

the finding of pyuria. In the sediment from clean-voided midstream specimens from men and those obtained by suprapubic aspiration or catheterization in women, a finding of more than five leukocytes per high-power field is generally considered abnormal (pyuria). If the patient has symptoms of a urinary tract infection as well as pyuria and bacteriuria, one is justified in making a diagnosis of infection and initiating empiric therapy. However, in female patients with symptoms of urinary tract infection, 60% of those with pyuria will have no bacterial growth from bladder urine obtained by catheterization or suprapubic aspiration emphasizing the need for confirmation by bacterial cultures.

Renal tuberculosis can cause "sterile" acid pyuria and should be considered in any patient with persistent pyuria and negative results on routine bacterial cultures. Specific fluorescent staining of the urinary sediment for acid-fast bacteria can be diagnostic; however, results will be positive from the sediment of spot specimens in only approximately 50% of patients with renal tuberculosis, whereas they are positive in the sediment of 24-hour specimens in 70–80% of such cases. *Mycobacterium smegmatis*, a commensal organism, may be present in the urine (particularly in uncircumcised men) and can give false-positive results on acid-fast stains.

Urolithiasis can also cause pyuria. In patients with persistent pyuria, the physician should consider obtaining at least a plain x-ray of the abdomen and possibly a CT urogram to determine whether urolithiasis is present. Similarly, a retained foreign body such as a self-induced bladder object or a forgotten internal ureteral stent can cause pyuria. A plain x-ray (KUB film) of the abdomen should reveal the offender.

3. Erythrocytes—The presence of even a few erythrocytes in the urine (hematuria) is abnormal and requires further investigation. Although gross hematuria is more alarming to the patient, microscopic hematuria is no less significant. Infrequent causes of hematuria include strenuous exercise (long-distance running), vaginal bleeding, and inflammation of organs near or directly adjoining the urinary tract, for example, diverticulitis or appendicitis. Hematuria associated with cystitis or urethritis generally clears after treatment. Persistent hematuria in an otherwise asymptomatic patient of either sex and any age signifies disease and is an indication for further testing. Studies indicated that approximately 20% of patients with hematuria will eventually be diagnosed with bladder cancer (Messing and Vaillancourt, 1990).

In patients with microscopic hematuria, a three-container method for collection of urine can provide information on the site of origin of erythrocytes. (1) Give the patient three containers, labeled 1, 2, and 3 (or initial, mid, and final). (2) Instruct the patient to urinate and to collect the initial portion of the urine stream (10–15 mL) in the first container, the middle portion (30–40 mL) in the second, and the final portion (5–10 mL) in the third. (3) Using methods described previously, centrifuge the three specimens individually, prepare slides of the urinary sediment (with or without staining), and examine the slides microscopically. If erythrocytes predominate in the initial portion of the specimen, they are usually from the anterior urethra; those in the final portion are generally from the bladder neck or posterior urethra; and the presence of equal numbers of erythrocytes in all three containers usually indicates a source above the bladder neck (bladder, ureters, or kidneys). It is important to collect the urine before physical examination (particularly before rectal examination in men) to avoid misleading results.

The three-container test may not be necessary in patients with gross hematuria, since the patients (men in particular) can usually tell the physician which portion of the stream contains the darkest urine (ie, the most erythrocytes). A specific dysmorphic erythrocyte configuration that can be detected with phase-contrast microscopy or by particle analyzer study of the urinary sediment and is highly indicative of active glomerular disease (Figure 5–2) can be useful. This dysmorphism is thought to be a result of extreme changes in osmolality and the high concentration of urinary chemical constituents affecting erythrocytes during passage through the kidney tubules. An automated system, iQ200, has been shown to be highly accurate for detecting, enumerating, and sizing erythrocytes in urine (Wah et al, 2005).

4. Epithelial cells—Squamous epithelial cells in the urinary sediment indicate contamination of the specimen from the distal urethra in males and from the introitus in females; no other significance should be placed on them. It is not uncommon to find transitional epithelial cells in the normal urinary sediment; however, if they are present in large numbers or clumps and are abnormal histologically (including large nuclei, multiple nucleoli, and an increased ratio of nucleus to cytoplasm), they are indicative of a malignant process affecting the urothelium (Figure 5–3).

5. Casts—Casts are formed in the distal tubules and collecting ducts, for the most part, are not seen in normal urinary sediment; therefore, they commonly signify intrinsic renal disease.

Although *leukocyte casts* have been considered suggestive of pyelonephritis, they are not an absolute indicator and should not be used as the sole criterion for diagnosis. Leukocyte casts must be distinguished from *epithelial cell casts*, because the latter have little significance when present in small numbers. The distinction can be made easily if a small amount of acetic acid is added under the coverslip to enhance nuclear detail. (Note that casts tend to congregate near the edges of the coverslip.) Epithelial cell or leukocyte casts in large numbers signify underlying intrinsic renal disease requiring further diagnostic workup. In renal transplant recipients, an increase in the number of epithelial cells or casts from the renal tubules may be an early indication of acute graft rejection.

Erythrocyte casts are pathognomonic of underlying glomerulitis or vasculitis. Hyaline casts probably represent a mixture of mucus and globulin congealed in the tubules; in small numbers, they are not significant. Hyaline casts are commonly seen in urine specimens taken after exercise and in concentrated or highly acidic urine specimens. Casts are rarely seen in alkaline urine and are therefore not usually present in urine specimens that have been left standing or in specimens from patients unable to acidify.

Granular casts most commonly represent disintegrated epithelial cells, leukocytes, or protein; they usually indicate intrinsic renal tubular disease.

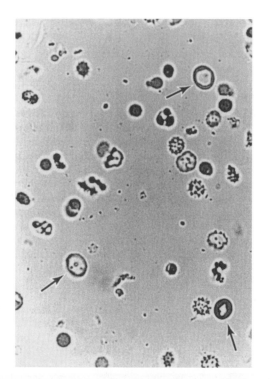 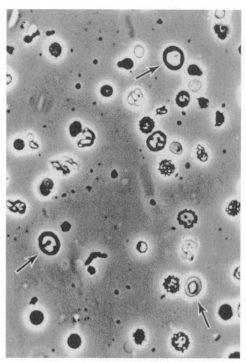

▲ **Figure 5–2.** *Left:* Dysmorphic erythrocytes in urine (*arrows*), viewed under light microscopy (magnification ×400). *Right:* Dysmorphic erythrocytes in urine (identical field), viewed under phase-contrast microscopy. (Reproduced, with permission, from Stamey TA, Kindrachuk RW: Urinary Sediment and Urinalysis: A Practical Guide for the Health Science Professional. WB Saunders, Philadelphia, PA, 1985.)

6. Other findings—The finding of crystals in urine can be helpful in some instances, but the mere presence of crystals does not indicate disease. Crystals form in normal urine below room temperature. Cystine, leucine, tyrosine, cholesterol, bilirubin, hematoidin, and sulfonamide crystals are abnormal findings of varying importance. Several types of crystals that may be found on microscopic examination of urinary sediment are shown in Figure 5–1.

The use of protease inhibitors for treatment of human immunodeficiency virus (HIV) has resulted in urolithiasis due to indinavir crystal formation in urine. The characteristic crystals are flat, rectangular plates, often in a fan or starburst pattern. The presence of trichomonads or yeast cells in the stained or unstained smear of sediment from a properly obtained urine specimen establishes a diagnosis and the need for treatment.

Artifacts present in the urine sediment can be difficult to differentiate from real abnormalities. Dirt and small pieces of vegetable fiber or hair are frequently found, but the most common artifacts are starch granules from examination gloves.

▶ Bacteriuria

A. Microscopic Examination

A presumptive diagnosis of bacterial infection may be made on the basis of results of microscopic examination of the urinary sediment. If several bacteria per high-power field are found in a urine specimen obtained by suprapubic aspiration or catheterization in a woman or in a properly obtained clean-voided midstream specimen from a man, a provisional diagnosis of bacterial infection can be made and empiric treatment started. The findings should be confirmed by bacterial culture. Finding several bacteria per high-power field in a voided specimen from a woman is of little significance. Methods using flow cytometry-based urine analysis (UF-50) can detect bacteria with nearly 80% accuracy.

B. Bacterial Cultures

The presumptive diagnosis of bacterial infection based on microscopic examination of the urinary sediment should be confirmed by culture.

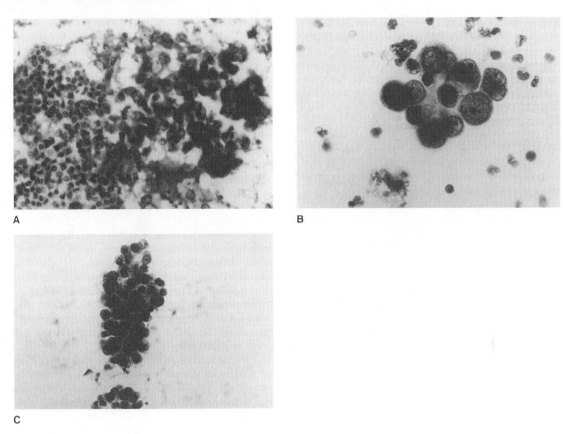

▲ **Figure 5–3.** Papanicolaou-stained bladder cytology specimens. **A:** Normal cells (left) and malignant cells (right). **B:** High-power view of malignant cells. **C:** Papillary cluster of malignant cells. (Courtesy of Larry Kluskens, MD, Cytopathology Laboratory, University of Iowa.)

1. Indications and interpretation—Cultures can be used to estimate the number of bacteria in the urine (quantitative cultures), to identify the exact organism present, and to predict which drugs will be effective in treating the infection. Cultures are particularly important in patients with recurrent or persistent infections, renal insufficiency, or drug allergies.

The number of bacteria present in the urine (colony count) is influenced by the method used to collect the urine specimen, the patient's hydration status, and whether the patient has been taking antimicrobial drugs. The concept that urinary tract infection is present only when the urine specimen contains 10^5 or more bacteria per milliliter is not an absolute rule; a lower count does not exclude the possibility of an infection, particularly in a symptomatic patient. Cultures with growth of multiple organisms usually signify contamination. The presence of a few organisms in a specimen with a low specific gravity is more significant than the same finding in a specimen with a high specific gravity, because the former is more dilute.

Identifying the drugs to which the bacteria are sensitive may or may not be necessary. *Escherichia coli*, which causes 85% of "routine" urinary tract infections, is known to be sensitive to numerous oral antimicrobial drugs. However, in patients with septicemia, renal insufficiency, diabetes mellitus, or suspected enterococcal, *Proteus*, or *Pseudomonas* infections, it is important to determine the antibiotic sensitivity of the organism and the drug concentration necessary for efficacious treatment. Monitoring antibiotic levels in blood and urine during treatment may be indicated, especially in severely ill patients and those receiving highly toxic drugs. These measurements can be done by most hospital laboratories.

2. Rapid tests for bacteriuria—In general, seriously ill or hospitalized patients with urinary tract infections should have cultures processed by an accredited bacteriology laboratory. However, for "routine" infections encountered in office practice, there are many satisfactory, cost-effective testing methods.

Rapid methods to screen for bacteria include growth-independent systems and growth-dependent systems. Several growth-dependent systems are available. One measures the turbidity of urine incubated in a broth medium for several hours. Positive results can be determined in as short a time period as 4 hours; however, 12 hours of growth is required before a test sample can be regarded as negative. A single non–growth-dependent screening test uses the leukocyte esterase test and the nitrite test. If both tests are positive, the specificity increases to 98–99.5%, which indicates probable urinary tract infection (Young and Soper, 2001).

Reliable culture methods involve use of small strips or glass slides coated with eosin–methylene blue agar on one side and nutrient agar on the other. The strips or slides are dipped in the urine specimen and then incubated for 24 hours. Although these methods are easy to use, their disadvantages are that (1) not all bacteria will grow under these conditions and (2) the accuracy of colony counts is debatable.

Perhaps, preferable for the physician's office (but still subject to some of the same limitations) is use of a divided plastic culture plate with blood agar on one side and deoxycholate agar on the other. A known amount of urine is inoculated onto the agar on each side of the plate, and colony counts are determined at 24–48 hours. The numbers of bacteria in 1 mL of the original urine specimen can be determined by multiplying the number of colonies by the volume (in milliliters) and dilution (if any) of the inoculum. If antibiotic sensitivity testing is also desired, an additional culture plate can be inoculated and small antibiotic-impregnated disks placed on the agar. Zones of growth inhibition seen around the disks at 12–24 hours indicate sensitivity.

3. Cultures for tuberculosis—A microscopic examination (fluorescent stain) that shows acid-fast bacilli can give a presumptive diagnosis of urinary tuberculosis. The rapidity of recovering mycobacteria in culture depends somewhat on the patient's bacillary load. Thus, if the smear is highly positive (3–4[+]), cultures would become positive in 1–2 weeks. At that time, a DNA culture probe can be done for tuberculosis. It should be noted that the probe cannot distinguish between tuberculosis and patients treated with bacillus Calmette-Guérin (BCG); if the patient had not received BCG treatment, then *Mycobacterium tuberculosis* infection is likely. The total time from receipt of the specimen to presumptive diagnosis is typically about 2 weeks. Susceptibility tests, if positive for tuberculosis, would require another week.

▶ Other Urine Tests

Many other tests of urine can be helpful in determining the presence of urologic disease.

A. Urothelial Cancer Tests

1. Urine cytology—The evaluation of voided or bladder wash (barbotage) urine for bladder urothelial cancer cells has been quite successful for high-grade tumors and carcinoma in situ with sensitivity ranging from 38% to 51% and specificity between 81% and 100% (Konety, 2006; Mowatt, 2010). Lower grade tumors less commonly shed abnormal cells and cytology is relatively insensitive in this setting. Urinary cytology is fairly interpreter dependent and detection of cancer can be improved by collection of fresh urine samples that are not given in the early morning, barbotage samples, and collection of multiple samples (at least three consecutive specimens). Cystoscopy remains the standard diagnostic test for initial diagnosis and surveillance of bladder cancer.

2. Bladder tumor antigen test—The bladder tumor antigen test (BTA; Bard Diagnostic Sciences, Inc, Redmond, WA, and Polymedco, Inc, Cortland Manor, NY) is an assay for the detection of bladder tumor antigen (human complement factor H related protein) in the urine. The BTA-TRAK test is quantitative assay and the BTA-STAT test is its qualitative, point of care counterpart. Both are more sensitive than cytology (especially for low-grade cancers) but less specific. The greatest utility of these tests is in surveillance of patients already diagnosed with bladder cancer, although they are Food and Drug Administration (FDA) approved for diagnostic use. The BTA test is unreliable in patients with active infection and those that have received intravesical therapy.

3. Nuclear matrix protein 22—The nuclear matrix protein 22 test (NMP22; Matritech, Inc, Newton, MA) is an immunoassay. Normal subjects will have low levels of NMP22 in the urine, whereas patients with active transitional cell carcinoma may have high levels of urinary NMP22 (Grossman et al, 2005). Like BTA testing, other urologic conditions can increase NMP22 levels in the absence of bladder cancer (Boman et al, 2002). Compared with cytology, NMP22 is more sensitive for detecting low-grade tumors but is equivalent in the detection of high-grade cancers. It is FDA approved for the diagnosis of bladder cancer (most effective in high-risk populations) and surveillance for known bladder cancer. NMP22 is unable to accurately detect recurrent disease in patients with urinary diversion.

4. ImmunoCyt—The ImmunoCyt test (Diagnocure, Quebec City, Canada) is an immunocytochemical test using fluorescent labeled antibodies to three markers found on exfoliated malignant urothelial cells: 19A211 a high-molecular-weight carcinoembryonic antigen and mucins LDQ10 and M344. It is done in conjunction with cytology to improve sensitivity in detection of low-grade urothelial tumor recurrence.

5. UroVysion Florescence in situ hybridization (FISH)—The UroVysion FISH test (Abbott Laboratories, Abbott Park, IL) detects increased copy numbers of chromosomes 3, 7, 17,

Table 5–1. Comparison of different urine tests for bladder transitional cell carcinoma.

Test	Sensitivity (%)	Specificity (%)
Hemoglobin dipstick	71	67
NMP22	68	79
BTA-TRAK	62	74
BTA-STAT	69	74
FDP	68	78
Telomerase	75	86
ImmunoCyt	84	75
UroVysion FISH	76	85
Flow cytometry	59	84
BLCA-4	96	100
Lewis X	80	86
Hyaluronidase	100	89
Hyaluronic acid	92	93
Survivin	100	87
Microsatellite DNA	72	80
Cytology	44	96

BTA, bladder tumor antigen; FDP, fibrin/fibrinogen degradation products; NMP22, nuclear matrix protein 22.

Source: Modified from Konety BR, Getzenberg RH: Urine-based markers of urological malignancy. J Urol 2001;165:600.

and deletions at 9p21. Using a panel of abnormalities, it is useful in the diagnosis of bladder cancer (especially in patients with hematuria) and for surveillance in patients with known cancer. Like other bladder tumor markers, it can improve upon the sensitivity of urine cytology. Unlike other tests, UroVysion FISH can be used in monitoring patients who have undergone intravesical chemotherapy (Mengual et al, 2007) Additionally, barbotage should be avoided because of an increase in false-positive readings and only voided urine samples should be sent for analysis.

The characteristics of these bladder cancer tests and others are compared in Table 5–1 (Konety, 2006; Konety and Getzenberg, 2001; Mowatt, 2010).

B. Prostate Cancer Tests

Recent studies have identified a novel biomarker, prostate cancer antigen 3 (PCA3), that is measured in voided urine sediment after prostate massage. PCA3 is a noncoding messenger RNA (mRNA) overexpressed in prostate cancer cells by 60–100-fold, and its use is currently experimental. At this time, it appears to be useful in helping to decide if men with

a negative first biopsy and high suspicion of prostate cancer should undergo repeat biopsy (Remzi et al, 2010). The role of PCA3 as a population-based screening test and its ability to predict prostate cancer in men with an elevated prostate-specific antigen (PSA) is currently under investigation.

C. Hormonal Studies

Tests for abnormalities in adrenal hormone secretion are important in the workup of patients with suspected adrenal tumors. Pheochromocytoma and neuroblastoma can be detected by measuring the excretion of vanillylmandelic acid. However, serum and urinary levels of metanephrine, epinephrine, and norepinephrine are more sensitive indicators, particularly in cases of pheochromocytoma. Although high levels of aldosterone in urine usually indicate an aldosterone-secreting tumor, drug interference may cause false-positive or false-negative results. Other adrenocortical tumors may be detected by their production of elevated levels of urinary 17-ketosteroids.

D. Studies of Stone Constituents

Patients with recurrent urolithiasis may have an underlying abnormality of excretion of calcium, uric acid, oxalate, magnesium, or citrate. Samples of 24-hour urine collections can be tested to determine abnormally high levels of each. A few patients may have elevated cystine levels in urine. The nitroprusside test, a simple *qualitative* screening test for cystine, may indicate the need for quantifying cystine levels in timed urine collections. Whenever a stone is recovered, a formal stone analysis is recommended.

E. Miscellaneous Studies

In patients with suspected fistulas of the urinary tract and bowel (eg, cancer of the colon, diverticulitis, and regional ileitis), discoloration of the urine after ingestion of a poorly absorbed dye such as phenol red will confirm the diagnosis. In an equally satisfactory test for fistulas, the patient is instructed to ingest gelatin capsules filled with granulated charcoal and to submit a urine sample several days later. Examination of the centrifuged urinary sediment will reveal the typical black granules if a fistula is present. In patients with suspected vesicovaginal fistulas, intravesical instillation of methylene blue or indigo carmine dye with resultant blue staining of a vaginal tampon can assist in diagnosis.

EXAMINATION OF URETHRAL DISCHARGE AND VAGINAL EXUDATE

▶ Urethral Discharge

Examination of urethral discharge in males can be particularly helpful in establishing a diagnosis. The following procedure, although exacting, provides proper specimens for determining the site of origin of bacteriuria or pyuria. Four sterile containers are labeled VB_1, VB_2, EPS, and VB_3 (VB = voided bladder urine; EPS = expressed prostatic secretions). The patient is instructed to retract the foreskin and cleanse the meatus with benzalkonium chloride or hexachlorophene and to collect the urine specimens, capping the containers immediately afterward. The initial 10–15 mL of urine is collected in container VB_1 and the subsequent 15–30 mL in container VB_2. The prostate is then massaged, and secretions are collected in container EPS. The patient voids a final time, collecting the specimen in container VB_3. An aliquot of each specimen is tested for nitrite and leukocyte esterase and then centrifuged, and the sediment is prepared for microscopic examination as described previously. A separate aliquot of each VB specimen and the EPS specimen are saved for subsequent culture if necessary. The presence of leukocytes or bacteria (or both) only in VB_1 indicates anterior urethritis; if present in all three VB specimens, they may indicate cystitis or upper urinary tract infection; if present in EPS or VB_3 only, they indicate a prostatic source of infection. Quantitative cultures can be similarly interpreted. Patients with positive results should be treated with appropriate antimicrobial drugs.

If the patient presents with the thick yellowish discharge typical of *Neisseria gonorrhoeae* infection, the discharge should be stained with Gram's stain and examined for gram-negative intracellular diplococci. It is important to remember that commensal bacteria in smegma may produce false-positive results.

If the patient presents with clear or whitish urethral discharge, a smear of the discharge obtained by milking the urethra or from VB_1 should be stained with methylene blue or Gram's stain and examined microscopically. The presence of trichomonads, yeast cells, or bacteria in properly collected specimens indicates disease requiring treatment.

In cases of acute epididymitis, urinalysis and urine culture are often helpful in establishing the cause. Epididymitis is most commonly caused by *Chlamydia* species in young men and by *E. coli* in men older than 35 years. Culturing chlamydiae is time consuming and expensive. Although a rapid immunofluorescence method of identifying *Chlamydia* is available, it is usually best to proceed with therapy based on the age of the patient and guided by clinical results.

The diagnosis of any sexually transmitted disease should raise the question of acquired immunodeficiency syndrome (AIDS). A recent study from the U.S. Centers for Disease Control and Prevention, in which a national sample of 12,571 males and females 15–44 years of age in 2002 were interviewed, demonstrated that one-half of this population reported that they had been tested at least once for HIV (other than through blood donation), and just over 15% had been tested within the past 12 months (Anderson et al, 2005). However, of those in this population deemed at high risk for HIV infection, one-third reported that they had never had an HIV test. This translates to an equivalent of 4.1–5.5 million, at-risk persons, aged 15–44 years, in the general population, having not been tested in the past year.

▶ Vaginal Exudate

The underlying cause of vaginitis is often a viral, yeast, or protozoal infection or the presence of a foreign body (eg, retained tampon), and a simple physical examination may be all that is required for diagnosis.

Vaginal secretions obtained by use of a swab can be examined either stained or unstained. A drop of saline is added to a drop of specimen on a glass slide, mixed thoroughly, and covered with a coverslip. Examination under a low- or high-power lens may reveal yeast cells or trichomonads, thus suggesting appropriate therapy. Since bacteria are always present in the vagina, they generally are not significant findings in a wet smear.

RENAL FUNCTION TESTS

▶ Urine Specific Gravity

With diminished renal function, the ability of the kidneys to concentrate urine lessens progressively until the specific gravity of urine reaches 1.006–1.010. However, the ability to dilute urine tends to be maintained until renal damage is extreme. Even in uremia, although the concentrating power of the kidneys is limited to a specific gravity of 1.010, dilution power in the specific gravity range of 1.002–1.004 may still be found. Determination of urine osmolality is undoubtedly a more meaningful measurement of renal function, but determination of specific gravity lends itself to office diagnosis.

▶ Serum Creatinine

Creatinine, the end product of the metabolism of creatine in skeletal muscle, is normally excreted by the kidneys. Because individual daily creatinine production is constant, the serum level is a direct reflection of renal function. Serum creatinine levels remain within the normal range (0.8–1.2 mg/dL in adults; 0.4–0.8 mg/dL in young children) until approximately 50% of renal function has been lost. Unlike most other excretory products, the serum creatinine level generally is not influenced by dietary intake or hydration status.

▶ Endogenous Creatinine Clearance

Because creatinine production is stable and creatinine is filtered through the glomerulus (although a small amount is probably secreted), its renal clearance is essentially equal to the glomerular filtration rate. The endogenous creatinine clearance test has thus become the most accurate and reliable measure of renal function available without resorting to infusion of exogenous substances such as radionuclides. Determination of creatinine clearance requires only the collection of a timed (usually 24-hour) urine specimen and a serum specimen. The resulting clearance is expressed in milliliters per minute, with 90–110 mL/min considered normal.

Because muscle mass differs among individuals, further standardization has been achieved and a corrected clearance level of 70–140 mL/min is considered normal.

Although creatinine is highly reliable as an estimate of renal function, values may be falsely low, particularly if only part of the urine is collected over the time period or if a serum specimen is not collected concurrently.

Blood Urea Nitrogen

Urea is the primary metabolite of protein catabolism and is excreted entirely by the kidneys. The blood urea nitrogen (BUN) level is therefore related to the glomerular filtration rate. However, unlike creatinine, BUN is influenced by dietary protein intake, hydration status, and gastrointestinal bleeding. Approximately two-thirds of renal function must be lost before a significant rise in BUN level becomes evident. For these reasons, an elevated BUN level is less specific for renal insufficiency than an elevated serum creatinine level. However, the BUN–creatinine (BUN–Cr) ratio can provide specific diagnostic information. It is normally 10:1; in dehydrated patients and those with bilateral urinary obstruction or urinary extravasation, the ratio may range from 20:1 to 40:1; patients with advanced hepatic insufficiency and overhydrated patients may exhibit a lower than normal BUN level and BUN–Cr ratio. In patients with renal insufficiency, extremely high BUN levels may develop that can be partially controlled by a decrease in dietary protein.

EXAMINATION OF BLOOD, SERUM, AND PLASMA

Complete Blood Count

Normochromic normocytic anemia is often seen with chronic renal insufficiency. Chronic blood loss from microscopic hematuria is usually not sufficient to cause anemia, although gross hematuria certainly can be. A specific increase in the number of erythrocytes, as manifested by elevated hemoglobin and hematocrit levels (erythrocytosis, not polycythemia), may be indicative of a paraneoplastic syndrome associated with renal cell cancer. The leukocyte count is usually nonspecific, although marked elevations may indicate an underlying leukemia that may be the cause of urologic symptoms.

Blood Clotting Studies

Clotting studies are generally not necessary unless an insidious disorder such as von Willebrand disease, hepatic disease, or sensitivity to ingested salicylates is suspected in a patient with unexplained hematuria. The determination of prothrombin time and bleeding time (and perhaps partial thromboplastin time) is usually sufficient. A platelet count is important in patients receiving chemotherapy and those who have received extensive radiation therapy.

Electrolyte Studies

Serum sodium and potassium determinations may be indicated in patients taking diuretics or digitalis preparations and in patients who have just undergone transurethral prostatectomy. Serum calcium determinations are useful in patients with calcium urolithiasis. Elevated calcium levels are occasionally indicative of a paraneoplastic syndrome in patients with renal cell cancer. Serum albumin levels should be measured simultaneously with calcium levels to adequately assess the significance of the latter.

Prostate Cancer Markers

PSA is an important, if controversial, prostate cancer marker. PSA is prostate specific but not cancer specific. Levels vary with prostate volume, inflammation, and amount of cancer within the gland. PSA has become useful as a screening tool and is most useful as a marker of effective treatment (falls to zero following removal of organ-confined cancer) and early recurrence (Hernandez et al, 2005). The percentage of free PSA (ratio of unbound to total PSA) in the serum is useful for increasing the specificity of PSA for diagnosing prostate cancer. If the percentage of free PSA is <10%, approximately 60% of men will have prostate cancer, whereas if the percentage of free PSA is >25%, only 8% will have it. The use of PSA for prostate cancer screening is a topic of considerable debate and will be explored more in Chapter 23.

Hormonal Studies

Serum parathyroid hormone studies are useful in determining the presence of a parathyroid adenoma in patients with urolithiasis and an elevated serum calcium level. Measurement of parathyroid hormone is not reliable, however, as a sole screening test for parathyroid adenoma and should not be used routinely in all patients with urolithiasis. Serum renin levels may be elevated in patients with renal hypertension, although many conditions can cause false-positive results. Studies of adrenal steroid hormones (eg, aldosterone, cortisol, epinephrine, and norepinephrine) are useful in determining adrenal function or the presence of adrenal tumors. Determinations of serum levels of the beta-subunit of human chorionic gonadotrophin (hCG) and of alpha-fetoprotein are indispensable in staging and in treatment follow-up for testicular tumors. One of these tumor markers is usually elevated in up to 85% of patients with nonseminomatous testicular tumors and can predict the recrudescence of tumor several months before disease is clinically evident. Serum testosterone studies can help to establish the cause of impotence or infertility.

▶ Other Studies

The finding of elevated fasting plasma glucose levels in patients with urologic disease can establish the diagnosis of diabetes mellitus and, thus, indicate a possible cause of renal insufficiency, neurovesical dysfunction, impotence, or recurrent urinary tract infection. Serum uric acid levels are often elevated in patients with uric acid stones. Elevated serum complement levels may be diagnostic of underlying glomerulopathies.

LABORATORY VALUES IN ELDERLY PATIENTS

Clearly, some laboratory values change as patients age, others stay the same, and the effects of aging on some are as yet unknown. Laboratory values that do not change with increasing age include complete blood count, serum electrolytes, and hepatic function tests, among others (Table 5–2).

Table 5–2. Laboratory values that do not change with age.

Hepatic function tests
Serum bilirubin
AST
ALT
GGTP
Coagulation tests
Biochemical tests
Serum electrolytes
Total protein
Calcium
Phosphorus
Serum folate
Arterial blood tests
pH
$PaCO_2$
Renal function tests
Serum creatinine
Thyroid function tests
T_4
Complete blood count
Hematocrit
Hemoglobin
Erythrocyte indices
Platelet count

AST, aspartate aminotransferase; ALT, alanine aminotransferase; GGTP, gamma-glutamyltransferase.

Table 5–3. Laboratory values that do change with age.

Value	Degree of Change
Alkaline phosphatase	Increases by 20% between third and eighth decades
Biochemical tests	
Serum albumin	Slight decline
Uric acid	Slight increase
Total cholesterol	Increases by 30–40 mg/dL by age 55 in women and age 60 in men
HDL cholesterol	Increases by 30% in men; decreases by 50% in women
Triglycerides	Increases by 30% in men and 50% in women
Serum B_{12}	Slight decrease
Serum magnesium	Decreases by 15% between third and eighth decades
PaO_2	Decreases by 25% between third and eighth decades
Creatinine clearance	Decreases by 10 mL/min/1.73 sq m/decade
Thyroid function tests	
T_3	Possible slight decrease
TSH	Possible slight increase
Glucose tolerance tests	
Fasting blood sugar	Minimal increase (within normal range)
1-Hour postprandial blood sugar	Increases by 10 mg/dL/decade after age 30
2-Hour postprandial blood sugar	Increases up to 100 plus age after age 40
Leukocyte count	Decreases

HDL, high-density lipoprotein; TSH, thyroid-stimulating hormone.
Note: Other factors that may make laboratory interpretation more difficult include atypical disease presentation, multiple concurrent diseases, and prescription and nonprescription drug use.

Laboratory values that change as patients age include creatinine clearance, alkaline phosphatase, uric acid, and cholesterol (Table 5–3).

BIBLIOGRAPHY

Anderson JE et al: HIV testing in the United States, 2002. Adv Data 2005;8:1–32.

Boman H et al: Four bladder tumor markers have a disappointingly low sensitivity for small size and low grade recurrence. J Urol 2002;167:80.

Godbole P, Johnstone JM: Routine urine microscopy and culture in paediatric surgical outpatients: Is it necessary? Pediatr Surg Int 2004;20:130.

Grossman HB et al: Detection of bladder cancer using a point-of-care proteomic assay. JAMA 2005;16:293.

Hernandez J et al: Biomarkers for the detection and prognosis of prostate cancer. Curr Urol Rep 2005;6:171.

Konety BR. Molecular markers in bladder cancer: A critical appraisal. Urol Oncol 2006;24(4):326–337.

Konety BR, Getzenberg RH: Urine based markers of urological malignancy. J Urol 2001;165:600.

Mengual L et al: Clinical utility of fluorescence in situ hybridization for the surveillance of bladder cancer patients treated with bacillus Calmette-Guerin therapy. Eur Urol 2007;52:752.

Messing EM, Vaillancourt A: Hematuria screening for bladder cancer. J Occup Med 1990;32:838.

Mowatt G et al: Systematic review of the clinical effectiveness and cost-effectiveness of photodynamic diagnosis and urine biomarkers (FISH, Immunocyt, NMP22) and cytology for the detection and follow-up of bladder cancer. Health Technol Assess 2010;14(4):1–331.

Remzi M et al: Follow-up of men with an elevated PCA3 score and a negative biopsy: Does an elevated PCA3 score indeed predict the presence of prostate cancer? BJU Int 2010;106:1138–1142.

Simerville JA et al: Urinalysis: A comprehensive review. Am Fam Physician 2005;71:1153.

Wah DT et al: Analytic performance of the iQ200 automated urine microscopy analyzer. Clin Chim Acta 2005;358:167.

Young JL, Soper DE: Urinalysis and urinary tract infection: Update for clinicians. Infect Dis Obstet Gynecol 2001;9:249.

Radiology of the Urinary Tract

6

Scott Gerst, MD, & Hedvig Hricak, MD, PhD

The pace of innovation in diagnostic radiology has increased exponentially, in tandem with computer advances and the rapid evolution of microprocessing power. Imaging of the urinary tract, as a result, has become more flexible and precise, with new procedures offering a great selection of options, and new imaging algorithms being implemented. Ultrasonography, computed tomography (CT), and magnetic resonance imaging (MRI) provide higher soft-tissue contrast resolution than conventional radiography, as well as multiplanar imaging capability, resulting in significant advances in almost all areas of uroradiology. In academic centers, metabolic and molecular imaging techniques have become the focus of new research, and have begun to enter the realm of daily clinical practice. While imaging advances have produced new algorithms for approaching diagnostic evaluation, appropriate use of imaging in each particular case also depends greatly on the equipment and professional talent available. One imaging modality or protocol may offer specific advantages over another depending on the clinical question, and the importance of a collaborative approach from the medical team cannot be overemphasized.

In summary, ever changing uroradiology remains indispensable in the diagnosis and treatment of patients with urologic disorders. This chapter will discuss the imaging techniques used in uroradiology, with summaries of the advantages and disadvantages of the various techniques, and will end with a brief discussion comparing imaging methods.

RADIOGRAPHY

X-rays are electromagnetic waves with photon energies that typically fall between those of gamma rays and ultraviolet radiation. Radiography is possible because tissues differ in their ability to absorb x-rays. A radiopaque contrast medium is frequently employed to enhance soft-tissue contrast.

Although newer imaging techniques have largely replaced conventional radiography for diagnosis of many urologic problems, general radiography remains useful for some urologic disorders; therefore, the urologist should be familiar with x-ray equipment and uroradiologic techniques. The basic types of uroradiologic studies are plain (conventional) abdominal films, (also known as KUB, which stands for kidney, ureter, bladder) intravenous urograms (IVUs), cystourethrograms, urethrograms, and angiograms. These studies are described separately in sections that follow.

▶ Basic Equipment and Techniques

1. Radiography fluoroscopy—Many conventional x-ray units contain both radiographic and fluoroscopic capabilities. These require a high voltage power supply, an x-ray tube, a collimating device, and an x-ray detector or film. Fluoroscopic units also use an electronic image intensifier and an image display system. Today, more radiology departments have become completely "filmless" as digital recording, displaying, and archiving of images are replacing film-based techniques.

2. Image intensification—Image intensifiers, coupled to video cameras, electronically augment the ordinary dim fluoroscopic image.

3. Image recording—Conventional recording of an x-ray image uses film and intensifying screens. The image intensifier and camera can be used to capture dynamic and static images. Real-time images are now typically recorded using conventional or digital video. Conventional spot or cine images may be acquired on x-ray film or digitally recorded.

4. Contrast media—Radiographic contrast media used in uroradiography are water-soluble iodinated compounds that are radiopaque. Similar compounds are used for basic radiographic techniques and CT, though iodine concentrations will differ depending on preference and route of administration. In general, intravenous administration for CT or IVU is performed with iodine 200 mg/ lb body weight in adults, and direct instillation to the collecting system or bladders uses similar media diluted to 15–45% concentration. The extracellular distribution of these agents results in improved contrast resolution and conspicuity of various structures.

Significant advances in water-soluble contrast media occurred with the introduction of low-osmolality, nonionic organic iodine-containing compounds. These nonionic agents significantly improve patient tolerance and decrease the incidence of adverse reactions, and at many institutions the use of nonionic agents is standard. Whether they reduce the mortality associated with the use of contrast media has not been proven. The major obstacle to their use is higher cost.

5. Adverse reactions—All procedures using intravascular contrast media carry a small but definite risk of adverse reactions. The overall incidence of adverse reactions is about 5%. Reactions in nonintravenous use (ie, cystograms) are extremely rare but have been reported.

Most reactions are minor, for example, nausea, vomiting, hives, rash, or flushing, and usually require only reassurance. Cardiopulmonary and anaphylactoid reactions can occur with little warning and can be life threatening or fatal. In a large meta-analysis, the incidence of death due to intravascular injection of contrast media was 0.9 deaths/100,000 injections. There are no reliable methods for pretesting patients for possible adverse reactions. The risks and benefits of contrast use should be carefully evaluated for each patient before the procedure is initiated. Treatment of adverse reactions involves the use of antihistamines, epinephrine, vascular volume expanders, bronchodilators, and other cardiopulmonary drugs as well as ancillary procedures indicated by the nature and severity of the reaction. In some cases a radiographic examination using intravascular contrast media is critical even if the patient has had a prior moderate or severe reaction. Such patients are given nonionic contrast agents and pretreated with corticosteroids, sometimes in combination with antihistamines, in an effort to prevent recurrence. This preventive treatment is not always successful, so any decision to administer contrast under these circumstances should be carefully weighed against the risks.

Nephrotoxicity caused by intravascular contrast agents is another concern. The pathogenesis of contrast nephropathy (CN) likely involves medullary ischemia due to contrast-induced vasoconstriction and direct tubular injury. Patients at higher risk are those with preexisting renal insufficiency, diabetes, dehydration, or patients who receive higher volumes of contrast material. Alternative procedures can be selected in high-risk patients. If contrast use is deemed necessary in a high-risk individual, CN can be minimized through attention to proper hydration, discontinuation of drugs that may exacerbate toxic effects, adequate hydration in the 24 hours prior to scanning, reduction of contrast volume, and possibly administration of oral N-acetylcysteine.

▶ Advantages and Disadvantages

Radiography produces anatomic images of almost any body part. Costs are moderate compared with cross-sectional imaging systems. Space requirements are modest, and portable equipment is available for use in hospital wards, operating rooms, and intensive care units. Because there are a great many specialists trained in radiography, its use is not confined to large medical centers. The major disadvantage of radiographic imaging is the use of ionizing radiation and relatively poor soft-tissue contrast. The evaluation of the urinary tract almost always requires opacification by iodine contrast media.

1. Plain film of the abdomen (Figures 6–1 through 6–3)—A plain film of the abdomen, frequently called a KUB film, is the simplest uroradiologic examination. It is generally the preliminary radiograph in extended radiologic examinations, such as intravenous urography, and is usually taken with the patient supine. It may demonstrate osseous abnormalities, abnormal calcifications, or large soft-tissue masses.

Kidney outlines usually can be seen on the plain film, so that their size, number, shape, and position can be assessed. The size of normal adult kidneys varies widely. The long diameter (the length) of the kidney is the most widely used and most convenient radiographic measurement. The average adult kidney is about 12–14 cm long. In children older than 2 years of age, the length of a normal kidney is approximately equal to the distance from the top of the first to the bottom of the fourth lumbar vertebral body. Patterns of calcification in the urinary tract (Figures 6–1 and 6–2) may help to identify specific diseases.

2. Urography (Figures 6–4 through 6–8)—The collecting structures of the kidneys, ureters, and bladder can be demonstrated radiologically with contrast media by the following methods:

▶ Intravenous Urography

The IVU, also known as excretory urography (EU) (Figure 6–4), or intravenous pyelography (IVP), can demonstrate a wide variety of urinary tract lesions (Figures 6–4 and 6–5), is simple to perform, and is well tolerated by most patients.

CT, sonography and MRI have replaced urography in the vast majority of cases. Nevertheless, urography is occasionally used and is useful for demonstrating small lesions in the urinary tract (eg, papillary necrosis, medullary sponge kidney, uroepithelial tumors, pyeloureteritis cystica).

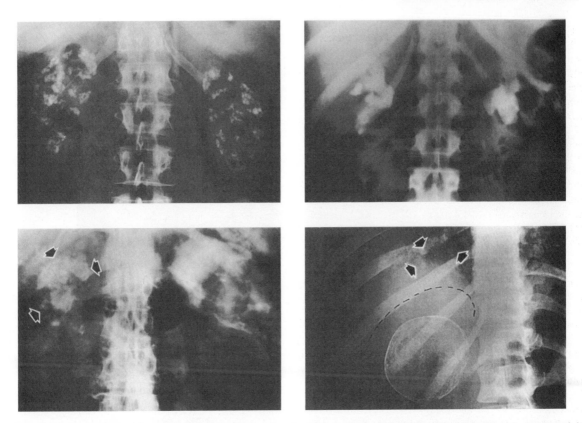

▲ **Figure 6–1.** Plain films of the abdomen with abnormal radiopacities. ***Upper left:*** Bilateral nephrocalcinosis. Young adult male with renal tubular acidosis. ***Upper right:*** Bilateral staghorn calculi. 37-year-old woman with chronic pyelonephritis and history of previous right staghorn pyelolithotomy. ***Lower left:*** Renal tuberculosis. Shrunken, autonephrectomized, and calcified right tuberculous kidney (*arrows*). 74-year-old man with history of renal and thoracolumbar spinal tuberculosis. ***Lower right:*** Papillary adenocarcinoma of right kidney. Remarkable tumor surface calcifications. Multiple pulmonary metastases (*arrows*) from the renal cancer. 22-year-old woman with painless soft tissue mass in the neck.

A. Patient Preparation

At one time dehydration was advocated as optimal preparation for intravenous urography (EU). This is no longer required. Furthermore, dehydration is to be avoided in infants, debilitated and elderly patients, and patients with diabetes mellitus, renal failure, multiple myeloma, or hyperuricemia.

It is controversial whether preliminary bowel cleansing is beneficial. The choice may be made according to individual preference.

B. Standard Technique

Following a preliminary plain film of the abdomen, additional radiographs are taken at timed intervals after the intravenous injection of iodine-containing contrast medium. Normal kidneys promptly excrete contrast agents, almost entirely by glomerular filtration.

The volume and speed of injection of the contrast medium, as well as the number and type of films taken, vary by preference, patient tolerance, and the particular clinical scenario.

C. Technique Modifications

Radiographic tomography, x-ray imaging of a selected plane in the body, permits recognition of kidney structures that otherwise are obscured on standard radiograms by extrarenal shadows, for example, those due to bone or feces (Figure 6–6). Image-intensified fluoroscopy permits study of urinary tract dynamics. "Immediate" films, which are taken immediately after the rapid (bolus) injection of contrast, typically show a dense nephrogram and permit better visualization of renal outlines. Abdominal (ureteral) compression devices temporarily obstruct the upper urinary tract during EU and improve the filling of renal collecting structures. "Delayed"

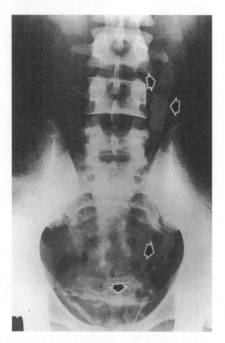
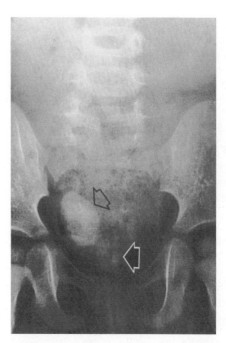

▲ **Figure 6–2.** Plain films of the abdomen with abnormal radiopacities. ***Left:*** Schistosomiasis calcification (*arrows*) in bladder and left ureter. 19-year-old male native of Aden with weight loss and hematuria. ***Right:*** Large vaginolith (*open arrow*) and small, barely visible bladder calculus (*solid arrow*). 4-year-old girl with common urogenital sinus.

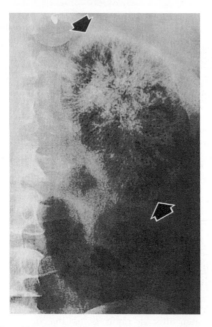
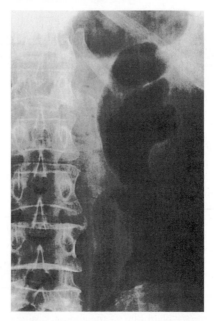

▲ **Figure 6–3.** Plain films of the abdomen with abnormal radiolucencies. ***Left:*** Emphysematous pyelonephritis. Interstitial striated pattern of radiolucent gas throughout the entire left kidney. Similar changes were present in the right kidney. 58-year-old diabetic man with pyuria and septic shock. ***Right:*** Gas pyelogram. No interstitial gas, but gas fills dilated left kidney calices, pelvis, and ureter. 50-year-old diabetic woman with sepsis and left upper urinary tract infection due to gas-forming micro-organisms.

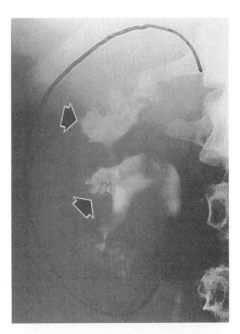
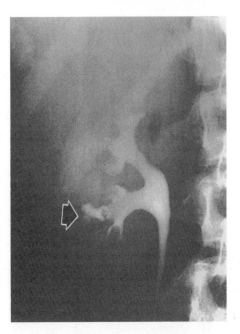

▲ **Figure 6–4.** Abnormal excretory urograms. ***Left:*** Medullary sponge kidney. Pronounced medullary tubular ectasia (*arrows*) of entire right kidney. Similar findings were present in upper pole pyramids of left kidney, and small medullary calculi were present in some areas of tubular ectasia in both kidneys. 34-year-old woman with repeated bouts of chills, fever, and left flank pain. ***Right:*** Renal tuberculosis. Irregular cavitation of lower pole pyramid (*arrow*). 22-year-old woman with positive urine culture for tuberculosis.

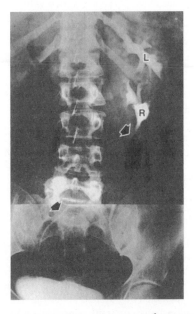
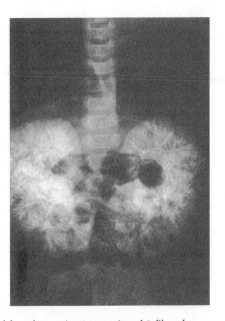

▲ **Figure 6–5.** Abnormal excretory urograms. ***Left:*** Crossed fused ectopia. Composite of 2 films from an excretory urogram shows ectopic right kidney (R) fused to left kidney (L). Right ureter (*arrows*) crosses midline and enters normally into right side of bladder. Healthy 31-year-old female potential kidney donor. ***Right:*** Infantile polycystic kidney disease. Very large kidneys with radiopaque spoke pattern radiating out to cortex. 26 hours after administration of intravenous contrast medium. 4-month-old girl with bilateral abdominal masses.

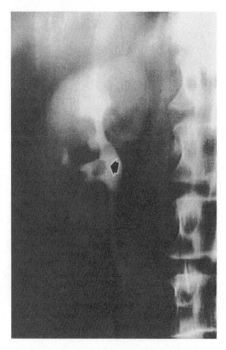 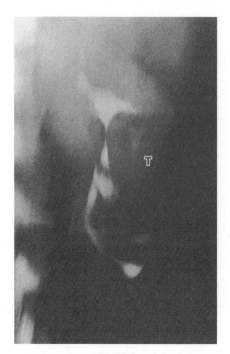

▲ **Figure 6–6.** Radiographic tomography. Tomography is used to image a plane in the body. The technique was widely used in uroradiology, often permitting demonstration of lesions otherwise hidden by overlying soft tissues or obscuring bowel shadows. However, computed tomography (CT) is rapidly replacing conventional excretory urograms, and thus tomography is declining in its use as well. **Left:** Transitional cell carcinoma. The tumor in the pelvis (*arrow*) is clearly shown free of obscuring gas shadows present on the nontomographic films. 56-year-old man with history of renal calculi. **Right:** Renal cell carcinoma (T). Displacement of mid-kidney collecting structures and a nephrogram defect are seen free of obscuring splenic flexure fecal shadows that were present on the nontomographic films. 44-year-old woman with fever, weight loss, anemia, and history of contralateral nephrectomy for carcinoma 15 years earlier.

films, taken hours later or on the following day, can contribute useful information. "Upright" films, taken with the patient standing or partially erect, reveal the degree of mobility and drainage of the kidneys and, if taken immediately after the patient has voided ("postvoiding" film), show any residual urine in the bladder.

▶ Retrograde Urograms

Retrograde urography is a minimally invasive procedure that requires cystoscopy and the placement of catheters in the ureters. A radiopaque contrast medium is introduced into the ureters or renal collecting structures through the ureteral catheters (Figures 6–7 and 6–8), and radiographs of the abdomen are taken. This study must be performed by a urologist or experienced interventional uroradiologist. Some type of local or general anesthesia should be used, and the

procedure occasionally causes later morbidity or urinary tract infection.

Retrograde urograms may be necessary if excretory urograms or CT urogram (CTU) are unsatisfactory, if the patient has a history of adverse reaction to intravenous contrast media, or if other methods of imaging are unavailable or inappropriate.

▶ Percutaneous Urograms

Outlining the renal collecting structures and ureters by percutaneous catheter is occasionally done when excretory or retrograde urography has failed or is contraindicated, or when there is a nephrostomy tube in place and delineation of the collecting system is desired. For antegrade studies, contrast medium is introduced either through nephrostomy tubes (nephrostogram) or by direct injection into the renal

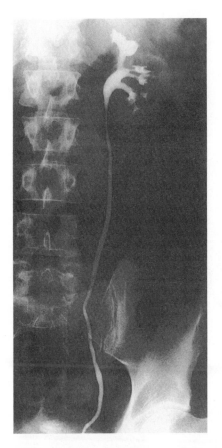

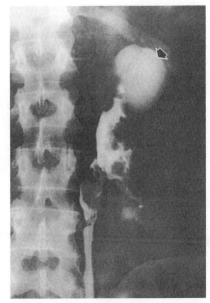

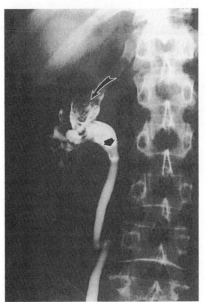

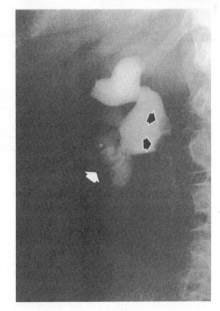

▲ **Figure 6–7.** Retrograde urograms and nephrostograms; lower ureters not all shown. ***Upper left:*** Normal retrograde urogram. Intrarenal collecting structures, pelvis, and ureter are normal. Adult male with microscopic hematuria and previous technically unsatisfactory excretory urogram. ***Upper right:*** Squamous cell carcinoma. Marked irregular filling defects involving calices, pelvis, and proximal ureter, with communicating abscess cavity in upper pole (*arrow*). Kidney also showed squamous meta-plasia and contained calculi. 51-year-old woman with 2-week history of left flank cellulitis and tenderness. ***Lower left:*** Transitional cell carcinoma. Severe deformity with filling defects in right upper pole calices (*curved arrow*) and blood clots in lower calices and at ureteropelvic junction (*straight arrow*). 65-year-old man with gross hematuria and right flank pain. ***Lower right:*** Fungus balls. Nephrostogram revealing 2 filling defects (*arrows*) in renal pelvis. Copious fungal matter aspirated through nephrostomy catheter. 65-year-old diabetic woman who had undergone left nephrectomy, with percutaneous nephrostomy catheter (*white arrow*) for obstruction of right kidney.

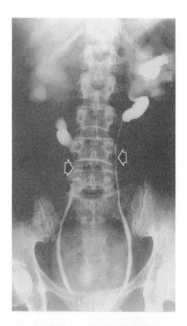
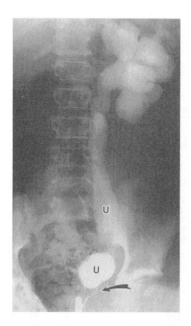
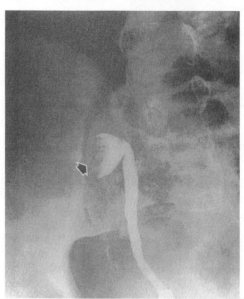
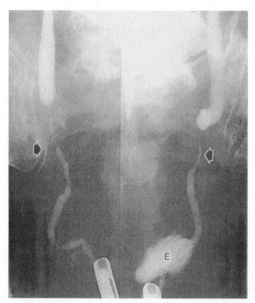

▲ **Figure 6–8.** Abnormal retrograde urograms. **Upper left:** Idiopathic retroperitoneal fibrosis. Smooth narrowing of both mid ureters (*arrows*), with bilateral proximal ureterectasis and hydronephrosis. 51-year-old woman with no urinary tract symptoms. **Upper right:** Functional ureteral obstruction. Obstruction was due to congenitally abnormal muscle arrangements in the affected very distal ureter (*curved arrow*). Pronounced hydronephrosis and dilatation of ureter (U) proximal to the short segment of abnormal ureter. 13-year-old boy with repeated urinary tract infections. **Lower left:** Transitional cell carcinoma of the ureter. No contrast medium has passed beyond the large, bulky, right ureteral tumor (*arrow*). The ureteral widening below the tumor is distinctive and is sometimes referred to as the "champagne glass" sign (in this instance, the glass is tipped on its side). 76-year-old man with nonfunctioning right kidney. **Lower right:** Ureteral constrictions secondary to extension of carcinoma of the colon. Bilateral distal ureteral narrowings (*arrows*) with upper tract obstruction. Composite of separate retrograde urograms. E = unintended extravasation about tip of left ureteral catheter. 76-year-old man with cancer of the sigmoid colon.

collecting structures via a percutaneous puncture through the patient's back. Percutaneous retrograde urograms of the upper urinary tract are made by retrograde injection of contrast medium through the opening of a skin ureterostomy or pyelostomy (skin ureterogram, skin urogram) or through the ostium of an interposed conduit, usually a segment of small bowel (loopogram).

3. Cystography, voiding, cystourethrography, and urodynamics (Figures 6–9 through 6–12)—Direct instillation of contrast media into the urinary bladder (cystography) allows a more focused examination of the bladder. Contrast is usually instilled via a transurethral catheter, but when necessary can be administered via percutaneous suprapubic bladder puncture. For urodynamic studies, pressure transducers are used within the bladder lumen and rectum for dynamic measurement of intraluminal and intra-abdominal pressures, respectively. Radiographs can be taken using standard overhead x-rays, or during fluoroscopy. Voiding cystourethrograms are radiographs of the bladder and urethra obtained during micturition. Cystography and cystourethrography are important radiologic techniques for detecting vesicoureteral reflux and may be used in the workup of patients with urinary stress incontinence. CT cystography (CT of the pelvis after the instillation of dilute contrast medium into the bladder) has been shown useful in the evaluation of traumatic bladder rupture.

4. Urethrography (Figures 6–13 through 6–15)—The urethra can be imaged radiographically by retrograde injection of radiopaque fluid or in antegrade fashion with voiding cystourethrography, or with voiding following EU. The antegrade technique is required when lesions of the posterior urethra, for example, posterior urethral valves, are suspected; the retrograde technique is more useful for examining the anterior (penile) urethra. The urethra may also be evaluated by tailored MRI examinations using thin-section imaging with a small field of view. Urethral tumor or diverticula, for example, may be readily demonstrated with MRI (Ryu and Kim, 2001).

5. Vasography (Figure 6–16)—Vasoseminal vesiculography is most often used in the investigation of male sterility. The radiopaque contrast medium is introduced into the ductal system by direct injection into an ejaculatory duct following panendoscopy or, more commonly, by injection into the vas deferens after it has been surgically exposed through a small incision in the scrotal neck.

6. Lymphangiography—Lymphangiography has been largely abandoned and replaced by CT and MRI.

7. Angiography—Nearly 50 years after Seldinger described techniques for percutaneous arteriography, catheter angiography maintains a limited role in treatment of some urologic disorders but is being replaced by CT or MRI for diagnostic

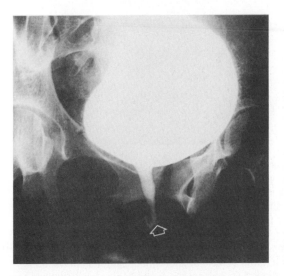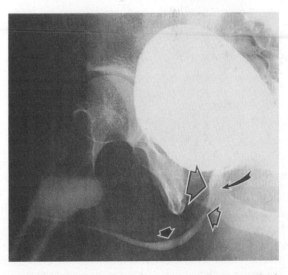

▲ **Figure 6–9.** Normal voiding cystourethrograms. **Left:** Normal female bladder and urethra. Arrow indicates urethral meatus. 22-year-old woman with voiding symptoms. **Right:** Normal male penile urethra. Large open arrow = prostatic urethra; small open arrow = membranous urethra; closed arrow = penile urethra; curved arrow = verumontanum. 27-year-old man with vague right lower abdominal and testicular pain.

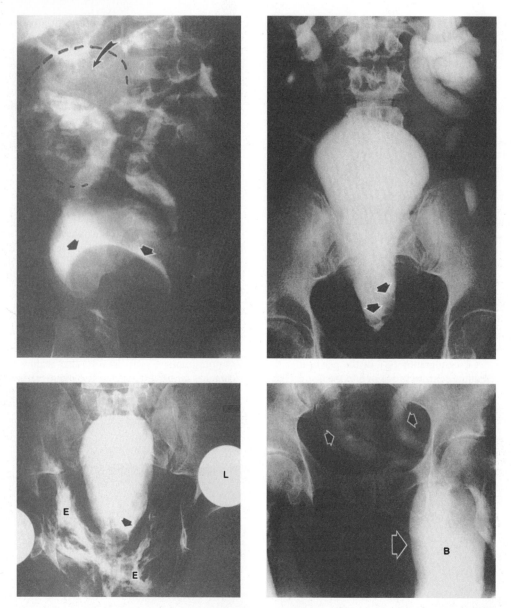

▲ **Figure 6–10.** Abnormal cystograms: retrograde cystograms or "cystograms" as part of excretory urogram studies. ***Upper left:*** Ectopic ureterocele. Giant ureterocele (*straight arrows*) to hydronephrotic, nonfunctioning upper portion (*curved arrow*) of duplex right kidney. 9-month-old-girl with urinary tract infections. ***Upper right:*** Pelvic lipomatosis. Pear-shaped bladder and increased radiolucency of the pelvic soft tissues secondary to pelvic lipomatosis of severity sufficient to produce obstructive dilatation of the upper urinary tracts. Filling defects (*arrows*) at bladder base due to cystitis glandularis. 62-year-old man with intermittent left flank pain. ***Lower left:*** Rupture of the membranous urethra. Pear-shaped bladder secondary to extraperitoneal extravasation (E) and perivesical hematoma. Arrow = inflated balloon of Foley catheter. 41-year-old man with renal transplant, after a motor vehicle accident that resulted in pelvic bone fractures, separation of the sacroiliac joints, and dislocation of the left (L) but not the right hip prosthesis (patient has bilateral hip prostheses). ***Lower right:*** Bladder hernia. Bilateral obstructive ureterectasis (*small arrows*) secondary to remarkable herniation of the entire bladder (*large arrow,* B) into the inguinal region, 5" 5′ , 225 lb, 53-year-old man with panniculus reaching to mid thigh, complaining of difficulty voiding.

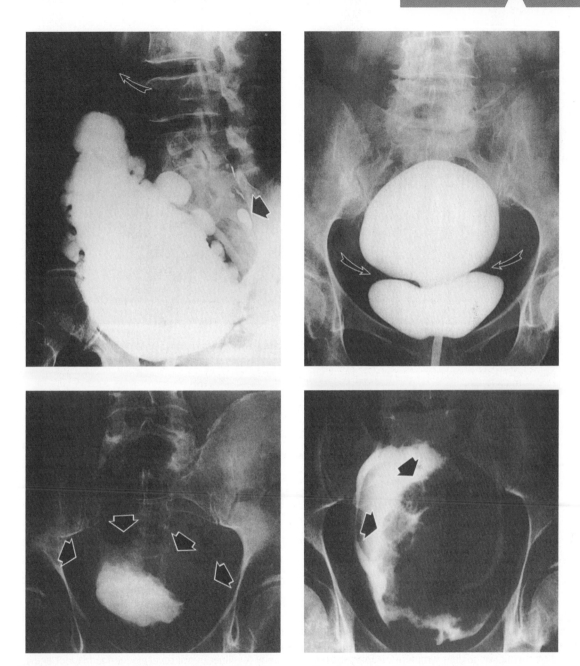

▲ **Figure 6–11.** Abnormal cystograms: retrograde cystograms or "cystograms" as part of excretory urogram studies. ***Upper left:*** Neurogenic bladder. This neurogenic bladder has a "Christmas-tree" shape, with gross trabeculation and many diverticula. Residual myelographic contrast medium in spinal canal (*straight arrow*). Right vesicoureteral reflux (*curved arrow*). 70-year-old man with urinary incontinence. ***Upper right:*** Congenital "hourglass" bladder. Transverse concentric muscular band (*arrows*) separates upper and lower bladder segments, both of which contracted and emptied simultaneously and completely with voiding. 66-year-old woman with urinary stress incontinence. ***Lower left:*** Hodgkin's disease of bladder. Global thickening of the bladder wall (*arrows*), more apparent on the left. 54-year-old man with generalized Hodgkin's disease. ***Lower right:*** Papillary transitional cell bladder carcinoma. Huge (12 cm) cauliflower-like bladder mass (*arrows*) filling almost the entire bladder. "Cystogram" film of an excretory urogram in a 40-year-old man with recurrent bladder tumor.

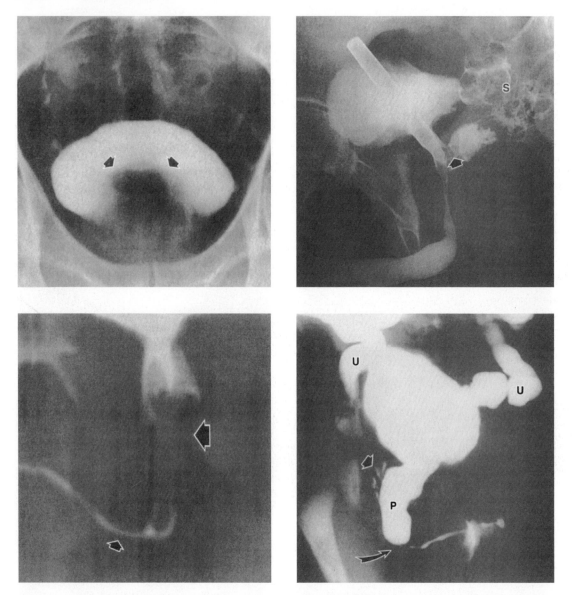

▲ **Figure 6–12.** Abnormal prostate and posterior urethra: cystograms and urethrograms. ***Upper left:*** Benign prostatic hyperplasia. Gross enlargement of prostate gland producing marked elevation (*arrows*) of the bladder base. The bladder shows small diverticula and slight trabeculation. Excretory urogram (cystogram) in a 65-year-old man with history of obstructive voiding symptoms. ***Upper right:*** Foreign body (eyeliner pencil cover) lodged in bladder and prostatic urethra, with urethrorectal fistula. Radiopaque medium enters rectum and sigmoid colon (S) through fistula (*arrow*) from prostatic urethra. Retrograde urethrogram in a 43-year-old man. ***Lower left:*** Rhabdomyosarcoma of prostate. Lobulated filling defects (*large arrow*) encroaching on widened prostatic urethra. Voiding cystourethrogram in a 5-year-old boy with voiding difficulties. Small arrow = penile urethra. ***Lower right:*** Posterior urethral valves. Marked dilatation and elongation of prostatic urethra (P), with reflux into prostatic ducts (*straight arrow*) secondary to posterior urethral valves (*curved arrow*) with bilateral vesicoureteral reflux into dilated ureters (U). Voiding cystourethrogram in a 10-day-old boy.

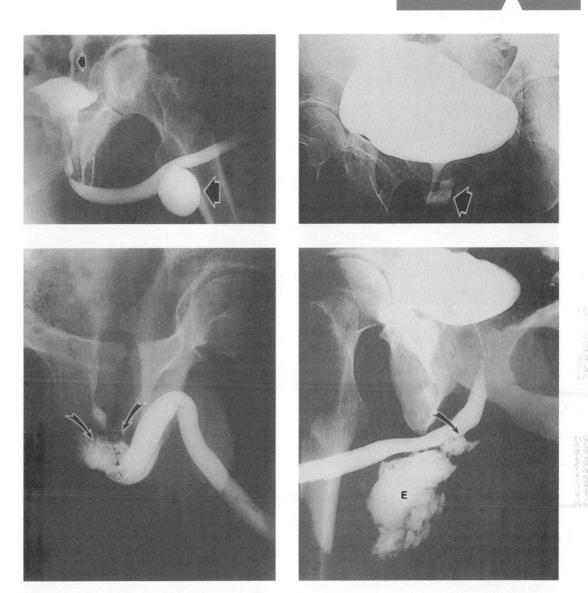

▲ **Figure 6–13.** Abnormal anterior urethras: voiding cystourethrograms and retrograde urethrograms. ***Upper left:*** Voiding cystourethrogram in a 78-year-old man with a history of urethral diverticulum of unknown etiology. 4-cm anterior urethral diverticulum (*large arrow*) and left vesicoureteral reflux (*small arrow*). ***Upper right:*** Urethral diverticulum in a woman. Large irregular diverticulum (*arrow*). Voiding cystourethrogram in a 51-year-old woman with voiding difficulties and suspected urethral stricture. ***Lower left:*** Ruptured urethra. Extravasation of contrast medium around the membranous urethra (*arrows*). Retrograde urethrogram in a 16-year-old boy in whom blunt perineal trauma was followed by bloody urethral discharge and inability to void. ***Lower right:*** Urethroscrotal fistula. Extravasation (E) into extraurethral tissues from fistula in bulbous urethra (*arrow*). Retrograde urethrogram in a 26-year-old man after end-to-end urethroplasty for stricture.

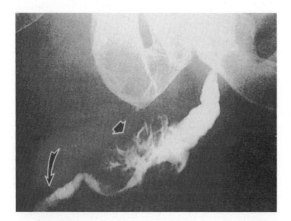
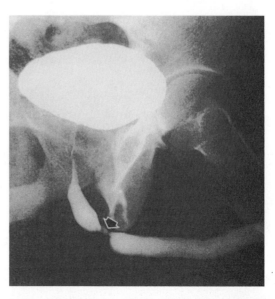

▲ **Figure 6–14.** Abnormal anterior urethras: retrograde urethrograms. **Left:** Urethral carcinoma. Filling of irregular sinus tracts and channels in a large epidermoid carcinoma of the bulbocavernous urethra (*straight arrow*). There are multiple thin transverse strictures of the penile urethra (*curved arrow*). 75-year-old man with obstructive voiding symptoms and 30-year history of urethral strictures requiring dilatations. **Right:** Focal urethral stricture (*arrow*). Middle-aged man with obstructive voiding symptoms who denied previous urethritis.

examinations. Although an established imaging technique with proven value and an acceptable incidence of complications and morbidity, angiography is moderately invasive and relatively expensive.

▶ Aortorenal and Selective Renal Arteriography (Figure 6–17)

Conventional arteriographic studies are performed almost exclusively by percutaneous needle puncture and catheterization of the common femoral arteries. Rapid sequence images are obtained during injection of nonionic contrast. Aortograms at the level of the renal vessels are followed by selective catheterization of renal arteries. CT and MR angiography involve peripheral injection of contrast media with breath hold rapid image acquisition through the targeted region of interest. CT angiography offers higher spatial resolution than magnetic resonance angiography (MRA), but carries the risks of radiation exposure and iodinated contrast usage.

Indications for renal arteriography include suspected renal artery stenosis (renovascular hypertension), vascular malformations, tumor embolization to minimize surgical blood loss or treat bleeding tumors, and trauma. Diagnostic renal angiography to demonstrate renal vascular anatomy is uncommon, as this information may be obtained noninvasively. Complications from conventional catheter

angiography include bleeding at the puncture site, contrast allergy or nephrotoxicity, and renal or distal emboli.

▶ Inferior Venacavography and Selective Venography (Figures 6–18 and 6–19)

The common femoral veins, or less commonly the internal jugular veins, are catheterized for angiography of the inferior vena cava, renal, and adrenal veins. Venography is rarely used today since the information can be obtained at cross-sectional imaging (CT or MRI) in almost all cases. Adrenal and renal venography is performed occasionally for venous sampling to localize hormone secretion in patients with indeterminate noninvasive imaging studies.

▶ Miscellaneous Urologic Angiography

Although angiography has little or no value in examination of the ureter, bladder, adrenals, and prostate, angiograms of these structures may be indicated in particular clinical situations, in which case the studies are usually "tailored" to the clinical problem. In this era of multiple cross-sectional methods, these procedures are rarely used.

Although uncommon, corpus cavernosograms are made by direct injection of suitable contrast material into the corpora cavernosa of the penis. They can be useful in examining

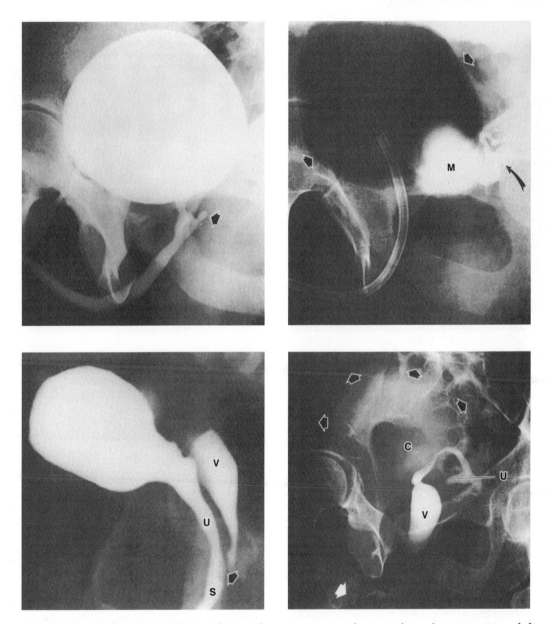

▲ **Figure 6–15.** Congenital genitourinary anomalies: voiding cystograms and retrograde urethrograms. ***Upper left:*** Utricle. Midline outpouching (*arrow*) from verumontanum between orifices of ejaculatory ducts, representing Müllerian duct cyst. ***Upper right:*** Gas cystogram combined with injection of utricle, oblique view. M = grossly dilated utricle (Müllerian duct cyst); straight arrows = bladder distended with air; curved arrow = coincident partial filling of left seminal vesicle and vas deferens. 34-year-old man with urgency, frequency, and suspected retrograde ejaculation. ***Lower left:*** Common urogenital sinus. Vagina (V) and urethra (U) join (at *arrow*) into a common urogenital sinus (S). Voiding cystourethrogram in a 3-week-old female pseudohermaphrodite with ambiguous genitalia and congenital adrenal hyperplasia. ***Lower right:*** Male pseudohermaphrodite. Bladder is distended with urine (*black arrows*). Retrograde urethrogram via hypospadiac meatus has fortuitously and selectively filled with contrast medium an extensive müllerian duct remnant consisting of vagina (V), cervix and cervical canal (C), and retroverted uterus (U). Residual contrast medium in hypoplastic anterior urethra (*white arrow*). 27-year-old man with small external genitalia, hypospadias, and perineal pain.

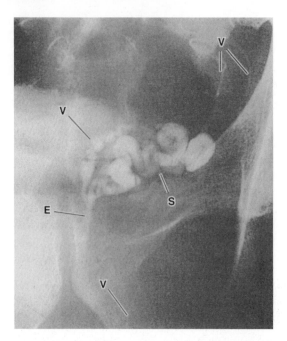

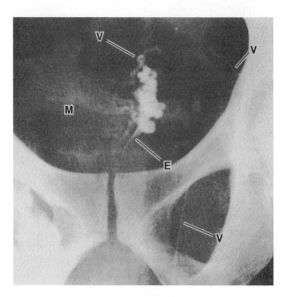

▲ **Figure 6–16.** Vasoseminal vesiculography (vasography). ***Left:*** Normal left vasoseminal vesiculogram. V = vas deferens; S = seminal vesicle; E = ejaculatory duct. 40-year-old man with hypospermia. ***Right:*** Seminal vesiculitis. Bilateral vasogram. Mass (M) produced by the swollen, nonfilling right seminal vesicle has displaced both ejacula-tory ducts (E) toward the left and indented the medial aspect of the proximal left seminal vesicle and vas deferens (V). 33-year-old man with painful ejaculations after repair of right varicocele.

for Peyronie's disease or fibrosis, impotence, priapism, and traumatic penile lesions.

SONOGRAPHY (FIGURES 6–20 THROUGH 6–26)

▶ Basic Principles

Sound is the mechanical propagation of pressure changes, or waves, through a deformable medium. A wave frequency of 1 cycle/s (cps) is called a hertz (Hz). Sound frequencies greater than 20 kHz are beyond the range of human hearing and are called **ultrasound**. Medical sonography uses ultrasound to produce images. The frequencies commonly used in medical sonography are between 3.5 and 15 MHz.

Ultrasound waves for imaging are generated by transducers, devices that convert electrical energy to sound energy and vice versa. These transducers act as both sonic transmitters and detectors. Ultrasound images are reflection images formed when part of the sound that was emitted by the transducer bounces back from tissue interfaces to the transducer. The sound reflected by stationary tissues forms anatomic gray-scale images. The sound reflected by moving structures has an altered frequency due to the Doppler effect. By determining the Doppler shift, vascular flow direction and velocity can be encoded graphically (spectral Doppler) or by color (color Doppler). A more sensitive method of detecting flow, called power mode Doppler, is available on modern equipment. This technique displays the integrated power of the Doppler signal rather than the mean Doppler frequency shift. Direction or velocity of flow is not displayed in power mode. Newer intravascular microbubble contrast agents provide more exquisite imaging of vascularity, and their use will likely increase in coming years (Ascenti et al, 2007, Fan et al, 2008).

Ultrasound images are rapidly updated on a video display, giving an integrated cross-sectional anatomic depiction of the site studied. Individual frames may be frozen during an examination for motion-free analysis and recording, or cine images may be rapidly recorded as digital video.

▶ Clinical Applications

Ultrasound is commonly used for the evaluation of the kidney, urinary bladder, prostate, testis, and penis.

Ultrasound is useful for assessing renal size and growth. It is also helpful in triaging patients with renal failure. For example, small echogenic kidneys suggest renal parenchymal

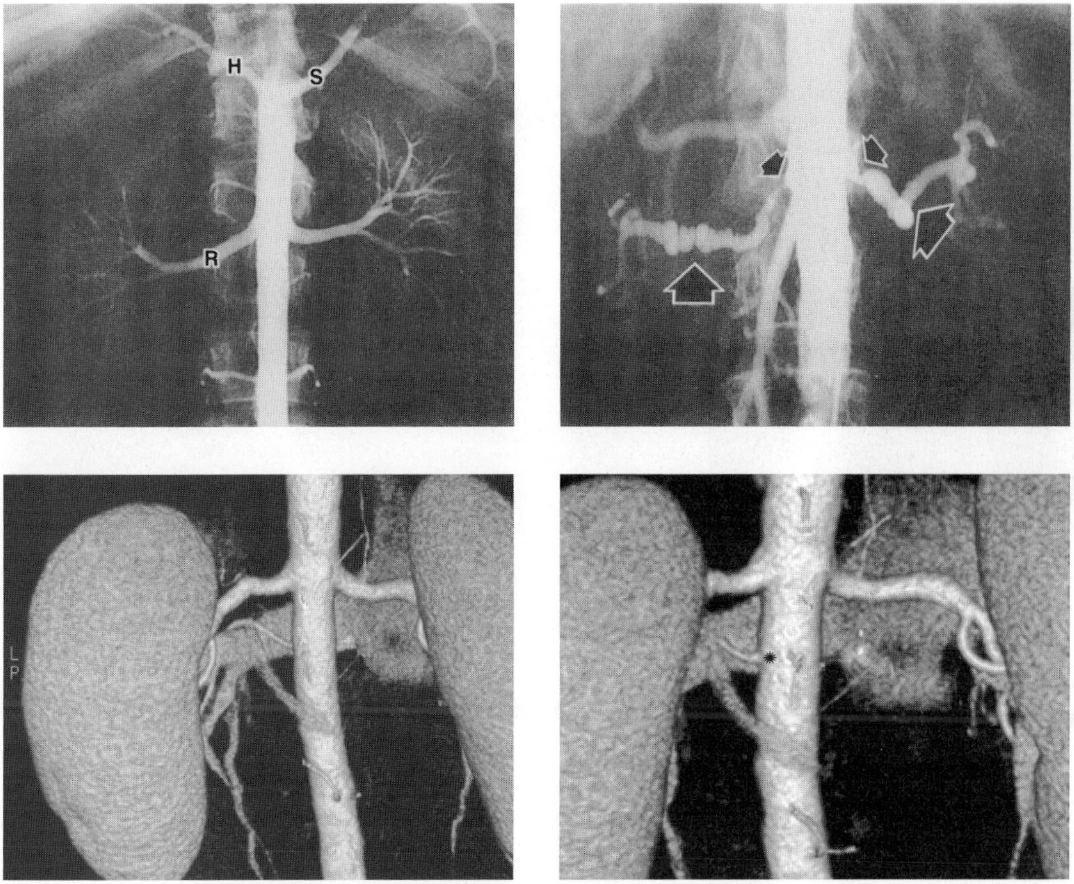

▲ **Figure 6–17.** Angiography: aortorenal arteriography. **Upper left:** Normal abdominal aortogram. The aortic catheter is hidden by the opacified normal aorta. Right (R) and left renal arteries and branches are well shown, as are the splenic (S) and hepatic (H) arteries arising from the celiac axis. The superior mesenteric artery is superimposed over the aortic silhouette and is not visible here. 28-year-old healthy female potential kidney donor. **Upper right:** Bilateral renal artery stenoses. Typical angiographic appearance and location of stenoses caused by atherosclerosis (*small arrows*) and fibromuscular dysplasia (*large arrows*). 58-year-old woman with abdominal bruits and a 16-year history of hypertension. **Lower left:** 3D coronal CT angiography image demonstrates an inferior accessory left renal artery (posterior view). **Lower right:** The left accessory renal artery origin (*asterisk*) is better demonstrated rotating the model in the axial plane. 65-year-old man undergoing preoperative evaluation for laparoscopic partial nephrectomy.

(medical) disease, whereas a dilated pelvocaliceal system indicates an obstructive, and potentially reversible, cause of renal failure.

Renal ultrasound is useful in detection and characterization of renal masses. Ultrasound provides an effective method of distinguishing benign cortical cysts from potentially malignant solid renal lesions. Since the most common renal lesion is a simple cortical cyst, ultrasound is a cost-effective method to confirm this diagnosis. Ultra-sound may also be used to follow up mildly complicated cysts detected on CT, for example, hyperdense cysts or cysts with thin septations.

The differential diagnosis for echogenic renal masses includes renal stones, angiomyolipomas, renal cortical neoplasms (including carcinoma), and, less commonly, abscesses and hematomas. All echogenic renal masses should be correlated with clinical history and, if necessary, confirmed with another imaging modality or follow-up ultrasound. Thin-section CT showing fat within the renal lesion characterizes it as a benign angiomyolipoma, and no

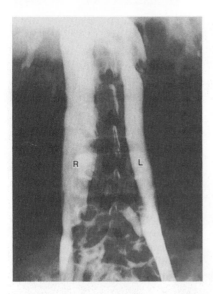
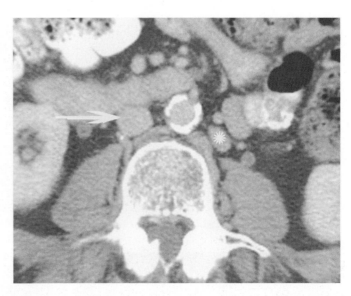

▲ **Figure 6–18.** Angiography: inferior venacavography. **Left:** Double inferior vena cava (R, L). Persistent left supracardinal vein anomaly. 23-year-old man after orchiectomy for testicular teratocarcinoma. **Right:** Example of duplicated IVC on IV contrast enhanced axial CT. Normal IVC (*arrow*) and duplicated IVC (*asterisk*).

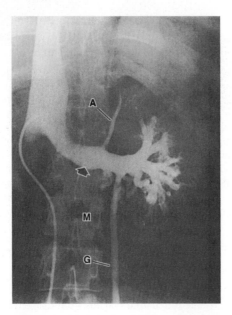
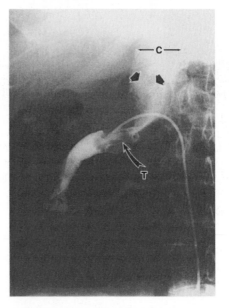

▲ **Figure 6–19.** Angiography: renal venography. **Left:** Normal left renal vein. On the left side, the adrenal (A) and gonadal (G) veins enter the renal vein (*arrow*). M = radiographic localization marker. Young woman with proteinuria. **Right:** Tumor thrombus. Straight arrows = upper margin of filling defect of the renal vein tumor thrombus (T) that extends into the vena cava (C). 68-year-old man with gross hematuria from adenocarcinoma of the right kidney.

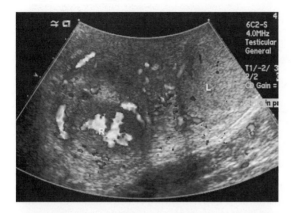

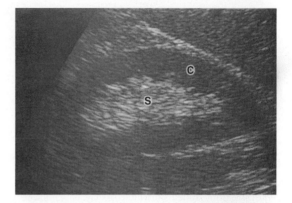

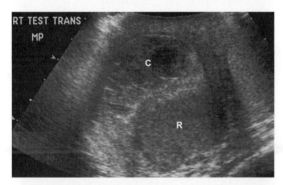

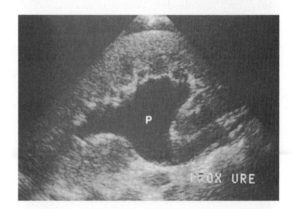

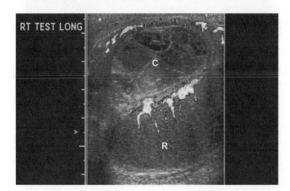

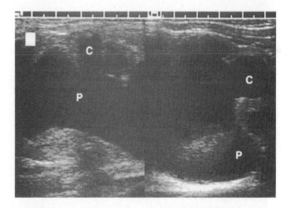

▲ **Figure 6–20.** 67-year-old man recently hospitalized for urosepsis. **Upper:** Transverse color Doppler image of the right (R) and left (L) testicles reveals right-sided hyperemia with associated hypoechoic echotexture and surrounding hypoechoic mass. **Middle:** Transverse grayscale right hemiscrotal image confirms hypoechoic right testicle (R) and extratesticular complex collection within the epididymal tail (C). **Lower:** Color Doppler confirms lack of flow within the complex collection. Pathology confirmed chronic granulomatous orchitis, epididymitis and periorchitis.

▲ **Figure 6–21.** Sonography of the kidney. **Upper:** Normal kidney. Renal cortex (C), normal renal sinus echoes (S). **Middle:** Moderate hydronephrosis and hydroureter; dilated renal pelvis (P). Dilated proximal ureter (proxure). **Lower:** Severe hydronephrosis of the transplanted kidney, compound sagittal scans, dilated clubbed calices (C), dilated renal pelvis (P).

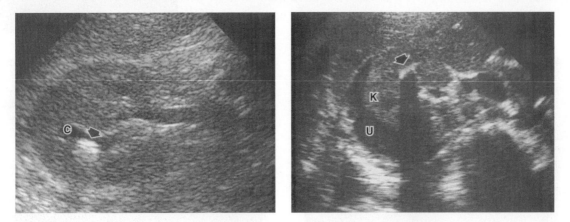

▲ **Figure 6–22.** Renal calculus and the consequences of obstruction as detected by sonography. **Upper left:** Transverse scan of the right kidney showing calicectasis (C) and renal calculus (*arrow*). **Upper right:** Acute obstruction of the right kidney (K) with spontaneous urine (U) extravasation into the perirenal space. Renal calculus (*arrow*).

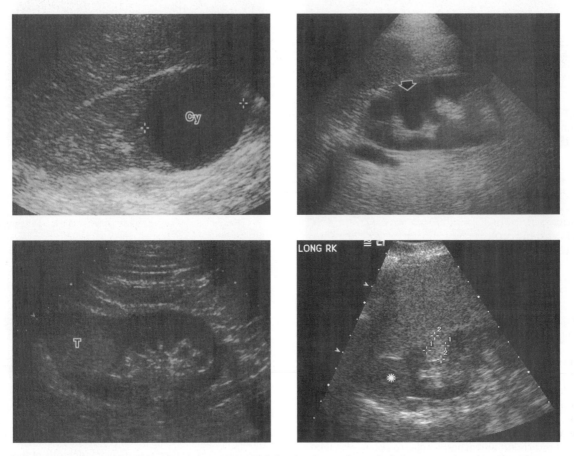

▲ **Figure 6–23.** Sonography of renal neoplasms. **Upper left:** Simple renal cyst (Cy) demonstrating sharp interfaces toward the renal parenchyma, no internal echoes, and increase through transmission. **Upper right:** Complex renal cyst (*arrow*) with lobulated margins and thick wall. **Lower left:** Solid tumor (T) in upper pole of left kidney with increased echogenicity relative to adjacent renal parenchyma. Pathology was oncocytoma. **Lower right:** Solid renal tumor (*asterisk*) in the right kidney (K) with separate hyperechoic interpolar partially exophytic mass. The interpolar mass represented a known angiomyolipoma, while the upper pole mass represented renal cell carcinoma.

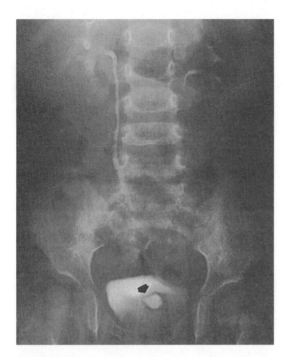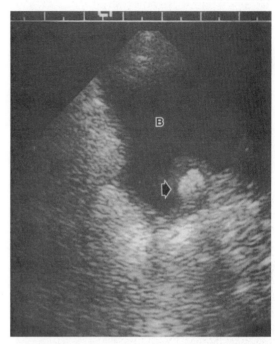

▲ **Figure 6-24.** Sonography with comparative study. Film from IVP (*left*) and transabdominal ultrasound (*right*) of the urinary bladder in a patient with duplication of the left kidney, ectopic ureterocele, and a calculus (*arrow*) within it. Urinary bladder (B).

further investigation is required. Echogenic lesions smaller than 1 cm are more difficult to characterize by CT owing to partial volume averaging; in the correct clinical setting, follow-up ultrasound rather than repeat CT may be more useful.

Doppler sonography is useful for the evaluation of renal vessels, vascularity of renal masses, and complications following renal transplant. It can detect renal vein thrombosis, renal artery stenosis, and ureteral obstruction prior to the development of hydronephrosis, arteriovenous fistulas, and pseudoaneurysms. Perinephric fluid collections following renal transplantation, extracorporeal shockwave lithotripsy, or acute obstructions are reliably detected by ultrasound.

Developments in other imaging modalities have decreased the use of ultrasound in several clinical scenarios. Most patients with suspected renovascular hypertension are evaluated with CTA or MRA rather than Doppler ultrasonography. Unenhanced helical CT is now the initial procedure of choice for the evaluation of the patient with acute flank pain and suspected urolithiasis. Helical CT also has the potential for identifying other causes of flank pain such as appendicitis and diverticulitis. For the evaluation of hematuria, recent studies indicate that CT (or CTU) is the preferred modality. A balance between optimizing

imaging quality and minimizing radiation exposure is advocated.

Applications of bladder sonography include assessment of bladder volume, wall thickness, and detection of bladder calculi and tumors. The suprapubic transabdominal approach is most commonly used. The transurethral approach during cystoscopy has been recommended for tumor detection and staging.

Ultrasound examination of the testis and scrotum is performed with a high-frequency transducer (10–15 MHz) for excellent spatial resolution. The addition of color and spectral Doppler sonography provides simultaneous display of morphology and blood flow. Sonography is highly accurate in differentiating intratesticular from extratesticular disease, and in the detection of intratesticular pathology. Ultrasound is commonly used to evaluate acute conditions of the scrotum. It can distinguish between inflammatory processes, inguinal hernias, and acute testicular torsion (Hart et al, 2008; Sparano et al, 2008). Epididymitis not responding to antibiotics within 2 weeks should be investigated further with scrotal ultrasonography.

▶ **Advantages and Disadvantages**

The main advantages of ultrasound are ease of use, high patient tolerance, noninvasiveness, lack of ionizing radiation,

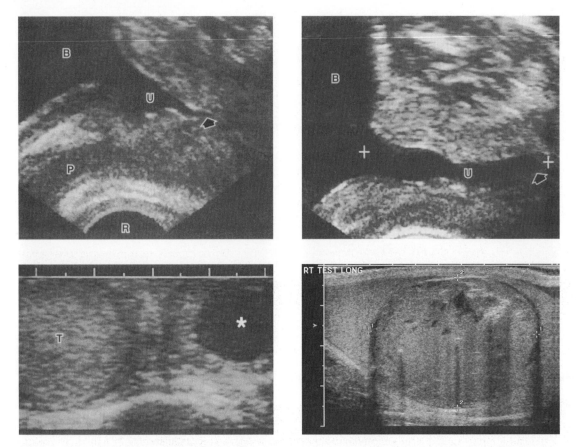

▲ **Figure 6–25.** The use of transrectal ultrasound in the evaluation of the prostatic urethra. ***Upper left:*** Sonographic appearance of the prostatic urethra (U) following transurethral resection as seen on transrectal ultrasound in the sagittal plane of scanning. Urinary bladder (B). The urethra (U) is dilated to the level of the verumontanum (*arrow*). Peripheral zone (P), rectum (R). ***Upper right:*** The prostatic urethra (U) is dilated to the level to the membranous urethra (*arrow*). Urinary bladder (B). The cursors are placed to measure the length of the prostatic urethra. ***Lower left and lower right:*** Examples of testicular ultrasound. ***Lower left:*** The right testis (T) is normal. There is a hypoechoic lesion within the left testis (*asterisk*). At surgery, it was a seminoma. ***Lower right:*** A large mixed solid and cystic intratesticular mass with foci of echogenic calcifications. Benign epidermoid cyst. This mass did not show concentric lamellation sometimes associated with epidermoid cysts. Ultrasound cannot always differentiate epidermoid cysts from malignant germ cell neoplasms.

low relative cost, and wide availability. Disadvantages include a relatively low signal-to-noise level, tissue nonspecificity, limited field of view, and dependence on the operator's skill and the patient's habitus.

COMPUTED TOMOGRAPHY SCANNING (FIGURES 6–27 THROUGH 6–33)

▶ Basic Principles

In CT scanning, a thin, collimated beam of x-rays is passed through the patient and captured by an array of solid-state or gas detectors.

The interconnected x-ray source and detector system are rapidly rotated in the gantry around the recumbent patient. Computers integrate the collected x-ray transmission data to reconstruct a cross-sectional image (tomogram).

Spiral (or helical) CT uses a slip-ring gantry that rotates continuously while the patient moves constantly through the collimated x-ray beam. Spiral CT technology affords the ability to image during specific phases of contrast bolus enhancement, including the ability to perform CT angiography, and allows improved image reformations. Multidetector, or multislice, helical CT scanners have an array of multiple rows of detectors in a helical scanner such that multiple scan images can be acquired per gantry rotation, and as a by-product

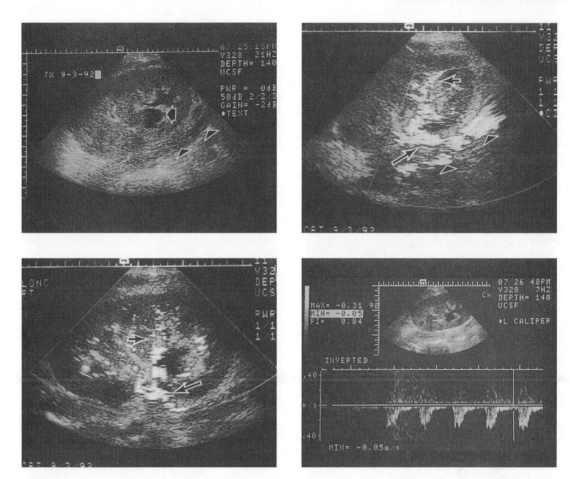

▲ **Figure 6–26.** Gray-scale and Doppler sonography: acute rejection in a renal transplant. **Upper left:** Gray-scale ultrasound image of transplant kidney shows poor corticomedullary differentiation. A small fluid collection is seen within the renal pelvis (*arrow*). Native external iliac vessels are seen as tubular hypoechoic structures (*arrowheads*). **Upper right and lower left:** Color Doppler images demonstrate flow within the native external iliac artery (*arrowheads*), the transplant renal artery (*long arrow*), and the interlobar arteries (*short arrow*). **Lower right:** Spectral Doppler analysis reveals an elevated resistive index of 0.84. These findings are compatible with, but not specific for, acute rejection. In the nonacute setting, cyclosporin toxicity or chronic rejection may also show elevated arterial resistive indices.

thinner sections and higher resolution achieved. Such systems are optimally paired with powerful computer workstations so that high-quality three-dimensional (3D) and multiplanar reformations can be quickly generated and analyzed.

▷ Clinical Applications

Renal CT is most commonly used in the evaluation of acute flank pain, hematuria, renal infection (search for abscess) or trauma, and in the characterization and staging of renal neoplasm. CT evaluation of renal anatomy and pathology generally requires intravenous injection of iodinated contrast media; noncontrast scans are needed, however, when renal or perirenal calcification, hemorrhage, or urine extravasation is suspected, since scans obtained after the administration of contrast media may mask these abnormalities. Also, pre- and postcontrast scans are required to determine whether a mass is solid or cystic.

Contrast media is usually administered as a rapid intravenous bolus for assessment of renal anatomy or measurement of aortorenal transit time. Using a bolus injection and rapid

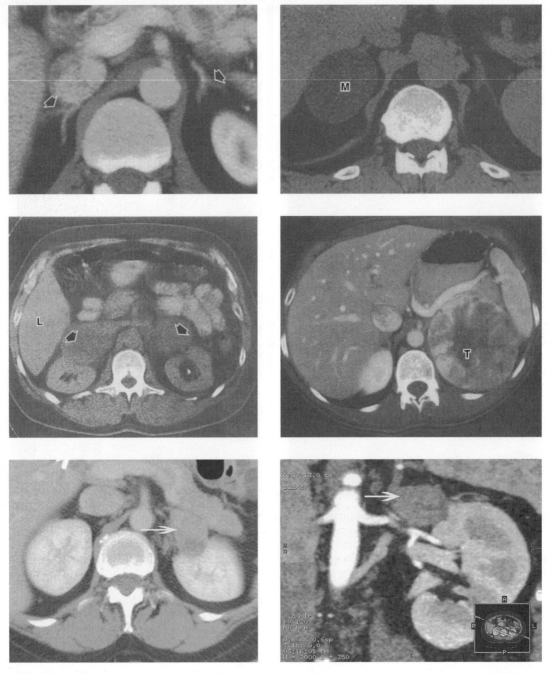

▲ **Figure 6–27.** CT scans: adrenal glands. ***Upper left:*** Normal adrenal glands (*arrows*) have inverted arrowhead or Y shape ***Upper right:*** CT densitometry. Thin section CT of incidental right adrenal mass (M) performed without intravenous contrast. Region of interest density measurement was below 10 Hounsfield Units (near zero), compatible with adrenal adenoma, confirmed by pathology. ***Mid left:*** Bilateral adrenal lymphoma. Enlarged adrenal glands (*arrows*) anterior to normal kidneys. L = liver. 53-year-old man with abdominal pain and histiocytic lymphoma of the central nervous system. ***Mid right:*** Left adrenal carcinoma. Large tumor (T) in left upper retroperitoneum with necrotic or cystic changes. Differential for CT included exophytic renal carcinoma. 52-year-old female with pulmonary nodules (metastases). ***Lower left:*** Axial CT image reveals a predominant solid mass (*arrow*) abutting the left kidney, with areas of cystic change. ***Lower right:*** Coronal oblique reformatted image from the same patient shows the mass (*arrow*) to be inseparable from the inferior left adrenal limb (*asterisk*). Pathologically proven adrenal carcinoma.

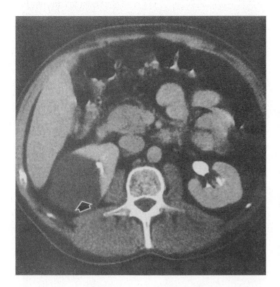
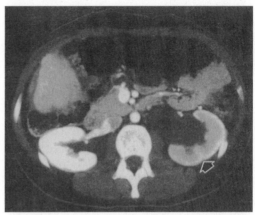

▲ **Figure 6–28.** CT scans: kidneys. *Left:* Simple renal cyst. Cyst (*arrow*) has a CT number close to that of water. 49-year-old man with flank pain. ***Right:*** New Hydronephrosis, severe on left and mild on right. Dilated left renal pelvis and delayed left nephrogram (*arrow*). 40-year-old female with ovarian carcinoma and peritoneal metastases.

sequence scanning, renal arterial opacification is followed immediately by enhancement of the cortex. A nephrogram phase with medullary enhancement is reached within 60 seconds. Excretion of contrast material into the collecting structures can be expected within 2–3 minutes after initiation of contrast administration.

Although CT can detect ureteral tumors, the current role of CT in the evaluation of the ureters is predominantly for tumor staging and evaluation of the cause and level of obstruction. Helical CT without oral or intravenous contrast is the preferred imaging modality for patients with renal colic or suspected urolithiasis (Figure 6–32).

In the evaluation of the urinary bladder, CT is used primarily in staging bladder tumors and in diagnosing bladder rupture following trauma (Shin et al, 2007). Performing CT after filling the bladder with dilute contrast medium (CT cystography) improves the sensitivity of this modality for detecting tumors and bladder rupture. For prostate diseases, CT is used for detection of lymphadenopathy, gross extraprostatic tumor extension, and to delineate prostatic abscesses. Newer, multidetector CT angiography may also have a role in prostate cancer localization. CT is used for detection of the abdominal location of suspected undescended testes, for staging of testicular tumors, and in the search for nodal or distant metastasis.

The addition of delayed CT imaging 10–15 minutes after intravenous contrast-enhanced CT shows high sensitivity and specificity in characterizing adrenal lesions. Benign adenomas, including lipid poor adenomas, show brisk contrast washout.

CTA or MRA are replacing conventional angiography for diagnostic examinations. New, dual-energy CT using dual or alternating sources of scan energy offers added benefits for postcontrast evaluation and allows virtual noncontrast imaging. Dual-energy CT will likely play an increasing role in evaluation for incidental renal (Brown et al, 2009; Graser et al, 2009) and adrenal masses, as well as in evaluation for urolithiasis, including stone composition determination (e.g., for urate stones) (Boll et al, 2009; Graser et al, 2008; Primak et al, 2007).

▶ **Advantages and Disadvantages**

The main advantages of CT include a wide field of view, the ability to detect subtle differences in the x-ray attenuation properties of various tissues, good spatial resolution, anatomical cross-sectional images, and relative operator independence. Carefully tailored examinations are essential. Reformatted helical image data in different planes and in 3D has made renal CT imaging, with renal angiography and urography, valuable in preoperative planning, such as for partial nephrectomy. Limitations of CT include restriction to the transaxial plane for direct imaging, tissue nonspecificity, low soft-tissue contrast resolution, and the need for contrast media (both oral and intravenous). Even with careful use of contrast media, tissue contrast is sometimes unsatisfactory. Finally, radiation exposure is a consideration with multisequence CT imaging (Newfal et al, 2004). Ongoing studies evaluating reduced exposure, and modifying protocols are under way.

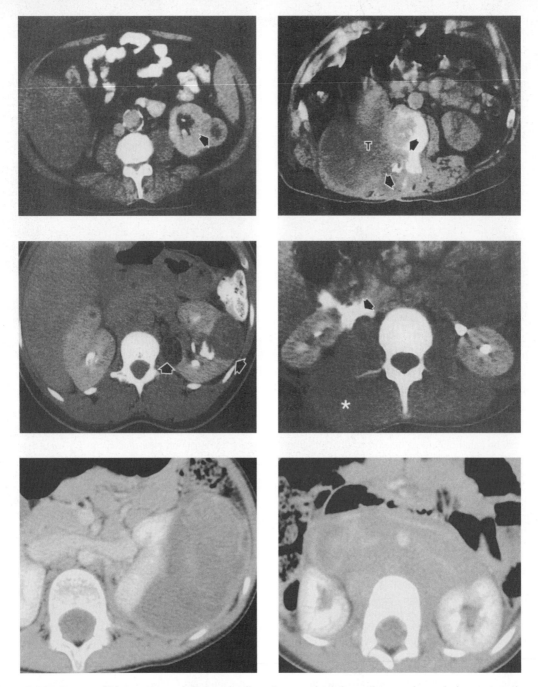

▲ **Figure 6–29.** CT scans: kidneys. ***Upper left:*** Renal cell carcinoma. The left renal tumor (*arrow*) shows central necrosis. Note calcification in the arteriosclerotic abdominal aorta. 61-year-old man with previous right nephrectomy for renal carcinoma. ***Upper right:*** Recurrent renal adenocarcinoma. Massive recurrence in right renal fossa (T), with extensive invasion of posterior soft tissues and destruction of vertebral bodies (*arrows*). 51-year-old man after right nephrectomy for carcinoma. ***Mid left:*** Renal angiomyolipomas. Bilateral heterogeneous renal masses. The larger lesions all showed areas of macroscopic fat density (*arrows*). 35-year-old female with probable lymphangioleiomyomatosis. ***Mid right:*** Right renal pelvic laceration. Enhanced CT scan through the kidneys showing extravasation of radiopaque material (*arrow*). Hemorrhage into the psoas and back muscles has enlarged their image (*asterisk*). 22-year-old man with laceration of the right renal pelvis due to a stab wound. ***Lower left:*** Large palpable heterogeneous left renal mass, with confirmed hemorrhage with subcapsular extension. Wilm's tumor in a 9-year-old female with acute onset fever and abdominal pain. ***Lower right:*** Large retroperitoneal neuroblastoma, encasing vessels.

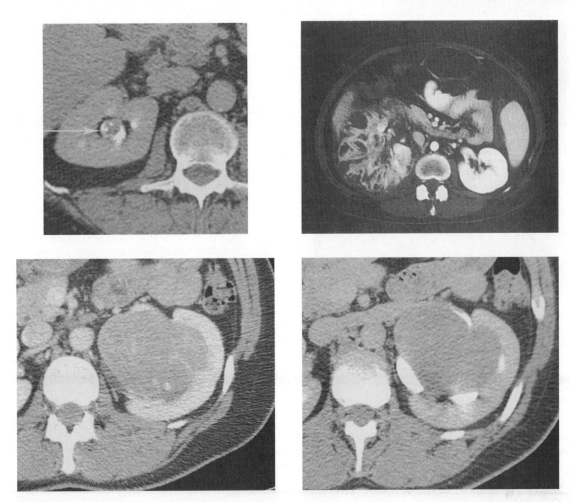

▲ **Figure 6–30.** CT scans: kidneys. **Upper left:** Transitional cell carcinoma. Delayed image CT urogram demonstrates an irregular nodular filling defect in the right upper collecting system (*arrow*). **Upper right:** 42-year-old woman with severe right pyelonephritis. An image through the mid pole of the right kidney reveals an enlarged kidney with marked destruction and striation of the renal parenchyma. Note the multiple low-density fluid collections. **Lower left:** Exophytic renal cell carcinoma. An image through the mid left kidney shows a mass that may be of renal cortical or collecting system origin. **Lower right:** A lower image in the same patient reveals that the mass arises from the kidney, as the contrast-containing collecting system is splayed by the mass. The renal vein is displaced anteriorly by the mass, but was free of thrombus.

MAGNETIC RESONANCE IMAGING (FIGURES 6–34 THROUGH 6–41)

▶ Basic Principles

Clinical MRI has its basis in the nuclear properties of the hydrogen atoms in the body. Hydrogen nuclei, when considered as aggregates, sometimes referred to as "protons," behave like tiny magnets, with net polarity (positive one direction, negative opposite) oriented along an axis at any given point in space. Ordinarily, the axes of the hydrogen nuclei in the body are randomly oriented. However, if the nuclei are placed in a strong magnetic field (like that produced in an MRI scanner), they precess and wobble like a spinning top around the lines of magnetic force.

When hydrogen nuclei in a strong magnetic field are additionally stimulated by short, pulsed radio waves of appropriate frequency, they absorb energy and invert their orientation with respect to the magnetic field. At the termination of radiofrequency pulses, the hydrogen nuclei return at various

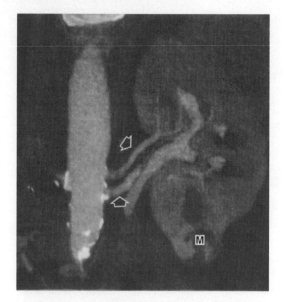

▲ **Figure 6–31.** 3D computed tomography (CT) and CT angiography (CTA) for renal mass, performed on multidetector CT scanner. Coronal oblique reformatted image with volume rendering shows a small enhancing mass (M) in the lower pole of the left kidney. The kidney has 2 renal arteries (*arrows*). The lower one, which serves the tumor, is the primary artery. 69-year-old male with solitary kidney and indeterminate lesion on prior CT.

rates to their original orientation within the magnetic field, emitting energy in the form of radio waves. This phenomenon is called **nuclear magnetic resonance (NMR)**. The emitted weak radio signals from the resonating hydrogen nuclei are received by sophisticated antenna, or coils, and transformed with various computer programs into cross-sectional images.

Different MR signal intensities reflect different hydrogen densities in body tissues, as well as differing physical, cellular, and chemical microenvironments and also flow (fluid) characteristics. The signals emitted from nuclei contain no innate spatial information. Spatial localization is achieved through varying magnetic field gradients and timing. There are biologically important nuclei other than hydrogen that are MR-sensitive, including those of phosphorus, sodium, and potassium, but these occur in lower physiologic concentrations than hydrogen. Imaging of these nuclei for tissue typing and mapping and as biologic tracers (MR spectroscopy) is undergoing intense research and development.

▶ Clinical Applications

Applications for MR in renal imaging include demonstration of congenital anomalies, diagnosis of renal vein thrombosis, and diagnosis and staging of renal cell carcinoma. MR angiography is useful in evaluating renal transplant vessels, renal vein tumor or thrombosis, and renal artery stenosis.

The use of contrast media in MRI of the kidney has broadened clinical applications. Using bolus injection of

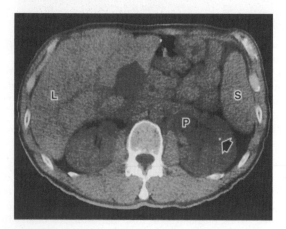

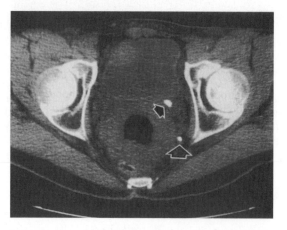

▲ **Figure 6–32.** Helical computed tomography (CT) without oral or intravenous contrast in a 42-year-old man with left flank pain. **Left:** CT image through the kidneys shows enlargement of the left kidney compared with the right, left pelvocaliectasis (P), and a stone in the mid pole of the left kidney (*arrow*). L = liver, S = spleen. **Right:** CT image through the base of the bladder shows an 8-mm stone (*arrow*) at the left ureterovesical junction with associated edema involving the left hemitrigone. Posterior to the ureteral stone is a 5-mm phlebolith (*open arrow*) within a pelvic vein.

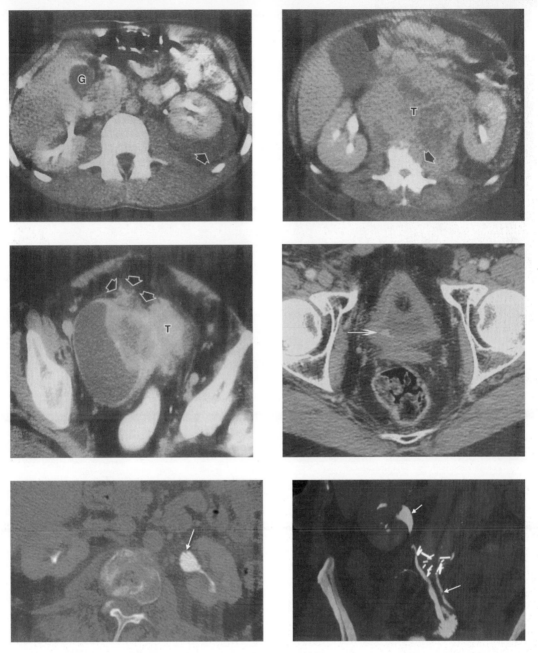

▲ **Figure 6–33.** CT scans: retroperitoneum, bladder, prostate. **Upper left:** Perirenal hematoma. Hematoma (*arrow*) displaces the left kidney anteriorly. G = gallbladder. 16-year-old boy with acute glomerulonephritis; low-grade fever and left flank pain following left renal biopsy. **Upper right:** Retroperitoneal metastatic seminoma. Large retroperitoneal mass of metastatic nodes (T) destroying vertebral body (*arrow*), obliterating outlines of central abdominal and retroperitoneal structures, and displacing kidneys laterally and bowel anteriorly. 46-year-old man with metastatic anaplastic testicular seminoma. **Middle left:** CT scan, transitional cell carcinoma of the urinary bladder with tumor (T) extension into the bladder diverticulum. There is tumor extension into the perivesical fat (*arrows*). **Middle right:** CT urogram in arterial phase, enhancing 5-mm transitional cell carcinoma of the urinary bladder (*arrow*). **Lower left:** Ureteritis cystica on CT urogram. Punctate rounded filling defect (*arrow*) in left renal pelvis on 12-minute delayed excretion images after intravenous contrast administration. **Lower right:** Coronal delayed reformat demonstrates other similar punctate collecting system filling defects. 77-year-old female after cystectomy on surveillance with stable, multiple punctate rounded filling defects bilaterally and negative urine cytology.

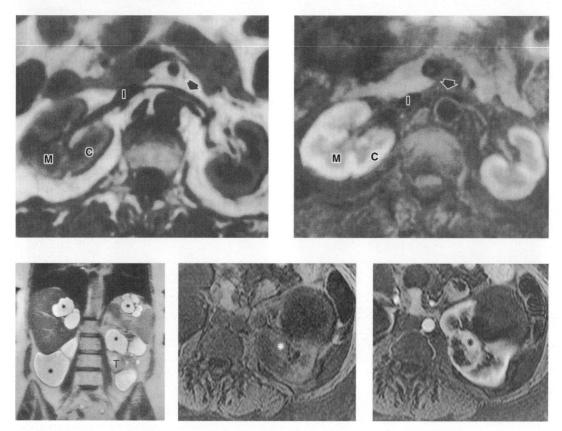

▲ **Figure 6–34.** Magnetic resonance imaging (MRI) appearance of the normal kidney. **Upper left:** T1-weighted conventional spin-echo image showing detailed anatomy of the kidney with differentiation between higher signal intensity cortex (C) and lower signal intensity medulla (M). Left renal vein (*arrow*), inferior vena cava (I). **Upper right:** T1-weighted spin-echo image using fat saturation technique. Because the fat signal has been suppressed, the computer automatically adjusts the gray scale of the signal intensity rendering even better contrast between higher signal intensity cortex (C) and lower signal intensity medulla (M). **Lower left:** Coronal T2-weighted image shows multiple renal and hepatic cysts (*asterisk*), as well as a partially solid and cystic left renal mass (T) in this adult female with polycystic kidney disease. **Lower mid:** Noncontrast T1-weighted fat saturation volume acquisition scan, used for dynamic imaging. The left renal mass is subtle on this precontrast scan (*asterisk*). **Lower right:** Arterial phase scan obtained following gadolinium-DTPA injection of contrast medium. The left renal mass (*asterisk*) shows avid enhancement of solid components. The addition of gadolinium adds significant soft tissue contrast.

gadolinium and rapid sequence imaging, both anatomy and function of the kidney can be assessed. Gadolinium, similar to iodine contrast media, is an extracellular contrast agent primarily excreted by glomerular filtration. Compared to iodinated contrast media, gadolinium has superior renal tolerance in patients with preexisting renal failure. Iodinated contrast agents used in radiography and CT increase attenuation linearly with their concentration. The effect of gadolinium on MR tissue signal intensity is more complex, though in general, at lower concentrations gadolinium causes an increase in signal intensity. Cases of nephrogenic system fibrosis (NSF) have

been reported in patients with renal failure who have received gadolinium. Recent studies have suggested that patients on dialysis or with estimated glomerular filtration rates of ≤30 mL/min are at higher risk for developing NSF after gadolinium administration (Wertman et al, 2008).

The use of gadolinium has extended the application of MRI to the evaluation of renal obstruction (MRU may be used when other studies are inconclusive) and the detection and characterization of renal tumors. Although MRI is capable of imaging blood vessels without contrast media, gadolinium bolus followed by rapid imaging is less susceptible to

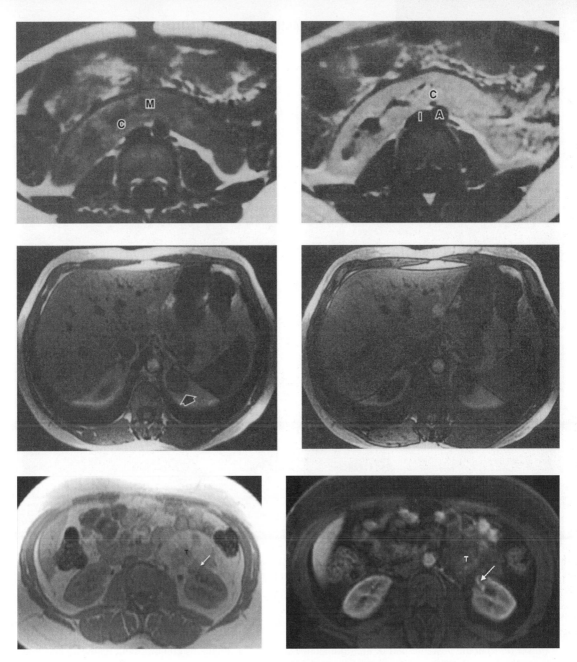

▲ **Figure 6–35.** Magnetic resonance (MR) images *Upper left and upper right:* Horseshoe kidney. Nonenhanced T1-weighted image (*upper left*); m, medulla; c, renal cortex. Gadolinium-DTPA-enhanced T1-weighted image (*upper right*). Following injection of the contrast medium, there is uniform enhancement of the renal cortex (C). The addition of the contrast enhancement shows that the part of the kidney in front of the aorta (A) and the inferior vena cava (I) is functioning renal parenchyma. *Middle left and lower right:* Chemical shift imaging, adrenal adenoma. On in-phase gradient T1-weighted image (*left*) there is a soft tissue intensity 2.7-cm mass in the left adrenal gland (*arrow*). Opposed phase T1-weighted image (*right*) shows marked signal loss in the lesion consistent with intracellular lipid; and therefore, a benign adenoma. 30-year-old female with indeterminate adrenal lesion noted on prior computed tomography (CT). *Lower left:* Biopsy-proven angiomyolipoma. Axial T1-weighted gradient echo in-phase imaging reveals a mass (T) arising off anterior interpolar left kidney. Renal contour defect (*arrow*) noted where mass originates. *Lower right:* Postintravenous gadolinium fat saturation T1-weighted image reveals a large amount of low-signal-intensity fat within the mass as well as vascular supply (*arrow*) arising via vessels extending from a defect in the renal cortex.

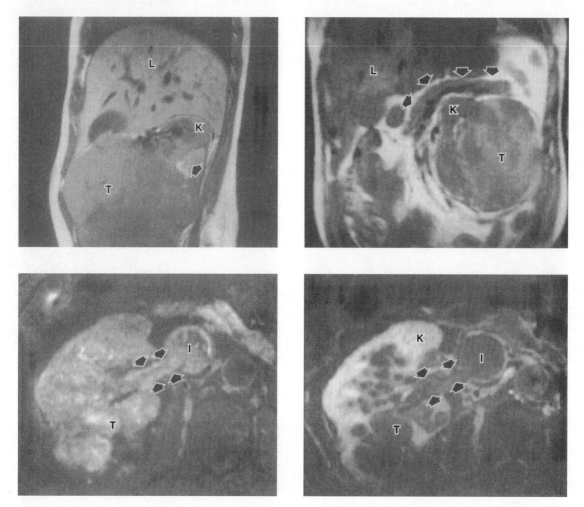

▲ **Figure 6–36.** Magnetic resonance imaging (MRI) appearance of renal cell carcinoma. The advantages of MRI are multiplanar imaging and the use of contrast media for better tumor characterization. *Upper left:* Sagittal T1-weighted image demonstrating a large renal cell carcinoma (T) arising from the inferior pole of the right kidney (K). Tumor extension in the posterior perirenal space (*arrow*). Liver (L). *Upper right:* Coronal image of a large renal cell carcinoma (T) replacing almost entire parenchyma of the left kidney (K). Superior displacement of the pancreas (*arrows*). Liver (L). *Lower left and lower right:* Fat saturation images before and after injection of the contrast medium. Heterogeneous tumor (*lower right*) in the posterior part of the right kidney shows heterogeneous enhancement following injection of gadolinium. The tumor is extending into the renal vein (*arrows*) and to the inferior vena cava (I).

flow direction and overestimation of stenosis, which can be seen in noncontrast MRA imaging. Gadolinium-enhanced MRA is useful for assessing renal artery stenosis and for evaluating potential renal donors (Figure 6–39).

MRI is used primarily to stage bladder tumors and to differentiate between benign bladder wall hypertrophy and infiltrating malignant neoplasm. There may be a potential advantage for combined endorectal and surface coil MR staging for bladder carcinoma as well. In imaging the prostate

gland, MRI is principally used to stage patients with prostate cancer (Claus et al, 2004; Coakley et al, 2002; Mazaheri et al, 2008). MR spectroscopy increases specificity and reduces interobserver variability in this setting (Shukla-Dave et al, 2007). MRI of the testis is appropriate when other imaging studies are inconclusive and is applicable to the evaluation of undescended testis, trauma, epididymo-orchitis, and tumors.

A modification of the MRI technique, called **chemical shift** imaging, can detect microscopic amounts of fat within lesions

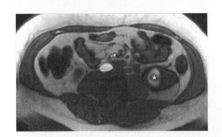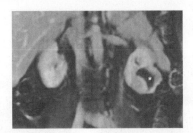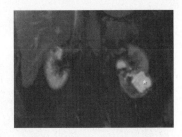

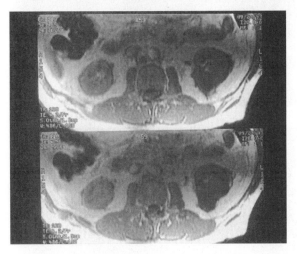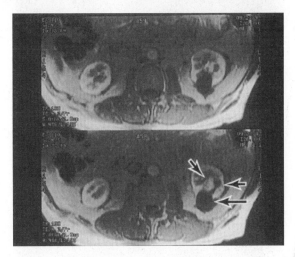

▲ **Figure 6–37.** 42-year-old female with abdominal pain after karate kick with gross hematuria. ***Upper left:*** Axial T1-weighted out-of-phase gradient echo image reveals high T1 signal intensity indicative of hemorrhage within a left renal lesion (*asterisk*), confirmed as cystic on other sequences. ***Upper middle:*** Coronal T1 fat saturation image after intravenous gadolinium administration shows lack of cyst enhancement (*asterisk*). ***Upper right:*** Delayed postcontrast imaging confirms communication with collecting system, showing cyst contents filling with high signal gadolinium (*asterisk*). Hemorrhage within a calyceal diverticulum after trauma. ***Lower images:*** Pre- and postcontrast and magnetic resonance imaging (MRI) of a renal cell carcinoma adjacent to a cyst in another patient ***Lower left:*** Precontrast T1-weighted image shows similar intensities for the cyst, tumor, and normal renal parenchyma. ***Lower right:*** Postcontrast T1-weighted image. The cyst (*long arrow*) is nonenhancing. The margins of the enhancing renal cell carcinoma (*short arrows*) are seen. The central fluid collection does not enhance.

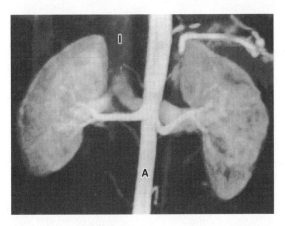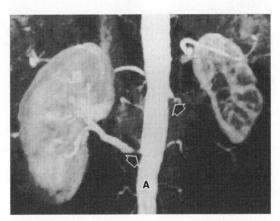

▲ **Figure 6–38.** Gadolinium-enhanced renal magnetic resonance angiography (MRA). ***Left:*** Maximum intensity projection (MIP) image from a renal MRA in a 22-year-old potential renal donor. The renal arteries are normal. ***Right:*** MIP image from a renal MRA in a 56-year-old man with suspected renovascular hypertension shows an atrophic left kidney with an occluded left renal artery (*arrow*) and a severely stenotic right renal artery (*open arrow*). The collateral capsular renal vessels are not seen. A = aorta, I = inferior vena cava.

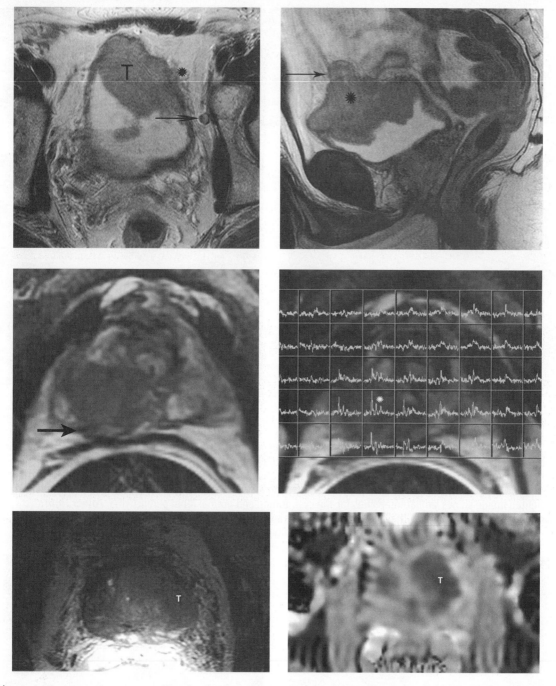

▲ **Figure 6–39.** Magnetic resonance imaging (MRI) examination of the pelvis. The upper images are examples of the ability of MRI to evaluate bladder neoplasms. **Upper left:** Axial T2-weighted image. A large anterior bladder tumor (T) shows associated perivesicular fat stranding (*asterisk*), raising the suspicion for extension through the muscularis. A prominent vessel (*arrow*) in the left obturator region exited through the obturator foramen on more inferior images. **Upper right:** T2-weighted sagittal image. The tumor (*asterisk*) extends into the urachal remnant (*arrow*). **Middle and lower rows:** Prostate cancer. Axial T2-weighted image (*middle left*) shows dominant right mid-gland peripheral and transition zone tumor with gross posterior extracapsular extension (*arrow*). Superimposed spectroscopy confirms depleted citrate (*asterisk*) compared to the adjacent choline and creatine peaks in the region of tumor (*middle right*). **Lower left:** Axial T2-weighted image in another patient demonstrates a large left mid-gland lesion (T) with associated capsular indistinctness and irregularity. **Lower right:** Apparent diffusion coefficient mapping confirms restricted diffusion within the tumor (T). Gleason 4 + 3 biopsy proven tumor in up to 75% of cores.

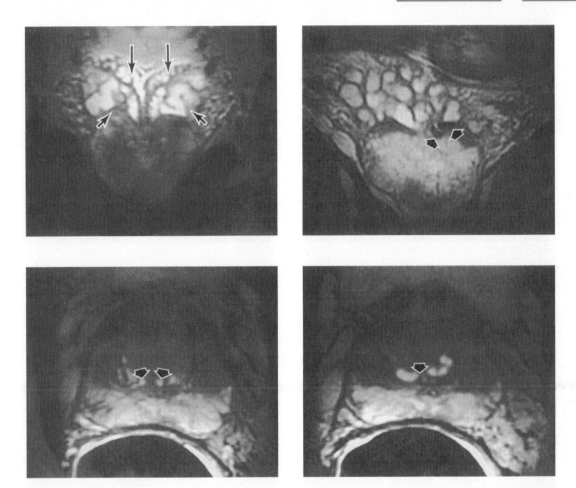

▲ **Figure 6–40.** Magnetic resonance imaging (MRI) of seminal vesicles, ductus deferens, and ejaculatory ducts. ***Upper left:*** T2-weighted image, normal seminal vesicles, and ductus deferens, and ejaculatory ducts. The ampullae of the ductus deferens (*long arrows*) are normally of high signal intensity on T2-weighted images and are immediately medial to the seminal vesicles (*short arrows*). The seminal vesicles are also of high signal intensity and are draped over the prostate gland. ***Upper right:*** Seminal vesicle and ductus deferens calculi. Coronal T2-weighted images show low-signal calculi within the proximal ductus deferens and medial aspect of the seminal vesicle on the left side (*arrows*). The patient had a history of prostatitis, prostatic pain, and hemorrhagic ejaculate. ***Lower left:*** Axial T2-weighted image through the prostate. The peripheral zone is of normal high signal intensity. The normal ejaculatory ducts (*arrows*) are identified as two small foci ducts of high-signal-intensity within the lower signal central zone. ***Lower right:*** Axial T2-weighted image through the prostate reveals a low-signal-intensity calculus (*arrow*) within the right ejaculatory duct (same patient as in upper right image).

(Figure 6–35, middle images). This technique is commonly used to characterize adrenal masses. Adrenal masses containing fat are either adrenal adenomas or myelolipomas, so the CT or MRI demonstration of fat in an adrenal lesion characterizes it as a benign lesion, even in the oncologic patient.

MR urography utilizes the sensitivity of MR imaging to demonstrate fluid (urine), producing urogram-like pictures without the need for contrast media. This technique is sensitive in the detection of ureterohydronephrosis and is

particularly useful in patients in whom contrast material is contraindicated, such as patients with prior contrast reactions or renal failure. Upper tract tumor can also be demonstrated (Takahashi et al, 2008, 2009).

Diffusion-weighted imaging, a technique under active investigation for urologic imaging with recent clinical implementation, exploits restricted water diffusion in diseased tissue. This technique has shown added benefit and promise, particularly for lesion detection in oncologic

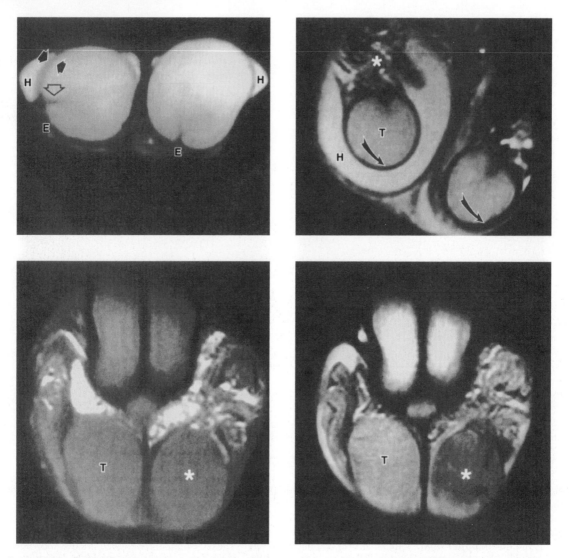

▲ **Figure 6–41.** Magnetic resonance imaging (MRI) appearance of scrotal contents. ***Upper left:*** Normal testis, T2-weighted image. The testicular tissue is of homogeneous high signal intensity. The tunica albuginea (*arrows*) demonstrates low signal intensity as does the mediastinum testis (*open arrowhead*). A small amount of fluid-hydrocele (H). Epididymis (E) is of low signal intensity. ***Upper right:*** Hydrocele of the right scrotum (T2-weighted image). Hydrocele (H) demonstrates high signal intensity. Testis (T). Tunica albuginea (*curved black arrows*). Varicocele (*asterisk*). ***Lower left and lower right:*** Images of a testicular tumor. On the proton density image (*lower left*), the signal intensity from both testicles is similar. On the T2-weighted image (*lower right*), testicular tumor (*asterisk*) demonstrates lower signal intensity as compared with the higher signal intensity of the normal testicular tissue (T).

imaging (Lim et al, 2009; Mazaheri et al, 2008; Seitz et al, 2009).

▶ Advantages and Disadvantages

Advantages of MRI include direct imaging in any plane desired (though transverse, sagittal, and coronal are most standard), choice of large or small field of view, excellent soft-tissue contrast, imaging without exposure to ionizing radiation, and (as compared to ultrasound) less operator dependence. MRI can image blood vessels and the urinary tract without contrast material. MR scanning, however, is not without drawbacks. The scanning time is relatively slow and as a result image clarity is often inferior compared with CT.

Absolute contraindications to MRI include the presence of (1) intracranial aneurysm clips, unless the referring physician is certain that the clip is made of a nonferromagnetic material (such as titanium); (2) intra-orbital metal fragments; and (3) any electrically, magnetically, or mechanically activated implants (including cardiac pacemakers, biostimulators, neurostimulators, cochlear implants, and hearing aids). Relative contraindications such as pregnancy should always be viewed in the light of risk versus benefit of the examination.

COMPARISON OF IMAGING METHODS (FIGURES 6–42 THROUGH 6–45)

As new imaging methods have been developed, changes have occurred in patterns of use for each type of imaging. For example, increased familiarity with and confidence in sonography and CT scanning have resulted in a substantial decrease in the use of many long-established conventional uroradiologic studies such as EU (Lang et al, 2003).

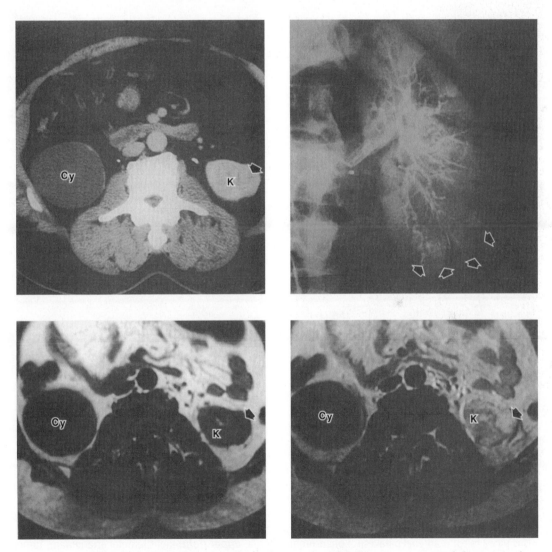

▲ **Figure 6–42.** Comparison of imaging methods in the evaluation of renal cell carcinoma. ***Upper left:*** Computed tomography (CT) scan showing a renal cyst (Cy) in the right kidney. There is bulging (*arrow*) in the contour of the left kidney (K), but it is difficult to discern if the lesion represents a neoplasm. ***Upper right:*** Angiogram showing small vascular lesions in the inferior pole of the left kidney (*arrows*). ***Lower left and lower right:*** MRI scans. ***Lower left:*** T1-weighted noncontrast scan. ***Lower right:*** T1-weighted postcontrast scan. The renal cyst (Cy) in the right kidney does not show any enhancement. The lesion (*arrow*) in the left kidney (K) shows marked enhancement, indicating that it is solid in nature. In this example, the contrast-enhanced MRI is superior to CT in the detection and characterization of the left renal mass.

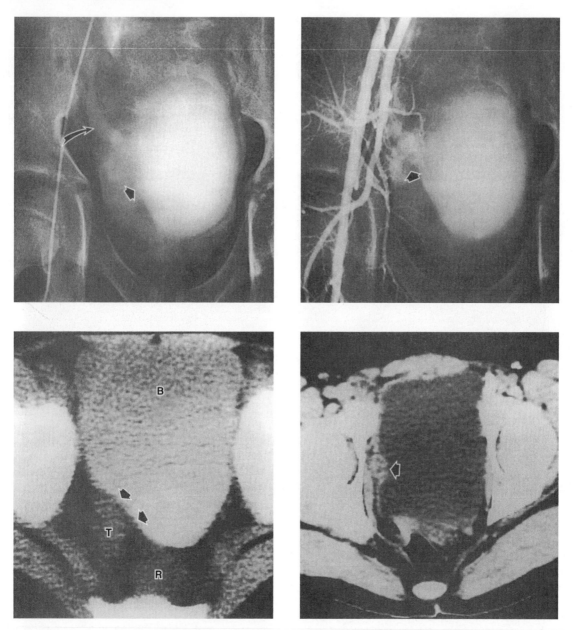

▲ **Figure 6–43.** Comparison of imaging methods: metastatic extra-adrenal familial pheochromocytoma. 10-year-old boy with hypertension and seizures precipitated by abdominal palpation. Family history of multiple extra-adrenal pheochromocytomas in the mother. ***Upper left:*** Excretory urogram. The right ureter is dilated and elevated (*curved arrow*), with the right posterior portion of the bladder displaced toward the left (*straight arrow*). The urographic diagnosis is possible extra-adrenal paravesical pheochromocytoma. ***Upper right:*** Right femoral arteriogram. Tumor stain (*arrow*) in right paravesical location. The angiographic diagnosis is extra-adrenal paravesical pheochromocytoma. ***Lower left:*** Computed tomography (CT) scan. Transverse tomogram through bladder (B) shows the tumor (T) indenting the bladder (*arrows*). R = rectum. ***Lower right:*** CT scan. Transverse tomogram through bladder. Recurrence of symptoms following removal of the right paravesical pheochromocytoma prompted another CT study, which shows recurrent tumor (*arrow*) in the bladder wall. Each imaging study complemented or supplemented the previous one. None, however, diagnosed the small liver metastases discovered at surgery.

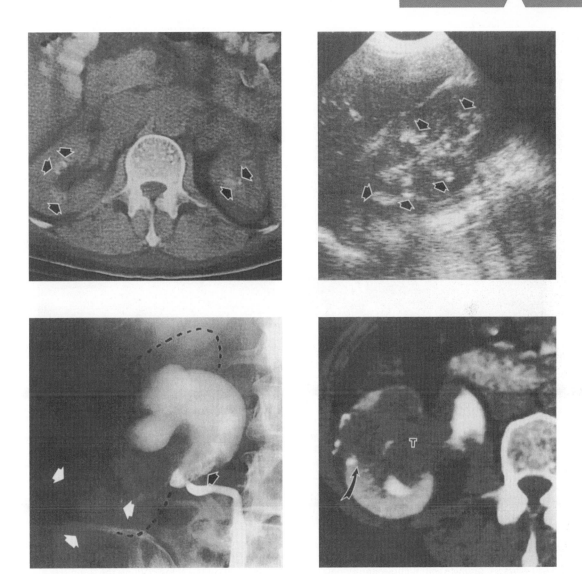

▲ **Figure 6–44.** Comparison of imaging methods. ***Upper left*** is an example of a nonenhanced computed tomography (CT), and upper right is an ultrasound study in the demonstration of renal calcifications. Fine calcifications in the medullary region indicate medullary nephrocalcinosis. They are of high density on CT (*arrows*) and are shown as echogenic foci (*arrows*) on an ultrasound scan. ***Lower left and lower right:*** Example of images of a transitional cell carcinoma and the calcified renal cyst. Retrograde urogram (*lower left*) shows filling defects due to tumor in the renal pelvis (*black arrow*) at ureteropelvic junction, and also seen are the calcifications in a lower pole mass (*white arrows*). Note that the infundibulum and calices of the lower pole failed to opacify in this 45-year-old woman with hematuria. On the CT scan (*lower right*) the cystic nature of the calcified renal mass (*curved arrow*) is well demonstrated and the CT scan shows better the extent of the tumor (T), which involves the entire lower pole of the kidney and extends into the dilated renal pelvis.

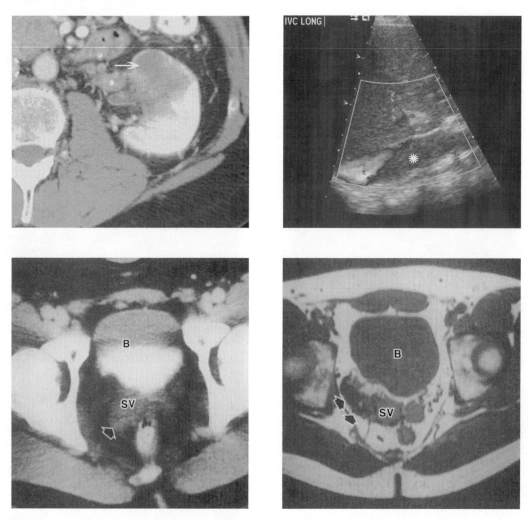

▲ **Figure 6–45.** Comparison of imaging methods. ***Upper left and upper right:*** Renal sarcoma with vascular invasion. Axial CT (*upper left*) reveals a left renal mass (*arrow*). The visualized left renal vein is invaded and expanded with thrombus (*asterisk*). On this sagittal ultrasound Doppler image (*upper right*) in the same patient, the thrombus extends across the midline from the left renal vein into the inferior vena cava (IVC) (*asterisk*). ***Lower left and lower right:*** Demonstration of an arterial venous malformation to the seminal vesicles. On the CT scan (*lower left*), the right seminal vesicle (SV) is enlarged, but the nature of the enlargement (*arrow*) is difficult to discern. On a magnetic resonance imaging (MRI) scan (*lower right*), the enlarged vessels (*arrows*) are demonstrated as the flowing blood within the vessel, lack signal intensity in contrast to the medium signal intensity of the seminal vesicles (SV). Urinary bladder (B).

Several factors are involved in these changes: (1) the increased effectiveness of newer imaging methods over older ones for some aspects of urodiagnosis; (2) the availability of equipment, trained technical personnel to operate it, and physicians to interpret the results; (3) increased awareness of the hazards of ionizing radiation (Nawfel et al, 2004); and (4) the desire to use noninvasive examinations if possible.

Because so many different types of imaging are available, each with different costs, risks, and areas of effectiveness, it

may be difficult for the clinician to decide which method will yield the most information with the least cost and risk. A particular study may be critical in one diagnostic situation but useless in another. For example, sonography is an excellent noninvasive, relatively inexpensive method for differentiating simple cysts from other mass lesions in the kidney but is much less effective in imaging the adrenal glands and ureters than is CT scanning. Sonography also relies considerably on the skill of the operator. CT scanning produces excellent images and is currently the preferred imaging method for the examination of the retroperitoneum. MRI rivals CT scanning in imaging capability for some structures, for example, the kidney, but has surpassed CT in imaging the pelvis. With advances in equipment and techniques, the use of MRI in urology will likely grow.

The patient and the clinician both benefit from careful consultation with the radiologist to ensure that the methods of imaging chosen are of value in diagnosis and treatment planning, and do not duplicate or merely confirm established findings, with loss of time and additional expense.

BIBLIOGRAPHY

Contrast Agents

Bettmann MA: Frequently asked questions: Iodinated contrast agents. Radiographics 2004;24(Suppl 1):S3–S10. [PMID: 15486247]

Caro JJ et al: The risks of death and of severe nonfatal reactions with high- vs low-osmolality contrast media: A meta-analysis. AJR Am J Roentgenol 1991;156(4):825–832. [PMID: 1825900]

Freed KS et al: Breakthrough adverse reactions to low-osmolar contrast media after steroid premedication. AJR Am J Roentgenol 2001;176(6):1389–1392. [PMID: 11373198]

Remy-Jardin M et al: Safety and effectiveness of gadolinium-enhanced multi-detector row spiral CT angiography of the chest: Preliminary results in 37 patients with contraindications to iodinated contrast agents. Radiology 2005;235(3):819–826. [PMID: 15845797]

Violon D: Renal failure and iodinated contrast media. A review. JBR-BTR 1999;82(2):57–62. [PMID: 10874391]

Weese DL et al: Contrast media reactions during voiding cystourethrography or retrograde pyelography. Urology 1993;41(1):81–84. [PMID: 8420087]

Radiography

Amis ES Jr: Epitaph for the urogram. Radiology 1999;213(3):639–640.

Chan DY et al: Image-guided therapy in urology. J Endourol 2001;15(1):105–110. [PMID: 11248911]

Dyer RB et al: Intravenous urography: Technique and interpretation. Radiographics 2001;21(4):799–821; discussion 822–794.

McFarlane JP et al: Outpatient ureteric procedures: A new method for retrograde ureteropyelography and ureteric stent placement. BJU Int 2001;87(3):172–176. [PMID: 11167637]

Morey AF et al: Bladder rupture after blunt trauma: Guidelines for diagnostic imaging. J Trauma 2001;51(4):683–686. PMID: 11586159]

Ultrasound

Agrawal A et al: Clinical and sonographic findings in carcinoma of the penis. J Clin Ultrasound 2000;28(8):399–406. [PMID: 10993967]

Ascenti G et al: Complex cystic renal masses: Characterization with contrast-enhanced US. Radiology 2007;243(1):158–165.

Bateman GA, Cuganesan R: Renal vein Doppler sonography of obstructive uropathy. AJR Am J Roentgenol 2002;178(4):921–925. [PMID: 11906873]

Carmignani L et al: High incidence of benign testicular neoplasms diagnosed by ultrasound. J Urol 2003;170(5):1783–1786. [PMID: 14532776]

Caoili EM et al: Evaluation of sonographically guided percutaneous core biopsy of renal masses. AJR Am J Roentgenol 2002;179(2):373–378. [PMID: 12130435]

Chow L et al: Power Doppler imaging and resistance index measurement in the evaluation of acute renal transplant rejection. J Clin Ultrasound 2001;29(9):483–490. [PMID: 11745858]

Datta SN et al: Urinary tract ultrasonography in the evaluation of haematuria—a report of over 1,000 cases. Ann R Coll Surg Engl 2002;84(3):203–205. [PMID: 12092877]

Fan L et al: Diagnostic efficacy of contrast-enhanced ultrasonography in solid renal parenchymal lesions with maximum diameters of 5 cm. J Ultrasound Med 2008;27(6):875–885.

Frauscher F et al: Comparison of contrast enhanced color Doppler targeted biopsy with conventional systematic biopsy: Impact on prostate cancer detection. J Urol 2002;167(4):1648–1652. [PMID: 11912381]

Hart JL et al: Ultrasound imaging of the scrotum. Br J Hosp Med (Lond) 2008;69(2):M18–M21.

Ragheb D, Higgins JL Jr: Ultrasonography of the scrotum: Technique, anatomy, and pathologic entities. J Ultrasound Med 2002;21(2):171–185. [PMID: 11833873]

Sellars ME, Sidhu PS: Ultrasound appearances of the testicular appendages: Pictorial review. Eur Radiol 2003;13(1):127–135. [PMID: 12541120]

Sparano A et al: Using color power Doppler ultrasound imaging to diagnose the acute scrotum. A pictorial essay. Emerg Radiol 2008;15(5):289–294.

Computed Tomography Scanning

Abramson S et al: Impact in the emergency department of unenhanced CT on diagnostic confidence and therapeutic efficacy in patients with suspected renal colic: A prospective survey. 2000 ARRS President's Award. American Roentgen Ray Society. AJR Am J Roentgenol 2000;175(6):1689–1695. [PMID: 11090405]

Boll DT et al: Renal stone assessment with dual-energy multidetector CT and advanced postprocessing techniques: Improved characterization of renal stone composition—pilot study. Radiology 2009;250(3):813–820.

Brown CL et al: Dual-energy CT iodine overlay technique for characterization of renal masses as cyst or solid: A phantom feasibility study. Eur Radiol 2009;19(5):1289–1295.

Caoili EM et al: Delayed enhanced CT of lipid-poor adrenal adenomas. AJR Am J Roentgenol 2000;175(5):1411–1415. [PMID: 11044054]

Caoili EM et al: Urinary tract abnormalities: Initial experience with multi-detector row CT urography. Radiology 2002;222(2):353–360.

Caoili EM et al: Optimization of multi-detector row CT urography: Effect of compression, saline administration, and prolongation of acquisition delay. Radiology 2005;235(1):116–123. [PMID: 15716388]

Graser A et al: Dual energy CT characterization of urinary calculi: Initial in vitro and clinical experience. Invest Radiol 2008;43(2):112–119.

Graser A et al: Dual-energy CT in patients suspected of having renal masses: Can virtual nonenhanced images replace true nonenhanced images? Radiology 2009; 252(2):433–440.

Israel GM, Bosniak MA. How I do it: Evaluating renal masses. Radiology 2005;236(2):441–450. [PMID: 16040900]

Joffe SA et al: Multi-detector row CT urography in the evaluation of hematuria. Radiographics 2003;23(6):1441–1455; discussion 1446–1455. [PMID: 14615555]

Kawashima A et al: Imaging evaluation of posttraumatic renal injuries. Abdom Imaging 2002;27(2):199–213. [PMID: 11847582]

Primak AN et al: Noninvasive differentiation of uric acid versus non-uric acid kidney stones using dual-energy CT. Acad Radiol 2007;14(12):1441–1447.

Shin SS et al: The sentinel clot sign: A useful CT finding for the evaluation of intraperitoneal bladder rupture following blunt trauma. Korean J Radiol 2007;8(6):492–497.

Szolar DH et al: Adrenocortical carcinomas and adrenal pheochromocytomas: Mass and enhancement loss evaluation at delayed contrast-enhanced CT. Radiology 2005;234(2):479–485. [PMID: 15671003]

Vaccaro JP, Brody JM: CT cystography in the evaluation of major bladder trauma. Radiographics 2000;20(5):1373–1381. [PMID: 10992026]

Magnetic Resonance Imaging

Claus FG et al: Pretreatment evaluation of prostate cancer: Role of MR imaging and 1H MR spectroscopy. Radiographics 2004;24(Suppl 1):S167–S180. [PMID: 15486239]

Coakley FV et al: Prostate cancer tumor volume: Measurement with endorectal MR and MR spectroscopic imaging. Radiology 2002;223(1):91–97. [PMID: 11930052]

Harisinghani MG et al: Noninvasive detection of clinically occult lymph-node metastases in prostate cancer. N Engl J Med 2003;348(25):2491–2499. [PMID: 12815134]

Hricak H et al: The role of preoperative endorectal magnetic resonance imaging in the decision regarding whether to preserve or resect neurovascular bundles during radical retropubic prostatectomy. Cancer 2004;100(12):2655–2663. [PMID: 15197809]

Lim HK et al: Prostate cancer: Apparent diffusion coefficient map with T2-weighted images for detection—a multireader study. Radiology 2009;250(1):145–151.

Mazaheri Y et al: Prostate cancer: Identification with combined diffusion-weighted MR imaging and 3D 1H MR spectroscopic imaging—correlation with pathologic findings. Radiology 2008;246(2):480–488.

Muglia V et al: Magnetic resonance imaging of scrotal diseases: When it makes the difference. Urology 2002;59(3):419–423. [PMID: 11880084]

Mullerad M et al: Comparison of endorectal magnetic resonance imaging, guided prostate biopsy and digital rectal examination in the preoperative anatomical localization of prostate cancer. J Urol 2005;174(6):2158–2163. [PMID: 16280755]

Pretorius ES et al: MR imaging of the penis. Radiographics 2001;21:S283–S298; discussion S298–289. [PMID: 11598264]

Ryu J, Kim B: MR imaging of the male and female urethra. Radiographics 2001;21(5):1169–1185. [PMID: 11553824]

Seitz M et al: Functional magnetic resonance imaging in prostate cancer. Eur Urol 2009;55(4):801–814.

Shukla-Dave A et al: Detection of prostate cancer with MR spectroscopic imaging: An expanded paradigm incorporating polyamines. Radiology 2007;245(2):499–506.

Takahashi N et al: Small (<2-cm) upper-tract urothelial carcinoma: Evaluation with gadolinium-enhanced three-dimensional spoiled gradient-recalled echo MR urography. Radiology 2008;247(2):451–457.

Takahashi N et al: MR urography for suspected upper tract urothelial carcinoma. Eur Radiol 2009;19(4):912–923.

Wertman R et al: Risk of nephrogenic systemic fibrosis: Evaluation of gadolinium chelate contrast agents at four American universities. Radiology 2008;248(3):799–806.

Comparison of Imaging Methods

Andrews SJ et al: Ultrasonography and abdominal radiography versus intravenous urography in investigation of urinary tract infection in men: Prospective incident cohort study. BMJ 2002;324(7335):454–456. [PMID: 11859046]

Bigongiari LR et al: Trauma to the bladder and urethra. American College of Radiology. ACR Appropriateness Criteria. Radiology 2000;215(Suppl):733–740. [PMID: 11429965]

Heidenreich A et al: Modern approach of diagnosis and management of acute flank pain: Review of all imaging modalities. Eur Urol 2002;41(4):351–362. [PMID: 12074804]

Jaffe JS et al: A new diagnostic algorithm for the evaluation of microscopic hematuria. Urology 2001;57(5):889–894. [PMID: 11337288]

Kawashima A et al: Imaging of renal trauma: A comprehensive review. Radiographics 2001;21(3):557–574. [PMID: 11353106]

Lang EK et al: Computerized tomography tailored for the assessment of microscopic hematuria. J Urol 2002;167(2 Pt 1):547–554. [PMID: 11792916]

Lang EK et al: Improved detection of renal pathologic features on multiphasic helical CT compared with IVU in patients presenting with microscopic hematuria. Urology 2003;61(3):528–532.

Nawfel RD et al: Patient radiation dose at CT urography and conventional urography. Radiology 2004;232(1):126–132. [PMID: 15220498]

Sourtzis S et al: Radiologic investigation of renal colic: Unenhanced helical CT compared with excretory urography. AJR Am J Roentgenol 1999;172(6):1491–1494. [PMID: 10350278]

Sudah M et al: Patients with acute flank pain: Comparison of MR urography with unenhanced helical CT. Radiology 2002;223(1):98–105.

Wefer AE et al: Advances in uroradiological imaging. BJU Int 2002;89(5):477–487; Quiz i-iii. [PMID: 11929470]

Vascular Interventional Radiology*

Roy L. Gordon, MD

7

Interventional uroradiologic procedures can be divided into two major groups: vascular and percutaneous nonvascular. Percutaneous nonvascular interventional procedures are discussed elsewhere. The intravascular route is used, as the therapy of choice, for the embolization of arteriovenous fistulas (AVFs) or malformations, and for bleeding sites. Transcatheter embolization is used for tumor embolization, for the ablation of renal function, for the treatment of testicular vein and ovarian vein varices, and for the treatment of high-flow priapism (Ginat et al, 2009). Balloon angioplasty and stenting of stenotic renal arteries are frequently performed endovascular techniques for the treatment of ischemic nephropathy and secondary hypertension. Renal artery aneurysms may also be treated using catheter-directed techniques such as stent grafting and selective embolization. Occasionally, fibrinolytic agents are delivered via an endovascular catheter to thrombosed renal arteries. Mechanical devices are also available for endovascular treatment of thrombosed renal vessels. This chapter will review these intravascular interventions.

TRANSCATHETER EMBOLIZATION

▶ Renal AVFs and Malformations

Transcatheter embolization is the treatment of choice for renal AVFs, which may be congenital, spontaneous, or acquired. Iatrogenic AVFs are the type most commonly treated by transcatheter embolization. These occur as a complication of such procedures as percutaneous renal biopsy (Libicher et al, 2006), nephrostomy placement, and pyelolithotomy. Trauma or surgery can also result in AVFs. AVF occurring in the transplant kidney is successfully managed by embolization. The classical angiographic finding of spontaneous or acquired AVF is a feeding artery with an early

draining vein. Ancillary findings include pseudoaneurysm and extravasation of contrast material. Congenital AVMs (AV malformations) consist of a group of multiple coiled communicating vessels that may be associated with enlarged feeding arteries and draining veins.

The modes of clinical presentation include hematuria; retroperitoneal or intraperitoneal hemorrhage; and congestive heart failure, cardiomegaly, or both. Hypertension can occur as a consequence of ischemia secondary to venous shunting of blood away from the affected area. A bruit may be heard on physical examination. Duplex Doppler ultrasound is the most useful diagnostic study, performed before angiographic intervention.

Successful intervention requires the angiographic identification, selective catheterization, and embolization of the feeding artery (Figures 7–1A, B). Using a transfemoral approach, an abdominal aortogram is performed to identify the arterial supply to the bleeding kidney. In the case of a renal transplant, an initial pelvic angiogram is performed in a steep oblique projection. The artery supplying the bleeding site is selectively catheterized. A 3 French (3F) coaxial microcatheter is then used for subselective catheterization and embolization of the feeding artery. The use of a microcatheter allows accurate placement of the embolic material. Microcoils are used for the occlusion of iatrogenic AVFs because they can be deployed very precisely, thereby minimizing the loss of renal parenchyma due to resultant ischemia (Figures 7–2A through C). The procedure is usually performed without significant complications. Very rarely, inadvertent nontarget embolization or thrombosis of the renal artery can occur.

▶ Bleeding Sites

Transcatheter embolization plays a key role in the management of hemorrhage in the urinary tract originating in the kidney, ureter, bladder, and pelvis (Ginat et al, 2009). Acute life-threatening hemorrhage can occur as a consequence of

*The authors wish to thank Dr. Anthony Verstandig, Hadassah University Hospital, Jerusalem, Israel, for providing the clinical information and images of the patient depicted in Figures 7–4A and 7–4B.

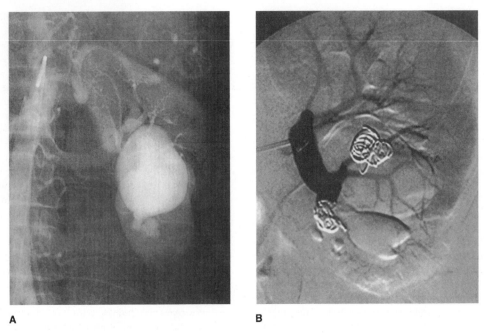

A   B

▲ **Figure 7–1.** Transcatheter embolization of a large arteriovenous malformation (AVM) in a 64-year-old woman with hematuria. **A:** A conventional film midstream aortogram. An enlarged left renal artery is seen. There is a large serpiginous AVM arising from the lower pole renal artery branch with aneurysmal dilatation of the draining renal vein. **B:** Selective left renal digital subtraction arteriogram (DSA) after coil embolization shows cessation of flow in the AVM. Coils have been placed in the terminal portion of the lower pole artery and within the AVM. Embolization resulted in resolution of the hematuria.

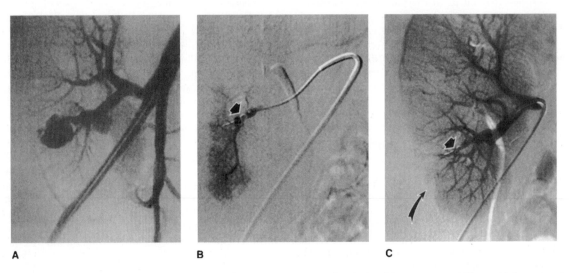

A   B   C

▲ **Figure 7–2.** Transcatheter embolization of a postbiopsy arteriovenous fistula (AVF) in a 14-year-old boy with hypertension and prior renal transplantation. A bruit was heard on examination. **A:** Pelvic arteriogram (DSA) shows an AVF arising from a lower pole branch artery. There is aneurysmal dilatation of the draining vein. **B:** DSA shows that the renal artery has been selectively catheterized, and a 3F coaxial catheter is positioned peripherally within the lower pole branch artery supplying the AVF. Several microcoils have been placed (*arrow*) and no flow is seen in the AVF. **C:** Completion DSA of the main renal artery shows absent flow in the AVF (*arrow*) with minimal devascularization of lower pole parenchyma (*curved arrow*).

trauma, instrumentation, and tumors. Chronic intractable hemorrhage is associated with radiation cystitis, tumors, prostatectomy, and infiltrative disorders. Hemodynamically stable patients undergo a noninvasive diagnostic study such as contrast-enhanced computed tomography (CT), before embolization.

Pelvic fractures resulting in life-threatening hemorrhage require embolization for control if resuscitation and external pelvic fixation have been ineffective. Embolization has been shown to be very effective at arresting hemorrhage. Using a transfemoral approach, the practitioner performs a nonselective pelvic arteriogram before selective catheterization and embolization of the hypogastric arteries. Because of contralateral crossover blood supply, pelvic lesions are treated by bilateral embolization. Gelfoam pledgets are frequently used. They can be deployed rapidly, are immediately effective if the patient has a normal coagulation profile, and produce temporary vascular occlusion. Gelfoam sponge is easily cut into pieces appropriate to the caliber of the vessel to be embolized. Coils may be used with, or instead of, Gelfoam. However, if used, they may hamper future access to the hypogastric artery in the event of rebleeding. Small embolic materials such as Gelfoam powder or Ivalon particles are not used to treat hemorrhage from pelvic trauma. They produce very peripheral occlusion of small vessels, thereby risking ischemia of nontarget organs. Complications specific to pelvic embolization are extremely uncommon. Nontarget embolization is rare.

▶ Tumors

A. Renal Cell Carcinoma

Primary renal cell carcinoma (RCC) is treated by surgical excision. In some cases, preoperative occlusive embolization of the renal artery is used as an adjunct to surgery. Embolization reduces intraoperative hemorrhage and allows immediate ligation of the renal vein. It is used in patients with very large tumors and also in tumors supplied by many parasitized vessels. Embolization accentuates cleavage planes and therefore facilitates nephrectomy. The optimal time delay between embolization and surgery is probably 1 day. Embolization may also favorably impact patient survival (Zielinski et al, 2000). A new application is to use selective embolization of a renal tumor as an adjunctive measure prior to radiofrequency or cryoablation of the tumor (Yamakado et al, 2006).

Palliation of nonresectable disease that causes pain and hematuria can be achieved by transcatheter embolization (Munro et al, 2003). Patients with bilateral RCC, and those with RCC in a single kidney, can undergo subselective embolization as an alternative to surgery, thereby sparing normal parenchyma. Embolization of RCC metastases to bone is performed before surgical resection to decrease intraoperative blood loss (Chatziioannou et al, 2000). CT or magnetic resonance imaging (MRI) may be used for tumor evaluation before and after intervention.

A transfemoral aortogram and selective arteriogram are performed to determine the blood supply to the kidney and tumor. An occlusive balloon catheter may be placed within the vessel and inflated before embolization to prevent reflux of embolic material and inadvertent nontarget embolization. However, many physicians use a simple selective catheter. Gelfoam pledgets are used for preoperative embolization (Figures 7–3A, B). Coils are not used because they can be dislodged during surgery when the kidney is manipulated. Absolute ethanol is the preferred embolic material for ablative palliative embolization of nonresectable tumor. Bone metastases are embolized by positioning a microcatheter in the vessel(s) supplying the tumor and injecting particles of polyvinyl alcohol (PVA) or other embolic agents such as embospheres until maximal obliteration of the angiographic tumor stain is achieved.

Tumor embolization is a safe procedure. Complications such as puncture-site hematoma and inadvertent nontarget embolization occur in <2% of patients. Almost all patients, however, experience postembolization syndrome (PES). PES consists of severe pain, nausea and vomiting, fever, and leukocytosis. It is probably caused by tissue necrosis that results from successful embolization. Transient ileus, transient hypertension, sepsis, and reversible renal failure have also been described. PES occurs within a few hours of the procedure and may last for several days. Its occurrence should not delay surgical intervention. Tissue swelling and tissue gas formation are seen on imaging studies. The severity of PES is related to the quantity of infarcted tissue. Analgesics and antibiotics are used for treatment. Administration of steroids and antibiotics before embolization may reduce the severity of PES.

B. Angiomyolipoma

Selective embolization has proved to be an effective method of controlling hemorrhage from benign renal lesions while preserving normal parenchyma (Kothary et al, 2005). This technique has been used in the treatment of active bleeding from angiomyolipoma and for the elective prevention of hemorrhage, especially if the tumors are multiple or bilateral, as in patients with tuberous sclerosis. Current guidelines suggest electively embolizing any tumors that are larger than 4 cm in diameter. The procedure is effective in decreasing tumor size and in preventing or treating hemorrhage in 85–90% of patients. CT can clearly identify the fat component of the tumor and is therefore used for diagnosis before intervention and for follow-up (Halpenny et al, 2009).

The technique for embolization is similar to that described for RCC. Through a transfemoral approach, angiography is used to define the arterial supply to the kidney and tumor. The feeding vessels are then selectively catheterized using a

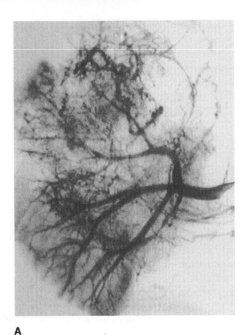
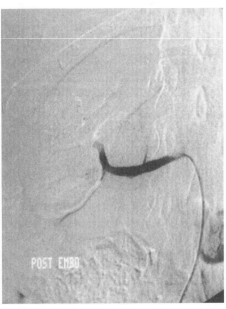

A

B

▲ **Figure 7–3.** Preoperative embolization of a large right renal cell carcinoma (RCC) in a 28-year-old woman. **A:** Digital subtraction arteriogram (DSA) of the right renal artery shows a large hypervascular mass involving most of the right kidney. There is tumor thrombus within the renal vein. **B:** Completion DSA of the right renal artery after Gelfoam embolization shows complete cessation of flow within the tumor and kidney. Contrast is seen within the main renal artery only.

coaxial microcatheter. The tumor volume is estimated, and an equal amount of absolute ethanol admixed with iodized oil is carefully injected until the flow ceases. Ethanol is easy to handle, is inexpensive, and produces permanent occlusion of the vascular bed. Iodized oil is radiopaque and therefore is useful for visualizing the flow of the embolic material during the embolization. It remains within the tumor, thereby allowing measurement of tumor response on follow-up CT. An occlusion balloon is reserved for more proximal embolization in a main renal artery when the risk of nontarget embolization is greatest.

The reported complications are similar to those seen after RCC embolization. Recurrence of tumor hemorrhage occurs in approximately 10–15% of patients and is treated by repeat embolization. A short-term tapered dose of prednisone may reduce PES after the procedure (Bissler et al, 2002).

▶ Ablation of Renal Function

Total renal infarction using transcatheter embolization may be indicated in certain circumstances: namely, abolition of urine production to assist in healing or palliation of terminal patients with urinary fistulas; prevention of excessive proteinuria; management of uncontrollable hypertension; rarely for benign obstructive uropathy in patients who are poor surgical candidates (De Baere et al, 2000; Toussi et al, 2001);

and for ablation of failed renal allografts causing the graft intolerance syndrome (Delgado et al, 2005). For patients with end-stage renal disease and intractable hypertension or nephrotic syndrome, the advantages of ablation must be weighed against the loss of production of vitamin D_3 and erythropoietic factors and, occasionally, the loss of the ability to eliminate some water. Total renal ablation must be achieved so that perfusion of surviving parenchyma via pericapsular branches cannot occur. The embolic agent must perfuse the entire renal substance but be safe if it passes through the kidney into the venous circulation. The technique is applicable in adults and children and in both native and allograft kidneys. Renal ablation appears to be a safe procedure, which is successful in most patients (De Baere et al, 2000).

Initially, a midstream aortogram is performed to identify the arterial supply to the kidneys. This is followed by renal artery catheterization and selective arteriography. An occlusion balloon catheter is placed in the vessel and contrast medium is injected to measure the volume of embolic agent needed to fill the vascular tree of the kidney. Absolute ethanol is the embolic agent of choice for the reasons mentioned above. An equal volume is carefully injected with the balloon inflated to prevent reflux to nontarget regions. The contents are then aspirated and an angiogram is performed to assess flow. The procedure is repeated as many times as necessary until complete cessation of blood flow is achieved.

PES of several days' duration occurs in all patients and is managed with antibiotics and analgesics. Inadvertent embolization of the adrenal artery and other visceral vessels is a rare but serious complication that can be avoided by using the occlusion balloon technique. Systemic toxicity from ethanol injection is not a clinical problem. Morbidity and mortality from the procedure is less than that from surgical nephrectomy.

▶ Embolization of Primary Varicocele

The subject of varicocele and male infertility is discussed in another chapter. A recent Cochrane analysis concludes that: "There is no evidence that treatment of varicoceles in men from couples with otherwise unexplained subfertility improves the couple's chance of conception" (Evers et al, 2009). The basis for intervention is the presence of a varicocele on physical examination; most varicoceles are left sided. Color Doppler sonography is usually performed routinely before intervention. Several reports have suggested a positive association between improvement of seminal parameters and pregnancy. Surgery and percutaneous transvenous embolization appear to be equally effective (Bechara et al, 2009). However, advantages of the percutaneous route include greater patient comfort, ease of bilateral treatment, and reduced recovery time.

The procedure is performed with conscious intravenous sedation and local anesthesia. The transjugular venous approach is preferred by many physicians, although the procedure can be performed transfemorally. Direct ultrasound guidance is used to access the jugular vein; a catheter is then guided fluoroscopically into the left gonadal vein. The left gonadal vein usually drains into the left renal vein, whereas the right gonadal vein usually drains directly into the inferior vena cava. The patient is placed in reverse Trendelenburg position and left gonadal venography is performed. A positive venogram result demonstrates incompetence with filling of collateral vessels. Embolization is achieved by placing coils within the gonadal vein, commencing at the region of the inguinal ligament, and continuing cranially toward the renal vein, until the gonadal vein and collateral vessels have been occluded. If a right-sided varicocele is also present, the right gonadal vein is then interrogated and embolized.

The recurrence rate of varicocele after embolization is approximately 4%. Minor complications include contrast extravasation from perforation of the vein, nontarget embolization, venospasm, and hematoma. Rarely, cardiac arrhythmia and contrast allergy can occur.

▶ Embolization of Ovarian Vein Varices (Pelvic Congestion Syndrome)

Pelvic congestion syndrome is a recognized cause of chronic pelvic pain in women that has been associated with lumbo-ovarian vein varices. Dyspareunia, when present, may be a poor prognostic indicator. Symptoms are often worse with fatigue, before menstruation, and in the upright position.

Occasionally, vulval and thigh varicosities are present on examination. The cause is probably multifactorial. The diagnosis of varicosed pelvic veins is confirmed by duplex Doppler ultrasound that is also used for postintervention follow-up. CT venography or magnetic resonance venography are alternative noninvasive diagnostic tests.

Transvenous embolization has produced durable relief of symptoms in most patients (>70%). Most responses occur within 2 weeks of treatment; however, continued improvement has been reported up to 12 months after the procedure (Kim et al, 2006). Using either a transfemoral or a transjugular approach, the ovarian veins are individually catheterized, and embolic agents such as coils or synthetic glue are deployed in the vessel at the level of the pelvic inlet (Figures 7–4A, B). Occasionally, embolization of internal iliac vein tributaries may be necessary. Reported complications are similar to those for varicocele embolization. The procedure does not appear to have a deleterious effect on fertility or the menstrual cycle.

▶ Treatment of High-Flow Priapism

High-flow priapism is a fairly rare condition resulting from increased arterial flow into the lacunar spaces of the cavernous tissue. The "arteriocavernous fistula" most often results from penile or perineal trauma. In some cases, the cause is unknown. Color Doppler sonography demonstrates the abnormality.

Transcatheter embolization is a minimally invasive, successful treatment for this condition (Kojima et al, 2009). A nonselective transfemoral pelvic angiogram is performed to demonstrate the fistula that originates from the pudendal artery. This procedure is followed by superselective catheterization of the injured artery using a microcatheter. The fistula is then closed by accurately deploying microcoils (Figures 7–5A, B). This technique preserves blood flow to the penis, thereby allowing normal erectile function in most cases. The use of microcoils prevents possible ischemic injury to the perineum. In the event of recurrence after embolization, repeat embolization is successful in nearly all patients. Surgery should be reserved for patients in whom embolization fails.

RENAL ARTERY ANGIOPLASTY AND STENTING

Ischemic nephropathy due to atherosclerotic vascular disease and renal artery stenosis is a leading cause of progressive renal failure. Renal artery stenosis is the most common cause of secondary hypertension. Surgical revascularization is an established method of treatment, with reported success rates of >70%. In recent years, percutaneous transluminal angioplasty (PTA) and stent placement have become an established alternative to surgery. These endovascular techniques are now the most common means of revascularization. However, there is great controversy over the relative benefits of revascularization compared to best medical treatment (Uder and Humke, 2005; White, 2006). In 2009, a randomized unblinded trial of treatment of over 800 patients with atherosclerotic renovascular disease by revascularization and medical

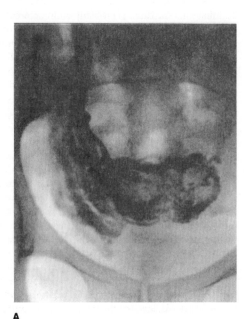
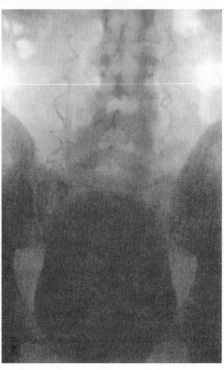

A   **B**

▲ **Figure 7–4.** Embolization of ovarian vein varices in a 30-year-old multiparous woman with pelvic congestion syndrome. She complained of increasing pelvic pain and dyspareunia. On examination there were prominent vulval varicosities. **A:** Transjugular right ovarian venography demonstrates multiple large ovarian vein varices. **B:** Radiograph taken after coil embolization of both ovarian veins and tributaries of the internal iliac veins. The varices have been occluded. The patient's symptoms resolved after the procedure.

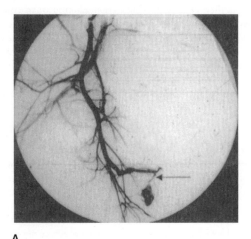
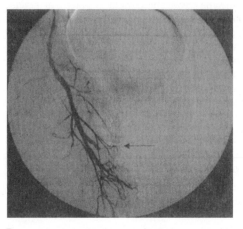

A   **B**

▲ **Figure 7–5.** A 17-year-old male had normal erectile function before a skateboard straddle injury. He had a painless partial erection for 13 months and was unable to achieve full erection for intercourse. **A:** A right internal iliac arteriogram shows a cavernosal arteriosinusoidal fistula arising from the internal pudendal artery (*arrow*). **B:** Repeat angiography after selective microcoil embolization for the fistula shows occlusion of the fistula (*arrow*). After the procedure there was complete detumescence, with return of normal sexual function over the next 3 months.

therapy was compared with medical treatment alone. The conclusion of this "ASTRAL" trial was: "We found substantial risks but no evidence of a worthwhile clinical benefit from revascularization in patients with atherosclerotic renovascular disease" (ASTRAL investigators 2009). The trial has been heavily criticized for its inclusion bias and selection of end points and it is likely that properly selected patients do benefit from revascularization (White, 2010).

Streichen et al (2010) reviewed the literature on primary stenting for atherosclerotic renal artery stenosis (ARAS). They concluded, "Recent evidence shows that impaired renal function associated with ARAS is more stable over time than previously observed. Optimal medical treatment should be the preferred option for most patients with ARAS. Only low-level evidence supports compelling indications for revascularization in ARAS, including rapidly progressive hypertension or renal failure and flash pulmonary edema."

However, other authors continue to emphasize the value of stenting: "ARAS may result in progressive renal impairment, renovascular hypertension, and/or cardiac disturbance syndromes. Because medical therapy does not affect the progressive nature of this disease process, more aggressive treatments are needed to definitively treat ARAS. When performed correctly, renal artery stenting has been shown to stabilize or improve renal function and/or renovascular hypertension in 65–70% of carefully selected patients with ARAS. Therefore, percutaneous renal artery stenting should be considered the primary treatment for patients with symptomatic ARAS (Carr et al, 2010).

PTA is the treatment of choice in the management of fibromuscular dysplasia occurring in a subset of hypertensive patients. The technique involves the use of an inflatable balloon catheter that is positioned endoluminally across the stenosis and then inflated (angioplasty).

Several diagnostic imaging modalities are used for patient selection and for postprocedure follow-up, including captopril radioisotope assay, duplex Doppler ultrasound, CT angiography, magnetic resonance angiography, and arteriography. The advantages and disadvantages of these techniques are beyond the scope of this chapter, but noncatheter angiography by CT or MR is replacing catheter angiography for diagnostic purposes.

Renal artery stenosis is described as ostial, nonostial, or branch vessel stenosis. An ostial lesion is located within 3 mm of the aortic lumen and is typical of atherosclerotic vascular disease. In fibromuscular dysplasia, nonostial and branch vessel lesions are more typically seen. The initial technical success rate of PTA varies. It may be as low as 35% for some atherosclerotic vascular disease ostial lesions, but in most series the overall rate approximates 95–100%. PTA results in stabilization or improvement of renal function in most patients with ischemic nephropathy and also leads to durable improvement or cure in most of those with hypertension. The best results after PTA have been achieved in hypertensive patients with fibromuscular dysplasia, in whom improvement or cure is achieved in approximately 90%.

Stent placement is usually the method of choice for endoluminal recanalization. Previously, stenting had been reserved for immediate failure or complication of PTA, such as elastic recoil or flow limiting intimal dissection, for residual stenoses of >30%, for a >20 mm Hg peak systolic pressure gradient after PTA, for early restenosis, and for ostial lesions that are difficult to treat by PTA alone. Renal artery stenting results in stabilization (38% of patients) or improvement (30% of patients) of renal function and in durable improvement (49%) or cure (20%) of hypertension (Leertouwer et al, 2000). PTA and stenting have also been used successfully to treat renal allograft artery stenosis. Primary patency rates vary after stenting. The average restenosis rate is approximately 17% after 6–12 months' follow-up. However, the rate increased to 20–30% with longer follow-up. Secondary patency may be achieved in >90% of patients.

Usually, the transfemoral approach is used, although a transaxillary approach may be required. Initially, a midstream aortogram is performed to identify the renal arteries, followed by a selective injection to evaluate the morphology and location of the stenosis, the diameter of the vessel, and the percentage of stenosis. In the presence of altered renal function with elevated creatinine levels, alternatives to iodinated contrast agents include gadolinium and carbon dioxide gas. Indicators of a significant stenosis include a reduction of cross-sectional diameter of at least 50%, poststenotic dilatation, collateral vessels to the affected kidney, and a transstenotic systolic pressure gradient of >20 mm Hg across the lesion. Before intervention, an oral antiplatelet agent such as clopidogrel is administered. The patient is heparinized and a vasodilating agent (eg, nitroglycerine) is given via the arterial catheter. Initially, the lesion is crossed with a guidewire. If a high-grade stenosis is present, predilatation with a small balloon may be necessary before definitive angioplasty or stent placement. An outer guiding catheter or sheath is used to facilitate contrast injection during the procedure and to improve catheter stability. Continuous fluoroscopic guidance and "vascular road-mapping" are also used to ensure precision. Frequently, a small tear in the vessel intima is seen after PTA. We prefer to use a balloon expandable stent because it can be very accurately deployed. The minimal recommended vessel diameter for stenting is 5 mm. A 10- to 20-mm-long stent is used, and approximately 1–2 mm should protrude into the aortic lumen when ostial lesions are treated (Figures 7–6A, B).

Success of the procedure is defined by <30% residual stenosis and by the resolution of a significant transstenotic pressure gradient. We frequently use a percutaneous closure device to achieve hemostasis. Antiplatelet medication is continued for 6 weeks after the procedure, and the patient is carefully followed up by clinical evaluation and repeat imaging.

The reported complication rate after PTA and stenting varies considerably but ranges from 3% to 10% in experienced operators. Complications include puncture-site hematoma; femoral artery pseudoaneurysm; contrast nephropathy; cholesterol embolization; stent malpositioning; and injury to the renal artery such as dissection, thrombosis, and rupture.

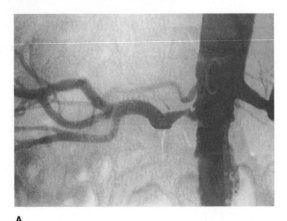

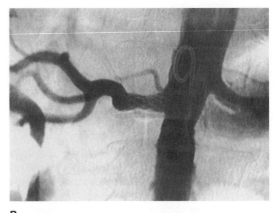

A   B

▲ **Figure 7–6.** Renal artery stenting in an 80-year-old woman with labile hypertension and right renal artery stenosis due to atherosclerotic vascular disease. Her hypertension was poorly controlled on three antihypertensive medications. **A:** A midstream aortogram at the level of the renal arteries demonstrates a high-grade ostial right renal artery stenosis. **B:** Repeat midstream aortogram after placement of a 20-mm-long Palmaz stent, dilated to 6 mm. A widely patent renal artery is seen. The stent protrudes slightly into the aortic lumen. The patient's hypertension improved after the procedure.

Rarely, procedure-related deaths have occurred. The use of endovascular distal protection devices when stenting the carotid arteries may provide benefits for renal artery stenting. These devices are usually small filters that trap micro emboli that may be dislodged during stent placement. They limit end-organ embolization (Dubel and Murphy, 2008).

OTHER ENDOVASCULAR PROCEDURES

▷ Catheter-Based Renal Sympathetic Denervation for Treatment of Resistant Hypertension

A recently developed catheter can be used by a standard transarterial endovascular route to deliver radiofrequency energy in the lumen of the renal artery. This causes selective renal denervation and reduction of sympathetic activity, resulting in a sustained reduction in hypertension. Patients with normal renal arteries and essential hypertension resistant to antihypertensive drug therapy have been successfully treated using this new technique with excellent results and minimal complications. There are very encouraging initial reports of a randomized prospective trial covering a 6-month period and a more recent publication with good results at 2 years follow-up (Esler et al, 2010; Sapoval et al, 2012; Symplicity HTN-1 Investigators, 2011).

▷ Renal Artery Aneurysms

Renal artery aneurysms are rare and are usually not symptomatic. They carry the risk of rupture, with associated life-threatening hemorrhage. Occasionally, they are associated with renovascular hypertension. Distal embolization may occur, leading to parenchymal infarction. The indications for treatment of renal artery aneurysms include diameter >2.5 cm, interval enlargement, renovascular hypertension, pain, hematuria, intrarenal thromboemboli, and lesions in women of childbearing age. The diagnosis is made by color Doppler sonography, CT, or MRI.

In the high-risk surgical patient, endovascular techniques may be well suited to aneurysm repair, by excluding the aneurysm while preserving flow to the kidney. Depending on the location of the aneurysm, its relationship to branch vessels, and the presence or absence of a "neck," either a stent graft or transcatheter embolization are possible treatment options (Horowitz et al, 2005; Eskandari and Resnick, 2005; Saltzberg et al, 2005). A stent graft is a metallic stent that is covered by surgical graft material. Its deployment across the aneurysm results in internal reconstruction of the vessel, with exclusion of blood flow to the aneurysm due to the impervious graft material. The cavity of the aneurysm may then thrombose.

Selective embolization of an aneurysm that is supplied by a branch vessel is performed by occluding blood flow proximally using coils. This approach results in distal parenchymal infarction and therefore can only be safely performed if there is sufficient renal functional reserve. If there is an identifiable neck separating the aneurysm from the native vessel, coils may be used to pack the aneurysm cavity, thereby resulting in thrombosis of the aneurysm while at the same time preserving distal flow. The risks of the procedure are similar to those reported above. Long-term results of endovascular repair are not yet available.

CATHETER-DIRECTED FIBRINOLYSIS

This procedure has been used extensively in the peripheral vasculature but only with limited success in the management of native renal artery or aortorenal bypass graft thrombosis.

Small series or individual case reports have suggested a possible role in the treatment of recent renal artery occlusion before PTA and for the treatment of acute renal artery thromboembolic disease (Nakayama et al, 2006).

There is a variety of mechanical devices to remove clot in addition to or as an alternative to pharmacologic thrombolysis (Siablis et al, 2005). The diagnosis is made by noninvasive imaging such as duplex Doppler ultrasound, MRI, or CT angiography and is then confirmed by angiography, at which time fibrinolytic therapy is begun. A diagnostic arteriogram is performed from a transfemoral approach, after which an infusion catheter or wire is embedded within the thrombosed segment. Tissue plasminogen activator (t-PA) is currently the most frequently used fibrinolytic agent in the United States. Several infusion protocols exist. Our preferred technique is continuous infusion of 1–2 mg t-PA/hour. Prophylactic antibiotics are administered. The patient is monitored for puncture site and systemic bleeding in the intensive care or step-down unit throughout the infusion therapy. A repeat arteriogram is performed 12–24 hours after the initiation of therapy. When recanalization has been achieved, an underlying stenotic lesion is usually identified, at which time PTA or stenting is performed.

Complications include puncture site and systemic hemorrhage and infection. Bleeding may be severe enough to require transfusion or to discontinue the infusion. The incidence of complications is related to the duration of therapy and the dose administered.

BIBLIOGRAPHY

ASTRAL Investigators, Wheatley K et al: Revascularization versus medical therapy for renal-artery stenosis. N Engl J Med 2009;361(20):1953–1962.

Bechara CF et al: Percutaneous treatment of varicocele with microcoil embolization: Comparison of treatment outcome with laparoscopic varicocelectomy. Vascular 2009;17(Suppl 3): S129–S136.

Bissler JJ et al: Reduction of postembolization syndrome after ablation or renal angiomyolipoma. Am J Kidney Dis 2002;39(5):966.

Carr TM III et al: Stenting for atherosclerotic renal artery stenosis. Tech Vasc Interv Radiol 2010;13(2):134–145.

Chatziioannou AN et al: Preoperative embolization of bone metastases from renal cell carcinoma. Eur Radiol 2000;10(4):593.

De Baere T et al: Transcatheter ethanol ablation in 20 patients with persistent urine leaks: An alternative to surgical nephrectomy. J Urol 2000;164(4):1148.

Delgado P et al: Intolerance syndrome in failed renal allografts: Incidence and efficacy of percutaneous embolization. Am J Kidney Dis 2005;46(2):339–344.

Dubel GJ, Murphy TP: Distal embolic protection for renal arterial interventions. Cardiovasc Intervent Radiol 2008;31(1):14–22.

Eskandari MK, Resnick SA: Aneurysms of the renal artery. Semin Vasc Surg 2005;18(4):202–208.

Esler MD et al: Symplicity HTN-2 Investigators: Renal sympathetic denervation in patients with treatment-resistant hypertension

(The Symplicity HTN-2 Trial): A randomised controlled trial. Lancet 2010;376(9756):1903–1909.

Evers JH et al: Surgery or embolisation for varicoceles in subfertile men. Cochrane Database Syst Rev 2009;(1):CD000479.

Ginat DT et al: Transcatheter renal artery embolization: Clinical applications and techniques. Tech Vasc Interv Radiol 2009; 12(4):224–239.

Halpenny D et al: The radiological diagnosis and treatment of renal angiomyolipoma-current status. Clin Radiol 2010;65(2):99–108. Epub 2009 Dec 3.

Horowitz MD et al: Renal artery pseudoaneurysm following partial nephrectomy treated with stent-graft. Br J Radiol 2005;78(926): 161–163.

Kim HS et al: Embolotherapy for pelvic congestion syndrome: Long-term results. J Vasc Interv Radiol 2006;17(2 Pt 1):289–297.

Kojima H et al: High-flow priapism undergoing arterial embolization: Review of literature following American Urological Association guideline on the management of priapism. Minim Invasive Ther Allied Technol 2009;18(1):1–5.

Kothary N et al: Renal angiomyolipoma: Long-term results after arterial embolization. J Vasc Interv Radiol 2005;16(1):45–50.

Leertouwer TC et al: Stent placement for renal arterial stenosis: Where do we stand? A meta-analysis. Radiology 2000;216(1):78–85.

Libicher M et al: Interventional therapy of vascular complications following renal transplantation. Clin Transplant 2006;20(Suppl 17):55–59.

Munro NP et al: The role of transarterial embolization in the treatment of renal cell carcinoma. BJU Int 2003;92(3):240–244.

Nakayama T et al: Thrombolytic therapy for traumatic unilateral renal artery thrombosis. Int J Urol 2006;13(2):168–170.

Saltzberg SS et al: Is endovascular therapy the preferred treatment for all visceral artery aneurysms? Ann Vasc Surg 2005;19(4):507–515.

Sapoval M et al: Endovascular renal artery denervation: Why, when, and how? [Published online ahead of print February 8, 2012]. Cardiovasc Intervent Radiol 2012. [PMID: 22314774.]

Siablis D et al: Percutaneous rheolytic thrombectomy for treatment of acute renal-artery thrombosis. J Endourol 2005;19(1):68–71.

Steichen O et al: Primary stenting for atherosclerotic renal artery stenosis. J Vasc Surg 2010;51(6):1574–1580.

Symplicity HTN-1 Investigators: Catheter-based renal sympathetic denervation for resistant hypertension: Durability of blood pressure reduction out to 24 months. Hypertension 2011;57(5):911–917.

Toussi H et al: Renal artery embolization for benign obstructive uropathy. J Urol 2001;165(4):1162.

Uder M, Humke U: Endovascular therapy of renal artery stenosis: Where do we stand today? Cardiovasc Intervent Radiol 2005;28(2): 139–147.

White CJ: Catheter-based therapy for atherosclerotic renal artery stenosis. Circulation 2006;113(11):1464–1473.

White CJ: Kiss my astral: One seriously flawed study of renal stenting after another. Catheter Cardiovasc Interv 2010;75(2):305–307.

Yamakado K et al: Radiofrequency ablation combined with renal arterial embolization for the treatment of unresectable renal cell carcinoma larger than 3.5 cm: Initial experience. Cardiovasc Intervent Radiol 2006;29(3):389–394.

Zielinski H et al: Comparison of preoperative embolization followed by radical nephrectomy with radical nephrectomy alone for renal cell carcinoma. Am J Clin Oncol 2000;23(1):6.

Percutaneous Endourology & Ureterorenoscopy

Joachim W. Thüroff, MD, & Rolf Gillitzer, MD

Retrograde instrumentation of the upper urinary tract, such as ureterorenoscopy, uses under endoscopic guidance the anatomically predestined access via the urethra and ureter, while techniques of antegrade instrumentation require a percutaneous puncture. This approach must respect the intrarenal anatomy just as in open surgical nephrotomy, and imaging techniques are required to guide the procedure.

First, and most important, a puncture direction must be determined that will provide straight access to the target and safe, bloodless instrumentation. Visualization of both the puncture needle and the target and precise guidance of the needle tip to the target require imaging techniques such as ultrasound, fluoroscopy, and, in selected cases, computed tomography (CT).

Contraindications to percutaneous kidney puncture are blood-clotting anomalies due to coagulopathies or pharmacologic anticoagulation. Preparation and draping of the surgical field are required as for open surgery, and the same standards of asepsis must be followed. Local anesthesia only is sufficient for puncture of the kidney and small-bore tract dilation (6–12F), for antegrade insertion of a ureteral stent or nephrostomy catheter. Lidocaine hydrochloride 2% USP, 10 mL, can be given for infiltration of the skin and tissues along the intended tract of puncture down to the renal capsule. During dilation of the tract, administration of a local anesthetic in lubricant (eg, lidocaine hydrochloride jelly 2%) serves the dual purpose of anesthetization and lubrication. Dilation of nephrostomy tracts up to 30F and extraction of small renal stones can be done under local anesthesia.

Percutaneous nephrolithotomy (PNL) remains indicated for treatment of large stones, staghorn calculi, and stones in caliceal diverticula. The extent of intrarenal instrumentation for stone disintegration and extraction usually requires epidural or general anesthesia. Because puncture, tract dilation, and stone disintegration and removal are preferably performed as a one-stage procedure, the use of local anesthesia in PNL is limited.

IMAGING AND PUNCTURE TECHNIQUES

Percutaneous puncture of the renal collecting system may be performed for diagnostic procedures (eg, antegrade pyelography, pressure/perfusion studies) or to establish access for therapeutic interventions (Table 8–1).

Both ultrasonic scanning and fluoroscopy provide visualization and guidance for a safe, accurate percutaneous puncture, but ultrasound has the following definite advantages:

1. No intravenous or retrograde administration of contrast dye

2. No radiation exposure

3. Continuous real-time control of puncture

4. Imaging of radiolucent, non–contrast-enhancing renal and extrarenal structures (eg, renal cyst, retroperitoneal tumor) for puncture

5. Imaging of all tissues along an intended nephrostomy tract (eg, bowel, lung)

6. Imaging in numerous planes simply by shifting, tilting, and rotating the scanning head

7. Three-dimensional information during puncture

Once the puncture needle has entered the renal collecting system, fluoroscopy is required for control and guidance of subsequent steps (eg, guidewire insertion, tract dilation, and catheter insertion). In selected cases, insertion and placement of a nephrostomy catheter in a dilated renal system may be possible with ultrasonic control only. Fluoroscopy provides a two-dimensional summation image with integration of all information from the third (anterior-posterior) dimension so that the entire length of a radiopaque catheter, wire, and so on can be visualized.

For percutaneous puncture of the renal collecting system, the patient should be placed on the fluoroscopy table in the prone position. Radiolucent bolsters may be placed under the abdomen to correct for lumbar lordosis and to

Table 8-1. Indications for percutaneous puncture of the renal collecting system.

Diagnostic indications
    Antegrade pyelography
    Pressure/perfusion study (Whitaker test)
Therapeutic indications
    Nephrostomy catheter drainage
    Antegrade ureteral stenting
    Dilation of ureteral strictures
    Percutaneous endopyeloplasty
    PNL
    Percutaneous resection and coagulation of urothelial tumors

PNL, percutaneous nephrolithotomy.

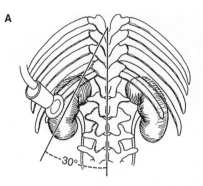

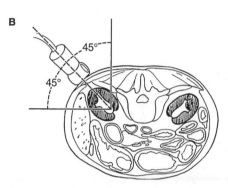

▲ **Figure 8–1.** Renal ultrasound. **A:** The longitudinal axis of the kidney forms a 30° angle with the midline. **B:** The transverse axis of the kidney forms a 45° angle with both a horizontal and a vertical line.

support the kidney. A standard puncture site is in the posterior axillary line midway between the 12th rib and the ileal crest; this site ensures that later the patient does not lie on the nephrostomy catheter in the supine position. Morbidly obese patients can be placed in a lateral decubitus position in order to minimize respiratory distress. Ultrasonic scanning is performed below the 12th rib to obtain a median longitudinal scan through the kidney. For optimal coupling of the ultrasonic beam to the skin, sterile gel (eg, K-Y jelly) is applied to the skin at the scanning site. In the frontal view of an intravenous pyelogram, the long axis of the kidney usually follows the psoas muscle, forming about a 30° angle with the midline (Figure 8–1A). In the transverse view of a CT scan, the transverse axis of the kidney forms about a 45° angle with both a horizontal and a sagittal line (Figure 8–1B). The position and direction of the transducer should be oriented roughly to the following marks: below the 12th rib (if possible), cranial to the puncture site, with a 30° caudal-lateral rotation, and with a 45° lateral tilt of the scanning head.

Factors that may influence the choice of scanning technique and puncture site include patient size; position and rotation of the kidney; anomalies of bony structures; positions of the colon, spleen, liver, and lung relative to the kidney; and the target of puncture (upper, middle, or lower calyx; caliceal diverticulum). The scanning head can be positioned to provide the best visualization and optimum puncture site for each patient. Thus, a puncture site as high as above the 11th rib may be chosen if the lung is not visualized in the puncture direction. A different puncture site must be chosen if bowel gas or the liver or spleen is visualized within the intended puncture direction.

The puncture direction should always aim through a pyramid into a dorsal calyx; puncture into an infundibulum may result in bleeding from segmental and interlobar vessels in the renal sinus, and direct puncture of the renal pelvis renders dilation of the nephrostomy tract and insertion of catheters and instruments difficult, with increased risk of

accidental catheter displacement after successful entry. For large, complete staghorn calculi, when PNL is to be performed for debulking the stone volume (followed by extracorporeal shockwave lithotripsy [ESWL] for disintegrating retained caliceal stones), puncture is usually performed through a lower dorsal calyx, a position from which the lower caliceal group, the renal pelvis, and part of the upper caliceal group can be reached easily with rigid instruments. However, for staghorn stones that are intended to be removed by PNL only (without ESWL), another access (eg, middle or upper calyx puncture) may be chosen. Stones in caliceal diverticula are approached by direct puncture of the diverticulum.

Once chosen, the target for access to the renal collecting system must be visualized ultrasonically. The cutaneous puncture site should be chosen in a virtual caudal extension of the perpendicular orientation (width) of the scanning plane. Skin and fascia are incised with a no. 11 blade. At this time, the scanning head may be shifted over the incision to measure the exact distance between the incision and the target. A 16- to 18-gauge puncture needle (Figure 8–2) may then be inserted blindly through the incision and aimed in the

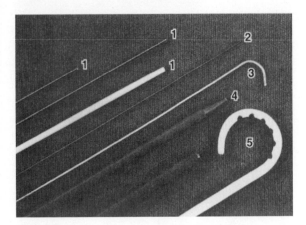

▲ **Figure 8–2.** Universal nephrostomy set (Bard-Angiomed), containing (1) coaxial 17.5-gauge needle with obturator/6F plastic sheath; (2) fine needle (22 gauge); (3) 0.035-in stiff guidewire with floppy J-tip (Lunderquist); (4) coaxial 10F dilator/12F introducer sheath system; and (5) 10F pigtail nephrostomy catheter.

direction previously determined by ultrasound. However, the needle should never be advanced blindly farther than through the abdominal fascia.

The scanning head is now placed in such a way that both the target and the puncture needle are visualized in the same scanning plane, and the needle is aligned so that its tip can be clearly seen. Vibrating the needle makes the tip more visible while the position of the scanning head is being adjusted. The needle can be safely moved back and forth down to the renal capsule as often as necessary, but the renal parenchyma ideally should be punctured only once.

A needle guide attached to the scanning head can be used to direct the needle exactly within the ultrasonic scanning plane. With some needle guides, the angle of puncture relative to the longitudinal axis of the scanning plane (depth) is also fixed and is shown on the monitor by an electronically generated line. If a steeper or flatter angle of puncture is desired, the entire scanning head and attached needle guide must be tilted, and the choice of puncture site is therefore limited. Another drawback of a needle guide is that it does not allow for independent adjustment of the puncture and scanning direction if the needle deviates from its intended direction after being advanced through the skin. This frequently occurs in patients with scars from previous operations and becomes more of a problem the farther the target is from the cutaneous puncture site. Freehand puncture with individual adjustment of puncture and scanning direction is preferable in these cases.

Movement of the kidney during respiration may complicate puncture if the target is small and is visible on the monitor only during a specific respiratory phase. If the direction of the needle and the position of the target are aligned and both are clearly seen on the monitor, the needle is advanced through the renal capsule during the appropriate phase of respiration (Figure 8–3). In this phase, the kidney is usually pushed to some extent by the puncture needle so that visualization of needle and target may be momentarily impaired. However, as soon as the tip of the needle has penetrated the fibrous renal capsule, it is seen even more clearly. If both the tip of the needle and the target are visualized clearly at the same spot on the scanning plane, the needle is in the desired space.

Antegrade injection of a small amount of contrast dye for fluoroscopy outlines the renal collecting system after successful puncture. However, if the collecting system has not been

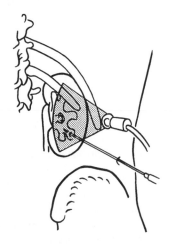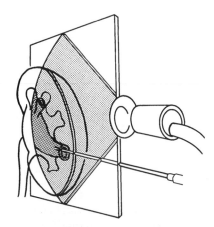

▲ **Figure 8–3.** Ultrasonically guided puncture of a dorsal lower calyx. Needle must be in the scanning plane to be visualized.

successfully punctured at the first attempt, contrast dye may fill the interlobar veins, which form a basket-like structure around the calyx, or may extravasate. In rare cases in which contrast dye is injected into the adventitia of the renal collecting system, extravasation may assume the configuration of the collecting system, mimicking successful puncture. Care must be taken to inject the least amount of dye necessary so that further fluoroscopic and ultrasonic orientation will not be hindered. A larger amount of dye injected outside the collecting system may compress the calyx to be entered and render puncture more difficult. If the position of the needle tip on ultrasound is close to its destination (ascertained by a small vibratory movement), the needle should be retracted a few millimeters only and readvanced at the appropriate angle and tilt. Once the collecting system is entered (Figure 8–4A), fluoroscopy alone is used to guide the subsequent steps of the procedure.

If fluoroscopy is used instead of ultrasound for guiding renal puncture, a fine-needle (20–22 gauge) puncture technique may be used. Intravenous or retrograde administration of contrast dye is needed. With retrograde injection, a ureteral balloon occlusion catheter can be inserted and blocked in the ureteropelvic junction (UPJ) to cause slight distention of the renal collecting system; this facilitates puncture of a nondilated system. First, a 16- to 18-gauge needle is inserted through the abdominal wall only, and a longer fine needle is inserted coaxially through the larger needle (Figure 8–4B). This technique improves control of the fine needle. As soon

as the fine needle has entered the collecting system, the larger needle can be advanced over the fine needle, which serves as a guide. After withdrawal of the fine needle, a regular guidewire can be inserted through the large needle into the collecting system.

Urine aspirated from the collecting system should be cultured, especially if there is suspicion of a urinary tract infection.

ANTEGRADE PYELOGRAPHY AND PRESSURE/PERFUSION STUDIES

Renal puncture is rarely indicated for diagnostic antegrade pyelography only, because less invasive radiographic techniques are available (eg, intravenous pyelography, ultrasound, CT, magnetic resonance imaging [MRI], retrograde pyelography). However, obtaining a radiograph after antegrade injection of contrast dye should be an integral part of every percutaneous puncture for any indication. Before contrast dye is injected, urine must be aspirated to decompress an obstructed collecting system. The contrast dye should be diluted to 20–30% for better visualization of details; antegrade pyelography then provides images of the collecting system with about the same resolution of detail as retrograde pyelography.

Antegrade pyelography is also performed in conjunction with a percutaneous pressure/perfusion study (Whitaker test) to assess pyeloureteral resistance. Percutaneous urodynamic studies of the dilated upper urinary tract are indicated only in the 10–30% of cases in which noninvasive radioisotope studies (diuresis renogram) fail to differentiate an obstructed dilated system from a nonobstructed dilated system. (This is more likely in cases of ureterovesical obstruction than in pelvic–ureteral obstruction, in which diuresis renograms are reliable.)

The Whitaker test provides simultaneous measurements of intrapelvic and intravesical pressures during antegrade perfusion, with flow rates of 5, 10, 15, and 20 mL/min. Puncture of the renal collecting system is performed with a coaxial needle/catheter system with an outer 6F catheter for the renal pressure/perfusion study; thus, puncture and catheter insertion can be done as a one-step procedure. Perfusion is started with flow rates of 5–10 mL/min until steady-state equilibrium of pressure readings is reached and the entire upper urinary tract is opacified (Figure 8–5). Pressure readings may be obtained intermittently from the perfusion catheter via a three-way stopcock, or continuously, if a double-lumen nephrostomy catheter or two separate catheters for perfusion and pressure measurement are used. Continuous recordings during perfusion from a single-lumen perfusion catheter via a T connection yield erroneous pressure readings (the smaller the lumen of the nephrostomy catheter and the higher the perfusion rate, the higher the pressure reading), unless the resistance of the entire system was previously calibrated for each rate of perfusion. To obtain accurate pressure readings, the positions of the intrapelvic and intravesical pressure

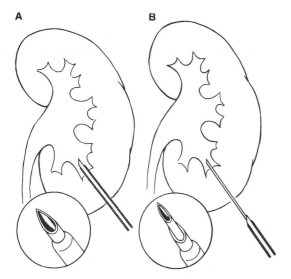

▲ **Figure 8–4.** Percutaneous puncture techniques. **A:** Ultrasonically guided technique: puncture with a 16- to 18-gauge coaxial needle/plastic sheath system. **B:** Fluoroscopically guided technique: coaxial fine-needle puncture through a larger needle/sheath system.

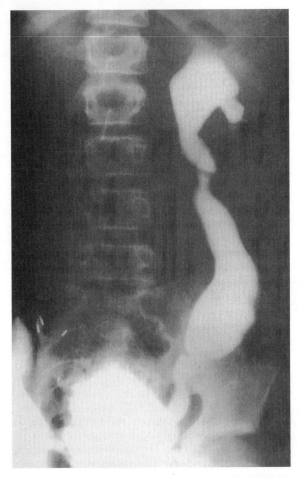

▲ **Figure 8–5.** Whitaker test in a dilated upper tract after vesicoureteral reimplantation (prune belly syndrome). Antegrade perfusion with 10 mL/min results in a vesicopelvic pressure gradient of 10 cm of water, with unobstructed flow.

manometers must be adjusted to the level of the renal pelvis and bladder, respectively. At a flow rate of 10 mL/min, differential pressures (renal pelvic pressure minus bladder pressure) below 13 cm water are normal, between 14 and 22 cm water suggest mild obstruction, and above 22 cm water suggest moderate to severe obstruction. At flow rates of 15 and 20 mL/min, upper limits of normal pressure are 18 and 21 cm water, respectively.

PERCUTANEOUS CATHETER PLACEMENT

Percutaneous nephrostomy catheter placement for drainage and decompression of the upper urinary tract is indicated if retrograde ureteral catheterization is not advisable (eg, in

sepsis secondary to ureteral obstruction) or proves to be impossible (eg, impassable ureteral obstruction due to stone, tumor, or stricture). After percutaneous endourologic procedures, a nephrostomy catheter is usually left indwelling for a few days. To convert a nephrostomy catheter diversion into internal stent drainage, antegrade ureteral stenting through the nephrostomy tract may be attempted even in cases in which previous attempts at retrograde stenting have failed. The antegrade approach to stenting can be expected to be successful if failure of retrograde stenting was not related to mere mechanical ureteral obstruction but rather to ureteral tortuosity, false passage (ureterovaginal fistula, urinoma after open surgery), or inability to identify the orifice endoscopically (ureterointestinal anastomosis).

For diagnostic procedures such as pressure/perfusion studies (Whitaker test), a 6F catheter is sufficient. Catheters of this size can be placed in a one-step procedure of puncture if coaxial needle/catheter systems are used (Figure 8–2). For therapeutic interventions such as nephrostomy drainage or antegrade ureteral stenting, softer, larger catheters must be inserted, and puncture tract dilation is necessary before catheter insertion. For dilation of a puncture tract, a 0.035- or 0.038-in guidewire must be inserted into the collecting system, either directly through the puncture needle or through the outer catheter of a coaxial needle/catheter system. Curved-tip (J) guidewires are less likely to cause damage to the mucosa of the renal pelvis than are straight guidewires. One of the most common problems of tract dilation is kinking of the guidewire during insertion of fascial dilators; therefore, guidewires with a floppy tip and a stiff proximal section (Lunderquist wire) are preferable over floppy guidewires. If the tip of the guidewire cannot be advanced into the renal pelvis because it is trapped in a dilated calyx with a narrow infundibulum or because an obstructing stone hinders passage, the outer catheter of a coaxial needle/catheter system can be used to manipulate the guidewire into the collecting system (Figure 8–6A), or angiographic catheters with different curved-tip configurations may be inserted over the guidewire for this purpose. Once the guidewire is in the correct position (upper calyx, renal pelvis, upper ureter), radiopaque fascial dilators can be inserted under fluoroscopic control with rotating movement of the dilator during advancement. If flexible plastic fascial dilators are used, sequential insertion of dilators of increasing size (usually in 2F steps) is necessary. If stiff metal or Kevlar dilators are used, dilation from 6F to 10–12F is possible in a one-step procedure.

After tract dilation, relatively stiff nephrostomy catheters (eg, polyethylene catheters) can be introduced easily over the guidewire. However, if softer catheters (eg, silicone or polyurethane catheters) are to be inserted, use of an introducer sheath is helpful. An introducer sheath is also helpful for antegrade ureteral stenting and for insertion of nephrostomy catheters with various self-retaining configurations of the tip (eg, pigtail). These catheters can be stretched into a straight configuration while being inserted through the introducer

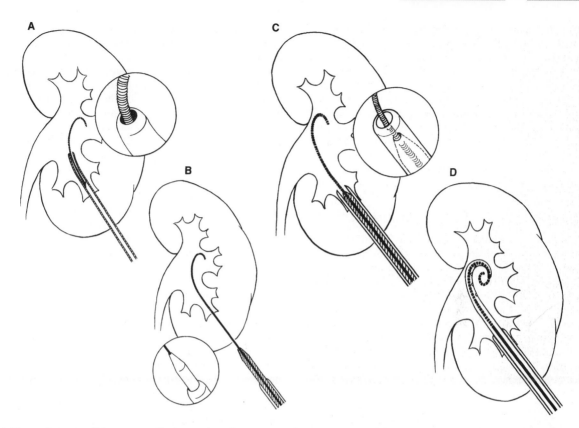

▲ **Figure 8–6.** Small-bore tract dilation and nephrostomy catheter insertion. ***A:*** J-guidewire inserted through the needle-sheath system and advanced with assistance of the plastic sheath into the renal pelvis. ***B:*** Insertion of a coaxial dilator/introducer sheath system over the guidewire. Stiff proximal section of the Lunderquist guidewire prevents extrarenal kinking. ***C:*** After the dilator has entered the collecting system, the introducer sheath is advanced over its tip. ***D:*** Pigtail nephrostomy catheter is inserted into the renal pelvis over the guidewire and through the introducer sheath.

sheath and over a guidewire; the tip resumes its original configuration due to the memory function of the material once the guidewire is withdrawn. The introducer sheath can be inserted with the last fascial dilator in a one-step procedure if a coaxial dilator/introducer sheath system is used (Figures 8–6B and C). The use of an introducer sheath provides universal access to the renal collecting system for placement of all types of catheters (nephrostomy catheters [Figure 8–6D], ureteral stents, balloon dilation catheters) and safety and working wires for different systems of large-bore nephrostomy tract dilation required for insertion of endoscopic instruments.

Nephrostomy catheters should be soft to avoid discomfort and irritation of the renal pelvis and should have a self-retaining mechanism or should be placed with enough slack to prevent dislodgment from the collecting system during movement of the kidney. Standard nephrostomy catheters are Malecot catheters, pigtail catheters, and loop catheters.

Loop catheters have a very effective retaining mechanism; they may cause serious complications, however, if the catheter is accidentally pulled out of the kidney.

Antegrade ureteral stenting can be done through the introducer sheath using either open- or closed-tip stents. Catheters with open-tip configuration are advanced with a pusher catheter over a guidewire, which must be inserted through the introducer sheath down the ureter and into the bladder as a first step. Catheters with closed-tip configuration are advanced by pushing the indwelling wire. In either technique, a thread through the proximal side hole of the catheter ensures that the catheter can be pulled back into the renal pelvis if it is advanced too far. The thread must be pulled out before the guidewire is withdrawn so that the pusher catheter can still hold the double-J stent in place.

An introducer sheath may also be used for insertion of a 7F balloon dilation catheter over a guidewire into the ureter to dilate ureteral strictures to 12–18F with balloon pressures of up to 15 atm. After successful dilation, an 8–10F stent is usually left indwelling for several weeks. This technique is most successful in ureteral strictures that are a complication of recent surgery for benign disorders, except ureteropelvic obstruction. Long-standing strictures or strictures due to tumor compression of the ureter, radiation damage, or ischemic ureteral necrosis after radical pelvic surgery are not likely to respond favorably to balloon dilation. Long-term results of ureteral balloon dilation cannot be determined from published data, either because the periods of follow-up were too short or because balloon dilations were repeated periodically.

ENDOSCOPIC INTRARENAL INSTRUMENTATION

Nephroscopes are endoscopic instruments with sheaths of 15–26F that are inserted percutaneously through a nephrostomy tract. Standard rigid instruments are available in sizes 18–26F; these have telescopes with offset eyepieces (Figure 8–7, left). Rigid instruments such as graspers and ultrasound probes can be inserted through a central working channel (Figure 8–7, right). Flexible fiberoptic nephroscopes may be used as well. These have a deflecting mechanism for the tip that allows inspection of otherwise difficult-to-reach calyces. A smaller working channel allows insertion of flexible instruments such as stone baskets, wire graspers, and electrohydraulic or laser probes. However, instrumentation through flexible nephroscopes is limited by the size and flexibility of working instruments such as stone forceps, and flexible endoscopes do not offer the optical quality and durability of rigid nephroscopes.

Nephroscopy is rarely indicated for diagnostic purposes only; in most cases, it is performed for percutaneous lithotripsy and extraction of renal stones (PNL). However, ESWL has gradually replaced PNL for treatment of renal stones and is now used in >90% of cases. PNL is still indicated in cases for which ESWL is not the primary choice of treatment. Such cases include urinary obstruction not caused by the stone itself, large-volume stones, and stones that cannot be positioned within the focus of the shock wave apparatus. PNL can achieve stone-free rates of >90%. Nephroscopes also may be used for direct-vision internal incision of ureteropelvic stenosis and for endoscopic treatment of urothelial tumors of the upper urinary tract.

Insertion of a nephroscope into the renal collecting system requires dilation of the puncture tract to 18–30F. A safety wire should be inserted parallel to the working wire and advanced into an upper calyx or the upper ureter to guide the way back into the collecting system in case the dilator and working wire become displaced accidentally. Insertion of an introducer sheath during small-bore tract dilation to 10–12F facilitates parallel insertion of safety and working wires. The central metal catheter of a coaxial metal dilator system (Figure 8–8, left), the central plastic catheter for insertion of sequential plastic dilators, or a balloon dilator can be inserted over the working wire. Balloon dilators of 9F size can dilate a nephrostomy tract to a diameter of 30F under pressure up to 10–12 atm in a one-step procedure. This may prove difficult or impossible if perirenal scar tissue from previous surgery prevents complete expansion of the balloon over its entire length. Sequential plastic dilators allow stepwise dilation of the tract under fluoroscopic control; however, on withdrawal

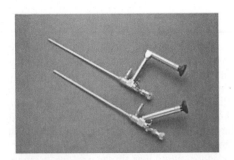
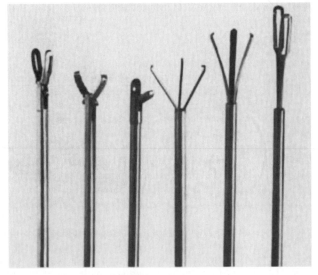

▲ **Figure 8-7.** Rigid nephroscopes. **Left:** Continuous-flow sheath telescopes with offset eyepieces for central access to a straight working channel. **Right:** Graspers and forceps for percutaneous endoscopic stone extraction.

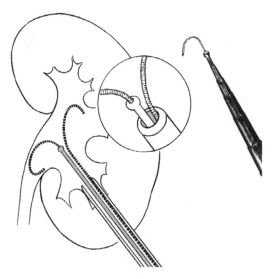

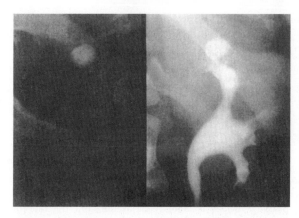

▲ **Figure 8–9.** Stone in upper caliceal diverticulum requiring percutaneous nephrolithotomy. ***Left:*** Plain abdominal radiograph. ***Right:*** Intravenous pyelogram.

▲ **Figure 8–8.** Large-bore tract dilation for nephroscopy. ***Left:*** Insertion of the central catheter of the Alken dilator system over a working wire through the introducer sheath (see also Figure 8–6). An introducer sheath allows parallel insertion of a safety wire into the collecting system. ***Right:*** Alken coaxial metal dilators for sequential tract dilation without loss of tract compression. Final step is coaxial insertion of a plastic working sheath or the metal nephroscope sheath.

▶ **Renal Stones**

In the era of ESWL, indications for PNL are limited to four types of stone disease:

1. Urinary obstruction not caused by the stone itself (eg, stone in a caliceal diverticulum [Figure 8–9, left and right], stone in association with ureteropelvic stenosis). These stones could be broken up by ESWL, but gravel would not pass spontaneously.

2. Large-volume stones (>3 cm, stone surface >500 mm^2) (Figure 8–10, left and right) (eg, staghorn stones). These stones can be treated by several sessions of ESWL, but only about 30% of patients become stone free. However,

for insertion of the next larger dilator, compression of the tract is lost intermittently and bleeding occurs into the collecting system, sometimes hindering subsequent endoscopy. Reusable Alken coaxial metal dilators (Figure 8–8, right) (each dilator slides over the next smaller one) allow stepwise tract dilation even in the presence of severe scarring with continuous nephrostomy tract compression for improved hemostasis.

With any dilation technique, the last step is insertion of a working sheath, which can be either the metal working sheath of the nephroscope or a larger Amplatz plastic sheath. With the balloon dilation technique, the Amplatz working sheath must be introduced over a plastic dilator; with use of serial plastic or coaxial metal dilators, the working sheath slides over the last dilator. The Pathway Access Sheath is a balloon dilator with coaxial external expandable sheath. It allows for balloon tract dilation and percutaneous access sheath placement in one step. A 28–30F Amplatz plastic working sheath is preferable to the metal nephroscope sheath in all cases in which extensive, prolonged instrumentation is anticipated (eg, staghorn stones). Larger plastic sheaths not only provide better drainage of irrigation fluid with lower intrapelvic pressures than do continuous-flow nephroscope sheaths but also allow easier extraction of large stone fragments.

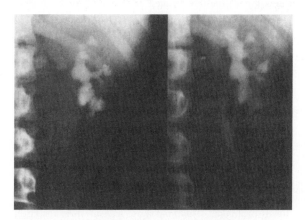

▲ **Figure 8–10.** Staghorn stone requiring combined percutaneous nephrolithotomy and extracorporeal shockwave lithotripsy. ***Left:*** Plain abdominal radiograph. ***Right:*** Intravenous pyelogram.

problems associated with passing large quantities of gravel (eg, ureteral obstruction, pain, fever, sepsis) can be prevented by first percutaneously debulking the stone and then performing ESWL for endoscopically inaccessible stones.

3. Stones that cannot be positioned within the focus of the shock wave apparatus (eg, stones in kidneys with abnormal position due to anomalies of the urinary tract or skeleton, stones in transplanted kidneys, kidney stones in very obese patients that cannot be positioned into the focus of the shock wave source due to the increased distance from skin to stone, or when the weight limit of the ESWL table is exceeded).

4. PNL may be of benefit for lower pole caliceal calculi even under the 2–3-cm range. The overall stone-free rate for these stones with ESWL is only about 60%.

Large-volume staghorn stones are a much more common indication for PNL than stones that can be extracted in toto. Small stones can be extracted with a variety of rigid forceps and graspers (Figure 8–7, right). Stones may be retrieved from difficult-to-reach calyces with flexible wire baskets and graspers inserted through flexible nephroscopes. Large stones must be disintegrated using mechanical, ultrasonic, electrohydraulic, or laser energy. Hollow ultrasonic probes allow for controllable, systematic stone disintegration under continuous suction for removal of sand and smaller fragments. Electrohydraulic probes are more powerful than ultrasonic probes and may be used through flexible nephroscopes, but they do not provide continuous suction and are associated with a higher risk of scattering stone fragments into inaccessible calyces and of damaging the mucosa of the renal pelvis. However, with electrohydraulic probes and the holmium: YAG laser, disintegration of hard or large stones is faster.

For soft stones, continuous disintegration and evacuation of fragments with ultrasound probes is most time efficient. Hard stones should be broken up into the largest possible fragments that can be extracted through the working sheath. The ureteropelvic portion of a staghorn stone should be left in place until the procedure is nearly completed, as it will act like a plug in a drain to prevent the loss of fragments into the ureter. An antegradely or retrogradely positioned ureteral balloon occlusion catheter might serve the same purpose; however, the extra procedure of retrograde ureteral catheterization is rarely indicated.

Normal saline should be used as the irrigation fluid except in the case of electrohydraulic lithotripsy, in which one-sixth normal saline is more appropriate. However, even with the low-pressure system provided by a large plastic working sheath, considerable amounts of irrigation fluid may be absorbed if small veins are opened and intrarenal manipulation is prolonged. This may cause transurethral resection (TUR) syndrome with use of hypotonic fluids. Intraoperative administration of diuretics (eg, mannitol, 12.5 g) is advisable and also has proved effective in preventing intrarenal reflux. If there is suspicion of extravasation, contrast dye must be injected and a diagnostic radiograph obtained. On completion of the procedure, a plain film should be obtained and a nephrostomy catheter placed. A Foley catheter with a 5-mL balloon may be inserted through a fenestrated trocar or through the plastic working sheath, which then is withdrawn and cut lengthwise for removal from the Foley catheter. Malecot catheters or straight polyethylene catheters (eg, chest tubes) may be used as well and should be secured to the skin with sutures. A final nephrostogram documents appropriate position of the catheter.

Nephrostomy catheters may be removed 1–4 days after antegrade pyelography to check for unobstructed upper urinary tract drainage. In cases of postoperative profuse hemorrhage, the nephrostomy catheter can be occluded for 1–2 days to allow for tamponade formation. Blood clots usually dissolve later spontaneously due to urokinase activity without problems. If ESWL is to be performed, it can be done 1–4 days after the percutaneous procedure. The nephrostomy catheter should be left in place during and after ESWL to provide drainage for urine and stone gravel and to allow for a second endoscopic procedure if some of the stone fragments do not pass spontaneously after ESWL.

After removing a large bore nephrostomy catheter (22–24F), urinary discharge from the nephrostomy tract can persist for several days and be bothersome and concerning to the patient. To prevent this, the nephrostomy tube can be exchanged over a guidewire under fluoroscopic guidance for a smaller caliber catheter. Leaving this smaller tube in place for a few days will permit the tissues around the tract to contract and minimize leakage.

Some experienced endourologists have propagated percutaneous stone treatment and endopyelotomy without standard placement of a nephrostomy catheter. Major advantages are marked reduction in analgesia requirements and length of hospitalization. Prerequisites are a small to moderate stone burden and no residual fragments, not more than two percutaneous tracts in one session, and no significant bleeding. Bleeding arising from the nephrostomy tract can be stopped nephroscopically by punctual electrocoagulation during withdrawal of the working sheath. However, this "tubeless" percutaneous renal surgery is best performed with intraoperative placement of a double-J ureteral stent to secure unobstructed urinary drainage. Expected patient discomfort from the nephrostomy catheter is traded against possible discomfort from the double-J ureteral stent and from cystoscopy to remove the stent later.

▶ Ureteropelvic Stenosis

With the advent of PNL and ureterorenoscopy, other endosurgical techniques have been developed that are similar to procedures used in the lower urinary tract. Direct-vision internal incision of ureteropelvic stenosis (pyelolysis, endopyelotomy, endopyeloplasty) seems to be a natural outgrowth of endoscopic techniques in the upper urinary tract.

Compared with the retrograde techniques of endopyelotomy (incision with a cold knife, Acucise catheter, Greenwald electrode, or laser) and the endoballoon dilation, the antegrade technique offers the advantage of an incision under direct vision. The cold-knife incision must be extended into the perirenal fat and is stented for 4–6 weeks to allow for healing, according to the principle of Davis' intubated ureterotomy.

Success rates of antegrade endopyelotomy of up to 65–95% are reported for primary cases and up to 89% for secondary cases after failed open-surgical pyeloplasty.

The success rates for retrograde endopyelotomy with fewer patients and less follow-up than in antegrade endopyelotomy range between 73% and 90%; for the Acucise endopyelotomy, between 76% and 81% (see Section "Ureteropelvic Stenosis"). The candidates for best endoscopic (antegrade and retrograde) outcome are those with less than grade II hydronephrosis and good renal function.

In most reports on endopyelotomy, the criteria of success differ from those of open pyeloplasty; relief of subjective symptoms is given priority over results of imaging studies such as decompression of a dilated collecting system on intravenous pyelography or renal ultrasound. Inadequate results after endopyelotomy may be related to a crossing vessel or to redundancy of the renal pelvis, which would be resected during open pyeloplasty. According to the law of Laplace, wall tension of a renal pelvis is, at the same intrapelvic pressures, higher in a more dilated collecting system with a larger diameter than in a less dilated system with a smaller diameter. A rise in tension supposedly represents a more important pathogenetic factor for developing progressive dilatation than elevated intrapelvic pressures due to anatomic obstruction of outflow. Secondary open pyeloplasty after failed endopyelotomy may be a more tedious operation with less satisfactory results in cases with extensive periureteral scarring due to extravasation of urine after endopyelotomy than primary open pyeloplasty.

▶ Renal Pelvis Tumor

Another technique of endoscopic surgery in the upper urinary tract is use of electroresection, electrocoagulation, electrovaporization, and neodymium:YAG laser coagulation for treatment of urothelial tumors of the renal pelvis. However, with the limited reports of treatment of upper urinary tract urothelial cancer endoscopically, recurrence rates are yet to be compared with those of standard surgical treatment.

Ensuring a strict follow-up, percutaneous management of transitional cell carcinoma of the collecting system may be an alternative to nephroureterectomy for patients with low-grade/low-stage tumors and for palliative treatment.

PERCUTANEOUS ASPIRATION AND BIOPSY

Percutaneous puncture of cystic or solid lesions of the kidney and the adjacent retroperitoneum is usually performed for diagnostic purposes, in some cases in combination with

Table 8–2. Indications for puncture of renal and retroperitoneal lesions.

Diagnostic indications
Fluid aspiration
Fluid chemistry
Bacteriology and sensitivity
Cytology
Radiography with percutaneously injected contrast dye
Histology (core biopsy)
Therapeutic indications
Catheter drainage
Urinoma, lymphocele
Abscess, hematoma
Fluid evacuation and injection of sclerosing agent
Simple renal cyst

therapeutic intentions such as drainage of fluid collections or obliteration of renal cysts (Tables 8–2 and 8–3). Because most of these lesions are radiolucent and are not enhanced with intravenously administered contrast dye, they cannot be visualized by fluoroscopy. Thus, ultrasound or CT scans are the imaging techniques of choice to depict these lesions and guide percutaneous puncture. The technique of ultrasonically guided puncture is the same whether the target is the renal collecting system or a cystic or solid renal or extrarenal lesion. For cytologic aspiration, a fine-needle (20–22 gauge) aspiration technique is used that is comparable with fine-needle aspiration biopsy of the prostate. There is no evidence that one type of needle is preferable to the others. For aspiration and evacuation of renal cysts or extrarenal fluid collections (urinoma, lymphocele), the same coaxial needle/

Table 8–3. Differential diagnosis of renal and retroperitoneal lesions.

Renal cystic lesion
Benign cyst
Hydrocalix
Abscess
Hematoma
Cystic tumor
Tumor in cyst
Retroperitoneal fluid collection
Urinoma
Lymphocele
Hematoma
Abscess
Cystic tumor
Solid renal and retroperitoneal lesions
Benign tumor
Malignant primary tumor
Metastatic tumor

catheter system can be used as for percutaneous puncture of the renal collecting system. A small catheter (6–10F) is placed for a few days to ensure complete drainage of fluid. When fluids of high viscosity (abscess, hematoma) are to be drained, large-bore catheters (14–20F) must be inserted, necessitating dilation of the percutaneous tract. Percutaneous renal biopsy for histologic diagnosis and classification of renal disease is performed with 14- to 16-gauge needles (eg, Franklin–Silverman, Tru-Cut) at the lower pole of the kidney.

▶ Renal Cysts

Renal cysts are found in about 50% of autopsy specimens in persons older than 50 years and are a frequent accidental finding on ultrasound or CT studies. Only a few cases require diagnostic percutaneous puncture. Indications for diagnostic puncture of a cystic lesion are an irregular, thick wall and internal echoes on ultrasound examination; density numbers on CT higher than those of serous fluid; and hematuria. Puncture for therapeutic procedures (evacuation of fluid and instillation of a sclerosing agent) is indicated only if, due to its size or location, the cyst causes compression and urinary obstruction of the neck of a calyx or the ureter, or discomfort and pain.

Various tests may be performed on aspirated fluid. No one test is pathognomonic except cytologic findings of malignant cells. However, neoplasms within a cyst are exceedingly rare, and cystic degeneration of a renal neoplasm can usually be easily identified by ultrasound and CT. Benign cysts contain clear, straw-colored fluid with low fat and protein content and lactic acid dehydrogenase levels of <250 mIU/mL. Cancer is suspected if the fluid is bloody or murky and has a high content of fat, protein, and lactic acid dehydrogenase. After aspiration of 20–30% of the cystic fluid, the same amount of 60% contrast dye is injected, and diagnostic radiographs are obtained in the prone, supine, upright, decubitus, and Trendelenburg positions. If necessary, another 20–30% of the cystic fluid may be replaced by air for obtaining double-contrast radiographs.

For therapeutic obliteration of cysts, sclerosing agents such as Pantopaque or 95% ethanol can be injected after complete evacuation of the cystic fluid. A volume of 10–100 mL of 95% ethanol, approximating 10–20% of the original volume of cystic fluid, is injected into the cyst and should be drained after 30 minutes.

▶ Retroperitoneal Fluid Collections

Low-viscosity retroperitoneal fluid collections (urinoma, lymphocele) are usually a complication of surgical procedures. However, urinoma may also be caused by exogenous trauma or by fornix rupture due to acute ureteral obstruction. Percutaneous techniques of catheter drainage eliminate the need for open surgical revision in most cases.

Insertion of a small (8–10F) catheter (with numerous side holes) is usually sufficient. Adjuvant measures are required to allow for sealing of a fluid leak or obliteration of a cyst. In

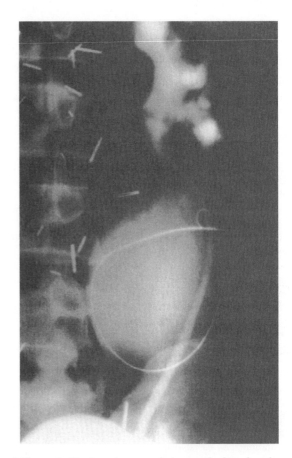

▲ **Figure 8–11.** Percutaneous drainage of a lymphocele causing ureteral displacement and compression.

cases of urinoma, the upper urinary tract must also be drained by a ureteral catheter or percutaneous nephrostomy catheter until drainage from the urinoma stops. Lymphoceles that develop following pelvic or retroperitoneal lymphadenectomy or renal transplantation often undergo spontaneous regression and usually do not require puncture and drainage. However, large lymphoceles developing after retroperitoneal lymphadenectomy may cause pain and even ureteral obstruction (Figure 8–11). Patients should be treated with parenteral nutrition, systemic administration of somatostatin, and abdominal compression by bandaging, but if lymph drainage after percutaneous puncture and catheter placement persists for >1 week, surgical intervention with intraperitoneal marsupialization of the lymphocele and ligation or electrocoagulation of lymphatic vessels is indicated.

High-viscosity fluid collections (hematoma, abscess) usually require a large-bore (14–20F) percutaneous catheter for sufficient drainage. Perirenal hematomas are most frequently caused by surgical or exogenous trauma and rarely develop spontaneously in the presence of a bleeding disorder or due to rupture of a renal tumor. Indications for percutaneous drainage are rare, as most small hematomas resolve spontaneously and should be followed by ultrasound or CT only. A hematoma that increases in size requires surgical intervention rather than percutaneous drainage. Secondary infection of a hematoma may be an indication for percutaneous drainage.

A perirenal abscess is mostly a complication of surgery; hematogenic renal abscess (renal carbuncle) is less frequent. Indications for puncture and drainage should be based on CT finding of a unifocal process that can be effectively and safely drained percutaneously. Multifocal renal abscess formation is not amenable to percutaneous drainage.

▶ Renal and Retroperitoneal Tumors

Percutaneous aspiration biopsy of renal and retroperitoneal tumors is indicated if less invasive radiographic studies are inconclusive and if cytologic findings may have an impact on further medical or surgical therapy (Figure 8–12). If curative treatment by open surgery seems to be feasible, aspiration biopsy is generally not indicated. If the identity of a renal lesion is questionable or if conservative, organ-sparing surgery is technically feasible, surgical excision of the lesion with intraoperative frozen sections is preferable over percutaneous aspiration biopsy. However, aspiration biopsy may be indicated to avoid radical nephrectomy of a possibly benign lesion. In multifocal or possibly metastatic lesions, cytologic evaluation can be crucial for planning surgical or medical therapy, and in these cases, aspiration biopsy is usually indicated. Interpretation of cytologic findings is limited by a 10–25% incidence of false-negative findings and the difficulty in discriminating normal renal tubular cells from low-grade renal cell cancer. As a rare complication, tumor seeding in the puncture tract has been described. The aspirate is immediately spread on glass slides. For standard Papanicolaou stains, alcohol fixation must be used.

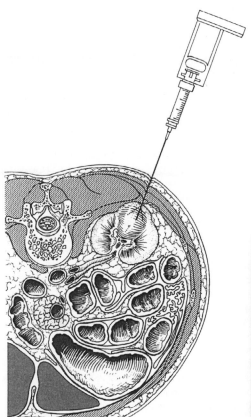

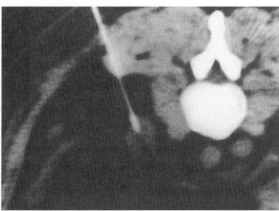

▲ **Figure 8–12.** Percutaneous fine-needle biopsy. **Left:** Aspiration biopsy of a renal lesion. **Right:** Guidance with computed tomography scanning for fine-needle aspiration biopsy of an exophytic renal cell carcinoma.

The widespread use of ultrasound has led to an increased rate of incidental diagnosis of small renal tumors, which account for 48–66% of renal cell carcinoma diagnoses. With the advent of minimally invasive techniques and improved radiodiagnostic possibilities, nonresectional renal tumor ablation has emerged and is gaining increased attention. However, cryotherapy, radiofrequency ablation (RFA), and high-intensity focused ultrasound (HIFU) are still considered experimental procedures in the clinical setting. However, cryotherapy and RFA are proving to be viable strategies for the treatment of small renal masses based on short-term and intermediate-term oncological outcomes. In a meta-analysis by treatment modality, 77.8% of tumors were treated by partial nephrectomy, 7.7% by cryoablation, 9.4% by RFA, and 5.1% by active surveillance. The therapeutic strategies of local energy application aim at selective tumor destruction with minimal injury to the surrounding normal kidney parenchyma and reduced morbidity. Cryotherapy is the most evaluated probe ablative method for the treatment of small renal masses. The biological principle of cryotherapy is tissue destruction by repeated rapid freeze and thaw cycles down to temperatures below −20°C. Liquid argon and liquid nitrogen are the two most commonly used freezing agents. The cell destruction mechanism comprises intra- and extracellular ice crystal formation leading to intracellular dehydration and ultimately cell disruption. This is followed by a delayed cell death, which occurs during the thaw phase owing to vasoconstriction and microcirculatory failure. Repeating the freeze–thaw cycle intensifies tissue damage. However, since the freezing effect decreases with increasing distance from the freezing probe, the "iceball" has to extend approximately 1 cm beyond the tumor margin to ensure complete tumor destruction. RFA involves coagulation of tumors by directly applying temperatures of 50–100°C throughout the tumor via needle electrodes. Since tissue carbonization at the electrode tip increases the impedance for radiofrequency transmission, tissue conductivity can be maintained by simultaneously irrigating saline through the tissue ("wet" RFA), resulting in larger RFA lesions for therapy of larger renal tumors. This can also be accomplished by multiple electrodes, which create overlapping ablation fields. The vicinity of larger caliber vessels results in dissipation of heat ("heat sink effect") and influences the efficacy of RFA negatively. Thus, peripheral exophytic tumors seem to be controlled better than central tumors in the vicinity of larger vessels.

Indications are similar for both techniques and are presently restricted to patients with comorbidity and/or advanced age who are not suitable to surgical treatment, impaired renal function, multiple bilateral tumors as in von Hippel–Lindau disease, and renal tumors in a solitary kidney. Guidelines for cryotherapy do not recommend treatment of tumors >3 cm in size and for RFA not >5 cm. Further relative contraindications for both procedures include hilar or central tumors and cystic tumors. An absolute contraindication is untreated coagulopathy.

The tumor mass can be approached by open surgery, laparoscopy, or percutaneously using fine probes and high-resolution imaging techniques. However, the minimally invasive character of the procedure itself ideally deserves a less invasive approach than open surgery. Proponents of laparoscopy emphasize the advantage of mobilizing the tumor and providing excellent exposure, thus avoiding damage to adjacent structures. It also allows for precise confirmation of probe positioning and monitoring the progress of the procedure such as development of the iceball in cryotherapy under direct vision. Percutaneous management requires MRI, CT scan with technical capabilities to construct three-dimensional pictures, or real-time ultrasound guidance for monitoring probe placement and progress of therapy. The percutaneous approach may be performed as an outpatient procedure, and it is typically reserved for posterior tumors. Special patients requiring multiple procedures as in von Hippel–Lindau disease thus may benefit from a percutaneous treatment. In contrast to cryoablation, which has the advantage of intraoperative laparoscopic and sonographic monitoring of the ice ball, RFA lacks reliable real-time monitoring of the therapeutic progress. However, the introduction of real-time MRI guidance and monitoring of RFA may overcome this difficulty.

Both methods, cryotherapy and RFA, have shown promising results in carefully selected patients. Cryotherapy is associated with 93% and 81% 5- and 10-year cancer-specific survival, respectively. However, significantly increased local progression rates were calculated for cryoablation (relative risk = 7.45) and RFA (relative risk = 18.23) as compared with partial nephrectomy. And follow-up of partial nephrectomy series is still considerably longer than for ablative techniques. It must be emphasized that a significant selection bias exists in the application of these techniques. Published series of ablative treatment options include statistically significant older patients and smaller tumors as compared with the standard of partial nephrectomy. Also, a significant number of tumors treated with ablative techniques have unknown or indeterminate histology that could influence oncological results as a confounding factor. Furthermore, it is important to consider that different criteria may be used to define disease recurrence for ablative and for resectional techniques, hampering comparison of results. In contrast to cryotherapy, where tumor size decreases with time, tumor size after RFA remains mostly constant. Tumor size after successful cryotherapy can decrease up to 75% over 3 years, and tumors may even completely disappear on MRI in some cases. This fact is important for posttreatment surveillance. A major drawback of ablative techniques is the lack of reliable histologic confirmation of complete tumor ablation. Assessment is commonly done by CT scan. After RFA, a successfully ablated lesion becomes fibrotic and nonperfused and does not show contrast enhancement as compared with a viable tumor.

Complication rates (major and minor) of cryotherapy are 1.4% and 12.2%, and complication rates of RFA are 2.2% and 6%, respectively. The most commonly observed complications of cryotherapy and RFA are pain, paresthesia, and hemorrhage at the probe insertion site, occurring in approximately 5% of all patients. Rare complications include perinephric hematoma, renal rupture, UPJ obstruction, and damage to adjacent organs. Anteriorly or centrally located tumors that abut the UPJ pose an increased risk for complications, especially colonic injuries or lesions of the renal collecting system and ureter. Bleeding complications have decreased with the use of ultrathin probes (1.5 mm diameter). Specifically for RFA, bleeding can be minimized by active coagulation of the puncture tract while removing the probe. Conversion rates for cryoablation (3.5%) are similar to laparoscopic partial nephrectomy rates (3.9%) and higher than RFA rates (1.6%).

Ablative methods are still constantly evolving. Uncertainties exist regarding the exact amount of energy required, duration of treatment, mode of energy delivery, and types of electrodes used and render comparison of published results difficult. The adjunctive use of chemotherapeutic agents such as cyclophosphamide, 5-fluorouracil, and bleomycin or radiotherapy may have a synergistic effect on cryoablation and intensify its ablative capabilities. Further development of imaging techniques and combination with new technologies, such as single-port laparoscopic and natural orifice transluminal endoscopic surgery (NOTES), may potentially expand the indication range for ablative surgery.

Other techniques with limited animal and clinical experience that remain experimental include HIFU, microwave thermotherapy (MT), laser interstitial thermotherapy (LITT), pulsed cavitational ultrasound, chemoablation with or without radiofrequency, and radiosurgery.

▶ Renal Biopsy

Renal biopsy for diagnosis and classification of medical renal disease can be performed percutaneously or by open surgery. Because specimens, rather than aspirates, are needed for diagnostic histologic study, large-bore (14–16 gauge) Franklin–Silverman or Tru-Cut needles are used. Ultrasonic or fluoroscopic guidance is preferable to blind renal puncture. However, even with puncture aimed precisely at the dorsal aspect of the lower pole of the kidney, where accidental injury to large vessels is less likely, bleeding is to be expected because of the vascularity of the parenchyma and is the major complication of this procedure (about 5% of cases, with a mortality rate of 0.1%). Hematoma can usually be followed conservatively by ultrasound or CT scan, but transvascular embolization, open surgical revision, and even nephrectomy have been required following diagnostic renal biopsy.

Therefore, open surgical biopsy rather than percutaneous biopsy is indicated in patients with solitary kidneys or uncontrolled hypertension.

URETERORENOSCOPY

Ureterorenoscopy is endoscopy of the ureter up to the renal pelvis for both diagnostic evaluation and therapeutic intervention (Table 8–4).

Ureterorenoscopes (Figure 8–13) are endoscopes for retrograde insertion into the ureter; however, they may also be used in an antegrade fashion via a percutaneously established nephrostomy tract. Technical improvements in the last decade have led to the introduction of smaller caliber, more versatile instruments. As a consequence of this progress, the ureterorenoscopic approach is used more widely, not only for management of urinary calculi but also for treatment of urothelial tumors. Rigid ureterorenoscopes are available in sizes 7–12F, and semirigid fiberoptic ureterorenoscopes and flexible ureterorenoscopes in sizes 6–9F. The smallest instruments are for diagnostic procedures only. Larger instruments, with a 3–6F working channel, can accept stone baskets, wire graspers, stone forceps, biopsy forceps, and ultrasonic, electrohydraulic, or laser probes for stone disintegration. Flexible ureterorenoscopes follow the topographic anatomy of the ureter more easily and facilitate inspection of middle and lower renal calyces if a deflecting mechanism for the tip of the instrument is provided. Newer state-of-the-art flexible ureterorenoscopes have 270° deflecting tips (dual active deflection) that allow access to virtually every calyx of the collecting system. However, the use of instrumentation through flexible nephroscopes is limited by the size and flexibility of working instruments such as stone forceps, and flexible ureterorenoscopes do not offer the optical quality and durability of rigid instruments.

Insertion of a ureterorenoscope into the ureteral orifice may be facilitated by dilation of the intramural ureter, either with sequential plastic dilators of increasing size, which are slid over a guidewire, or with a balloon dilator catheter (Figure 8–14). Dilation of the ureter is often unnecessary if a small (3–4F) ureteral catheter is inserted through the working channel of the ureterorenoscope into the ureter as a guide, and the ureterorenoscope is then rotated 180° and

Table 8–4. Indications for ureterorenoscopy.

Diagnostic indications
    Lesions of ureter or renal pelvis
    Hematuria from the upper tract
Therapeutic indications
    Ureteral stone treatment
    Direct vision internal ureterotomy of ureteral strictures
    Endoscopic resection and coagulation of ureteral tumors

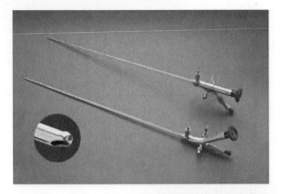

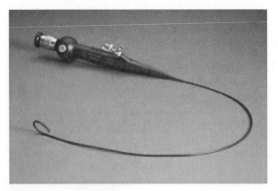

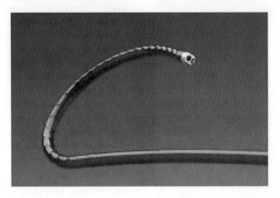

▲ **Figure 8–13.** Ureterorenoscopes: 8F telescopes with center and offset eyepieces. 7.5F flexible ureteroscope with 270° tip deflection.

introduced in an upside-down orientation (Figure 8–15). In this position, the ureteral catheter will spread the roof of the intramural ureter like a tent and the nose of the instrument will slide flat on the trigone into the orifice. The orifice and intramural ureter will thus be dilated only to the extent necessary for insertion of the instrument.

▶ **Diagnostic Ureterorenoscopy**

Indications for diagnostic ureterorenoscopy are those rare lesions of the ureter or renal pelvis whose nature cannot be determined with less invasive diagnostic procedures such as retrograde pyelography, selective urinary cytology, CT, or MRI. If a small ureterorenoscope without a working channel is used for a diagnostic procedure, a biopsy of a lesion cannot be obtained. If ureterorenoscopy is performed for evaluation of hematuria from the upper tract, the source of bleeding can rarely be identified during gross hematuria because of limited irrigation through ureterorenoscopes, resulting in poor visibility. If the urine has cleared, the chances of identifying a lesion that could not be detected on radiographic studies are small as well.

▶ **Ureteral Stones**

Ureterorenoscopy is most frequently performed for treatment of ureteral stones, although >90% of ureteral stones can be treated by ESWL either in situ or after repositioning the ureteral stone into the renal pelvis using a ureteral catheter (push-back or flush-back procedures). For the remaining indications of ureteral stone treatment, ureterorenoscopy is used for extraction of stones, repositioning of stones into the renal pelvis for subsequent ESWL, and intraureteral stone disintegration. Growing experience in general ureteroscopic techniques and the use of smaller caliber instruments have also rendered the procedure practicable and safe in the pediatric population, with no evidence of decreasing renal function, and/or renal growth or initiation of vesicoureteral reflux after the procedure.

For extraction of a distal ureteral stone that is unresponsive to ESWL, a short rigid ureterorenoscope and alligator forceps or Dormia basket approach are most helpful. Ureteroscopic clearance rates for distal ureteral stones approach 93–100%. Impacted proximal ureteral stones that did not respond to in situ ESWL and could not be mobilized with a

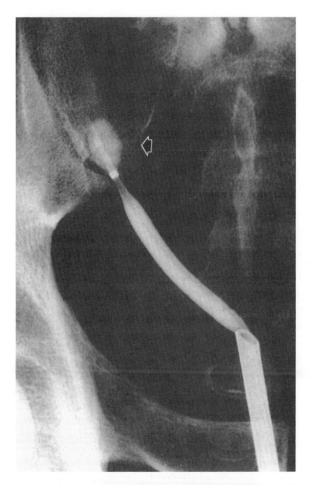

▲ **Figure 8–14.** Ureteral dilation with balloon catheter before ureterorenoscopic removal of a distal ureteral stone (*arrow*).

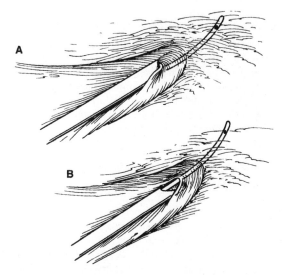

▲ **Figure 8–15.** Ureterorenoscopy. **A:** Straightforward advancement of the instrument over a thin ureteral catheter or guidewire can catch the mucosa of the orifice. **B:** With 180° upside-down rotation of the instrument, the ureteral catheter holds the orifice open like a tent.

ureteral catheter usually can be repositioned into the renal pelvis under direct vision for subsequent ESWL using a small semirigid or rigid ureterorenoscope. If the stones are too large or impacted, intraureteral lithotripsy for stone disintegration may become necessary. Flexible ureteroscopic instrumentation in the upper ureter and the necessity to pass and withdraw the ureteroscope repeatedly to extract stone fragments bear an increased risk of injury to the ureter. Hence, in skilled hands, stone clearance rates for proximal ureteral calculi range from 82% to 87%. The "ureteral access sheath" has been developed to facilitate ureteral reentry and to allow multiple reinsertions of the ureterorenoscope into the upper urinary tract while reducing trauma to the distal ureter. The introducer sheath is available in sizes 12–16F. The better drainage of irrigation fluid from the introducer sheath allows

endoscopy to be performed with increased irrigation flow rates, thus enhancing visualization of the upper urinary tract while maintaining low (<40 cm) intrapelvic pressures. Use of an introducer sheath is also supposed to decrease wear on the ureteroscope and reduce operative time. However, controversy still exists regarding a possible risk of ureteral injury from placement of the working sheath resulting in ureteral stricture rates of 1.4%, which, however, are still in the range of modern series of flexible ureteroscopy without the introducer sheath.

To prevent pushing back of stones or fragments into the renal pelvis during lithotripsy, a 3F wire basket can be used to hold the stone during disintegration or a 3F balloon catheter can be passed alongside the stone and blocked proximally. The Dretler stone cone (Microvasive; Boston Scientific, Natick, MA) is a nitinol device that applies the same principle. It can be coiled proximal to the stone, preventing upward ureteral migration of stone fragments during lithotripsy and facilitating stone fragment retrieval after successful disintegration. Ultrasound probes allow safe stone disintegration under continuous suction, but they are not as effective as electrohydraulic and laser probes and can be used through rigid ureterorenoscopes only. Pneumatic probes are thinner, very effective, and require rather inexpensive equipment, but can only be used through rigid and semirigid ureterorenoscopes. Both electrohydraulic and laser probes can be used through rigid or flexible ureterorenoscopes. Laser probes for intraureteral lithotripsy have the smallest diameter (<1F) and do not harm the mucosa of the ureter if used under direct vision. Several pulsed lasers such as holmium:YAG laser, pulsed-dye laser, and Alexandrite laser are available for intraureteral lithotripsy. The holmium:YAG laser is most widely used for ureteroscopic lithotripsy because of its high efficiency. It can successfully disintegrate stones of any composition with stone fragmentation rates approaching 100%. Moreover, it can be used to coagulate, ablate, and incise tissues. Laser probes are flexible and as small as 200 μm in core diameter so that they can be easily passed through flexible ureteroscopes without hindering tip deflection and, thus, maximize their durability. Electrohydraulic probes, which are available in sizes 1.6–5F, require less expensive equipment, but they bear the risk of ureteral damage if used inappropriately. The combination of flexible ureteroscopy with atraumatic ancillary tools, such as nitinol tipless baskets and thin holmium laser fibers (200 μm), permits ureteroscopic treatment of renal stones when ESWL or percutaneous treatment are not an option or have failed. A 79–90% success rate has been reported for lower pole stones treated ureteroscopically. However, success is highly dependent on number of stones and stone size and multiple procedures may be required. If ureteral perforation occurs as a complication of intraureteral instrumentation, ureteral stenting using a 6–8F double-J stent for 2–6 weeks usually allows healing without late sequelae. Stents should be used for a few days even after uncomplicated ureterorenoscopy to prevent pain from urinary stasis because of edema of the intramural ureter after instrumentation. If there is ureteral perforation and a stent has been placed, the bladder should be on continuous drainage for a few days using a transurethral Foley catheter or a suprapubic cystostomy catheter to prevent urinoma formation from vesicoureteral reflux via the double-J stent.

Ureteropelvic Stenosis

Ureteroscopic endopyelotomy of UPJ obstruction is feasible with cold knife, electrocautery, or holmium laser. Success rates range between 73% and 90% in different series. However, subsequent repeat balloon dilation of the UPJ may be required in 10% of cases, and 3% may even require repeat incision. At least 10% of recurrences are treated by open or laparoscopic surgery. Thus, the advantages of this minimally invasive procedure such as a reduced hospitalization time and convalescence are at the cost of poorer outcomes compared with open or laparoscopic pyeloplasty. Also, the risk of complications of ureteroscopy, which range between 1% and 15%, such as ureteral perforation, stricture, false passage, ureteral avulsion, bleeding, and sepsis must be weighed against the possible benefits.

In recent years, Acucise endopyelotomy has gained increased attention as an alternative treatment of UPJ obstruction and other postoperative ureteral strictures in selected patients. It is simple and a truly minimally invasive method that can be performed in an ambulatory setting, but it relies on fluoroscopic rather than visual ureteroscopic guidance. The device permits combining balloon dilatation and incision by electrocautery in one step. Overall success rates for UPJ range between 76% and 81%, and even better outcomes are reported in secondary UPJ obstruction. Prognosticators of treatment failure of UPJ are a stricture length >2 cm, <20% split renal function, the presence of either anterior or posterior crossing vessels, and massive hydronephrosis.

Ureteral Strictures

Cold-knife, electrocautery, or laser incision of a stenosis into the periureteral fat should be followed by stenting of the ureter for 4–6 weeks according to Davis' principle of intubated ureterotomy. The intraoperative use of an endoscopic ultrasound probe can provide important information about the exact stricture location and its relation to adjacent structures and, thus, help to direct the incision.

Best results are obtained in ureteral strictures that are a complication of surgery for benign disorders if treatment is established early. Proximal and distal ureteral strictures respond better to endoureterotomy than midureteral strictures. However, long-term results of this technique as compared with open surgical repair remain to be determined. Long-standing strictures or strictures due to external ureteral compression, radiation damage, or ischemic ureteral necrosis after surgery are not satisfactorily treated by internal ureterotomy. Acucise treatment of ureteral strictures should be reserved for short strictures (<1.5 cm) in a good functioning kidney.

Ureteral Tumors

Endoscopic electroresection and laser coagulation of ureteral tumors are the ureterorenoscopic variants of percutaneous endoscopic treatment of renal pelvis tumors (see Sections "Endoscopic Intrarenal Instrumentation" and "Renal Pelvis Tumor"). Endoscopic treatment of urothelial tumors of the upper urinary tract with curative intent is still confined to low-grade/low-stage small tumors in a solitary kidney, bilateral disease, or chronic renal failure. Follow-up ureterorenoscopy allows surveillance of patients after organ-sparing treatment and simultaneous biopsy, if necessary. Although rare, benign fibroepithelioma of the ureter (Figure 8–16) is sufficiently treated by ureterorenoscopic techniques. The same precautions and limitations apply for endoscopic treatment of urothelial cancer of the ureter as listed previously for percutaneous endoscopic treatment of renal pelvis tumors.

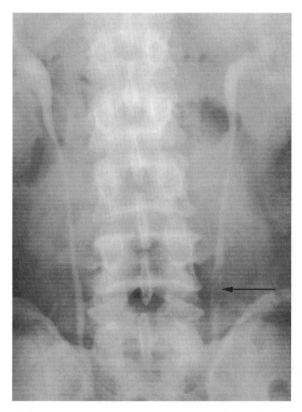

▲ **Figure 8–16.** Intravenous pyelogram revealing a fibro-epithelioma in the midleft ureter (*arrow*) without urinary obstruction.

BIBLIOGRAPHY

Percutaneous Catheter Placement

Dyer RB et al: Update on interventional uroradiology. Urol Clin North Am 1997;24:623.

Gofrit ON et al: Lateral decubitus position for percutaneous nephrolithotripsy in the morbidly obese or kyphotic patient. J Endourol 2002;16(6):383.

Goodwin WE et al: Percutaneous trocar (needle) nephrostomy in hydronephrosis. JAMA 1955;157:891.

Kaye KW, Goldberg ME: Applied anatomy of the kidney and ureter. Urol Clin North Am 1982;9:3.

Lau MWM et al: Urinary tract obstruction and nephrostomy drainage in pelvic malignant disease. Br J Urol 1995;76:565.

Pedersen JF: Percutaneous nephrostomy guided by ultrasound. J Urol 1974;112:157.

See WA: Continuous antegrade infusion of Adriamycin as adjuvant therapy for upper tract urothelial malignancies. Urology 2000;56(2):216.

Seldinger SI: Catheter replacement of the needle in percutaneous arteriography. Acta Radiol 1953;39:368.

Smith AD, Badlani GH: Special use of retrograde percutaneous nephrostomy in endourology. J Endourol 1987;1:23.

Tekin MI et al: Practical approach to terminate urinary extravasation: Percutaneous fistula tract embolization with *N*-butyl cyanoacrylate in a case with partial nephrectomy. Tech Urol 2001;7(1):67.

Thüroff JW, Alken P: Ultrasound for renal puncture and fluoroscopy for tract dilatation and catheter placement: A combined approach. Endourology 1987;2:1.

Thüroff JW, Becht E: Urologist's ultrasound. In: Lytton B et al (eds) Advances in Urology, Vol. 1. Year Book Medical Publishers, 1988.

Antegrade Pyelography and Pressure/Perfusion Studies

Ahlawat R, Basarge N: Objective evaluation of the outcome of endopyelotomy using Whitaker's test and diuretic renography. Br J Urol 1995;76:686.

Jones A et al: Compliance studies, pressure flow measurements and renal function assessment in patients with upper urinary tract dilatation. J Urol 1987;138:571.

Kashi SH et al: Does the Whitaker test add to antegrade pyelography in the investigation of collecting system dilatation in renal allografts? Br J Radiol 1993;66:877.

Pagne S, Ramsay J: The effect of double-J-stents on renal pelvic dynamics in the pig. J Urol 1988;140:637.

Whitaker RH: Methods of assessing obstruction in dilated ureters. Br J Urol 1973;45:15.

Whitaker RH, Buxton-Thomas MS: A comparison of pressure flow studies and renography in equivocal upper urinary tract obstruction. J Urol 1984;131:446.

Woodburg P et al: Constant pressure perfusion: A method to determine obstruction in the upper urinary tract. J Urol 1989;142:632.

Percutaneous Renal Stone Treatment

Albala DM et al: Lower pole I: A prospective randomized trial of extracorporeal shock wave lithotripsy and percutaneous nephrostolithotomy for lower pole nephrolithiasis: Initial results. J Urol 2001;166(6):2072.

Alken P et al: Percutaneous nephrolithotomy: A routine procedure? Br J Urol 1983;51(Suppl):1.

Calvert RC, Burgess NA: Urolithiasis and obesity: Metabolic and technical considerations. Curr Opin Urol 2005;15(2):113.

Cato AR, Tulloch AGS: Hypermagnesemia in a uremic patient during renal pelvis irrigation with Renacidin. J Urol 1974;111:313.

Chatham JR et al: Effect of percutaneous nephrolithotomy on differential renal function as measured by mercaptoacetyl triglycine nuclear renography. Urology 2002;59(4):522, discussion 525.

Desai MR et al: A prospective randomized comparison of type of nephrostomy drainage following percutaneous nephrostolithotomy: Large bore versus small bore versus tubeless. J Urol 2004;172(2):565.

el-Damanhoury H et al: Surgical aspects of urolithiasis in children. Pediatr Nephrol 1991;5:339.

Feng MI et al: Prospective randomized study of various techniques of percutaneous nephrolithotomy. Urology 2001;58(3):345.

Fernström I, Johansson B: Percutaneous pyelolithotomy: A new extraction technique. Scand J Urol Nephrol 1976;10:257.

Heimbach D et al: Percutaneous chemolysis: An important tool in the treatment of urolithiasis. Int Urol Nephrol 1998;30(6):655.

Holman E et al: Simultaneous bilateral compared with unilateral percutaneous nephrolithotomy. BJU Int 2002;89(4):334.

Jou YC et al: Nephrostomy tube-free percutaneous nephrolithotomy for patients with large stones and Staghorn stones. Urology 2006;67(1):30.

Lahme S et al: Minimally invasive PCNL in patients with renal pelvic and calyceal stones. Eur Urol 2001;40(6):619.

Limb J, Bellman GC: Tubeless percutaneous renal surgery: Review of first 112 patients. Urology 2002;59(4):527, discussion 531.

Minon Cifuentes J et al: Percutaneous nephrolithotomy in transplanted kidney. Urology 1991;38:232.

Osman M et al: Percutaneous nephrolithotomy with ultrasonography-guided renal access: Experience from over 300 cases. BJU Int 2005;96(6):875.

Pathak AS, Bellman GC: One-step percutaneous nephrolithotomy sheath versus standard two-step technique. Urology 2005; 66(5):953.

Ramakumar S, Segura JW: Renal calculi: Percutaneous management [review]. Urol Clin North Am 2000;27(4):617.

Rao PN et al: Prediction of septicemia following endourological manipulation for stones in the upper urinary tract. J Urol 1991; 146:955.

Schwartz BF, Stoller M: Percutaneous management of caliceal diverticula [review]. Urol Clin North Am 2000;27(4):635.

Segura JW et al: Percutaneous removal of kidney stones: Review of 1000 cases. J Urol 1985;134:1077.

Segura JW: The role of percutaneous surgery in renal and ureteral stone removal. J Urol 1989;141(Pt 2 of 2):780.

Segura JW: Role of percutaneous procedures in the management of renal calculi. Urol Clin North Am 1990;17:207.

Suby HI, Albright F: Dissolution of phosphatic urinary calculi by the retrograde introduction of citrate solution containing magnesium. N Engl J Med 1943;228:81.

Thüroff JW, Alken P: Stones in caliceal diverticula: Removal by percutaneous nephrolithotomy. In: Jonas U et al (eds) Endourology: New and Approved Techniques. Springer-Verlag, 1988.

Wong MY: An update on percutaneous nephrolithotomy in the management of urinary calculi [review]. Curr Opin Urol 2001; 11(4):367.

Percutaneous Endoscopic Surgery

American Urological Association: Guideline for Management of the Clinical Stage 1 Renal Mass. Available at: http://www.auanet.org/content/guidelines-and-quality-care/clinical-guidelines/main-reports/renalmass09.pdf. Accessed: September 22, 2009.

Aron M, Gill IS: Renal tumor ablation. Curr Opin Urol 2005;15(5):298.

Aslan P, Preminger GM: Retrograde balloon cautery incision of ureteropelvic junction obstruction. Urol Clin North Am 1998;25:295.

Berger A et al: Cryoablation for renal tumors: current status. Curr Opin Urol 2009;19:138.

Bernardo NO, Smith AD: Percutaneous endopyelotomy. Urology 2000;56:322.

Chow WH et al: Rising incidence of renal cell cancer in the United States. JAMA 1999;281(17):1628.

Danuser H et al: Endopyelotomy for primary ureteropelvic junction obstruction: Risk factors determine the success rate. J Urol 1998;159(1):56.

Danuser H et al: Influence of stent size on the success of antegrade endopyelotomy for primary ureteropelvic junction obstruction: Results of 2 consecutive series. J Urol 2001;166(3):902.

Davis DM: Intubated ureterotomy: A new operation for ureteral and ureteropelvic strictures. Surg Gynecol Obstet 1943;76:513.

Delakas D et al: Long-term results after percutaneous minimally invasive procedure treatment of symptomatic simple renal cysts. Int Urol Nephrol 2001;32(3):321.

Delvecchio FC et al: Combined antegrade and retrograde endoscopic approach for the management of urinary diversion-associated pathology. J Endourol 2000;14(3):251.

Figenshau RS, Clayman RV: Endourologic options for management of ureteropelvic junction obstruction in the pediatric patient. Urol Clin North Am 1998;25:199.

Gill IS: Renal cryotherapy: Pro. Urology 2005;65(3):415.

Gill IS, et al: Renal cryoablation: Outcome at 3 years. J Urol 2005;173(6):1903.

Goldfischer ER, Smith AD: Endopyelotomy revisited. Urology 1998;51:855.

Hauser S, Studer UE: Therapy of carcinoma of the kidney pelvis. Urologe A 2001;40(6):452.

Hibi H et al: Retrograde ureteroscopic endopyelotomy using the holmium:YAG laser. Int J Urol 2002;9(2):77.

Hulbert JC et al: Percutaneous intrarenal marsupialization of a perirenal cystic collection: Endocystolysis. J Urol 1988;139:1039.

Hvarness H et al: Long-term remission of transitional cell carcinoma after Bacillus Calmette-Guérin instillation in the renal pelvis. J Urol 2001;166(5):1829.

Jabbour ME et al: Percutaneous management of grade II upper urinary tract transitional cell carcinoma: The long-term outcome. J Urol 2000;163:1105.

Kapoor R et al: Endopyelotomy in poorly functioning kidney: Is it worthwhile? J Endourol 2001;15(7):725.

Kumar R et al: Optimum duration of splinting after endopyelotomy. J Endourol 1999;13(2):89.

Kunkle DA et al: Excise, ablate or observe: The small renal mass dilemma—A meta-analysis and review. J Urol 2008;179:1227.

McAchran SE et al: Radiofrequency ablation of renal tumors: Past, present, and future. Urology 2005;66(5A):15.

Meretyk I et al: Endopyelotomy: Comparison of ureteroscopic retrograde and antegrade percutaneous techniques. J Urol 1992;148:775.

Nakada SY et al: Retrospective analysis of the effect of crossing vessels on successful retrograde endopyelotomy outcomes using spiral computerized tomography angiography. J Urol 1998;159:62.

Okubo K et al: Intrarenal bacillus Calmette-Guérin therapy for carcinoma in situ of the upper urinary tract: Long-term follow-up and natural course in cases of failure. BJU Int 2001;88(4):343.

Potter SR et al: Percutaneous endoscopic management of urothelial tumors of the renal pelvis. Urology 2001;58(3):457.

Rosdy E: Percutaneous transrenal ureteroneocystostomy. J Endourol 1999;13(5):369.

Savage SJ, Streem SB: Simplified approach to percutaneous endopyelotomy. Urology 2000;56:848.

Schenkman EM, Terry WF: Comparison of percutaneous endopyelotomy with open pyeloplasty for pediatric ureteropelvic junction obstruction. J Urol 1998;159:1013.

Schwartz BF et al: Treatment of refractory kidney transplant ureteral strictures using balloon cautery endoureterotomy. Urology 2001;58(4):536.

Segura JW: Antegrade endopyelotomy. Urol Clin North Am 1998;25:311.

Shalhav AL et al: Adult endopyelotomy: Impact of etiology and antegrade versus retrograde approach on outcome. J Urol 1998; 160:685.

Shalhav AL et al: Endopyelotomy for high-insertion ureteropelvic junction obstruction [review]. J Endourol 1998;12(2):127.

Sterrett SP et al: Renal thermal ablative therapy. Urol Clin North Am 2008;35:397

Streem SB: Percutaneous endopyelotomy [review]. Urol Clin North Am 2000;27(4):685, ix.

Van Cangh PJ, Nesa S: Endopyelotomy. Urol Clin North Am 1998;25:281.

Watterson JD et al: Holmium:YAG laser endoureterotomy for ureterointestinal strictures. J Urol 2002;167(4):1692.

Weizer AZ et al: Complications after percutaneous radiofrequency ablation of renal tumors. Urology 2005;66(6):1176.

Wolf JS: Retrograde Acucise endopyelotomy. Urology 1998;51:859.

Yohannes P, Smith AD: The endourological management of complications associated with horseshoe kidney. J Urol 2002;168(1):5.

Percutaneous Aspiration and Biopsy

Bodner L et al: The role of interventional radiology in the management of intra- and extra-peritoneal leakage in patients who have undergone continent urinary diversion. Cardiovasc Intervent Radiol 1997;20:274.

Bush WH Jr et al: Needle tract seeding of renal cell carcinoma. AJR Am J Roentgenol 1977;129:725.

Coptcoat MJ et al: Endoscopic tissue liquidization and surgical aspiration. J Endourol 1988;2:321.

De Dominicis C et al: Percutaneous sclerotization of simple renal cysts with 95% ethanol followed by 24–48 h drainage with nephrostomy tube. Urol Int 2001;66(1):18.

Diaz-Buxo JA, Donadio JV Jr: Complications of percutaneous renal biopsy: An analysis of 1,000 consecutive biopsies. Clin Nephrol 1975;4:223.

Ferrucci JT et al: Malignant seeding of the tract after thin-needle aspiration biopsy. Radiology 1979;130:345.

Gibbons RP et al: Needle tract seeding following aspiration of renal cell carcinoma. J Urol 1977;118:865.

Hara I et al: Role of percutaneous image-guided biopsy in the evaluation of renal masses. Urol Int 2001;67(3):199.

Michael JM et al: Angiomyolipoma of the renal sinus: Diagnosis by percutaneous biopsy. Urology 2000;55(2):286.

Sadi MV et al: Percutaneous drainage of retroperitoneal abscesses. J Endourol 1988;2:293.

Stiles KP et al: The impact of bleeding times on major complication rates after percutaneous real-time ultrasound-guided renal biopsies. J Nephrol 2001;14(4):275.

Wehle MJ, Grabstald H: Contraindications to needle aspiration of a solid renal mass: Tumor dissemination by renal needle aspiration. J Urol 1986;136:446.

Stone Basketing, Ureterorenoscopy

Abrahams HM, Stoller ML: The argument against the routine use of ureteral access sheaths. Urol Clin North Am 2004;31(1):83.

Al-Awadi KA et al: Steinstrasse: A comparison of incidence with and without 'J' stenting and the effect of 'J' stenting on subsequent management. BJU Int 1999;84:618.

Bagley DH: Ureteroscopic surgery: Changing times and perspectives. Urol Clin North Am 2004;31(1):1.

Borboroglu PC et al: Ureteral stenting after ureteroscopy for distal ureteral calculi: A multi-institutional prospective randomized controlled study assessing pain, outcomes and complications. J Urol 2001;166(5):1651.

Busby JE, Low RK: Ureteroscopic treatment of renal calculi. Urol Clin North Am 2004;31(1):89.

Chen CL, Bagley DH: Ureteroscopic management of upper tract transitional cell carcinoma in patients with normal contralateral kidneys. J Urol 2000;164:1173.

Conlin MJ et al: Ureteroscopy, development and instrumentation. Urol Clin North Am 1997;24:25.

Delvecchio FC et al: Assessment of stricture formation with the ureteral access sheath. Urology 2003;61(3):518.

Denstedt JD et al: A prospective randomized controlled trial comparing nonstented versus stented ureteroscopic lithotripsy. J Urol 2001;165(5):1419.

Dourmashkin RL: Cystoscopic treatment of stones in the ureter with special reference to large calculi: Based on a study of 1550 cases. J Urol 1945;54:245.

Dretler SP: Clinical experience with electromechanical impactor. J Urol 1993;150:1402.

Dretler SP: The stone cone: A new generation of basketry. J Urol 2001;165(5):1593.

El-Anany FG et al: Retrograde ureteropyeloscopic holmium laser lithotripsy for large renal calculi. BJU Int 2001;88(9):850.

Gettman MT, Segura JW: Management of ureteric stones: Issues and controversies. BJU Int 2005;95(Suppl 2):85.

Goldfischer ER, Gerber GS: Endoscopic management of ureteral strictures. J Urol 1997;157:770.

Grasso M et al: Ureteropyeloscopic diagnosis and treatment of upper urinary tract urothelial malignancies. Urology 1999;54:240.

Grasso M, Ficazzola M: Retrograde ureteropyeloscopy for lower pole caliceal calculi. J Urol 1999;162(11):1904.

Hafner C et al: Evidence for oligoclonality and tumor spread by intraluminal seeding in multifocal urothelial carcinomas of the upper and lower urinary tract. Oncogene 2001;20(35):4910.

Hara I et al: Usefulness of ureteropyeloscopy for diagnosis of upper urinary tract tumors. J Endourol 2001;15(6):601.

Hollenbeck BK et al: Flexible ureteroscopy in conjunction with in situ lithotripsy for lower pole calculi. Urology 2001;58(6):859.

Hosking DH et al: Is stenting following ureteroscopy for removal of distal ureteral calculi necessary? J Urol 1999;161(1):48.

Krambeck AE et al: The evolution of ureteroscopy: A modern single-institution series. Mayo Clin Proc 2006;81(4):468.

Kourambas J et al: Dose a ureteral access sheath facilitate ureteroscopy? J Urol 2001;165(3):789.

Lam JS, Gupta M: Ureteroscopic management of upper tract transitional cell carcinoma. Urol Clin North Am 2004;31(1):115.

Larizgoitia I, Pons JMV: A systematic review of the clinical efficacy and effectiveness of the holmium:YAG laser in urology. BJU Int 1999;84:1.

Lechevallier E et al: Retrograde Acucise endopyelotomy: Long term results. J Endourol 1999;13:575.

Mendez-Torres FR et al: Retrograde ureteroscopic endopyelotomy. Urol Clin North Am 2004;31(1):99.

Nakada SY et al: Long-term outcome of flexible ureterorenoscopy in the diagnosis and treatment of lateralizing essential hematuria. J Urol 1997;157:776.

Nakada SY: Acucise endopyelotomy. Urology 2000;55(2):277.

Netto NR et al: Ureteroscopic stone removal in the distal ureter. Why change? J Urol 1997;157:2081.

Patel RC, Newman RC: Ureteroscopic management of ureteral and ureteroenteral strictures. Urol Clin North Am 2004;31(1):107.

Richter F et al: Endourologic management of benign ureteral strictures with and without compromised vascular supply. Urology 2000;55:652.

Schuster TG et al: Ureteroscopy for the treatment of urolithiasis in children. J Urol 2002;167(4):1813.

Seseke F et al: Treatment of iatrogenic postoperative ureteral strictures with Acucise endoureterotomy. Eur Urol 2002;42(4):370.

Singal RK, Denstedt JD: Contemporary management of ureteral stones. Urol Clin North Am 1997;24:59.

Sofer M et al: Holmium:YAG laser lithotripsy for upper urinary tract calculi in 598 patients. J Urol 2002;167:31.

Thomas R et al: Safety and efficacy of pediatric ureteroscopy for management of calculous disease. J Urol 1993;149:1082.

Vanlangendonck R, Landman J: Ureteral access strategies: pro-access sheath. Urol Clin North Am 2004;31(1):71.

Zheng W, Denstedt JD: Intracorporeal lithotripsy: Update on technology. Urol Clin North Am 2000;27:301.

Laparoscopic Surgery

9

J. Stuart Wolf Jr., MD, FACS, & Marshall L. Stoller, MD

Laparoscopy plays a prominent role in urology. Current residents finish their training with considerable exposure to the techniques, and a plethora of courses educate physicians already in practice. Alternatives to standard laparoscopy, including hand assistance and robotic assistance, further enhance capabilities.

PHYSIOLOGY OF LAPAROSCOPY

Laparoscopy with pneumoperitoneum exposes the patient to physiologic challenges that differ from that of open surgery, but can be met successfully with proper preparation and awareness (Ost et al, 2005).

▶ Physiology: Cardiovascular

As intra-abdominal pressure increases with pneumoperitoneum, the systemic vascular resistance increases and venous return decreases. A small increase in intra-abdominal pressure augments venous return and cardiac output. As intra-abdominal pressure rises, the increase in resistance exceeds the increase in pressure, and venous return and cardiac output fall (Figure 9–1). This transition point occurs at a lower intra-abdominal pressure in the hypovolemic compared with the normovolemic state. Given normovolemia, an intra-abdominal pressure of 15 mm Hg is associated with tolerable reduction of cardiac output.

The absorption of insufflated carbon dioxide (CO_2) has direct cardio-inhibitory effects, but CO_2 also stimulates the sympathetic nervous system. If acidosis develops then there are parasympathetic effects as well. Moderate hypercapnia (excess CO_2 in blood) produces an increase in cardiac output and blood pressure and a decrease in systemic vascular resistance, which counteract the effect of intra-abdominal pressure.

Overall, an intra-abdominal pressure of 15 mm Hg and moderate hypercapnia in healthy patients produce a hyperdynamic state (increased central venous pressure, systemic vascular resistance, heart rate, and blood pressure) without significant alteration of cardiac output (Junghans et al, 2005).

▶ Physiological Complications: Cardiovascular

The cardiovascular complications of laparoscopy include tension pneumoperitoneum, cardiac dysrhythmias, fluid overload, and venous thrombosis.

When the intra-abdominal pressure is excessive, usually >40 mm Hg, the overwhelming increase of vascular resistance can produce "tension pneumoperitoneum." Venous return, cardiac output, and blood pressure drop precipitously. Volume status must be optimized to prevent tension pneumoperitoneum at lower pressures. In general, the intra-abdominal pressure should be kept below 15–20 mm Hg. The response to "tension pneumoperitoneum" should be immediate desufflation.

Tachycardia and ventricular extrasystoles due to hypercapnia are usually benign, but fatal dysrhythmias can occur with very high arterial partial pressure of CO_2 ($PaCO_2$). Vagal stimulation by peritoneal distention can produce bradydysrhythmias (Valentin et al, 2004).

Because insensible fluid losses and urine output are less during laparoscopy than during open surgery, after optimizing volume status before insufflation intraoperative fluid administration should be limited to appropriate replacement for blood loss plus a maintenance rate of 5 mL/kg/h to avoid volume overload.

Since increased abdominal pressure during laparoscopy restricts lower extremity venous return, sequential compression devices may be the best choice for venous thrombosis prophylaxis during major laparoscopic procedures (Montgomery and Wolf, 2005).

▶ Physiology: Pulmonary, Acid–Base, and Insufflant Related

Increased intra-abdominal volume elevates the diaphragm, which reduces lung capacity and compliance. Insufflated CO_2 diffuses into the bloodstream. The amount of CO_2 absorbed during intraperitoneal CO_2 laparoscopy at typical

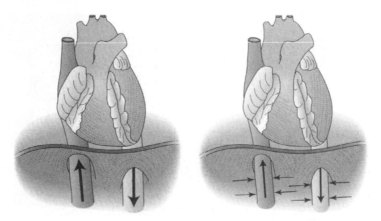

▲ **Figure 9–1.** Reduction of venous return and cardiac output during laparoscopy. (Borrowed with permission from Wolf JS Jr, Stoller ML: The physiology of laparoscopy: Basic principles, complications, and other considerations. J Urol 1994; 152:294.)

pressures is equivalent to adding 5–25% to the body's baseline production of CO_2. Subcutaneous emphysema, elevated intra-abdominal pressure, extraperitoneal insufflation, and increased duration of insufflation all increase the rate of CO_2 absorption.

▶ Physiological Complications: Pulmonary, Acid–Base, and Insufflant Related

The pulmonary, acid–base, and insufflant-related complications of laparoscopy include hypercapnia, acidosis, extraperitoneal gas collections, and venous gas embolism (VGE).

Moderate hypercapnia is stimulatory overall, but if $PaCO_2$ exceeds 60 mm Hg, then potentially lethal cardiodepressive effects predominate. Increasing ventilation rate and tidal volume adequately eliminates excess CO_2 in most patients. $PaCO_2$ is estimated intraoperatively by the partial pressure of end-tidal CO_2 ($P[et]CO_2$) measured with capnometry, which generally is 3–5 mm Hg lower than $PaCO_2$ during general anesthesia. During prolonged operations or in patients with pulmonary disease, the gradient may widen unpredictably, and arterial blood gases should be obtained for accurate monitoring (Kim, 2008).

Absorption of insufflated CO_2 causes a mild respiratory acidosis. With gas insufflation pressures >20 mm Hg, a metabolic acidosis also can develop, likely related to retained acids from decreased urine output.

Gases insufflated into the peritoneal cavity may leak into several extraperitoneal spaces. Subcutaneous emphysema is the most common site of extraperitoneal gas. Although generally innocuous, it increases the risk of hypercapnia (Saggar et al, 2008). Pneumopericardium, pneumomediastinum, and pneumothorax can inhibit cardiac filling and/or lung excursion. A CO_2 pneumothorax will usually resolve sponta-

neously, but thoracostomy should be performed for a symptomatic pneumothorax (Msezane et al, 2007).

VGE is the passage of gas bubbles through the venous system into the heart and pulmonary circulation (Min et al, 2007). When clinically significant, right heart outflow is impeded, producing hypoxemia, hypercapnia, and depressed cardiac output. Many VGEs during laparoscopy have been fatal. VGE is indicated by hypoxemia, pulmonary edema, increased airway pressure, hypotension, jugular venous distention, facial plethora, dysrhythmias, and a mill-wheel murmur. The capnometer will register a sudden fall in $P(et)CO_2$ if the CO_2 embolus is large. Swift response is required, including immediate desufflation, rapid ventilation with 100% oxygen, steep head-down tilt with the right side up, and general resuscitative maneuvers.

SELECTION OF LAPAROSCOPIC APPROACH

There are a number of alternative approaches to laparoscopic surgery. Access can be transperitoneal or retroperitoneal. Options for surgical manipulation include standard laparoscopy, hand assistance, and robotic assistance. Additional modifications are being developed, such as microlaparoscopy, laparoendoscopic single-site surgery (LESS), and natural orifice translumenal endoscopic surgery (NOTES) (Kommu et al, 2009; Raman et al, 2008). Only the most common alternatives are described here.

▶ Transperitoneal Versus Retroperitoneal

The transperitoneal route provides a capacious working space and allows direct visualization of familiar intraperitoneal anatomy. It is the most common route for most procedures. Transperitoneal access may be difficult, however, in patients who have had extensive abdominal surgery. The retroperitoneal approach allows easier and more rapid access to the retroperitoneal structures and avoidance of intra-abdominal organs and adhesions. The disadvantage of the retroperitoneal technique is the limited working space. Comparisons of the two routes for a variety of procedures have shown no consistent difference in operative times, cost, length of stay, or postoperative convalescence (Desai et al, 2005). The approach therefore is dictated by the familiarity of the surgeon and the patient's condition.

▶ Hand Assistance

Hand-assisted laparoscopic surgery (HALS) entails the insertion of a hand through a 7–9-cm incision into the laparoscopic field, while maintaining pneumoperitoneum with a hand-assistance device that employs a compressive mechanism to affix to the abdomen and prevent leakage of pneumoperitoneum around the intra-abdominal hand (Figure 9–2). The intra-abdominal hand is used for dissection, tissue identification, retraction, and control of injuries. The benefits of HALS include shorter operative times than for similar standard laparoscopic transperitoneal procedures in many series, ease of learning by inexperienced surgeons, and enhanced ability to manage difficult surgical situations. Additionally, conversion from standard laparoscopy to hand assistance is an alternative to conversion to open surgery. Disadvantages of HALS include problems with the devices (gas leakage or interference with port placement), physical strain on the hand, interference of the hand in the operative field, and the creation of a larger incision (and likely more wound complications) than for a standard laparoscopic procedure (Wolf, 2005). Numerous comparative studies between standard and hand-assisted laparoscopy show generally similar convalescence (Silberstein and Parsons, 2009).

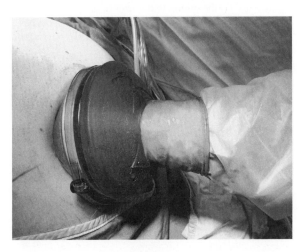

▲ **Figure 9–2.** Surgeon's hand inside Gelport. (Applied Medical, Rancho Santa Margarita, CA.)

▶ Robotic Assistance

The robot for laparoscopic surgery (da Vinci Surgical System; Intuitive Surgical, Sunnyvale, CA) has a three-dimensional camera and arms that are directed by the surgeon seated at the control console (Figure 9–3). It has achieved great popularity for application to radical prostatectomy and cystectomy, and it is being increasingly used for renal surgery as well. The advantages of robotic assistance include easier transference of open surgical skills to laparoscopic surgery, instrument tips with multiple degrees of freedom, and better ergonomics than standard laparoscopy. Disadvantages include the cost of the system and disposables and the need for a trained assistant at the bedside (Nelson, 2007).

LAPAROSCOPIC INSTRUMENTATION AND BASIC TECHNIQUES

▶ Preoperative Preparation

Although any operation in a patient with obesity, previous abdominal surgery, or abnormal anatomy is difficult, laparoscopy is relatively more challenged by these factors than is open surgery. In addition, open surgery may be favored physiologically over laparoscopy in patients with severe pulmonary disease or congestive heart failure. The patient being offered laparoscopy should be fully informed of the risks and benefits, most appropriately in the context of a comparison with the spectrum of risks and benefits of the corresponding open surgery. Inform the patient of the surgeon's experience with the particular laparoscopic procedure, and advise that conversion to open surgery may be required. For transperitoneal laparoscopic surgery without intended bowel resection, patient preparation with a clear liquid diet and oral magnesium citrate on the preoperative day is adequate. For retroperitoneoscopic surgery, bowel preparation is not necessary.

The primary laparoscopic cart (see later) is positioned opposite the surgeon. For an upper abdominal or retroperitoneal procedure, a secondary monitor for nursing staff or assistants placed on the opposite side of the patient is useful. Operating rooms with equipment booms from the ceiling minimize clutter and reduce setup time. After induction of anesthesia and endotracheal intubation, insert a urethral catheter and orogastric tube. For pelvic surgery, position the patient supine (or in some cases, dorsal lithotomy), with the chest securely taped to allow steep Trendelenburg tilt of the table. For transperitoneal procedures into the retroperitoneum, place the patient in partial flank position (45°) without flexion of the table. Direct retroperitoneoscopic procedures benefit from full flank position with table flexion.

▶ Entry: Obtaining Pneumoperitoneum

Initial access is commonly obtained with the closed (Veress needle) or open (Hasson cannula) techniques. Either is acceptable, but if the Veress needle is the first choice then the

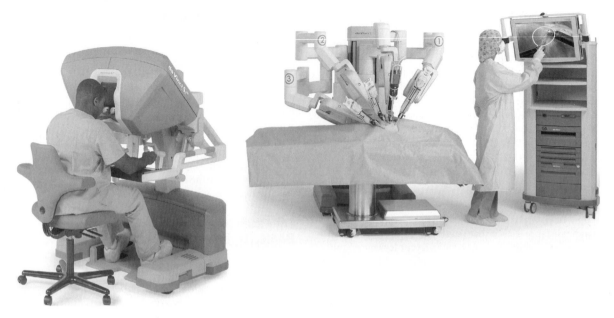

▲ **Figure 9–3.** da Vinci Surgical System. (Intuitive Surgical, Sunnyvale, CA.)

open technique should be learned as well, since sometimes the former is contraindicated or fails.

The Veress needle has a spring-loaded stylet that retracts back only under pressure from firm tissue (ie, fascia) to expose the sharp cannula; once the tip is free in the intraperitoneal space, the stylet springs forward and protects against visceral injury. The needle is usually placed at the location of the first port, although the site should be moved away from any prior incisions (extensive abdominal surgery or suspected dense adhesions are a relative contraindication for Veress needle use). The needle is inserted almost perpendicular to the abdominal wall, tilting slightly away from the large midline vessels. An exception is when the needle is being placed at the umbilicus in thin individuals, in which case it needs to be angled more acutely.

After inserting the needle, attach a 10-cc syringe half-filled with saline and aspirate back. There should be no aspirated gas or liquid. Next, inject saline through the needle and attempt to aspirate. Fluid should flow in easily and not return. Finally, the saline in the hub of the Veress needle should drop rapidly into the abdomen. These maneuvers assess for the possibility that the needle tip is in a luminal structure (bowel, blood vessel, etc), but all will be "normal" if the needle is preperitoneal—which is the most common erroneous placement (Figure 9–4). This possibility is assessed by the final test, the "opening pressure" as gas is insufflated. The pressure should not rise above 8 mm Hg within the first one-half liter of gas, or if it does, it should only be momentary and quickly correctable by a twist, slight withdrawal, and

tilting up of the needle (which will free the needle tip from omental or mesenteric fat). If these conditions are met, then continue insufflation, but if not, then disconnect the insufflation tubing, allow the gas to escape, and withdraw the needle.

The Hasson technique is placement of a laparoscopic port through a small incision under direct vision. Make a 1.5–3-cm incision down to and through the peritoneal membrane. Place stay sutures and then insert the Hasson port (10/12 cannula containing a blunt obturator, with a conical adjustable sleeve, Figure 9–5). Tie the sutures to the arms of the device to secure the conical sleeve within the fascia. An alternative port has a retaining balloon that inflates intra-abdominally and is held

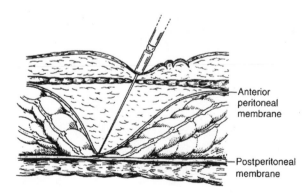

▲ **Figure 9–4.** Preperitoneal location of the tip of Veress needle.

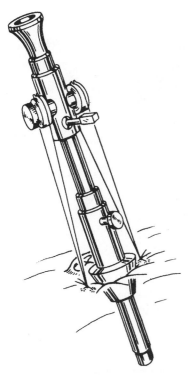

▲ **Figure 9–5.** Hasson cannula.

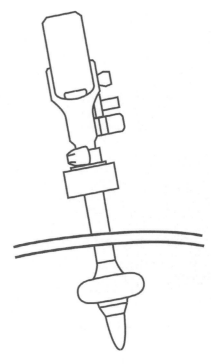

▲ **Figure 9–6.** Self-retaining port. (AutoSuture Co, Norwalk, CT.)

up tight against the fascia by an adjustable retaining ring (Figure 9–6). Another alternative is to make a smaller incision in the fascia and peritoneal membrane and insert a blunt port that dilates rather than cuts the fascia (see later). Finally, a visualizing trocar (see later) can be used without prior insufflation.

▶ Entry: Port Placement

The general scheme of port placement is to surround the site with the necessary number of instruments placed widely enough apart that they do not "sword fight" in the abdomen and with the laparoscope situated so that a good visual angle can be attained.

Standard port sizes range from 5 to 12 mm. "Needlescopic" ports (3 mm) as well as extra-wide ports (18 and 30 mm) are available for specialized use. Ports can be disposable, reusable, or "reposable." The third contains both reusable and disposable components. The trocars inside the ports can be cutting or noncutting. Disposable sharp trocars are shielded (Figure 9–7). Some reusable trocars have nonshielded sharp tips. The

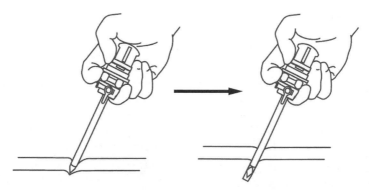

▲ **Figure 9–7.** Insertion of port with shielded sharp tip. A blunt shield moves forward to shield the blade once resistance decreases. (AutoSuture Co, Norwalk, CT.)

Hasson-type ports employ blunt tips. There are ports with clear plastic tips (Figure 9–8) that allow visualization with the laparoscope as the port is being inserted. The Step system (AutoSuture, Norwalk, CT; Figure 9–9) employs an expandable sheath that is inserted with a Veress needle. The needle is removed and a dilating trocar is used to insert the port. This and other ports that dilate or screw into the fascia make a smaller fascial defect and pose less risk of injury than sharp-tipped ports.

If the Veress needle has been used for abdominal entry, the next step is to place the first port, which is usually for the laparoscope and inserted at the site of Veress needle placement. To avoid inadvertent removal of the port during the procedure, anchor it to the skin with suture. Alternatively, special sheaths can secure the port. Subsequent ports are placed under visual control through the laparoscope.

▶ Entry: Extraperitoneal Approach

For flank retroperitoneoscopic surgery, make a 2-cm incision near the tip of the 12th rib down through the lumbodorsal fascia under direct vision. Explore the retroperitoneal space with a finger, and then dilate the space with a balloon

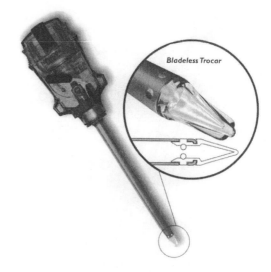

▲ **Figure 9–8.** Nonbladed trocar, with clear plastic tip that allows visualization as the abdominal wall is penetrated. (Ethicon Endo-Surgery, Cincinnati, OH.)

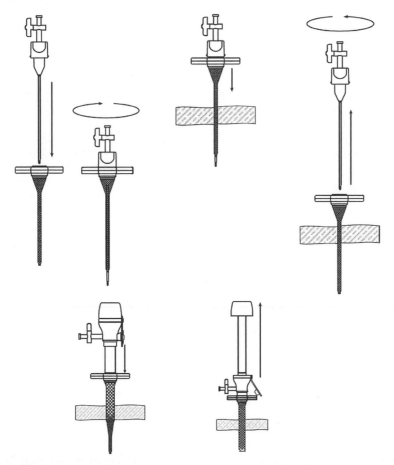

▲ **Figure 9–9.** Step system port. (AutoSuture Co, Norwalk, CT.)

images and many surgeons now use them routinely. For pediatric surgery, a 5-mm laparoscope typically is used, but 2-mm laparoscopes are also available. Most laparoscopes employ a 0° or 30° lens, with the latter providing more viewing angles, and laparoscopes with flexible tips are also available. In some laparoscopes, the camera chip is placed on the tip, which removes an interface and enhances resolution. One or two large monitors, a strong light source with cables in good condition, and the digital image converter (camera box) complete the video apparatus. Still-image and video-capture devices provide documentation. Other equipment on the laparoscopic cart includes the insufflator and additional energy sources.

▶ Laparoscopic Instrumentation

Laparoscopic operating instruments provide grasping and dissection, cutting, hemostasis, retraction, irrigation and aspiration, suturing, clipping or stapling, specimen entrapping, morcellating, and intraoperative imaging. Many are available in both disposable and reusable versions. Most standard instruments are 5 or 10 mm in diameter and 35 cm in length, but there are longer, narrow, or wider devices for particular uses.

▶ Exiting the Abdomen

After a laparoscopic procedure is completed, inspect the operative field at 5 mm Hg pressure to allow exposure of bleeding that may have been tamponaded by the working pneumoperitoneum pressure. Remove the ports under vision so that any bleeding from the abdominal wall can be detected. Close the fascial defect of all port sites ≥10 mm. The Carter-Thomason needle-suture passer (Figure 9–11) (Inlet Medical Inc., Eden Prairie, MN) or similar devices simplify this step. In children, close even 5-mm port sites. Because retained CO_2 may contribute to postoperative discomfort, attempt to

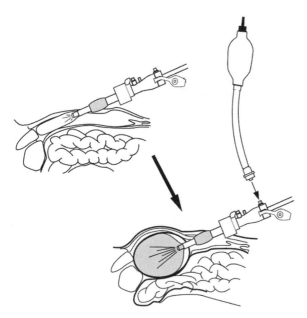

▲ **Figure 9–10.** Preperitoneal distention balloon. (Auto-Suture Co, Norwalk, CT.)

(commercially available, Figure 9–10, or self-made). Insert a self-retaining port at this location, and place additional ports as needed. For pelvic extraperitoneal surgery, direct the balloon through an infraumbilical incision toward the pubic bone and dilate the preperitoneal space.

▶ Laparoscopic Video Instrumentation and Cart

The standard adult laparoscope is 10 mm in diameter, although the newer 5-mm laparoscopes provide excellent

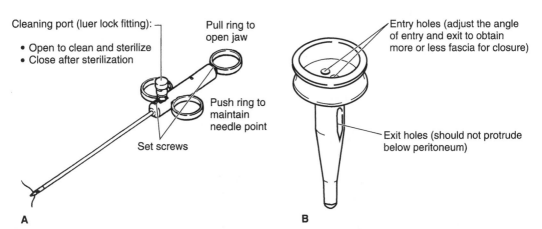

Cleaning port (luer lock fitting):
- Open to clean and sterilize
- Close after sterilization

Pull ring to open jaw

Push ring to maintain needle point

Set screws

Entry holes (adjust the angle of entry and exit to obtain more or less fascia for closure)

Exit holes (should not protrude below peritoneum)

A   **B**

▲ **Figure 9–11.** Carter-Thomason device (Inlet Medical Inc., Eden Prairie, MN). **A:** Needle point-suture passer. **B:** Fascial closure guide.

remove all gas. Close the port incisions with a subcuticular stitch or wound glue and apply sterile tape.

Postoperative Care

For urologic laparoscopic procedures that do not involve bowel resection, hospital stay can be limited to 1 or 2 days in most patients with aggressive postoperative management. Offer parenteral narcotics the afternoon and evening after the procedure. Unless contraindicated, use intravenous ketorolac around the clock for the first 24 hours, including a dose at skin closure in the operating room (Breda et al, 2007). Start a clear liquid diet postoperatively, but if nausea develops, then delay for a few hours before trying again. On the morning of postoperative day 1, advance to a regular diet as tolerated and switch from parenteral to oral pain medication. Get the patient up to a chair on the day of the operation, and start ambulation in the hallway the next day.

SPECIFIC PROCEDURES

Pelvic Lymph Node Dissection

Laparoscopic pelvic lymph node dissection (LPLND) in the setting of prostate cancer was the first adult laparoscopic urologic procedure to gain widespread acceptance. The technique was initially described prior to widespread prostate-specific antigen testing, and LPLND had positive results in up to one-third of prostate cancer patients. Due to lower positive node rates associated with stage migration, interest in stand-alone LPLND has waned. With the rise of laparoscopic/robotic radical prostatectomies and cystectomies, however, the utility of LPLND (as part of these procedures) remains.

There are no contraindications specific to LPLND other than those general to laparoscopy, although intraperitoneal laparoscopic hernia repair, other pelvic surgery, or radiotherapy can result in adhesions.

The patient is positioned supine with Trendelenburg tilt. LPLND can be performed transperitoneal or extraperitoneal (Figure 9–12). Initial access is typically through an umbilical port followed by two to three additional ports in a diamond- or fan-shaped pattern (Figure 9–13). Key landmarks are the obliterated umbilical ligament, gonadal vessels, and internal inguinal ring (Figure 9–14), with the limits of the nodal dissection for prostate cancer usually being the iliac bifurcation, the pubis, the obturator nerve, the pelvic side wall, and the medial umbilical ligament. Dissection for bladder, penile, or urethral cancer usually involves a more extended field, bounded by the common iliac artery, the genitofemoral nerve, and the bladder.

Complications of LPLND are similar to those of open PLND. Specifically, injuries to the obturator nerve, iliac and epigastric vessels, and ureter have been reported but are uncommon. Other potential complications include lymphocele, bowel or bladder injury, subcutaneous emphysema,

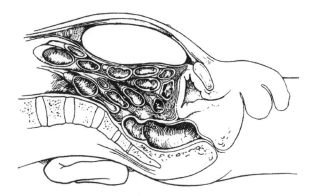

▲ **Figure 9–12.** Balloon device inflated in the preperitoneal space for extraperitoneal laparoscopic pelvic lymph node dissection.

thromboembolic events, and scrotal swelling. Open surgical pelvic lymphadenectomy and LPLND provide similar nodal yield.

Varicocelectomy

Laparoscopic varicocelectomy is rarely performed today due to refinements in the subinguinal microsurgical technique (Ahmed et al, 2007).

Orchidopexy

Laparoscopy has been judged by many pediatric urologists to be the gold-standard diagnostic tool for nonpalpable testes. Although not as firmly established, laparoscopic orchidopexy appears to be comparable with, if not better than, open orchidopexy (Baker et al, 2001). Laparoscopy may be used for intersex evaluation as well.

Positioning is usually supine with the legs frog legged. A small laparoscope is inserted through a periumbilical site. One to three port sites have been utilized. The first step involves identifying the inguinal ring with the corresponding gonadal vessels and vas deferens. If the vas deferens and vessels are seen entering the inguinal ring, the laparoscope is removed and an open inguinal exploration is performed as would be for a palpable cryptorchid testis. If the gonadal vessels are blind ending, the procedure is terminated. If an unsalvageable testis is identified, laparoscopic orchiectomy can be performed. If a salvageable testis is identified intra-abdominally, working ports are placed and the testis is freed from its nonvital attachments (Figure 9–15). If sufficient cord length can be gained, a scrotal incision is made and the testis is fixed in a scrotal location. If there is insufficient cord length, a one- or two-stage Fowler–Stephens procedure may be performed. A multi-institutional review found decreased testicular atrophy and a higher rate of postoperative scrotal testicular positioning after the two-stage procedure. Fifteen

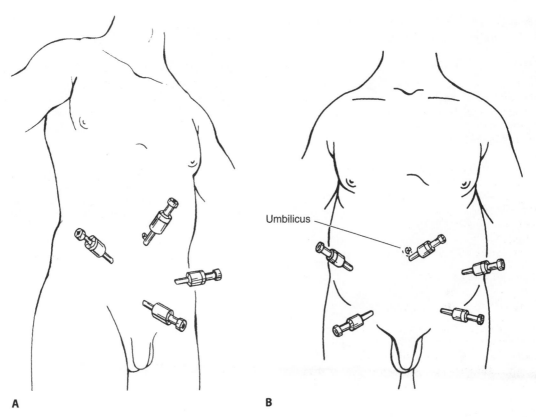

▲ **Figure 9–13.** Port placements for laparoscopic pelvic lymph node dissection. **A:** Diamond configuration typically used. **B:** Fan configuration for use in obese patients.

complications were noted in 310 procedures, with an overall success rate of 93%.

▶ **Renal Cyst Decortication**

Although simple renal cysts are common, they rarely require intervention. Occasionally, pain, infection, early satiety, or secondary obstruction can develop that prompts active treatment, although in many cases, percutaneous aspiration and sclerosis of the cyst will suffice. Even less frequently, a cystic mass may need to be explored for diagnostic purposes. Cyst decortication also can be performed for pain relief in patients with polycystic kidney disease who still have adequate renal function.

Via a three- or four-port approach (usually transperitoneal), the colon is reflected medially to expose the kidney, and Gerota's fascia is incised to expose the cyst(s). Laparoscopic ultrasound may be useful. If there is suspicion of a connection to the collecting system, or if the collecting system is in close proximity and at risk for injury, instillation of dyed saline through a previously placed retrograde ureteral catheter may be useful. The roof of the cyst is excised,

without incising into surrounding renal parenchyma. A biopsy of any suspicious areas should be obtained. Perirenal fat may be fixed to the cyst base to help prevent cyst reaccumulation. Long-term success is high (Yoder and Wolf, 2004). Complications specific to renal cyst decortication include cyst regrowth and injury of renal parenchyma or collecting system.

▶ **Simple and Radical Nephrectomy**

Laparoscopy has become a well-accepted technique for a number of benign and malignant renal conditions, including nonfunctioning kidneys, chronic infections, symptomatic polycystic kidney disease, and tumors. Initially, large tumor size was considered a contraindication for laparoscopic nephrectomy, but with experience, tumor size has become less of an issue. The only limitation is the expertise of the urologist. Laparoscopic radical nephrectomy including renal vein thrombus is feasible. Relative contraindications include profound perirenal inflammation, bulky lymphadenopathy that limits hilar access, large venous thrombus, and adjacent organ involvement.

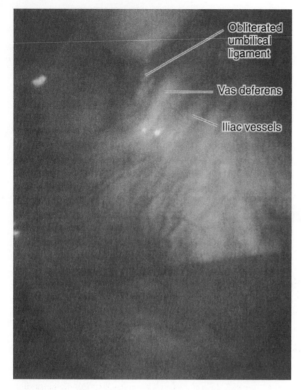

▲ **Figure 9–14.** Key landmarks for laparoscopic pelvic lymph node dissection are the obliterated umbilical ligament, gonadal vessels, and internal inguinal ring.

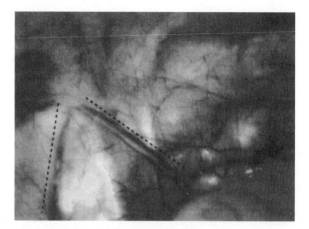

▲ **Figure 9–15.** *Dashed lines* indicate incisions into posterior peritoneum for orchidopexy of a left intra-abdominal testis.

The patient is placed in a lateral decubitus position, padded, and secured. Table flexion and variation in decubitus position from 45° to 90° varies with the specific approach and surgeon preference. The surgeon and assistant both stand toward the patient's anterior body wall for the transperitoneal approach.

The techniques for a laparoscopic nephrectomy will be discussed in detail as a template for other common laparoscopic upper retroperitoneal procedures. There are many variations on port placement. For transperitoneal laparoscopic nephrectomy, a three- to four-port "L"-shaped configuration for left nephrectomy and a reversed "L"-shaped pattern for right nephrectomy are commonly used. The initial port is placed two fingerbreadths below the costal margin at the lateral edge of the rectus muscle and the abdomen is insufflated initially to 15–18 mm Hg. Intra-abdominal organs are inspected for inadvertent injury. Another port is placed in the midaxillary line two fingerbreadths above the iliac crest. One to two additional ports are placed along the lateral edge of the rectus muscle including one able to accept the endoscopic stapler if use is anticipated. Depending on the patient's body habitus and relative position of the kidney and spleen/liver, other configurations may be chosen (Figure 9–16).

For left-sided lesions, the left colon is mobilized from the splenic flexure toward the iliac vessels, leaving the anterior fascicle of Gerota's fascia intact. The lienophrenic ligament is incised, allowing medial rotation of the spleen. Further medial rotation is achieved by mobilizing the lateral edge of the pancreas, thus revealing the renal hilum. The ureter is identified and transected. Following the gonadal vein superiorly will help identify the renal vein. The renal vein is dissected over the aorta to help avoid damage to the adrenal or lumbar veins. One should be careful using clips on vascular branches near the renal hilum because these can interfere with subsequent utilization of the endoscopic stapler. The renal artery is

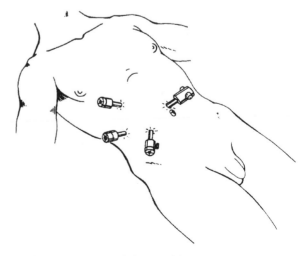

▲ **Figure 9–16.** One of the possible port configurations for right transperitoneal laparoscopic nephrectomy.

typically found posterior to the renal vein and is transected after securing it with clips or an endoscopic stapler. Once the artery is transected, the renal vein is secured and transected in a similar fashion. If the hilar dissection is difficult and the vein and artery cannot be separated, the endoscopic stapler can be used to transect the artery and vein en bloc. The superior border of the kidney is dissected, either incorporating the adrenal gland or more medially if adrenal sparing is intended. The lateral renal attachments are the last to be transected, because they help suspend the kidney and ease hilar dissection.

The kidney can be removed intact or morcellated after being placed into a specimen retrieval bag. If intact extraction is desired, a premarked incision is utilized, or a port site may be extended for extraction. For morcellation, the neck of the bag is brought through the port site. Appropriate drapings should be used to prevent potential tumor seeding. Blunt forceps are used to remove the specimen piecemeal, and laparoscopic monitoring is used to help prevent injuries. These instruments are then considered contaminated and are removed from the field. As with all laparoscopic procedures, insufflation pressures should be reduced to 5 mm Hg for final evaluation of hemostasis. Port sites >5 mm that utilized cutting trocars require fascial closure.

For right-sided transperitoneal nephrectomy, the ascending colon is mobilized from the hepatic flexure toward the iliac bifurcation. The triangular ligament is incised, with care not to injure the diaphragm. The liver is retracted with a blunt-tipped instrument. The duodenum is mobilized medially to help expose the inferior vena cava (IVC). Entering the plane of Leriche directly anterior to the IVC will guide dissection to the renal vein. Dissection lateral to the lower edge of the IVC will reveal the psoas muscle and ureter. Although the right renal vein is shorter, it rarely has veins draining into it as on the left side. The remainder of the technique is similar to that previously described.

Retroperitoneal nephrectomy begins with the patient in a full lateral decubitus position with similar padding and bed adjustments. In contrast to the transperitoneal approach, the surgeon and the assistant stand on the dorsal side of the patient. After an incision is made over Petit's triangle, blunt dissection through the lumbodorsal fascia is performed and a plane is developed over the psoas muscle. A dissecting balloon trocar is placed into this space. There are commercially available dissecting balloon trocars for this purpose, or a "homemade" version can be constructed by attaching a glove to a catheter. The commercially available dissecting trocar has the advantage of allowing direct visual monitoring of the dissection. Pneumoretroperitoneum is created and two to three additional port sites are placed according to surgeon preference (Figure 9–17). The kidney is retracted anteriorly to allow direct access to the hilum. Blunt dissection easily exposes the artery, which is clipped and transected. Anterior to the arterial stump, the vein is dissected and controlled. After hilar control, the ureter is identified and transected. Further dissection is similar to that of transperitoneal techniques. Many laparoscopists remove the specimen intact when performing retroperitoneoscopic nephrectomy due to the limited working space. If morcellation is preferred, specimen-bag entrapment may require incising the peritoneum if the specimen is large. The final steps of ensuring hemostasis under low-pressure insufflation and inspecting the port sites remain the same.

The technique for hand-assisted laparoscopic nephrectomy is similar to that for transperitoneal laparoscopic nephrectomy. If hand assistance is chosen, port placement is altered to allow room for the hand-assistance device. For left-sided lesions, the hand-assistance device is typically placed in the midline and may incorporate the umbilicus. For obese patients, the device may be placed paramedian, closer to the pathology. For right-sided lesions, the device may be placed in the midline or alternatively in the right lower quadrant using a muscle-splitting diagonal incision (Gibson). Placement of the hand-assistance device is dependent on the surgeon's arm length, desired position of the nondominant hand, and the

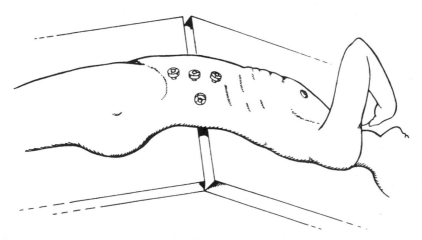

▲ **Figure 9–17.** One of the possible port configurations for left retroperitoneal laparoscopic nephrectomy.

patient's body habitus. Two or three ports are placed according to surgeon preference. Dissection is similar to the transperitoneal description mentioned earlier. Lateral renal attachments can be transected earlier because the hand can provide counter traction, facilitating hilar dissection. Specimen extraction is rapidly performed through the hand-assist incision.

The major and minor complication rates from laparoscopic nephrectomy are approximately 5% and 10%, respectively, and approximately 3% of cases are converted to open surgery (Permpongkosol et al, 2007). Minor complications include ileus, mild hemorrhage, urinary tract infection, hernia, and wound infection. Major complications include pulmonary embolus, pneumothorax, injury to various viscera, and hemorrhage from the aorta, IVC, or iliac, gonadal, lumbar, or renal vessels. Technical complications are more common during the first 30–50 cases of a surgeon's experience.

Comparisons of laparoscopic and open surgical nephrectomy reveal shorter and less intense convalescence with laparoscopy and similar complication and cancer-control rates (Columbo et al, 2008). Operative times are longer for laparoscopy initially, but with experience, operative times may even be shorter than with open surgery. Studies comparing different laparoscopic techniques show similar outcomes, suggesting that no approach is uniformly superior (Gabr et al, 2009). The surgeon should be familiar with the various techniques so that the optimal procedure can be performed.

Nephroureterectomy

Nephroureterectomy is the gold-standard treatment for upper tract urothelial carcinoma. The open surgical procedure is performed through a long curved flank incision or two separate incisions, leading to significant postoperative morbidity. Laparoscopic nephroureterectomy incorporates the benefits of cancer control with less postoperative pain and earlier return to normal activity. Transperitoneal, retroperitoneal, hand-assisted, and robotic-assisted techniques have been described. The kidney dissection is similar to a laparoscopic radical nephrectomy except that the ureter is left intact prior to the distal transection.

Optimal management of the distal ureter remains controversial. The technique of transurethral resection of the intramural ureter, leaving the distal ureter free in the retroperitoneum, has been largely abandoned owing to risk of local recurrence. A number of alternative minimally invasive approaches have been described, including one- or two-port transvesical dissection of the distal ureter (Figure 9–18) with (two-port) or without (one-port) transvesical closure of the ureteral orifice, endoscopic stapling or energy ablation of the tented up ureter from an extravesical approach, and others. Some simply perform the nephrectomy laparoscopically and excise the bladder cuff and remove the specimen through a lower abdominal incision. Even in cases without open surgical bladder cuff, the nephroureterectomy specimen should always be removed intact. Cancer-control rates appear adequate, and complication rates are similar to those for laparoscopic radical nephrectomy (Manabe et al, 2007).

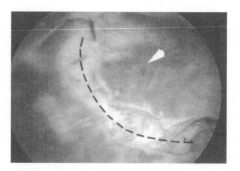

▲ **Figure 9–18.** Transvesical dissection of the distal ureter performed with a Colling's knife on a resectoscope placed through a 10-mm port inserted suprapubically into the bladder. After the nephrectomy portion of the procedure and clipping of the ureter, incision (*dotted black line*) is gradually made around the ureteral orifice (*white arrowhead*) until the distal ureter can be pulled free of the bladder.

▶ Partial Nephrectomy and Renal Mass Ablation

Partial nephrectomy is performed for imperative, relative, and elective indications. Some patients who are candidates for open surgical partial nephrectomy have been treated inappropriately with laparoscopic radical nephrectomy because of the more favorable postoperative convalescence. The laparoscopic approach to partial nephrectomy, however, provides both nephron-sparing and improved convalescence. Widespread adoption of the procedure has been limited by its technical difficulty.

Transperitoneal, retroperitoneal, hand-assisted, and robotic-assisted techniques have been described. Although the overall technique is similar to that for laparoscopic radical nephrectomy, a few modifications are required. Some physicians perform preoperative ureteral catheterization to assess collecting system closure. Laparoscopic ultrasound may be useful to delineate tumor margins and multifocality. The kidney is dissected from perirenal fat as needed to expose the lesion (leaving a cap of fatty tissue over the tumor) and bring it into the operative field. The renal artery may be occluded with a laparoscopic bulldog or Satinsky clamp, or direct manual compression using hand assistance can be used. Superficial lesions can be excised without hilar clamping, and methods for "clampless" partial nephrectomy for deeper lesions have been reported. Parenchymal cooling using a variety of methods has been described, but it is not standard, although other maneuvers to minimize reperfusion injury (intravenous fluids, mannitol, etc) are frequently used. Tumors are resected with "cold" scissors or energy devices (Figure 9–19). The use of biopsies and frozen section is variable. Vessels and collecting system entry sites are closed using intracorporeal suturing techniques and/or tissue glues. The overlying parenchyma is frequently coagulated using the laparoscopic argon beam coagulator. Tissue glues and bulking agents (collagen, gelatin,

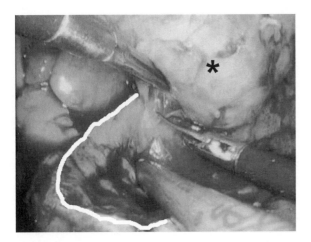

▲ **Figure 9–19.** Partial nephrectomy. Tumor (*black asterisk*) is being elevated by a grasper (entering from top of figure), as it is excised with scissors. An irrigator–aspirator depresses the tumor bed and helps maintain visualization. The peripheral resection margin is indicated with the white line.

etc) may be placed on the resection bed to help optimize hemostasis. Bolstering sutures can be placed to compress and reconstruct the remaining renal tissue.

Complications of laparoscopic partial nephrectomy include hemorrhage and urinary leak, generally at a rate somewhat greater than for open surgical partial nephrectomy (Gill et al, 2007). Cancer-control rates appear to be equivalent to those of open partial nephrectomy.

An alternative to tumor resection is cryoablation or radiofrequency ablation of small peripheral renal lesions. The dissection techniques are similar to that for laparoscopic partial nephrectomy. A biopsy should be taken to confirm malignancy. For cryoablation, the probe is passed into the tumor and the lesion is frozen to less than −20°C, thawed, and then refrozen. This process can be monitored by laparoscopic ultrasound. For radiofrequency ablation, the probe is introduced into the lesion after adequate mobilization and biopsy and is used to deliver a preset amount of energy based on tumor volume. Temperature at the tip of the probe is 100°C. After treatment, the lesion may be resected, or the coagulated mass can be left in situ. Cryoablation and radiofrequency coagulation techniques may decrease blood loss and operative times compared with partial nephrectomy. Renal arterial clamping is unnecessary, thus avoiding the risk of ischemia and reperfusion injury. The spectrum of complications is similar to that of laparoscopic partial nephrectomy. Long-term data are scant, and close follow-up is required (Kunkle and Uzzo, 2008).

▶ Donor Nephrectomy

Laparoscopy has become the standard for donor nephrectomy in the United States. Most laparoscopic procedures are left-sided, single-artery kidneys for technical reasons, but multiple arteries and right-sided donation can be addressed with excellent outcomes. The positioning and dissection technique is similar to that of laparoscopic nephrectomy, except that the ligation of the vasculature is the last step before intact extraction. For the pure laparoscopic technique, a premarked low transverse incision is carried down to the peritoneum. The renal artery and vein are then ligated and transected. To optimize renal vein length, especially on the right side, an endoscopic stapler that lays down three rows of staples without cutting can be used, in place of the more commonly used stapler that lays down six rows of staples and cuts in between rows 3 and 4. A peritoneotomy is made and the kidney is passed to the recipient team.

Many centers use hand-assisted laparoscopic techniques for live renal donation. Proponents of hand-assisted approaches argue that the incision should be made at the beginning of the procedure and utilized for assistance in dissection. Others use the retroperitoneal approach for laparoscopic donor nephrectomy, claiming decreased operative times. Surgeon experience and comfort level will dictate the laparoscopic technique. Laparoscopic donor nephrectomy produces renal units that function as well as those from open surgical procedures, with similar complication rates (Nanidis et al, 2008).

▶ Pyeloplasty

Laparoscopic pyeloplasty is increasingly utilized to address ureteropelvic junction obstruction. Transperitoneal, retroperitoneal, and hand-assisted techniques have been described. Common to all approaches is the need to be well skilled in laparoscopic suturing, and as such robotic assistance has become popular. Port placement is similar to that for laparoscopic transperitoneal or retroperitoneal nephrectomy. Dissection and reconfiguration of the ureteropelvic junction is similar to that of open surgery and is dependent on intraoperative findings. The Anderson-Hynes dismembered pyeloplasty, Y-V plasty, Heineke-Mikulicz reconstruction, Davis intubated ureterotomy, Hellstrom vascular relocation, and tubularized flap pyeloplasty have all been described laparoscopically. The procedure has been performed in infants, children, adults, and the elderly. If there is an anterior crossing vessel, it is optimal to transect and anastomose the ureter anterior to the crossing vessel (Figure 9–20). A large redundant renal pelvis may be reduced and tapered. A ureteral stent may be placed before or during the repair.

Open surgical and laparoscopic pyeloplasty appear to offer equivalent pain relief, activity level improvement, and relief of obstruction. The outcomes are better than with other minimally invasive approaches such as endopyelotomy or balloon dilation (Dimarco et al, 2006). Complications are similar to that for laparoscopic nephrectomy, with the addition of urinary leak and failure of the procedure to correct the obstruction.

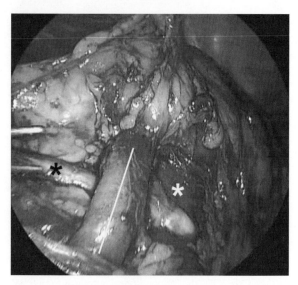

▲ **Figure 9–20.** Ureteropelvic junction obstruction of left kidney associated with crossing vessel (*white line*) before laparoscopic pyeloplasty. Renal pelvis is marked with *white asterisk* and ureter is indicated by a *black asterisk*.

▶ **Adrenalectomy**

On the basis of shorter operative time, reduced complications and convalescence, and equivalent surgical outcome compared with open surgery, laparoscopic adrenalectomy is the standard approach for most surgical adrenal lesions, including aldosteronomas, pheochromocytomas, Cushing's adenomas, incidentalomas, metastatic lesions, symptomatic myelolipomas, and feminizing/virilizing tumors (Lee et al, 2008). Large (>6 cm), invasive carcinomas are considered by most to be the only contraindication to laparoscopic adrenalectomy. Experienced laparoscopists have reported successful laparoscopic adrenalectomy for up to 15-cm lesions. Transperitoneal (anterior or lateral), retroperitoneal (posterior or lateral), hand-assisted, and transthoracic laparoscopic approaches have been reported. Bilateral synchronous adrenalectomy and partial adrenalectomy have been performed.

The laparoscopic approach to the adrenal gland is similar to that previously described for transperitoneal laparoscopic nephrectomy, although the ports are placed in a subcostal location (Figure 9–21). The dissection can be compared to opening a book. For left-sided lesions, the spleen is mobilized medially while the characteristic yellow adrenal tissue is mobilized to the right. Dissection continues in a counterclockwise direction. The main adrenal vein enters the renal vein. Proceed cautiously at the superomedial aspect because the superior adrenal vein (from the inferior phrenic vein) can be substantial. After controlling the adrenal vein, blunt and sharp dissection is used to mobilize the adrenal gland from the psoas

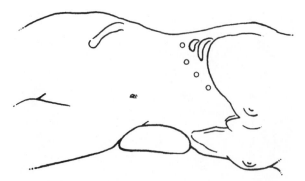

▲ **Figure 9–21.** One of the possible port configurations for right transperitoneal laparoscopic adrenalectomy.

muscle and superior aspect of the kidney. On the right side, the surgical approach is again analogous to opening a book, and dissection proceeds in a clockwise direction. The triangular ligament is incised with the posterior peritoneum, allowing medial retraction of the liver and colon. This exposes the IVC, and the adrenal gland is gently mobilized laterally. The adrenal vein emptying into the IVC is ligated and transected.

Complication and conversion rate of laparoscopic adrenalectomy are lower than for nephrectomy (Permpongkosol et al, 2007). Vascular and visceral injuries, cardiovascular complications related to pheochromocytoma, pneumothorax, and other typical complications have been reported. Suppression of contralateral adrenal function by a cortisol-producing tumor (Cushing's syndrome) may result in an Addisonian crisis, typically within the first 10 postoperative days.

▶ **Retroperitoneal Lymph Node Dissection**

Open surgical retroperitoneal lymph node dissection (RPLND) involves a xiphoid-to-pubis midline incision and significant morbidity related to ileus, blood loss, and postoperative pain. Laparoscopic RPLND offer a considerably less intense experience for the patient. The dissection template is the same as with the open approach. For left-sided lesions, the para-aortic, preaortic, and retroaortic nodes are removed (Figure 9–22). The boundaries are the renal vessels, the medial edge of the aorta, and the ureter inferiorly down to the iliac vessels. For right-sided lesions, the interaortocaval, precaval, retrocaval, and preaortic nodes are removed. The boundaries are the renal vessels, the aorta, and the ureter inferiorly down to the iliac vessels. Additionally, the para-aortic nodes between the renal hilum and the inferior mesenteric artery are removed. Laparoscopic RPLND should be approached with caution in patients with bulky nodal disease.

The patient is positioned in a modified lateral decubitus fashion. The initial port is placed near the umbilicus. Additional ports are placed to optimize dissection and retraction. The dissection is similar to the previously described

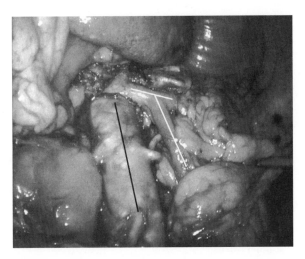

▲ Figure 9–22. Left-sided laparoscopic retroperitoneal lymph node dissection. *Black line* indicates aorta and *white lines* indicate renal and gonadal veins.

transperitoneal laparoscopic nephrectomy except that on the left side, the spleen and pancreas are rotated further medially and the descending colon is mobilized lower into the pelvis. On the right side, the posterior peritoneum is incised under the liver to reveal the superior margin of the IVC, and the colon and duodenum are mobilized further medially to expose the retroperitoneal area of interest. A methodical approach, using the same split-and-roll technique as in open RPLND, is performed. Nerve-sparing techniques are similar to the open approach in hopes of preserving ejaculatory function.

Complications of laparoscopic RPLND include hemorrhage, lymphocele, chylous ascites, injury to renal and lumbar veins, and bowel injury. Postchemotherapy dissections are more difficult, with higher morbidity and conversion rates. Follow-up studies suggest oncologic efficacy comparable with that of open techniques (Rassweiler et al, 2008).

▶ Radical Prostatectomy

Interest in laparoscopic urologic surgery intensified with successful laparoscopic techniques for radical prostatectomy. Laparoscopic prostatectomy has become routine in most centers with the availability of robotic assistance, with operative times similar to those for open prostatectomy. The indications for laparoscopic radical prostatectomy are similar to the open approach, and contraindications are the same as those for general laparoscopy.

A transperitoneal approach is most popular. The patient is positioned in a modified lithotomy fashion with the thighs abducted for access to the perineum and the table in steep Trendelenburg position. A periumbilical insufflation port is placed with four to five additional ports in a fan-shaped pattern. Laparoscopic dissection begins by incising the

peritoneum posterior to the bladder to expose the seminal vesicles and vas deferentia, or by incising the peritoneum anterior to the bladder to open the space of Retzius. One major difference from the open procedure is that dissection of the prostate is often performed from the bladder neck distally to the prostatic apex. The lateral pedicles can be controlled with electrocautery or coagulating shears, or if nerve sparing is desired, then clips are used. The laparoscopic approach has the advantage of performing the anastomosis under magnified vision (and in three dimensions with the robot).

Once adequate experience has been gained, oncologic results (as measured by margins and prostate-specific antigen recurrence) are comparable with those with open radical prostatectomy (Ficarra et al, 2009). Similarly, incontinence and sexual dysfunction rates are comparable. Blood loss is less than with open techniques because the pneumoperitoneum helps reduce venous hemorrhage. Conversion to open surgery is rare after the initial learning curve.

▶ Radical Cystectomy with Urinary Diversion

The laparoscopic approach to radical cystectomy with urinary diversion, although growing in popularity, has not achieved the dominance as in prostatectomy. The cystectomy portion of the procedure is often considered less technically demanding than prostatectomy; it is the urinary diversion with bowel that makes the procedure so difficult.

The cystectomy/cystoprostatectomy portion of the procedure is similar to that of laparoscopic radical prostatectomy. The urinary diversion with bowel can be performed through a "mini-laparotomy" after first harvesting the bowel laparoscopically, or it can be performed totally intracorporeally. Data on oncologic efficacy and complications are still sparse (Nix et al, 2010). Certainly, though, these techniques will continue to evolve.

▶ Miscellaneous Laparoscopic Procedures

Numerous other laparoscopic procedures have been described. Interesting examples include laparoscopic ureteroneocystostomy for vesicoureteral reflux, psoas hitch with or without a Boari flap, augmentation enterocystoplasty, parapelvic cyst resection, lumbar sympathectomy, ileal ureter, anatrophic nephrolithotomy, pyelolithotomy, ureterolithotomy, flank herniorrhaphy, and catheterizable cecal tubes (ACE Malone). Continued improvement in technology, surgical skills, and patient demand will likely further expand laparoscopic urologic surgery.

COMPLICATIONS

During the first decade of urologic laparoscopy, much attention was paid to its "steep learning curve." Reports from pioneering centers indicated complication rates that were high initially but then fell markedly with experience (Kumar and Gill, 2006). For surgeons with laparoscopic experience during training, however, this "learning curve" is less dramatic

(Cadeddu et al, 2001). In general, the rates of minor and major complications of laparoscopy are similar to those in open surgery. The intraoperative complications that are most feared during laparoscopy, just as in open surgery, are vascular and viscus injury. The problem in laparoscopy is that such injuries may require an emergent change in the approach (ie, conversion to hand assistance or open surgery), whereas in open surgery, the problem can be managed right there. As such, maneuvers during laparoscopic surgery must be more deliberate and careful, not because complications are easier to create but because they may be harder to manage.

FUTURE OF LAPAROSCOPY

Laparoscopy is now well established in urology, although for some applications, laparoscopy has not yet reached its fullest potential. Evolving technologies likely will enhance not only laparoscopy but also all surgical endeavors. LESS, NOTES, microlaparoscopy, and robotic assistance continue to develop. The greatest challenge is to integrate laparoscopy into urologic practice such that it is a technique not only for specialists but also for all urologists with a surgical practice.

BIBLIOGRAPHY

Ahmed MA et al: Comparison of outcomes of different varicocelectomy techniques: Open inguinal, laparoscopic, and subinguinal microscopic varicocelectomy: A randomized clinical trial. Urology 2007;69(3):417–420.

Baker LA et al: A multi-institutional analysis of laparoscopic orchidopexy. BJU Int 2001;87(6):484–489.

Breda A et al: Association of bowel rest and ketorolac analgesia with short hospital stay after laparoscopic donor nephrectomy. Urology 2007;69(5):828–831.

Cadeddu JA et al: Complications of laparoscopic procedures after concentrated training in urologic laparoscopy. J Urol 2001;166: 2109–2111.

Columbo JR et al: Seven years after laparoscopic radical nephrectomy: Oncologic and renal functional outcomes. Urology 2008;71(6):1149–1154.

Desai MM et al: Prospective randomized comparison of transperitoneal versus retroperitoneal laparoscopic radical nephrectomy. J Urol 2005;173:38–41.

Dimarco DS et al: Long-term success of antegrade endopyelotomy compared with pyeloplasty at a single institution. J Endourol 2006;20:707–712.

Ficarra V et al: Retropubic, laparoscopic, and robot-assisted radical prostatectomy: A systematic review and cumulative analysis of comparative studies. Eur Urol 2009;55(5):1037–1063.

Gabr AH et al: Approach and specimen handling do not influence oncological perioperative and long-term outcomes after laparoscopic radical nephrectomy. J Urol 2009;182(3):874–880.

Gill IS et al: Comparison of 1,800 laparoscopic and open partial nephrectomies for single renal tumors. J Urol 2007;178(1):41–46.

Junghans T et al: Effect of increasing cardiac preload, sympathetic antagonism, or vasodilation on visceral blood flow during pneumoperitoneum. Langenbecks Arch Surg 2005;390(6):538–543.

Kim YS: Arterial and end-tidal carbon dioxide pressure differences during laparoscopic colorectal surgery. Eur J Anaesthesiol 2008;25(1):74–75.

Kommu SS et al: Laparo-endoscopic single-site surgery: Preliminary advances in renal surgery. BJU Int 2009;103(8):1034–1037.

Kumar U, Gill IS: Learning curve in human laparoscopic surgery. Curr Urol Rep 2006;7(2):120–124.

Kunkle DA, Uzzo RG: Cryoablation or radiofrequency ablation of the small renal mass. Cancer 2008;113(10):2671–2680.

Lee J et al: Open and laparoscopic adrenalectomy: Analysis of the national surgical quality improvement program. J Am Coll Surg 2008;206(5):953–959.

Manabe D et al: Comparative study of oncologic outcome of laparoscopic nephroureterectomy and standard nephroureterectomy for upper urinary tract transitional cell carcinoma. Urology 2007; 69(3):457–461.

Min SK et al: Carbon dioxide and argon gas embolism during laparoscopic hepatic resection. Acta Anaesthesiol Scand 2007;51(7): 949–953.

Montgomery JS, Wolf JS Jr: Venous thrombosis prophylaxis for urological laparoscopy: Fractionated heparin versus sequential compression devices. J Urol 2005;173(5):1623–1626.

Msezane LP et al: Case report: conservative management of a large capnothorax following laparoscopic renal surgery. J Endourol 2007;21(12):1445–1447.

Nanidis TG et al: Laparoscopic versus open live donor nephrectomy in renal transplantation: A meta-analysis. Ann Surg 2008; 247(1):58–70

Nelson JB: Debate: Open radical prostatectomy vs. laparoscopic vs. robotic. Urol Oncol 2007;25(6):490–493.

Nix J et al: Prospective randomized controlled trial of robotic versus open radical cystectomy for bladder cancer: Perioperative and pathologic results. Eur Urol 2010;57(2):196–201.

Ost MC et al: Urological laparoscopy: Basic physiological considerations and immunological consequences. J Urol 2005;174(4, pt 1):1183–1188.

Permpongkosol S et al: Complications of 2,775 urological laparoscopic procedures: 1993 to 2005. J Urol 2007;177(2):580–585.

Raman JD et al: Single-incision laparoscopic surgery: Initial urological experience and comparison with natural-orifice transluminal endoscopic surgery. BJU Int 2008;101(12):1493–1496.

Rassweiler JJ et al: Laparoscopic retroperitoneal lymph node dissection: Does it still have a role in the management of clinical stage I nonseminomatous testis cancer? A European perspective. Eur Urol 2008;54(5):1004–1019.

Saggar VR et al: Factors influencing development of subcutaneous carbon dioxide emphysema in laparoscopic totally extraperitoneal inguinal hernia repair. J Laparoendosc Adv Surg Tech A 2008; 18(2):213–216.

Silberstein J, Parsons JK: Hand-assisted and total laparoscopic nephrectomy: A comparison. J Soc Laparoendosc Surg 2009;13:36–43.

Valentin MD et al: Recurrent asystolic cardiac arrest and laparoscopic cholecystectomy: A case report and review of the literature. J Soc Laparoendosc Surg 2004;8(1):65–68.

Wolf JS Jr: Devices for hand-assisted laparoscopic surgery. Expert Rev Med Devices 2005;2(6):725–730.

Yoder BM, Wolf JS Jr: Long-term outcome of laparoscopic decortication of peripheral and peripelvic renal and adrenal cysts. J Urol 2004;171(2):583–587.

Robotic Surgery in Urology

10

Maxwell V. Meng, MD, MPH

Minimally invasive surgery has played an important role in urologic surgery, with the widespread and frequent application of extracorporeal (shock wave lithotripsy), endoscopic, and laparoscopic techniques. Over the past decade, the introduction of robotic assistance has significantly altered the landscape of laparoscopic surgery in urology and will likely continue to play an important role in the future.

BACKGROUND

▶ History

Despite the variety and complexity of operations achievable with traditional laparoscopy, major limitations included the two-dimensional vision and instrumentation with restricted degrees of freedom as well as reduced tactile feedback (haptics). Thus, initial efforts were limited to extirpative or ablative procedures while technically demanding reconstruction requiring suturing and intracorporeal knot tying was primarily limited to highly experienced or specialized surgeons.

The concept of having an apparatus to aid or augment what is possible with the human hand is not new. The term "robot" is derived from the Czech word *robota* meaning "work" or "forced labor" and was introduced by the writer Karel Capek. Isaac Asimov coined the term robotics, although the definition of a robot is quite varied. Critical elements of a robot include programmability, flexibility, and ability to interact with the environment. Thus, most robots are computerized systems with mechanical capabilities.

With respect to surgical robots, there are those that are shared control (robot is primarily an assistant, such as camera holder), telesurgical, and supervisory controlled. The first robot utilized in urology was the PROBOT, an example of the last type where the robot performed transurethral resection of the prostate based on directions programmed into the controlling computer. The currently used robots are telesurgical or master–slave systems, wherein the surgeon controls the robotic arms during the procedure from a remote console and the robot is merely an instrument; thus, given the lack of automation, procedures performed with these machines may be better categorized as robotic-assisted surgery.

Computer Motion Inc. developed both AESOP, which controlled the endoscope using either voice or hand/foot control, and the ZEUS surgical system, consisting of three robotic arms attached to the operating table controlled remotely by the surgeon. In 2003, the company was acquired by Intuitive Surgical Inc., which was founded in 1995 and had developed the da Vinci surgical system, composed of a surgeon console, video tower and computer, and patient-side cart with three or four robotic arms.

▶ da Vinci System

Figure 10–1 shows the da Vinci system. It is currently the most widely utilized surgical robot with nearly 1500 units in operation worldwide. The surgeon sits at the console where an immersive, three-dimensional view of the surgical field is provided. Control of the instruments is achieved via freemoving finger controls, which translate the physical motion of the fingers and wrists into electrical signals and computerized such that the robotic arms mirror these movements (Figure 10–2). The surgical cart consists of either three or four arms, depending on the generation. True binocular vision is provided by a 12-mm scope with two separate video channels. A variety of inter-changeable instruments are available and attached to the robotic arms, which are introduced into the body through 8 mm or 5 mm ports. The ends of the instruments have seven degrees of freedom and are able to mimic the surgeon's hand after tremor filtration and motion scaling, if desired. Unlike traditional laparoscopy, the da Vinci system incorporates (1) three-dimensional vision, (2) articulation of the instruments at the wrist, (3) improved surgeon ergonomics, and (4) natural translation of surgeon movements to instrument tips. It

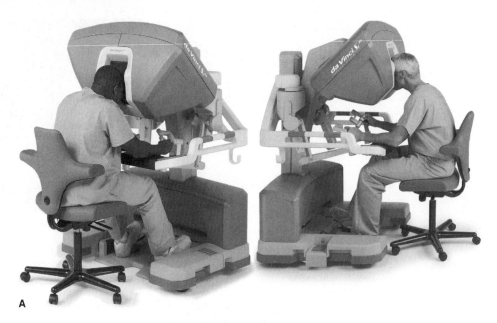

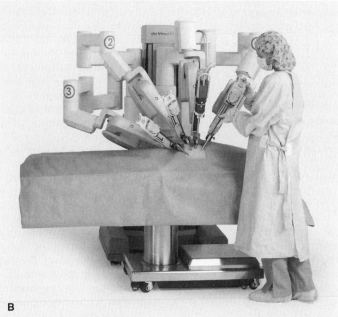

▲ **Figure 10–1.** The da Vinci Si robotic surgical system made by Intuitive Surgical Inc. It consists of the **(A)** surgeon console (here with the dual console HD Si) and **(B)** patient-side surgical cart, in this model with four arms (Images courtesy of Intuitive Surgical Inc.).

remains to be determined whether incorporation of robotics into traditional urologic procedures improves patient outcomes, but it is clear that for most surgeons, complex and reconstructive tasks are likely facilitated by robotic assistance. Although nearly every imaginable urologic operation, ranging from vasovasostomy to renal transplantation, has been performed with the aid of the robot, the remainder of the chapter will discuss the most common and well-established applications of robotic surgery within urology.

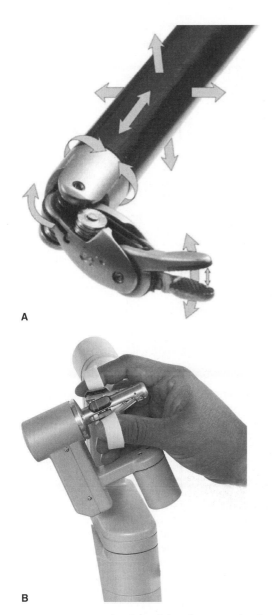

A

B

▲ **Figure 10–2.** Example of the **(A)** EndoWrist technology, with seven degrees of freedom at the tip of the instrument and **(B)** surgeon's hand control at the console.

LOWER URINARY TRACT OPERATIONS

▷ Radical Prostatectomy

The initial target market for the da Vinci system was cardiothoracic surgery, attempting to minimize morbidity by avoiding a sternotomy and taking advantage of the precision and fine instrument movement afforded by the robot. Both coronary revascularization and mitral valve repair are currently performed with robotic assistance, but the operations are technically demanding and have not expanded as rapidly as the application to radical prostatectomy. The first laparoscopic radical prostatectomy was performed in 1991 and several centers reported their experiences with the minimally invasive approach in the late 1990s. Despite refinements in techniques and outcomes comparable with those of traditional open prostatectomy, laparoscopic radical prostatectomy remained a challenging operation, with significant learning curve, and was performed by relatively few surgeons. However, the operation ultimately proved to be the ideal application of robotic assistance and over the past decade, it has largely supplanted both open and laparoscopic prostatectomy; in 2010 it is estimated that 80% of radical prostatectomy operations in the United States will be performed with robotic assistance. Moreover the robot is widely available and has been rapidly adopted by surgeons throughout the country, in both community and academic medical centers.

The operation is fundamentally no different than open or laparoscopic radical prostatectomy, with the goals of complete removal of the prostate and seminal vesicles, performing lymphadenectomy when indicated, and preservation of urinary and sexual function. Various approaches have been described including transperitoneal versus extraperitoneal, and for the transperitoneal technique, the initial dissection can proceed either anteriorly (ie, retropubic space and through the bladder neck) or posteriorly (ie, dissection of the seminal vesicles and through the plane between the prostate and rectum). Regardless of technique, the patient must be placed in a steep Trendelenburg position in order to displace the bowels cranially, away from the pelvis. Some patients with underlying cardiac or pulmonary disease or obesity may not tolerate being in this position for a prolonged period. In addition, the abdomen is insufflated with carbon dioxide typically to 15 mm Hg pressure, further affecting pulmonary and cardiac function and requiring carefully monitoring by the anesthesia team. Meticulous attention to patient positioning is critical to prevent neuropraxia in the dark operating room environment; it may also be difficult to assess the patient with the additional equipment and bulk of the robotic system. Once the robot is docked in position with the camera and instruments inserted through the ports, the patient and operating room table cannot be moved until the instruments and robot are disengaged. Factors that make the robotic approach challenging include prior complex abdominal or pelvic surgery, morbid obesity, large prostate or median lobe, and prior radiation or prostate surgery; nevertheless, these are not absolute contraindications and surgery is often feasible despite these factors.

In assessing the success of robotic-assisted laparoscopic radical prostatectomy, the relevant outcomes of cancer control, urinary continence, and sexual function must be evaluated. Compared with open retropubic prostatectomy, robotic-assisted prostatectomy is associated with decreased risks of operative blood loss and need for transfusion.

Table 10–1. Perioperative and oncologic outcomes of robotic-assisted laparoscopic radical prostatectomy from select published series.

Series	No.	OR time (mean)	EBL (mean)	Hospital stay (d)	Positive margins			Biochemical recurrence (%)
					pT2 (%)	pT3 (%)	Overall (%)	
Ahlering et al (2004)	60	231	103	—	9	—	16.7	—
Joseph et al (2006)	325	180	196	—	11	—	13	—
Smith et al (2007)	100	208[a]	141[a]	1.1	9	50	15	16[b,c]
Badani et al (2007)	2766	154	142	1.14	13	35	12	7.3
Zorn et al (2007a)	744	234	222	1.4	13	45	19	6.9
Patel et al (2008)	1500	105	111	1	4	33	9	5
Murphy et al (2009)	400	186	[d]	3.1	10	42	19	13

[a]Chan RC et al: Effect of a large prostate gland on open and robotically assisted laparoscopic radical prostatectomy. BJU Int 2008;101:1140.
[b]Barocas DA et al: Robotic assisted laparoscopic prostatectomy versus radical retropubic prostatectomy for clinically localized prostate cancer: Comparison of short-term biochemical recurrence-free survival. J Urol 2010;183:990.
[c]Actuarial survival.
[d]Transfusion rate 2.5%.

With respect to oncologic outcomes, open radical retropubic prostatectomy is the gold standard against which new techniques must be compared. Large series of men undergoing surgery at high-volume centers have been published with long-term follow-up and include both pathologic outcomes and biochemical outcomes (Table 10–1). Smith et al (2007) reported lower rates of positive surgical margins in the robotic group compared with the open group (15% vs 35%, $p < .001$). Similar rates of positive surgical margins have been reported by Ahlering et al (2004) (16.7%), Menon et al (2007) (11%), and Patel et al (2010) (10.6%) and are likely not significantly different when compared with radical retropubic prostatectomy. In two large robotic series, the risk of positive margin was 4% and 13% in pT2 and 34% and 35% in pT3 (Badani et al, 2007; Patel et al, 2008). The risk of biochemical recurrence after robotic prostatectomy appears to be low and comparable with that of open prostatectomy. At median follow-up of 22 months, Badani et al (2007) reported 5-year actuarial biochemical-free survival of 84%. Longer follow-up is required to evaluate if there are significant differences in recurrence-free, and more importantly, cancer-specific survival. Using the SEER-Medicare Linked Database, Hu et al (2009) did not find a difference in rates of utilization of secondary cancer treatments, such as androgen deprivation and radiation therapy, for men undergoing minimally invasive versus open surgery, suggesting that cancer outcomes were similar.

After open prostatectomy, continence rates 1 year after surgery are expected to be ≥90%. Most single institution series of robotic prostatectomy report comparable results, with ≥93% of men being continent 12 months after surgery (Table 10–2). Although there do not appear to be significant differences, men undergoing robotic prostatectomy may have

more rapid return of continence. However, data from Hu et al (2009) suggest that men undergoing minimally invasive prostatectomy may have worse urinary outcomes compared with open prostatectomy. The population-based study found an increase in diagnosis of both incontinence and erectile dysfunction. It is important to note that the study did not differentiate between laparoscopic and robotic surgery, covered the early period of minimally invasive prostatectomy (2003–2007), and relied on Medicare claims rather than validated surveys to assess outcomes.

The enhanced three-dimensional and magnified visualization of the da Vinci system has led to a better appreciation and renewed consideration of the neuroanatomy of the prostate and parasympathetic innervation responsible for male erections. Techniques developed during the evolution of robotic prostatectomy to improve preservation of nerve bundles include high anterior release of the periprostatic fascia (coined the Veil of Aphrodite) and minimizing the use of thermal energy during dissection around the neurovascular bundles. Whether these maneuvers ultimately improve erectile function is unclear, but the reexamination of technique and anatomy has led to alterations in both minimally invasive and open surgical operations; it is difficult to determine which approach yields the best sexual function. Overall rates of potency after open prostatectomy have been reported to approach 70%, but are largely dependent on baseline function and age (Table 10–3). Approximately 60–70% of patients undergoing bilateral nerve-sparing robotic prostatectomy can be expected to have erections 12 months after surgery. As mentioned, Hu et al (2009) reported an increased diagnosis of erectile dysfunction (26.8 vs 19.2 per 100 person-years) in men undergoing minimally invasive prostatectomy. They also

Table 10–2. Urinary outcomes after robotic-assisted laparoscopic radical prostatectomy from select series.

	No.	Urinary continence rate (months)				Anastomotic stricture rate (%)
		3	6	12	>12	
Joseph et al (2006)	325	93	96	—	—	2.1
Patel (2007)	500	89	95	97	—	—
Zorn et al (2007b)	300	47	68	90	92	1.4
Menon et al (2007)	1142	—	—	84	—	—
Murphy et al (2009)	395	—	—	91	95	3.8
Patel et al (2010)	1100	85	96	97	98	—

noted that the minimally invasive approach was associated with shorter hospitalization, lower rates of blood transfusion, fewer respiratory and surgical complications, and fewer anastomotic strictures. However, they noted an increased rate of genitourinary complications. Table 10–4 summarizes complications in published robotic prostatectomy series.

Radical Cystectomy

Similar to laparoscopic radical prostatectomy, laparoscopic cystectomy was reported to be feasible early in the evolution of laparoscopy (1992) but was infrequently performed due to the technical challenges and limitations in instrumentation, prolonged operative time, and need for complex reconstruction. With increasing laparoscopic skills and experience with radical prostatectomy, more reports of laparoscopic cystectomy emerged and the operation developed over the past decade, with robotic-assisted cystectomy a natural progression given the benefits provided by the robot. Nevertheless, it remains a difficult operation given the need for meticulous cancer excision, extended lymphadenectomy in all cases, and urinary tract reconstruction.

The primary indication for robotic cystectomy includes patients with muscle-invasive or high-risk/refractory noninvasive urothelial carcinoma of the bladder. The operation has been reported to be feasible in both men (cystoprostatectomy) and women (anterior pelvic exenteration), and it also includes removal of the pelvic lymph nodes. Most surgeons perform the extirpative portion of the operation using the robot, and then make a small lower abdominal incision to extract the specimens as well as perform the urinary diversion; however, a purely minimally invasive approach to the entire operation has been described and is feasible, but it is time consuming and potentially of little additional benefit.

Table 10–3. Sexual function outcomes after robotic-assisted laparoscopic radical prostatectomy from select series.

	No.	Mean age (years)	Follow-up (months)	Nerve-sparing (%)		Intercourse (%)		Overall potency % (months)			
				U	B	U	B	3	6	12	>18
Joseph et al (2006)	325	60	12	24	70	58	81	—	—	81	—
Patel (2007)	200	63	12	—	—	—	—	—	70	78	—
Zorn et al (2007b)	258	59	24	26	60	62	83	53	61	80	84
Menon et al (2007)	1142	60	12	25	33	74	97	—	—	70	100
Tewari et al (2008)	215	60	12	11	85	—	87	—	—	87	—
Murphy et al (2009)	248	60	12	28	65	—	—	—	—	62	—
Patel et al (2010)	404	58	12	0	100	—	97	69	82	92	97

U, unilateral; B, bilateral.

Table 10–4. Reported complications after robotic-assisted laparoscopic radical prostatectomy from select series.

	No.	Overall	Clavien ≥III	Death	Bowel injury	Blood transfusion	Neuropraxia	Urine leak	Thromboembolic event	Urinary retention
Joseph et al (2006)	325	10	—	0	0.3	1.3	0.6	1.2	1.5	—
Patel (2007)	1500	4.4	—	0	0.13	0.5	—	1.4	0.33	0.3
Zorn et al (2007b)	300	10.6	—	—	0	1.7	1.4	1.4	0.6	—
Badani et al (2007)	2766	12.2	0.6	<0.01	—	1.5	—	—	—	—
Murphy et al (2009)	400	15.8	5.3	0	1.2	2.5	—	4.5	—	—
Novara et al (2010)	415	21.6	3.2	—	1.2	5.3	0.9	6.7	0.2	1.4
Lasser et al (2010)	239	17	5.4	0.4	0.4	4.2	1.3	2.9	0.4	0.8
Coelho et al (2010)	2500	5.1	0.96	0	0.08	0.48	0	1.4	0.32	0.52

Most series regarding robotic cystectomy are single-institution, nonrandomized case series. Nix et al (2010) report the only prospective, randomized trial comparing robotic versus open radical cystectomy for bladder cancer in a total of 41 men. The primary endpoint evaluated was the lymph node yield, and the mean number removed in the robotic and open groups was 19 and 18, respectively. There were no significant differences with respect to positive surgical margins or perioperative outcomes, including length of hospitalization and overall complication rate. The same group reported no case of positive surgical margin in 100 consecutive cases of robotic radical cystectomy (Pruthi et al, 2010), while the International Robotic Cystectomy Consortium (Hellenthal et al, 2010) reported a rate of 6.8% in 513 patients—1.5% for stage ≤pT2, 8.8% for pT3, and 39% for pT4. Further evaluation, beyond surrogates such as lymph node number and margin status, is necessary to assess the oncologic efficacy of the operation.

Yuh et al. (2009) prospectively analyzed the impact of robotic cystectomy on quality of life in 34 patients undergoing surgery. Despite a significant number (38%) requiring chemotherapy, quality of life as assessed by the Functional Assessment of Cancer Therapy-Bladder instrument showed improvements at 3 months after surgery and total scores at 6 months exceeding preoperative scores.

Kauffman et al (2010) characterized the complications in 79 consecutive patients undergoing robotic radical cystectomy. Within 90 days of surgery, 49% experienced a complication of which 79% were low grade including infectious (41%) or gastrointestinal (27%). Sixteen percent of patients had a high-grade complication and were significantly associated with age older than 65 years, operative blood loss ≥500 mL, and intravenous fluids >5 L. These compare favorably with open radical cystectomy. Other studies suggest that advantages of the robotic approach include reduced blood loss, lower transfusion rate, shorter hospital stay, and earlier resumption of regular diet (Wang et al, 2008).

UPPER URINARY TRACT OPERATIONS

▶ Pyeloplasty

The management of ureteropelvic junction (UPJ) obstruction has evolved and various approaches have been attempted, including traditional open surgery, endoscopic, and laparoscopic/robotic. The open operation options include dismembered, flap, and incisional-intubated types, based on the specific ureteral anatomy, size of the renal pelvis, and the presence or absence of a crossing renal vessel. All of these have been applied using either pure laparoscopy or robotic assistance, and the outcomes must be compared against the gold standard of open techniques, with contemporary series reporting success in >90% of cases.

The first laparoscopic adult pyeloplasty was reported in 1993, where a dismembered pyeloplasty was performed similar to the open technique. Since that time, larger series of laparoscopic pyeloplasty have been reported with resolution of UPJ obstruction in >90%. Many would consider it the gold standard in the management of cases of adult UPJ obstruction today. Nevertheless, it remained largely performed by experienced surgeons at academic referral centers given the low incidence of condition and technical challenges of the complex reconstruction, including cutting of the pelvis and ureter and subsequent suturing. Robotic assistance was first reported for pyeloplasty in 2002, given the potential to facilitate tailoring the pelvis and ureter, and suturing the anastomosis. Outcomes have been excellent, with short-term resolution of the UPJ obstruction to be >95%; many of these series have included cases of secondary UPJ obstruction after failed prior therapy (eg, endopyelotomy) (Singh et al, 2010). Hemal et al (2010) compared robotic and laparoscopic pyeloplasty in 60 patients. Advantages of the robotic method included faster operative time, less blood loss, and shorter hospitalization (2 vs 3.5 days), with similar success rates (97% robotic vs 100% laparoscopic).

Mufarrij et al (2008) reported the combined robotic pyeloplasty experience in 140 patients from three medical centers. The mean operative time was 217 minutes with length of stay 2.1 days. Resolution of UPJ obstruction on the first follow-up imaging study was 96% and the complication rate was 10%, and the mean follow-up was 29 months. Gupta et al (2010) reported similar outcomes in 85 patients, with 97% success at 14 months follow-up.

▶ Partial Nephrectomy

The management of renal tumors has evolved rapidly over the past 20 years, with the advent of laparoscopic techniques as well as the application of ablative technologies. The first laparoscopic radical nephrectomy, performed in 1990, represented a shift toward minimally invasive renal surgery, and subsequent data have proven that equivalent cancer control is achieved by the laparoscopic technique. The excellent oncologic outcomes combined with the ease of completely removing the kidney, even for small masses, have contributed to the relative underutilization of nephron-sparing surgery (Dulabon et al, 2010). Recent publications have suggested that greater efforts should be made to spare as much normal renal parenchyma as possible, and that partial nephrectomy needs to be performed more often (McKiernan et al, 2002; Huang et al, 2006). However, open partial nephrectomy has been viewed as a difficult operation because of patient morbidity, expectation of significant bleeding, and concerns surrounding surgical margins. All of these factors are relevant in the discussion of laparoscopic partial nephrectomy. Despite the fact that the first laparoscopic partial nephrectomy was reported in 1993, acceptance and dissemination were relatively slow, given the technical skills required to ensure complete tumor excision and to achieve hemostasis.

Large series from highly experienced laparoscopic surgeons confirm both the oncologic adequacy of laparoscopic partial nephrectomy as well as the safety and low risk of complications. Improved instrumentation, such as vascular and bulldog clamps, and application of energy sources facilitated tumor excision and renorrhaphy. However, concerns still surrounded renal injury given the ischemic time required for the procedure, most often performed without renal hypothermia. Thus, hand assistance was proposed as an aid to reduce warm ischemia time. Likewise, the robot may also facilitate minimally invasive partial nephrectomy by making specific aspects easier and thereby shorten the duration of vascular occlusion. Minimally invasive partial nephrectomy, either laparoscopic or robotic, is a challenging operation requiring meticulous tumor excision, control of bleeding, and closure of the collecting system with the simultaneous need for alacrity and underlying risk of significant bleeding.

Gettman et al (2004) reported the initial series of partial nephrectomy procedures using the da Vinci robot. They demonstrated that the operation was feasible, with no case of conversion to open, and operative time averaged 215 minutes. In 8 of the 13 cases, renal cooling was achieved by an intra-arterial catheter, while the remainder underwent partial nephrectomy with vascular clamping alone (warm ischemia). Another report compared outcomes between robotic partial nephrectomy performed by an experienced open surgeon and laparoscopic partial nephrectomy performed by experienced laparoscopic experts (Deane et al, 2008). There were no significant differences in operative time, operative blood loss, and warm ischemia time, suggesting that robotic assistance was able to help those less experienced with laparoscopy achieve good outcomes. A larger, contemporary single surgeon study found no difference in the techniques with respect to blood loss and positive surgical margins; however, the robotic approach had advantages of shorter operative and warm ischemia time as well as length of hospitalization (Wang et al, 2009).

Over the past 3 years, numerous publications have confirmed the feasibility of robotic partial nephrectomy with outcomes similar to laparoscopic partial nephrectomy (Scoll et al, 2010; Benway et al, 2009). Rates of positive surgical margin are <5% and complications typically occur in <10% of patients. Potential complications include wound infection, urinary leak/urinoma, and ileus. Major complications include bleeding and need for open surgical conversion.

Newer techniques have been developed and tested to obtain hemostasis, including the use of hemostatic agents, thermal energy devices, and novel sutures and suturing aids. In addition, selective clamping of renal artery branches or omission/early release of vascular occlusion has been performed to reduce the potential for renal injury. These modifications have allowed surgeons to approach more difficult tumors—those >4 cm, endophytic location, multiple masses, and those located adjacent to the renal helium and large vessels. Long-term data are required to confirm cancer control equivalent to radical nephrectomy and/or open partial nephrectomy and preservation of renal function. Most agree, however, that the availability of the robot permits surgeons with less experience with laparoscopy to perform the procedure and shortens the learning curve for the operation.

PEDIATRIC OPERATIONS

In urology, robotic assistance has been applied to nearly every pediatric operation that has been accomplished via laparoscopy. The advantages may be greater in this domain given the preponderance of reconstructive, rather than extirpative, procedures. Conversely, the pediatric population poses unique challenges—limited working space within the body, need for smaller ports and instruments, restricted access to the smaller patient by the large surgical cart, and limited haptics on delicate tissue. In addition, the relative benefits of minimally invasive surgery on postoperative recovery and morbidity may be less significant than in the adult. Although a survey of parental satisfaction of open and robotic pyeloplasty using a validated surgery demonstrated greater satisfaction with the robotic approach, the differences were not at great as anticipated (Freilich et al, 2010).

The most common robotic-assisted operation in children is pyeloplasty, and the early cumulative experience demonstrates that the outcomes are not significantly different from open pyeloplasty (Lee et al, 2006; Olsen et al, 2007). Success is expected in >95% of cases with complication rates <20%. Other applications of the robot include heminephrectomy for nonfunctioning polar moiety in a duplicated system, extravesical ureteral reimplantation, and bladder augmentation. The role of robotics in operations such as adrenalectomy and total nephrectomy are unclear, given the ease in performing the procedure via traditional laparoscopy and inability to take advantage of the added dexterity and precision provided by the robot.

SINGLE-SITE ROBOTIC SURGERY

The newest variation of minimally invasive urologic surgery is the use of only one incision through which all of the instruments and laparoscope are introduced and the procedure is performed, best termed laparoendoscopic single-site surgery (LESS). Tools have been developed to facilitate the ease of surgery and ergonomics, including smaller deflectable-tip laparoscopes, bent and articulating laparoscopic instruments, and single-port access systems. A major challenge of LESS is the need to adapt to new laparoscopic instruments and the "sword fighting" and crossing of instruments both inside and outside of the body. The da Vinci robot has been successfully applied to LESS in performing prostatectomy, radical and partial nephrectomy, and dismembered pyeloplasty (Kaouk et al, 2008). It is expected that further refinements of the robotic system will permit better adaptation to LESS, and these are currently being developed and tested.

COST-EFFECTIVENESS

A major criticism of the robotic system is the associated financial costs. Each da Vinci surgical system is approximately $1.5 million with annual maintenance requirements of over $100,000. In addition, the costs of disposables associated with the robot exceed those of traditional laparoscopy. Bolenz et al (2010) compared the costs associated with robotic, laparoscopic, and open prostatectomy for prostate cancer in 643 patients treated over a 6-year period. Robotic prostatectomy was associated with the highest cost, due to differences in surgical supply and operating room cost. Even with improvements in operative time, rapid time to discharge, and increase in surgical volume, robotic prostatectomy is likely to remain more expensive than other techniques (Lotan, 2010). Given the unproven improvement in outcomes with robotic assistance, physicians should be cautious in the wholesale application to all minimally invasive operations and attempts should be made to systematically study newer surgical technologies. In the future, these economic factors will only be more relevant for both surgeons and patients given the explosion of health care expenditure, greater scrutiny of outcome and quality of care, and inevitable cost cutting measures in the era of health care reform.

TRAINING IN ROBOTICS

The introduction and proliferation of new technology and surgical techniques has raised questions regarding how best to train both residents and practicing urologists. Currently, there are no established systems to ensure surgeon competency and safety with robotic urological surgery. These issues have been raised by a panel of experts (Zorn et al, 2009), and future guidelines should be expected to help standardize the process of robotic education, training, proctoring, and credentialing.

BIBLIOGRAPHY

Radical Prostatectomy

Ahlering TE et al: Robot-assisted versus open radical prostatectomy: A comparison of one surgeon's outcomes. Urology 2004;63:819. [PMID: 15134953]

Badani KK et al: Evolution of robotic radical prostatectomy: Assessment after 2766 procedures. Cancer 2007;110:1951. [PMID: 17893904]

Barocas DA et al: Robotic assisted laparoscopic prostatectomy versus radical retropubic prostatectomy for clinically localized prostate cancer: Comparison of short-term biochemical recurrence-free survival. J Urol 2010;183:990. [PMID: 20083261]

Chan RC et al: Effect of a large prostate gland on open and robotically assisted laparoscopic radical prostatectomy. BJU Int 2008; 101:1140. [PMID: 18399829]

Coelho RF et al: Early complication rates in a single-surgeon series of 2500 robotic-assisted radical prostatectomies: Report applying a standardized grading system. Eur Urol 2010;57(6):945–952. [PMID: 20181424]

Hu JC et al: Comparative effectiveness of minimally invasive vs. open radical prostatectomy. JAMA 2009;302:1557. [PMID: 19826025]

Joseph JV et al: Robotic extraperitoneal radical prostatectomy: An alternative approach. J Urol 2006;175:945. [PMID: 16469589]

Lasser MS et al: An unbiased prospective report on perioperative complications of robot-assisted laparoscopic radical prostatectomy. Urology 2010;75:1083. [PMID: 20110114]

Menon M et al: Vattikuti Institute prostatectomy: Contemporary technique and analysis of results. Eur Urol 2007;51:648. [PMID: 17097214]

Murphy DG et al: Operative details and oncological and functional outcome of robotic-assisted laparoscopic radical prostatectomy: 400 cases with a minimum of 12 months follow-up. Eur Urol 2009;55:1358. [PMID: 19147274]

Novara G et al: Prospective evaluation with standardized criteria for postoperative complications after robotic-assisted laparoscopic radical prostatectomy. Eur Urol 2010;57:363. [PMID: 19944519]

Patel VR et al: Robotic radical prostatectomy: Outcomes of 500 cases. BJU Int 2007;99:1109. [PMID:17437441]

Patel VR et al: Robot-assisted laparoscopic radical prostatectomy: Perioperative outcomes of 1500 cases. J Endourol 2008;22:2299. [PMID: 18837657]

Patel VR et al: Continence, potency and oncological outcomes after robotic-assisted radical prostatectomy: Early trifecta results of a high-volume surgeon. BJU Int 2010;106(5):696–702. [PMID: 20707793]

Smith JA Jr et al: A comparison of the incidence and location of positive surgical margins in robotic-assisted laparoscopic radical prostatectomy and open retropubic radical prostatectomy. J Urol 2007;178:2385. [PMID: 17936849]

Tewari A et al: Cancer control and the preservation of neurovascular tissue: How to meet the competing goals during robotic radical prostatectomy. BJU Int 2008;101:1013. [PMID: 18261153]

Zorn KC et al: da Vinci robot error and failure rates: Single institution experience on a single three-arm robot unit of more than 700 consecutive robot-assisted laparoscopic radical prostatecomies. J Endourol 2007a;21:1341. [PMID: 18042027]

Zorn KC et al: Robotic-assisted laparoscopic prostatectomy: Functional and pathologic outcomes with interfascial nerve preservation. Eur Urol 2007b;61:755. [PMID: 17084520]

Radical Cystectomy

Hellenthal NJ et al: Surgical margin status after robot assisted radical cystectomy: Results from the International Robotic Cystectomy Consortium. J Urol 2010;184:87. [PMID: 20478596]

Kauffman EC et al: Critical analysis of complications after robotic-assisted radical cystectomy with identification of preoperative and operative risk factors. BJU Int 2010;105:520. [PMID: 19735257]

Nix J et al: Prospective randomized controlled trial of robotic versus open radical cystectomy for bladder cancer: Perioperative and pathologic results. Eur Urol 2010;57:196. [PMID: 19853987]

Parra RO et al: Laparoscopic cystectomy: Initial report on a new treatment for the retained bladder. J Urol 1992;148:1140. [PMID: 1404624]

Pruthi RS et al: Robotic radical cystectomy for bladder cancer: Surgical and pathological outcomes in 100 consecutive cases. J Urol 2010;183:510. [PMID: 20006884]

Wang GJ et al: Robotic vs. open radical cystectomy: Prospective comparison of perioperative outcomes and pathological measures of early oncological efficacy. BJU Int 2008;101:89. [PMID: 17888044]

Yuh B et al: Short-term quality-of-life assessed after robot-assisted radical cystectomy: A prospective analysis. BJU Int 2009;103:800. [PMID: 19021613]

Pyeloplasty

Gupta NP et al: Outcome analysis of robotic pyeloplasty: A large single-centre experience. BJU Int 2010;105:980. [PMID: 19874304]

Hemal AK et al: Laparoscopic pyeloplasty versus robotic pyeloplasty for ureteropelvic junction obstruction: A series of 60 cases performed by a single surgeon. Can J Urol 2010;17:5012. [PMID: 20156381]

Mufarrij PW et al: Robotic dismembered pyeloplasty: A 6-year, multi-institutional experience. J Urol 2008;180:1391. [PMID: 18707739]

Singh I et al: Robot-assisted pyeloplasty: Review of the current literature, technique and outcome. Can J Urol 2010;17:5099. [PMID: 20398449]

Partial Nephrectomy

Benway BM et al: Robot assisted partial nephrectomy versus laparoscopic partial nephrectomy for renal tumors: A multi-institutional analysis of perioperative outcomes. J Urol 2009;182:866. [PMID: 19616229]

Deane LA et al: Robotic versus standard laparoscopic partial/wedge nephrectomy: A comparison of intraoperative and perioperative results from a single institution. J Endourol 2008;22:947. [PMID: 18397157]

Dulabon LM et al: Trends in renal tumor surgery delivery within the United States. Cancer 2010;116:2316. [PMID: 20225227]

Gettman MT et al: Robotic-assisted laparoscopic partial nephrectomy: Technique and initial clinical experience with DaVinci robotic system. Urology 2004;64:914. [PMID: 15533477]

Huang WC et al: Chronic kidney disease after nephrectomy in patients with renal cortical tumours: A retrospective cohort study. Lancet Oncol 2006;7:735. [PMID: 16945768]

McKiernan J et al: Natural history of chronic renal insufficiency after partial and radical nephrectomy. Urology 2002;59:816. [PMID: 12031359]

Scoll BJ et al: Robot-assisted partial nephrectomy: A large single-institutional experience. Urology 2010;75:1328. [PMID: 20080290]

Wang AJ et al: Robotic partial nephrectomy versus laparoscopic partial nephrectomy for renal cell carcinoma: Single-surgeon analysis of >100 consecutive procedures. Urology 2009;73:306. [PMID: 19038419]

Pediatric Operations

Freilich DA et al: Parental satisfaction after open versus robot assisted laparoscopic pyeloplasty: Results from modified Glasgow Children's Benefit Inventory Survey. J Urol 2010;183:704. [PMID: 20022046]

Lee RS et al: Pediatric robot assisted laparoscopic dismembered pyeloplasty: Comparison with a cohort of open surgery. J Urol 2006;175:683. [PMID: 16407025]

Olsen LH et al: Pediatric robot assisted retroperitoneoscopic pyeloplasty: A 5-year experience. J Urol 2007;178:2137. [PMID: 17870122]

Single-Site Robotic Surgery

Kaouk JH et al: Robotic single-port transumbilical surgery in humans: Initial report. BJU Int 2008;103:366. [PMID: 18778351]

Cost-Effectiveness

Bolenz C et al: Cost comparison of robotic, laparoscopic, and open radical prostatectomy for prostate cancer. Eur Urol 2010;57:453. [PMID: 19931979]

Lotan Y: Economics of robotics in urology. Curr Opin Urol 2010;20:92. [PMID: 19875963]

Training in Robotics

Zorn KC et al: Training, credentialing, proctoring and medicolegal risks of robotic urological surgery: Recommendations of the society of urologic robotic surgeons. J Urol 2009;182:1126. [PMID: 19625032]

Retrograde Instrumentation of the Urinary Tract

11

Marshall L. Stoller, MD

The ability to manipulate the urinary tract without the need for an open surgical incision differentiates urology from other disciplines. Such intervention may be required for diagnostic or therapeutic purposes (or both). Understanding the various catheters, guidewires, stents, endoscopes, and associated instrumentation is key in helping physicians accomplish their desired tasks. Manipulation of the urinary tract should be performed in a gentle fashion; instruments need not be forced. An understanding of anatomy and alternative instrumentation should allow physicians to accomplish their tasks with finesse. The patient should understand the proposed procedure and potential complications. For example, the attempt to place a retrograde ureteral catheter to drain an infected kidney may ultimately lead to a percutaneous nephrostomy if the surgeon is unable to achieve retrograde drainage. Knowing when to stop is as important as knowing when to start.

Many procedures are performed at the bedside or in a cystoscopy suite under local anesthesia. A patient who is comfortable, informed, and assured will more likely cooperate and tolerate the procedure. A physician who is familiar with the proposed instrumentation and understands its limitations and alternatives will win the patient's confidence.

Manipulation of the urinary tract can result in significant injury. Anticipated prolonged procedures should be covered with appropriate antibiotics directed by preoperative urine cultures and sensitivities. Generous use of a water-soluble lubricant and low-pressure irrigation decreases the likelihood of significant iatrogenic infections. Patient positioning is as important as proper choice of instrumentation. Pressure points must be identified and adequately padded, especially when the patient is placed in the dorsal lithotomy position. In addition, the legs should be secured in their stirrups to prevent accidental injury, such as those that might result from a leg hitting the surgeon after an unexpected obturator reflex during endoelectric surgery.

URETHRAL CATHETERIZATION

Urethral catheterization is the most frequent retrograde manipulation performed on the urinary tract. Catheters are placed to drain the bladder during and after surgical procedures requiring anesthetics, to assess urinary output in critically ill patients, to collect reliable urine specimens, for urodynamic evaluation, for radiographic studies (eg, cystograms), and to assess residual urine. Such catheters can be left indwelling with a self-retaining balloon, as is done with a Foley catheter. An in-and-out procedure to drain a bladder does not require a self-retaining device. Adequate lubrication and sufficient frequency to keep the bladder at reasonable volumes are critical and must be emphasized to the patient performing self-intermittent catheterization; sterility is secondary. In contrast, when a catheter is left indwelling it is important to use sterile technique.

▶ Technique of Catheterization

A. In Men

The penis should be positioned pointing toward the umbilicus to decrease the acute angulation as the catheter traverses the bulbar urethra. On most occasions, the catheter passes without difficulty. When difficulties arise, a careful history relating to previous urologic manipulations is critical. Strictures are not infrequent and can occur after endourologic surgery. Urethral strictures can be found from the meatus to the bladder neck. History of a straddle injury may suggest a bulbar urethral stricture. Adequate lubrication injected into the urethra and instruction of the patient to relax his pelvic floor eases the passage beyond the striated rhabdosphincter. A large-caliber catheter of approximately 18F should be used. Narrow, stiff, small catheters have greater potential of creating false passages and possible perforation. Coudé (elbowed) tipped catheters frequently help negotiate a high bladder neck, as seen with benign prostatic hyperplasia. With self-retaining Foley catheters, complete advancement until the elbowed valve is at the meatus or until the urine returns is important. Inflating the balloon prematurely (while it is in the urethra) may result in severe pain and possible urethral rupture. This must be emphasized to ancillary nursing personnel dealing with patients who are unable to communicate effectively, because under such circumstances, urethral rupture may present only after severe infection is evident.

B. In Women

It may be difficult to identify the meatus, especially in patients with obesity or hypospadias. Lateral and outward traction on the labia and the use of the posterior bill of a vaginal speculum may be helpful. With adequate instruction and a mirror to visualize the meatus, women can learn to catheterize themselves. For repeat catheterizations, a finger inserted into the vagina can help to guide the catheter.

C. Difficult Placement and Removal

When a urethral catheter cannot be placed, filiforms and followers may be used. The narrow filiform leaders are stiff and can puncture the urethra if too much force is used. Thus, gentle advancement should stop when resistance is encountered, and the initial filiform should be left in place. A second and third filiform, and possibly additional ones, should be placed next to the previously placed catheters in hope that the existing catheter occupies false passages or tortuous kinks. Eventually, one of the filiforms should pass and coil into the bladder. A screw adaptor at the end of the filiform can be used to connect progressively larger followers to dilate the narrowed urethra. After adequate dilatation, an open-tipped Council catheter can be placed over the filiform and into the bladder. If a problem or undue resistance is encountered at any stage, the procedure should be aborted and a suprapubic cystostomy should be placed to achieve adequate drainage.

Indwelling catheters should be secured to a closed gravity drainage system. Drainage tubing connected to catheters should be positioned to limit dependent curls and thereby limit airlocks that will frequently limit bladder evacuation. For long-term requirements in males, the catheter should be secured to the abdominal wall to decrease urethral traction pressure and potential stricture formation. Meatal care is needed to ensure adequate egress of urethral secretions.

Difficulty is much less common when removing indwelling urethral catheters. Here, the retention balloon is deflated prior to removal. On occasion, the balloon may not deflate. Inspection of the valve frequently reveals a problem. One may cut proximal to the valve in hopes of evacuating the balloon contents, but this is not always successful. Other options include transperineal or transabdominal balloon puncture (best with ultrasonographic guidance), or injection of an organic agent such as ether through the balloon port (with a full bladder to prevent chemical cystitis) to dissolve the balloon wall. If the catheter cannot be advanced, retracted, or twisted, one should suspect an unintended suture that could have been placed during prior surgery; such sutures can be cut via the small pediatric endoscope placed along the Foley catheter. Another complication of urethral catheters is incrustation, especially when a catheter is left indwelling for a long time.

▶ Catheter Design

Catheters differ in size, shape, type of material, number of lumens, and type of retaining mechanism (Figure 11–1). Standard sizes of external catheter diameters and most endoscopic instruments are given according to Charriére's French scale (units of 0.33 mm = 1 French [F] or 1 Charriére [Charr]). Thus, 3F equals 1 mm in diameter and 30F equals 10 mm in diameter.

The choice of catheter size is dependent on the patient and the purpose. Large-caliber catheters are used to evacuate blood clots or other debris. Other catheters are used to stabilize grafts after open urethroplasties, for stenting after endoscopic incisions of strictures, for support of external ureteral catheters, or to assess urinary output. Triple-lumen catheters (one port for balloon inflation and deflation, and one each for inflow and outflow) have smaller lumens than two-way catheters. Other catheter variables include balloon size and construction materials; smaller catheters typically have smaller balloons. Large balloons (eg, 30 mL) can be inflated well over 50 mL to decrease the likelihood of the balloon migrating into the prostatic fossa, especially after transurethral resection of the prostate (TURP). They can be used as traction devices against the bladder neck to control hemorrhage from the prostatic fossa after TURP.

The rigidity of the catheter, the ratio between internal and external diameters, and the biocompatibility depend on the material with which the catheter is made. The standard latex catheter can result in severe reactions in patients with latex allergies, most commonly seen in those with myelomeningoceles. Silicone varieties are good alternatives in such situations. Mucosal irritation is decreased when catheters with a low coefficient of friction are used. Hydromers are placed onto catheters to allow for transient coating, creating an interface between biologic tissues and the foreign catheter; this interface lasts for approximately 5 days. Permanent hydrogel coatings last the life of the catheter. Decreasing the coefficient of friction of these catheters brings about a decrease in mucosal irritation and better biocompatibility. Catheters with a longer lasting interface result in decreased incrustation.

URETHROSCOPY

To identify and aid in treating urethral pathology, endoscopic inspection via a urethroscope with a 0° lens is helpful. Stricture disease can be identified or confirmed after radiographic studies. Strictures are characterized by circumferential narrowing.

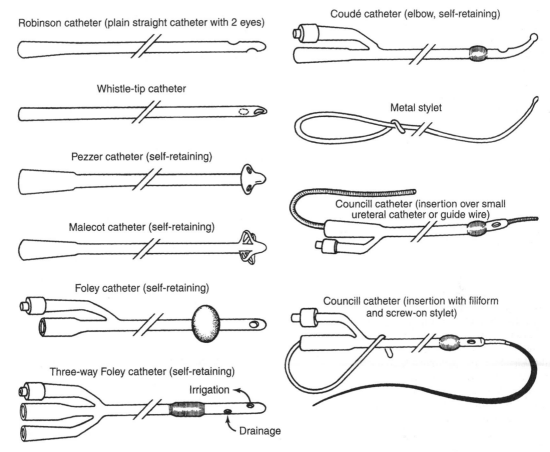

▲ **Figure 11–1.** Urethral catheters, metal stylet, catheter, and guidewire techniques for catheter insertion.

Sequential dilation of urethral strictures by inserting catheters of increasing size exerts shear and tear forces to the mucosa and is likely to produce extended scarring. Thus, stricture recurrence is common if periodic urethral dilation is terminated. Balloon dilation of a stricture with 7–9F balloon dilators (which can be passed over guidewires and inflated up to 30F with pressures of up to 15 atm) does not exert shear force, but the long-term results are varied. Limited circumferential strictures can be incised under direct vision with an endoscopic cold knife. The incision is usually made at the 12-o'clock position, adequate to allow passage of the urethroscope. The bladder then can be evacuated and adequate irrigation used if further incision results in hemorrhage. It is difficult to identify the true extent and depth of a stricture solely by vision because scarring can involve deeper tissues. Here, urethral ultrasonography is an adjunct.

Urethral diverticulum can be identified with urethroscopy. A catheter can be placed through the neck of the diverticulum to help confirm its location during definitive open surgical repair. Urethroscopy can be used to direct injection of dye into rare retained müllerian duct cysts, to identify and extract foreign bodies or rare calculi, and to access biopsy-suspicious lesions. Urethroscopy allows endoscopic treatment of urethral condylomata.

▶ **CYSTOSCOPY**

Endoscopic inspection of the lower urinary tract requires irrigation, illumination (fiberoptics), and optics. The optics and illumination are offset by the irrigating and working port. To optimize a complete examination, the rigid endoscope should be rotated, and 0°, 30°, 70°, and 120° lenses may be required. Suprapubic pressure facilitates inspection of the bladder dome, which frequently has an air bubble. A systematic approach is required when evaluating the urethra, prostate, bladder walls, dome and neck, and ureteral orifices (including location, number, shape, and character of efflux). The bladder should be evaluated at different levels of filling. It is only after full distention of the bladder that characteristic glomerulations and ecchymoses are seen in patients with interstitial cystitis. Rectal examination with the endoscope in place is informative, especially in assessing prostate size and length of prostatic urethra. Similarly, concurrent vaginal examination in women can be useful in evaluation of cystoceles.

Choice of irrigant during endoscopic manipulation is important. There are conductive and nonconductive irrigants. Conductive irrigants, which include saline and lactated Ringer's solution, would be inappropriate during traditional endoelectric surgery because the electrical charge would be diffused by the irrigant. Nonconductive irrigants include water and glycine. Water has a theoretic advantage of increasing visibility, and because it is hypotonic, it can lyse tumor cells. If the potential exists for increased intravascular absorption, iso-osmotic or other nonhemolyzing agents are preferred to hypotonic solutions.

Rigid endoscopy results in discomfort, which can be minimized with 1% lidocaine per urethra as a local anesthetic. Flexible endoscopes decrease patient discomfort and allow for instrumentation in the supine rather than the dorsal lithotomy position. They are now used routinely in an office setting for hematuria/tumor surveillance and double-J stent retrieval. Videoendoscopy with flexible scopes allows patients to visualize normal and abnormal anatomy and thus helps them understand their pathology. Videoendoscopy reduces fluid contact to the urologist and can help reduce potential cervical neck disease exacerbated with altered posture when endoscopy is performed without videoendoscopic monitoring. However, there are disadvantages. Flexible scopes have smaller irrigating ports, and they do not have a working sheath. As a result, changing lenses, assessing residual urine, and repeat evacuation of irrigant cannot be completed without entirely removing the endoscope. Rigid endoscopy allows for a greater variety of instrumentation, better optics, and increased durability.

Instrumentation similar to that used to evaluate the urethra and bladder can be used to inspect continent urinary reservoirs or conventional ileal loops. A Robinson or a Foley catheter placed prior to the endoscope gives the operator a visual landmark and an exit port for irrigation to keep the procedure at a low pressure. Alternatively, the Foley balloon can be inflated and the catheter plugged to transiently expand the intestinal segment in hopes of helping to identify landmarks or pathologic lesions. Endoscopic inspection allows for identification of calculi, foreign bodies and mucous plugs, and also has the potential for intubation of ureterointestinal anastomoses.

URETERAL CATHETERIZATION

Ureteral catheterization is required in performing retrograde pyelography, collecting urine for cytologic examination or cultures, and performing brush biopsies (Figure 11–2). Other procedures (Figure 11–3) that require ureteral

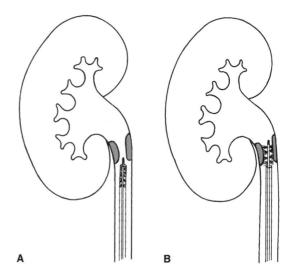

▲ **Figure 11–2.** Brushing of a proximal ureteral lesion. **A:** Insertion of the brush covered by a catheter. **B:** Advancement of the brush through the lesion.

catheterization include draining an obstructed kidney due to either intrinsic or extrinsic compressions and placement of an internal double-J stent. Finding the ureteral orifice can be difficult. Long-term indwelling Foley catheters, infection, history of ureteral reimplantation, or renal transplantation can hinder identification of the ureteral orifice. One must first try to identify the interureteric ridge and then look for a jet of urinary efflux. Varying bladder volumes and use of intravenous methylene blue may be helpful. However, it may take up to 5–20 minutes for intravenous agents to be excreted out of the ureteral orifice. Once the orifice is identified, catheters usually are placed uneventfully. However, in the setting of benign prostatic hyperplasia with J-hooking of the distal ureter, previous retroperitoneal surgery, reimplantation of the ureter, decreased lower extremity mobility or other skeletal abnormalities, or edema or kinking secondary to longstanding impacted ureteral calculi, catheterization procedures can be difficult or impossible. An Albiron bridge may help direct catheters and guidewires.

There are many configurations of catheter tips (Figure 11–4). Acorn or cone-tipped catheters are excellent for routine retrograde pyelography. Care should be taken to eliminate air in the catheter before injection to avoid confusing air with a filling defect. Fluoroscopy helps determine the appropriate volume of radiocontrast material to decrease the likelihood of pyelolymphatic or pyelovenous reflux or forniceal rupture. The average collecting system holds 7–9 mL of contrast material. If performed under local anesthesia, overdistention is recognized by severe ipsilateral flank pain. With low-pressure injections, there is no systemic absorption of contrast material. A Coudé-tipped catheter allows for

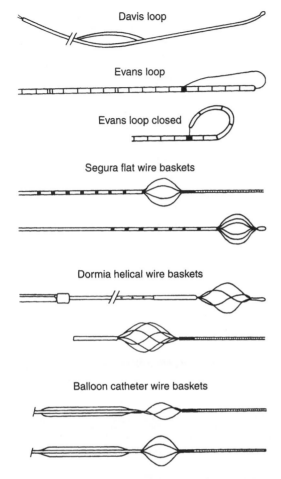

▲ Figure 11–3. Loops, wire baskets, and wire baskets with balloon catheters for extraction of ureteral stones.

dramatic mobility of the tip of the catheter by merely twisting it; there is no need for exaggerated motion of the endoscope. This is helpful in orifices that are difficult to identify because of edema or tumor infiltration.

To bypass severe angulations, passage of a guidewire must first be attempted. Straight guidewires can be made floppy if they have retractable cores, and this allows easy passage frequently. At times, hydrophilic coudé-tipped torque guidewires are helpful. If the orifice can be engaged with the tip of the guidewire but the guidewire cannot be advanced, the tip of the endoscope should be pivoted toward the contralateral orifice while the guidewire is advanced through the endoscope just enough to keep the guidewire engaged in the orifice. The guidewire should then be advanced against the back wall of the bladder, effectively changing the vector force so that the wire can be advanced through a severe J deformity (Figure 11–5). With the guidewire advanced, an exchange catheter can be advanced over the guidewire for injection of

contrast material, to be exchanged later for another guidewire or an open-ended catheter. A coudé-tipped guidewire or floppy-tipped guidewire (with a removable core guide) can be advanced through such exchange catheters to facilitate bypassing stones or severe kinks. A push–pull maneuver (pulling the exchange catheter while pushing the guidewire) frequently straightens the ureter as a result of resistance from the exchange catheter, allowing advancement of the guidewire. To increase resistance, an occlusion balloon ureteral catheter can be inflated and with gentle traction can help straighten a kinked or tortuous ureter. Additional helpful maneuvers include deep exhalation, thus elevating the diaphragm, external cephalad pressure by an assistant, or Trendelenburg patient positioning.

Double-J catheters are used to facilitate internal drainage due to obstruction from ureteral angulation and internal or external ureteral compression; they are also used to help decrease the likelihood of sepsis or obstruction in the presence of steinstrasse after extracorporeal shock wave lithotripsy. Double-J stents increase the internal lumen of the ureter. This increase may be used to one's advantage in the setting of a narrow ureter. Placing a double-J catheter and postponing the ureteroscopy for a few days significantly decreases the difficulty of the subsequent procedure. Double-J stents disrupt normal ureteral peristalsis. These stents can be placed over a guidewire or with a closed leading end. With proper placement of the proximal end into the renal pelvis, the J should project in the lateral position when seen on fluoroscopy or x-ray. Projecting in an anterior–posterior position suggests a proximal ureteral location. Proximal-J stent placement can be confirmed by renal ultrasonography during placement in pregnant patients. If it is too long, the distal end in the bladder can result in severe irritative voiding symptoms; if too short, it is more likely to migrate proximally beyond the ureteral orifice into the ureter. In the latter situations, drainage cannot be ensured, and the stent must be extracted with a ureteroscope or snared with a ureteral stone basket.

Patients must be informed that internalized stents have been placed. Frequently, they will not feel the stent. When the stent is left in place for prolonged periods, the likelihood of incrustations, poor drainage, and difficult extraction is increased. It is unclear whether double-J stents facilitate drainage because of drainage around the catheter or via the numerous side holes communicating with the internal lumen. New helically ridged double-J ureteral stents likely enhance ureteral stone passage through unidirectional ratchet-like motion over the external ridges during respiratory and body wall motion. Other complications include distal migration into the bladder, distal migration beyond the bladder neck (resulting in total urinary incontinence), and flank pain during micturition secondary to reflux. The catheter can be removed with forceps via a flexible or rigid cystoscope or by pulling a string that has been attached to the distal end of the catheter and left exiting through the meatus.

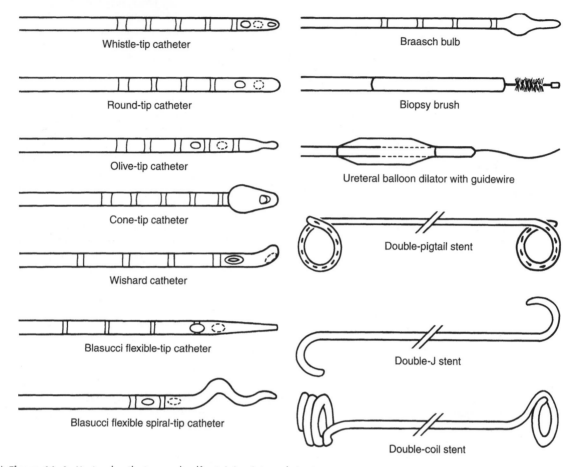

▲ **Figure 11–4.** Ureteral catheters and self-retaining internal stents.

Although double-J catheters have potential complications, they can help ensure internal urinary drainage.

Balloon dilators can be used to ease passage of ureteroscopes (rigid or flexible; see Chapter 8) and extract intact large calculi. Balloons are routinely passed over a guidewire. Woven balloons have a tight, unfolded outer surface that shortens in longitudinal length when inflated. In contrast, nonwoven varieties are folded and may be difficult to pass after initial inflation and deflation; however, they do not shorten in length with inflation. Balloons inflated alongside distal ureteral calculi can result in balloon perforation or extrusion of the calculus outside the ureteral lumen. Balloon inflation is best achieved with ratcheted or torqued syringe aids directed with pressure gauges. Ureteral access sheaths, frequently made with a hydrophilic coating, can be placed over a guidewire. They dilate the ureter without the need for a ureteral balloon and simplify multiple passages up the ureter.

Retrograde endopyelotomy is an alternative to laparoscopic and open surgical repair, and percutaneous antegrade approaches. After documentation of the exact location of the ureteropelvic junction obstruction under fluoroscopic control, a 150-cm superstiff Lunderquist guidewire is advanced into the renal pelvis. The endoscope is removed and the retrograde endopyelotomy device (Acucise) is advanced over the guidewire under fluoroscopic control. After the incising wire is directed laterally, the balloon is inflated during cautery. Successful results are seen in approximately 80% of patients. An internal endopyelotomy double-J stent, 14F at the proximal end, straddling the ureteropelvic junction, and tapered to 6–8F as it enters and coils in the bladder, or a routine 7F double-J ureteral stent is placed over the stiff guidewire and left in place for 6 weeks. Placing a standard double-J catheter before this procedure dilates the ureter and eases passage of the Acucise and the endopyelotomy double-J catheter.

A large selection of endoscopic baskets is available to entrap and remove material including calculi, sloughed papillae, bulky tumors, fungal bezoars, and foreign bodies. Baskets are designed with and without filiform leaders and can be advanced on their own or, more commonly, through the working ports of flexible and rigid ureteroscopes. Round

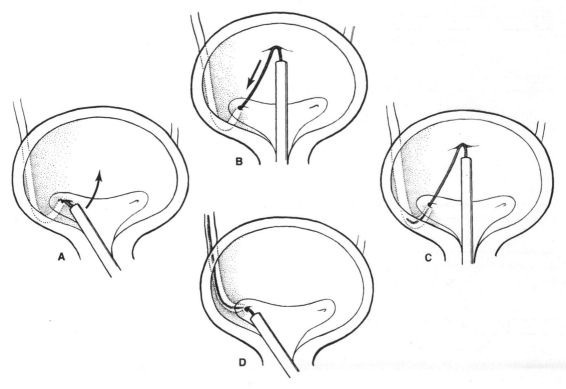

▲ **Figure 11–5.** Negotiating a difficult ureteral orifice. ***A:*** Guidewire engaged in orifice cannot be advanced. ***B:*** Endoscope is rotated toward contralateral orifice. Guidewire remains engaged in orifice. ***C:*** Guidewire is advanced against bladder wall. ***D:*** Guidewire negotiated beyond angulation.

wire baskets can be torqued to help entrap the target material. A few (2–3) wired baskets are used for large material, while numerous (4–6) wired baskets are used for small or numerous objects. Flat-wired baskets can engage stones effectively. If twisted, however, the wire can fold and transform into a knifelike edge. Once the basket is engaged, one should ensure that the endothelium is not entrapped. Gentle traction helps extract these foreign materials. Engaged baskets may be difficult to disengage. Occasionally, one must cut the handle and place a ureteroscope alongside the basket to facilitate stone and basket extraction. Nitinol baskets have rounded tops and decrease potential endothelial trauma.

Transurethral injections can be performed through a variety of endoscopes. Newer injectables include fibrin glue, Botox, and bulking agents for deflux procedures.

TRANSURETHRAL SURGERY

Resectoscopes are endoscopes with sheaths of 10–30F (Figure 11–6) designed for transurethral surgery; they allow urologists to excise, fulgurate, or vaporize tissue from the lower genitourinary tract. Applying an alternating current at high frequencies decreases muscular contractions and allows for cutting and coagulation properties. A pure sine wave is optimal for cutting, whereas dampened oscillating waveforms are best for coagulation. It is possible to combine the two waves to allow for simultaneous cutting and coagulation. A ground plate, as an indifferent electrode, usually applied over the hip, is required. The cutting current results in rapid vaporization of tissue, allowing the cutting loop to move easily through tissue with minimal resistance, and separates the chip, enabling easy flow into the bladder. Rapid succession of cutting sweeps allows rapid surgical excision. In contrast, a coagulation current results in less rapid vaporization and thus decreased separation of tissue from the cutting current. If a traditional resectoscope does not cut tissue, the operator should check for a broken resecting loop, a broken or disconnected cable or generator, or a conductive irrigant (as with saline) that diffuses the current. In contrast, plasmakinetic or bipolar resectoscopes send current from one edge of the endoscopic loop to the other. A high electrical current is generated locally at the loop and effectively vaporizes tissue on contact. Due to the bipolar design,

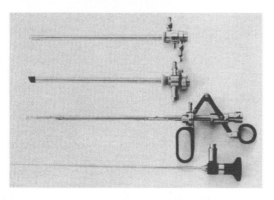

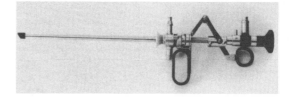

▲ **Figure 11–6.** Transurethral resectoscope. **Left:** Continuous-flow sheath, standard sheath, working element with cutting loop, telescope. **Right:** Instrument assembled.

conductive irrigants are used with these bipolar resectoscopes. Resection can also be performed with lasers in a similar fashion.

Before transurethral surgery, the urethra should be calibrated with sounds to ensure ease in placing the resectoscope. Urethral sounds and probes come in numerous varieties (Figure 11–7). An Otis urethrotome can be used to incise the urethra at the 12-o'clock position, thereby decreasing the potential for stricture disease in narrow urethras. Generous use of a water-soluble lubricant is indicated. Before placement of the resectoscope, the loop should be inspected for defects and for appropriate engagement to ensure complete retraction into the sheath, thereby allowing resected tissue to flow easily into the bladder. The endoscope can be placed under direct vision, especially if the patient has not recently been cystoscoped. Alternatively, a Timberlake obturator allows for blind placement of the resectoscope sheath. Older endoscopes require the operator to intermittently remove the working element to allow evacuation of bladder contents. Contemporary endoscopes have an additional channel for continuous operation. An alternative is a percutaneous suprapubic drainage catheter, which allows for maximal continuous flow. Orientation with identification of landmarks, such as the verumontanum and the ureteral orifices, before resection dramatically decreases the potential for complications. Bladder lesions are best resected with minimal bladder distention to decrease the likelihood of perforation. A Bugbee electrode can be used for point coagulation of bleeding points or pathologic lesions. A rollerball can be used to coagulate large areas. Transurethral resection can be used to resect an obstructing prostate gland, to drain prostatic abscesses, or to unroof the ejaculatory duct in select infertility patients.

TURP is a time-tested procedure for resecting prostatic tissue and decreasing symptoms of urinary obstruction. In experienced hands, this can be done with minimal complications. New, alternative procedures are being investigated, especially with patients who are poor anesthetic risks, whose

life expectancy is limited, or who are averse to TURP. Those with small glands or with bladder neck contractures have been treated by transurethral incision of the prostate from a point just distal to the ureteral orifices to the verumontanum. Transcystoscopic urethroplasty, also known as prostatic

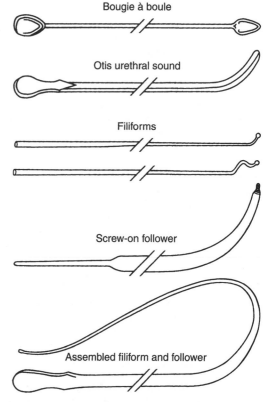

▲ **Figure 11–7.** Urethral probes and sounds.

balloon dilatation, dilates the prostatic urethra under visual and fluoroscopic control. Intraurethral coils can be placed in high-risk patients to avoid permanent catheter drainage. Thermotherapy treatment delivers temperatures of 41°C to 44°C for 60 minutes. Obstructing median lobes are unsuited for such techniques. Interstitial laser ablation of the prostate gland is another method for the management of prostatic enlargement. A variety of bipolar systems are available that allow for vaporization of prostatic tissue. Hemorrhage is limited compared to formal resection techniques, and takes longer to remove an equivalent amount of tissue. Long-term studies are required to compare a variety of newer techniques with TURP.

There are various cutting techniques for resecting an obstructing prostate gland during TURP. All require good vision, a comfortable operator, identification of the surgical capsule, and established goals that are met before starting additional stages of the procedure. Pulsatile arterial bleeders should be coagulated first and venous hemorrhage next. Occasionally, arterial bleeders cannot be coagulated without additional resection of tissue. An Ellik bulb or piston syringe should be available to evacuate resected tissue. At the conclusion of the procedure, one should ensure adequate resection and hemostasis, and perform an inspection for forgotten chips of tissue and possible injuries. A Foley catheter should be placed into the bladder and irrigated to confirm unobstructed flow and adequate hemostasis. If an undermined trigone is suspected, a coudé-tipped catheter, a finger in the rectum, or a stylet inserted into the catheter can help in proper placement. The Foley balloon should be inflated 20 mL + 1 mL for each gram of resected tissue. Gentle traction on the catheter can aid hemostasis.

Video cameras are routinely attached to the optical eyepiece while transurethral surgery is performed. Use of the camera helps to reduce the risk of cervical disc disease and distance the surgeon from blood products. It is an excellent resource to improve the teaching of endoscopic surgery.

Acute complications include intra- or extraperitoneal rupture of the bladder, rectal perforation, incontinence, incision of a ureteral orifice with possible reflux or stricture, hemorrhage, gas explosion (especially during resection of a bladder lesion at the dome in the presence of accumulated gas), epididymitis, sepsis, and transurethral resection syndrome. The transurethral resection syndrome is characterized by delusional hyponatremia resulting in possible confusion, congestive heart failure, or pulmonary edema. It is secondary to a large amount of fluid being absorbed, usually through a perforation of a low-pressure system such as the venous sinusoids. If perforations are noted, especially into a sinus, the height of the irrigating solution should be lowered, hemostasis achieved, and the procedure brought to a rapid conclusion. Other complications include impotence (with excessive coagulation) and urethral stricture disease. After an adequate TURP, retrograde ejaculation almost always occurs.

LOWER TRACT CALCULI

Most bladder calculi originating from the upper tract pass spontaneously through the urethra. In contrast, bladder calculi resulting from outlet obstruction may require endoscopic extraction. Many of these calculi can be washed out or extracted with the aid of various forceps or a resectoscope loop. Calculi too large to pass through an endoscopic sheath first require fragmentation. Visual lithotrites with crushing jaws or a punch-type mechanism are effective. Introduction of these bulky devices is potentially dangerous. A distended bladder facilitates effective engagements of the stone without injuring the bladder wall. Twisting the lithotrite before crushing ensures that the bladder wall is free from the instrument.

Other methods available to fragment bladder calculi include ultrasonic, electrohydraulic, laser, and pneumatic lithotrites. Ultrasonic lithotrites use vibratory energy delivered via a rigid metal transducer. An offset endoscopic lens is required. Gentle pressure of the transducer against the stone facilitates fragmentation; excessive pressure can erode or perforate the bladder wall. A hollow core with suction extracts the fragments. Electrohydraulic lithotripsy generates a spark gap, resulting in a shock wave. It is delivered at the end of a flexible catheter and can be applied as single or repetitive shocks. Fragmentation can be performed with normal saline. A rheostat can adjust the power output. A high setting can result in the stone caroming to various locations in the bladder; lower settings result in suboptimal fragmentation. To optimize fragmentation, the tip of the lithotrite should be a few millimeters away from the stone. To protect the endoscopic optics, the endoscope should be kept at a distance. Shock waves fragment brittle material, such as the stone or a lens. Biologic tissues are elastic and are unharmed as long as the spark gap does not touch them. Air-driven, jack-hammer-like devices (rigid and flexible) can be used for stone fragmentation. Pneumatic lithotrites are effective with minimal tissue trauma. They use reusable probes and are powered by compressed gas. The photothermal mechanism of holmium lasers is effective in fragmenting all types of stones, large, small and multiple bladder stones and is now the most popular lithotrite. Uric acid calculi produce small amounts of cyanide gas when fragmented with holmium lasers; no clinical sequelae have been documented.

ADVANCED INSTRUMENTATION

▶ Lasers

Lasers (light amplification by stimulated emission of radiation) have been used through flexible and rigid endoscopes. Carbon dioxide and argon lasers result in tissue penetration that is inadequate for the needs of urology. Neodymium:YAG lasers give adequate tissue coagulation and are useful for various lesions. The holmium:YAG system is excellent for stone fragmentation and tissue ablation and is now the most

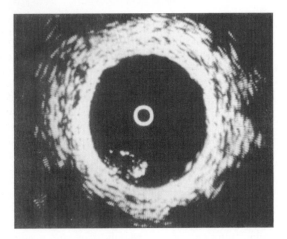

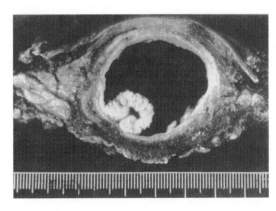

▲ **Figure 11–8.** Multifocal bladder cancer. **Left:** Transurethral ultrasound. **Right:** Cystectomy specimen.

popular system in use. Disadvantages are the lack of adequate tissue for histopathologic evaluation and the initial cost of machinery.

▶ Ultrasonography

Ultrasound has found increased application to the lower genitourinary tract. It results in minimal discomfort; gives a three-dimensional appreciation of the shape, size, and volume of organs and disease; and can provide direct intervention. Various transducers are available; high-megahertz transducers are required for superficial structures (for example, scrotal structures) to assess testicular disease (including tumors and torsion), while low-megahertz transducers are reserved for deep structures (for example, guiding percutaneous access for kidneys and bladders). Intervening tissue can significantly reduce image quality.

Transrectal ultrasound is valuable in evaluating the prostate to determine size and confirm digital information or survey the prostate based on an elevated prostate specific antigen to help determine the presence and stage of a suspected malignant tumor. Because of the low incidence of detecting malignancies (1.6–7%), mass screening programs are not cost effective. Direct needle biopsies, with automatic biopsy mechanisms, are quick, well tolerated, and result in reliable tissue cores and less pain than traditional needles (such as Tru-Cut) directed under digital palpation. Percutaneous drainage tubes, radioactive seed implants, and temperature coils used for cryosurgery of the prostate can be placed safely under transrectal ultrasonic guidance. Transrectal ultrasonography can yield unreliable images that often are misinterpreted by the novice. Pitfalls include faulty instrument settings, poor coupling caused by feces or gas, and unrecognized artifacts resulting from reverberation, deflection, shadowing, or enhancement.

Suprapubic ultrasonography can help to assess prostate anatomy, especially size and intravesical extension. It can help to evaluate the bladder for residual urine and for calculi that are questionable on plain abdominal radiographs. (Changing the patient's position can shift the position of a calculus.) Distal ureteral stones can be identified, especially when visualized through a full bladder used as an acoustic window. Double-J stents, incrustations, diverticula, and large malignant lesions can be identified. The procedure also can direct placement of suprapubic cystostomy drainage catheters.

Additional applications include endocavitary, color, Doppler, and dynamic ultrasonography. Endocavitary ultrasound, which includes transvaginal, transurethral (Figure 11–8), and transcystoscopic techniques, can delineate vaginal, urethral, and bladder disease. Endoureteral ultrasound can help in the identification of crossing vessels, preferably before an endopyelotomy. Color and Doppler ultrasound can assess blood flow as related to erectile dysfunction. Dynamic ultrasound can supplement urodynamic findings. Ultrasound applied to the lower genitourinary tract causes minimal discomfort and provides valuable information.

BIBLIOGRAPHY

Urethral Catheterization

Bloom DA et al: A brief history of urethral catheterization. J Urol 1994;151:317.

Cardenas DD et al: Intermittent catheterization with a hydrophilic-coated catheter delays urinary tract infections in acute spinal cord injury: A prospective, randomized, multicenter trial. PM R 2011;3(5):408–417.PM R. 2011 May;3(5):418.

Choong S et al: A prospective, randomized, double-blind study comparing lignocaine gel and plain lubricating gel in relieving pain during flexible cystoscopy. Br J Urol 1997;80:69.

Foxley S: Indwelling urinary catheters: Accurate monitoring of urine output. Br J Nurs 2011;20(9):564, 566–569.

Lapides J et al: Clean, intermittent self-catheterization in the treatment of urinary tract disease. J Urol 1972;107:458.

Lee EA, Malatt C: Making the hospital safer for older adult patients: A focus on the indwelling urinary catheter. Perm J 2011;15(1):49–52.

Mamoulakis C et al: Results from an international multicentre double-blind randomized controlled trial on the perioperative efficacy and safety of bipolar vs monopolar transurethral resection of the prostate. BJU Int 2012;109(2):240–248.

Stenzelius K et al: Noble metal alloy-coated latex versus silicone Foley catheter in short-term catheterization: A randomized controlled study. Scand J Urol Nephrol 2011;45(4):258–264.

Williams JC et al: Deflation techniques for faulty Foley catheter balloons: Presentation of a cystoscopic technique. Tech Urol 1996;2:174.

Transrectal and Transurethral Ultrasound

Demura T et al: Differences in tumor core distribution between palpable and nonpalpable prostate tumors in patients diagnosed using extensive transperineal ultrasound-guided template prostate biopsy. Cancer 2005;103(9):1826–1832.

Eisenberg ML et al: The importance of tumor palpability and transrectal ultrasonographic appearance in the contemporary clinical staging of prostate cancer. Urol Oncol 2011;29(2):171–176.

Huffman JL et al: Ureteral catheterization, retrograde ureteropyelography and self retaining ureteral stents. In: Bagley DH et al (eds) Urologic Endoscopy: A Manual and Atlas. Little, Brown and Company, Boston, Toronto, 1985, pp. 163–177.

Monga M: The dwell time of indwelling ureteral stents—the clock is ticking but when should we set the alarm? J Urol 2011;185(2):387.

Nash PA et al: Sono-urethrography in the evaluation of anterior urethral strictures. J Urol 1995;154:72.

Phan CN, Stoller ML: Helically ridged ureteral stent facilitates the passage of stone fragments in an experimental porcine model. Br J Urol 1993;72:17.

Stone Basketing

de la Rosette JJ et al: Handling and prevention of complications in stone basketing. Eur Urol 2006;50(5):991–998.

Dourmashkin RL: Cystoscopic treatment of stones in the ureter with special reference to large calculi: Based on a study of 1550 cases. J Urol 1945;54:245.

Leone NT et al: Changing trends in the use of ureteroscopic instruments from 1996 to 2008. J Endourol 2010;24(3):361–365.

Wang CJ et al: Randomized trial of NTrap for proximal ureteral stones. Urology 2011;77(3):553–557.

Wolf JS Jr et al: Cost-effectiveness vs. patient preference in the choice of treatment for distal ureteral calculi: A literature-based decision analysis. J Endourol 1995;9:243.

Cytology, Biopsy Histology

Dodd LG et al: Endoscopic brush cytology of the upper urinary tract: Evaluation of its efficacy and potential limitations in diagnosis. Acta Cytol 1997;41:377.

Endoscopy

Hopkins HH: The modern urological endoscope. In: Gow JG and Hopkins HH (eds) A Handbook of Urological Endoscopy. Churchill Livingstone, Edinburgh, London, New York, 1978, pp. 20–34.

Merkle EM et al: Virtual cystoscopy based on helical CT scan datasets: Perspectives and limitations. Br J Radiol 1998;71:262.

Reuter MA, Reuter HJ: The development of the cystoscope. J Urol 1998;159:638.

Lithotripsy

Bapat SS: Endoscopic removal of bladder stones in adults. Br J Urol 1977;49:527.

Hussein NS, Gohar MR: Pneumatic ureterolithotripsy in paediatric and adolescent patients: A ten-year experience at the Hospital Universiti Sains Malaysia. Singapore Med J 2011;52(1):42–46.

Kara C et al: Transurethral cystolithotripsy with holmium laser under local anesthesia in selected patients. Urology 2009;74(5):1000–1003.

Vassar GJ et al: Holmium:YAG lithotripsy efficiency varies with energy density. J Urol 1998;160:471.

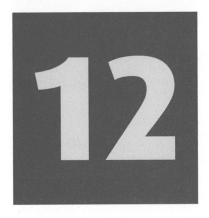

Urinary Obstruction & Stasis

Emil A. Tanagho, MD, & Tom F. Lue, MD, FACS, ScD (Hon)

Because of their potential damage on renal function, urinary obstruction and stasis are important urologic disorders. Ureteral obstruction leads to hydronephrosis, kidney atrophy that may terminate in renal failure. Furthermore, obstruction often is complicated by infection, which causes additional damage to the organs involved.

▶ Classification

Obstruction may be classified according to cause (congenital or acquired), duration (acute or chronic), degree (partial or complete), and level (upper or lower urinary tract).

▶ Etiology

Congenital anomalies, more common in the urinary tract than in any other organ system, are generally obstructive. In adult life, many types of acquired obstructions can occur.

A. Congenital

The common sites of congenital narrowing are the external meatus in boys (meatal stenosis) or just inside the external urinary meatus in girls, the distal urethra (stenosis), posterior urethral valves, ectopic ureters, ureteroceles, and the ureterovesical and ureteropelvic junctions (Beganović et al, 2007; Tan and Smith, 2004). Another congenital cause of urinary stasis is damage to sacral roots 2–4 as seen in spina bifida and myelomeningocele. Vesicoureteral reflux causes both vesical and renal stasis (see Chapter 13).

B. Acquired

Acquired obstructions are numerous and may be primary in the urinary tract or secondary to retroperitoneal lesions that invade or compress the urinary passages. Among the common causes are (1) urethral stricture secondary to infection or injury; (2) benign prostatic hyperplasia or cancer of the prostate; (3) vesical tumor involving the bladder neck or one or both ureteral orifices; (4) local extension of cancer of the prostate or cervix into the base of the bladder, occluding the ureters; (5) compression of the ureters at the pelvic brim by metastatic nodes from cancer of the prostate or cervix; (6) ureteral stone; (7) retroperitoneal fibrosis or malignant tumor; and (8) pregnancy.

Neurogenic dysfunction affects principally the bladder. The upper tracts are damaged secondarily by ureterovesical obstruction or reflux and, often, by complicating infection. Severe constipation, especially in children, can cause bilateral hydroureteronephrosis from compression of the lower ureters.

Elongation and kinking of the ureter secondary to vesicoureteral reflux commonly lead to ureteropelvic obstruction and hydronephrosis. Unless a voiding cystourethrogram is obtained in children with this lesion, the primary cause may be missed and improper treatment given.

▶ Pathogenesis and Pathology

Obstruction and neuropathic vesical dysfunction have the same effects on the urinary tract. These changes can best be understood by considering the effects of (1) a severe meatal stricture on the lower tract (distal to the bladder neck), (2) a large obstructing prostate on the midtract (bladder), and (3) an impacted stone in the ureter on the upper tract (ureter and kidney).

A. Lower Tract (eg, Urethral Stricture)

Hydrostatic pressure proximal to the obstruction causes dilation of the urethra. The wall of the urethra may become thin, and a diverticulum may form. If the urine becomes infected, urinary extravasation may occur, and periurethral abscess can result. The prostatic ducts may become widely dilated.

B. Midtract (eg, Prostatic Hyperplasia)

In the earlier stages (compensatory phase), the muscle wall of the bladder becomes hypertrophied and thickened. With decompensation, it becomes less contractile and, therefore, weakened (Lieber et al, 2010).

1. Stage of compensation—To balance the increasing outlet resistance, the bladder musculature hypertrophies. Its thickness may double or triple. Complete emptying of the bladder is thus made possible.

Hypertrophied muscle may be seen endoscopically. With secondary infection, the effects of infection are often superimposed. There may be edema of the submucosa, which may be infiltrated with plasma cells, lymphocytes, and polymorphonuclear cells. At cystoscopy, surgery, or autopsy, the following evidence of this compensation may be visible (Figure 12–1):

A. TRABECULATION OF THE BLADDER WALL—The wall of the distended bladder is normally quite smooth. With hypertrophy, muscle bundles with deposit of interstitial collage fibers become taut and give a coarsely interwoven appearance to the mucosal surface commonly described as trabeculation. The trigonal muscle and the interureteric ridge, which normally are only slightly raised above the surrounding tissues, respond to obstruction by hypertrophy of their smooth musculature. The ridge then becomes prominent. This trigonal

hypertrophy causes increased resistance to urine flow in the intravesical ureteral segments. It is this mechanism that causes relative functional obstruction of the ureterovesical junctions, leading to back pressure on the kidney and hydroureteronephrosis. The obstruction increases in the presence of significant residual urine, which further stretches the ureterotrigonal complex (Tanagho and Meyers, 1965). (A urethral catheter relieves the obstruction somewhat by eliminating the trigonal stretch. Definitive prostatectomy leads to permanent release of stretch and gradual softening of trigonal hypertrophy with relief of the obstruction.)

B. CELLULES—Normal intravesical pressure is about 30 cm of water at the beginning of micturition. Pressures two to four times as great may be reached by the trabeculated (hypertrophied) bladder in its attempt to force urine past the obstruction. This pressure tends to push mucosa between the superficial muscle bundles, causing the formation of small pockets, or cellules (Figure 12–1).

C. DIVERTICULA—If cellules force their way entirely through the musculature of the bladder wall, they become saccules, then actual diverticula, which may be embedded in perivesical fat or covered by peritoneum, depending on their

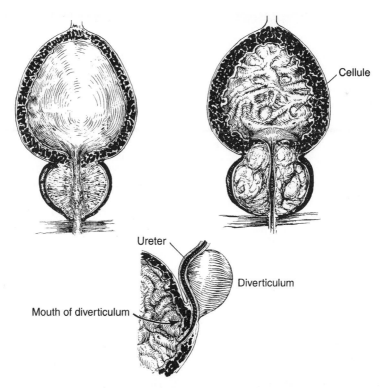

▲ **Figure 12–1.** Changes in the bladder developing from obstruction. ***Upper left:*** Normal bladder and prostate. ***Upper right:*** Obstructing prostate causing trabeculation, cellule formation, and hypertrophy of the interureteric ridge. ***Bottom:*** Marked trabeculation (hypertrophy) of the vesical musculature; diverticulum displacing left ureter.

location. Diverticula have no muscle wall and are therefore unable to expel their contents into the bladder efficiently even after the primary obstruction has been removed. When secondary infection occurs, it is difficult to eradicate; surgical removal of the diverticula may be required. If a diverticulum pushes through the bladder wall on the anterior surface of the ureter, the ureterovesical junction will become incompetent (see Chapter 13).

D. Mucosa—In the presence of acute infection, the mucosa may be reddened and edematous. This may lead to temporary vesicoureteral reflux in the presence of a "borderline" junction. The chronically inflamed membrane may be thinned and pale. In the absence of infection, the mucosa appears normal.

2. Stage of decompensation—The compensatory power of the bladder musculature varies greatly. One patient with prostatic enlargement may have only mild symptoms of prostatism but a large obstructing gland that can be palpated rectally and observed cystoscopically; another may suffer acute retention and yet have a gland of normal size on rectal palpation and what appears to be only a mild obstruction cystoscopically.

In the face of progressive outlet obstruction, possibly aggravated by prostatic infection with edema or by congestion, decompensation of the detrusor may occur, resulting in the presence of large amount of residual urine after voiding. The amount may range up to 500 mL or more.

C. Upper Tract

1. Ureter—In the early stages of obstruction, intravesical pressure is normal while the bladder fills and is increased only during voiding. The pressure is not transmitted to the ureters and renal pelves because of the competence of the ureterovesical "valves." (A true valve is not present; the ureterotrigonal unit, by virtue of its intrinsic structure, resists the retrograde flow of urine.) However, owing to trigonal hypertrophy (see Section "Trabeculation of the bladder wall") and to the resultant increase in resistance to urine flow across the terminal ureter, there is progressive back pressure on the ureter and kidney, resulting in ureteral dilatation and hydronephrosis. Later, with the phase of decompensation accompanied by residual urine, there is an added stretch effect on the already hypertrophied trigone that increases appreciably the resistance to flow at the lower end of the ureter and induces further hydroureteronephrosis. With decompensation of the ureterotrigonal complex, the valve-like action may be lost, vesicoureteral reflux occurs, and the increased intravesical pressure is transmitted directly to the renal pelvis, aggravating the degree of hydroureteronephrosis (Riccabona, 2010; Routh et al, 2010).

Secondary to the back pressure resulting from reflux or from obstruction by the hypertrophied and stretched trigone or by a ureteral stone, the ureteral musculature thickens in its

attempt to push the urine downward by increased peristaltic activity (stage of compensation). This causes elongation and some tortuosity of the ureter (Figure 12–2). At times, this change becomes marked, and bands of fibrous tissue develop. On contraction, the bands further angulate the ureter, causing secondary ureteral obstruction. Under these circumstances, removal of the obstruction below may not prevent the kidney from undergoing progressive obstruction due to the secondary ureteral obstruction.

Finally, because of increasing pressure, the ureteral wall becomes attenuated and therefore loses its contractile power (stage of decompensation). Dilatation may be so extreme that the ureter resembles a loop of bowel (Gimpel et al, 2010) (Figures 12–3 and 13–8, upper right).

2. Kidney—The pressure within the renal pelvis is normally close to zero. When this pressure increases because of obstruction or reflux, the pelvis and calyces dilate. The degree of hydronephrosis that develops depends on the duration, degree, and site of the obstruction (Figure 12–4). The higher the obstruction, the greater effect on the kidney. If the renal pelvis is entirely intrarenal and the obstruction is at the ureteropelvic junction, all the pressure will be exerted on the parenchyma (Klein et al, 2010). If the renal pelvis is extrarenal, only part of the pressure produced by a ureteropelvic stenosis is exerted on the parenchyma; this is because the extrarenal pelvis is embedded in fat and dilates more readily, thus "decompressing" the calyces (Figure 12–2).

In the earlier stages, the renal pelvic musculature undergoes compensatory hypertrophy in its effort to force urine past the obstruction. Later, however, the muscle becomes stretched and atonic (and decompensated).

The progression of hydronephrotic atrophy is as follows (Chevalier, 2010; Rodriguez, 2004):

1. The earliest changes in the development of hydronephrosis are seen in the calyces. The end of a normal calyx is concave because of the papilla that projects into it; with increase in intrapelvic pressure, the fornices become blunt and rounded. With persistence of increased intrapelvic pressure, the papilla becomes flattened, then convex (clubbed) as a result of compression enhanced by ischemic atrophy (Figure 12–5). The parenchyma between the calyces is affected to a lesser extent. The changes in the renal parenchyma are due to (a) compression atrophy from increase in intrapelvic pressure (more accentuated with intrarenal pelves) and (b) ischemic atrophy from hemodynamic changes, mainly manifested in arcuate vessels that run at the base of the pyramids parallel to the kidney outline and are more vulnerable to compression between the renal capsule and the centrally increasing intrapelvic pressure.

2. This spotty atrophy is caused by the nature of the blood supply of the kidney. The arterioles are "end arteries"; therefore, ischemia is most marked in the areas farthest from the interlobular arteries. As the back pressure

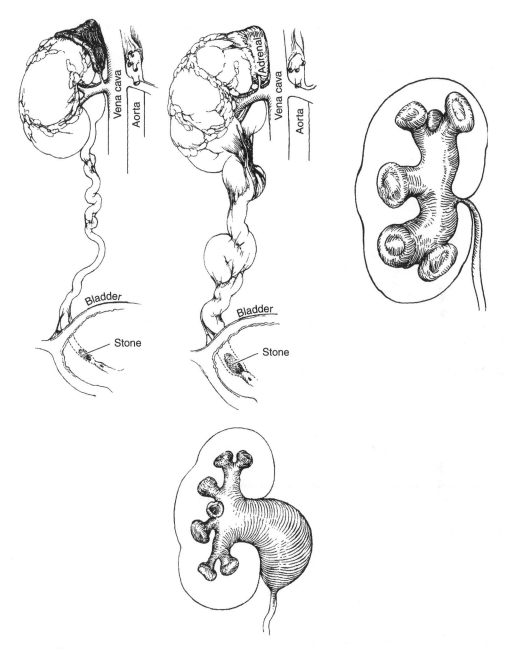

▲ **Figure 12–2.** Mechanisms and results of obstruction. ***Upper left:*** Early stage. Elongation and dilatation of ureter due to mild obstruction. ***Upper center:*** Later stage. Further dilatation and elongation with kinking of the ureter; fibrous bands cause further kinking. ***Upper right:*** Intrarenal pelvis. Obstruction transmits all back pressure to parenchyma. ***Lower:*** Extrarenal pelvis, when obstructed, allows some of the increased pressure to be dissipated by the pelvis.

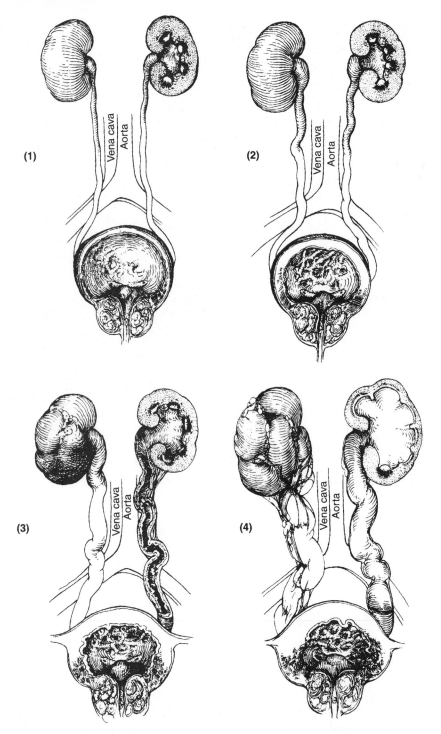

▲ **Figure 12–3.** Pathogenesis of bilateral hydronephrosis. Progressive changes in bladder, ureters, and kidneys from obstruction of an enlarged prostate: thickening of bladder wall, dilatation and elongation of ureters, and hydronephrosis.

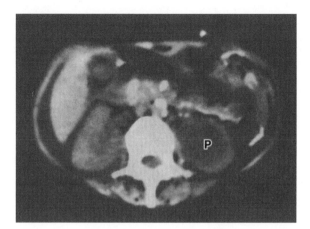

▲ **Figure 12–4.** Hydronephrotic left renal pelvis. Low-density mass (P) in left renal sinus had attenuation value similar to that of water, suggesting the correct diagnosis. Unless intravenous contrast material is used, differentiation from peripelvic cyst may be difficult.

increases, hydronephrosis progresses, with the cells nearest the main arteries exhibiting the greatest resistance.

3. This increased pressure is transmitted up the tubules. The tubules become dilated, and their cells atrophy from ischemia. It should be pointed out that a few instances of dilated renal pelves and calyces are not due to the presence of obstruction. Rarely, the renal cavities are congenitally capacious and thus simulate hydronephrosis. More commonly, hydronephrosis may occur in childhood owing to the back pressure associated with vesicoureteral reflux. If the valvular incompetence resolves (and this is common), some degree of the hydronephrotic changes may persist. These persisting changes may cause the physician to suspect the presence of obstruction, which may lead to unnecessary surgery. A radioisotope renogram to assess ureteral drainage function can be performed to determine whether organic obstruction is present.

4. Only in unilateral hydronephrosis are the advanced stages of hydronephrotic atrophy seen. Eventually, the kidney is completely destroyed and appears as a thin-walled sac filled with clear fluid (water and electrolytes) or pus (Figure 12–6).

If obstruction is unilateral, the increased intrarenal pressure causes some suppression of renal function on that side. The closer the intrapelvic pressure approaches the glomerular filtration pressure (6–12 mm Hg), the less urine can be secreted. Glomerular filtration rate and renal plasma flow are reduced, concentrating power is gradually lost, and the urea–creatinine concentration ratio of urine from the hydronephrotic kidney is lower than that of urine from the normal kidney.

Hydronephrotic atrophy is an unusual type of pathologic change. Other secretory organs (eg, the submaxillary gland) cease secreting when their ducts are obstructed. This causes

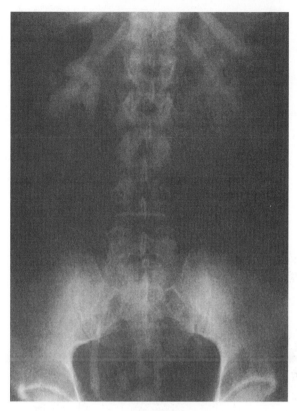

▲ **Figure 12–5.** Lower right ureteral obstruction. Mild-to-moderate dilatation of the collecting system with rounded blunting of the calyces.

primary (disuse) atrophy. The completely obstructed kidney, however, continues to secrete urine. (If this were not so, hydronephrosis could not occur, since it depends on increased intrarenal pressure.) As urine is excreted into the renal pelvis, fluid and, particularly, soluble substances are reabsorbed, through either the tubules or the lymphatics. This has been demonstrated by injecting phenolsulfonphthalein (PSP) into the obstructed renal pelvis. It disappears (is reabsorbed) in a few hours and is excreted by the other kidney. If the intrapelvic pressure in the hydronephrotic kidney rapidly increases to a level approaching filtration pressure (resulting in cessation of filtration), a safety mechanism is activated that produces a break in the surface lining of the collecting structure at the weakest point—the fornices. This leads to escape and extravasation of urine from the renal pelvis into the parenchymal interstitium (pyelointerstitial backflow). The extravasated fluid is absorbed by the renal lymphatics, and the pressure in the renal pelvis drops, allowing further filtration of urine. This explains the process by which the markedly hydronephrotic kidney continues to function. Further evidence of the occurrence of extravasation and reabsorption is

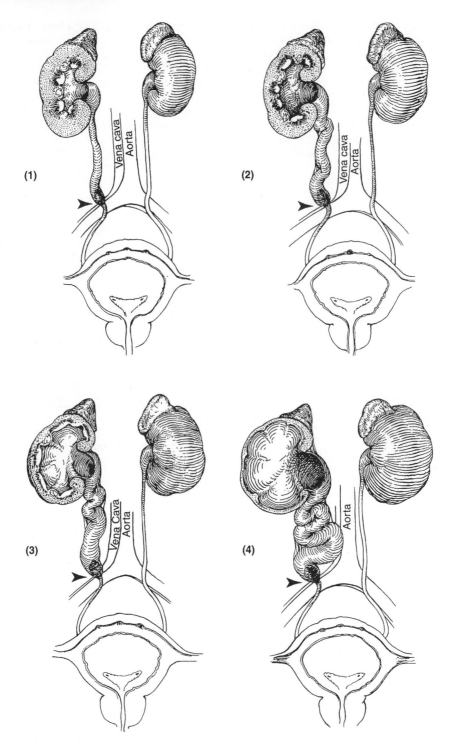

▲ **Figure 12–6.** Pathogenesis of unilateral hydronephrosis. Progressive changes in ureter and kidney secondary to obstructing calculus (*arrowheads*). As the right kidney undergoes gradual destruction, the left kidney gradually enlarges (compensatory hypertrophy).

that the markedly hydronephrotic kidney does not contain urine in the true sense; only water and a few salts are present.

Functional impairment in unilateral hydronephrosis, as measured by excretory urograms or renal scans, is greater and increases faster than that seen in bilateral hydronephrotic kidneys showing comparable damage on urography. As unilateral hydronephrosis progresses, the normal kidney undergoes compensatory hypertrophy (particularly in children) of its nephrons (renal counterbalance), thereby assuming the function of the diseased kidney in order to maintain normal total renal function. For this reason, successful anatomic repair of the ureteral obstruction of such a kidney may fail to improve its powers of waste elimination.

If both kidneys are equally hydronephrotic, a strong stimulus is continually being exerted on both to maintain maximum function. This is also true of a hydronephrotic solitary kidney. Consequently, the return of function in these kidneys after repair of their obstructions is at times remarkable.

The extent of recovery after partial obstruction is difficult to determine preoperatively. Renal scanning with dimercaptosuccinic acid (DMSA) is most helpful. Temporary drainage, especially by nephrostomy, followed by tests to assess renal function is the best measure.

▶ Physiologic Explanation of Symptoms of Bladder Neck Obstruction

The following hypothesis has been proposed to explain the syndrome known as "prostatism," which occurs with progressive vesical obstruction:

The bladder, like the heart, is a hollow muscular organ that receives fluid and forcefully expels it. And, like the heart, it reacts to an increasing workload by going through the successive phases of compensation and finally decompensation.

Normally, contraction of the detrusor muscle in the presence of urine pulls the bladder neck open and the urine is expelled. The intravesical pressure generated in this instance varies between 20 and 40 cm of water.

With bladder neck obstruction, hypertrophy of the vesical musculature develops, allowing the intravesical voiding pressure to rise to 50–100 cm or more of water in order to overcome the increased outlet resistance. Despite this, the encroaching prostate appears to interfere with the mechanisms that ordinarily open the internal orifice. Also, the contraction phase may not last long enough for all of the urine to be expelled; "exhaustion" of the muscle occurs prematurely. The refractory phase then sets in, and the detrusor is temporarily unable to respond to further stimuli. A few minutes later, voiding may be initiated again and completed.

A. Compensation Phase

1. Stage of irritability—In the earliest stages of obstruction of the bladder neck, the vesical musculature begins to hypertrophy. The force and size of the urinary stream remain normal because the balance is maintained between the expelling power of the bladder and urethral resistance. During this phase, however, the bladder appears to be hypersensitive. As the bladder is distended, the need to void is felt. In patients with a normal bladder, these early urges can be inhibited, and the bladder relaxes and distends to receive more urine. However, in patients with a hypertrophied detrusor, the contraction of the detrusor is so strong that it virtually goes into spasm, producing the symptoms of an irritable bladder. The earliest symptoms of bladder neck obstruction, therefore, are urgency (even to the point of incontinence) and frequency, both day and night. Needs to mention C fibers here.

2. Stage of compensation—As the obstruction increases, further hypertrophy of the muscle fibers of the bladder occurs, and the power to empty the bladder completely is thereby maintained. During this period, in addition to urgency and frequency, the patient notices hesitancy in initiating urination while the bladder develops contractions strong enough to overcome resistance at the bladder neck. The obstruction causes some loss in the force and size of the urinary stream and the stream becomes slower as vesical emptying nears completion (exhaustion of the detrusor as it nears the end of the contraction phase).

B. Decompensation Phase

If vesical tone becomes impaired or if urethral resistance exceeds detrusor power, some degree of decompensation occurs. The contraction phase of the vesical muscle becomes too short to completely expel the contents of the bladder, and some urine remains in the bladder (residual urine).

1. Acute decompensation—The tone of the compensated vesical muscle can be temporarily impaired by rapid filling of the bladder (high fluid intake) or by overstretching of the detrusor (postponement of urination though the urge is felt). This may cause increased difficulty of urination, with marked hesitancy and the need for straining to initiate urination; a very weak and small stream; and termination of the stream before the bladder completely empties (residual urine). Acute and sudden complete urinary retention may also occur.

2. Chronic decompensation—As the degree of obstruction increases, a progressive imbalance between the power of the bladder musculature and urethral resistance develops. Therefore, it becomes increasingly difficult to expel all the urine during the contraction phase of the detrusor. The symptoms of obstruction become more marked. The amount of residual urine gradually increases, and this diminishes the functional capacity of the bladder. Progressive frequency of urination is noted. On occasion, as the bladder decompensates, it becomes overstretched and attenuated. It may contain 1000–3000 mL of urine. It loses its power of contraction, and overflow (paradoxic) incontinence results.

▶ Clinical Findings

A. Symptoms

1. Lower and midtract (urethra and bladder)—Symptoms of obstruction of the lower and midtract are typified by the symptoms of urethral stricture, benign prostatic hyperplasia, neurogenic bladder, and tumor of the bladder involving the vesical neck. The principal symptoms are hesitancy in starting urination, lessened force and size of the stream, and terminal dribbling. Hematuria, which may be partial (eg with stricture); initial or terminal (eg with prostatic congestion); or total (eg with vesical tumor). Other symptoms are burning on urination, cloudy urine (due to complicating infection), and occasionally acute urinary retention (Elbadawi, 1998a and 1998b).

2. Upper tract (ureter and kidney)—Symptoms of obstruction of the upper tract are typified by the symptoms of ureteral stricture or ureteral or renal stone. The principal complaints are pain in the flank radiating along the course of the ureter, gross total hematuria (from stone), gastrointestinal symptoms, chills, fever, burning on urination, and cloudy urine with onset of infection, which is the common sequel to obstruction or vesicoureteral reflux. Nausea, vomiting, loss of weight and strength, and pallor are due to uremia secondary to bilateral hydronephrosis. A history of vesicoureteral reflux in childhood may be significant (Aslan and Kogan, 2003). Obstruction of the upper tract may be silent even when uremia supervenes.

B. Signs

1. Lower and midtract—Palpation of the urethra may reveal induration about a stricture. Rectal examination may show atony of the anal sphincter (damage to the sacral nerve roots) or benign or malignant enlargement of the prostate. Vesical distention may be found.

Although observation of the force and caliber of the urinary stream affords a rough estimate of maximum flow rate, the rate can be measured accurately with a urine flowmeter or, even more simply, by the following technique: Have the patient begin to void. When observed maximum flow has been reached, interpose a container to collect the urine and simultaneously start a stopwatch. After exactly 5 seconds, remove the container. The flow rate in milliliters per second can easily be calculated. The normal urine flow rate is 20–25 mL/s in males and 25–30 mL/s in females. Any flow rate <15 mL/s should be regarded with suspicion. A flow rate <10 mL/s is indicative of obstruction or weak detrusor function. Flow rates associated with an atonic neurogenic bladder (diminished detrusor power), or with urethral stricture or prostatic obstruction (increased urethral resistance), may be as low as 3–5 mL/s. A cystometrogram can differentiate between these two causes of impaired flow rate. After definitive treatment of the cause, the flow rate should return to normal.

In the presence of a vesical diverticulum or vesicoureteral reflux, although detrusor power is normal, the urinary stream may be impaired because of the diffusion of intravesical pressure into the diverticulum and vesicoureteral junction as well as the urethra. Excision of the diverticulum or repair of the vesicoureteral junctions leads to efficient expulsion of urine via the urethra.

2. Upper tract—An enlarged kidney may be discovered by palpation or percussion. Renal tenderness may be elicited if infection is present. Cancer of the cervix may be noted; it may invade the base of the bladder and occlude one or both ureteral orifices, or its metastases to the iliac lymph nodes may compress the ureters. A large pelvic mass (tumor, pregnancy) can displace and compress the ureters. Children with advanced urinary tract obstruction (usually due to posterior urethral valves) may develop ascites. Rupture of the renal fornices allows leakage of urine retroperitoneally; with rupture of the bladder, urine may pass into the peritoneal cavity through a tear in the peritoneum (Kibar et al, 2010).

C. Laboratory Findings

Anemia may be found secondary to chronic infection or in advanced bilateral hydronephrosis (stage of uremia). Leukocytosis is to be expected in the acute stage of infection. Little, if any, elevation of the white blood count accompanies the chronic stage.

Large amounts of protein are usually not found in the obstructive uropathies. Casts are not common from hydronephrotic kidneys. Microscopic hematuria may indicate renal or vesical infection, tumor, or stone. Pus cells and bacteria may or may not be present. In the presence of significant bilateral hydronephrosis, both urea and creatinine are elevated.

D. Urinary Tract Imaging (Figure 12–7)

A plain film of the abdomen may show enlargement of renal shadows, calcific bodies suggesting ureteral or renal stone, or tumor metastases to the bones of the spine or pelvis. Metastases in the spine may be the cause of spinal cord damage (neuropathic bladder); if they are osteoblastic, they are almost certainly from cancer of the prostate.

Excretory urograms reveal almost the entire story unless renal function is severely impaired. They are more informative when partial obstruction is present because the radiopaque material is retained. These urograms demonstrate the degree of dilatation of the pelves, calyces, and ureters. The point of ureteral stenosis is revealed. Segmental dilatation of the lower end of a ureter implies the possibility of vesicoureteral reflux (Figure 12–7), which can be revealed by voiding cystography. The cystogram may show trabeculation as an irregularity of the vesical outline and may show diverticula. Vesical tumors, nonopaque stones, and large intravesical prostatic lobes may cause radiolucent shadows. A film taken immediately after voiding will show residual urine.

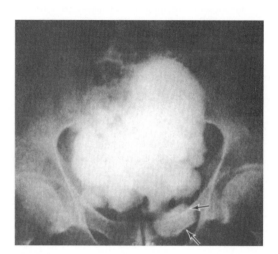

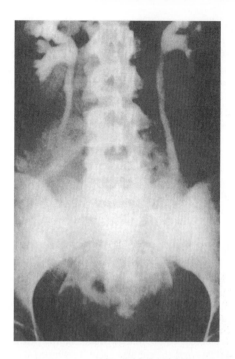

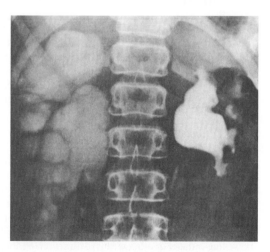

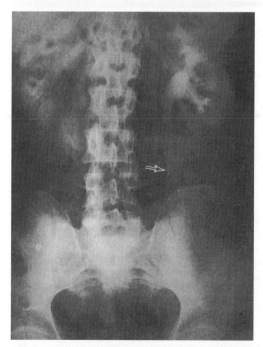

▲ **Figure 12–7.** Changes in bladder, ureters, and kidneys caused by obstruction. ***Upper left:*** Cystogram showing benign prostatic enlargement and multiple diverticula. Arrows point to femoral hernia that probably developed as a result of straining to urinate. ***Upper right:*** Pregnancy. Significant dilatation and elongation of upper right ureter due to compression at the pelvic line. Left side normal. ***Lower left:*** Excretory urogram, 70 minutes after injection. Advanced right hydronephrosis secondary to ureteropelvic obstruction. Mild ureteropelvic obstruction on left. ***Lower right:*** Stone in left ureter (at *arrow*) with mild hydronephrosis.

Retrograde cystography shows changes of the bladder wall caused by distal obstruction (trabeculation, diverticula) or demonstrates the obstructive lesion itself (enlarged prostate, posterior urethral valves, cancer of the bladder). If the ureterovesical valves are incompetent, ureteropyelograms may be obtained by reflux.

Retrograde urograms may show better detail than the excretory type, but care must be taken not to overdistend the passages with too much opaque fluid; small hydronephroses can be made to look quite large. The degree of ureteral or ureterovesical obstruction can be judged by the degree of delay of drainage of the radiopaque fluid instilled.

Computed tomography (CT), magnetic resonance imaging (MRI), and sonography can also help determine the extent of dilatation and parenchymal atrophy (Silverman et al, 2009). CT scan with and without contrast is the best modality when stone obstruction is suspected (Kennish et al, 2010). To avoid irradiation in pregnant women, MRI and sonography are the preferred tests. However, both tests have limited value in delineating ureteral anatomy if it is not dilated.

E. Isotope Scanning (Nuclear Renography)

The glomerular agent Tc 99m **diethylenetriaminepentaacetic acid** (DTPA) and the tubular agent Tc 99m MAG3 are most commonly used in the evaluation of obstruction. However, to predict functional recovery, **DMSA**, a cortical agent, has been shown to be superior to tubular selective agents DTPA or MAG3. In the presence of obstruction, the radioisotope renogram may show depression of both the vascular and secretory phases and a rising rather than a falling excretory phase due to retention of the isotope-containing urine in the renal pelvis. Furosemide is often given 20 minutes after the tracer is given to induce diuresis, which helps the interpretation of the clearance curve.

F. Instrumental Examination

Exploration of the urethra with a catheter or other instrument is a valuable diagnostic measure. Passage may be blocked by a stricture or tumor. Spasm of the external sphincter may make passage difficult. Passage of the catheter immediately after voiding allows estimation of the amount of residual urine in the bladder. Bladder ultrasound can also accurately measure the amount of postvoid residual urine and determine outlet obstruction (Housami et al, 2009). Residual urine is common in bladder neck obstruction (enlarged prostate), cystocele, and neurogenic (neuropathic) bladder.

Measurement of vesical tone by means of cystometry is helpful in diagnosing neurogenic bladder and in differentiating between bladder neck obstruction and vesical atony. Inspection of the urethra, bladder, ureter, and renal pelvis by means of panendoscopy, cystoscopy, or ureteroscopy may reveal the primary obstructive cause (Van Cangh et al, 2001). Catheters may be passed to the renal pelves and urine specimens obtained.

The function of each kidney may be measured, and retrograde ureteropyelograms can be obtained (Whitaker and Buxton-Thomas, 1984).

▶ Differential Diagnosis

A thorough examination usually leaves no doubt about the diagnosis. The differential diagnosis under these circumstances is rarely difficult. If seemingly simple infection does not respond to medical therapy or if infection recurs, obstruction, a foreign body, or vesicoureteral reflux is the probable cause, and complete study of the urinary tract is indicated.

▶ Complications

Stagnation of urine leads to infection, which then may spread throughout the entire urinary system. Once established, infection is difficult and at times impossible to eradicate even after the obstruction has been relieved.

Often, the invading organisms are urea splitting (*Proteus,* staphylococci), which causes the urine to become alkaline. Calcium salts precipitate and form bladder or kidney stones more easily in alkaline urine. If both kidneys are affected, the result may be renal insufficiency. Secondary infection increases renal damage.

Pyonephrosis is the end stage of a severely infected and obstructed kidney. The kidney is functionless and filled with thick pus. At times, a plain film of the abdomen may show an air urogram caused by gas liberated by infecting organisms.

▶ Treatment

A. Relief of Obstruction

Treatment of the main causes of obstruction and stasis (benign prostatic hyperplasia, cancer of the prostate, neurogenic bladder, ureteral stone, posterior urethral valves, and ureteral stenosis) is described in detail elsewhere in this book (Glassberg, 2001; Hashim and Abrams, 2010; Myers and McAninch, 2009).

1. Lower tract obstruction (distal to the bladder)—With patients in whom secondary renal or ureterovesical damage (reflux in the latter) is minimal or nonexistent, correction of the obstruction is sufficient. If significant reflux is demonstrated and does not subside spontaneously after relief of obstruction, surgical repair may be needed. Repair becomes imperative if there is considerable hydronephrosis in addition to reflux. Preliminary drainage of the bladder by an indwelling catheter or other means of diversion (eg, loop ureterostomy) is indicated in order to preserve and improve renal function. If, after a few months of drainage, reflux persists, the incompetent ureterovesical junction should be surgically repaired. Persistent obstruction from prostatic enlargement of urethral stricture may also require surgical intervention (Andrich and Mundy, 2008; Robert et al, 2011; Roehrborn, 2011).

2. Upper tract obstruction (above the bladder)—If tortuous, kinked, dilated, or atonic ureters have developed secondary to lower tract obstruction (so that they are themselves obstructive), vesical drainage will not protect the kidneys from further damage; the urine proximal to the obstruction must be diverted by nephrostomy or ureterostomy. The kidneys then may regain some function. Over a period of many months, the ureter may become less tortuous and less dilated; its obstructive areas may open up. If radiopaque material instilled into the nephrostomy tube passes readily to the bladder, it may be possible to remove the nephrostomy tube. If obstruction or reflux persists, surgical repair is indicated. Permanent urinary diversion (eg, ureteroileal conduit) may be necessary.

If one kidney has been irreversibly damaged, as measured by kidney function tests, urography, sonography, CT scan, or scintigraphy, nephrectomy may be necessary.

B. Eradication of Infection

Once the obstruction is removed, every effort should be made to eradicate infection. If the infection has been severe and prolonged, antibiotics may fail to sterilize the urinary tract. On the other hand, the incidence of urinary tract infection is low in children whose upper tract obstruction is diagnosed prenatally (Roth et al, 2009).

▶ Prognosis

No simple statement can be made about the prognosis in this group of patients. The outcome depends on the cause, site, degree, and duration of the obstruction. The prognosis is also definitely influenced by complicating infection, particularly if the infection has been present for a long time.

If renal function is fair to good, if the obstruction or other causes of stasis can be corrected, and if complicating infection can therefore be eradicated, the prognosis is generally excellent.

BIBLIOGRAPHY

Andrich DE, Mundy AR: What is the best technique for urethroplasty? Eur Urol 2008;54(5):1031–1041.

Aslan AR, Kogan BA: The effect of bladder outlet obstruction on the developing kidney. BJU Int 2003;92(Suppl 1):38.

Beganović A et al: Ectopic ureterocele: Long-term results of open surgical therapy in 54 patients. J Urol 2007;178(1):251–254.

Chevalier RL et al: Mechanisms of renal injury and progression of renal disease in congenital obstructive nephropathy. Pediatr Nephrol 2010;25(4):687–697.

Elbadawi A: Voiding dysfunction in benign prostatic hyperplasia: Trends, controversies and recent revelations. I. Symptoms and urodynamics. Urology 1998a;51(Suppl 5A):62.

Elbadawi A: Voiding dysfunction in benign prostatic hyperplasia: Trends, controversies and recent revelations. II. Pathology and pathophysiology. Urology 1998b;51(Suppl 5A):73.

Glassberg KI: The valve bladder syndrome: 20 years later. J Urol 2001;166:1406.

Gimpel C et al: Complications and long-term outcome of primary obstructive megaureter in childhood. Pediatr Nephrol 2010; 25(9):1679–1686.

Hashim H, Abrams P: Emerging drugs for the treatment of benign prostatic obstruction. Expert Opin Emerg Drugs 2010;15(2):159–174.

Housami F et al: The use of ultrasound-estimated bladder weight in diagnosing bladder outlet obstruction and detrusor overactivity in men with lower urinary tract symptoms. Indian J Urol 2009; 25(1):105–109.

Kennish SJ et al: Unenhanced CT for the evaluation of acute ureteric colic: The essential pictorial guide. Postgrad Med J 2010;86 (1017):428–436.

Kibar Y et al: Timing of posterior urethral valve diagnosis and its impact on clinical outcome. J Pediatr Urol 2010;7(5):538–842.

Klein J et al: Congenital ureteropelvic junction obstruction: Human disease and animal models. Int J Exp Pathol 2010;92(3):168–192.

Lieber MM et al: Natural history of benign prostatic enlargement: Long-term longitudinal population-based study of prostate volume doubling times. BJU Int 2010;105(2):214–219.

Myers JB, McAninch JW: Management of posterior urethral disruption injuries. Nat Clin Pract Urol 2009;6(3):154–163.

Riccabona M: Obstructive diseases of the urinary tract in children: Lessons from the last 15 years. Pediatr Radiol 2010;40(6):947–955.

Robert G et al: Lower urinary tract symptoms suggestive of benign prostatic hyperplasia: Who are the high-risk patients and what are the best treatment options? Curr Opin Urol 2011;21(1):42–48.

Rodriguez MM: Developmental renal pathology: Its past, present, and future. Fetal Pediatr Pathol 2004;23:211.

Roehrborn CG: Male lower urinary tract symptoms (LUTS) and benign prostatic hyperplasia (BPH). Med Clin North Am 2011; 95(1):87–100.

Roth CC et al: Occurrence of urinary tract infection in children with significant upper urinary tract obstruction. Urology 2009;73(1): 74–78.

Routh JC et al: Predicting renal outcomes in children with anterior urethral valves: A systematic review. J Urol 2010;184(4, Suppl): 1615–1619.

Silverman SG et al: What is the current role of CT urography and MR urography in the evaluation of the urinary tract? Radiology 2009;250(2):309–323.

Tan BJ, Smith AD: Ureteropelvic junction obstruction repair: When, how, what? Curr Opin Urol 2004;14:55.

Tanagho EA, Meyers FH: Trigonal hypertrophy: A cause of ureteral obstruction. J Urol 1965;93:678.

Van Cangh PJ et al: The role of endourology in ureteropelvic junction obstruction. Curr Urol Rep 2001;2:149.

Vecchioli-Scaldazza C, Morosetti C: Effect of aging on urinary incontinence in woman. Arch Ital Urol Androl 2010;82(3):167–171.

Whitaker RH, Buxton-Thomas M: A comparison of pressure flow studies and renography in equivocal upper urinary tract obstruction. J Urol 1984;131:446.

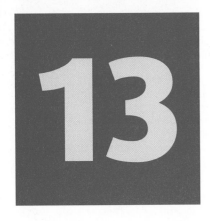

13

Vesicoureteral Reflux

Emil A. Tanagho, MD, & Hiep T. Nguyen, MD

Under normal circumstances, the ureterovesical junction allows urine to enter the bladder but prevents urine from regurgitating into the ureter, particularly at the time of voiding. In this way, the kidney is protected from high pressure in the bladder and from contamination by infected vesical urine. When this valve is incompetent, the chance for development of urinary infection is significantly enhanced, and pyelonephritis may occur. In significant cases especially in children, pyelonephritis—acute, chronic, or healed—is secondary to vesicoureteral reflux (VUR).

ANATOMY OF THE URETEROVESICAL JUNCTION

An understanding of the causes of VUR requires knowledge of the anatomy of the ureterovesical valve. Anatomic studies performed by Hutch (1972) and by Tanagho and Pugh (1963) (Figure 13–1) are incorporated into the following discussion.

▶ Mesodermal Components

The mesodermal component, which arises from the Wolffian duct, is made up of two parts that are innervated by the sympathetic nervous system:

A. The Ureter and the Superficial Trigone

The smooth musculature of the renal calyces, pelvis, and extravesical ureter is composed of helically oriented fibers that allow for peristaltic activity. As these fibers approach the vesical wall, they are reoriented into the longitudinal plane. The ureter passes obliquely through the vesical wall; the intravesical ureteral segment is thus composed of longitudinal muscle fibers only and therefore cannot undergo peristalsis. As these smooth-muscle fibers approach the ureteral orifice, those that form the roof of the ureter swing to either side to join those that form its floor. They then spread out and join equivalent muscle bundles from the other ureter and also continue caudally, thus forming the superficial trigone. The trigone passes over the neck of the bladder, ending at the

verumontanum in the male and just inside the external urethral meatus in the female. Thus, the ureterotrigonal complex is one structure. Above the ureteral orifice, it is tubular; below that point, it is flat.

B. Waldeyer's Sheath and the Deep Trigone

Beginning at a point about 2–3 cm above the bladder, an external layer of longitudinal smooth muscle surrounds the ureter. This muscular sheath passes through the vesical wall, to which it is connected by a few detrusor fibers. As it enters the vesical lumen, its roof fibers diverge to join its floor fibers, which then spread out, joining muscle bundles from the contralateral ureter and forming the deep trigone, which ends at the bladder neck.

▶ Endodermal Component

The vesical detrusor muscle bundles are intertwined and run in various directions. As they converge on the internal orifice of the bladder, however, they tend to become oriented into three layers.

A. Internal Longitudinal Layer

The internal longitudinal layer continues into the urethra submucosally and ends just inside the external meatus in the female and at the caudal end of the prostate in the male.

B. Middle Circular Layer

The middle circular layer is thickest anteriorly and stops at the vesical neck.

C. Outer Longitudinal Layer

The muscle bundles of the outer longitudinal layer take a circular and spiral course about the external surface of the female urethra and are incorporated within the peripheral prostatic tissue in the male. They constitute the true vesicourethral sphincter.

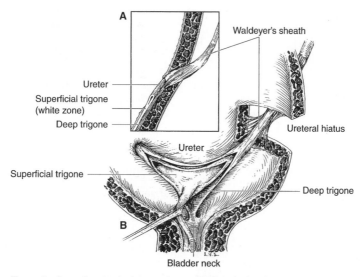

▲ **Figure 13–1.** Normal ureterotrigonal complex. **A:** Side view of ureterovesical junction. Waldeyer's muscular sheath invests the juxtavesical ureter and continues downward as the deep trigone, which extends to the bladder neck. The ureteral musculature becomes the superficial trigone, which extends to the verumontanum in the male and stops just short of the external meatus in the female. **B:** Waldeyer's sheath is connected by a few fibers to the detrusor muscle in the ureteral hiatus. This muscular sheath, inferior to the ureteral orifices, becomes the deep trigone. The musculature of the ureters continues downward as the superficial trigone. (Redrawn and modified, with permission, from Tanagho EA, Pugh RCB: The anatomy and function of the ureterovesical junction. Br J Urol 1963;35:151.)

The vesical detrusor muscle is innervated by the parasympathetic nerves (S_2–S_4).

PHYSIOLOGY OF THE URETEROVESICAL JUNCTION

Although many investigators had suspected that normal trigonal tone tended to occlude the intravesical ureter, it remained for Tanagho et al (1965) to prove it. Using nonrefluxing dogs, they demonstrated the following:

1. Interruption of the continuity of the trigone resulted in reflux. An incision was made in the trigone 3 mm below the ureteral orifice, resulting in an upward and lateral migration of the ureteral orifice with shortening of the intravesical ureter. Reflux was demonstrable. After the incision healed, reflux ceased.

2. Unilateral lumbar sympathectomy resulted in paralysis of the ipsilateral trigone. This led to lateral and superior migration of the ureteral orifice and reflux.

3. Electrical stimulation of the trigone caused the ureteral orifice to move caudally, thus lengthening the intravesical ureter. This maneuver caused a marked rise in resistance to flow through the ureterovesical junction.

Ureteral efflux of urine ceased. Intravenous injection of epinephrine caused the same reaction. On the other hand, isoproterenol caused the degree of occlusion to drop below normal. If the trigone was incised, however, electrical stimulation of the trigone or the administration of epinephrine failed to increase ureteral occlusive pressure.

4. During gradual filling of the bladder, intravesical pressure increased only slightly, whereas pressure within the intravesical ureter rose progressively—owing, apparently, to increasing trigonal stretch. A few seconds before the expected sharp rise in intravesical pressure generated for voiding, the closure pressure in the intravesical ureter rose sharply and was maintained for 20 seconds after detrusor contraction had ceased. This experiment demonstrated that ureterovesical competence is independent of detrusor action and is governed by the tone of the trigone, which contracts vigorously just before voiding, thus helping to open and funnel the vesical neck. At the same time, significant pull is placed on the intravesical ureter so that it is occluded during the period when intravesical pressure is high. During the voiding phase, there is naturally no efflux of ureteral urine.

One may liken this function to the phenomenon of the Chinese thimble: The harder the finger (trigone) pulls, the tighter the thimble (intravesical ureter) becomes. Conversely, a deficient pull may lead to incomplete closure of the uretero-vesical junction.

It was concluded from these experiments that normal ureterotrigonal tone prevents VUR. Electrical or pharmacologic stimulation of the trigone caused increased occlusive pressure in the intravesical ureter and increased resistance to flow down the ureter, whereas incision or paralysis of the trigone led to reflux. The theory that ureterovesical competence was maintained by intravesical pressure compressing the intravesical ureter against its backing of detrusor muscle was thereby disproved.

Biopsy of the trigone (and the intravesical ureter) in patients with primary reflux revealed marked deficiency in the development of its smooth muscle (Figure 13–2). Electrical stimulation of such a trigone caused only a minor contraction of the ureterotrigonal complex. This work led to the conclusion that the common cause of reflux, particularly in children, is congenital attenuation of the ureterotrigonal musculature.

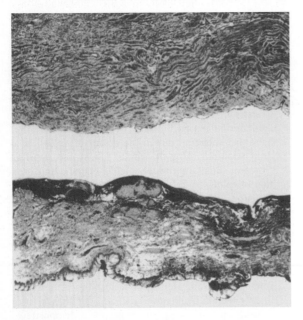

▲ **Figure 13–2.** Histology of the trigone in primary reflux. **Top:** Normal trigone demonstrating wealth of closely packed smooth-muscle fibers. **Bottom:** The congenitally attenuated trigonal muscle that accompanies vesicoureteral reflux. Note the absence of inflammatory cell. (Reproduced, with permission, from Tanagho EA et al: Primary vesicoureteral reflux: Experimental studies of its etiology. J Urol 1965;93:165.)

VESICOURETERAL REFLUX

CAUSES

The major cause of VUR is attenuation of the trigone and its contiguous intravesical ureteral musculature. Any condition that shortens the intravesical ureter may also lead to reflux, but this is less common. Familial VUR has been observed by a number of authors. It appears to be a genetic trait.

▶ Congenital Causes

A. Trigonal Weakness (Primary Reflux)

Trigonal weakness is by far the most common cause of ureteral reflux. It is most often seen in young children, more common in girls than in boys. Reflux in adults—usually women—probably represents the same congenital defect. Weakness of one side of the trigone leads to a decrease in the occlusive pressure in the ipsilateral intravesical ureter. Diffuse ureterotrigonal weakness causes bilateral reflux.

It is postulated that ureteral trigonal weakness is related to the development of the ureteral bud on the mesonephric duct. It is known that the ureter acquires its musculature from its cranial end caudally so that if a segment is muscularly deficient, it is deficient in its most caudal part. It is also postulated that if the ureter is too close to the urogenital sinus on the mesonephric duct, it will join the latter relatively early in embryonic life, before acquiring adequate mesenchymal tissue around itself to be differentiated later into proper trigonal musculature as well as lower ureter. This embryologic hypothesis explains all the known features of refluxing ureters: their muscular weakness, their lateral placement on the bladder base with a very short submucosal segment, and their usual association with weak ureteral musculature and gaping ureteral orifices (which, in severe cases, ensures a golf-hole endoscopic appearance at their junction with the bladder wall). It also explains why, in duplicated systems, if there is only one refluxing unit, it is the upper orifice (which originated closer to the urogenital sinus on the mesonephric duct and thus has the least muscular development).

In the normal state, the intravesical ureterotrigonal muscle tone exerts a downward pull, whereas the extravesical ureter tends to pull cephalad (Figure 13–3). If trigonal development is deficient, not only is its occlusive power diminished but the ureteral orifice tends to migrate upward toward the ureteral hiatus. The degree of this retraction relates to the degree of incompetence of the junction (Figure 13–4). If the ureteral orifice lies over the ureteral hiatus in the bladder wall (so-called golf-hole orifice), it is completely incompetent. The degree of incompetence is judged by the findings on excretory urography and cystography and the cystoscopic appearance of the ureteral orifices.

B. Familial Reflux

There appears to be genetic predisposition for reflux. The reported prevalence of VUR among siblings of index patients

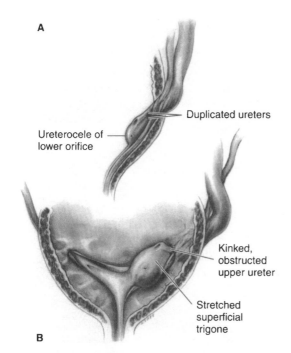

A

Ureterocele of lower orifice

Duplicated ureters

Kinked, obstructed upper ureter

Stretched superficial trigone

B

▲ **Figure 13–3.** **A:** Small ureterocele developing in a duplicated system (where it always involves a lower ureteral orifice). **B:** Expansion of submucosal segment leads to lifting and angulation of ipsilateral lower pole ureteral orifice. Duplicated system ureteroceles are rarely so small. (Diagrammatic representation.) (Reproduced, with permission, from Tanagho EA: Ureteroceles: Embryogenesis, pathogenesis and management. J Cont Educ Urol 1979;18:13.)

with reflux has ranged from 4.7% to 51%, which is significantly higher than the incidence of reflux in the general population (1%) (Ataei et al, 2004). In addition, the incidence of reflux varies among nationalities and races. Studies involving genotype screening of specific subgroups of patients suggest that there is heterogeneity in the genetics of VUR (reviewed by Carvas et al, 2010). Several genes have been associated with VUR, including uroplakin-3, SLIT2/ROBO2, and TGF-β. In addition, several chromosomal regions (on chromosomes 1, 2, 3, 5, 13, and 18) have also been identified. Despite extensive analysis, the exact form of genetic transmission has yet to be delineated.

C. Ureteral Abnormalities

1. Complete ureteral duplication (Figure 13–5)—The intravesical portion of the ureter to the upper renal segment is usually of normal length, whereas that of the ureter to the lower pole is abnormally short; this orifice is commonly incompetent.

However, Stephens (1957) demonstrated that the musculature of the superiorly placed orifice is attenuated, which further contributes to its weakness.

2. Ectopic ureteral orifice—Single ureter or one of a pair may open well down on the trigone, at the vesical neck, or in the urethra. In this instance, VUR is the rule. This observation makes it clear that the length of the intravesical ureter is not the sole factor in reflux. Such intravesical ureteral segments are usually devoid of smooth muscle. Thus, they have no occlusive force.

3. Ureterocele—A ureterocele involving a single ureter rarely allows reflux, but this lesion usually involves the ureter that drains the upper pole of a duplicated kidney. Because the ureteral orifice is obstructed, the intramural ureter becomes dilated. This increases the diameter of the ureteral hiatus, further shortening the intravesical segment of the other ureter, which therefore may become incompetent. Resection of the ureterocele usually causes its ureter to reflux freely as well.

▶ Voiding Dysfunction

Abnormal voiding habits have been associated with reflux. Toilet-trained children, in particular girls, may alter their bladder function by inhibiting their urge to void. This can result in abnormally high voiding pressure, bladder overactivity, and poor bladder compliance. These changes in bladder dynamics can either induce the development of primary reflux or prevent its resolution (Greenfield and Wan, 2000). In addition, alterations in the bowel function (eg, constipation) can cause further deterioration in bladder function and consequently the development or persistence of primary reflux (Bower et al, 2005).

▶ Vesical Trabeculation

Occasionally, a heavily trabeculated bladder may be associated with reflux. The causes include spastic neurogenic bladder and severe obstruction distal to the bladder. These lesions, however, are associated with trigonal hypertrophy as well; the resultant extra pull on the ureterotrigonal muscle tends to protect the junction from incompetence. In a few such cases, however, the vesical mucosa may protrude through the ureteral hiatus just above the ureter to form a diverticulum, or saccule (Figure 13–6). The resulting dilatation of the hiatus shortens the intravesical segment; reflux may then occur.

▶ Edema of the Vesical Wall Secondary to Cystitis

As noted previously, valves vary in their degrees of incompetence. A "borderline" junction may not allow reflux when the urine is sterile, but valvular function may be impaired when cystitis causes associated edema involving the trigone and

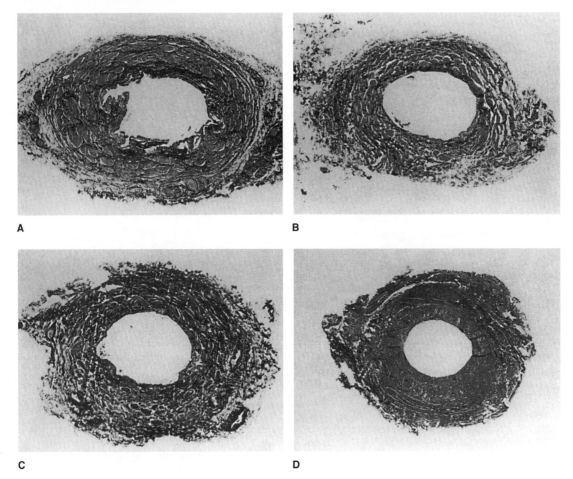

▲ **Figure 13–4.** Histology of the various grades of submucosal muscular weakness of the ureteral orifice. (See also Figure 13-9.) **A:** Normal. Minimal deficiency. (Cone orifice.) **B:** More marked muscular weakness. (Stadium orifice.) **C:** Marked muscular deficiency. (Horseshoe orifice.) **D:** Extreme muscular deficiency. Only a few muscle fibers can be seen; the rest is collagen tissue.

intravesical ureter. In addition, the abnormally high voiding pressure may lead to reflux, in which case, secondary pyelonephritis may ensue. After cure of the infection, cystography again reveals no reflux. It is believed that a completely normal junction will not decompensate even under these circumstances.

It has been shown that pyelonephritis of pregnancy is associated with VUR. Many patients give a history of urinary tract infections during childhood. The implication is that they "outgrew" reflux at puberty, but if bacteriuria becomes established during pregnancy, their "borderline" valves may become incompetent. This condition may be aggravated by the hormones of pregnancy, which may contribute to a further loss of tone of the ureterotrigonal complex. After delivery, reflux is usually no longer demonstrable (Hutch and Amar, 1972).

▶ Eagle–Barrett (Prune Belly) Syndrome

The Eagle–Barrett syndrome is a relatively rare condition in which there is failure of normal development of the abdominal muscles and the smooth muscle of the ureters and bladder. Bilateral cryptorchidism is the rule. At times, talipes equinovarus and hip dislocation are also noted. Because the smooth muscle of the ureterotrigonal complex is deficient, reflux is to be expected; advanced hydroureteronephrosis is therefore found.

▶ Iatrogenic Causes

Certain operative procedures may lead to either temporary or permanent ureteral regurgitation.

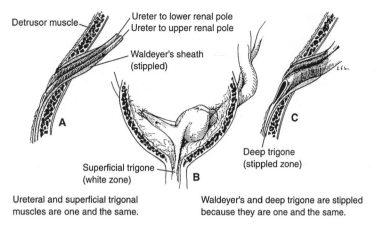

▲ **Figure 13–5.** Ureteral duplication and ureterocele as causes of vesicoureteral reflux. *A:* Ureteral duplication showing juxtavesical and intravesical ureters encased in common sheath (Waldeyer's). The superior ureter, which always drains the lower renal pole, has a shorter intravesical segment; in addition, it is somewhat devoid of muscle. It therefore tends to allow reflux. *B:* Duplication with ureterocele that always involves caudal ureter, which drains upper renal pole. Pinpoint orifice is obstructive, causing hydroureteronephrosis. Resulting wide dilatation of ureter and ureteral hiatus shortens the intravesical segment of the other ureter, often causing it to reflux. *C:* Resection of ureterocele allows reflux into that ureter.

A. Prostatectomy

With any type of prostatectomy, the continuity of the superficial trigone is interrupted at the vesical neck. If the proximal trigone moves upward, temporary reflux may occur. This mechanism may account for the high fever (and even bacteremia) that is sometimes observed when the catheter is finally removed. Fortunately, in 2–3 weeks, the trigone again becomes anchored and reflux ceases.

Preexisting trigonal hypertrophy (due to prostatic obstruction) helps to compensate for the effect of trigonal interruption; thus, reflux may never occur.

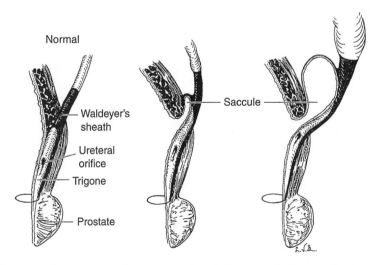

▲ **Figure 13–6.** Development of ureteral saccule, seen occasionally in cases of primary reflux but more commonly in obstructed or neurogenic bladders with marked trabeculation. Note that the vesical mucosa herniates through the ureteral hiatus, pulling the ureteral orifice upward with it. The orifice may ultimately open in the saccule rather than in the bladder.

B. Wedge Resection of the Posterior Vesical Neck

Wedge resection of the posterior vesical neck, often ill advised when performed in conjunction with plastic revision of the vesical neck for supposed vesical neck stenosis or dysfunction, may also upset trigonal continuity and allow reflux.

C. Ureteral Meatotomy

Extensive ureteral meatotomy may be followed by reflux. Fortunately, however, limited incision of the roof of the intravesical ureter divides few muscle fibers, since the fibers have left the roof to join muscle fibers on the floor. Wide resection for treatment of vesical cancer is often followed by ureteral reflux.

D. Resection of Ureterocele

If the ureteral hiatus is widely dilated, this procedure is often followed by reflux.

▶ Contracted Bladder

A bladder that is contracted secondary to interstitial cystitis, tuberculosis, radiotherapy, carcinoma, or schistosomiasis may be associated with ureteral reflux.

COMPLICATIONS

VUR damages the kidney through one or both of two mechanisms: (1) pyelonephritis and (2) hydroureteronephrosis.

▶ Pyelonephritis

VUR is one of the common contributing factors leading to the development of cystitis, particularly in females. When reflux is present, bacteria reach the kidney and the urinary tract cannot empty itself completely, so infection is perpetuated. Pyelonephritis is discussed in more detail in Chapter 14.

▶ Hydroureteronephrosis (See also Chapter 12)

Dilation of the ureter, renal pelvis, and calyces is usually observed in association with reflux (Figure 13–7), sometimes to an extreme degree (Figure 13–8). In males, because they have a relatively long segment of sterile urethra, such changes are often seen in the absence of infection. Sterile reflux is less damaging than infected reflux.

There are three reasons for the dilatation:

1. **Increased work load:** The ureter is meant to transport the urine secreted by the kidney to the bladder only once. In the presence of reflux, variable amounts of urine go back and forth, and the work load may be doubled, quadrupled, or increased 10-fold or even more. Eventually, the ureter is not able to transport the increased volume of urine, and stasis and dilatation result.

2. **High hydrostatic pressure:** The ureter is protected from the high pressures of the urinary bladder by a competent ureterovesical junction. If there is free reflux, the high intravesical pressure is directly transmitted to the ureteral and pelvic walls, which results in marked stretching and dilation.

3. **Weak ureteral musculature:** In reflux, the ureteral wall is invariably deficient in musculature to some degree. The more severe the reflux, the more apparent the muscular deficiency. Some cases show more massive dilatation than others. The properly muscularized ureter is better able to resist and compensate for overwork and hydrostatic pressure than the muscularly deficient ureter. The latter tends to undergo further dilatation once it is subjected to any increased intraluminal pressure.

Whether sterile reflux is harmful is the subject of controversy. My colleagues and I believe there is conclusive evidence that severe sterile reflux can lead to parenchymal damage. Pyelointerstitial backflow or pyelotubular backflow under the high pressures of reflux (not infrequently seen during cystographic studies) leads to extravasation of urine in the interstitium of the kidney. The presence of urine in any interstitium will result in a marked inflammatory response with cellular infiltration, resulting finally in fibrosis and scarring. On a long-term basis, this can lead to parenchymal changes indistinguishable from pyelonephritic scarring caused by inflammation due to bacterial infection. This damage may be termed **reflux nephropathy**. If severe, it will produce parenchymal damage serious enough to lead to end-stage kidney disease.

Ransley's studies (1976) indicate that intrarenal reflux is more likely to occur in the presence of flat, concave, or compound papillae, because their collecting ducts tend to open with an increase in intrapelvic pressure and reflux. Papillae prone to reflux are more commonly seen in the polar segments of the kidney. Normal papillae might also permit intrarenal reflux if flattened as a result of the changes due to reflux.

Intravesical pressure is transmitted through the incompetent ureteral orifice. This back pressure is quite high at the time of voiding. Furthermore, the ureteropelvic and ureterovesical junctions are less distensible than the rest of the ureter. Either junction may have trouble passing the normal amount of secreted urine plus the refluxed urine; functional obstruction may result. A common cause of ureteropelvic and ureterovesical "obstruction" is VUR. Such changes indicate the need for cystography.

INCIDENCE

VUR occurs in 25–40% (Fanos and Cataldi, 2004) of children with urinary tract infection but in only 8% of adults with bacteriuria. This discrepancy is explained by the fact that girls usually have pyelonephritis, whereas women usually have cystitis only. Bacteriuria does not always imply pyelonephritis.

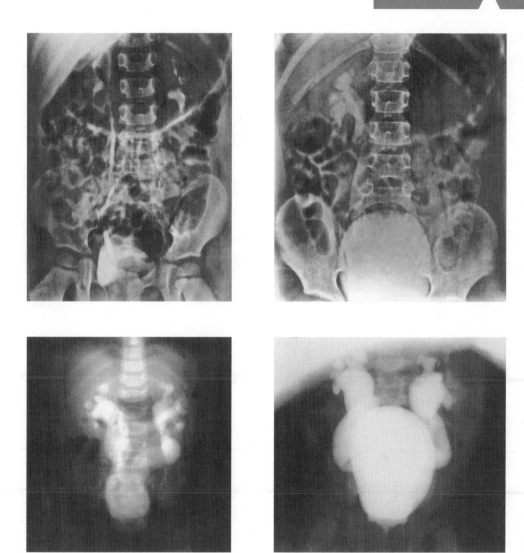

▲ **Figure 13–7.** Excretory urogram with changes that imply right vesicoureteral reflux. ***Upper left:*** Excretory urogram showing normal right urogram and a ureter that is mildly dilated and remains full through its entire length. The ureteral change implies reflux. ***Upper right:*** Cystogram demonstrates the reflux. Note, now, the degree of dilatation of the ureter, pelvis, and calyces. ***Lower left:*** Excretory urogram shows bilateral hydroureteronephrosis with pyelonephritic scarring. These findings imply the presence of reflux. ***Lower right:*** Voiding cystourethrogram. Free reflux bilaterally.

The fairly competent (borderline) valve refluxes only during an acute attack of cystitis. Since cystography is performed in such cases only after the infection has been eradicated, the incidence of reflux found on cystography is abnormally low. On the other hand, reflux is demonstrable in 85% of patients whose excretory urograms reveal significant changes typical of healed pyelonephritis.

When infection associated with reflux occurs during the first few weeks of life, many patients are septic and uremic.

Most are boys with posterior urethral valves. After 1 year of age, the female:male ratio of children with infection and reflux is approximately 3:1–4:1.

CLINICAL FINDINGS

A history compatible with acute pyelonephritis implies the presence of VUR. This is most commonly seen in females, particularly young girls. Persistence of recurrent "cystitis"

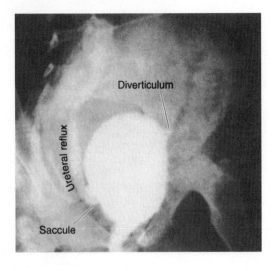

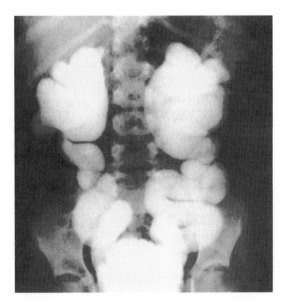

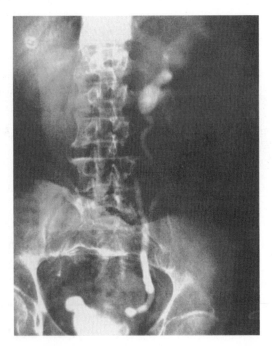

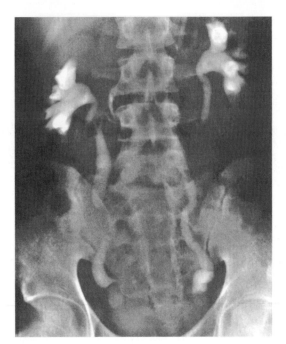

▲ Figure 13–8. Cystograms revealing vesicoureteral reflux. **Upper left:** Saccule at right ureterovesical junction. **Upper right:** Meningomyelocele. Reflux with severe bilateral hydroureteronephrosis; serum creatinine, 0.6 mg/dL; phenolsulfon-phthalein excretion, 5% in 1 hour. **Lower left:** Postprostatectomy patient with reflux on left and bilateral saccules. **Lower right:** Ten-year-old boy with meningomyelocele. Bladder has been emptied. Impairment of drainage at ureterovesical junctions is demonstrated. (Courtesy of Hutch JA, Amar AD: *Vesicoureteral Reflux and Pyelonephritis.* Appleton-Century-Crofts, 1972.)

may suggest the possibility of reflux. Such patients often have asymptomatic low-grade pyelonephritis.

▶ Symptoms Related to Reflux

A. Symptomatic Pyelonephritis

The usual symptoms in adults are chills and high fever, renal pain, nausea and vomiting, and symptoms of cystitis. In children, only fever, vague abdominal pains, and sometimes diarrhea are apt to occur.

B. Asymptomatic Pyelonephritis

The patient may have no symptoms whatsoever. The incidental findings of pyuria and bacteriuria may be the only clues. This fact points up the need for a screening urinalysis in all children.

C. Symptoms of Cystitis Only

In cases of symptoms of cystitis only, bacteriuria is resistant to antimicrobial drugs, or infection quickly recurs following treatment. These patients may have reflux with asymptomatic chronic pyelonephritis.

D. Renal Pain on Voiding

Surprisingly, renal pain on voiding is a rare complaint in patients with VUR.

E. Uremia

The last stage of bilateral reflux is uremia due to destruction of the renal parenchyma by hydronephrosis or pyelonephritis (or both). The patient often adjusts to renal insufficiency and may appear quite healthy. Many renal transplants are performed in patients whose kidneys have deteriorated secondarily to reflux and accompanying infection. Early diagnosis, based on careful urinalysis, would have led to the proper diagnosis in childhood. Progressive pyelonephritis is, with few exceptions, preventable.

F. Hypertension

In the later stages of atrophic pyelonephritis, a significant incidence of hypertension is observed.

▶ Symptoms Related to the Underlying Disease

The clinical picture is often dominated by the signs and symptoms of the primary disease.

A. Urinary Tract Obstruction

Young girls may have hesitancy in initiating the urinary stream and an impaired or intermittent stream secondary to spasm of the periurethral striated muscle (see "Distal Urethral Stenosis" in Chapter 41). In males, the urinary stream may be slow as a result of posterior urethral valves (infants) or prostatic enlargement (men older than 50 years).

B. Spinal Cord Disease

The patient may have a serious neurogenic disease such as paraplegia, quadriplegia, multiple sclerosis, or meningomyelocele. Symptoms may be limited to those of neurogenic bladder: incontinence of urine, urinary retention or large residual volume, and vesical urgency.

▶ Physical Findings

During an attack of acute pyelonephritis, renal tenderness may be noted. Its absence, however, does not rule out chronic renal infection. Palpation and percussion of the suprapubic area may reveal a distended bladder secondary to obstruction or neurogenic disease. The finding of a hard midline mass deep in the pelvis in a male infant is apt to represent a markedly thickened bladder caused by posterior urethral valves. Examination may reveal a neurologic deficit compatible with a paretic bladder.

▶ Laboratory Findings

The most common complication of reflux, particularly in females, is infection. Bacteriuria without pyuria is not uncommon. In males, the urine may be sterile because of the long, sterile urethra.

The serum creatinine may be elevated in the advanced stage of renal damage, but it may be normal even when the degree of reflux and hydronephrosis is marked (Figure 13–8, upper right).

▶ X-Ray Findings

The plain film may reveal evidence of spina bifida, meningomyelocele, or the absence of the sacrum and thus point to a neurologic deficit. Even in VUR, excretory urograms may be normal, but usually, one or more of the following clues to the presence of reflux is noted (Figure 13–7): (1) a persistently dilated lower ureter, (2) areas of dilatation in the ureter, (3) ureter visualized throughout its entire length, (4) the presence of hydroureteronephrosis with a narrow juxtavesical ureteral segment, or (5) changes of healed pyelonephritis (caliceal clubbing with narrowed infundibula or cortical thinning). A normal intravenous urogram does not rule out reflux.

The presence of ureteral duplication suggests the possibility of reflux into the lower pole of the kidney. In this case, hydronephrosis or changes compatible with pyelonephritic scarring may be seen. Abnormality of the upper segment of a duplicated system can be caused by the presence of an ectopic ureteral orifice with reflux or by obstruction secondary to a ureterocele.

Reflux is diagnosed by demonstration of its existence with one of the following techniques: simple or delayed cystography, voiding cystourethrography, or voiding cinefluoroscopy. Radionuclide scanning can be used: 1 mCi of ^{99m}Tc is instilled into the bladder along with sterile saline solution, and the gamma camera will reveal ureteral reflux.

Reflux can be demonstrated by a technique using indigotindisulfonate sodium (indigo carmine), a blue dye. The bladder is filled with sterile water containing 5 mL of indigo carmine per 100 mL, after which the patient voids and the bladder is thoroughly flushed out with sterile water. The ureteral orifices are then viewed cystoscopically for blue-tinged efflux. This technique has the advantage that no ionizing radiation is used, and its efficiency is equal to that of voiding cystourethrography. In general, reflux demonstrable only with voiding implies a more competent valve than does reflux that occurs at low pressures. As has been pointed out, failure to demonstrate reflux on one study does not rule out intermittent reflux.

The voiding phase of the cystogram may reveal changes compatible with distal urethral stenosis with secondary spasm of the voluntary periurethral muscles in girls (Figure 39–1) or changes diagnostic of posterior urethral valves in young boys.

▶ Instrumental Examination

A. Cystoscopy

Most young girls with reflux have smooth-walled or only slightly trabeculated bladders. Chronic cystitis, ureteral duplication, or ureterocele may be evident. An orifice may be ectopic and be found at the bladder neck or even in the urethra. As the bladder is filled, a small diverticulum may form on the roof of the ureteral orifice (Figure 13–6). These findings imply the possibility of reflux. The major contribution of cystoscopy is to allow study of the morphologic characteristics of the ureteral orifice and its position in relation to the vesical neck (Figure 13–9). However, cystoscopy should not be performed as a part of the workup for reflux. Rather, it can be performed prior to surgical correction to help define the anatomic and rule out other bladder and ureteral anomalies.

1. Morphology—The orifice of a normal ureter has the appearance of a volcanic cone. That of a slightly weaker valve looks like a football stadium; an even weaker one has the appearance of a horseshoe with its open end pointing toward the vesical neck. The completely incompetent junction has a golf-hole orifice that lies over the ureteral hiatus.

2. Position—By and large, the more defective the appearance of the ureteral orifice, the farther from the vesical neck it lies. The degree of lateralization of the orifice reflects the degree of ureterotrigonal deficiency.

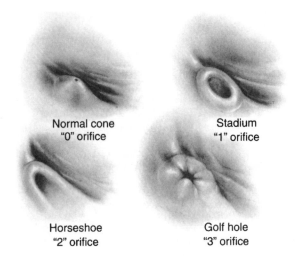

Normal cone "0" orifice

Stadium "1" orifice

Horseshoe "2" orifice

Golf hole "3" orifice

▲ **Figure 13–9.** Cystoscopic appearance of the normal ureteral orifice and 3° of incompetence of the ureterovesical junction. (See also Figure 13–4.) (Reproduced, with permission, from Lyon RP et al: The ureteral orifice: Its configuration and competency. J Urol 1969;102:504.)

DIFFERENTIAL DIAGNOSIS

Functional (nonocclusive) vesicoureteral obstruction may cause changes similar to those suggesting the presence of reflux on excretory urography. Multiple cystograms fail to show reflux. Tanagho et al (1970) showed that this congenital obstruction is due to an abundance of circularly oriented smooth-muscle fibers in the ureteral musculature at this point. Its action is sphincteric.

Significant obstruction distal to the vesical neck leads to hypertrophy of both the detrusor and trigonal muscles. The latter exert an exaggerated pull on the intravesical ureter and thus cause functional obstruction (Tanagho and Meyers, 1965). Hydroureteronephrosis is therefore to be expected; VUR is uncommon.

Other lesions that may cause hydroureteronephrosis without reflux include low ureteral stone, occlusion of the ureter by cervical or prostatic cancer, urinary tract tuberculosis, and schistosomiasis.

TREATMENT

It is impossible to give a concise and definitive discourse on the treatment of VUR because of the many factors involved and because there is no unanimity of opinion among urologists on this subject. In general, probably more than half of the cases of primary reflux that occur in children can be controlled by nonsurgical means; the rest require some form of operative procedure. Adults with reflux usually require vesicoureteroplasty.

▶ Medical Treatment

A. Indications

In the majority of the cases, children with primary reflux are initially treated medically, since there is a chance of spontaneous resolution. Positive predictors for reflux resolution include unilateral reflux, the lower grades of reflux, the earlier age of presentation, and male gender (Estrada et al, 2009). A boy with posterior urethral valves may cease to have reflux once these valves are destroyed.

In a woman who occasionally develops acute pyelonephritis following intercourse but whose urine quickly clears on antimicrobial therapy, reflux will probably be controlled if she takes steps to prevent vesical infections. This is particularly true if reflux cannot be demonstrated cystographically when her urine is sterile. The maintenance of sterile urine allows her "borderline" valve to remain competent.

B. Methods of Treatment

Urinary infection should be definitively treated with antimicrobial drugs, after which chronic suppressive therapy should be continued until the reflux has resolved or surgically corrected. However, recent studies have challenged the effectiveness of prophylactic antibiotics in the treatment of children with VUR (reviewed by Koyle and Caldamone, 2007). A similar urinary tract infection rate of approximately 23% was seen in those receiving and not receiving prophylactic antibiotics. In addition, no difference was observed in the renal damage among VUR patients randomized to receive antibiotic prophylaxis or no antibiotics. Current prospective, randomized trials have been instituted to more definitively evaluate the effectiveness of prophylactic antibiotics in the treatment of patients with primary VUR.

Children with reflux often have voiding dysfunction due to thin-walled bladders and do not perceive the normal urge to void when the bladder is full. Further detrusor tone is lost with overfilling, increasing the likelihood of residual urine. Such children should "void by the clock" every 3–4 hours whether they have the urge or not. Vesical residual urine may then be minimized.

C. Evaluation of Success of Medical Treatment

Cystograms should be repeated every 12–18 months. Excretory urography or nuclear renal scan should be performed periodically to be sure that renal deterioration does not occur. About half of children with reflux resolve their reflux during observation.

▶ Surgical Treatment

A. Indications

Reflux caused by the following abnormalities will not disappear spontaneously: (1) ectopic ureteral orifice, (2) ureteral duplication, (3) ureterocele associated with ureteral duplication and reflux into the uninvolved ureter, and (4) low-pressure reflux with significant hydroureteronephrosis.

Absolute indications for surgery include the following conditions: (1) if it is not possible to keep the urine sterile and reflux persists, (2) if acute pyelonephritis recurs despite a strict medical regimen and chronic suppressive antimicrobial therapy, (3) if increased renal damage is demonstrated by serial excretory urograms or nuclear scan, or (4) if noncompliance with medical treatment. Relative indications for surgery include failure to resolve after prolonged observation period (ie, >3 years), parental decision (avoidance of chronic antibiotic usage or radiologic evaluation), or the presence of a diverticulum.

B. Types of Surgical Treatment

In cases of markedly impaired kidney function and massively dilated ureters, preliminary urinary diversion may be required to improve renal function and to allow dilated ureters to regain tone, after which definitive relief of obstruction (eg, posterior urethral valves) and ureterovesicoplasty can be performed at the optimum time. Some patients with irreversible lesions causing reflux (eg, meningomyelocele) or badly damaged and atonic ureters may require permanent diversion of the urine (ie, ureteroileocutaneous anastomosis).

1. Temporary urinary diversion—If refluxed urine drains freely into the bladder, cystostomy (or an indwelling urethral catheter in girls) may prove helpful. If the ureters are dilated and kinked, a low redundant loop can be brought to the skin. The ureter is opened at this point and urine collected into an ileostomy bag. Later, the loop and the section of ureter distal to it can be resected and the ureter proximal to the loop reimplanted into the bladder. Nephrostomy may be necessary if there is no ureteral redundancy.

2. Permanent urinary diversion—If it is felt that successful ureterovesicoplasty cannot be accomplished, a Bricker type of diversion is indicated. If renal function is poor and the ureters are widely dilated and atonic, ureterocutaneous diversion may be the procedure of choice.

3. Other surgical procedures

a. If reflux is unilateral, with the affected kidney badly damaged and the other kidney normal, nephrectomy is indicated.

b. If one renal pole of a duplicated system is essentially functionless, heminephrectomy with removal of its entire ureter should be done. If there is moderate hydronephrosis of one renal pole with duplication, an alternative is anastomosis of the dilated ureter or pelvis to the normal ureter or pelvis. The remainder of the dilated refluxing ureter should be removed.

c. In unilateral reflux, anastomosis of the lower end of the refluxing ureter into the side of its normal mate (transureteroureterostomy) has a few proponents.

4. Definitive repair of ureterovesical junction (ureterovesicoplasty)

a. **Principles of repair (Tanagho, 1970)**

1. Resect the lower 2–3 cm of the ureter in which the muscle is underdeveloped.

2. Free up enough extravesical ureter so that an intravesical segment 2.5 cm long can be formed.

3. Place the intravesical ureter in a submucosal position.

4. Suture the wall of the new ureteral orifice to the cut edge of the trigonal muscle.

b. **Types of operation**—The following procedures satisfy the preceding principles and have been successful in a high percentage of cases: suprahiatal repair, increasing the length of intravesical ureter above the level of the ureteral hiatus (Paquin, 1959; Politano and Leadbetter, 1958); infrahiatal repair, the advancement procedures of Hutch (1963) and Glenn and Anderson (1967); combined supra- and infrahiatal repair, which is the most attractive; and transtrigonal repair (Cohen, 1975).

If the ureters are unduly tortuous, the redundant portions must be resected. If they are widely dilated, the lower ends must be tailored to a more normal size.

c. **Results of ureterovesicoplasty**—About 93% of patients no longer show reflux after ureterovesicoplasty. About 3% develop ureterovesical stenosis that requires reoperation. At least 75% have and maintain sterile urine without antimicrobial drugs 3–6 months after surgery. Many patients in whom bacteriuria persists have cystitis only. This has been demonstrated by the finding that renal urine specimens collected by ureteral catheters are sterile. Febrile attacks cease. Considering that only the most severe and advanced cases are submitted to surgical repair, these are impressive results, and they exceed by far the cure rates reported when only antimicrobial drugs are used (10–15%). This operation is rightly considered one of the most significant accomplishments of modern urology.

C. Subureteric Transurethral Injection (STING)

More recently, endoscopic treatment of reflux has become popular treatment for reflux. A biocompatible material such as Deflux (a mixture of dextranomer microspheres and non-animal-stabilized hyaluronic acid) can be injected into the intramural ureter. The bulking agent allows for the coaptation of the ureteral orifice and intramural ureter (Aaronson, 2005) in order to prevent reflux. The success rate for the STING procedure varies from 70% to 90%, depending upon the grade of the reflux treated. While it does not approximate the cure rate from open surgery, technical improvements and risk factors for failure are gradually being identified that are aimed at improving performance (reviewed by Routh et al, 2010). More recent studies have suggested that VUR may recur following successful endoscopic injection, warranting

long-term follow-up (Yucel et al, 2007; Holmdahl et al, 2010).

PROGNOSIS

In patients with reflux who are judged to have fairly competent valves, conservative therapy as outlined previously is highly successful in the cure of the reflux and therefore of infection.

Patients with very incompetent ureterovesical valves subjected to surgical repair also have an excellent prognosis. A few children, however, have such badly damaged urinary tracts when finally submitted to diagnostic procedures that little help other than permanent urinary diversion can be offered.

BIBLIOGRAPHY

Aaronson IA: Does deflux alter the paradigm for the management of children with vesicoureteral reflux? Curr Urol Rep 2005;6(2):152–156.

Agarwal S: Vesicoureteral reflux and urinary tract infections. Curr Opin Urol 2000;10:587.

Ataei N et al: Screening for vesicoureteral reflux and renal scars in siblings of children with known reflux. Pediatr Nephrol 2004;19(10):1127–1131.

Atwell JD, Cox PA: Growth of the kidney following unilateral antireflux surgery. Eur Urol 1981;7:257.

Bailey RR, Rolleston GL: Vesicoureteric reflux and reflux nephropathy: The Christchurch contribution. N Z Med J 1997;110:266.

Bakshandeh K et al: Vesicoureteral reflux and end stage renal disease. J Urol 1976;116:557.

Belman AB: Vesicoureteral reflux. Pediatr Clin North Am 1997;44:1171.

Birmingham Reflux Study Group: Operative versus non-operative treatment of severe vesicoureteric reflux in children: Five years' observation. Br Med J Clin Res 1987;295:237.

Blake NS, O'Connell E: Endoscopic correction of vesicoureteric reflux by subureteric Teflon injection: Follow-up ultrasound and voiding cystography. Br J Radiol 1989;62:443.

Bomalaski MD et al: Vesicoureteral reflux and ureteropelvic junction obstruction: Association, treatment options and outcome. J Urol 1997;157:969.

Bourne HH et al: Intrarenal reflux and renal damage. J Urol 1976;115:304.

Bower WF et al: Dysfunctional elimination symptoms in childhood and adulthood. J Urol 2005;174(4, Pt 2):1623–1627; discussion 1627–1628.

Carvas F et al: The genetics of primary, nonsyndromic vesicoureteral reflux. Curr Opin Urol 2010;20:336–342.

Cohen SJ: Ureterocystoneostomie: Eine neue antireflux Technik. [Ureterocystoneostomy: A new technique for reflux prevention.] Aktuelle Urologie 1975;6:1.

Darge K: Diagnosis of vesicoureteral reflux with ultrasonography. Pediatr Nephrol 2002;17:52.

de Klerk DP et al: Vesicoureteral reflux and ureteropelvic junction obstruction: Late occurrence of ureteropelvic obstruction after successful ureteroneocystostomy. J Urol 1979;121:816.

Devriendt K et al: Vesico-ureteral reflux: A genetic condition? Eur J Pediatr 1998;157:265.

Dewan PA: Ureteric reimplantation: A history of the development of surgical techniques. BJU Int 2000;85:1000.

Dewan PA, Anderson P: Ureterocystoplasty: The latest developments. BJU Int 2001;88:744.

Duckett JW Jr: Ureterovesical junction and acquired vesicoureteral re-flux. J Urol 1982;127:249.

Duckett JW, Bellinger MF: A plea for standardized grading of vesicoureteral reflux. Eur Urol 1982;8:74.

Estrada CR Jr et al: Nomograms for predicting annual resolution rate of primary vesicoureteral reflux: Results from 2462 children. J Urol 2009;182(4):1535–1541.

Fanos V, Cataldi L: Antibiotics or surgery for vesicoureteric reflux in children. Lancet 2004;364(9446):1720–1722.

Garin EH et al: Primary vesicoureteral reflux: Review of current concepts. Pediatr Nephrol 1998;12:249.

Glenn JF, Anderson EE: Distal tunnel ureteral reimplantation. J Urol 1967;97:623.

Greenfield SP, Wan J: The relationship between dysfunctional voiding and congenital vesicoureteral reflux. Curr Opin Urol 2000; 10(6):607–610.

Hendren WH: Complications of megaureter repair in children. J Urol 1975;113:228.

Holland NH et al: Relation of urinary tract infection and vesicoureteral reflux to scars: Follow-up of thirty-eight patients. J Pediatr 1990;116:S65.

Holmdahl G et al: The Swedish reflux trial in children: II. Vesicoureteral reflux outcome. J Urol 2010;184(1):280–285.

Huland H et al: Vesicoureteral reflux in end stage renal disease. J Urol 1979;121:10.

Hutch JA: Ureteric advancement operation: Anatomy, technique, and early results. J Urol 1963;89:180.

Hutch JA: The mesodermal component: Its embryology, anatomy, physiology and role in prevention of vesicoureteral reflux. J Urol 1972;108:406.

Hutch JA, Amar AD: *Vesicoureteral Reflux and Pyelonephritis.* Appleton-Century-Crofts, New York, 1972.

Jodal U et al: Medical or surgical management for children with vesico-ureteric reflux? Acta Paediatr Suppl 1999;88:53.

Johnston JH: Vesicoureteric reflux with urethral valves. Br J Urol 1979;51:100.

Kershen RT, Atala A: New advances in injectable therapies for the treatment of incontinence and vesicoureteral reflux. Urol Clin North Am 1999;26:81.

Koff SA: Relationship between dysfunctional voiding and reflux. J Urol 1992;148:1703.

Koff SA, Murtagh DS: The uninhibited bladder in children: Effect of treatment of recurrence of urinary infection and on vesicoureteral reflux resolution. J Urol 1983;130:1138.

Koo HP, Bloom DA: Lower ureteral reconstruction. Urol Clin North Am 1999;26:167.

Koyle MA, Caldamone AA: Part 4: Considerations regarding the medical management of VUR: What have we really learned? Curr Med Res Opin 2007;23(Suppl 4):S21–S25.

Lerner GR et al: Reflux nephropathy. Pediatr Clin North Am 1987; 34:747.

Lyon RP et al: Treatment of vesicoureteral reflux: Point system based on 20 years of experience. Trans Am Assoc Genitourin Surg 1979;71:146.

Lyon RP et al: The ureteral orifice: Its configuration and competency. J Urol 1969;102:504.

Mundy AR et al: Improvement in renal function following ureteric reimplantation for vesicoureteric reflux. Br J Urol 1982;53:542.

O'Donnell B: Management of urinary tract infection and vesicoureteric reflux in children. 2. The case for surgery. Br Med J 1990;300:1393.

Paltiel HJ, Lebowitz RL: Neonatal hydronephrosis due to primary vesicoureteral reflux: Trends in diagnosis and treatment. Radiology 1989;170:787.

Paquin AJ Jr: Ureterovesical anastomosis: The description and evaluation of a technique. J Urol 1959;82:573.

Politano VA, Leadbetter WF: An operative technique for correction of vesicoureteral reflux. J Urol 1958;79:932.

Pope JC IV et al: How they begin and how they end: Classic and new theories for the development and deterioration of congenital anomalies of the kidney and urinary tract, CAKUT. J Am Soc Nephrol 1999;10:2018.

Ransley PG: The renal papilla and intrarenal reflux. In: Williams PI, Chisholm GD (eds) *Scientific Foundations of Urology.* Year Book Medical Publishers, Chicago, 1976.

Ransley PG: Vesicoureteral reflux: Continuous surgical dilemma. Urology 1978;12:246.

Roberts JA: Experimental pyelonephritis in the monkey. 4. Vesicoureteral reflux and bacteria. Invest Urol 1976;14:198.

Rolleston GL et al: Intrarenal reflux and the scarred kidney. Arch Dis Child 1974;49:531.

Rose JS et al: Intrarenal reflux and its relationship to renal scarring. J Urol 1975;113:400.

Routh JC et al: Dextranomer/hyaluronic acid for pediatric vesicoureteral reflux: Systematic review. Pediatrics 2010;125(5):1010–1019.

Salvatierra O Jr et al: Primary vesicoureteral reflux and end-stage renal disease. JAMA 1973;226:1454.

Salvatierra O Jr, Tanagho EA: Reflux as a cause of end stage kidney disease: Report of 32 cases. J Urol 1977;117:441.

Seruca H: Vesicoureteral reflux and voiding dysfunction: A prospective study. J Urol 1989;142:494.

Shimada K et al: Renal growth and progression of reflux nephropathy in children with vesicoureteral reflux. J Urol 1988;140:1097.

Sillen U: Bladder dysfunction in children with vesico-ureteric reflux. Acta Paediatr Suppl 1999;88:40.

Skoog SJ et al: A nonsurgical approach to the management of primary vesicoureteral reflux. J Urol 1987;138:941.

Smellie JM: Vesico-ureteric reflux. Acta Paediatr 1999;88:1182.

Stephens FD: Treatment of megaloureters by multiple micturition. Aust N Z J Surg 1957;27:130.

Tanagho EA: Surgical revision of the incompetent ureterovesical junction: A critical analysis of techniques and requirements. Br J Urol 1970;42:410.

Tanagho EA: Ureteral tailoring. J Urol 1971;106:194.

Tanagho EA: The pathogenesis and management of megaureter. In: Johnston JH, Goodwin WE (eds) *Reviews in Paediatric Urology.* Excerpta Medica, North Holland, The Netherlands, 1974.

Tanagho EA et al: Primary vesicoureteral reflux: Experimental studies of its etiology. J Urol 1965;93:165.

Tanagho EA et al: The intravesical ureter in primary reflux. J Urol 1969;101:824.

Tanagho EA et al: Pathophysiology of functional ureteral obstruction. J Urol 1970;104:73.

Tanagho EA, Jonas U: Reduced bladder capacity: Cause of ureterovesical reflux. Urology 1974;4:421.

Tanagho EA, Meyers FH: Trigonal hypertrophy: A cause of ureteral obstruction. J Urol 1965;93:678.

Tanagho EA, Pugh RCB: The anatomy and function of the ureterovesical junction. Br J Urol 1963;35:151.

Van den Abbeele AD et al: Vesicoureteral reflux in asymptomatic siblings of patients with known reflux: Radionuclide cystography. Pediatrics 1987;79:147.

Verber IG et al: 99mTc dimercaptosuccinic acid (DMSA) scan as first investigation of urinary tract infection. Arch Dis Child 1988; 63:1320.

Weiss RA: Update on childhood urinary tract infections and reflux. Semin Nephrol 1998;18:264.

Weiss RM, Biancani P: Characteristics of normal and refluxing ureterovesical junctions. J Urol 1983;129:858.

Whitaker RH: Reflux induced pelvi-ureteric obstruction. Br J Urol 1976;48:555.

White RH: Vesicoureteric reflux and renal scarring. Arch Dis Child 1989;64:407.

White RH: Management of urinary tract infection and vesicoureteric reflux in children. 1. Operative treatment has no advantage over medical management. Br Med J 1990;300:1391.

Williams DI: The natural history of reflux. Urol Int 1971;26:350.

Woodard JR, Rushton HG: Reflux uropathy. Pediatr Clin North Am 1987;34:1349.

Woodard JR, Zucker I: Current management of the dilated urinary tract in prune belly syndrome. Urol Clin North Am 1990; 17:407.

Yucel S et al: Durability of a single successful endoscopic polytetrafluoroethylene injection for primary vesicoureteral reflux: 14 year followup results. J Urol 2007;178(1):265–268.

Bacterial Infections of the Genitourinary Tract

14

Hiep T. Nguyen, MD

Urinary tract infection (UTI) is a term that is applied to a variety of clinical conditions ranging from the asymptomatic presence of bacteria in the urine to severe infection of the kidney with resultant sepsis. UTI is one of the more common medical problems. It is estimated that 150 million patients are diagnosed with a UTI yearly, resulting in at least $6 billion in health care expenditures (Stamm and Norrby, 2001). UTIs are at times difficult to diagnose; some cases respond to a short course of a specific antibiotic, while others require a longer course of a broad-spectrum antibiotic. Accurate diagnosis and treatment of a UTI is essential to limit its associated morbidity and mortality and avoid prolonged or unnecessary use of antibiotics. Advances in our understanding of the pathogenesis of UTI, the development of new diagnostic tests, and the introduction of new antimicrobial agents have allowed physicians to appropriately tailor specific treatment for each patient.

EPIDEMIOLOGY

The epidemiology of UTI grouped by age and sex is shown in Table 14–1. In newborns up to 1 year of age, bacteriuria is present in 2.7% of boys and 0.7% in girls (Wettergren et al, 1985). The incidence of UTI in uncircumcised males is higher than in circumcised males (1.12% compared with 0.11%) during the first 6 months of life (Wiswell and Roscelli, 1986). In children between 1 and 5 years of age, the incidence of bacteriuria in girls increases to 4.5%, while it decreases in boys to 0.5% (Randolph and Greenfield, 1964). Most UTIs in children younger than 5 years are associated with congenital abnormalities of the urinary tract, such as vesicoureteral reflux or obstruction. The incidence of bacteriuria remains relatively constant in children 6–15 years of age. However, the UTIs in these children are more likely to be associated with functional abnormalities of the urinary tract, such as dysfunctional voiding. During adolescence, the incidence of UTI significantly increases (to 20%) in young women, while remaining constant in young men (Sanford, 1975).

Approximately 7 million cases of acute cystitis are diagnosed yearly in young women (Schappert, 1999); this likely is an underestimate of the true incidence of UTI because at least 50% of all UTIs do not come to medical attention. The major risk factors for women 16–35 years of age are related to sexual intercourse and diaphragm use. Later in life, the incidence of UTI increases significantly for both males and females. For women between 36 and 65 years of age, gynecologic surgery and bladder prolapse appear to be important risk factors. In men of the same age group, prostatic hypertrophy/obstruction, catheterization, and surgery are relevant risk factors. For patients older than 65 years, the incidence of UTI continues to increase in both sexes. Incontinence and chronic use of urinary catheters are important risk factors in these patients. In those younger than 1 year and those older than 65 years, the morbidity and mortality of UTI are the greatest (Shortliffe and McCue, 2002).

Based on data from the Urologic Diseases in North America Project, the overall lifetime prevalence of UTI was estimated to be 14,000 per 100,000 men (Griebling, 2005a) and 53,000 per 100,000 women (Griebling, 2005b). Overall medical expenditures for the treatment of UTIs in the United States were estimated to be $1 billion for men (Griebling, 2005a) and $2.5 billion for women (Griebling, 2005b). The increased cost in treatment of UTIs for women is primarily due to an increase in the trend toward using fluoroquinolones as a first-line therapy for UTI. UTIs occurred in 2.4–2.8% of children. In this patient population, UTIs resulted in more than 1.1 million physician visits annually, accounting for 0.7% of the doctor visits (Freedman, 2005).

PATHOGENESIS

▶ Bacterial Entry

Understanding of the mode of bacterial entry, host susceptibility factors, and bacterial pathogenic factors is essential to tailoring appropriate treatment for the diverse

Table 14–1. Epidemiology of UTI by age, group, and sex.

Age (y)	Incidence (%)		Risk factors
	Female	Male	
<1	0.7	2.7	Foreskin, anatomic GU abnormalities
1–5	4.5	0.5	Anatomic GU abnormalities
6–15	4.5	0.5	Functional GU abnormalities
16–35	20	0.5	Sexual intercourse, diaphragm use
36–65	35	20	Surgery, prostate obstruction, catheterization
>65	40	35	Incontinence, catheterization, prostate obstruction

UTI, urinary tract infection; GU, genitourinary.

clinical manifestations of UTI. There are four possible modes of bacterial entry into the genitourinary tract. It is generally accepted that periurethral bacteria ascending into the urinary tract causes most UTI. Most cases of pyelonephritis are caused by the ascent of bacteria from the bladder, through the ureter and into the renal parenchyma. Consequently, the short nature of the female urethra combined with its close proximity to the vaginal vestibule and rectum likely predisposes women to more frequent UTIs than men (Nicolle et al, 1982).

Other modes of bacterial entry are uncommon causes of UTI. Hematogenous spread can occur in immunocompromised patients and in neonates. *Staphylococcus aureus*, *Candida* species, and *Mycobacterium tuberculosis* are common pathogens that travel through the blood to infect the urinary tract. Lymphatogenous spread through the rectal, colonic, and periuterine lymphatics has been postulated as a cause for UTI; however, currently, there is little scientific support to suggest that dissemination of bacteria through lymphatic channels plays a role in the pathogenesis of UTI. Direct extension of bacteria from adjacent organs into the urinary tract can occur in patients with intraperitoneal abscesses or vesicointestinal or vesicovaginal fistulas. Relapsing infection from an inadequately treated focus in the prostate or kidney may seed other parts of the urinary tracts.

▶ Host Defenses

Host factors have an essential role in the pathogenesis of UTI. Unobstructed urinary flow with the subsequent washout of ascending bacteria is essential in preventing UTI. In addition, the urine itself has specific characteristics (its osmolality, urea concentration, organic acid concentration, and pH) that inhibit bacterial growth and colonization (Sobel, 1997). It also contains factors that inhibit bacterial adherence, such as

Tamm–Horsfall glycoprotein (THG; Duncan, 1988; Pak et al, 2001; Wagenlehner et al, 2005). Is has been observed that the severity of the bacteriuria and the degree of inflammatory changes in the urinary tract were much greater in THG-deficit mice, suggesting that THG helps eliminate bacterial infection from the urinary tract and acts as a general host-defense factor against UTI (Raffi et al, 2005). Urinary retention, stasis, or reflux of urine into the upper urinary tract can promote bacterial growth and subsequent infection. Consequently, any anatomic or functional abnormalities of the urinary tract that impede urinary flow can increase the host's susceptibility to UTI. These abnormalities include obstructive conditions at any level of the urinary tract, neurologic diseases affecting the function of the lower urinary tract, diabetes, and pregnancy. Similarly, the presence of foreign bodies (such as stones, catheters, and stents) allows the bacteria to hide from these host defenses.

The epithelium lining the urinary tract not only provides a physical barrier to infection but also has the capacity to recognize bacteria in order to innate host defenses. The urothelial cells express toll-like receptors (TLRs) that upon engagement by specific bacterial components lead to production of inflammatory mediators (Chowdhury et al, 2004). In response to the presence of bacteria, cells lining the urinary tract secrete chemoattractants such as interleukin-8 to recruit neutrophils to the area and limit tissue invasion (Frendeus et al, 2001). Specific serum and urinary antibodies are produced by the kidney to enhance bacterial opsonization and phagocytosis and to inhibit bacterial adherence. The protective role of both cellular and humoral-mediated immunity in preventing UTIs remains unclear; deficiency in B-cell or T-cell function has not been associated with the increased frequency of UTI or altered the course of the infection (Schaeffer, 2001; Svanborg Eden et al, 1988). However, it should be noted that the same host-defense mechanisms that help to prevent/limit the infection (such as the inflammatory responses) can lead to cell and tissue damage. In the kidneys, cell damage and subsequent development of scarring may lead to pathological conditions such as hypertension, preeclampsia during pregnancy, and renal dysfunction and failure (Jahnukainen et al, 2005).

Many studies have demonstrated that there is selectivity in bacterial adherence to cells lining the urinary tract, and the degree of adherence correlates with colonization and infection. Women with recurrent UTIs have higher adherence of bacteria to their mucosal cells in vitro compared with women who never had an infection (Navas et al, 1994). The increased adherence may be due to having more binding sites for bacterial adhesins on their mucosal cells. Alternatively, these patients may not secrete soluble compounds, which normally compete for the same receptors that bind bacterial adhesins. Blood group antigens may constitute one group of these soluble compounds that inhibit bacterial adherence (Lomberg et al, 1986). These findings would suggest a genetic predisposition for UTI.

Other important host factors include the normal flora of the periurethral area or the prostate and the presence of vesicoureteral reflux. In women, the normal flora of the periurethral area composed of organisms such as lactobacillus provides a defense against the colonization of uropathogenic bacteria (Osset et al, 2001). Alterations in the periurethral environment (such as changes in the pH or estrogen levels or the use of antibiotics) can damage the periurethral flora, allowing uropathogens to colonize and subsequently to infect the urinary tract (Schaeffer et al, 1999). In men, the prostate secretes fluid containing zinc, which has potent antimicrobial activity (Fair et al, 1976). Finally, in children, the presence of vesicoureteral reflux does not increase their susceptibility to UTI but does allow bacteria to be inoculated into the upper tract and the infection to progress.

Aging is associated with an increased susceptibility to UTI, in part because of the increased incidence of obstructive uropathy in men (Matsumoto, 2001; Nicolle, 2002) and alteration in the vaginal and periurethral flora from menopause in women (Foxman et al, 2001). Other causes include soiling of the perineum from fecal incontinence, neuromuscular diseases, increased instrumentation, and bladder catheterization (Ronald, 2002).

▶ Bacterial Pathogenic Factors

Not all bacteria are capable of adhering to and infecting the urinary tract. Of the many strains of *Escherichia coli*, the uropathogens belong to a limited number of O, K, and H serogroups. They have increased adherence properties to uroepithelial cells (Blanco et al, 1996; Hovanec and Gorzynski, 1980; Orskov et al, 1982), resistance to the bactericidal activity of human serum (Bjorksten and Kaijser, 1978), production of hemolysin (Hughes et al, 1983; Koronakis and Hughes, 1996), and the increased expression of K capsular antigen (Whitfield and Roberts, 1999). The ability of *E. coli* to adhere to epithelial cells is mediated by ligands located on the tips of the bacterial fimbriae (pili). The ligands bind to glycolipids or glycoprotein receptors on the surface membrane of uroepithelial cells. The pili are classified by their ability to cause hemagglutination and the type of sugar that can block this process. P pili, which can agglutinate human blood, bind to glycolipid receptors on uroepithelial cells, erythrocytes (P blood group antigens), and renal tubular cells (Svenson et al, 1983). Type 1 pili, which can agglutinate guinea pig blood, bind to mannoside residues on uroepithelial cells (Ofek et al, 2000). P pili are observed in >90% of the *E. coli* strains causing pyelonephritis but <20% of the strains causing lower UTIs (Kallenius et al, 1981; Roberts et al, 1997a). In contrast, type 1 pili may help bacteria to adhere to bladder mucosa (Connell et al, 1996; Martinez et al, 2000). Most uropathogenic *E. coli* have both types of pili. Once attachment to the uroepithelial cells occurs, other bacterial pathogenic factors become important. Most uropathogenic *E. coli* strains produce hemolysin, which initiates tissue invasion and makes iron available for the infecting pathogens (Hughes et al, 1983; Koronakis and Hughes, 1996). The presence of K antigen on the invading bacteria protects them from phagocytosis by neutrophils (Bortolussi et al, 1979; Evans et al, 1981). These factors allow the infecting pathogens to escape the various host defenses (Svanborg et al, 1996).

It has been observed that many bacteria such as *E. coli* have the ability to invade into the host cells, acting as opportunistic intracellular pathogens (Bower et al, 2005). Cytotoxic necrotizing factor, Afa/Dr adhesions, and type 1 pili have been shown to promote invasion into the host cells. Binding of FimH adhesin at the distal tip of type 1 pili to the host membrane leads to the recruitment of focal adhesin kinase, phosphoinositide-3-kinases, α-actinin, and vinculin, which results in localized actin rearrangements and engulfment of the bound bacterium by zippering of the membrane around the bacteria (reviewed by Anderson et al, 2004). The intracellular bacteria mature into biofilms, creating pod-like bulges on the urothelial surface. The pods contain bacteria encased in a polysaccharide-rich matrix surrounded by a protective shell of uroplakin. The ability of the uropathogenic bacteria to transiently invade, survive, and multiply within the host cells and to create biofilms on genitourinary tract tissues may provide a mechanism for the persistence and recurrence of UTIs.

CAUSATIVE PATHOGENS

Most UTIs are caused by a single bacterial species. At least 80% of the uncomplicated cystitis and pyelonephritis are due to *E. coli*, with most of pathogenic strains belonging to the O serogroups (Orskov et al, 1982). Other less common uropathogens include *Klebsiella, Proteus,* and *Enterobacter* spp. and enterococci. In hospital-acquired UTIs, a wider variety of causative organisms is found, including *Pseudomonas* and *Staphylococcus* spp. (Wagenlehner and Naber, 2000); UTIs caused by *S. aureus* often result from hematogenous dissemination. Group B beta-hemolytic streptococci can cause UTIs in pregnant women (Wood and Dillon, 1981). *Staphylococcus saprophyticus*, once often thought of as urinary contaminants, can cause uncomplicated UTIs in young women (Hovelius and Mardh, 1984). In children, the causative bacterial spectrum is slightly different from that of adults, with *Klebsiella* and *Enterobacter* spp. being more common causes of UTI (Jeena et al, 1996; Ronald, 2002; Schlager, 2001). Anaerobic bacteria, lactobacilli, corynebacteria, streptococci (not including enterococci), and *Staphylococcus epidermidis* are found in normal periurethral flora. They do not commonly cause UTIs in healthy individuals and are considered common urinary contaminants.

DIAGNOSIS

The diagnosis of UTI is sometimes difficult to establish and relies on urinalysis and urine culture. Occasionally, localization studies may be required to identify the source of the infection. Most often, the urine is often obtained from a voided specimen. In children who are not toilet trained, a urine collection device, such as a bag, is placed over the genitalia, and the urine is cultured from the bagged specimen. These two methods of urine collection are easy to obtain, but potential contamination from the vagina and perirectal area may occur. There is a high false-positive rate, especially from bagged specimens (Al-Orifi et al, 2000). Suprapubic aspiration avoids potential contamination; however, due to its invasiveness, it is rarely used except in children and selected patients. Urine obtained from a urinary catheter is less invasive than a suprapubic aspiration and is less likely to be contaminated than that obtained from a voided specimen. If a patient has an indwelling catheter, a urine specimen should be obtained from the collection port on the catheter.

Urinalysis

The urine can be immediately evaluated for leukocyte esterase, a compound produced by the breakdown of white blood cells (WBCs) in the urine. Urinary nitrite is produced by reduction of dietary nitrates by many gram-negative bacteria. Esterase and nitrite can be detected by a urine dipstick and are more reliable when the bacterial count is >100,000 colony-forming units (CFUs) per milliliter. Microscopic examination of the urine for WBCs and bacteria is performed after centrifugation. When bacteria counts are >100,000 CFU/mL, bacteria can be detected microscopically (Jenkins et al, 1986). More than three WBCs per high-power field suggest a possible infection. The sensitivity and specificity of these tests are shown in Table 14–2 (Williams et al, 2010). The urinary nitrite test is highly specific but not sensitive, whereas the other three tests have a sensitivity and specificity approximately 80%. A combination of these tests may help to identify those patients in whom urine culture will be positive. Conversely, when esterase, nitrite, blood, and protein are absent in a urine sample, <2% of the urine samples will be positive by culture, providing a >98% negative predictive value and a sensitivity of 98% (Patel et al, 2005). A recent systematic review of the literature indicates that urinalysis is more effective in the diagnosis of UTI as determined by urine culture in children older than 2 years than for younger children (Mori et al, 2010).

Urine Culture

The gold standard for identification of UTI is the quantitative culture of urine for specific bacteria. The urine should be collected in a sterile container and cultured immediately after collection. When this is not possible, the urine can be stored in the refrigerator for up to 24 hours. The sample is then diluted and spread on culture plates. Each bacterium will form a single colony on the plates. The number of colonies is counted and adjusted per milliliter of urine (CFU/mL). Defining the CFU/mL that represents clinically significant infection can be difficult. It is dependent on the method of collection, the sex of the patient, and the type of bacteria isolated (Table 14–3). Traditionally, >100,000 CFU/mL is used to exclude contamination. However, studies have clearly demonstrated that clinically significant UTI can occur with <100,000 CFU/mL bacteria in the urine (Stamm et al, 1982).

Localization Studies

Occasionally, it is necessary to localize the site of infection. For upper urinary tract localization (Lorentz, 1979), the bladder is irrigated with sterile water and a ureteral catheter is placed into each ureter. A specimen is collected from the

Table 14–2. Sensitivity and specificity of urinalysis.

Tests	Sensitivity (%)	Specificity (%)
Esterase (E)	79 (73-84)	87 (80-92)
Nitrite (N)	49 (41-57)	98 (96-99)
E or N	88 (82-91)	79 (69-87)
E + N	45 (30-61)	98 (96-99)
WBC	74 (67-80)	86 (82-90)
Bacteria	88 (75-94)	92 (83-96)

WBC, white blood cell.

Table 14–3. Probability of UTIs based upon urine culture.

Collection	CFU	Probability of infection (%)
Suprapubic	Gram negative any Gram positive >1000	>99
Catheterization	>10^5 10^4-5 10^3-4 <10^3	95 Likely Repeat Unlikely
Clean catch		
Male	>10^4	Likely
Female	3 specimens: >10^5 2 specimens: >10^5 1 specimen: >10^5 5 × 10^4-10^5 1-5 × 10^4 symptomatic 1-5 × 10^4 nonsymptomatic <10^4	95 90 80 Repeat Repeat Unlikely Unlikely

UTIs, urinary tract infections; CFU, colony-forming unit.

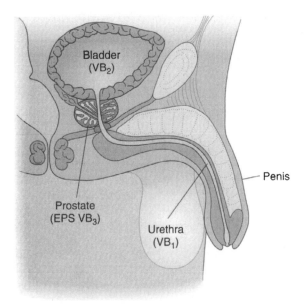

▲ **Figure 14–1.** Localization of lower urinary tract infection. A positive culture in the voided bladder urine specimen VB_1 suggests infection of the urethra, while in VB_2, an infection of the bladder, and in EPS or VB_3, an infection of the prostate.

Table 14–4. Antibiotics that require dosage adjustments for liver and renal diseases.

Renal diseases (Cr clearance <30 mL/min)
Aminoglycosides
Beta-lactams
Cefoxitin, ceftizoxime
Cefonicid, ceftazidime
Cefuroxime, cefepime
Cefpirome, moxalactam
Carbenicillin, ticarcillin, ticarcillin-clavulanate
Vancomycin
Tetracyclines (except doxycycline)
Sulfonamides
Hepatic diseases (with elevated bilirubin)
Chloramphenicol
Tetracyclines
Clindamycin, rifampin, pefloxacin
Renal-hepatic diseases
Ceftriaxone
Cefoperazone
Carbenicillin
Ticarcillin
Azlocillin
Mezlocillin
Piperacillin

renal pelvis. Culture of this specimen will indicate whether infection in the upper urinary tract is present. In men, infection in the lower urinary tract can be differentiated (Figure 14–1) (Meares and Stamey, 1968). A specimen is collected at the beginning of the void and represents possible infection in the urethra. A midstream specimen is next collected and represents possible infection in the bladder. The prostate is then massaged and the patient is asked to void again. This specimen represents possible infection of the prostate.

ANTIBIOTICS

Treatment with antimicrobial agents has minimized the morbidity and mortality associated with UTIs. The goal in treatment is to eradicate the infection by selecting the appropriate antibiotics that would target specific bacterial susceptibility. However, choosing the appropriate antimicrobial agents is often difficult. Many antibiotics are available, and the lowest effective dose and length of therapy are not well defined. Many conventions for the treatment of UTI are arbitrary. The general principles for selecting the appropriate antibiotics include consideration of the infecting pathogen (antibiotic susceptibility, single-organism vs poly-organism infection, pathogen vs normal flora, community vs hospital-acquired infection); the patient (allergies,

underlying diseases, age, previous antibiotic therapy, other medications currently taken, outpatient vs inpatient status, pregnancy); and the site of infection (kidney vs bladder vs prostate). Because most antibiotics are cleared from the body by the liver or the kidney, certain antimicrobial agents need to be adjusted in the presence of liver or renal diseases (Table 14–4). Table 14–5 lists the common uropathogens and the recommended oral and intravenous antimicrobial agents for treatment. Table 14–6 lists the common sites of UTI, the recommended treatment, and the duration of therapy. In patients with recurrent UTIs or those who are at risk for UTI (such as children with vesicoureteral reflux), prophylactic antibiotics may be used. Table 14–7 lists common prophylactic regimens.

▶ Trimethoprim–Sulfamethoxazole

Trimethoprim–sulfamethoxazole (TMP–SMX) is commonly used to treat many UTIs, except those caused by *Enterococcus* and *Pseudomonas* spp. It interferes with the bacterial metabolism of folate. TMP–SMX is highly effective and relatively inexpensive. Adverse reactions occur in 6–8% of patients using this medication; they include hypersensitivity reactions, rashes, gastrointestinal upset, leukopenia, thrombocytopenia, and photosensitivity. TMP–SMX should not be used in patients who have a folic

Table 14–5. Recommended antimicrobial agents for common genitourinary pathogens.

Bacteria	Oral therapy	Parenteral therapy
Gram-positive cocci		
Staphylococcus aureus	Nafcillin, nitrofurantoin, ciprofloxacin	Nafcillin, vancomycin
Staphylococcus epidermidis	Ampicillin, nitrofurantoin, ciprofloxacin	Ampicillin, penicillin G
Staphylococcus saprophyticus	Ampicillin, nitrofurantoin, ciprofloxacin	Ampicillin, penicillin G

Streptococcus, group D
  S. faecalis (enterococci)
  S. bovis
	Ampicillin, nitrofurantoin
	Penicillin G, ampicillin
		Ampicillin plus gentamicin
		Ampicillin, vancomycin

Streptococcus, group B	Ampicillin, cephalosporin	Ampicillin, cephalosporin
Gram-negative cocci		
Neisseria gonorrhoeae	Ciprofloxacin plus doxycycline	Ceftriaxone
Gram-negative rods		
Escherichia coli	TMP-SMX, ciprofloxacin, nitrofurantoin	Gentamicin
Enterobacter spp.	TMP-SMX, ciprofloxacin, nitrofurantoin	Gentamicin plus piperacillin
Gardnerella vaginalis	Metronidazole, ampicillin	Metronidazole
Klebsiella spp.	TMP-SMX, ciprofloxacin	Gentamicin plus cephalosporin
Proteus spp.	Ampicillin, TMP-SMX, ciprofloxacin	Ampicillin, gentamicin
Pseudomonas aeruginosa	Carbenicillin, tetracycline, ciprofloxacin	Gentamicin plus piperacillin
Serratia spp.	TMP-SMX, carbenicillin	TMP-SMX, amikacin
Other pathogens		
Chlamydiae	Tetracycline, erythromycin	Tetracycline, erythromycin
Mycoplasmas, ureaplasmas	Tetracycline, erythromycin	Tetracycline, erythromycin
Obligate anaerobes	Metronidazole, clindamycin	Metronidazole, clindamycin

TMP-SMX, trimethoprim plus sulfamethoxazole.

acid deficiency state, glucose-6-phosphate dehydrogenase deficiency, or acquired immunodeficiency syndrome (AIDS), or in pregnant patients. It is the most frequently prescribed antibiotic for uncomplicated UTI (Huang and Stafford, 2002). Recently, the use of TMP–SMX has declined due to the increased incidence of bacterial resistance (Brown et al, 2002) and physicians' preference for other newer antibiotics (Huang and Stafford, 2002). TMX can be use as monotherapy in the treatment of uncomplicated UTI without significant lost in antibacterial coverage (Nguyen et al, 2010).

▶ Fluoroquinolones

Fluoroquinolones have a broad spectrum of activity, especially against gram-negative bacteria. Although they have adequate activity against *Staphylococci* species, fluoroquinolones do not have good activity against *Streptococci* species and anaerobic bacteria. They interfere with the bacterial DNA gyrase, preventing bacterial replication. Although they are highly effective in the treatment of UTI, fluoroquinolones are relatively expensive. Adverse reactions are infrequent and include mild gastrointestinal effects, dizziness, and lightheadedness. Fluoroquinolones should not be used in patients who are pregnant and should be used judiciously in children because of potential damage to developing cartilage. Due to their broad spectrum of activity, fluoroquinolones have gained popularity in the empiric treatment of both uncomplicated and complicated UTIs (Schaeffer, 2002).

▶ Nitrofurantoin

Nitrofurantoin has good activity against most gram-negative bacteria (except for *Pseudomonas* and *Proteus* spp.), *Staphylococci,* and *Enterococci* species. It inhibits bacterial

Table 14–6. Recommended antimicrobial agents and duration of therapy based upon the type of UTI.

Diagnosis	Pathogen	Choice of antibiotics	Duration of therapy
Cystitis	E. coli Klebsiella Proteus	1st: TMP-SMX 2nd: Fluoroquinolone	1–3 days
Pyelonephritis	E. coli Proteus Klebsiella Enterobacteria	1st: Gluoroquinolone 2nd: 2nd generation cephalosporin 3rd: Aminopenicillin/BLI	7–10 days
Complicated UTI	E. coli Enterococci Pseudomonas Staphylococci	1st: Fluoroquinolone 2nd: Aminopenicillin/BLI 3rd: 3rd generation cephalosporin Aminoglycosides	3–5 days after afebrile
Prostatitis	E. coli Enterobacteria Pseudomonas Enterococci	1st: Fluoroquinolone 2nd: 2nd generation cephalosporin 3rd: 3rd generation cephalosporin	Acute: 2 weeks Chronic: 4–6 weeks
Epididymitis	E. coli Enterobacteria Enterococci Chlmaydia Ureaplasma	1st: Fluoroquinolone 2nd: 2nd generation cephalosporin 1st: Doxycycline 2nd: Macrolide	2 weeks

BLI, beta-lactamase inhibitor; TMP-SMX, trimethoprim plus sulfamethoxazole.
(Adapted from Table 2 from Wagenlehner and Naber: Hospital acquired urinary tract infections. J Hosp Infect 2000:46:171.)

enzymes and DNA activity. Nitrofurantoin is highly effective in the treatment of UTI and is relatively inexpensive. Adverse reactions are relatively common and include gastrointestinal upset, peripheral polyneuropathy, and hepatotoxicity. Long-term use may result in pulmonary hypersensitivity reaction and interstitial changes. With increasing awareness of this antibiotic and its activity against common uropathogens, nitrofurantoin usage in the treatment of uncomplicated UTIs has increased from 14% to 30% in the past 5 years (Huang and Stafford, 2002).

Table 14–7. Prophylactic antibiotics regimen.

Nitrofurantoin, 50 or 100 mg daily
Nitrofurantoin macrocrystals, 100 mg daily
TMP-SMX, 40/200 mg daily
Cephalexin, 250 mg daily
Ciprofloxacin, 250 mg daily
Trimethoprim, 100 mg daily

▶ **Aminoglycosides**

Aminoglycosides are commonly used in the treatment of complicated UTI. They are highly effective against most gram-negative bacteria. When combined with ampicillin, they are effective against enterococci. They inhibit bacterial DNA and RNA synthesis. The principal adverse effects of aminoglycosides are nephrotoxicity and ototoxicity. Aminoglycosides are primarily used in patients with complicated UTIs who require intravenous antibiotics (Santucci and Krieger, 2000). Aminoglycosides can be given as a single daily dosing; this regimen is directed toward obtaining higher peak and lower trough levels in order to achieve more effective microbial killing while reducing toxicity (Carapetis et al, 2001).

▶ **Cephalosporins**

Cephalosporins have good activity against most uropathogens (Garcia-Rodriguez and Munoz Bellido, 2000). First-generation cephalosporins have good activity against gram-positive bacteria, E. coli, and Proteus and Klebsiella spp. Second-generation cephalosporins have increased activity against anaerobes and *Haemophilus influenzae*. Third-generation cephalosporins have broader coverage against gram-negative bacteria but less against gram-positive bacteria. The cephalosporins inhibit bacterial cell wall synthesis. Adverse reactions include hypersensitivity and gastrointestinal upset. Oral cephalosporins have been used effectively in the empiric treatment of uncomplicated UTIs (Lawrenson and Logie, 2001); in children with febrile UTI/pyelonephritis, oral third-generation cephalosporins such as cefixime have been shown to be safe and effective (Hoberman et al, 1999).

▶ Penicillins

First-generation penicillins are ineffective against most uropathogens and are not commonly used in the treatment of UTI. However, the aminopenicillins (amoxicillin and ampicillin) have good activity against *Enterococci*, *Staphylococci*, *E. coli*, and *Proteus mirabilis*. However, gram-negative bacteria can quickly develop resistance to many aminopenicillins. The addition of beta-lactamase inhibitors such as clavulanic acid makes the aminopenicillins more active against the gram-negative bacteria. Although penicillins and aminopenicillins are inexpensive, the addition of the beta-lactamase inhibitors makes them more expensive. Adverse reactions include hypersensitivity (which can be immediate or delayed), gastrointestinal upset, and diarrhea. In general, penicillins are not commonly used in the treatment of UTI unless they are combined with beta-lactamase inhibitors (Sotto et al, 2001).

▶ Antibiotic Resistance

The use of antibiotics has significant consequences for the treatment of future infection. Drug resistance among uropathogens has increased steadily during the past several years (Miller and Tang, 2004) and has much geographical variability. The use of broad-spectrum antibiotics has long been associated with the development of methicillin-resistant *Staphylococcus aureus* (MRSA) and *Clostridium difficile* superinfection. More recently, it is recognized that antibiotic use selects for and maintains antibiotic resistance as well as enhances its spread. Individuals prescribed an antibiotic in the primary care setting for a urinary infection develop bacterial resistance to that antibiotic (reviewed by Costelloe et al, 2010). The effect appears to be the greatest in the first month following treatment but may persist up to 12 months. Local hospital antibiograms, which quantifies drug resistance seen at the hospital microbiology laboratory during a particular year, can provide information regarding local antibiotic resistance among bacteria for a specific locale. Evaluating these antibiograms together, some important trends in drug resistance can be seen (Kahlmeter, 2003). Among uropathogens particularly *E. coli*, resistance to Ampicillin (18–54%),

trimethoprim (9–27%), and sulfamethoxazole (16–49%) were high. Resistance to nitrofurantoin and fluoroquinolones were generally lower (<3%). However, with more extensive usage, resistance to these drugs is increasing (Johnson et al, 2008; Karaca et al, 2005). Even aminoglycosides that are considered to be effective, first-line choice for the treatment of complicated UTIs are not immune to the development of resistance (Lau et al, 2004). To limit the development of antibiotic resistance among uropathogens, judicial usage of antibiotics (duration and selection of the antibiotics) will be required. An uncomplicated first time cystitis does not require a 14-day course of treatment with a fluoroquinolone but simply a 3-day course of treatment with TMP–SMX.

▶ Probiotics

The intestinal microbial flora consists of diverse bacterial species that inhabit the gastrointestinal tract. These bacteria are integral to the ontogeny and regulation of the immune system and protection of the body from infection. The interaction of the gut microbial flora with intestinal epithelial cells and immune cells exerts beneficial effects on the urinary tract. Intermittent and chronic antibiotic usage damages the intestinal flora. Probiotics such as lactic acid bacteria and bifidobacteria can restore normal intestinal flora and promote good host defense (Abad and Safdar, 2009). Probiotics are commonly consumed as part of fermented foods with specially added active live cultures; such as in yogurt, soy yogurt, or as dietary supplements. Their benefits remain to be definitively proven but has minimal side effects. However, probiotics should be avoided in critically ill and immunocompromised patients for the risk of sepsis.

CLINICAL PRESENTATION

KIDNEY INFECTION

▶ Acute Pyelonephritis

Acute pyelonephritis is defined as inflammation of the kidney and renal pelvis, and its diagnosis is usually made clinically.

A. Presentation and Findings

Patients with acute pyelonephritis present with chills, fever, and costovertebral angle tenderness. They often have accompanying lower-tract symptoms such as dysuria, frequency, and urgency. Sepsis may occur, with 20–30% of all systemic sepsis resulting from a urine infection. Urinalysis commonly demonstrates the presence of WBCs and red blood cells in the urine. Leukocytosis, increased erythrocyte sedimentation, and elevated levels of C-reactive protein are commonly seen on blood analysis. Bacteria are cultured from the urine when the culture is obtained before antibiotic treatment is instituted. *E. coli* is the most common causative organism, accounting for 80% of the cases. *Klebsiella, Proteus, Enterobacter, Pseudomonas, Serratia,* and *Citrobacter* spp. account for the remaining cases. Of the gram-positive bacteria, *Streptococcus faecalis* and *S. aureus* can be important causes of pyelonephritis. In reproductive-age women, sexual activity and patient and family history of UTI are associated with an increased risk of developing pyelonephritis. Diabetes and urinary incontinence also independently increase this risk (Scholes et al, 2005).

B. Radiographic Imaging

Contrast-enhanced computed tomography (CT) scans can accurately demonstrate findings, confirming the diagnosis of pyelonephritis (Dacher et al, 1993). Acute bacterial infection causes constriction of peripheral arterioles and reduces perfusion of the affected renal segments. Perfusion defects, which can be segmental, multifocal, or diffuse, are seen as areas of reduced signal density (Figure 14–2). Renal enlargement, attenuated parenchyma, and a compressed collecting system are other characteristic findings on CT scan. However, CT scan is not necessary unless the diagnosis is unclear or the patient is not responding to therapy. Radionuclide study with ^{99m}Tc-dimercaptosuccinic acid is equally sensitive in detecting the perfusion defects of pyelonephritis (Levtchenko et al, 2001). In patients with acute pyelonephritis, renal ultrasonography is important to rule out concurrent urinary tract obstruction but cannot reliably detect inflammation or infection of the kidney.

C. Management

The management of acute pyelonephritis depends on the severity of the infection (Ghiro et al, 2002; Nickel, 2001). In patients who have toxicity because of associated septicemia,

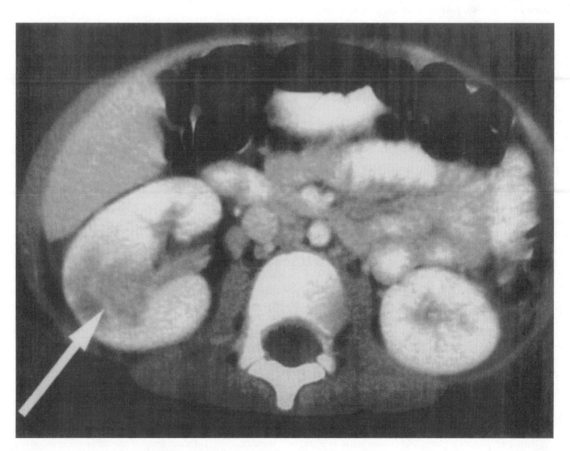

▲ **Figure 14–2.** Acute pyelonephritis. Computed tomography scan with intravenous contrast demonstrates a perfusion defect (*white arrow*) and enlargement of the affected kidney.

hospitalization is warranted. Approximately 10–30% of all adult patients with acute pyelonephritis require hospitalization, with incidence of 11.7 per 10,000 for women and 2.4 per 10,000 for men (Brown et al, 2005). Empiric therapy with intravenous ampicillin and aminoglycosides is effective against a broad range of uropathogens, including enterococci and *Pseudomonas* species. Alternatively, amoxicillin with clavulanic acid or a third-generation cephalosporin can be used. In a recent study of community-acquired UTIs in children hospitalized in a tertiary center (Marcus et al, 2005), it was noted that 40% of the culture-proved UTIs were caused by non–*E. coli* pathogens. Non–*E. coli* infections were more commonly found in males who had renal abnormalities and who had received antibiotic therapy in the prior month. Non–*E. coli* uropathogens were often resistant to cephalosporins and aminoglycosides. About 19% of the patients were initially treated with inappropriate empiric intravenous antibiotics. Fever from acute pyelonephritis may persist for several days despite appropriate therapy. Parenteral therapy should be maintained until the patient defervesces. If bacteremia is present, parenteral therapy should be continued for an additional 7–10 days and then the patient should be switched to oral treatment for 10–14 days. In patients who are not severely ill, outpatient treatment with oral antibiotics is appropriate. For adults, treatment with fluoroquinolones or TMP–SMX is well tolerated and effective. Therapy should continue for 10–14 days. Some patients in whom acute pyelonephritis develops will require follow-up radiologic examination such as voiding cystourethrogram or cystoscopy.

▶ Emphysematous Pyelonephritis

Emphysematous pyelonephritis is a necrotizing infection characterized by the presence of gas within the renal parenchyma or perinephric tissue. About 80–90% of patients with emphysematous pyelonephritis have diabetes; the rest of the cases are associated with urinary tract obstruction from calculi or papillary necrosis (Shokeir et al, 1997; Tseng et al, 2005).

A. Presentation and Findings

Patients with emphysematous pyelonephritis present with fever, flank pain, and vomiting that fails initial management with parenteral antibiotics (Tang et al, 2001). Pneumaturia may be present. Bacteria most frequently cultured from the urine include *E. coli, Klebsiella pneumoniae,* and *Enterobacter cloacae.*

B. Radiographic Imaging

The diagnosis of emphysematous pyelonephritis is made after radiographic examination. Gas overlying the affected kidney may be seen on a plain abdominal radiograph [kidneys, ureters, bladder (KUB)]. CT scan is much more sensitive in detecting the presence of gas in the renal parenchyma than renal ultrasonography.

C. Management

In the management of emphysematous pyelonephritis, prompt control of blood glucose and relief of urinary obstruction are essential, in addition to fluid resuscitation and parenteral antibiotics. The mortality rate is 11–54% (Michaeli et al, 1984). Poor prognostic factors include high serum creatinine level, low platelet count, and the presence of renal/perirenal fluid in association with a bubbly/loculated gas pattern or gas in the collecting system (Wan et al, 1998). In combination with medical treatment, percutaneous drainage appears to be helpful in accelerating resolution of the infection and minimizing the morbidity and mortality of the infection (Chen et al, 1997). Nephrectomy may be required if there is no function in the affected kidney. About 3–4 weeks of parenteral antibiotic therapy is usually required.

▶ Chronic Pyelonephritis

Chronic pyelonephritis results from repeated renal infection, which leads to scarring, atrophy of the kidney, and subsequent renal insufficiency. The diagnosis is made by radiologic or pathologic examination rather than from clinical presentation.

A. Presentation and Findings

Many individuals with chronic pyelonephritis have no symptoms, but they may have a history of frequent UTIs. In children, there is a strong correlation between renal scarring and recurrent UTIs (Wennerstrom et al, 2000). The developing kidney appears to be very susceptible to damage, and this susceptibility appears to be age dependent. Renal scarring induced by UTIs is rarely seen in adult kidneys. Because patients with chronic pyelonephritis are often asymptomatic, the diagnosis is made incidentally when radiologic investigation is initiated to evaluate for the complications associated with renal insufficiency, such as hypertension, visual impairments, headaches, fatigue, and polyuria. In these patients, urinalysis may show leukocytes or proteinuria but is likely to be normal. Serum creatinine levels reflect the severity of the renal impairment. Urine cultures are only positive when there is an active infection.

B. Radiographic Imaging

Intravenous pyelogram or CT scan can readily demonstrate a small and atrophic kidney on the affected side. Focal coarse renal scarring with clubbing of the underlying calyx is characteristic. Ultrasonography similarly can demonstrate these findings. Dimercaptosuccinic acid (DMSA) is the best imaging modality to look for renal scarring (Figures 14–3A and B;

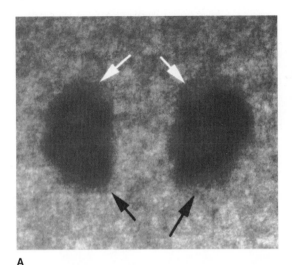
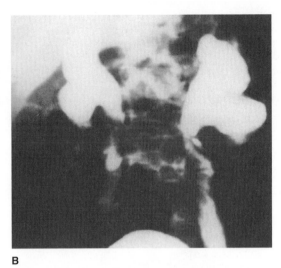

A   **B**

▲ **Figure 14–3.** Chronic pyelonephritis. Multiple parenchymal defects (*white and black arrows*) are seen on DMSA scan **(A)**, suggestive of scarring from recurrent infection. Voiding cystourethrogram **(B)** revealed high-grade reflux in this patient.

Stoller and Kogan, 1986). Areas of scarring can be seen as photopenic areas.

C. Management

The management of chronic pyelonephritis is somewhat limited because renal damage incurred by chronic pyelonephritis is not reversible. Eliminating recurrent UTIs and identifying and correcting any underlying anatomic or functional urinary problems such as obstruction or urolithiasis can prevent further renal damage. In children, evaluation for vesicoureteral reflux with a voiding cystourethrogram is important to eliminate a risk factor for recurrent pyelonephritis and renal scarring. Long-term use of continuous prophylactic antibiotic therapy may be required to limit recurrent UTIs and renal scarring. Rarely, removal of the affected kidney may be necessary due to hypertension or having a large stone burden in a nonfunctioning kidney.

▷ Renal Abscesses

Renal abscesses result from a severe infection that leads to liquefaction of renal tissue; this area is subsequently sequestered, forming an abscess. They can rupture out into the perinephric space, forming **perinephric abscesses**. When the abscesses extend beyond the Gerota's fascia, **paranephric abscesses** develop. Historically, most renal/perinephric abscesses result from hematogenous spread of staphylococci, in particular from infected skin lesions. Patients with diabetes, those undergoing hemodialysis, or intravenous drug abusers were at high risk for developing renal abscesses. With the development of effective antibiotics and better

management of diseases such as diabetes and renal failure, renal/perinephric abscesses due to gram-positive bacteria are less prevalent; those caused by *E. coli* or *Proteus* species are becoming more common (Merimsky and Feldman, 1981; Thorley et al, 1974). Abscesses that form in the renal cortex are likely to arise from hematogenous spread, whereas those in the corticomedullary junction are caused from gram-negative bacteria in conjunction with some other underlying urinary tract abnormalities, such as stones or obstruction.

A. Presentation and Findings

The most common presenting symptoms in patients with renal/perinephric abscesses include fever, flank or abdominal pain, chills, and dysuria. Many of the symptoms have lasted for more than 2 weeks. A flank mass may be palpated in some patients. Urinalysis usually demonstrates WBCs; however, it may be normal in approximately 25% of the cases (Thorley et al, 1974). Urine cultures only identify the causative organisms in about one-third of cases and blood cultures in only about half of cases (Edelstein and McCabe, 1988).

B. Radiographic Imaging

Renal abscesses can be accurately detected using ultrasonography or CT scans. There is a wide range of ultrasonographic findings ranging from an anechoic mass within or displacing the kidney to an echogenic fluid collection that tends to blend with the normally echogenic fat within Gerota's fascia (Corriere and Sandler, 1982). With high sensitivity, CT scans can demonstrate an enlarged kidney with focal areas of hypoattenuation early on during the course of the infection.

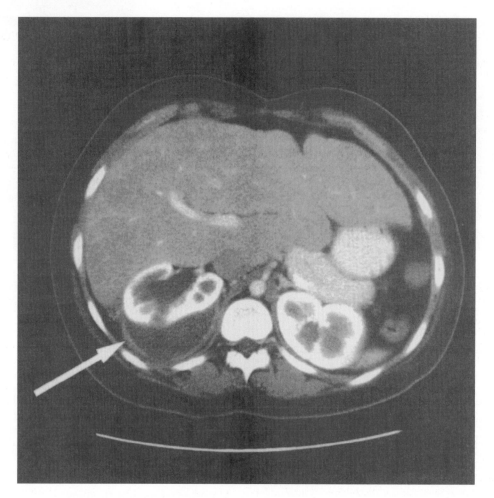

▲ **Figure 14–4.** Renal abscess. CT scan with intravenous contrast demonstrates a large perinephric fluid collection with rim enhancement (*white arrow*). The parenchyma defect in the right kidney is suggestive of pyelonephritis.

Once the inflammatory wall forms around the fluid collection, the abscess appears as a mass with a rim of contrast enhancement, the "ring" sign (Figure 14–4). CT scans may also demonstrate thickening of Gerota's fascia, stranding of the perinephric fat, or obliteration of the surrounding soft-tissue planes (Dalla Palma et al, 1999). Intravenous pyelogram and kidneys, ureter, and bladder tests are less sensitive tests in detecting renal/perinephric abscesses, with results being normal in about 20% of the cases (Thorley et al, 1974).

C. Management

The appropriate management of renal abscess first must include appropriate antibiotic therapy. Because it is often very difficult to identify the correct causative organisms from the urine or blood, empiric therapy with broad-spectrum antibiotics (ampicillin or vancomycin in combination with an aminoglycoside or third-generation cephalosporin) is usually recommended. If the patient does not respond within 48 hours of treatment, percutaneous drainage under CT scan or ultrasound guidance is indicated (Siegel et al, 1996). The drained fluid should be cultured for the causative organisms. If the abscess still does not resolve, then open surgical drainage or nephrectomy may be necessary. Follow-up imaging is needed to confirm resolution of the abscesses. These patients will also require evaluation for underlying urinary tract abnormalities such as stone or obstruction after the infection has resolved.

▶ Xanthogranulomatous Pyelonephritis

Xanthogranulomatous pyelonephritis (XGP) is a form of chronic bacterial infection of the kidney. The affected kidney is almost always hydronephrotic and obstructed. In most cases, XGP occurs unilaterally. Severe inflammation and necrosis obliterate the kidney parenchyma. Characteristically, foamy lipid-laden histiocytes (xanthoma cells) are present and may be mistaken for renal clear cell carcinoma (Iskandar et al, 1993; Lorentzen and Nielsen, 1980).

A. Presentation and Findings

Patients with XGP commonly present with flank pain, fever, chills, and persistent bacteriuria. A history of urolithiasis is present in about 35% of the patients (Malek and Elder, 1978). On physical examination, a flank mass can often be palpated. Urinalysis commonly demonstrates WBCs and protein. Serum blood analysis reveals anemia and may show hepatic dysfunction in approximately 50% of the patients (Malek and Elder, 1978). Because XGP primarily occurs unilaterally, azotemia or renal failure is not often seen (Goodman et al, 1979). *E. coli* or *Proteus* species are commonly cultured from the urine. However, one-third of patients with XGP have no growth in their urine, most likely because they have recently received antibiotic therapy. Approximately 10% of the patients with XGP have mixed organisms or anaerobic bacteria identified in their urine. Culture of the affected renal tissue can reliably identify the causative organism.

B. Radiographic Imaging

CT scan is the most reliable method in imaging patients suspected of having XGP. It usually demonstrates a large heterogeneous, reniform mass. The renal parenchyma is often marked with multiple water-density lesions, representing dilated calyces or abscesses (Figures 14–5A and B; Goldman et al, 1984). On contrast-enhanced images, these lesions will have a prominent blush peripherally, while the central areas, which are filled with pus and debris, do not enhance. An area of central calcification surrounded by a contracted pelvis may also be seen (Eastham et al, 1994). The inflammatory process may be seen extending to the perinephric fat, the retroperitoneum, and adjacent organs such as the psoas muscle, spleen, colon, or the great vessels. Because of the association of urolithiasis and XGP, renal calculi may be seen (Parsons, 1993). Renal ultrasonography can also be used in performing imaging on patients with XGP (Tiu et al, 2001). It usually reveals an enlarged kidney with a large central echogenic area and anechoic parenchyma. However, ultrasonography does not provide comparable anatomic details with those obtained from CT scan. It is not uncommon for XGP to be misdiagnosed as a renal tumor because of their similar appearances on radiologic imaging (Zorzos et al, 2002).

C. Management

The management of XGP is dependent on accurate diagnosis. In some cases, XGP is misdiagnosed as a renal tumor. A nephrectomy is performed and a diagnosis is made pathologically. In those in whom a diagnosis of XGP is suspected, kidney-sparing surgery such as a partial nephrectomy is indicated. However, when the infection is extensive, a nephrectomy

with excision of all involved tissue is warranted. There are reported cases of treating XGP with antibiotic therapy alone (Brown et al, 1996) or in combination with percutaneous drainage; however, these treatments are not likely to be curative in most patients and may lead to complications such as renal cutaneous fistula.

▶ Pyonephrosis

Pyonephrosis refers to bacterial infection of a hydronephrotic, obstructed kidney, which leads to suppurative destruction of the renal parenchyma and potential loss of renal function. Because of the extent of the infection and the presence of urinary obstruction, sepsis may rapidly ensue, requiring rapid diagnosis and management.

A. Presentation and Findings

Patients with pyonephrosis are usually very ill, with high fever, chills, and flank pain. Lower tract symptoms are not usually present. Bacteriuria and pyuria may not be present when there is complete obstruction of the affected kidney.

B. Radiographic Imaging

Imaging with renal ultrasonography can be performed to rapidly diagnose pyonephrosis. Ultrasonographic findings include persistent echoes in the inferior portion of the collecting system, fluid–debris level with dependent echoes that shift with positional changes (Figure 14–6), strong echoes with acoustic shadowing from air in the collecting system, and weak echoes throughout a dilated collecting system. Renal or ureteral calculi may also be identified on ultrasonography.

C. Management

Management of pyonephrosis includes immediate institution of antibiotic therapy and drainage of the infected collecting system. Broad-spectrum antimicrobials are indicated to prevent sepsis while the causative organism is being identified; antibiotics should be started before manipulation of the urinary tract. Performing drainage of the obstruction through the lower urinary tract (such as using a ureteral stent) should be reserved for patients who are not septic. Extensive manipulation may rapidly induce sepsis and toxemia. In the ill patient, drainage of the collecting system with a percutaneous nephrostomy tube is preferable. Once the infection is treated, additional imaging evaluation is required to identify the cause of the urinary obstruction, such as urolithiasis or ureteropelvic junction obstruction.

BLADDER INFECTION

▶ Acute Cystitis

Acute cystitis refers to urinary infection of the lower urinary tract, principally the bladder. Acute cystitis more commonly affects women than men. The primary mode of infection is

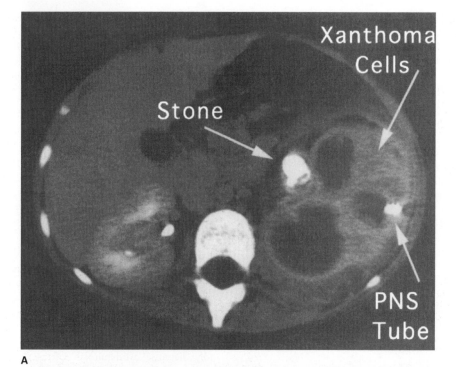

▲ **Figure 14–5.** Xanthogranulomatous pyelonephritis. **A:** CT scan demonstrates a large heterogeneous left kidney, with dilated calyces and areas filled with lipid-laden macrophages. Xanthogranulomatous pyelonephritis is often associated with the presence of renal stones. **B:** Pathology specimen better demonstrated the pockets of intraparenchymal abscesses and deposition of macrophages (*arrows*). PNS, percutaneous nephrostomy.

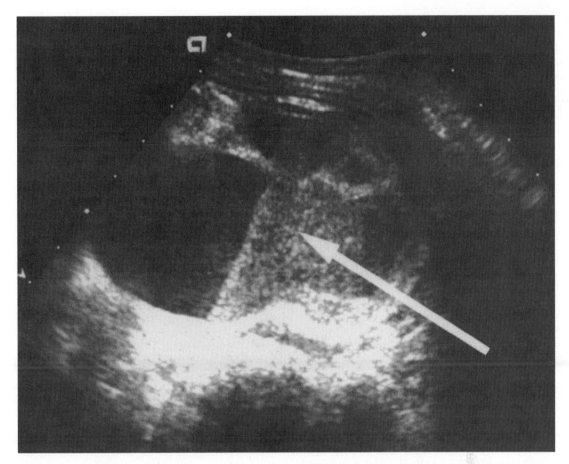

▲ **Figure 14–6.** Pyonephrosis. Ultrasonography demonstrates fluid–debris level (*white arrow*) within the dilated renal pelvis.

ascending from the periurethral/vaginal and fecal flora. The diagnosis is made clinically. In children, the distinction between upper and lower UTI is important. In general, those in whom acute cystitis developed do not usually require any extensive radiologic investigation (such as a voiding cysto-urethrogram), but those in whom pyelonephritis developed do (American Academy of Pediatrics, 1999).

A. Presentation and Findings

Patients with acute cystitis present with irritative voiding symptoms such as dysuria, frequency, and urgency. Low back and suprapubic pain, hematuria, and cloudy/foul-smelling urine are also common symptoms. Fever and systemic symptoms are rare. Typically, urinalysis demonstrates WBCs in the urine, and hematuria may be present. Urine culture is required to confirm the diagnosis and identify the causative organism. However, when the clinical picture and urinalysis are highly suggestive of the diagnosis of acute cystitis, urine culture may not be needed. *E. coli* causes most of the acute

cystitis. Other gram-negative (*Klebsiella* and *Proteus* spp.) and gram-positive (*S. saprophyticus* and enterococci) bacteria are uncommon pathogens (Gupta et al, 1999a). Diabetes and lifetime history of UTI are risk factors for acute cystitis. Of interest, the use of oral or vaginal estrogen was not protective in postmenopausal women with recurrent acute cystitis (Jackson et al, 2004).

B. Radiographic Imaging

In uncomplicated infection of the bladder, radiologic evaluation is often not necessary.

C. Management

Management for acute cystitis consists of a short course of oral antibiotics (reviewed by Falagas et al, 2009). TMP–SMX, nitrofurantoin, and fluoroquinolones have excellent activity against most pathogens that cause cystitis. TMP–SMX and nitrofurantoin are less expensive and thus are recommended for the treatment of uncomplicated cystitis (Huang and Stafford, 2002). However, it is estimated that resistance to TMP–SMX by *E. coli* isolates causing uncomplicated acute cystitis is approximately 20%, compared with <2% to nitrofurantoin (Gupta et al, 1999a). In adults and children, the duration of treatment is usually limited to 3–5 days (Abrahamsson et al, 2002; Naber, 1999). Longer therapy is not indicated. Single-dose therapy for the treatment of recurrent cystitis/UTI appears to be less effective (Philbrick, 1986); however, fluoroquinolones with long half-lives (fleroxacin, pefloxacin, and rufloxacin) may be suitable for single-dose therapy (Naber, 1999). Resistance to penicillins and aminopenicillins is high and thus they are not recommended for treatment.

▶ Recurrent Cystitis/UTI

A. Presentation and Findings

Recurrent cystitis/UTI is caused either by bacterial persistence or reinfection with another organism. Identification of the cause of the recurrent infection is important, because the management of bacterial persistence and reinfection are distinct. If bacterial persistence is the cause of recurrent UTI, the removal of the infected source is often curative, whereas preventative therapy is effective in treating reinfection.

B. Radiographic Imaging

When bacterial persistence is the suspected cause, radiologic imaging is indicated. Ultrasonography can be obtained to provide a screening evaluation of the genitourinary tract. More detailed assessment with intravenous pyelogram, cystoscopy, and CT scans may occasionally be necessary. In patients who have frequent, recurrent UTI, bacterial localization studies and more extensive radiologic evaluation (such as retrograde pyelograms) are warranted. When bacterial reinfection is the suspected cause of recurrent cystitis, the patient should be carefully evaluated for evidence of vesicovaginal or vesicoenteric fistula. Otherwise, radiologic examination is often not necessary in these patients.

C. Management

Management of recurrent cystitis, again, depends on its cause. Surgical removal of the infected source (such as urinary calculi) is needed to treat bacterial persistence. Similarly, fistulas need to be repaired surgically to prevent bacterial reinfection. In most cases of bacterial reinfection, medical management with prophylactic antibiotics is indicated. Low-dose continuous prophylactic antibiotic has been shown to reduce the recurrences of UTI by 95% compared with placebo or historical controls (Mangiarotti et al, 2000; Nicolle and Ronald, 1987). Alternatively, intermittent self-start antibiotic therapy can be used in treating recurrent cystitis in some women. Motivated patients self-identify episodes of infection on the basis of their symptoms and treat themselves with a single dose of antibiotics such as TMP–SMX. This

regimen has been shown to be effective and economical in selected patients (Pfau and Sacks, 1993; Raz et al, 1991). When the recurrent cystitis/UTI is related to sexual activity, frequent emptying of the bladder and a single dose of antibiotic taken after sexual intercourse can significantly reduce the incidence of recurrent infection (Pfau and Sacks, 1994). Alternatives to antibiotic therapy in the treatment of recurrent cystitis/UTI include intravaginal estriol (Raz and Stamm, 1993), lactobacillus vaginal suppositories (Reid and Burton, 2002), and cranberry juice taken orally (Lowe and Fagelman, 2001).

▶ Malakoplakia

Malakoplakia is an uncommon inflammatory disease of the bladder that can also affect other parts of the urinary tract, including the ureters and kidneys (Stanton and Maxted, 1981). In the bladder, it manifests as plaques or nodules made of large histiocytes (von Hansemann cells) with laminar inclusion bodies (Michaelis–Gutmann bodies) (McClure et al, 1981).

A. Presentation and Findings

Malakoplakia more commonly affects women than men (Stanton and Maxted, 1981) and is associated with a history of UTI. Patients with malakoplakia often have chronic illness or are immunosuppressed. In patients with malakoplakia of the bladder, irritative voiding symptoms (urgency and frequency) and hematuria are common (Curran, 1987). When the disease affects the ureter or kidney, the patient may present with fever, flank pain, or flank mass. When it affects both kidneys, signs or symptoms of azotemia or renal failure may be present (Dobyan et al, 1993). Treatment with fluoroquinolone has significantly decreased the mortality rate associated with renal malakoplakia (Tam et al, 2003).

B. Radiologic Imaging

Radiologic imaging with ultrasonography or CT may demonstrate a mass in the bladder and evidence of obstruction if the disease extends to the ureter (Vas et al, 1985). When the disease involves the kidney, focal or diffuse, hypodense, parenchymal masses may be seen on CT imaging (Frederic et al, 1981). It is often difficult to distinguish malakoplakia from malignancy (transitional cell or renal cell carcinoma) with radiologic imaging. The diagnosis is often established after biopsy.

C. Management

Management of malakoplakia primarily consists of antibiotic therapy, in particular those that produce high intracellular levels. Consequently, TMP–SMX and fluoroquinolones are recommended in the treatment of malakoplakia. Bethanecol and ascorbic acid, which enhance phagolysosomal activity, may have some benefits (Stanton and Maxted, 1981; Trujillo-Santos et al, 1999). In patients with malakoplakia limited to the lower urinary tract, antibiotic therapy alone is usually sufficient. However, when malakoplakia involves the ureter or kidney, surgical excision may be needed in addition to the antibiotic therapy (Dasgupta et al, 1999; Long and Althausen, 1989). The prognosis is poor and the mortality rate is high in patients who have bilateral renal involvement, regardless of treatment.

PROSTATE INFECTION

▶ Acute Bacterial Prostatitis

Acute bacterial prostatitis refers to inflammation of the prostate associated with a UTI. It is thought that infection results from ascending urethral infection or reflux of infected urine from the bladder into the prostatic ducts. In response to bacterial invasion, leukocytes (polymorphonuclear leukocytes, lymphocytes, plasma cells, and macrophages) are seen within and surrounding the acini of the prostate. Edema and hyperemia of the prostatic stroma frequently develop. With prolonged infection, variable degree of necrosis and abscess formation can occur.

A. Presentation and Findings

Acute bacterial prostatitis is uncommon in prepubertal boys but frequently affects adult men. It is the most common urologic diagnosis in men younger than 50 years (Collins et al, 1998). Patients with acute bacterial prostatitis usually present with an abrupt onset of constitutional (fever, chills, malaise, arthralgia, myalgia, lower back/rectal/perineal pain) and urinary symptoms (frequency, urgency, dysuria). They may also present with urinary retention due to swelling of the prostate. Digital rectal examination reveals tender, enlarged glands that are irregular and warm. Urinalysis usually demonstrates WBCs and occasionally hematuria. Serum blood analysis typically demonstrates leukocytosis. Prostate-specific antigen levels are often elevated. The diagnosis of prostatitis is made with microscopic examination and culture of the prostatic expressate and culture of urine obtained before and after prostate massage. In patients with acute prostatitis, fluid from the prostate massage often contains leukocytes with fat-laden macrophages. However, at the onset of acute prostatitis, prostatic massage is usually not suggested because the prostate is quite tender and the massage may lead to bacteremia. Similarly, urethral catheterization should be avoided. Culture of urine and prostate expressate usually identifies a single organism, but occasionally, polymicrobial infection may occur. E. coli is the most common causative organism in patients with acute prostatitis. Other gram-negative bacteria (*Proteus, Klebsiella, Enterobacter, Pseudomonas,* and *Serratia* spp.) and enterococci are less frequent pathogens. Anaerobic and other gram-positive bacteria are rarely a cause of acute prostatitis (Roberts et al, 1997b).

B. Radiologic Imaging

Radiologic imaging is rarely indicated in patients with acute prostatitis. Bladder ultrasonography may be useful in determining the amount of residual urine. Transrectal ultrasonography is indicated only in patients who do not respond to conventional therapy.

C. Management

Treatment with antibiotics is essential in the management of acute prostatitis. Empiric therapy directed against gram-negative bacteria and enterococci should be instituted immediately while awaiting the culture results. Trimethoprim and fluoroquinolones have high drug penetration into prostatic tissue and are recommended for 4–6 weeks (Wagenlehner et al, 2005). The long duration of antibiotic treatment is to allow complete sterilization of the prostatic tissue to prevent complications such as chronic prostatitis and abscess formation (Childs, 1992; Nickel, 2000). Patients who have sepsis, are immunocompromised or in acute urinary retention, or have significant medical comorbidities would benefit from hospitalization and treatment with parenteral antibiotics. Ampicillin and an aminoglycoside provide effective therapy against both gram-negative bacteria and enterococci. Patients with urinary retention secondary to acute prostatitis should be managed with a suprapubic catheter because transurethral catheterization or instrumentation is contraindicated.

▶ Chronic Bacterial Prostatitis

In contrast to the acute form, chronic bacterial prostatitis has a more insidious onset, characterized by relapsing, recurrent UTI caused by the persistence of pathogen in the prostatic fluid despite antibiotic therapy.

A. Presentation and Findings

Most patients with chronic bacterial prostatitis typically present with dysuria, urgency, frequency, nocturia, and low back/perineal pain. These patients usually are afebrile and not uncommonly have a history of recurrent or relapsing UTI, urethritis, or epididymitis caused by the same organism (Nickel and Moon, 2005). Others are asymptomatic, but the diagnosis is made after investigation for bacteriuria. In patients with chronic bacterial prostatitis, digital rectal examination of the prostate is often normal; occasionally, tenderness, firmness, or prostatic calculi may be found on examination. Urinalysis demonstrates a variable degree of WBCs and bacteria in the urine, depending on the extent of the disease. Serum blood analysis normally does not show any evidence of leukocytosis. Prostate-specific antigen levels may be elevated. Diagnosis is made after identification of bacteria from prostate expressate or urine specimen after a prostatic massage, using the four-cup test (Table 14–8). The causative organisms are similar to those of acute bacterial prostatitis. It is currently believed that other gram-positive

Table 14–8. Technique of localization cultures (four-cup test) for the diagnosis of prostatitis.

1. Preparation:
   - Require that the patient has a full bladder
   - Retract foreskin of uncircumcised men
   - Clean glans with soap/water or povidone-iodine

2. Collection:
   - Collect first 10 mL of voided urine (VB1)
   - Discard the next 100 mL
   - Collect the next 10 mL of voided urine (VB2)
   - Massage prostate and collect prostate expressate (EPS)
   - Collect first 10 mL of voided urine after massage (VB3)
   - Immediate culture and microscopic examination of all specimen

3. Interpretation:
   - All specimens <103 CFU/ mL → not bacterial prostatitis
   - VB3 or EPS >10× CFU of VB1 → chronic bacterial prostatitis
   - VB1 > other specimens → urethritis or specimen contamination
   - All specimens >10^3 CFU/mL → treat for UTI and repeat test

4. Caution:
   - Sensitivity of the test may not be high (Lipsky, 1999)
   - Time consuming and expensive

5. Alternative:
   - Voided specimen before and after prostate massage (Nickel, 1997)

CFU, colony-forming unit; UTI, urinary tract infection.

bacteria, *Mycoplasma, Ureaplasma,* and *Chlamydia* spp. are not causative pathogens in chronic bacterial prostatitis.

B. Radiologic Imaging

Radiologic imaging is rarely indicated in patients with chronic prostatitis. Transrectal ultrasonography is only indicated if a prostatic abscess is suspected.

C. Management

Antibiotic therapy is similar to that for acute bacterial prostatitis (Bjerklund Johansen et al, 1998). Interestingly, the presence of leukocytes or bacteria in the urine and prostatic massage does not predict antibiotic response in patients with chronic prostatitis (Nickel et al, 2001). In patients with chronic bacterial prostatitis, the duration of antibiotic therapy may be 3–4 months. Using fluoroquinolones, some patients may respond after 4–6 weeks of treatment. The addition of an alpha-blocker and anti-inflammatory agents to antibiotic therapy has been shown to reduce symptom recurrences (Barbalias et al, 1998; Murphy et al, 2009). Despite maximal therapy, cure is not often achieved due to poor penetration of antibiotic into prostatic tissue and relative isolation of the bacterial foci within the prostate. Third-line agents include 5α-reductase inhibitors, glycosaminoglycans, quercetin, cernilton (CN-009), and saw palmetto. When recurrent episodes of infection occur despite

antibiotic therapy, suppressive antibiotic (TMP–SMX 1 single-strength tablet daily, nitrofurantoin 100 mg daily, or ciprofloxacin 250 mg daily) may be used (Meares, 1987). Transurethral resection of the prostate has been used to treat patients with refractory disease; however, the success rate has been variable and this approach is not generally recommended (Barnes et al, 1982).

▶ Granulomatous Prostatitis

Granulomatous prostatitis is an uncommon form of prostatitis. It can result from bacterial, viral, or fungal infection, the use of bacillus Calmette-Guérin therapy (Rischmann et al, 2000), malakoplakia, or systemic granulomatous diseases affecting the prostate. Two-thirds of the cases have no specific cause. There are two distinct forms of nonspecific granulomatous prostatitis: noneosinophilic and eosinophilic. The former represents an abnormal tissue response to extravasated prostatic fluid (O'Dea et al, 1977). The latter is a more severe, allergic response of the prostate to some unknown antigen.

A. Presentation and Findings

Patients with granulomatous prostatitis often present acutely, with fever, chills, and obstructive/irritative voiding symptoms. Some may present with urinary retention. Patients with eosinophilic granulomatous prostatitis are severely ill and have high fevers. Digital rectal examination in patients with granulomatous prostatitis demonstrates a hard, indurated, and fixed prostate, which is difficult to distinguish from prostate carcinoma. Urinalysis and culture do not show any evidence of bacterial infection. Serum blood analysis typically demonstrates leukocytosis; marked eosinophilia is often seen in patients with eosinophilic granulomatous prostatitis. The diagnosis is made after biopsy of the prostate.

B. Management

Some patients respond to antibiotic therapy, corticosteroids, and temporary bladder drainage. Those with eosinophilic granulomatous prostatitis dramatically response to corticosteroids (Ohkawa et al, 2001). Transurethral resection of the prostate may be required in patients who do not respond to treatment and have significant outlet obstruction.

▶ Prostate Abscess

Most cases of prostatic abscess result from complications of acute bacterial prostatitis that were inadequately or inappropriately treated. Prostatic abscesses are often seen in patients with diabetes; those receiving chronic dialysis; or patients who are immunocompromised, undergoing urethral instrumentation, or who have chronic indwelling catheters.

A. Presentation and Findings

Patients with prostatic abscess present with similar symptoms to those with acute bacterial prostatitis. Typically, these

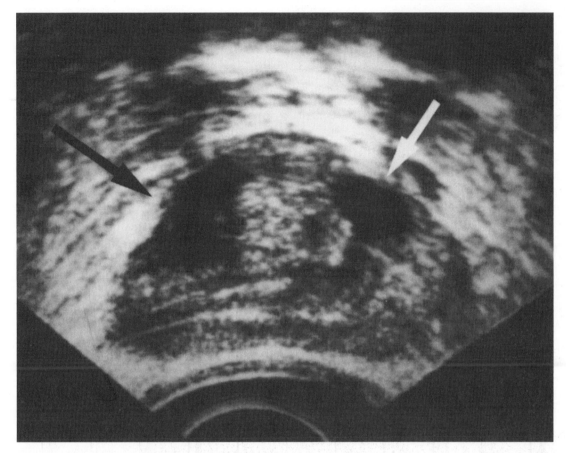

▲ **Figure 14–7.** Prostatic abscess. Transrectal ultrasonography demonstrates hypoechoic lesions (*black and white arrows*) in the prostate consistent with abscesses.

patients were treated for acute bacterial prostatitis previously and had a good initial response to treatment with antibiotics. However, their symptoms recurred during treatment, suggesting development of prostatic abscesses. On digital rectal examination, the prostate is usually tender and swollen. Fluctuance is only seen in 16% of patients with prostatic abscess (Weinberger et al, 1988).

B. Radiologic Imaging

Imaging with transrectal ultrasonography (Figure 14–7) or pelvic CT scan is crucial for diagnosis and treatment.

C. Management

Antibiotic therapy in conjunction with drainage of the abscess is required. Transrectal ultrasonography or CT scan can be used to direct transrectal drainage of the abscess (Barozzi et al, 1998). Transurethral resection and drainage may be required if transrectal drainage is inadequate. When

properly diagnosed and treated, most cases of prostatic abscess resolve without significant sequelae (Weinberger et al, 1988).

URETHRITIS

▶ Types of Urethritis

Infection/inflammation of the urethra can be categorized into those types caused by *Neisseria gonorrhoeae* and by other organisms (*Chlamydia trachomatis, Ureaplasma urealyticum, Trichomonas vaginalis,* and herpes simplex virus) (Dixon et al, 2002). Most cases are acquired during sexual intercourse.

A. Presentation and Findings

Patients with urethritis may present with urethral discharge and dysuria. The amount of discharge may vary significantly, from profuse to scant amounts. Obstructive voiding symptoms are primarily present in patients with recurrent infection, in whom urethral strictures subsequently develop. It is important to note that approximately 40% of patients with gonococcal urethritis are asymptomatic (John and Donald, 1978). The diagnosis is made from examination and culture of the urethra. It is important to obtain the specimen from within the urethra, rather than from just the discharge. Approximately 30% of men infected with *N. gonorrhoeae* will have concomitant infection with *C. trachomatis.*

B. Radiologic Imaging

Retrograde urethrogram is indicated only in patients with recurrent infection and obstructive voiding symptoms. Most patients with uncomplicated urethritis do not require any radiologic imaging.

C. Management

Pathogen-directed antibiotic therapy is required. In patients with gonococcal urethritis, ceftriaxone (250 mg intramuscularly) or fluoroquinolones (ciprofloxacin 250 mg) (David et al, 2000) or norfloxacin (800 mg) may be used. For patients with nongonococcal urethritis, treatment is with tetracycline or erythromycin (500 mg four times daily) or doxycycline (100 mg twice daily) for 7–14 days (O'Mahony, 1999). However, the most essential component of treatment is prevention. Sexual partners of the affected patients should be treated, and protective sexual practices (such as using condoms) are recommended.

EPIDIDYMITIS/ORCHITIS

▶ Causes of Epididymitis/Orchitis

Infection and inflammation of the epididymis most often result from an ascending infection from the lower urinary tract. The infection in the epididymis may spread to involve the testis. Most cases of epididymitis/orchitis in men younger than 35 years are due to sexually transmitted organisms (*N. gonorrhoeae* and *C. trachomatis*); those in children and older men are due to urinary pathogens such as *E. coli*. Other causes of epididymitis/orchitis in young children are due to a postinfectious inflammatory reaction to pathogens such as mycoplasma pneumoniae, enteroviruses, and adenoviruses, which often follows a more benign course. In homosexual men who practice anal intercourse, *E. coli* and other coliform bacteria are common causative organisms.

A. Presentation and Findings

Patients with epididymitis/orchitis present with severe scrotal pain that may radiate to the groin or flank. Scrotal enlargement due to the inflammation of the epididymis/testis or a reactive hydrocele may develop rapidly. Other symptoms of urethritis, cystitis, or prostatitis may be present before or concurrent with the onset of scrotal pain. On physical examination, an enlarged and red scrotum is present, and it is often difficult to distinguish the epididymis from the testis during the acute infection. A thickened spermatic cord can occasionally be palpated. Urinalysis typically demonstrates WBCs and bacteria in the urine or urethral discharge. Serum blood analysis often reveals leukocytosis.

B. Radiologic Imaging

Frequently, it is difficult to distinguish epididymitis from acute testicular torsion based on the history and physical examination alone (Petrack and Hafeez, 1992). Scrotal Doppler ultrasonography or radionuclide scanning can be used to confirm the diagnosis (Paltiel et al, 1998). The presence of blood flow in the testis on Doppler ultrasonography or uptake of the tracers into the center of the testis on radionuclide scanning rules out torsion. On scrotal ultrasonography, patients with epididymitis/orchitis commonly have an enlarged epididymis or testis with increased blood flow. A reactive hydrocele may also be seen. Prepubertal children who are diagnosed with epididymitis will require radiologic investigation for urinary tract anomalies such as reflux or ureteral ectopia (Likitnukul et al, 1987). Postpubertal children who are diagnosed with epididymitis should be educated about sexually transmitted diseases and safe sexual practices.

C. Management

Oral antibiotic treatment is directed against specific causative organisms, as mentioned in the previous sections on urethritis and UTI. In addition, bed rest, scrotal elevation, and the use of nonsteroidal anti-inflammatory agents are helpful in reducing the duration of the symptoms. In patients with epididymitis/orchitis caused by sexually transmitted organisms, treatment of their sexual partners is recommended to prevent reinfection. For patients with sepsis or severe infection, hospitalization and parenteral antibiotic therapy may be needed. Open drainage is indicated in cases in which an abscess develops. Occasionally, patients with chronic, relapsing epididymitis and scrotal pain may require epididymectomy/orchiectomy for relief of their symptoms.

SPECIAL CIRCUMSTANCES

▶ UTI Related to Pregnancy

With pregnancy, there are anatomic and physiologic changes to the urinary tract due to compression by the gravid uterus and alterations in the hormonal milieu. Renal length increases approximately by 1 cm during normal pregnancy as a result of increased vascular and interstitial volume (Waltzer, 1981). The glomerular filtration rate increases by 30–50%, most likely secondary to the increase in cardiac output (Waltzer, 1981). Typically, there is significant ureteral dilation with resultant urinary stasis during the second and third trimesters of gestation. This hydroureter is attributed to the smooth muscle–relaxing effects of progesterone and the mechanical compression of the ureters by the uterus at the level of the pelvic brim (Waltzer, 1981). The bladder is also affected, both physically and physiologically. The enlarged uterus displaces the bladder superiorly and anteriorly. The bladder becomes hyperemic, and its capacity is increased, most likely due to the effects of progesterone (Waltzer, 1981).

Because of these changes in the urinary tract during normal pregnancy, bacteriuria is a clinically relevant finding in pregnant women. It is estimated that the prevalence of bacteriuria is 4–6% (Sweet, 1977), which is not significantly different from that in nonpregnant women of comparable age. Interestingly, approximately 30% of those who have bacteriuria on screening evaluation later have pyelonephritis, compared with only 1–2% in those who do not have bacteriuria (Sweet, 1977). Treatment of bacteriuria decreases the incidence of pyelonephritis during pregnancy to approximately 3% (Christensen, 2000; Sweet, 1977). A history of previous UTIs and low socioeconomic status are risk factors for bacteriuria in pregnancy (Schnarr and Smaill, 2008).

Overall, the incidence of acute bacterial pyelonephritis is 1–4% in pregnant women (Gilstrap et al, 1981; Wing, 1998). About 60–70% of the episodes of pyelonephritis occur during the second and third trimesters of pregnancy, when urinary stasis is the greatest. In 10–20%, recurrent episodes of pyelonephritis develop before delivery (Gilstrap et al, 1981). Significant maternal risk factors include diabetes and history of UTI. When left untreated, pyelonephritis during pregnancy is associated with a high rate of infant prematurity and its associated perinatal mortality (Locksmith and Duff, 2001; McGregor and French, 1998; Schieve et al, 1994). It remains unclear whether treated pyelonephritis during pregnancy has any effects on the developing fetus (Gilstrap and Ramin, 2001).

Consequently, it is recommended that women be screened for bacteriuria during pregnancy to prevent the development of pyelonephritis. A voided urine specimen should be obtained at the first prenatal visit and at 16 weeks of gestation (Stenqvist et al, 1989). For asymptomatic individuals, significant bacteriuria is defined as two voided urine cultures with >10^5 CFU/mL of a single organism. For symptomatic pregnant women, >10^3 CFU/mL is considered to be significant (Rubin et al, 1992). Pregnant women who are found to have bacteriuria should be treated with penicillins, oral cephalosporins (Christensen, 2000; Wing et al, 1999), or fosfomycin trometamol (Minassian et al, 1998). Table 14–9 lists the antibiotics and their effects on pregnancy. However, amoxicillin is not recommended because of the rate of bacterial resistance (Hart et al, 2001). A 3-day course is suggested, although single-dose therapy may be effective in some patients (Tincello and Richmond, 1998). Repeat urine culture to document eradication of bacteriuria is necessary in all patients. Patients with acute bacterial pyelonephritis should be treated with parenteral cephalosporins, penicillins with beta-lactamase inhibitors, or monobactams (Rubin et al, 1992).

Table 14–9. Antibiotics and their effects on pregnancy.

Drugs	Side effects on the developing fetus
Sulfonamides	Kernicterus
Trimethoprim	Interferes with neural tube development
Tetracyclines	Dysplasia and discoloration of teeth and bones
Nitrofurantoin	Hemolysis and G6PD deficiency
Aminoglycosides	Nerve damage
Fluoroquinolones	Interferes with cartilage formation
Penicillins	Safe
Cephalosporins	Safe
Beta-lactamase inhibitors	Safe
Monobactams	Safe
Fosfomycin trometamol	Safe

Periodic surveillance urine culture is recommended because many of these women will have recurrent episodes of pyelonephritis.

▶ UTI in Patients with Human Immunodeficiency Virus or Acquired Immunodeficiency Syndrome

Human immunodeficiency virus (HIV) alters the normal host defense against bacterial infection. When the CD4 lymphocyte count falls to <200 per mm^3, the risk of bacterial and opportunistic UTI increases dramatically (Evans et al, 1995; Hoepelman et al, 1992). In addition, antiretroviral medications used to treat HIV (eg, zidovudine) can further suppress normal immune response and increase the risk of UTI in these patients.

A. UTI/Cystitis

Hoepelman et al (1992) obtained urine cultures from HIV-positive men prospectively and when they had symptoms suggestive of a UTI. They observed that positive urine cultures were identified in 30% of HIV-infected men with CD4 < 200 per mm^3 and in 11% with CD4 = 200–500 per mm^3, while none with CD4 > 500 per mm^3 had evidence of a urine infection. Gugino et al (1998) similarly observed that the incidence of bacteriuria in asymptomatic HIV-infected women was the same as that in uninfected women. Causative organisms include common uropathogens such as *E. coli* and *Klebsiella* and *Enterococcus* spp. Urinary infection with *S. aureus* and *Pseudomonas aeruginosa* is more common in HIV-infected patients (Schonwald et al, 1999). Because of the common prophylactic use of TMP–SMX to prevent *Pneumocystis carinii* pneumonia in AIDS patients, the incidence of UTI in this group is decreased. However, when a UTI develops in these patients, the infecting organism is typically resistant to TMP–SMX (van Dooyeweert et al, 1996).

B. Prostatitis

In HIV patients, the incidence of bacterial prostatitis is approximately 3% and it is 14% in patients with AIDS, compared with 1–2% in noninfected men of similar age (Leport et al, 1989). Causative organisms include common prostatitis pathogens such as *E. coli* and *Proteus* spp. and other less common organisms such as *Salmonella typhi, S. aureus, P. aeruginosa, and N. gonorrhoeae* (Staiman and Lowe, 1995). Prolonged treatment (4–6 weeks) with fluoroquinolones may be necessary because of a high risk of reinfection and lower immunity status in these patients. Prostatic abscess is more common in patients with AIDS compared with that in the general population (Staiman and Lowe, 1995; Trauzzi et al, 1994). Causative organisms include *E. coli* and other gram-negative bacteria or opportunistic fungus or mycobacterial infection (Lee et al, 2001). Effective drainage and prolonged antimicrobial or antifungal therapy are needed.

C. Epididymitis and Urethritis

In HIV-infected men, epididymitis may be caused by *N. gonorrhoeae* and *C. trachomatis*. However, infection by coliform bacteria such as *E. coli* is more common, especially in patients having unprotected anal intercourse (Berger et al, 1987). In HIV-infected patients with suppurative or antibiotic-resistant epididymitis, infection with fungi or mycobacteria should be considered (Desmond et al, 1993). In HIV-infected men who present with urethritis, treatment for both *Chlamydia* and *N. gonorrhoeae* is indicated even when gonococcus is isolated only from culture. Due to increased viral shedding with genital infections, it is recommended that HIV-infected patients abstain from sexual intercourse until 7 days after treatment is completed.

D. Infection by Uncommon Organisms

Urinary infection with *Mycobacterium* species can develop in HIV-infected patients. The kidneys are first infected and the infection spreads to the lower urinary tract. In patients with AIDS, it is estimated that 6–23% have renal tuberculosis (Marques et al, 1996). *M. tuberculosis* is the most common pathogen, with *Mycobacterium avium and Mycobacterium intracellulare* being less common (Sepkowitz et al, 1995). In HIV-infected patients who present with irritative/obstructive voiding symptoms but have no evidence of bacterial infection on culture, infection of the lower urinary tract by *Mycobacterium* species should be considered. Treatment with at least two antituberculosis agents is needed for 6–9 months.

▶ UTIs in Patients with Diabetes Mellitus

UTIs are more common and tend to have more complicated course in patients with diabetes mellitus (reviewed by Chen et al, 2009). There is a two- to fivefold increase in the incidence of acute pyelonephritis in diabetic patients compared with nondiabetic patients. Complications such as emphysematous pyelonephritis and renal and perirenal abscesses are more frequently seen in the diabetic patients (Williams and Schaeffer, 2004). Interestingly, the mortality and risk of hospitalization for UTI were not increased in patients with diabetes; however, the length of hospitalization may be prolonged. Asymptomatic bacteriuria occurs in diabetic women more commonly than in nondiabetics. It is associated with an increased risk of UTI among patients with type-2 diabetes. However, treatment of asymptomatic bacteriuria with antimicrobial therapy has not been shown to reduce symptomatic UTIs, pyelonephritis, or hospitalization for UTI (Ooi et al, 2004).

The risk for UTI correlated with the degree of glycemia as measured by HBA_{1c}. Autonomic neuropathy resulting in dysfunctional voiding and urinary retention can prevent bacterial clearance through micturition and thereby promoting bacterial growth. Defects in the local urinary cytokine secretions and an increased adherence of the microorganisms to the uroepithelial cells are also potential mechanisms that may contribute to the increased prevalence of both asymptomatic and symptomatic bacteriuria in these patients (Hoepelman et al, 2003; Nicolle, 2005). No relationship between specific uropathogen prevalence and diabetes status have been found; however, diabetic patients with asymptomatic bacteriuria are more likely to be infected with by *Klebsiella* and *Enterococcus* than by *E. coli*.

Although resistant bacteria are more frequently found in diabetic patients with UTI, empiric treatment with antibiotic therapy for a diabetic patient with complicated UTIs is similar to that of the nondiabetic patient. One important exception is that staphylococcal infection is not uncommon in the diabetic patients and can lead to urinary tract sepsis. This should be considered especially when a diabetic patient presents with a renal carbuncle. Oral outpatient therapy is not recommended for the diabetic patient with a complicated UTI. Treatment with TMP–SMX should be avoided if possible, because it can potentiate the hypoglycemic effects of the oral hypoglycemic drugs. Fluoroquinolones are safe and effective (ie, low resistance) in the treatment of diabetic patients with complicated UTIs (Williams and Schaeffer, 2004).

BIBLIOGRAPHY

Abad CL, Safdar N: The role of lactobacillus probiotics in the treatment or prevention of urogenital infections—a systematic review. J Chemother 2009;21(3):243–252.

Abrahamsson K et al: Antibiotic treatment for five days is effective in children with acute cystitis. Acta Paediatr 2002;91:55.

Al-Orifi F et al: Urine culture from bag specimens in young children: Are the risks too high? J Pediatr 2000;137:221.

American Academy of Pediatrics. Committee on Quality Improvement. Subcommittee on Urinary Tract Infection: Practice parameter: The diagnosis, treatment, and evaluation of the initial urinary tract infection in febrile infants and young children. Pediatrics 1999;103:843.

Anderson GG et al: Host subversion by formation of intracellular bacterial communities in the urinary tract. Microbes Infect 2004; 6(12):1094–1101.

Barbalias GA et al: Alpha-blockers for the treatment of chronic prostatitis in combination with antibiotics. J Urol 1998;159:883.

Barnes RW et al: Transurethral resection of the prostate for chronic bacterial prostatitis. Prostate 1982;3:215.

Barozzi L et al: Prostatic abscess: Diagnosis and treatment. AJR Am J Roentgenol 1998;170:753.

Berger RE et al: Etiology and manifestations of epididymitis in young men: Correlations with sexual orientation. J Infect Dis 1987; 155:1341.

Bjerklund Johansen TE et al: The role of antibiotics in the treatment of chronic prostatitis: A consensus statement. Eur Urol 1998; 34:457.

Bjorksten B, Kaijser B: Interaction of human serum and neutrophils with Escherichia coli strains: Differences between strains isolated from urine of patients with pyelonephritis or asymptomatic bacteriuria. Infect Immun 1978;22:308.

Blanco M et al: Virulence factors and O groups of Escherichia coli isolates from patients with acute pyelonephritis, cystitis and asymptomatic bacteriuria. Eur J Epidemiol 1996;12:191.

Bortolussi R et al: Capsular K1 polysaccharide of Escherichia coli: Relationship to virulence in newborn rats and resistance to phagocytosis. Infect Immun 1979;25:293.

Bower JM et al: Covert operations of uropathogenic Escherichia coli within the urinary tract. Traffic 2005;6(1):951–954.

Brown PD et al: Prevalence and predictors of trimethoprim-sulfamethoxazole resistance among uropathogenic Escherichia coli isolates in Michigan. Clin Infect Dis 2002;34:1061.

Brown P et al: Acute pyelonephritis among adults: Cost of illness and considerations for the economic evaluation of therapy. Pharmacoeconomics 2005;23(11):1123–1142.

Brown PS Jr et al: Xanthogranulomatous pyelonephritis: Report of nonsurgical management of a case and review of the literature. Clin Infect Dis 1996;22:308.

Carapetis JR et al: Randomized, controlled trial comparing once daily and three times daily gentamicin in children with urinary tract infections. Pediatr Infect Dis J 2001;20:240.

Chen MT et al: Percutaneous drainage in the treatment of emphysematous pyelonephritis: 10-year experience. J Urol 1997;157:1569.

Chen SL et al: Diabetes mellitus and urinary tract infection: Epidemiology, pathogenesis and proposed studies in animal models. J Urol 2009;182(6, Suppl):S51–S56.

Childs S: Current diagnosis and treatment of urinary tract infections. Urology 1992;40:295.

Christensen B: Which antibiotics are appropriate for treating bacteriuria in pregnancy? J Antimicrob Chemother 2000;46:29;discussion 63.

Chowdhury P et al: Minireview: Functions of the renal tract epithelium in coordinating the innate immune response to infection. Kidney Int 2004;66(4):1334–1344.

Collins MM et al: How common is prostatitis? A national survey of physician visits. J Urol 1998;159:1224.

Connell I et al: Type 1 fimbrial expression enhances Escherichia coli virulence for the urinary tract. Proc Natl Acad Sci USA 1996; 93:9827.

Corriere JN Jr, Sandler CM: The diagnosis and immediate therapy of acute renal and perirenal infections. Urol Clin North Am 1982; 9:219.

Costelloe C et al: Effect of antibiotic prescribing in primary care on antimicrobial resistance in individual patients: Systematic review and meta-analysis. BMJ 2010;18:34.

Curran FT: Malakoplakia of the bladder. Br J Urol 1987;59:559.

Dacher JN et al: Rational use of CT in acute pyelonephritis: Findings and relationships with reflux. Pediatr Radiol 1993;23:281.

Dalla Palma L et al: Medical treatment of renal and perirenal abscesses: CT evaluation. Clin Radiol 1999;54:792.

Dasgupta P et al: Malakoplakia: von Hansemann's disease. BJU Int 1999;84:464.

David N et al: Ciprofloxacin 250 mg for treating gonococcal urethritis and cervicitis. Sex Transm Infect 2000;76:495.

Desmond N et al: Tuberculous epididymitis: A case report in an HIV seropositive male. Int J STD AIDS 1993;4:178.

Dixon L et al: Chlamydia trachomatis infection and non-gonococcal urethritis in homosexual and heterosexual men in Edinburgh. Int J STD AIDS 2002;13:425.

Dobyan DC et al: Renal malakoplakia reappraised. Am J Kidney Dis 1993;22:243.

Duncan JL: Differential effect of Tamm-Horsfall protein on adherence of Escherichia coli to transitional epithelial cells. J Infect Dis 1988;158:1379.

Eastham J et al: Xanthogranulomatous pyelonephritis: Clinical findings and surgical considerations. Urology 1994;43:295.

Edelstein H, McCabe RE: Perinephric abscess: Modern diagnosis and treatment in 47 cases. Medicine (Baltimore) 1988;67:118.

Evans DJ Jr et al: Hemolysin and K antigens in relation to serotype and hemagglutination type of Escherichia coli isolated from extraintestinal infections. J Clin Microbiol 1981;13:171.

Evans JK et al: Incidence of symptomatic urinary tract infections in HIV seropositive patients and the use of cotrimoxazole as prophylaxis against Pneumocystis carinii pneumonia. Genitourin Med 1995;71:120.

Fair WR et al: Prostatic antibacterial factor: Identity and significance. Urology 1976;7:169.

Falagas ME et al: Antibiotics versus placebo in the treatment of women with uncomplicated cystitis: A meta-analysis of randomized controlled trials. J Infect 2009;58(2):91–102.

Foxman B et al: Urinary tract infection among women aged 40 to 65: Behavioral and sexual risk factors. J Clin Epidemiol 2001;54:710.

Frederic N et al: Renal malakoplakia: Ultrasonic and computed appearances. J Belge Radiol 1981;64:361.

Freedman AL: Urologic diseases in North America Project: Trends in resource utilization for urinary tract infections in children. J Urol 2005;173(3):949–954.

Frendeus B et al: Interleukin-8 receptor deficiency confers susceptibility to acute pyelonephritis. J Infect Dis 2001;183:S56.

Garcia-Rodriguez JA, Munoz Bellido JL: Oral cephalosporins in uncomplicated urinary tract infections. Clin Microbiol Infect 2000;6:73.

Ghiro L et al: Retrospective study of children with acute pyelonephritis: Evaluation of bacterial etiology, antimicrobial susceptibility, drug management and imaging studies. Nephron 2002;90:8.

Gilstrap LC III et al: Acute pyelonephritis in pregnancy: An anterospective study. Obstet Gynecol 1981;57:409.

Gilstrap LC III, Ramin SM: Urinary tract infections during pregnancy. Obstet Gynecol Clin North Am 2001;28:581.

Goldman SM et al: CT of xanthogranulomatous pyelonephritis: Radiologic–pathologic correlation. AJR Am J Roentgenol 1984; 142:963.

Goodman M et al: Xanthogranulomatous pyelonephritis (XGP): A local disease with systemic manifestations. Report of 23 patients and review of the literature. Medicine (Baltimore) 1979;58:171.

Griebling, TL: Urologic diseases in America project: Trends in resource use for urinary tract infections in men. J Urol 2005a;173 (4):1288–1294.

Griebling TL: Urologic diseases in America project: Trends in resource use for urinary tract infections in women. J Urol 2005b;173(4):1281–1287.

Gugino L et al: Asymptomatic bacteriuria in human immunodeficiency (HIV)-infected women. Prim Care Update Ob Gyns 1998;5:146.

Gupta K et al: Increasing prevalence of antimicrobial resistance among uropathogens causing acute uncomplicated cystitis in women. JAMA 1999a;281:736.

Gupta K et al: The prevalence of antimicrobial resistance among uropathogens causing acute uncomplicated cystitis in young women. Int J Antimicrob Agents 1999b;11:305.

Hart A et al: Ampicillin-resistant Escherichia coli in gestational pyelonephritis: Increased occurrence and association with the colonization factor Dr adhesin. J Infect Dis 2001;183:1526.

Hoberman A et al: Oral versus initial intravenous therapy for urinary tract infections in young febrile children. Pediatrics 1999;104:79.

Hoepelman AI et al: Bacteriuria in men infected with HIV-1 is related to their immune status (CD4+ cell count). AIDS 1992;6:179.

Hoepelman AI et al: Pathogenesis and management of bacterial urinary tract infections in adult patients with diabetes mellitus. Int J Antimicrob Agents 2003;22(Suppl 2):35–43.

Hovanec DL, Gorzynski EA: Coagglutination as an expedient for grouping Escherichia coli associated with urinary tract infections. J Clin Microbiol 1980;11:41.

Hovelius B, Mardh PA: Staphylococcus saprophyticus as a common cause of urinary tract infections. Rev Infect Dis 1984;6:328.

Huang ES, Stafford RS: National patterns in the treatment of urinary tract infections in women by ambulatory care physicians. Arch Intern Med 2002;162:41.

Hughes C et al: Hemolysin production as a virulence marker in symptomatic and asymptomatic urinary tract infections caused by Escherichia coli. Infect Immun 1983;39:546.

Iskandar SS et al: Lipid-laden foamy macrophages in renal cell carcinoma: Potential frozen section diagnostic pitfall. Pathol Res Pract 1993;189:549.

Jackson SL et al: Predictors of urinary tract infection after menopause: A prospective study. Am J Med 2004;117(12):903–911.

Jahnukainen T et al: Mechanisms of renal damage owing to infection. Pediatr Nephrol 2005;20(8):1043–1053.

Jeena PM et al: Bacteriuria in children attending a primary health care clinic: A prospective study of catheter stream urine samples. Ann Trop Paediatr 1996;16:293.

Jenkins RD et al: Review of urine microscopy for bacteriuria. JAMA 1986;255:3397.

John J, Donald WH: Asymptomatic urethral gonorrhoea in men. Br J Vener Dis 1978;54:322.

Johnson L et al: Emergence of fluoroquinolone resistance in outpatient urinary Escherichia coli isolates. Am J Med 2008;121(10):876–884.

Kahlmeter G: An international survey of the antimicrobial susceptibility of pathogens from uncomplicated urinary tract infections: The ECO.SENS Project. J Antimicrob Chemother 2003;51(1): 69–76.

Kallenius G et al: Occurrence of P-fimbriated Escherichia coli in urinary tract infections. Lancet 1981;2:1369.

Karaca Y et al: Co-trimoxazole and quinolone resistance in Escherichia coli isolated from urinary tract infections over the last 100 years. Int J Antimicrob Agents 2005;26(1):75–77.

Koronakis V, Hughes C: Synthesis, maturation and export of the E. coli hemolysin. Med Microbiol Immunol (Berl) 1996;185:65.

Lau SM et al: Resistance rates to commonly used antimicrobials among pathogens of both bacteremic and non-bacteremic community-acquired urinary tract infection. J Microbiol Immunol Infect 2004;37(3):185–191.

Lawrenson RA, Logie JW: Antibiotic failure in the treatment of urinary tract infections in young women. J Antimicrob Chemother 2001;48:895.

Lee LK et al: The urologist and the patient infected with human immunodeficiency virus or with acquired immunodeficiency syndrome. BJU Int 2001;88:500.

Leport C et al: Bacterial prostatitis in patients infected with the human immunodeficiency virus. J Urol 1989;141:334.

Levtchenko EN et al: Role of Tc-99m DMSA scintigraphy in the diagnosis of culture negative pyelonephritis. Pediatr Nephrol 2001;16:503.

Likitnukul S et al: Epididymitis in children and adolescents: A 20-year retrospective study. Am J Dis Child 1987;141:41.

Lipsky BA: Prostatitis and urinary tract infection in men: What's new; what's true? Am J Med 1999;106:327.

Locksmith G, Duff P: Infection, antibiotics, and preterm delivery. Semin Perinatol 2001;25:295.

Lomberg H et al: Influence of blood group on the availability of receptors for attachment of uropathogenic Escherichia coli. Infect Immun 1986;51:919.

Long JP Jr, Althausen AF: Malakoplakia: A 25-year experience with a review of the literature. J Urol 1989;141:1328.

Lorentz WB: Localization of urinary tract infection. Urol Clin North Am 1979;6:519.

Lorentzen M, Nielsen HO: Xanthogranulomatous pyelonephritis. Scand J Urol Nephrol 1980;14:193.

Lowe FC, Fagelman E: Cranberry juice and urinary tract infections: What is the evidence? Urology 2001;57:407.

Malek RS, Elder JS: Xanthogranulomatous pyelonephritis: A critical analysis of 26 cases and of the literature. J Urol 1978;119:589.

Mangiarotti P et al: Antibiotic prophylaxis in children with relapsing urinary tract infections: Review. J Chemother 2000;12:115.

Marcus N et al: Non-Escherichia coli versus Escherichia coli community-acquired urinary tract infections in children hospitalized in a tertiary center: Relative frequency, risk factors, antimicrobial resistance and outcome. Pediatr Infect Dis J 2005; 24(7):581–585.

Marques LP et al: AIDS-associated renal tuberculosis. Nephron 1996;74:701.

Martinez JJ et al: Type 1 pilus-mediated bacterial invasion of bladder epithelial cells. Embo J 2000;19:2803.

Matsumoto T: Urinary tract infections in the elderly. Curr Urol Rep 2001;2:330.

McClure J et al: The ultrastructural features of malakoplakia. J Pathol 1981;134:13.

McGregor JA, French JI: Prevention of preterm birth. N Engl J Med 1998;339:1858; discussion 1860.

Meares EM Jr: Acute and chronic prostatitis: Diagnosis and treatment. Infect Dis Clin North Am 1987;1:855.

Meares EM, Stamey TA: Bacteriologic localization patterns in bacterial prostatitis and urethritis. Invest Urol 1968;5:492.

Merimsky E, Feldman C: Perinephric abscess: Report of 19 cases. Int Surg 1981;66:79.

Michaeli J et al: Emphysematous pyelonephritis. J Urol 1984;131:203.

Miller LG, Tang AW: Treatment of uncomplicated urinary tract infections in an era of increasing antimicrobial resistance. Mayo Clinic Proc 2004;79(8):1048–1053; quiz 1053–1054.

Minassian MA et al: A comparison between single-dose fosfomycin trometamol (Monuril) and a 5-day course of trimethoprim in the treatment of uncomplicated lower urinary tract infection in women. Int J Antimicrob Agents 1998;10:39.

Mori R et al: Diagnostic performance of urine dipstick testing in children with suspected UTI: A systematic review of relationship with age and comparison with microscopy. Acta Paediatr 2010; 99(4):581–584.

Murphy AB et al: Chronic prostatitis: Management strategies. Drugs 2009;69(1):71–84.

Naber KG: Short-term therapy of acute uncomplicated cystitis. Curr Opin Urol 1999;9:57.

Navas EL et al: Blood group antigen expression on vaginal cells and mucus in women with and without a history of urinary tract infections. J Urol 1994;152:345.

Nickel JC: The Pre and Post Massage Test (PPMT): A simple screen for prostatitis. Tech Urol 1997;3:38.

Nickel JC: Antibiotics for bacterial prostatitis. J Urol 2000;163:1407.

Nickel JC: The management of acute pyelonephritis in adults. Can J Urol 2001;8:29.

Nickel JC et al: Predictors of patient response to antibiotic therapy for the chronic prostatitis/chronic pelvic pain syndrome: A prospective multicenter clinical trial. J Urol 2001;165:1539.

Nickel JC, Moon T: Chronic bacterial prostatitis: An evolving clinical enigma. Urology 2005;66(1):2–8.

Nicolle LE: Urinary tract infection in geriatric and institutionalized patients. Curr Opin Urol 2002;12:51.

Nicolle LE, Ronald AR: Recurrent urinary tract infection in adult women: Diagnosis and treatment. Infect Dis Clin North Am 1987;1:793.

Nicolle LE et al: The association of urinary tract infection with sexual intercourse. J Infect Dis 1982;146:579.

Nicolle LE: Urinary tract infection in diabetes. Curr Opin Infect Dis 2005;18(1):49–53.

O'Dea MJ et al: Non-specific granulomatous prostatitis. J Urol 1977;118:58.

Nguyen HT et al: Trimethoprim in vitro antibacterial activity is not increased by adding sulfamethoxazole for pediatric Escherichia coli urinary tract infection. J Urol 2010;184(1):305–310.

Ofek I et al: Role of bacterial lectins in urinary tract infections: molecular mechanisms for diversification of bacterial surface lectins. Adv Exp Med Biol 2000;485:183.

Ohkawa M et al: Non-specific eosinophilic granulomatous prostatitis responded favorably to an antimicrobial agent and a hydrocortisone. Int J Urol 2001;8:578.

O'Mahony C: Treatment of non-specific urethritis should be two weeks, not 1. Sex Transm Infect 1999;75:449.

Ooi ST et al: Management of asymptomatic bacteriuria in patients with diabetes mellitus. Ann Pharmacother 2004;38(3):490–493.

Orskov I et al: O, K, H and fimbrial antigens in Escherichia coli serotypes associated with pyelonephritis and cystitis. Scand J Infect Dis Suppl 1982;33:18.

Osset J et al: Assessment of the capacity of Lactobacillus to inhibit the growth of uropathogens and block their adhesion to vaginal epithelial cells. J Infect Dis 2001;183:485.

Pak J et al: Tamm-Horsfall protein binds to type 1 fimbriated Escherichia coli and prevents E. coli from binding to uroplakin Ia and Ib receptors. J Biol Chem 2001;276:9924.

Paltiel HJ et al: Acute scrotal symptoms in boys with an indeterminate clinical presentation: Comparison of color Doppler sonography and scintigraphy. Radiology 1998;207:223.

Parsons MA: Xanthogranulomatous gastritis: An entity or a secondary phenomenon? J Clin Pathol 1993;46:580.

Patel HD et al: Can urine dipstick testing for urinary tract infection at point of care reduce laboratory workload? J Clin Pathol 2005;6(1):18–31.

Petrack EM, Hafeez W: Testicular torsion versus epididymitis: A diagnostic challenge. Pediatr Emerg Care 1992;8:347.

Pfau A, Sacks TG: Single dose quinolone treatment in acute uncomplicated urinary tract infection in women. J Urol 1993;149:532.

Pfau A, Sacks TG: Effective postcoital quinolone prophylaxis of recurrent urinary tract infections in women. J Urol 1994;152: 136.

Philbrick JT: Single dose for urinary tract infections. J Gen Intern Med 1986;1:207.

Raffi HS et al: Tamm-Horsfall protein acts as a general host-defense factor against bacterial cystitis. Am J Nephrol 2005;20(8):1043–1053.

Randolph MF, Greenfield M: The incidence of asymptomatic bacteriuria and pyuria in infancy: A study of 400 infants in private practice. J Pediatr 1964;65:57.

Raz R, Stamm WE: A controlled trial of intravaginal estriol in postmenopausal women with recurrent urinary tract infections. N Engl J Med 1993;329:753.

Raz R et al: Comparison of single-dose administration and three-day course of amoxicillin with those of clavulanic acid for treatment of uncomplicated urinary tract infection in women. Antimicrob Agents Chemother 1991;35:1688.

Reid G, Burton J: Use of Lactobacillus to prevent infection by pathogenic bacteria. Microbes Infect 2002;4:319.

Rischmann P et al: BCG intravesical instillations: Recommendations for side-effects management. Eur Urol 2000;37:33.

Roberts JA et al: Epitopes of the P-fimbrial adhesin of E. coli cause different urinary tract infections. J Urol 1997a;158:1610.

Roberts RO et al: A review of clinical and pathological prostatitis syndromes. Urology 1997b;49:809.

Ronald A: The etiology of urinary tract infection: Traditional and emerging pathogens. Am J Med 2002;113:14.

Rubin RH et al: An approach to evaluating antibacterial agents in the treatment of urinary tract infection. Clin Infect Dis 1992;14:S246; discussion S253.

Sanford JP: Urinary tract symptoms and infections. Annu Rev Med 1975;26:485.

Santucci RA, Krieger JN: Gentamicin for the practicing urologist: Review of efficacy, single daily dosing and "switch" therapy. J Urol 2000;163:1076.

Schaeffer AJ et al: Role of vaginal colonization in urinary tract infections (UTIs). Adv Exp Med Biol 1999;462:339.

Schaeffer AJ: What do we know about the urinary tract infection-prone individual? J Infect Dis 2001;183:S66.

Schaeffer AJ: The expanding role of fluoroquinolones. Am J Med 2002;113:45.

Schappert SM: Ambulatory care visits to physician offices, hospital outpatient departments, and emergency departments: United States, 1997. Vital Health Stat 13 1999;i–iv:1–39.

Schieve LA et al: Urinary tract infection during pregnancy: Its association with maternal morbidity and perinatal outcome. Am J Public Health 1994;84:405.

Schlager TA: Urinary tract infections in children younger than 5 years of age: Epidemiology, diagnosis, treatment, outcomes and prevention. Paediatr Drugs 2001;3:219.

Schnarr J, Smaill F: Asymptomatic bacteriuria and symptomatic urinary tract infections in pregnancy. Eur J Clin Invest 2008;38(Suppl 2):50–57.

Scholes D et al: Risk factors associated with acute pyelonephritis in healthy women. Ann Intern Med 2005;142(1):20–27.

Schonwald S et al: Urinary tract infections in HIV disease. Int J Antimicrob Agents 1999;11:309.

Sepkowitz KA et al: Tuberculosis in the AIDS era. Clin Microbiol Rev 1995;8:180.

Shokeir AA et al: Emphysematous pyelonephritis: A 15-year experience with 20 cases. Urology 1997;49:343.

Shortliffe LM, McCue JD: Urinary tract infection at the age extremes: Pediatrics and geriatrics. Am J Med 2002;113:55.

Siegel JF et al: Minimally invasive treatment of renal abscess. J Urol 1996;155:52.

Sobel JD: Pathogenesis of urinary tract infection: Role of host defenses. Infect Dis Clin North Am 1997;11:531.

Sotto A et al: Risk factors for antibiotic-resistant Escherichia coli isolated from hospitalized patients with urinary tract infections: A prospective study. J Clin Microbiol 2001;39:438.

Staiman VS, Lowe FC: Prostatic disease in HIV-infected patients. AIDS Read 1995;5:165.

Stamm WE et al: Diagnosis of coliform infection in acutely dysuric women. N Engl J Med 1982;307:463.

Stamm WE, Norrby SR: Urinary tract infections: Disease panorama and challenges. J Infect Dis 2001;183:S1.

Stanton MJ, Maxted W: Malakoplakia: A study of the literature and current concepts of pathogenesis, diagnosis and treatment. J Urol 1981;125:139.

Stenqvist K et al: Bacteriuria in pregnancy: Frequency and risk of acquisition. Am J Epidemiol 1989;129:372.

Stoller ML, Kogan BA: Sensitivity of 99m technetium-dimercaptosuccinic acid for the diagnosis of chronic pyelonephritis: Clinical and theoretical considerations. J Urol 1986;135:977.

Svanborg C et al: Bacterial adherence and mucosal cytokine responses: Receptors and transmembrane signaling. Ann N Y Acad Sci 1996;797:177.

Svanborg Eden C et al: Host-parasite interaction in the urinary tract. J Infect Dis 1988;157:421.

Svenson SB et al: P-fimbriae of pyelonephritogenic Escherichia coli: Identification and chemical characterization of receptors. Infection 1983;11:61.

Sweet RL: Bacteriuria and pyelonephritis during pregnancy. Semin Perinatol 1977;1:25.

Tam VK et al: Renal parenchymal malakoplakia: A rare cause of ARF with a review of recent literature. Am J Kidney Dis 2003;41(6):E13–E17.

Tang HJ et al: Clinical characteristics of emphysematous pyelonephritis. J Microbiol Immunol Infect 2001;34:125.

Thorley JD et al: Perinephric abscess. Medicine (Baltimore) 1974;53:441.

Tincello DG, Richmond DH: Evaluation of reagent strips in detecting asymptomatic bacteriuria in early pregnancy: Prospective case series. BMJ 1998;316:435.

Tiu CM et al: Sonographic features of xanthogranulomatous pyelonephritis. J Clin Ultrasound 2001;29:279.

Trauzzi SJ et al: Management of prostatic abscess in patients with human immunodeficiency syndrome. Urology 1994;43:629.

Trujillo-Santos AJ et al: Therapeutic options for malakoplakia secondary to Escherichia coli infection. Clin Infect Dis 1999;29:444.

Tseng CC et al: Host and bacterial virulence factors predisposing to emphysematous pyelonephritis. Am J Kidney Dis 2005;46(3):432–439.

van Dooyeweert DA et al: The influence of PCP prophylaxis on bacteriuria incidence and resistance development to trimethoprim/sulfamethoxazole in HIV-infected patients. Neth J Med 1996;49:225.

Vas W et al: Computed tomography and ultrasound appearance of bladder malakoplakia. J Comput Tomogr 1985;9:119.

Wagenlehner FM et al: The role of antibiotics in chronic bacterial prostatitis. Int J Antimicrob Agents 2005;26(1):1–7.

Wagenlehner FM, Naber KG: Hospital-acquired urinary tract infections. J Hosp Infect 2000;46:171.

Waltzer WC: The urinary tract in pregnancy. J Urol 1981;125:271.

Wan YL et al: Predictors of outcome in emphysematous pyelonephritis. J Urol 1998;159:369.

Weinberger M et al: Prostatic abscess in the antibiotic era. Rev Infect Dis 1988;10:239.

Wennerstrom M et al: Primary and acquired renal scarring in boys and girls with urinary tract infection. J Pediatr 2000;136:30.

Wettergren B et al: Epidemiology of bacteriuria during the first year of life. Acta Paediatr Scand 1985;74:925.

Whitfield C, Roberts IS: Structure, assembly and regulation of expression of capsules in Escherichia coli. Mol Microbiol 1999;31:1307.

Williams GJ et al: Absolute and relative accuracy of rapid urine tests for urinary tract infection in children: A meta-analysis. Lancet Infect Dis 2010;10(4):240–250.

Williams DH, Schaeffer AJ: Current concepts in urinary tract infections. Minerva Urol Nefrol 2004:56(1):15–31.

Wing DA: Pyelonephritis. Clin Obstet Gynecol 1998;41:515.

Wing DA et al: Outpatient treatment of acute pyelonephritis in pregnancy after 24 weeks. Obstet Gynecol 1999;94:683.

Wiswell TE, Roscelli JD: Corroborative evidence for the decreased incidence of urinary tract infections in circumcised male infants. Pediatrics 1986;78:96.

Wood EG, Dillon HC Jr: A prospective study of group B streptococcal bacteriuria in pregnancy. Am J Obstet Gynecol 1981;140:515.

Zorzos I et al: Xanthogranulomatous pyelonephritis—The "great imitator" justifies its name. Scand J Urol Nephrol 2002;36:74.

Specific Infections of the Genitourinary Tract

15

Emil A. Tanagho, MD, & Christopher J. Kane, MD

Specific infections are those caused by particular organisms, each of which cause a clinically unique disease with identifiable pathologic tissue reactions.

TUBERCULOSIS

Tubercle bacilli may invade one or more (or even all) of the organs of the genitourinary tract and cause a chronic granulomatous infection that shows the same characteristics as tuberculosis in other organs. Urinary tuberculosis is a disease of young adults (60% of patients are between the ages of 20 and 40) and is more common in males than in females.

▶ Etiology

The infecting organism is *Mycobacterium tuberculosis*, which reaches the genitourinary organs by the hematogenous route from the lungs. The primary site is often not symptomatic or apparent.

The kidney and possibly the prostate are the primary sites of tuberculous infection in the genitourinary tract. All other genitourinary organs become involved by either ascent (prostate to bladder) or descent (kidney to bladder, prostate to epididymis). The testis may become involved by direct extension from epididymal infection.

▶ Pathogenesis (Figure 15–1)

A. Kidney and Ureter

When a shower of tubercle bacilli hits the renal cortex, the organisms may be destroyed by normal tissue resistance. Evidence of this is commonly seen in autopsies of persons who have died of tuberculosis; only scars are found in the kidneys. However, if enough bacteria of sufficient virulence become lodged in the kidney and are not overcome, a clinical infection is established.

Tuberculosis of the kidney progresses slowly; it may take 15–20 years to destroy a kidney in a patient who has good resistance to the infection. As a rule, therefore, there is no

renal pain and little or no clinical disturbance of any type until the lesion has involved the calyces or the pelvis, at which time, pus and organisms may be discharged into the urine. It is only at this stage that symptoms (of cystitis) are manifested. The infection then proceeds to the pelvic mucosa and the ureter, particularly its upper and vesical ends. This may lead to stricture and obstruction (hydronephrosis).

As the disease progresses, a caseous breakdown of tissue occurs until the entire kidney is replaced by cheesy material. Calcium may be laid down in the reparative process. The ureter undergoes fibrosis and tends to be shortened and therefore straightened. This change leads to a "golf-hole" (gaping) ureteral orifice, typical of an incompetent valve.

B. Bladder

Vesical irritability develops as an early clinical manifestation of the disease as the bladder is bathed by infected material. Tubercles form later, usually in the region of the involved ureteral orifice, and finally coalesce and ulcerate. These ulcers may bleed. With severe involvement, the bladder becomes fibrosed and contracted; this leads to marked frequency. Ureteral reflux or stenosis and, therefore, hydronephrosis may develop. If contralateral renal involvement occurs later, it is probably a separate hematogenous infection.

C. Prostate and Seminal Vesicles

The passage of infected urine through the prostatic urethra ultimately leads to invasion of the prostate and one or both seminal vesicles. There is no local pain.

On occasion, the primary hematogenous lesion in the genitourinary tract is in the prostate. Prostatic infection can ascend to the bladder and descend to the epididymis.

D. Epididymis and Testis

Tuberculosis of the prostate can extend along the vas or through the perivasal lymphatics and affect the epididymis.

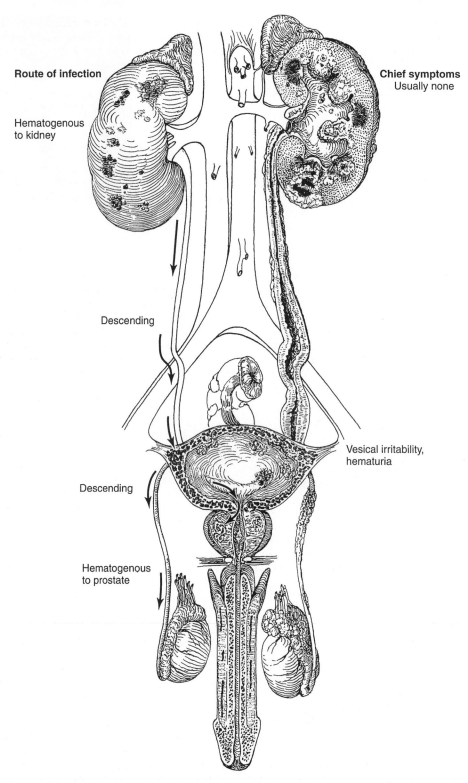

▲ **Figure 15–1.** Pathogenesis of tuberculosis of the urinary tract.

Because this is a slow process, there is usually no pain. If the epididymal infection is extensive and an abscess forms, it may rupture through the scrotal skin, thus establishing a permanent sinus, or it may extend into the testicle.

▶ Pathology

A. Kidney and Ureter

The gross appearance of the kidney with moderately advanced tuberculosis is often normal on its outer surface, although the kidney is usually surrounded by marked perinephritis. Usually, however, there is a soft, yellowish localized bulge. On section, the involved area is seen to be filled with cheesy material (caseation). Widespread destruction of parenchyma is evident. In otherwise normal tissue, small abscesses may be seen. The walls of the pelvis, calyces, and ureter may be thickened, and ulceration appears frequently in the region of the calyces at the point at which the abscess drains. Ureteral stenosis may be complete, causing "autonephrectomy." Such a kidney is fibrosed and functionless. Under these circumstances, the bladder urine may be normal and symptoms absent.

Tubercle foci appear close to the glomeruli. These are an aggregation of histiocytic cells possessing a vesicular nucleus and a clear cell body that can fuse with neighboring cells to form a small mass called an epithelioid reticulum. At the periphery of this reticulum are large cells with multiple nuclei (giant cells). This pathologic reaction, which can be seen macroscopically, is the basic lesion in tuberculosis. It can heal by fibrosis or coalesce and reach the surface and ulcerate, forming an ulcerocavernous lesion. Tubercles might undergo a central degeneration and caseate, creating a tuberculous abscess cavity that can reach the collecting system and break through. In the process, progressive parenchymal destruction occurs. Depending on the virulence of the organism and the resistance of the patient, tuberculosis is a combination of caseation and cavitation and healing by fibrosis and scarring.

Microscopically, the caseous material is seen as an amorphous mass. The surrounding parenchyma shows fibrosis with tissue destruction, small round cell and plasma cell infiltration, and epithelial and giant cells typical of tuberculosis. Acid–fast stains will usually demonstrate the organisms in the tissue. Similar changes can be demonstrated in the wall of the pelvis and ureter.

In both the kidney and ureter, calcification is common. It may be macroscopic or microscopic. Such a finding is strongly suggestive of tuberculosis but, of course, is also observed in bilharzial infection. Secondary renal stones occur in 10% of patients.

In the most advanced stage of renal tuberculosis, the parenchyma may be completely replaced by caseous substance or fibrous tissue. Perinephric abscess may develop, but this is rare.

B. Bladder

In the early stages, the mucosa may be inflamed, but this is not a specific change. The bladder is quite resistant to actual invasion. Later, tubercles form and can be easily seen endoscopically as white or yellow raised nodules surrounded by a halo of hyperemia. With mural fibrosis and severe vesical contracture, reflux may occur.

Microscopically, the nodules are typical tubercles. These break down to form deep, ragged ulcers. At this stage, the bladder is quite irritable. With healing, fibrosis develops that involves the muscle wall.

C. Prostate and Seminal Vesicles

Grossly, the exterior surface of these organs may show nodules and areas of induration from fibrosis. Areas of necrosis are common. In rare cases, healing may end in calcification. Large calcifications in the prostate should suggest tuberculous involvement.

D. Spermatic Cord, Epididymis, and Testis

The vas deferens is often grossly involved; fusiform swellings represent tubercles that in chronic cases are characteristically described as beaded. The epididymis is enlarged and quite firm. It is usually separate from the testis, although occasionally it may adhere to it. Microscopically, the changes typical of tuberculosis are seen. Tubular degeneration may be marked. The testis is usually not involved except by direct extension of an abscess in the epididymis.

E. Female Genital Tract

Infections are usually carried by the bloodstream; rarely, they are the result of sexual contact with an infected male. The incidence of associated urinary and genital infection in women ranges from 1% to 10%. The uterine tubes may be affected. Other presentations include endarteritis, localized adnexal masses (usually bilateral), and tuberculous cervicitis, but granulomatous lesions of the vaginal canal and vulva are rare.

▶ Clinical Findings

Tuberculosis of the genitourinary tract should be considered in the presence of any of the following situations: (1) chronic cystitis that refuses to respond to adequate therapy; (2) the finding of sterile pyuria; (3) gross or microscopic hematuria; (4) a nontender, enlarged epididymis with a beaded or thickened vas; (5) a chronic draining scrotal sinus; or (6) induration or nodulation of the prostate and thickening of one or both seminal vesicles (especially in a young man). A history of present or past tuberculosis elsewhere in the body should cause the physician to suspect tuberculosis in the genitourinary tract when signs or symptoms are present.

The diagnosis rests on the demonstration of tubercle bacilli in the urine by culture or positive polymerase chain reaction (PCR). The extent of the infection is determined by (1) the palpable findings in the epididymides, vasa deferentia, prostate, and seminal vesicles; (2) the renal and ureteral lesions as revealed by imaging; (3) involvement of the bladder as seen through the cystoscope; (4) the degree of renal damage as measured by loss of function; and (5) the presence of tubercle bacilli in one or both kidneys.

A. Symptoms

There is no classic clinical picture of renal tuberculosis. Most symptoms of this disease, even in the most advanced stage, are vesical in origin (cystitis). Vague generalized malaise, fatigability, low-grade but persistent fever, and night sweats are some of the nonspecific complaints. Even vesical irritability may be absent, in which case only proper collection and examination of the urine will afford the clue. Active tuberculosis elsewhere in the body is found in less than half of patients with genitourinary tuberculosis.

1. Kidney and ureter—Because of the slow progression of the disease, the affected kidney is usually completely asymptomatic. On occasion, however, there may be a dull ache in the flank. The passage of a blood clot, secondary calculi, or a mass of debris may cause renal and ureteral colic. Rarely, the presenting symptom may be a painless mass in the abdomen.

2. Bladder—The earliest symptoms of renal tuberculosis may arise from secondary vesical involvement. These include burning, frequency, and nocturia. Hematuria is occasionally found and is of either renal or vesical origin. At times, particularly in a late stage of the disease, the vesical irritability may become extreme. If ulceration occurs, suprapubic pain may be noted when the bladder becomes full.

3. Genital tract—Tuberculosis of the prostate and seminal vesicles usually causes no symptoms. The first clue to the presence of tuberculous infection of these organs is the onset of a tuberculous epididymitis.

Tuberculosis of the epididymis usually presents as a painless or only mildly painful swelling. An abscess may drain spontaneously through the scrotal wall. A chronic draining sinus should be regarded as tuberculous until proved otherwise. In rare cases, the onset is quite acute and may simulate an acute nonspecific epididymitis.

B. Signs

Evidence of extragenital tuberculosis may be found (lungs, bone, lymph nodes, tonsils, intestines).

1. Kidney—There is usually no enlargement or tenderness of the involved kidney.

2. External genitalia—A thickened, nontender, or only slightly tender epididymis may be discovered. The vas deferens often is thickened and beaded. A chronic draining sinus through the scrotal skin is almost pathognomonic of tuberculous epididymitis. In the more advanced stages, the epididymis cannot be differentiated from the testis on palpation. This may mean that the testis has been directly invaded by the epididymal abscess.

Hydrocele occasionally accompanies tuberculous epididymitis. The idiopathic hydrocele should be tapped so that underlying pathologic changes, if present, can be evaluated (epididymitis, testicular tumor). Involvement of the penis and urethra is rare.

3. Prostate and seminal vesicles—These organs may be normal to palpation. Ordinarily, however, the tuberculous prostate shows areas of induration, even nodulation. The involved seminal vesicle is usually indurated, enlarged, and fixed. If epididymitis is present, the ipsilateral seminal vesicle usually shows changes as well.

C. Laboratory Findings

Proper urinalysis affords the most important clue to the diagnosis of genitourinary tuberculosis.

1. Persistent pyuria without organisms on culture means tuberculosis until proved otherwise. Acid–fast stains done on the concentrated sediment from a 24-hour specimen are positive in at least 60% of cases. However, this must be corroborated by a positive culture.

   If clinical response to adequate treatment of bacterial infection fails and pyuria persists, tuberculosis must be ruled out by bacteriologic and imaging.

2. Cultures for tubercle bacilli from the first morning urine are positive in a very high percentage of cases of tuberculous infection. If positive, sensitivity tests should be ordered. In the face of strong presumptive evidence of tuberculosis, negative cultures should be repeated. Three to five first morning voided specimens are ideal.

   It can also be infected with tubercle bacilli, or it may become hydronephrotic from fibrosis of the bladder wall (ureterovesical stenosis) or vesicoureteral reflux.

   If tuberculosis is suspected, the tuberculin test should be performed. A positive test, particularly in an adult, is hardly diagnostic, but a negative test in an otherwise healthy patient speaks against a diagnosis of tuberculosis.

D. X-Ray Findings (Figure 15–2)

A plain film of the abdomen may show enlargement of one kidney or obliteration of the renal and psoas shadows due to perinephric abscess. Punctate calcification in the renal parenchyma may be due to tuberculosis. Renal stones are found in 10% of cases. Calcification of the ureter may be noted, but this is rare (Figure 15–2).

Excretory urograms can be diagnostic if the lesion is moderately advanced. The typical changes include (1) a "moth-eaten" appearance of the involved ulcerated calyces; (2) obliteration of one or more calyces; (3) dilatation of the calyces due to ureteral stenosis from fibrosis; (4) abscess cavities that connect with calyces; (5) single or multiple ureteral strictures, with secondary dilatation, with shortening and

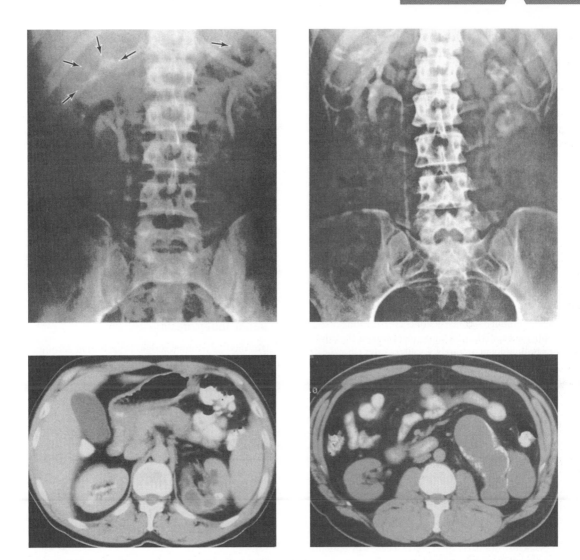

▲ **Figure 15–2.** Radiologic evidence of tuberculosis. ***Upper left:*** Excretory urogram showing "moth-eaten" calyces in upper renal poles. Calcifications in upper calyces; right upper ureter is straight and dilated. ***Upper right:*** Excretory urogram showing ulcerated and dilated calyces on the left. ***Lower left:*** Abdominal computed tomography (CT) with contrast showing left renal tuberculosis with calcification, poor parenchymal perfusion, and surrounding inflammation. ***Lower right:*** Noncontrast abdominal CT showing late effects of renal TB with calyceal dilation, loss of parenchyma, and urothelial calcifications. (CT images courtesy of Fergus Coakley, MD, UCSF Radiology.)

therefore straightening of the ureter; and (6) the absence of function of the kidney due to complete ureteral occlusion and renal destruction (autonephrectomy). Ultrasound and computed tomography (CT) also show the calcifications, renal contractions and scars, and ureteral and calyceal strictures suggestive of genitourinary tuberculosis. Ultrasound has the advantage of low cost and low invasiveness. Contrast CT scan is highly sensitive for calcifications and the characteristic anatomic changes.

E. Cystoscopic Examination

Thorough cystoscopic study is indicated even when the offending organism has been found in the urine and excretory urograms show the typical renal lesion. This study clearly demonstrates the extent of the disease. Cystoscopy may reveal the typical tubercles or ulcers of tuberculosis. Biopsy can be done if necessary. Severe contracture of the bladder may be noted. A cystogram may reveal ureteral reflux.

▶ Differential Diagnosis

Chronic nonspecific cystitis or pyelonephritis may mimic tuberculosis perfectly, especially since 15–20% of cases of tuberculosis are secondarily invaded by pyogenic organisms. If nonspecific infections do not respond to adequate therapy, a search for tubercle bacilli should be made. Painless epididymitis points to tuberculosis. Cystoscopic demonstration of tubercles and ulceration of the bladder wall means tuberculosis. Urograms are usually definitive.

Acute or chronic nonspecific epididymitis may be confused with tuberculosis, since the onset of tuberculosis is occasionally quite painful. It is rare to have palpatory changes in the seminal vesicles with nonspecific epididymitis, but these are almost routine findings in tuberculosis of the epididymis. The presence of tubercle bacilli on a culture of the urine is diagnostic. On occasion, only the pathologist can make the diagnosis by microscopic study of the surgically removed epididymis.

Multiple small renal stones or nephrocalcinosis seen by x-ray may suggest the type of calcification seen in the tuberculous kidney. In renal tuberculosis, the calcium is in the parenchyma, although secondary stones are occasionally seen.

Necrotizing papillitis, which may involve all of the calyces of one or both kidneys or, rarely, a solitary calyx, shows caliceal lesions (including calcifications) that simulate those of tuberculosis. Careful bacteriologic studies fail to demonstrate tubercle bacilli.

Medullary sponge kidneys may show small calcifications just distal to the calyces. The calyces are sharp, however, and no other stigmas of tuberculosis can be demonstrated.

In disseminated coccidioidomycosis, renal involvement may occur. The renal lesion resembles that of tuberculosis. Coccidioidal epididymitis may be confused with tuberculous involvement.

Urinary bilharziasis is a great mimic of tuberculosis. Both present with symptoms of cystitis and often hematuria. Vesical contraction, seen in both diseases, may lead to extreme frequency. Schistosomiasis must be suspected in endemic areas; the typical ova are found in the urine. Cystoscopic and urographic findings are definitive for making the diagnosis.

▶ Complications

A. Renal Tuberculosis

Perinephric abscess may cause an enlarging mass in the flank. A plain film of the abdomen shows obliteration of the renal and psoas shadows. Sonograms and CT scans may be more helpful. Renal stones may develop if secondary nonspecific infection is present. Uremia is the end stage if both kidneys are involved.

B. Ureteral Tuberculosis

Scarring with stricture formation is one of the typical lesions of tuberculosis and most commonly affects the juxtavesical portion of the ureter. This may cause progressive hydronephrosis.

Complete ureteral obstruction may cause complete nonfunction of the kidney (autonephrectomy).

C. Vesical Tuberculosis

When severely damaged, the bladder wall becomes fibrosed and contracted. Stenosis of the ureters or reflux occurs, causing hydronephrotic atrophy.

D. Genital Tuberculosis

The ducts of the involved epididymis become occluded. If this is bilateral, sterility results. Abscesses of the epididymis may invade the testes and even involve the scrotal skin.

▶ Treatment

Genitourinary tuberculosis is extrapulmonary tuberculosis. The primary treatment is medical therapy. Surgical excision of an infected organ, when indicated, is merely an adjunct to overall therapy.

A. Renal Tuberculosis

A strict medical regimen should be instituted. A combination of drugs is usually desirable. The following drugs are effective in combination: (1) isoniazid (INH), 200–300 mg orally once daily; (2) rifampin (RMP), 600 mg orally once daily; (3) ethambutol (EMB), 25 mg/kg daily for 2 months, then 15 mg/kg orally once daily; (4) streptomycin, 1 g intramuscularly once daily; and (5) pyrazinamide, l.5–2 g orally once daily. It is preferable to begin treatment with a combination of isoniazid, rifampin, and ethambutol. The European Association of Urology guidelines recommends 2 or 3 months of intensive triple drug therapy (INH, RMP, and EMB) daily followed by 3 months of continuation therapy with INH and RMP two or three times per week. If resistance to one of these drugs develops, one of the others listed should be chosen as a replacement. The following drugs are usually considered only in cases of resistance to first-line drugs and when expert medical personnel are available to treat toxic side effects, should they occur: aminosalicylic acid (PAS), capreomycin, cycloserine, ethionamide, pyrazinamide, viomycin. *Pyrazinamide may cause serious liver damage.*

B. Vesical Tuberculosis

Tuberculosis of the bladder is always secondary to renal or prostatic tuberculosis; it tends to heal promptly when definitive treatment for the "primary" genitourinary infection is given. Vesical ulcers that fail to respond to this regimen may require transurethral electrocoagulation. Vesical instillations of 0.2% monoxychlorosene (Clorpactin) may also stimulate healing.

Should extreme contracture of the bladder develop, it may be necessary to divert the urine from the bladder or perform augmentation cystoplasty with ileum or colon.

C. Tuberculosis of the Epididymis

This condition never produces an isolated lesion; the prostate is always involved and usually the kidney as well. Only rarely does the epididymal infection break through into the testis. Treatment is medical. If after months of treatment an abscess or a draining sinus exists, epididymectomy is indicated.

D. Tuberculosis of the Prostate and Seminal Vesicles

Although a few urologists advocate removal of the entire prostate and the vesicles when they become involved by tuberculosis, the majority opinion is that only medical therapy is indicated. Control can be checked by culture of the semen for tubercle bacilli.

E. General Measures for All Types

Optimal nutrition is no less important in treating tuberculosis of the genitourinary tract than in the treatment of tuberculosis elsewhere. Anticholinergic medications may help with bladder irritability.

F. Treatment of Other Complications

Perinephric abscess usually occurs when the kidney is destroyed, but this is rare. The abscess must be drained, and nephrectomy should be done either then or later to prevent development of a chronic draining sinus. Prolonged antimicrobial therapy is indicated. If ureteral stricture develops on the involved side, ureteral dilatations offer a better than 50% chance of cure. The severely involved bladder may cause incompetence of the ureterovesical junction on the uninvolved side. Ureteroneocystostomy cannot be done in such a bladder; some form of urinary diversion may be required. For this reason, serial imaging and assessments of renal function are necessary even when the treatment is medical.

CANDIDIASIS

Candida albicans is a yeast-like fungus that is a normal inhabitant of the respiratory and gastrointestinal tracts and the vagina. The intensive use of potent modern antibiotics is apt to disturb the normal balance between normal and abnormal organisms, thus allowing fungi such as *Candida* to overwhelm an otherwise healthy organ. The bladder and, to a lesser extent, the kidneys have proved vulnerable; candidemia has been observed (Table 15–1).

The patient may present with vesical irritability or symptoms and signs of pyelonephritis. Fungus balls may be passed spontaneously. The diagnosis is made by observing mycelial or yeast forms of the fungus microscopically in a properly collected urine specimen. The diagnosis may be confirmed

Table 15–1. Risk factors for fungal UTI.

Indwelling catheters
Antimicrobials
Diabetes mellitus
Impaired host immunity including malignancy, steroids, malnutrition
Genitourinary tract abnormalities

UTI, urinary tract infection.

by culture. Excretory urograms may show caliceal defects and ureteral obstruction (fungus masses).

Treatment of candiduria in asymptomatic catheterized patients is typically not of utility. Oral fluconazole may transiently clear funguria, but it typically recurs promptly and may recur with resistant candida species. Vesical candidiasis usually responds to alkalinization of the urine with sodium bicarbonate. A urinary pH of 7.5 is desired; the dose is regulated by the patient, who checks the urine with indicator paper. Candiduria should be treated in symptomatic patients, patients with neutropenia, renal transplant patients, and patients who will undergo urologic procedures.

Removing or changing urologic catheters, stent, and tubes may be beneficial. Treatment with fluconazole (200 mg/day for 7–14 days) or with amphotericin B deoxycholate at widely ranging doses (0.3–1.0 mg/kg per day for 1–7 days) has been successful. In the absence of renal insufficiency, oral flucytosine (25 mg/kg qid) may be valuable for eradicating candiduria in patients with urologic infection due to non-*albicans* species of *Candida*.

ACTINOMYCOSIS

Actinomycosis is a chronic granulomatous disease in which fibrosis tends to become marked and spontaneous fistulas are the rule. On rare occasions, the disease involves the kidney, bladder, or testis by hematogenous invasion from a primary site of infection. The skin of the penis or scrotum may become involved through a local abrasion. The bladder may also become diseased by direct extension from the appendix, bowel, or oviduct.

▶ Etiology

Actinomyces israelii is the causative organism.

▶ Clinical Findings

There is nothing specifically pathognomonic about the symptoms or signs in actinomycosis. Pelvic involvement can be confused with malignancy. The microscopic demonstration of the organisms, which are visible as yellow bodies called "sulfur granules," makes the diagnosis. If persistently sought, these may be found in the discharge from sinuses or in the urine. Definitive diagnosis is established by culture.

Urographically, the lesion in the kidney may resemble tuberculosis (eroded calyces) or tumor (space-occupying lesion).

▶ Treatment

Penicillin G is the drug of choice. The dosage is 10–20 million U/day parenterally for 4–6 weeks, followed by penicillin V orally for a prolonged period. If secondary infection is suspected, a sulfonamide is added; streptomycin is also efficacious. Broad-spectrum antibiotics are indicated only if the organism is resistant to penicillin. Surgical drainage of the abscess or, better, removal of the involved organ is usually indicated.

▶ Prognosis

Removal of the involved organ (eg, kidney or testis) may be promptly curative. Drainage of a granulomatous abscess may cause the development of a chronic draining sinus. Chemotherapy is helpful.

SCHISTOSOMIASIS (BILHARZIASIS)

Schistosomiasis, caused by a blood fluke, is a disease of warm climates. In its three forms, it affects about 350 million people. *Schistosoma mansoni* is widely distributed in Africa, South and Central America, Pakistan, and India; *Schistosoma japonicum* is found in the Far East; and *Schistosoma haematobium* (*Bilharzia haematobium*) is limited to Africa (especially along its northern coast), Saudi Arabia, Israel, Jordan, Lebanon, and Syria.

Schistosomiasis is on the increase in endemic areas because of the construction of modern irrigation systems that provide favorable conditions for the intermediate host, a freshwater snail. This disease principally affects the urogenital system, especially the bladder, ureters, seminal vesicles, and, to a lesser extent, the male urethra, and prostate gland. Because of emigration of people from endemic areas, the disease is being seen with increasing frequency in both Europe and the United States. Infection with *S. mansoni* and *S. japonicum* mainly involves the colon.

▶ Etiology

Humans are infected when they come in contact with larva-infested water in canals, ditches, or irrigation fields during swimming, bathing, or farming procedures. Fork-tailed larvae, the cercariae, lose their tails as they penetrate deep under the skin. They are then termed **schistosomules**. They cause allergic skin reactions that are more intense in people infected for the first time. These schistosomules enter the general circulation through the lymphatics and the peripheral veins and reach the lungs. If the infection is massive, they may cause

pneumonitis. They pass through the pulmonary circulation, to the left side of the heart, and to the general circulation. The worms that reach the vesicoprostatic plexus of veins survive and mature, whereas those that go to other areas die.

▶ Pathogenesis

The adult *S. haematobium* worm, a digenetic trematode, lives in the prostatovesical plexus of veins. The male is about 10 × 1 mm in size; is folded upon itself; and carries the long, slim 20 × 0.25 mm female in its "schist," or gynecophoric canal. In the smallest peripheral venules, the female leaves the male and partially penetrates the venule to lay her eggs in the subepithelial layer of the affected viscus, usually in the form of clusters that form tubercles. The ova are seen only rarely within the venules; they are almost always in the subepithelial or interstitial tissues. The female returns to the male, which carries her to other areas to repeat the process.

The living ova, by a process of histolysis and helped by contraction of the detrusor muscle, penetrate the overlying urothelium, pass into the cavity of the bladder, and are extruded with the urine. If these ova reach fresh water, they hatch, and the contained larvae—ciliated miracidia—find a specific freshwater snail that they penetrate. There, they form sporocysts that ultimately form the cercariae, which leave the snail hosts and pass into fresh water to repeat their life cycle in the human host.

▶ Pathology

The fresh ova excite little tissue reaction when they leave the human host promptly through the urothelium. The contents of the ova trapped in the tissues and the death of the organisms causes a severe local reaction, with infiltration of round cells, monocytes, eosinophils, and giant cells that form tubercles, nodules, and polyps. These are later replaced by fibrous tissue that causes contraction of different parts of the bladder and strictures of the ureter. Fibrosis and massive deposits of eggs in subepithelial tissues interfere with the blood supply of the area and cause chronic bilharzial ulcerations. Epithelial metaplasia is common, and squamous cell carcinoma is a frequent sequela. Secondary infection of the urinary tract is a common complication and is difficult to overcome. The trapped dead ova become impregnated with calcium salts and form sheets of subepithelial calcified layers in the ureter, bladder, and seminal vesicles.

▶ Clinical Findings

A. Symptoms

Penetration of the skin by the cercariae causes allergic reactions, with cutaneous hyperemia and itching that are more intense in people infected for the first time. During the stage of generalization or invasion, the patient complains of symptoms such as malaise, fatigue and lassitude, low-grade fever, excessive sweating, headache, and backache. When the ova are laid in the bladder wall and begin to be extruded, the patient complains of terminal, slightly painful hematuria that is occasionally profuse. This may remain the only complaint for a long time until complications set in, when vesical symptoms become exaggerated and progressive. Increasing frequency, suprapubic and back pain, urethralgia, profuse hematuria, pyuria, and necroturia are likely to occur, with secondary infection, ulceration, or malignancy. Renal pain may be due to ureteral stricture, vesicoureteral reflux, or secondary stones obstructing the ureter. Fever, rigor, toxemia, and uremia are manifestations of renal involvement.

B. Signs

In early uncomplicated cases, there are essentially no clinical findings. Later, a fibrosed, pitted, bilharzial glans penis; a urethral stricture or fistula; or a perineal fibrous mass may be found. A suprapubic bladder mass or a renal swelling may be felt abdominally. Rectal examination may reveal a fibrosed prostate, an enlarged seminal vesicle, or a thickened bladder base.

C. Laboratory Findings

Urinalysis usually reveals the terminal-spined dead or living ova, blood and pus cells, and bacteria. Malignant squamous cells may be seen. The hemogram usually shows leukocytosis with eosinophilia and hypochromic normocytic anemia. Serum creatinine and blood urea nitrogen measurements may demonstrate some degree of renal impairment.

A variety of immunologic methods have been used to confirm the diagnosis of schistosomiasis. Positive immunologic tests indicate previous exposure but not whether schistosomiasis is currently present. The cercariae, schistosomules, adult worms, and eggs are all potentially antigenic. Adult worms, however, acquire host antigen on their integument that circumvents the immunologic forces of the host. Antibody production may be manifested as hypergammaglobulinemia.

D. X-Ray Findings

A plain film of the abdomen may show areas of grayness in the flank (enlarged hydronephrotic kidney) or in the bladder area (large tumor). Opacifications (stones) may be noted in the kidney, ureter, or bladder. Linear calcification may be seen in the ureteral and bladder walls (Figure 15–3). Punctate calcification of the ureter (ureteritis calcinosa) and a honeycombed calcification of the seminal vesicle may be obvious (Figure 15–3).

Excretory urograms may show either normal or diminished renal function and varying degrees of dilatation of the upper urinary tracts (Figure 15–4). These changes include hydronephrosis, dilated and tortuous ureters, ureteral strictures, or a small contracted bladder having a capacity of only a few milliliters. Gross irregular defects of the bladder wall

may represent cancer (Figure 15–4). Abdominal and pelvic CT is replacing excretory urography as the initial imaging of choice in many centers.

Retrograde urethrography may reveal a bilharzial urethral stricture. Cystograms often reveal vesicoureteral reflux, particularly if the bladder is contracted.

E. Cystoscopic Examination

Cystoscopy may show fresh conglomerate, grayish tubercles surrounded by a halo of hyperemia, old calcified yellowish tubercles, sandy patches of mucous membrane, and a lusterless ground-glass mucosa that lacks the normal vascular pattern. Other obvious lesions include bilharzial polyps; chronic ulcers on the dome that bleed when the bladder is deflated (weeping ulcers); vesical stones; malignant lesions; stenosed or patulous ureteric orifices; and a distorted, asymmetric trigone. All are signs of schistosomal infestation.

▶ Differential Diagnosis

Bilharzial cystitis is unmistakable in endemic areas. The presence of schistosomal ova in the urine, together with radiographic and cystoscopic findings, usually confirms the diagnosis. Nonspecific cystitis usually responds to medical treatment unless there is a complicating factor. Tuberculous cystitis may mimic bilharzial cystitis; the detection of tubercle bacilli, together with the radiographic picture, is confirmatory, but tuberculosis may occur in a bilharzial bladder. Squamous cell tumors of the bladder are common. They are seen as early as the second or third decade of life and are much more common in men than in women.

▶ Treatment

A. Medical Measures

Praziquantel, metrifonate, and oxamniquine are the drugs of choice in treating schistosomiasis. These drugs do not have the serious side effects associated with the older drugs (eg, antimonials).

1. Praziquantel is unique in that it is effective against all human schistosome species. It is given orally and is effective in adults and children. Patients in the hepatosplenic stage of advanced schistosomiasis tolerate the drug well. The recommended dosage for all forms of schistosomiasis is 20 mg/kg three times in 1 day only.

2. Metrifonate is also a highly effective oral drug. It is the drug of choice for treatment of *S. haematobium* infections but is not effective against *S. mansoni* or *S. japonicum*. For treatment of *S. haematobium* infections, the dosage is 7.5–10 mg/kg (maximum 600 mg) once and then repeated twice at 2-week intervals.

3. Oxamniquine is a highly effective oral drug and is the drug of choice for treatment of *S. mansoni* infections. It is safe and effective in advanced disease. It is not effective in *S. haematobium* or *S. japonicum* infections. The dosage is

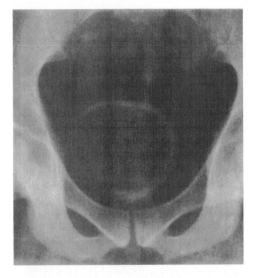

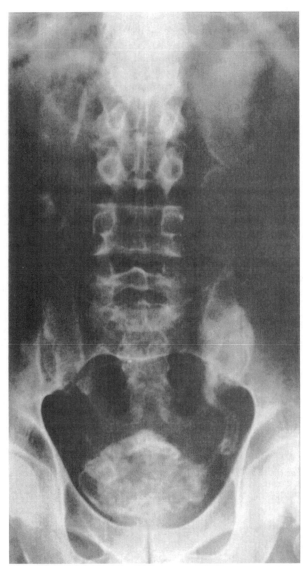

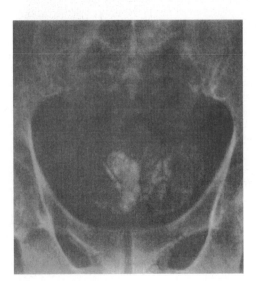

▲ **Figure 15–3.** Schistosomiasis. Plain films. ***Upper left:*** Extensive calcification in the wall of a contracted bladder. ***Right***: Extensive calcification of the bladder and both ureters up to the renal pelves. The ureters are dilated and tortuous. ***Lower left:*** Extensive calcification of seminal vesicles and ampullae of vasa.

12–15 mg/kg given once; for children <30 kg, 20 mg/kg is given in two divided doses in 1 day, with an interval of 2–8 hours between doses. Cure rates are 70–95%.

4. Niridazole, a nitrothiazole derivative, is effective in treating *S. mansoni* and *S. haematobium* infections. It may be tried against *S. japonicum* infections. It is given orally and should be administered only under close medical supervision. The dosage is 25 mg/kg (maximum, 1.5 g) daily in two divided doses for 7 days. Side effects may include nausea, vomiting, anorexia, headache, T-wave depression, and temporary suppression of spermatogenesis.

B. General Measures

Antibiotics or urinary antiseptics are needed to overcome or control secondary infection. Supportive treatment in the form of iron, vitamins, and a high-calorie diet is indicated in selected cases.

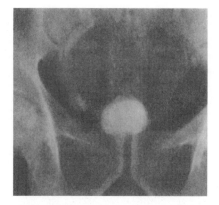

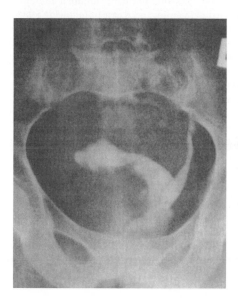

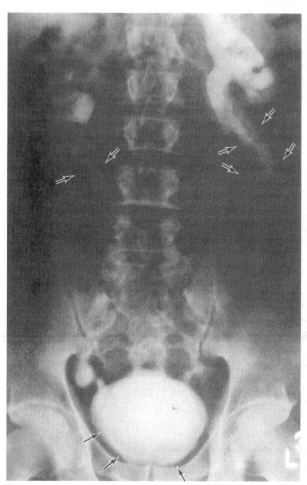

▲ **Figure 15–4.** Schistosomiasis. ***Upper left:*** Excretory urogram showing markedly contracted bladder. Lower right ureter dilated probably secondary to vesicoureteral reflux. ***Right:*** Excretory urogram at 2 hours showing a fairly normal right kidney. The upper ureter is distorted. *Arrows* point to calcified wall. The lower ureter is quite abnormal. The calyces and pelvis of the left kidney are dilated, but the kidney shows atrophy secondary to nonspecific infection. The upper ureter is dilated and displaced by elongation due to obstruction. *Arrows* show calcification. Linear calcification can be seen in the periphery of the lower half of the bladder wall (*arrows*). ***Lower left:*** Nodular squamous cell carcinoma of the bladder. Dilated left lower ureter probably secondary to obstruction by tumor. Nonvisualization of the right ureter caused by complete occlusion.

C. Complications

Treatment of the complications of schistosomiasis of the genitourinary tract makes demands on the skill of the physician. Juxtavesical ureteral strictures require resection of the stenotic segment with ureteroneocystostomy. If the ureter is not long enough to reimplant, a tube of bladder may be fashioned, turned cephalad, and anastomosed to the ureter. Vesicoureteral reflux requires a suitable surgical repair. A

contracted bladder neck may need transurethral anterior commissurotomy or a suprapubic Y-V plasty.

A chronic "weeping" bilharzial bladder ulcer necessitates partial cystectomy. The contracted bladder is treated by enterocystoplasty (placing a segment of bowel as a patch on the bladder). This procedure, which significantly increases vesical capacity, is remarkably effective in lessening the severity of symptoms associated with contracted bladder. Preoperative vesicoureteral reflux may disappear.

The most dreaded complication, squamous cell carcinoma, requires radical cystectomy with urinary diversion if the lesion is deemed operable. Unfortunately, late diagnosis is common.

Prognosis

With early diagnosis and treatment, mild and early cases of schistosomiasis can be effectively treated usually without complications. On the other hand, massive repeated infections undermine the function of the urinary tract to such an extent that patients are chronically ill and may have shortened life spans.

In many endemic areas, attempts have been made to control the disease by mass treatment of patients, proper education, mechanization of agriculture, and various methods of eradication or control of the snail population. All these efforts have failed to be fully effective.

FILARIASIS

Filariasis is endemic in the countries bordering the Mediterranean, in south China and Japan, the West Indies, and the South Pacific islands, particularly Samoa. Limited infection, as seen in American soldiers during World War II, gives an entirely different clinical picture from that seen in the frequent reinfections usually encountered among the native population.

Etiology

Wuchereria bancrofti is a threadlike nematode about 0.5 cm or more in length that lives in the human lymphatics. In the lymphatics, the female gives off microfilariae, which are found in the peripheral blood, particularly at night. The intermediate host (usually a mosquito) bites an infected person and becomes infested with microfilariae, which develop into larvae. These are in turn transferred to another human, in whom they reach maturity. Mating occurs, and microfilariae are again produced. *Brugia malayi*, a nematode that causes filariasis in Southeast Asia and adjacent Pacific islands, acts in a similar fashion.

Pathogenesis and Pathology

The adult nematode in the human host invades and obstructs the lymphatics; this leads to lymphangitis and lymphadenitis. In long-standing cases, the lymphatic vessels become thickened and fibrous; there is a marked reticuloendothelial reaction.

Clinical Findings

A. Symptoms

In mild cases (few exposures), the patient suffers recurrent lymphadenitis and lymphangitis with fever and malaise. Not infrequently, inflammation of the epididymis, testis, scrotum, and spermatic cord occurs. These structures then become edematous, boggy, and, at times, tender. Hydrocele is common. In advanced cases (many exposures), obstruction of major lymph channels may cause chyluria and elephantiasis.

B. Signs

Varying degrees of painless elephantiasis of the scrotum and extremities develop as obstruction to lymphatics progresses. Lymphadenopathy is common.

C. Laboratory Findings

Chylous urine may look normal if minimal amounts of fat are present, but in an advanced case or following a fatty meal, it is milky. On standing, the urine forms layers: the top layer is fatty, the middle layer is pinkish, and the lower layer is clear. In the presence of chyluria, large amounts of protein are to be expected. Hypoproteinemia is found, and the albumin–globulin ratio is reversed. Both white blood cells (leukocytes) and red blood cells (erythrocytes) are found.

Marked eosinophilia is the rule in the early stages. Microfilariae may be demonstrated in the blood, which should be drawn at night. The adult worm may be found by biopsy. When filariae cannot be found, an indirect hemagglutination titer of 1/128 and a bentonite flocculation titer of 1/5 in combination are considered diagnostic.

D. Cystoscopy

Following a fatty meal, endoscopy to observe the efflux of milky urine from the ureteral orifices may differentiate between unilateral and bilateral cases.

E. X-Ray Findings

Retrograde urography and lymphangiography may reveal the renolymphatic connections in patients with chyluria.

Prevention

In endemic areas, mosquito abatement programs must be intensively pursued.

Treatment

A. Specific Measures

Diethylcarbamazine 0.5–2 g/kg for 3 weeks or albendazole 400 mg orally twice daily are the treatments of choice. Antibiotics may be necessary to control secondary infection.

B. General Measures

Prompt removal of recently infected patients from the endemic area almost always results in regression of the symptoms and signs in early cases.

C. Surgical Measures

Elephantiasis of the external genitalia may require surgical excision.

D. Treatment of Chyluria

Mild cases require no therapy. Spontaneous cure occurs in 50% of cases. If nutrition is impaired, the lymphatic channels may be sealed off by irrigating the renal pelvis with 2% silver nitrate solution. Should this fail, renal decapsulation and resection of the renal lymphatics should be performed. This can now be performed laparoscopically with diminished morbidity.

▶ Prognosis

If exposure has been limited, resolution of the disease is spontaneous and the prognosis is excellent. Frequent reinfection may lead to elephantiasis of the scrotum or chyluria.

ECHINOCOCCOSIS (HYDATID DISEASE)

Involvement of the urogenital organs by hydatid disease is relatively rare in the United States. It is common in Australia, New Zealand, South America, Africa, Asia, the Middle East, and Europe. Livestock are the intermediate hosts. Canines, especially dogs, are the final hosts.

▶ Etiology

The adult tapeworm (*Echinococcus granulosus*) inhabits the intestinal tracts of carnivorous animals. Its eggs pass out with the feces and may be ingested by such animals as sheep, cattle, pigs, and occasionally humans. Larvae from these eggs pass through the intestinal wall of the various intermediate hosts and are disseminated throughout the body. In humans, the liver is principally involved, but about 3% of infected humans develop echinococcosis of the kidney.

If a cyst of the liver should rupture into the peritoneal cavity, the scoleces (tapeworm heads) may directly invade the retrovesical tissues, thus leading to the development of cysts in this area.

▶ Clinical Findings

If renal hydatid disease is closed (not communicating with the pelvis), there may be no symptoms until a mass is found. With communicating disease, there may be symptoms of cystitis, and renal colic may occur as cysts are passed from the kidney. X-ray films may show calcification in the wall of the cyst (Figure 15–5), and urograms often reveal changes typical of a space-occupying lesion. The cystic nature of the lesion may be demonstrated on sonograms and CT scans. Calcification in the cyst wall may be noted. Scintillation scanning or angiography can also suggest the presence of a cyst. Serologic tests that should be done include immunoelectrophoresis and indirect hemagglutination. The Casoni intracutaneous procedure is unreliable.

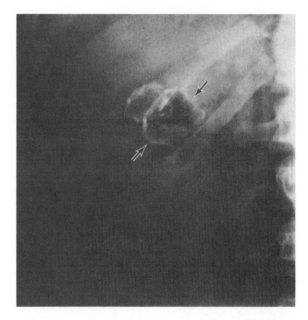

▲ **Figure 15–5.** Hydatid disease, right kidney. Plain film showing two calcified hydatid cysts.

Retroperitoneal (perivesical) cysts may cause symptoms of cystitis, or acute urinary retention may develop secondary to pressure. The presence of a suprapubic mass may be the only finding. It may rupture into the bladder and cause hydatiduria, which establishes the diagnosis.

▶ Treatment

Nephrectomy is generally the treatment of choice for renal hydatid disease. Medical treatment includes albendazole 400 mg twice daily or praziquantel 40 mg/kg/day (before surgery). Aspiration of the cyst is unwise; leakage or rupture may occur. Retroperitoneal cysts are best treated by marsupialization and curettage.

▶ Prognosis

Echinococcosis of the kidney usually has a good prognosis. The problem presented by perivesical cysts is more troublesome. After surgical intervention, drainage may be prolonged. It must be remembered, too, that involvement of other organs, especially the liver, is usually present.

BIBLIOGRAPHY

Tuberculosis

Carl P, Stark L: Indications for surgical management of genitourinary tuberculosis. World J Surg 1997;21:505.

Cek M et al: EAU guidelines for the management of genitourinary tuberculosis. Eur Urol 2005;48(3):353.

Chuang FR et al: Extrapulmonary tuberculosis in chronic hemodialysis patients. Ren Fail 2003;25:739.

Gokalp A et al: Genito-urinary tuberculosis: A review of 83 cases. Br J Clin Pract 1990;44:599.

Hamrick-Turner J et al: Tuberculosis of the lower genitourinary tract: Findings on sonography and MR. (Letter.) AJR Am J Roentgenol 1992;158:919.

Hemal AK et al: Polymerase chain reaction in clinically suspected genitourinary tuberculosis: Comparison with intravenous urography, bladder biopsy, and urine acid fast bacilli culture. Urology 2000;56:570.

Jung YY et al: Genitourinary tuberculosis: Comprehensive cross-sectional imaging. AJR Am J Roentgenol 2005;184(1):143.

Lenk S, Schroeder J: Genitourinary tuberculosis. Curr Opin Urol 2001;11:93.

Matos MJ et al: Genitourinary tuberculosis. Eur J Radiol 2005;55 (2):181.

Poulios C, Malovrouvas D: Progress in the approach of tuberculosis of the genitourinary tract: Remarks on a decade's experience over cases. Acta Urol Belg 1990;58:101.

Queipo JA et al: Mycobacterial infection in a series of 1261 renal transplant recipients. Clin Microbiol Infect 2003;9:518.

Skoutelis A et al: Serious complications of tuberculous epididymitis. Infection 2000;28:193.

Tikkakoski T et al: Tuberculosis of the lower genitourinary tract: Ultrasonography as an aid to diagnosis and treatment. J Clin Ultrasound 1993;21:269.

Valentini AL et al: Diagnostic imaging of genitourinary tuberculosis. Rays 1998;23:126.

Candidiasis

Pappas PG et al: Guidelines for treatment of Candidiasis. Clin Infect Dis 2004;38:165–167.

Priestley CJ et al: What is normal vaginal flora? Genitourin Med 1997;73:23.

Rivera L et al: Morphotypes of Candida albicans and their associations with underlying diseases and source of samples. New Microbiol 1996;19:335.

Rodgers CA, Beardall AJ: Recurrent vulvovaginal candidiasis: Why does it occur? Int J STD AIDS 1999;10:435.

Sobel JD et al: Candiduria: A randomized, double-blind study of treatment with fluconazole and placebo. Clin Infect Dis 2000; 30:19–24.

Wise GJ et al: Fungal infections of the genitourinary system: Manifestations, diagnosis, and treatment. Urol Clin North Am 1999;26:701.

Woolley PD, Higgins SP: Comparison of clotrimazole, fluconazole and itraconazole in vaginal candidiasis. Br J Clin Pract 1995; 49:65.

Actinomycosis

Jani AN et al: Disseminated actinomycosis presenting as a testicular mass: A case report. J Urol 1990;143:1012.

Lee YC et al: Computed tomography guided core needle biopsy diagnosis of pelvic actinomycosis. Gynecol Oncol 2000;79:318.

Lippes J: Pelvic actinomycosis: A review and preliminary look at prevalence. Am J Obstet Gynecol 1999;180(Pt 1):265.

Smego RA Jr et al: Actinomycosis. Clin Infect Dis 1998;26:1255.

Schistosomiasis (Bilharziasis)

Badawi AF et al: Role of schistosomiasis in human bladder cancer: Evidence of association, aetiological factors, and basic mechanisms of carcinogenesis. Eur J Cancer Prev 1995;4:45.

Bichler KH et al: Schistosomiasis: A critical review. Curr Opin Urol 2001;11:97.

Engels D et al: The global epidemiological situation of schistosomiasis and new approaches to control and research. Acta Trop 2002; 82:139.

Ghoneim MA: Bilharziasis of the genitourinary tract. BJU Int 2002; 89(Suppl 1):22.

Hardin BM et al: Urinary tract shistosomiasis J Urol 2010;184 (5):22136–22137.

Helling-Giese G et al: Schistosomiasis in women: Manifestations in the upper reproductive tract. Acta Trop 1996;62:225.

Mostafa MH et al: Relationship between schistosomiasis and bladder cancer. Clin Microbiol Rev 1999;12:97.

Naude JH: Reconstructive urology in the tropical and developing world: A personal perspective. BJU Int 2002;89(Suppl 1):31.

Shokeir AA: Renal transplantation: The impact of schistosomiasis. BJU Int 2001;88:915.

Stock JA et al: Urinary schistosomiasis in childhood. Urology 1994;44:305.

Filariasis

De Vries CR: The role of the urologist in the treatment and elimination of lymphatic filariasis worldwide. BJU Int 2002;89(Suppl 1): 37.

Kehinde EO et al: Parasites of urological importance. Urol Int 2008; 81(1):1–13.

Kohli V et al: Filarial chyluria. Indian Pediatr 1994;31:451.

Pool MO et al: Bilateral excision of perinephric fat and fascia (Gerota's fasciectomy) in the treatment of intractable chyluria. J Urol 1991;146:1374.

Punekar SV et al: Surgical disconnection of lymphorenal communication for chyluria: A 15-year experience. Br J Urol 1997;80:858.

Taylor MJ, Hoerauf A: A new approach to the treatment of filariasis. Curr Opin Infect Dis 2001;14:727.

Yagi S et al: Endoscopic treatment of refractory filarial chyluria: A preliminary report. J Urol 1998;159:1615.

Zhang X et al: Renal pedicle lymphatic disconnection for chyluria via retroperitoneoscopy and open surgery: Report of 53 cases with follow-up. J Urol 2005;174:1828.

Onchocerciasis

Kumate J: Infectious diseases in the 21st century. Arch Med Res 1997; 28:155.

Ottesen EA: Immune responsiveness and the pathogenesis of human onchocerciasis. J Infect Dis 1995;171:659.

Van Laethem Y, Lopes C: Treatment of onchocerciasis. Drugs 1996; 52:861.

Echinococcosis (Hydatid Disease)

Cagatay G et al: Isolated renal hydatidosis: Experience with 20 cases. J Urol 2003;169:186.

Cirenei A: Histopathology, clinical findings and treatment of renal hydatidosis. Ann Ital Chir 1997;68:275.

Migaleddu V et al: Imaging of renal hydatid cysts. AJR Am J Roentgenol 1997;169:1339.

Pasaoglu E et al: Hydatid cysts of the kidney, seminal vesicle and gluteus muscle. Australas Radiol 1997;41:297.

Ranzini AC et al: Ultrasonographic diagnosis of pelvic echinococcosis: Case report and review of the literature. J Ultrasound Med 2002; 21:207.

Yeniyol CO et al: Primary cyst hydatid of adrenal: A case report. Int Urol Nephrol 2000;32:227.

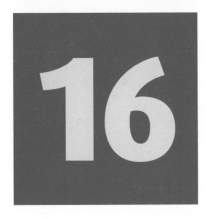

16

Sexually Transmitted Diseases

John N. Krieger, MD

The usual approach to sexually transmitted diseases (STDs) considers the causative agents, emphasizing different classes, genera, species, and microbiological characteristics. This fits with most medical school curricula since the causative agents span the full spectrum of medical microbiology (viruses, bacteria, protozoa, ectoparasites, and so on). This classical approach often proves difficult in clinical practice, where many different types of agents must be considered in the differential diagnosis of an individual patient.

This chapter takes a very selective and practical approach. Because patients present with symptoms and signs that may be caused by pathogens from different microbiological classes, we will emphasize diagnosis and treatment of clinical syndromes in contrast to traditional teaching (Table 16–1). This is a large subject with much active research and a huge literature. We stress the most important conditions encountered in urology: urethritis, epididymitis, genital ulcers, genital warts, plus a brief consideration of human immunodeficiency virus (HIV) infection.

URETHRITIS AND CERVICITIS

▷ Urethritis in Men

Definition. Urethritis, or urethral inflammation, is frequently caused by infection.

Clinical presentation. Characteristically, patients complain of urethral discharge and dysuria. On examination, the discharge may be purulent or mucopurulent. Asymptomatic infections are common (CDCP, 2006; McCormack and Rein, 2000). The most important pathogens are bacteria, *Neisseria gonorrhoeae*, and *Chlamydia trachomatis*.

Laboratory testing. Testing is recommended to document a specific disease because both of these infections are reportable to health departments, and because specific diagnosis may improve compliance and partner notification (CDCP, 2006). The traditional diagnostic algorithm includes microscopic examination of the Gram-stained urethral smear for gram-negative intracellular diplococci and culture for *N. gonorrhoeae*. New nucleic acid amplification tests have proved accurate for detection of *N. gonorrhoeae* and *C. trachomatis* in first-void urine in high-risk populations (CDCP, 2006; Gaydos et al, 2009; McCormack and Rein, 2000). If diagnostic testing is unavailable, patients should be treated empirically for both infections (CDCP, 2006).

Complications. Complications of urethritis in men include epididymitis (see later), disseminated gonococcal infection, and Reiter's syndrome (CDCP, 2006; McCormack and Rein, 2000). Complications of urethritis in female sexual partners include pelvic inflammatory disease, ectopic pregnancy, and infertility (CDCP, 2006; Mead, 2000). Complications in children include neonatal pneumonia and ophthalmia neonatorum (CDCP, 2006).

A. Etiology

Gonococcal and chlamydial infections. Gonorrhea is diagnosed when *N. gonorrhoeae* is detected by Gram stain, culture, or nucleic acid amplification testing. Nongonococcal urethritis (NGU) is diagnosed when gram-negative intracellular organisms cannot be diagnosed on microscopic examination or by diagnostic testing. *C. trachomatis*, the most common infectious cause of NGU, is responsible for 23–55% of cases in reported series, but the proportion of cases is substantially lower in urological practice. The prevalence of chlamydial infection differs by age group, with a lower prevalence among older men. In addition, the proportion of NGU caused by *C. trachomatis* has been declining. Documentation of chlamydial NGU is important because this diagnosis supports partner referral, evaluation, and treatment (CDCP, 2006; Krieger, 2000; McCormack and Rein, 2000).

Other infectious causes. The etiology of most cases of nonchlamydial NGU is unknown. The genital mycoplasmas, *Mycoplasma genitalium*, *Ureaplasma urealyticum*, and possibly *Mycoplasma hominis*, are implicated in 20–30% of cases in some series (Bradshaw et al, 2006; Gaydos et al, 2009; Ross

Table 16–1. Sexually transmitted disease (STD) syndromes.[a]

Urethritis and cervicitis[b]	Gonococcal infection Nongonococcal urethritis Chlamydial infection Mucopurulent cervicitis
Epididymitis[b]	
Genital ulcers[b]	Genital herpes simplex virus Syphilis Chancroid Lymphogranuloma venereum Granuloma inguinale (donovanosis)
Human papillomavirus (HPV) infections[b]	Genital warts Subclinical genital HPV
HIV infection[b]	
Vaginal discharge	Trichomoniasis Vulvovaginal candidiasis Bacterial vaginosis
Pelvic inflammatory disease	
Ectoparasitic infections	Pediculosis pubis Scabies
Vaccine-preventable STDs	Hepatitis A Hepatitis B
Proctitis, proctocolitis, and enteritis	
Sexual assault and STDs	

[a]According to Centers for Disease Control and Prevention: 2006 Sexually transmitted disease treatment guidelines. MMWR Morb Mortal Wkly Rep 2006:51(No. RR-11):1–100.
[b]Considered in this chapter.

et al, 2009; Stamm et al, 2007). Specific diagnostic tests for these organisms are not indicated routinely. *Trichomonas vaginalis*, a protozoan parasite, and herpes simplex virus (HSV) may also cause NGU (Gaydos et al, 2009; Hobbs et al, 2006; Martin, 2008). Testing and treatment for these organisms should be considered in situations where NGU is unresponsive to treatment (CDCP, 2006; McCormack and Rein, 2000; Shahmanesh et al, 2009).

B. Document Urethritis

It is important to document the presence of urethritis because some patients have symptoms in the absence of inflammation. Urethritis may be documented by the presence of any of the following clinical signs: mucopurulent urethral discharge on physical examination, ≥5 leukocytes per oil immersion microscopic field of the Gram-stained urethral secretions, a positive leukocyte esterase test on first-void urine, or ≥10 leukocytes per high-power microscopic field of the first-void urine (CDCP, 2006; McCormack and Rein, 2000). The Gram stain is the preferred diagnostic test for documenting urethritis and for evaluating the presence or absence of gonococcal infection because it is rapid, highly sensitive, and specific.

If none of the criteria for urethritis are met, then treatment should be deferred. The patient should be tested for both *N. gonorrhoeae* and *C. trachomatis* and followed up closely in the event of a positive test result.

Empiric treatment of symptoms without documenting the presence of urethritis is recommended only if the patient is at high risk for infection and is unlikely to return for follow-up. Empiric treatment should be appropriate for both gonococcal and chlamydial infection. Sex partners should be referred for appropriate evaluation and treatment.

C. Treatment of Gonococcal Infections

Epidemiology. There are an estimated 600,000 new gonococcal infections per year in the United States. In men, most infections cause symptoms that cause the patient to seek treatment soon enough to prevent serious sequelae. However, this may not be soon enough to prevent transmission of infection to sex partners. In contrast, many gonococcal (and also chlamydial) infections in women do not cause recognizable symptoms until the patient presents with complications, such as pelvic inflammatory disease (Mead, 2000). Symptomatic and asymptomatic pelvic inflammatory disease both result in tubal scarring, increased rates of ectopic pregnancy, and infertility.

Dual therapy for gonococcal and chlamydial infections. Dual therapy is recommended for both gonococcal and chlamydial infection because patients are often coinfected with both pathogens (CDCP, 2006; CDCP, 2007; McCormack and Rein, 2000). Quinolone-resistant *N. gonorrhoeae* have been reported from many geographic areas, and such infections are becoming widespread in parts of Asia (Ghanem et al, 2005; Perez-Losada et al, 2007; Rahman et al, 2002).

Antimicrobial resistance. Increasing antimicrobial resistance resulted in substantial changes in the gonorrhea treatment guidelines (CDCP, 2007). Fluoroquinolones (ie, ciprofloxacin, ofloxacin, or levofloxacin) were the most frequently used drugs for treating gonorrhea because of their high efficacy, ready availability, and convenience as a single-dose, oral therapy. Unfortunately, this practice resulted in increasing fluoroquinolone resistance in *N. gonorrhoeae*. Since 2000, quinolones could no longer be recommended for treating patients who acquired their infections in Asia, the Pacific Islands, or Hawaii. Progressive increases in resistance led to extension of these recommendations to patients in California in 2002, and to treatment of gonorrhea in men who have sex with men elsewhere in the United States in 2004. Recent increases in the prevalence of fluoroquinolone-resistant *N. gonorrhoeae* throughout the United States led to the conclusion that fluoroquinolones can no longer be recommended for treating gonococcal infections anywhere in the United States. Consequently, only one class of drugs, the cephalosporins, is still recommended and available for the treatment of gonorrhea (CDCP, 2007). Of the recommended cephalosporins, only cefixime is available in an oral formulation. Spectinomycin 2 g in a single dose is considered an effective alternative regime. But this drug is also not available in the United States. This means that there is only one available oral treatment recommended for gonorrhea in the United States.

Recommended regimens. Table 16–2 summarizes recommended treatment regimens for uncomplicated gonococcal infections, where the recommended treatments reliably cure ≥97% of infections (CDCP, 2006; CDCP, 2007). Pharyngeal infections are more difficult to treat, and few regimens reliably cure >90% of infections. Patients who cannot tolerate cephalosporins should be treated with spectinomycin (2 g as a single intramuscular dose). However, this regimen is only 52% effective for pharyngeal infections.

Routine test-of-cure cultures are no longer recommended for patients treated with the recommended regimens. Such patients should refer their sex partners for evaluation and treatment. However, patients should be reevaluated if their symptoms persistent after therapy. Any gonococci that persist should be evaluated for antimicrobial susceptibility. Infections identified after treatment are usually reinfections rather than treatment failures. Persistent inflammation may be caused by *C. trachomatis* or other organisms.

Complications. A few patients have complications such as disseminated gonococcal infection, perihepatitis, meningitis, or endocarditis. These infections result from gonococcal bacteremia. Disseminated gonococcal infection often causes petechial or pustular skin lesions, asymmetrical arthralgias, tenosynovitis, or septic arthritis. Occasionally, patients have perihepatitis, and rare patients have endocarditis or meningitis. *N. gonorrhoeae* strains that cause disseminated infection tend to cause minimal genital tract inflammation. The recommended treatment is ceftriaxone (1 g intramuscularly or intravenously every 24 hours for disseminated infection or 1 g intravenously every 12 hours for meningitis or endocarditis).

D. Treatment of Nongonococcal Urethritis

Treatment should be initiated as soon as possible after diagnosis (Table 16–2). Single-dose regimens are preferred because these treatments offer the advantages of improved compliance and directly observed therapy (CDCP, 2006). The recommended treatments employ either azithromycin or doxycycline. Alternative choices for patients who are allergic or cannot tolerate these drugs include a 7-day course of either erythromycin or ofloxacin. Routine follow-up and repeat testing are no longer recommended for patients taking the recommended regimens. However, patients should return for reevaluation if symptoms persist or recur after completion of treatment. The presence of symptoms alone without documentation of signs or laboratory findings of inflammation is not sufficient for retreatment. Patients should refer their sex partners for appropriate evaluation and treatment.

E. Treatment of Recurrent and Persistent Urethritis

Objective signs of urethritis should be documented before prescribing a repeat course of empirical therapy (CDCP, 2006; McCormack and Rein, 2000). Men with persistent or recurrent urethritis should be retreated with the initial regimen if they did not comply with treatment or if they were reexposed to an untreated sex partner. Other patients should have a wet mount and urethral culture for *T. vaginalis*. For patients who were compliant with the initial regimen and who were not reexposed, the regimen in Table 16–2 should be used. This provides treatment for both *T. vaginalis* and the genital mycoplasmas.

▶ Mucopurulent Cervicitis in Women

Clinical findings. Mucopurulent cervicitis holds many parallels to urethritis in men (CDCP, 2006; McCormack and Rein, 2000; Mead, 2000). Characteristically, patients have a purulent or mucopurulent endocervical exudate visible in

Table 16–2. Urethritis, cervicitis, and related infections: recommended treatment regimens.[a]

Gonococcal infections
Uncomplicated urethral, cervical, and rectal infections
Cefixime, 400 mg as a single oral dose; or ceftriaxone, 125 mg as a single IM dose; plus azithromycin, 1 g as a single oral dose; or doxycycline, 100 mg orally twice a day for 7 days
Uncomplicated pharyngeal infections[a]
Ceftriaxone, 125 mg as a single IM dose, plus azithromycin, 1 g as a single oral dose; or doxycycline, 100 mg orally twice a day for 7 days
Nongonococcal urethritis (chlamydial infections)
Azithromycin, 1 g as a single oral dose; or doxycycline, 100 mg orally twice a day for 7 days
Recurrent and persistent urethritis
Metronidazole, 2 g as a single oral dose, plus erythromycin base, 500 mg orally four times a day for 7 days; or erythromycin ethylsuccinate, 800 mg orally four times a day for 7 days

[a]According to Centers for Disease Control and Prevention: 2002 Sexually transmitted disease treatment guidelines. MMWR Morb Mortal Wkly Rep 2002;51:1; and Centers for Disease Control and Prevention. Sexually transmitted disease treatment guidelines 2006. MMWR Morb Mortal Wkly Rep 2006;51(No. RR-11)1–100.

the endocervical canal or on an endocervical swab sample. Easily induced endocervical bleeding is also common, as is an increased number of polymorphonuclear cells on the Gram-stained endocervical secretions. Patients may present with abnormal vaginal discharge or abnormal vaginal bleeding, for example, after intercourse, but many are asymptomatic.

Diagnosis and treatment. As is the case with urethritis in men, *N. gonorrhoeae* and *C. trachomatis* are the most important infectious causes of mucopurulent cervicitis. However, neither pathogen may be identified in many women. Treatment should be guided by the results of testing for gonococcal and chlamydial infection, unless the patient is considered unlikely to return for follow-up. In such cases, empirical therapy should be given for both *C. trachomatis* and *N. gonorrhoeae*.

EPIDIDYMITIS

Definition and classification. Epididymitis is a clinical syndrome characterized by pain, swelling, and epididymal inflammation. Arbitrarily, epididymitis syndromes have been classified as acute, if symptoms have been present for less than 6 weeks, or chronic if symptoms have been present for 3 months or longer. Some experts suggest that chronic epididymitis may be subcategorized by etiology into inflammatory chronic epididymitis, obstructive chronic epididymitis, and chronic epididymalgia (Nickel et al, 2002).

Etiology. Epididymitis is caused by sexually transmitted pathogens or by organisms causing urinary tract infection (CDCP, 2006; Krieger, 2000). Among sexually active men younger than 35 years, most cases of epididymitis are caused by sexually transmitted pathogens, particularly *C. trachomatis* and *N. gonorrhoeae*. Epididymitis may also be caused by *Escherichia coli* among men who are the insertive partners during anal intercourse. Sexually transmitted epididymitis is usually associated with urethritis, which is often asymptomatic. Patients with uncomplicated sexually transmitted epididymitis do not require thorough evaluation for anatomic abnormalities.

Most cases of epididymitis in men older than 35 years are associated with urinary tract infection. The most common pathogens are gram-negative enteric bacteria. Epididymitis associated with urinary infection is more common among men who have anatomic abnormalities or those who have recently had urinary tract instrumentation. Therefore, evaluation of genitourinary tract anatomy is indicated for men with epididymitis associated with urinary tract infection.

Clinical presentation and diagnosis. Epididymitis is typically associated with unilateral hemiscrotal pain and tenderness. An inflammatory hydrocele and palpable swelling of the epididymis are characteristic. Diagnostic recommendations include a Gram-stained smear for evaluation of urethritis and for presumptive identification of gonococcal infection, diagnostic testing for *N. gonorrhoeae* and *C. trachomatis*,

Table 16–3. Epididymitis: recommended treatment regimens.[a]

Gonococcal or chlamydial infection likely
Ceftriaxone, 250 mg in a single IM dose, plus doxycyline, 100 mg orally twice a day for 10 days
Enteric infection likely
Ofloxacin, 300 mg orally twice a day for 10 days, or levofloxacin, 500 mg orally once a day for 10 days

[a]According to Centers for Disease Control and Prevention: 2002 Sexually transmitted disease treatment guidelines. MMWR Morb Mortal Wkly Rep 2002;51:1; and Centers for Disease Control and Prevention: Sexually transmitted diseases treatment guidelines 2006. MMWR Morb Mortal Wkly Rep 2006;51(No. RR-11)1–100.

urine Gram stain and culture, syphilis serology, and HIV testing (if sexually transmitted epididymitis is likely).

Treatment. Outpatient management is appropriate for most patients with epididymitis. Hospitalization should be considered when severe pain suggests other possible diagnoses, such as testicular torsion, testicular infarction, or testicular abscess; when patients are febrile; or when noncompliance with medication regimens is likely (CDCP, 2006; Krieger, 2000). Empiric antimicrobial regimens are summarized in Table 16–3. Adjunctive measures include bed rest, scrotal elevation, and analgesics until fever and local inflammation subside.

Routine follow-up is recommended. Failure to respond within 3 days requires reevaluation of both the diagnosis and treatment. Swelling and tenderness that persist after completion of antimicrobial therapy should be reevaluated to consider other possible diagnoses. These conditions include testicular tumor, abscess, infarction, tuberculosis, fungal epididymitis, or collagen-vascular disorders (Cho et al, 2003; de Vries et al, 2001; Giannopoulos et al, 2001; Gul et al, 2009; Krieger, 2000; Yu-Hung Lai et al, 2009). HIV-infected patients with epididymitis should receive the same initial therapy as HIV-negative men. However, fungal infections, atypical mycobacteria, and other opportunistic infections are more likely than in nonimmunosuppressed patients.

GENITAL ULCER DISEASES

Etiology. In the United States, genital herpes (HSV) is the most common cause of genital ulcers. Other important considerations are syphilis and chancroid. In contrast, lymphogranuloma venereum (LGV) and granuloma inguinale (donovanosis) are uncommon causes of genital ulcers in this country. Each of these ulcerative STDs is associated with a two- to fivefold increased risk of HIV transmission.

Diagnostic testing. Diagnosis based solely on the history and physical findings is often inaccurate (CDCP, 2006). Patients may be infected with more than one agent simultaneously. Ideally, evaluation of patients with genital ulcers should include testing for the most common causes: HSV, syphilis, and chancroid. These tests include a culture or antigen test for HSV, a dark-field examination or direct immunofluorescence test for *Treponema pallidum* (syphilis), and a culture for *Haemophilus ducreyi* (chancroid). In the future, improved molecular detection tests may become available commercially for these organisms (Suntoke et al, 2009). After thorough diagnostic evaluation, 25% of patients with genital ulcers do not have a laboratory-confirmed diagnosis. HIV testing also should be recommended for patients who have genital ulcers (see later).

Often, patients must be treated before test results become available. In this situation, treatment is recommended for both syphilis and chancroid.

Genital Herpes Simplex Virus Infection

Clinical presentation. Genital HSV is an incurable and recurrent viral infection. Characteristic genital lesions start as painful papules or vesicles. Often, the genital lesions have evolved into pustules or ulcers when the patient is seen in the office.

Primary HSV infection. With primary genital herpes, the ulcerative lesions persist for 4–15 days until crusting or reepithelization, or both, occurs. Pain, itching, vaginal or urethral discharge, and tender inguinal adenopathy are the predominant local symptoms. Primary HSV infection is associated with a high frequency and prolonged duration of systemic and local symptoms. Fever, headache, malaise, and myalgias are common. The clinical symptoms of pain and irritation from genital lesions gradually increase over the first 6–7 days, reach maximum intensity between days 7 and 11 of disease, and then recede gradually during the second or third week.

Recurrent HSV infection. In contrast to first episodes, recurrent HSV infection is characterized by symptoms, signs, and anatomic sites localized to the genital region. Local symptoms, such as pain and itching, are mild compared with the symptoms of initial infection, and the duration of the usual episode ranges from 8 to 12 days or less.

Etiology. Two HSV serotypes cause genital ulcers, HSV-1 and HSV-2. Both viruses infect the genital tract. Studies suggest that 5–30% of first-episode cases of genital HSV infection are caused by HSV-1. However, recurrences of HSV-1 infection are substantially less likely than recurrences of HSV-2. Therefore, HSV-2 cases accumulate in the population of patients with recurrent genital lesions. Typing the infecting strain has prognostic importance and is useful for patient counseling. However, most commercially available antibody tests are not accurate enough to distinguish HSV-1 from HSV-2 infection. Better assays should become available in the future.

Epidemiology. Serologic studies suggest that 45 million people in the United States are infected with genital HSV-2. Most infections are mild or unrecognized. Therefore, most HIV-infected people do not receive this diagnosis. Such asymptomatic or mildly symptomatic persons shed virus intermittently in their genital tracts and can infect their sex partners. First-episode genital HSV infections are more likely to cause symptoms than recurrent infections. Occasional cases are severe enough to require hospitalization for complications such as disseminated infection, pneumonitis, hepatitis, meningitis, or encephalitis.

Treatment. Systemic antiviral therapy results in partial control of symptoms and signs of genital HSV infection. Treatment does not cure the infection or change the frequency or severity of recurrences after discontinuation of treatment. Three antiviral drugs have proved beneficial in randomized clinical trials: acyclovir, valacyclovir, and famciclovir (Table 16–4). Topical treatment with acyclovir has proved substantially less effective than systemic treatment.

Initial HSV episodes. Patients with first clinical episodes of genital HSV should receive antiviral treatment to speed healing of genital lesions and shorten the duration of viral shedding. Patients should also be counseled about the natural history of genital herpes, the risks for sexual and perinatal transmission, and methods to reduce transmission. Patients with severe disease should receive intravenous treatment with acyclovir.

Recurrent HSV episodes. Most persons with first clinical episodes of genital HSV-2 experience recurrent episodes. Treatment can shorten the duration of lesions and decrease recurrences. Thus, many patients can benefit from antiviral therapy, and this option should be discussed. There are two approaches to antiviral therapy for recurrent HSV: episodic treatment and daily suppressive treatment. Episodic therapy is beneficial for many patients with occasional recurrences. Such therapy is started during the prodrome or first day of lesions. Thus, patients receiving episodic therapy should receive the medication or a prescription so that they may initiate treatment at the first symptom or sign of lesions. Traditionally, 5 days of treatment has been recommended for recurrent HSV (Table 16–4), but recent data suggest that shorter (3-day) courses may work equally well (Corey et al, 2004; Wald et al, 2002; Wald et al, 2006).

Daily therapy. Daily suppressive therapy is useful for patients who experience frequent recurrences (six or more per year). Therapy reduces the frequency of recurrences by >75%. Such treatment has been shown to be safe and effective for as long as 6 years with acyclovir and for as long as 1 year with both valacyclovir and famciclovir. Daily therapy does not appear to be associated with clinically significant HSV-drug resistance. After 1 year, discontinuation of treatment should be considered, since the frequency of recurrences often decreases with time.

Syphilis

Clinical presentation. Syphilis may be the deepest and darkest subject in all of infectious diseases. This complex illness is caused by *T. pallidum*, a spirochete, and holds a special place

Table 16–4. Genital ulcers: recommended treatment regimens.[a]

Genital herpes
First episode
  Acyclovir, 400 mg orally three times a day for 7–10 days; or acyclovir, 200 mg orally five times a day for 7–10 days; or famciclovir, 250 mg orally three times a day for 7–10 days; or valacyclovir, 1 g orally twice a day for 7–10 days
Severe disease
  Acyclovir, 5–10 mg/kg body weight IV every 8 hours for 2–7 days or until clinical resolution

Recurrent episodes
Episodic recurrences
  Acyclovir, 400 mg orally three times a day for 5 days; or acyclovir, 200 mg orally five times a day for 5 days; or acyclovir, 800 mg orally twice a day for 5 days; or famciclovir, 125 mg orally twice a day for 5 days; or valacyclovir, 500 mg orally twice a day for 3–5 days; or valacyclovir, 1 g orally once a day for 5 days
Daily suppressive therapy
  Acyclovir, 400 mg orally twice a day; or famciclovir, 250 mg orally twice a day; or valacyclovir, 250 mg orally twice a day; or valacyclovir, 500 mg orally twice a day; or valacyclovir, 1 g orally once a day

Syphilis
Primary and secondary
  Benzathine penicillin G, 2.4 million units IM as a single dose
Tertiary (except neurosyphilis)
  Benzathine penicillin G, 2.4 million units IM weekly for 3 weeks
Neurosyphilis
  Aqueous crystalline penicillin G, 3–4 million units IV every 4 hours for 10–14 days; or procaine penicillin, 2.4 million units IM daily for 10–14 days, plus probenecid, 500 mg orally four times a day for 10–14 days
Latent syphilis
  Early
    Benzathine penicillin G, 2.4 million units IM as a single dose
  Late or of unknown duration
    Benzathine penicillin G, 2.4 million units IM weekly for 3 weeks

Chancroid
Azithromycin, 1 g as a single oral dose; or ceftriaxone, 250 mg as a single IM dose; or ciprofloxacin, 500 mg orally twice a day for 3 days; or erythromycin base, 500 mg orally four times a day for 7 days

Granuloma inguinale
Trimethoprim-sulfamethoxazole, 1 double-strength tablet orally twice a day for a minimum of 3 weeks; or doxycycline, 100 mg orally twice a day for a minimum of 3 weeks

Lymphogranuloma venereum
Doxycycline, 100 mg orally twice a day for 21 days

[a]According to Centers for Disease Control and Prevention: 2002 Sexually transmitted disease treatment guidelines. MMWR Morb Mortal Wkly Rep 2002;51:1; and Centers for Disease Control and Prevention: Sexually transmitted diseases treatment guidelines 2006. MMWR Morb Mortal Wkly Rep 2006;51(No. RR-11):1–100.

in the history of medicine as "the great impostor" and "the great imitator." Sir William Osler in 1897 said, "Know syphilis in all its manifestations and relations, and all other things clinical will be added unto you."

Syphilis is a systemic disease. Patients may seek treatment for symptoms of signs of primary, secondary, or tertiary infection. Primary infection is characterized by an ulcer, or chancre, at the site of infection. Secondary manifestations include rash, mucocutaneous lesions, and adenopathy. Tertiary infection may present with cardiac, neurologic, ophthalmic, auditory, or gummatous lesions. In addition, syphilis may be diagnosed by serologic testing of asymptomatic patients; this is termed latent syphilis. Latent syphilis acquired within the preceding year is classified as early latent syphilis. All other cases of latent syphilis are classified as late latent or syphilis of unknown duration.

Sexual transmission of syphilis occurs only when mucocutaneous lesions are present. These manifestations are uncommon after the first year of infection in untreated patients. However, all individuals exposed to a person with syphilis should be evaluated clinically and by serologic testing.

Diagnosis. Definitive diagnosis of early syphilis is done by dark-field examination or direct immunofluorescent antibody tests of lesion exudates, because antibodies may not be present. Presumptive diagnosis depends on serologic testing. Serologic tests are either nontreponemal, such as the Venereal Disease Research Laboratory (VDRL) and rapid plasma reagin (RPR) tests, or treponemal, such as the fluorescent treponemal antibody absorption (FTA-ABS) test and microagglutination assay for antibody to *T. pallidum* (MHA-TP). Use of only one type of serologic test is considered insufficient for diagnosis. False-positive nontreponemal tests occur with a variety of medical conditions. Nontreponemal tests correlate with disease activity, with results reported quantitatively. In general, a fourfold change in titer is considered significant. Most patients with reactive treponemal tests remain reactive for life. Treponemal test titers correlate poorly with disease activity. Thus, combination of both treponemal and nontreponemal tests is necessary for patient management.

Tremendous progress during the last decade has led to sequencing of the entire genome of *T. pallidum* and to correlation of functional activities with this genetic information (Matejkova et al, 2008; Radolf and Desrosiers, 2009). From an epidemiological perspective, the real news is that eradication of syphilis from the United States (CDCP, 2004) and from the world (Rompalo, 2001) has been established as an important public health goal, although this goal may prove difficult to achieve because of high rates of infection in certain at-risk populations (termed "core groups").

Treatment. For more than 40 years, penicillin has been the treatment of choice for syphilis (Table 16–4). Patients who are allergic to penicillin should receive a 2-week course of doxycycline (100 mg orally twice daily) or tetracycline (500 mg orally four times a day). Treatment results in healing of local lesions and prevents sexual transmission and late sequelae. Patients with syphilis should be tested for HIV infection. In areas with a high prevalence of HIV, this test should be repeated after 3 months if the initial HIV test is negative. Patients with syphilis and symptoms or signs of ophthalmic disease should have a slit-lamp examination and those with symptoms or signs of neurologic disease should have cerebrospinal fluid evaluation. Treatment failures occur with any regimen. Thus, serologic testing should be repeated 6 and 12 months after initial treatment.

Chancroid

Etiology and clinical presentation. Chancroid is an acute ulcerative disease, often associated with inguinal adenopathy ("bubo"). *H. ducreyi*, a gram-negative facultative bacillus, is the causative agent. The infection is endemic in parts of the United States and the disease also occurs in outbreaks. It is estimated that 10% of patients with chancroid are coinfected with either *T. pallidum* or HSV. Each of these ulcerative infections is associated with an increased rate of HIV transmission.

Diagnosis. Definitive diagnosis of chancroid requires identification of the causative bacterium, *H. ducreyi*, on specialized culture media that are not widely available. In addition, these media have an estimated sensitivity <80%. In practice, a probable diagnosis of chancroid may be based on the following: the patient has a painful genital ulcer; there is no evidence of *T. pallidum* by dark-field examination or by a negative syphilis serologic test at least 7 days before the onset of ulcers; an HSV test is negative; and the clinical appearance is typical. The combination of a painful genital ulcer and tender inguinal adenopathy suggests the diagnosis of chancroid. Unfortunately, this characteristic clinical appearance occurs in only one-third of cases. However, the combination of a painful genital ulcer and suppurative inguinal adenopathy is considered almost pathognomonic. The combination of a human model of infection with new molecular methods has resulted in improved understanding of *H. ducreyi* genes and virulence factors (Janowicz et al, 2009; Labandeira-Rey et al, 2009; Suntoke et al, 2009).

Treatment. Recommended antimicrobial regimens are summarized in Table 16–4. Appropriate treatment of chancroid cures the infection, resolves symptoms, and prevents transmission. Successful treatment results in dramatic resolution of ulcers and symptoms. However, scarring can continue in extensive cases despite successful treatment. Uncircumcised or HIV-infected patients may respond less well to treatment. Testing for HIV and syphilis is recommended at the time of diagnosis and again 3 months later, if the initial test results for syphilis or HIV were negative.

Follow-up evaluation is recommended after 3–7 days. If there is minimal or no clinical improvement, consider another diagnosis or the possibility of coinfection with another STD. A few *H. ducreyi* strains are resistant to antimicrobial agents. Large ulcers or fluctuant lymphadenopathy may take >2 weeks for resolution. Occasionally, patients require incision and drainage or needle aspiration of fluctuant inguinal nodes.

Lymphogranuloma Venereum

Etiology and clinical presentation. LGV is caused by the invasive serovars of *C. trachomatis* (L1, L2, and L3). The disease is a rare cause of genital ulcers in the United States.

Tender inguinal or femoral lymphadenopathy, or both, often unilateral, is the characteristic clinical presentation in heterosexual men. Women and homosexual men may present with inflammatory involvement of perirectal and perianal lymphatics, strictures, fistulas, or proctocolitis. The self-limited genital ulcers have usually healed when most patients seek medical care. In most cases, diagnosis is made by serologic testing plus exclusion of other causes of inguinal adenopathy or genital ulcers.

Treatment. Therapy causes microbiological cure and prevents ongoing tissue destruction (Table 16–4). Doxycycline is preferred. Erythromycin and azithromycin are alternatives. Prolonged therapy, for a minimum of 3 weeks, is necessary with each of these drugs. However, tissue reaction and scarring can progress after effective treatment. Inguinal adenopathy, known as "bubos," may require needle aspiration through intact skin or incision and drainage to prevent inguinal or femoral ulcerations. Patients should be followed up until clinical symptoms and signs are resolved.

Granuloma Inguinale (Donovanosis)

Etiology and epidemiology. Granuloma inguinale is caused by *Calymmatobacterium granulomatis*, a gram-negative intracellular bacillus that has many similarities to *Klebsiella* species (O'Farrell, 2002; O'Farrell et al, 2008). This infection is rare in the United States. Granuloma inguinale is an important cause of genital ulcers in tropical and developing countries, particularly India, Papua New Guinea, central Australia, and southern Africa.

Clinical presentation. Clinically, granuloma inguinale presents with painless, progressive genital ulcers. The genital lesions are highly vascular, with a "beefy red" appearance. Patients seldom have inguinal adenopathy. The causative organism cannot be cultured on standard microbiologic media. Diagnosis requires visualization of dark-staining Donovan bodies on tissue crush preparations or biopsy specimens. Molecular diagnostic tests should be available in the near future (Behets et al, 1999; O'Farrell et al, 2008). Secondary bacterial infections may develop in the lesions. In addition, coinfection with other STD agents may occur.

Treatment. Effective treatment halts progressive tissue destruction (Table 16–4). Trimethoprim–sulfamethoxazole or doxycycline is recommended. Alternative drugs are ciprofloxacin or erythromycin. Azithromycin also appears promising (O'Farrell, 2002). Prolonged duration of treatment is often necessary to facilitate granulation and reepithelization of the ulcers. Patients should be reevaluated after the first few days of treatment. Addition of an aminoglycoside, such as gentamicin, should be considered if lesions have not responded. Treatment should be continued until all lesions have healed. Relapse can occur 6–18 months after effective initial therapy.

▶ Genital Warts

Etiology. Genital warts are caused by human papillomavirus (HPV) infection. Of the more than 80 HPV genotypes, more than 20 infect the genital tract. Most of these genital HPV infections are asymptomatic, subclinical, or unrecognized. Depending on their size and anatomic locations, visible external warts can be painful, friable, pruritic, or all three. Most visible genital warts are caused by HPV types 6 or 11. These HPV types can also cause exophytic warts on the cervix and within the vagina, urethra, and anus. HPV types 6 and 11 are only rarely associated with development of invasive squamous cell carcinoma of the external genitalia.

HPV types 16, 18, 31, 33, and 35 are uncommon in visible, external genital warts. These HPV types are associated with cervical dysplasia, as well as vaginal, anal, and cervical squamous cell carcinoma. HPV types 16, 18, 31, 33, and 35 have also been associated with external genital intraepithelial neoplastic lesions, including squamous cell carcinoma, carcinoma *in situ*, bowenoid papulosis, erythroplasia of Queyrat, and Bowen's disease. Patients with external genital warts can be infected simultaneously with multiple HPV types.

Diagnosis. Most often, the diagnosis of genital warts can be made by inspection. Diagnosis can be confirmed by biopsy, if necessary, although biopsy is rarely necessary for diagnosis. Biopsy is indicated if the diagnosis is uncertain; if lesions do not respond to standard therapy; if the disease worsens during treatment; if the patient is immunocompromised; or if warts are pigmented, indurated, fixed, or ulcerated. Routine use of type-specific HPV nucleic acid tests is not indicated for diagnosis or management of visible genital warts (CDCP, 2006).

Treatment. For visible genital warts, the primary goal of treatment is removal of symptomatic lesions. Treatment can induce wart-free periods in most patients. Genital warts are often asymptomatic, and clinical lesions may resolve spontaneously. Currently, there are no data indicating that available therapy can eradicate HPV infection or change the natural history of infection. In theory, removal of exophytic warts may decrease infectivity, but there is no evidence that treatment changes the risk for development of dysplastic or cancerous lesions in the patient or in sexual partners.

Treatment decisions should be guided by the provider's experience and patient preferences. None of the recommended therapies is superior or ideal for every case. Current treatments can be considered as patient applied or provider administered (Table 16–5). Most patients with visible warts

Table 16–5. External genital warts: Recommended treatment regimens.[a]

Patient applied
Podofilox, 0.5% solution of gel to lesions twice a day for 3 days, followed by 4 days off therapy; repeat as needed for up to 4 cycles; or imiquimod, 5% cream to lesions at bedtime 3 times a week for up to 16 weeks; wash off after 6–10 hours

Provider administered
Cryotherapy with liquid nitrogen or cryoprobe; repeat as necessary every 1–2 weeks; or podophyllin resin, 10–25% in tincture of benzoin; repeat weekly as necessary; or trichlor/bichloracetic acid, 80–90%; apply until white "frosting"; repeat weekly as necessary; or surgical removal (laser surgery), or intralesional interferon

[a]According to Centers for Disease Control and Prevention: 2002 Sexually transmitted disease treatment guidelines. MMWR Morb Mortal Wkly Rep 2002;51:1; and Centers for Disease Control and Prevention: Sexually transmitted diseases treatment guidelines 2006. MMWR Morb Mortal Wkly Rep 2006;51(No. R-11):1–100.

have lesions that respond to most treatment modalities. Many patients require a course of therapy. In general, lesions on moist surfaces or in intertriginous areas respond better to topical treatments, such as trichloroacetic acid, podophyllin, or imiquimod, than do warts on drier surfaces.

Podofilox is an antimitotic drug that results in destruction of warts. Most patients experience pain or local irritation after treatment. Imiquimod is a topically active immune enhancer that stimulates production of cytokines, followed by local inflammation and resolution of warts (Cook and Brownell, 2008; Stefanaki et al, 2008). Effective use of cryotherapy requires training to avoid either overtreatment or undertreatment and poor results. Pain is common after application of the liquid nitrogen, followed by necrosis of the warts. Podophyllin resin contains several antimitotic compounds. Different resin preparations vary in the concentrations of active components and contaminants. Although both trichloroacetic acid and bichloracetic acid are recommended and are used widely, these treatments are associated with several potential problems. The acid can spread rapidly if applied excessively, with damage to normal adjacent tissues. These solutions should be applied sparingly and allowed to dry before the patient stands. If the patient experiences excessive discomfort, the acid can be neutralized by using soap or sodium bicarbonate (baking soda). Recent data suggest that the treatment approach should be changed if a patient has not improved substantially after three provider-administered treatments or if warts do not resolve completely after six treatments.

Surgical removal offers the advantage of rendering the patient wart free in a single visit. Several approaches are possible, including tangential scissor or shave excision, curettage, electrosurgery, or laser surgery. All of these methods require local anesthesia and are more time consuming and expensive than the methods discussed in the previous paragraph. Surgical approaches are most useful for patients who have a large number or a large volume of genital warts, if the diagnosis is uncertain, or if patients have been unresponsive to other treatments. Patients should be warned that scarring, hypopigmentation, and hyperpigmentation are common after ablative therapies. Occasionally, patients have chronic pain after such treatment.

Recurrence of warts is common after all therapies, with most recurrences occurring within the first 3 months. Women should be counseled about the need for regular cervical cytologic screening. Examination of sex partners is unnecessary for management of external genital warts, because the role of reinfection is probably minimal. However, sex partners of patients with genital warts may benefit from evaluation for genital warts and other STDs. Recent availability of highly effective, multivalent HPV vaccines offer the opportunity to substantially improve the clinical epidemiology of HPV infection by vaccinating adolescents prior to initiation of sexual activity (Koutsky et al, 2002; Munoz et al, 2009; Paavonen et al, 2009).

SUBCLINICAL GENITAL HPV INFECTION

Subclinical HPV infection (without visible genital warts) is more common than visible genital lesions. Most cases are diagnosed indirectly by cervical cytology, colposcopy, or biopsy of genital skin, or by routine use of acetic acid soaks and examination with magnification for "acetowhite" areas. The consensus of expert opinion is to discourage routine examination for "acetowhitening" (CDCP, 2006). This test has poor specificity for HPV infection. In addition, the acetowhite test has many false-positive results in low-risk populations. Definitive diagnosis of subclinical HPV infection requires detection of HPV nucleic acid or capsid protein, but these tests are not recommended outside of research settings.

Treatment of subclinical HPV infection is not recommended in the absence of dysplasia. Diagnosis is often questionable because many of the diagnostic tests (ie, cytology, acetowhitening, colposcopy) correlate poorly with detection of HPV, DNA, or RNA. Furthermore, no therapy has been proved to eradicate infection. HPV has been demonstrated in normal-appearing tissue adjacent to treated areas after aggressive surgical treatment.

HIV INFECTION: OVERVIEW OF DETECTION, INITIAL EVALUATION, AND REFERRAL

Infection with HIV includes a wide clinical spectrum, ranging from asymptomatic infection to AIDS. The rate of clinical progression is highly variable. Some persons progress from HIV infection to AIDS within a few months; others remain asymptomatic for decades. Overall, the median time from infection to AIDS is around 10 years. In general, adults with HIV infection remain asymptomatic for prolonged periods.

However, HIV viral replication continues during all stages of infection, with substantial increases in the viral burden during later stages of infection, accompanied by marked deterioration in immune functions.

Increasing awareness of risk factors for HIV infection has led to increased testing and earlier diagnosis for many patients. The primary risk factors for HIV infection are sexual contact with an HIV-infected person and sharing injecting-drug equipment.

Early diagnosis is important because treatment can slow down the decline in immune function (CDCP, 2006). HIV-infected persons with evidence of immune dysfunction are at risk for preventable infections. Prophylactic treatment can substantially reduce the risk for pneumonia (*Pneumocystis carinii* and bacterial), toxoplasma encephalitis, and mycobacterial disease (tuberculosis and *Mycobacterium avium* complex). Early diagnosis also facilitates patient counseling, which may reduce transmission. In addition, early diagnosis facilitates planning for referral to a health-care provider/facility experienced in care of HIV-infected persons.

▶ Testing for HIV

Diagnostic testing for HIV should be offered to anyone at risk for infection, especially those seeking evaluation for STDs. Appropriate pre- and posttest counseling and informed consent should be included in the test procedure. Some states required documentation of informed consent.

Usually, HIV infection is documented using HIV-1 antibody tests. HIV antibodies are detected in >95% of infected persons within 6 months of infection. In most laboratories, this is a two-stage procedure beginning with a sensitive screening test, such an enzyme immunoassay. Reactive screening test results are then confirmed by a supplemental test, such as the Western blot, or an immunofluorescence assay. Patients with positive results on both the screening and confirmatory tests are infected with HIV. Such infected persons can transmit HIV.

In the United States, almost all HIV infections are caused by HIV-1. Extremely rare cases are caused by a second virus, HIV-2. Thus, routine clinical testing for HIV-2 is not recommended. The only indications are in blood centers or for persons who have specific demographic or behavioral risk factors for HIV-2. These person's risk factors include those from countries where HIV-2 is endemic (West Africa, Angola, Mozambique, France, and Portugal) or their sex partners come from endemic areas. The possibility of HIV-2 infection should also be considered in situations where there is clinical suspicion of HIV disease in the absence of a positive HIV-1 antibody test.

▶ Acute Retroviral Syndrome

This syndrome occurs in many persons shortly after HIV infection, before antibody tests are positive. The syndrome is characterized by acute symptoms and signs, including fever, malaise, lymphadenopathy, and skin rash. Suspicion of acute retroviral syndrome should prompt nucleic acid testing to detect HIV. New data suggest that early initiation of treatment during this period can result in a lower HIV viral burden, delayed HIV-related complications, and perhaps immune reconstitution.

▷ Initial Management of HIV Infection

It is advisable to refer HIV-infected persons to a single clinical resource for comprehensive care (Centers for Disease Control and Prevention, 2006). Because of the limited availability of these facilities, it is often advisable to initiate evaluation and provide access to psychosocial services while planning for referral and continuation of medical care. Thus, brief consideration of initial management is in order.

Recently diagnosed HIV infection may not have been acquired recently. Persons with newly diagnosed HIV infection can be at any of the clinical stages of infection. Thus, it is important to be alert for signs and symptoms that suggest advanced infection, such as fever, weight loss, diarrhea, oral candidiasis, cough, or shortness of breath. These findings suggest the need for urgent referral.

In nonemergent situations, the recommended evaluation of a person with a newly diagnosed HIV infection includes a detailed medical history that emphasizes sexual and substance abuse history, previous STDs, and specific HIV-related symptoms or diagnoses. The physical examination should include a pelvic examination in women, with Pap smear and testing for gonorrhea and chlamydial infection. Recommended blood work includes complete blood count with platelet count; chemistry profile; testing for toxoplasma antibody and hepatitis viral markers; syphilis serologic test; and a $CD4^+$ T-lymphocyte count (Centers for Disease Control and Prevention, 2006). Other evaluations should include a tuberculin skin test and chest x-ray. Finally, provision should be made for evaluation and management of sex and injecting-drug partners.

HIV and circumcision. Three large, well-conducted randomized clinical trials showed that adult male circumcision reduces HIV infection rates by approximately 60% in high-risk heterosexual populations (Auvert et al, 2005; Bailey et al, 2007; Gray et al, 2007). These findings are consistent with substantial epidemiological data from the developing world and more limited data from the United States (Warner et al, 2009). Fortunately, the adult male circumcision procedures were done under local anesthesia with low complication rates (Auvert et al, 2005; Bailey et al, 2007; Gray et al, 2007; Krieger et al, 2007). Importantly, prospective data suggest that there was no adverse effect on male sexual function or satisfaction (Kigozi et al, 2008; Krieger et al, 2008). These data form the basis for implementation of programs to promote safe male circumcision in high-risk populations (Nagelkerke et al, 2007). This urological procedure is one of very few public health interventions that hold promise to reduce HIV infection rates.

BIBLIOGRAPHY

Auvert B et al: Randomized, controlled intervention trial of male circumcision for reduction of HIV infection risk: The ANRS 1265 Trial. PLoS Med 2005;2:e298.

Bailey RC et al: Male circumcision for HIV prevention in young men in Kisumu, Kenya: A randomised controlled trial. Lancet 2007;369:643–656.

Behets FM et al: Chancroid, primary syphilis, genital herpes, and lymphogranuloma venereum in Antananarivo, Madagascar. J Infect Dis 1999;180:1382–1385.

Bradshaw CS et al: Etiologies of nongonococcal urethritis: Bacteria, viruses, and the association with orogenital exposure. J Infect Dis 2006;193:336–345.

Centers for Disease Control and Prevention. Congenital syphilis—United States, 2002. MMWR Morb Mortal Wkly Rep 2004;53:716–719.

Centers for Disease Control and Prevention. Sexually transmitted diseases treatment guidelines 2006. MMWR Morb Mortal Wkly Rep 2006;51(No. RR-11):1–100.

Centers for Disease Control and Prevention. Update to CDC's sexually transmitted diseases treatment guidelines, 2006: Fluoroquinolones no longer recommended for treatment of gonococcal infections. MMWR Morb Mortal Wkly Rep 2007;56:332–336.

Cho YH et al: Clinical features of patients with Behcet's disease and epididymitis. J Urol 2003;170:1231–1233.

Cook K, Brownell I: Treatments for genital warts. J Drugs Dermatol 2008;7:801–807.

Corey L et al: Once-daily valacyclovir to reduce the risk of transmission of genital herpes. N Engl J Med 2004;350:11–20.

de Vries M et al: Polyarteritis nodosa presenting as an acute bilateral epididymitis. Arch Intern Med 2001;161:1008.

Gaydos CA et al: *Mycoplasma genitalium* compared to *Chlamydia*, Gonorrhea, and Trichomonas as an etiologic agent of urethritis in men attending STD clinics. Sex Transm Infect 2009;85:438–440.

Ghanem KG et al: Fluoroquinolone-resistant *Neisseria gonorrhoeae*: The inevitable epidemic. Infect Dis Clin North Am 2005;19: 351–365.

Giannopoulos A et al: Epididymitis caused by *Candida glabrata*: A novel infection in diabetic patients? Diabetes Care 2001;24:2003–2004.

Gray RH et al: Male circumcision for HIV prevention in men in Rakai, Uganda: A randomised trial. Lancet 2007;369:657–666.

Gul HC et al: Epididymoorchitis due to *Brucella melitensis*: Review of 19 patients. Urol Int 2009;82:158–161.

Hobbs MM et al: Methods for detection of *Trichomonas vaginalis* in the male partners of infected women: Implications for control of trichomoniasis. J Clin Microbiol 2006;44:3994–3999.

Janowicz DM et al: Experimental infection of human volunteers with *Haemophilus ducreyi*: Fifteen years of clinical data and experience. J Infect Dis 2009;199:1671–1679.

Kigozi G et al: The effect of male circumcision on sexual satisfaction and function, results from a randomized trial of male circumcision for human immunodeficiency virus prevention, Rakai, Uganda. BJU Int 2008;101:65–70.

Koutsky LA et al: A controlled trial of a human papillomavirus type 16 vaccine. N Engl J Med 2002;347:1645–1651.

Krieger JN: Prostatitis, epididymitis and orchitis. In: Mandell GL et al (eds) Mandell, Douglas, and Bennett's Principles and Practice of Infectious Diseases, 15th ed, Vol. 1. Churchill-Livingstone, Philadelphia, 2000, pp. 1243–1251.

Krieger JN et al: Adult male circumcision outcomes: Experience in a developing country setting. Urol Int 2007;78:235–240.

Krieger JN et al: Adult male circumcision: Effects on sexual function and sexual satisfaction in Kisumu, Kenya. J Sex Med 2008;5: 2610–2622.

Labandeira-Rey M et al: Inactivation of the *Haemophilus ducreyi* luxS gene affects the virulence of this pathogen in human subjects. J Infect Dis 2009;200:409–416.

Martin DH: Nongonococcal urethritis: New views through the prism of modern molecular microbiology. Curr Infect Dis Rep 2008;10: 128–132.

Matejkova P et al: Complete genome sequence of *Treponema pallidum* ssp. pallidum strain SS14 determined with oligonucleotide arrays. BMC Microbiol 2008;8:76.

McCormack WM, Rein M: Urethritis. In: Mandell GL et al (eds) Mandell, Douglas, and Bennett's Principles and Practice of Infectious Diseases, 5th ed, Vol. 1. Churchill-Livingstone, Philadelphia, 2000, pp. 1208–1218.

Mead PB: Infections of the female pelvis. In: Mandell GL et al (eds) Mandell, Douglas, and Bennett's Principles and Practice of Infectious Diseases, 5th ed, Vol. 1. Churchill-Livingstone, Philadelphia, 2000, pp. 1235–1243.

Munoz N et al: Safety, immunogenicity, and efficacy of quadrivalent human papillomavirus (types 6, 11, 16, 18) recombinant vaccine in women aged 24–45 years: A randomised, double-blind trial. Lancet 2009;373:1949–1957.

Nagelkerke NJ et al: Modelling the public health impact of male circumcision for HIV prevention in high prevalence areas in Africa. BMC Infect Dis 2007;7:16.

Nickel JC et al: The patient with chronic epididymitis: Characterization of an enigmatic syndrome. J Urol 2002;167:1701–1704.

O'Farrell N: Donovanosis. Sex Transm Infect 2002;78:452–457.

O'Farrell N et al: Genital ulcers and concomitant complaints in men attending a sexually transmitted infections clinic: Implications for sexually transmitted infections management. Sex Transm Dis 2008;35:545–549.

Paavonen J et al: Efficacy of human papillomavirus (HPV)-16/18 AS04-adjuvanted vaccine against cervical infection and precancer caused by oncogenic HPV types (PATRICIA): Final analysis of a double-blind, randomised study in young women. Lancet 2009;374(9686):301–314.

Perez-Losada M et al: Distinguishing importation from diversification of quinolone-resistant *Neisseria gonorrhoeae* by molecular evolutionary analysis. BMC Evol Biol 2007;7:84.

Radolf JD, Desrosiers DC: *Treponema pallidum*, the stealth pathogen, changes, but how? Mol Microbiol 2009;72:1081–1086.

Rahman M et al: Antimicrobial susceptibility of *Neisseria gonorrhoeae* isolated in Bangladesh (1997 to 1999): Rapid shift to fluoroquinolone resistance. J Clin Microbiol 2002;40:2037–2040.

Rompalo AM: Can syphilis be eradicated from the world? Curr Opin Infect Dis 2001;14:41–44.

Ross J et al: *Mycoplasma genitalium* in asymptomatic patients—implications for screening. Sex Transm Infect 2009;85(6): 436–437.

Shahmanesh M et al: 2009 European guideline on the management of male non-gonococcal urethritis. Int J STD AIDS 2009;20: 458–464.

Stamm WE et al: A randomized, double-blind study comparing single-dose rifalazil with single-dose azithromycin for the empirical treatment of nongonococcal urethritis in men. Sex Transm Dis 2007;34:545–552.

Stefanaki C et al: Comparison of cryotherapy to imiquimod 5% in the treatment of anogenital warts. Int J STD AIDS 2008;19: 441–444.

Suntoke TR et al: Evaluation of multiplex real-time PCR for detection of *Haemophilus ducreyi*, *Treponema pallidum*, herpes simplex virus type 1 and 2 in the diagnosis of genital ulcer disease in the Rakai District, Uganda. Sex Transm Infect 2009;85:97–101.

Wald A et al: Two-day regimen of acyclovir for treatment of recurrent genital herpes simplex virus type 2 infection. Clin Infect Dis 2002;34:944–948.

Wald A et al: Comparative efficacy of famciclovir and valacyclovir for suppression of recurrent genital herpes and viral shedding. Sex Transm Dis 2006;33:529–533.

Warner L et al: Male circumcision and risk of HIV infection among heterosexual African American men attending Baltimore sexually transmitted disease clinics. J Infect Dis 2009;199:59–65.

Yu-Hung Lai A et al: Tuberculous epididymitis presenting as huge scrotal tumor. Urology 2009;73:1163.e5–1163.e7.

Urinary Stone Disease

17

Marshall L. Stoller, MD

Urinary calculi are the third most common affliction of the urinary tract, exceeded only by urinary tract infections and pathologic conditions of the prostate. They are common in both animals and humans. The nomenclature associated with urinary stone disease arises from a variety of disciplines. Struvite stones, for example, composed of magnesium ammonium phosphate hexahydrate, are named in honor of H.C.G. von Struve (1772–1851), a Russian naturalist. Before the time of von Struve, the stones were referred to as guanite, because magnesium ammonium phosphate is prominent in bat droppings. Calcium oxalate dihydrate is frequently referred to as weddellite, because it was commonly found in floor samples collected from the Weddell Sea in Antarctica. The history of the nomenclature associated with urinary stone disease is as intriguing as that of the development of the interventional techniques used in their treatment.

Urinary stones have plagued humans since the earliest records of civilization. The etiology of stones remains speculative. If urinary constituents are similar from each kidney and if there is no evidence of obstruction, why do most stones present in a unilateral fashion? Why do not small stones pass uneventfully down the ureter early in their development? Why do some people form one large stone and others form multiple small calculi? There is much speculation concerning these and other questions.

Advances in the surgical treatment of urinary stones have outpaced our understanding of their etiology. As clinicians, we are concerned with an expedient diagnosis and efficient treatment. Equally important is a thorough metabolic evaluation directing appropriate medical therapy and lifestyle changes to help reduce recurrent stone disease. Without such follow-up and medical intervention, stone recurrence rates can be as high as 50% within 5 years. Uric acid calculi can recur even more frequently. Physicians look forward to gaining a better understanding of this multifactorial disease process in hopes of developing more effective prophylaxis.

RENAL AND URETERAL STONES

▶ Etiology

Mineralization in all biologic systems has a common theme in that the crystals and matrix are intertwined. Urinary stones are no exception; they are polycrystalline aggregates composed of varying amounts of crystalloid and organic matrix. Theories to explain urinary stone disease are incomplete.

Stone formation requires supersaturated urine. Supersaturation depends on urinary pH, ionic strength, solute concentration, and complexation. Urinary constituents may change dramatically during different physiologic states from a relatively acid urine in a first morning void to an alkaline tide noted after meals. Ionic strength is determined primarily by the relative concentration of monovalent ions. As ionic strength increases, the activity coefficient decreases. The activity coefficient reflects the availability of a particular ion.

The role of solute concentrations is clear: The greater the concentration of two ions, the more likely they are to precipitate. Low ion concentrations result in undersaturation and increased solubility. As ion concentrations increase, their activity product reaches a specific point termed the *solubility product (K_{sp})*. Concentrations above this point are metastable and are capable of initiating crystal growth and heterogeneous nucleation. As solutions become more concentrated, the activity product eventually reaches the formation product (K_{fp}). Supersaturation levels beyond this point are unstable, and spontaneous homogeneous nucleation may occur.

Multiplying two ion concentrations reveals the concentration product. The concentration products of most ions are greater than established solubility products. Other factors must play major roles in the development of urinary calculi, including complexation. Complexation influences the availability of specific ions. For instance, sodium complexes with oxalate and decreases its free ionic form, while sulfates can complex with calcium. Crystal formation is modified by a variety of other substances found in the urinary tract, including magnesium, citrate, pyrophosphate, and a variety of trace metals. These inhibitors may act at the active crystal growth sites or as inhibitors in solution (as with citrate).

The nucleation theory suggests that urinary stones originate from crystals or foreign bodies immersed in supersaturated urine. This theory is challenged by the same arguments that support it. Stones do not always form in patients who are hyperexcretors or who are at risk for dehydration. Additionally, up to a third of stone formers' 24-hour urine collections are completely normal with respect to stone-forming ion concentrations.

The crystal inhibitor theory claims that calculi form due to the absence or low concentration of natural stone inhibitors including magnesium, citrate, pyrophosphate, and a variety of trace metals. This theory does not have absolute validity, since many people lacking such inhibitors may never form stones, and others with an abundance of inhibitors may, paradoxically, form them.

A. Crystal Component

Stones are composed primarily of a crystalline component. Crystals of adequate size and transparency are easily identified under a polarizing microscope. X-ray diffraction is preferred to assess the geometry and architecture of calculi. A group of stones from the same geographic location or the same historical time period typically have crystalline constituents that are common.

Multiple steps are involved in crystal formation, including nucleation, growth, and aggregation. Nucleation initiates the stone process and may be induced by a variety of substances, including proteinaceous matrix, crystals, foreign bodies, and other particulate tissues. Heterogeneous nucleation (epitaxy), which requires less energy and may occur in less saturated urine, is a common theme in stone formation. It should be suspected whenever an oriented conglomerate is found. A crystal of one type thereby serves as a nidus for the nucleation of another type with a similar crystal lattice. This is frequently seen with uric acid crystals initiating calcium oxalate formation. It takes time for these early nidi to grow or aggregate to form a stone incapable of passing with ease through the urinary tract.

How these early crystalline structures are retained in the upper urinary tract without uneventful passage down the ureter is unknown. The theory of mass precipitation or intranephronic calculosis suggests that the distal tubules or collecting ducts, or both, become plugged with crystals, thereby establishing an environment of stasis, ripe for further stone growth. This explanation is unsatisfactory; tubules are conical in shape and enlarge as they enter the papilla (ducts of Bellini), thereby reducing the possibility of ductal obstruction. In addition, urine transit time from the glomerulus into the renal pelvis is only a few minutes, making crystal aggregation and growth within the uriniferous tubules unlikely.

The fixed particle theory postulates that formed crystals are somehow retained within cells or beneath tubular epithelium. Alexander Randall noted whitish-yellow precipitations of crystalline substances occurring on the tips of renal papillae as submucosal plaques. These plaques are associated with both the vasa recta and the urinary collecting ducts and grow deep within the papilla. The tips of the plaques can be appreciated during endoscopy of the upper urinary tract. Carr hypothesized that calculi form in obstructed lymphatics and then rupture into adjacent fornices of a calyx. Arguing against Carr's theory are the grossly visible early stone elements in areas remote from fornices.

B. Matrix Component

The amount of the noncrystalline, matrix component of urinary stones varies with stone type, commonly ranging from 2% to 10% by weight. It is composed predominantly of protein, with small amounts of hexose and hexosamine. An unusual type of stone called a matrix calculus can be associated with previous kidney surgery or chronic urinary tract infections and has a gelatinous texture (Figure 17–1). Histologic inspection reveals laminations with scant calcifications. On plain abdominal radiographs, matrix calculi are usually radiolucent and can be confused with other filling defects, including blood clots, upper-tract tumors, and fungal bezoars. Noncontrast computed tomography (CT) reveals calcifications and can help to confirm the diagnosis. The role of matrix in the initiation of ordinary urinary stones as well as matrix stones is unknown. It may serve as a nidus for crystal aggregation or as a naturally occurring glue to adhere small crystal components and thereby hinder uneventful passage down the urinary tract. Alternatively, matrix may have an inhibitory role in stone formation or may be an innocent bystander, playing no active role in stone formation.

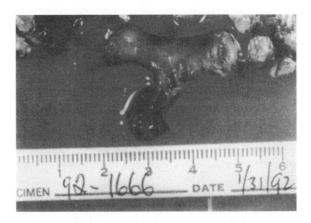

▲ **Figure 17–1.** Gross picture of matrix calculus percutaneously extracted after extracorporeal shock wave lithotripsy failure.

▶ Urinary Ions

A. Calcium

Calcium is a major ion present in urinary crystals. The risk of urinary stones increases as fractional calcium absorption from the gut increases; calcium absorption from the gut decreases with increased calcium intake. Only 50% of plasma calcium is ionized and available for filtration at the glomerulus. More than 95% of the calcium filtered at the glomerulus is reabsorbed at both the proximal and distal tubules and limited amounts in the collecting tube. Less than 2% is excreted in the urine. Diuretic medications may exert a hypocalciuric effect by further decreasing calcium excretion. Many factors influence the availability of calcium in solution, including complexation with citrate, phosphate, and sulfate. An increase in monosodium urates and a decrease in urinary pH further interfere with this complexation and therefore promote crystal aggregation.

B. Oxalate

Oxalate is a normal waste product of metabolism and is relatively insoluble. Normally, approximately 10–15% of oxalate found in the urine originates from the diet; the vast majority is a metabolic by-product. Most of the oxalate that enters the large bowel is consumed by bacterial decomposition. Oxalobacter formigenes may alter the availability of oxalate absorption. Diet, however, can have an impact on the amount of oxalate found in the urine. Once absorbed from the small bowel, oxalate is not metabolized and is excreted almost exclusively by the proximal tubule. The presence of calcium within the bowel lumen is an important factor influencing the amount of oxalate that is absorbed. The control of oxalate in the urine plays a pivotal role in the formation of calcium oxalate calculi. Normal excretion ranges from 20 to 45 mg/day and does not change significantly with age. Excretion is higher during the day when one eats. Small changes in oxalate levels in the urine can have a dramatic impact on the supersaturation of calcium oxalate. The important precursors of oxalate are glycine and ascorbic acid; however, the impact of ingested vitamin C (<2 g/day) is negligible.

Hyperoxaluria may develop in patients with bowel disorders, particularly inflammatory bowel disease, small-bowel resection, and bowel bypass. Renal calculi develop in 5–10% of patients with these conditions. Chronic diarrhea with fatty stools results in a saponification process. Intraluminal calcium binds to the fat, thereby becoming unavailable to bind to oxalate. The unbound oxalate is readily absorbed from the gut and increases urinary oxalate levels.

Excessive oxalate may occur secondary to the accidental or deliberate ingestion of ethylene glycol (partial oxidation to oxalate). This may result in diffuse and massive deposition of calcium oxalate crystals and may occasionally lead to renal failure.

C. Phosphate

Phosphate is an important buffer and complexes with calcium in urine. It is a key component in calcium phosphate and magnesium ammonium phosphate stones. The excretion of urinary phosphate in normal adults is related to the amount of dietary phosphate (especially in meats, dairy products, and vegetables). The small amount of phosphate filtered by the glomerulus is predominantly reabsorbed in the proximal tubule. Parathyroid hormone inhibits this reabsorption. The predominant crystal found in patients with hyperparathyroidism is phosphate, in the form of hydroxyapatite, amorphous calcium phosphate, and carbonate apatite.

D. Uric Acid

Uric acid is the by-product of purine metabolism. The pK_a of uric acid is 5.75. Undissociated uric acid predominates with pH values less than this. Elevated pH values increase urate, which is soluble. Approximately 10% of the filtered uric acid finds its way into the urine. Other defects in purine metabolism may result in urinary stone disease. Rarely, a defect in xanthine dehydrogenase results in increased levels of xanthine; the xanthine may precipitate in urine, resulting in stone formation. Unusual alterations in adenine metabolism may result in the production of 2,8-dihydroxyadeninuria, which is poorly soluble in urine and may develop into a urinary stone. This results from a deficiency of adenine phosphoribosyltransferase (APRT). Pure uric acid crystals and calculi are relatively radiolucent and may not be identified on plain abdominal films (Figure 17–2). They are visible on noncontrast CT images and are suggestive when found to have low Hounsfield units (HU). Some uric acid calculi may be partially radiopaque, however, because of associated calcium phosphate deposits.

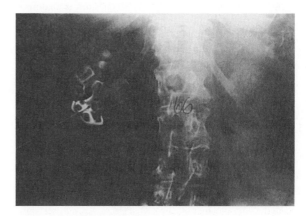

▲ **Figure 17–2.** Radiolucent right staghorn renal calculus appreciated after percutaneous injection of radiocontrast material. This uric acid stone was effectively removed in a single percutaneous procedure. Postoperative urinary alkalinization has been effective prophylaxis.

E. Sodium

Although not identified as one of the major constituents of most urinary calculi, sodium plays an important role in regulating the crystallization of calcium salts in urine. Sodium is found in higher than expected concentrations in the core of renal calculi and may play a role in initiating crystal development and aggregation. High dietary sodium intake increases urinary calcium excretion and increases the urinary levels of monosodium urates that promote stone growth. This reduces the ability of urine to inhibit calcium oxalate crystal agglomeration. These effects are thought to be due to a sodium-induced increase in bicarbonaturia and decrease in serum bicarbonate. Interestingly, increased dietary sodium intake increases ones thirst and increases voided volumes. Conversely, a reduction in dietary sodium helps to reduce recurrent calcium nephrolithiasis.

F. Citrate

Citrate is a key factor affecting the development of calcium urinary stones. A deficiency commonly is associated with stone formation in those with chronic diarrhea or renal tubular acidosis type I (distal tubular defect) and in patients prescribed chronic thiazide therapy. Citrate plays a pivotal role in the citric acid cycle in renal cells. Metabolic stimuli that consume this product (as with intracellular metabolic acidosis due to fasting, hypokalemia, or hypomagnesemia) reduce the urinary excretion of citrate. Estrogen increases citrate excretion and may be a factor that decreases the incidence of stones in women, especially during pregnancy. Alkalosis also increases citrate excretion.

G. Magnesium

Dietary magnesium deficiency is associated with an increased incidence of urinary stone disease. Magnesium is a component of struvite calculi. Experimentally, lack of dietary magnesium is associated with increased calcium oxalate stone formation and calcium oxalate crystalluria. The exact mechanism whereby magnesium exerts its effect is undefined. Dietary magnesium supplements typically do not protect against stone formation.

H. Sulfate

Urinary sulfates may help prevent urinary calculi. They can complex with calcium. These sulfates occur primarily as components of longer urinary proteins, such as chondroitin sulfate and heparin sulfate.

I. Other Urinary Stone Inhibitors

Inhibitors of urinary stone formation other than citrate, magnesium, and sulfates have been identified. These consist predominantly of urinary proteins and other macromolecules such as glycosaminoglycans, pyrophosphates, and uropontin. Although citrate appears to be the most active inhibitory component in urine, these substances demonstrate a substantial role in preventing urine crystal formation. The N-terminal amino acid sequence and the acidic amino acid content of these protein inhibitors, especially their high aspartic acid content, appear to play pivotal inhibitory roles. Fluoride may be an inhibitor of urinary stone formation.

▶ Stone Varieties

A. Calcium Calculi

Calcifications can occur and accumulate in the collecting system, resulting in nephrolithiasis. Eighty to eighty-five percent of all urinary stones are calcareous.

Calcium nephrolithiasis is most commonly due to elevated urinary calcium, elevated urinary uric acid, elevated urinary oxalate, or a decreased level of urinary citrate. Hypercalciuria is found as a solitary defect in 12% of patients and in combination with other defects in an additional 18%. Hyperuricosuria is identified as a solitary defect in 8% of patients and associated with additional defects in 16%. Elevated urinary oxalate is found as a solitary finding in 5% of patients and as a combined defect in 16%. Finally, decreased urinary citrate is found as an isolated defect in 17% of patients and as a combined defect in an additional 10%. Approximately one-third of patients undergoing a full metabolic evaluation will find no identifiable metabolic defect.

Symptoms from stones are secondary to obstruction, with resultant pain, infection, nausea, and vomiting, and rarely culminate in renal failure. Asymptomatic hematuria or repetitive urinary tract infections recalcitrant to apparently appropriate antibiotics should lead one to suspect a possible urinary stone. Calcifications within the parenchyma of the kidney, known as nephrocalcinosis, rarely cause symptoms, however, and usually are not amenable to traditional therapies appropriate for urinary stone disease (Figure 17–3). Nephrocalcinosis is frequently encountered with renal tubular acidosis and hyperparathyroidism. Nephrolithiasis and nephrocalcinosis frequently coexist. Most patients with nephrolithiasis, however, do not have obvious nephrocalcinosis.

Nephrocalcinosis may result from a variety of pathologic states. Ectatic collecting tubules, as seen with medullary sponge kidney, are common; this is frequently a bilateral process. Theoretically, obstructed collecting ducts may be a source of chronic flank pain. Increased calcium absorption from the small bowel is common with sarcoidosis, milk-alkali syndrome, hyperparathyroidism, and excessive vitamin D intake. Disease processes resulting in bony destruction, including hyperparathyroidism, osteolytic lesions, and multiple myeloma, are a third mechanism. Finally, dystrophic calcifications forming on necrotic tissue may develop after a renal insult.

1. Absorptive hypercalciuric nephrolithiasis—Normal calcium intake averages approximately 900–1000 mg/day. Approximately one-third is absorbed by the small bowel,

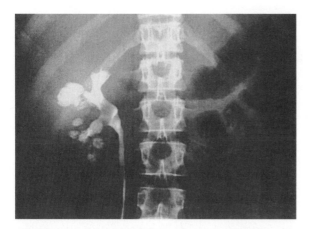

▲ **Figure 17–3.** Retrograde pyelogram demonstrating multiple punctate calcifications within the renal parenchyma establishing the diagnosis of nephrocalcinosis. Renal pelvis and infundibula are free of calculi.

and of that portion, approximately 150–200 mg is obligatorily excreted in the urine. A large reservoir of calcium remains in the bone. Most dietary calcium is excreted in the stool. Absorptive hypercalciuria is secondary to increased calcium absorption from the small bowel, predominantly from the jejunum. This results in an increased load of calcium filtered from the glomerulus. The result is suppression of parathyroid hormone, leading to decreased tubular reabsorption of calcium, culminating in hypercalciuria (>4 mg/kg). This physiologic cascade is in response to the primary defect, an increased absorption of calcium from the small bowel.

Absorptive hypercalciuria traditionally has been subdivided into three types. Type I absorptive hypercalciuria is independent of diet and represents 15% of all calcareous calculi. There is an elevated urinary calcium level (>150–200 mg/24 hour) even during a calcium-restricted diet. Cellulose phosphate is an effective nonabsorbable exchange resin. This effectively binds the calcium in the gut, preventing bowel absorption. Cellulose phosphate has no impact on the calcium transport defect. Urinary calcium excretion returns to normal values with therapy.

Cellulose phosphate must be taken with meals to be available when calcium is ingested. A typical dose is 10–15 g orally in three divided doses and is well tolerated. This therapy is relatively contraindicated in postmenopausal women and in children during their active growth cycles. Inappropriate use may lead to a negative calcium balance and a secondary hyperparathyroid state. As with all stone formers, long-term follow-up is required. Cellulose phosphate may bind other cations besides calcium, including magnesium. Secondary hyperoxaluria may develop owing to decreased calcium in the gut. See the section on hyperoxaluria for a more detailed discussion.

Hydrochlorothiazides are an alternative, more common treatment for type I absorptive hypercalciuria. Initially, there is a reduction in renal excretion of calcium. The increased absorbed calcium is likely deposited in bone. Eventually, the bone reservoir reaches its capacity and the drug becomes less effective. Hydrochlorothiazides have limited long-term efficacy (approximately 3–5 years). These drugs have no effect on the defective bowel transport system. Hydrochlorothiazides may be alternated with cellulose phosphate as an effective treatment regimen.

Type II absorptive hypercalciuria is dietary dependent. There is no specific medical therapy. Calcium excretion returns to normal on a calcium-restricted diet. These are the rare patients that should limit their calcium intake to 400–600 mg/day. Type II absorptive hypercalciuria is not as severe as type I.

Type III absorptive hypercalciuria is secondary to a phosphate renal leak and accounts for 5% of all urinary calculi. Decreased serum phosphate leads to an increase in 1,25-dihydroxyvitamin D synthesis. The physiologic cascade culminates in an increased absorption of phosphate, and calcium, from the small bowel and an increased renal excretion of calcium—hence its classification as absorptive hypercalciuria. Successful treatment replaces bioavailable phosphate. Orthophosphate (Neutra-Phos, now available over the counter) inhibits vitamin D synthesis and is best taken as 250 mg three to four times daily. It is best taken after meals and before bedtime. Orthophosphates do not alter intestinal calcium absorption.

2. Resorptive hypercalciuric nephrolithiasis—A subset (<10%) of patients with clinically obvious primary hyperparathyroidism present with nephrolithiasis. This group represents less than 5% of all patients with urinary stones and are more commonly seen in women. Patients with calcium phosphate stones, women with recurrent calcium stones, and those with both nephrocalcinosis and nephrolithiasis should be suspected of having hyperparathyroidism. Hypercalcemia and an elevated serum parathyroid level are the most consistent signs of hyperparathyroidism.

Parathyroid hormone results in a cascade of events starting with an increase in urinary phosphorus and a decrease in plasma phosphorus, followed by an increase in plasma calcium and a decrease in urinary calcium. Its action on the kidney and on the bone is independent of each other. Ultimately, renal damage is secondary to the hypercalcemia. It limits the concentrating ability of the kidney and impairs the kidney's ability to acidify urine. Surgical removal of the offending parathyroid adenoma is the most effective way of treating this disease. However, up to 25% of these patients will develop new urinary stones after successful surgery, most commonly seen in men. Attempts at long-term medical management are challenging.

3. Renal-induced hypercalciuric nephrolithiasis—Hypercalciuria of renal origin is due to an intrinsic renal tubular defect in calcium excretion. This creates a physiologically vicious cycle. Excessive urinary calcium excretion results in a relative decrease in serum calcium, which leads to a secondarily increased parathyroid hormone level that mobilizes calcium from the bone and increases calcium absorption from the gut. This step completes the pathologic cycle by delivering increased levels of calcium back to the kidney, whereby the renal tubules excrete large amounts of calcium. These patients have an elevated fasting urinary calcium level, normal serum calcium level, and a secondarily elevated parathyroid hormone level.

Renal hypercalciuria is effectively treated with hydrochlorothiazides. Unlike their role in type I absorptive hypercalciuria, in this setting hydrochlorothiazides have a durable long-term effect. As a diuretic, they decrease the circulating blood volume and subsequently stimulate proximal tubular absorption of calcium as well as other constituents. They also increase reabsorption at the distal tubule. Both mechanisms correct the secondary hyperparathyroid state.

Hypercalciuric states may result in elevated parathyroid levels. To help differentiate primary hyperparathyroidism from secondary hyperparathyroidism in patients with urinary stone disease, one can prescribe a hydrochlorothiazide challenge (50 mg twice a day for 7–10 days). Patients with secondary hyperparathyroidism will have a return to normal serum parathyroid levels, while those with primary hyperparathyroidism will continue to have elevated serum values.

4. Hyperuricosuric calcium nephrolithiasis—Hyperuricosuric calcium nephrolithiasis is due to either an excessive dietary intake of purines or an increase in endogenous uric acid production. In both situations, there is an increase in urinary monosodium urates. Monosodium urates absorb and adsorb urinary stone inhibitors and facilitate heterogeneous nucleation.

Patients have elevated urinary uric acid levels (>600 mg/24 hour in women and >750 mg/24 hour in men) and consistently have a urinary pH >5.5. The urinary pH helps to differentiate hyperuricosuric calcium from hyperuricosuric uric acid stone formation.

Patients with excessive purine oral intake can be successfully treated by changing to a low purine diet. Those with excessive endogenous uric acid production can be treated with allopurinol. Allopurinol is a xanthine oxidase inhibitor and reduces uric acid synthesis and renal excretion of uric acid. It also inhibits uric acid–calcium oxalate crystallization. Allopurinol has many potential side effects, including a variety of skin rashes and, rarely, liver toxicity. Potassium citrate is an alternative treatment, especially when associated with hypocitraturia.

5. Hyperoxaluric calcium nephrolithiasis—Hyperoxaluric calcium nephrolithiasis is secondary to increased urinary oxalate levels (>40 mg/24 hour). It is frequently found in patients with inflammatory bowel disease or other chronic diarrheal states that result in severe dehydration. It is rarely associated with excessive oxalate intake, as seen in poisoning with ethylene glycol or endogenous overproduction.

Chronic diarrheal states alter oxalate metabolism. Malabsorption leads to increased luminal fat and bile salts. Intraluminal gut calcium readily and preferentially binds to fat and bile resulting in a saponification process. The intraluminal gut calcium that normally would have bound to oxalate is thus decreased. The unbound oxalate is readily absorbed and is unaffected by the usual metabolic inhibitors of energy-dependent pumps. Bile salts may increase the passive bowel absorption of oxalate. A small increase in oxalate absorption and subsequent urinary excretion dramatically increases the formation product of calcium oxalate. This increases the potential for heterogeneous nucleation and crystal growth in this metastable environment. All patients with increased urinary excretion of oxalate do not necessarily form calcium oxalate calculi, other factors must be contributory.

Enteric hyperoxaluric calcium nephrolithiasis is successfully treated with oral calcium supplementation. The calcium binds to the intraluminal oxalate and thus limits its absorption. It must be given with meals when the oxalate is present. Other oral cations are effective binders including magnesium supplements. An alternative therapy includes a diet limited to medium-chain fatty acids and triglycerides; however, it is poorly tolerated by patients. Equally difficult is an attempt to alter oxalate intake. Unless large amounts of specific oxalate-rich foods can be excluded, an alternative diet may result in *increased* oxalate levels.

Primary hyperoxaluria is a rare hereditary disease. It is associated with calcium oxalate renal calculi, nephrocalcinosis, and other distant deposits of oxalate, culminating in progressive renal failure and eventual death. Type I is associated with an enzyme deficiency of 2-oxoglutarate:glyoxylate carboligase, resulting in elevated urinary levels of glycolic acid and oxalic acid. Type II has increased excretory levels of L-glyceric acid rather than elevated levels of glycolic acid. It is associated with a D-glycerate dehydrogenase enzyme deficiency. This ultimately results in the accumulation of hydroxy pyruvate, which is eventually converted to oxalate. Oxalate crystal deposits develop rapidly in transplanted kidneys. Combined liver and renal transplantation has cured this previously fatal rare disease.

6. Hypocitraturic calcium nephrolithiasis—Citrate is an important inhibitor of urinary stone disease. Increased metabolic demands on the mitochondria of proximal renal tubular cells decrease the excretion of citrate. Such conditions include intracellular metabolic acidosis, hypokalemia (as with thiazide therapy), fasting, hypomagnesemia, androgens, gluconeogenesis, and an acid-ash diet. Citrate may be consumed in the urine by bacteria during a urinary tract infection. The cause of hypocitraturia may be unknown in some cases. In contrast, alkalosis, alkaline-ash diet, estrogen, and vitamin D increase urinary citrate levels.

Citrate acts in solution and complexes with calcium. This decreases the ionic calcium concentration and thus the activity

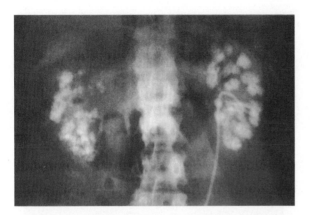

▲ **Figure 17–4.** Scout abdominal radiograph demonstrating bilateral, multiple renal calculi in a patient with renal tubular acidosis, type I.

product. Citrate decreases agglomeration, spontaneous nucleation, and crystal growth of calcium oxalate. It also decreases calcium oxalate calculi by decreasing monosodium urates that can absorb inhibitors and facilitate heterogeneous nucleation.

Hypocitraturic (<450 mg/24 h) calcium nephrolithiasis is associated commonly with renal tubular acidosis type I (distal tubule) (Figure 17–4), thiazide therapy (accompanied by potassium wastage), and chronic diarrhea. Treatment is successful with potassium citrate supplementation. Routine dosage is 20–30 mEq two to three times daily (tablet, crystal or liquid preparation) and is usually well tolerated. Six to eight glasses of lemonade can increase urinary citrate excretion by approximately 150 mg/24 h and thus either limit or eliminate the need for pharmacologic citrate supplementation.

B. Noncalcium Calculi

1. Struvite—Struvite stones are composed of magnesium, ammonium, and phosphate (MAP). They are found most commonly in women and may recur rapidly. They frequently present as renal staghorn configured calculi (branched with stones occupying the renal pelvis and at least to renal infundibuli) and rarely present as obstructing ureteral stones except after surgical intervention (Figure 17–5). Struvite stones are infection stones associated with urea-splitting organisms, including *Proteus, Pseudomonas, Providencia, Klebsiella, Staphylococci,* and *Mycoplasma*. The high ammonium concentration derived from the urea-splitting organisms results in an alkaline urinary pH. The urinary pH of a patient with a MAP stone rarely is <7.2 (normal urinary pH is 5.85). It is only at this elevated urinary pH (>7.19) that MAP crystals precipitate. MAP crystals are soluble in the normal urinary pH range of 5–7. Preoperative bladder cultures do not necessarily reflect the bacteriologic composition found in calculi. Foreign bodies and neurogenic bladders may predispose patients to urinary infections and subsequent struvite

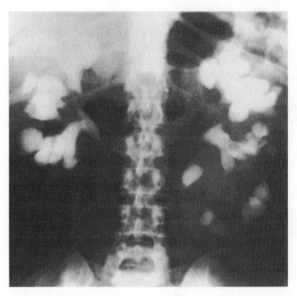

▲ **Figure 17–5.** Scout abdominal radiograph demonstrating large bilateral struvite staghorn calculi. Patient was treated for many years with numerous antibiotics for recurrent urinary tract infections. Only after this radiograph were calculi identified and removed and the infections resolved.

stone formation. Massive diuresis does not prevent struvite calculi. Women with recurrent non–*Escherichia coli* urinary infections despite apparently appropriate antibiotic therapy should be evaluated for struvite calculi with a conventional kidney–ureter–bladder (KUB) radiograph or renal ultrasound, or both. It is impossible to sterilize such calculi with antibiotics. Culture-specific antibiotics can reduce urease levels and help reduce stone recurrence. Stone removal is therapeutic.

Long-term management is optimized with the removal of all foreign bodies, including catheters of all varieties. A short ileal loop urinary diversion helps decrease the risk of stones in those with supravesical urinary diversion. All stone fragments should be removed with or without the aid of follow-up irrigations. Hemiacidrin (Renacidin) irrigations should be used with caution if at all. Rapid magnesium toxicity can result in death even with a low-pressure irrigation setup (<20 cm water pressure) and negative daily urine cultures. Acetohydroxamic acid inhibits the action of bacterial urease, thereby reducing the urinary pH and decreasing the likelihood of precipitation. Most patients have a difficult time tolerating this medication.

2. Uric acid—Uric acid stones comprise <5% of all urinary calculi and are usually found in men. Patients with gout, myeloproliferative diseases, or rapid weight loss and those treated for malignant conditions with cytotoxic drugs have an increased incidence of uric acid lithiasis. Most patients with uric acid calculi, however, do not have hyperuricemia. Elevated urinary uric acid levels are frequently due to dehydration and excessive purine intake. Patients present with a urinary pH consistently <5.5, in contrast to patients with hyperuricosuric calcium nephrolithiasis, who have a urinary pH >5.5. As the urinary pH increases above the dissociation constant pK_a of 5.75, it dissociates into a relatively soluble urate ion. Treatment is centered on maintaining a urine volume >2 L/day and a urinary pH >6.0. Reducing dietary purines or the administration of allopurinol also helps reduce uric acid excretion. Alkalinization, however, is the mainstay of therapy (with oral sodium bicarbonate, potassium bicarbonate, potassium citrate, or intravenous 1/6 normal sodium lactate) and may dissolve calculi (the rate of dissolution is dependent on the stone surface area). Stone fragments after lithotripsy have a dramatically increased surface area compared with intact stones and thus will dissolve more rapidly. Dissolution proceeds at approximately 1 cm of stone (as seen on KUB) per month, with compliant alkalinization.

3. Cystine—Cystine lithiasis is secondary to an inborn error of metabolism resulting in abnormal intestinal (small bowel) mucosal absorption and renal tubular absorption of dibasic amino acids, including cystine, ornithine, lysine, and arginine. The genetic defects associated with cystinuria have now been mapped to chromosome 2p.16 and more recently to 19q13.1. Cystine lithiasis is the only clinical manifestation of this defect. Classic cystinuria is inherited in an autosomal recessive fashion. Homozygous expression has a prevalence of 1:20,000, while the heterozygous expression is 1:2000. It represents 1–2% of all urinary stones, with a peak incidence in the second or third decade. Homozygous cystinurics excrete more than 250 mg/day, resulting in constant supersaturation. Heterozygous patients usually excrete 100–150 mg/day. Unaffected patients typically excrete <40 mg/day. Approximately 400 mg/L of cystine can remain in solution at a urinary pH of 7.0. As the urinary pH increases above 7.0, the amount of soluble cystine increases exponentially.

The solubility of cystine is pH dependent, with a pK of approximately 8.1. There is no difference in the solubility curves in normal versus patients with cystinuria. There is no known inhibitor for cystine calculi, and cystine stone formation is completely dependent on excessive cystine excretion. Cystine stones are frequently associated with calcium calculi and their related metabolic abnormalities. They may present as single, multiple, or staghorn configured stones. The diagnosis is suspected in patients with a family history of urinary stones and the radiographic appearance of a faintly opaque, ground-glass, smooth-edged stone (Figure 17–6). Urinalysis frequently reveals hexagonal crystals. The stones have an amber color. Stone analysis confirms the diagnosis. Quantitative urinary cystine evaluation helps confirm the diagnosis and differentiate heterozygous from homozygous states. It is also important to help titrate medical therapy.

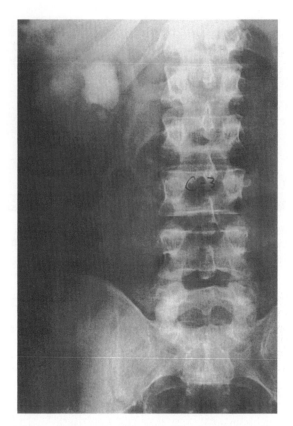

▲ **Figure 17–6.** Scout radiograph demonstrating a right cystine calculus. Note ground-glass appearance with smooth edges.

Medical therapy includes high fluid intake (>3 L/d, day and night) and urinary alkalinization. Patients should monitor their pH with Nitrazine indicator paper and keep their pH values above 7.5. It is difficult or impossible to maintain levels >8.0. A low-methionine (precursor to cystine) diet has limited impact, as most of the cystine is endogenous and most of the ingested methionine is incorporated into protein. Glutamine, ascorbic acid, and captopril are effective in some patients. Penicillamine can reduce urinary cystine levels. It complexes with the amino acid, and this complex is dramatically more soluble. Treatment should be titrated with quantitative urinary cystine values. Many patients poorly tolerate penicillamine, reporting skin rashes (discrete or confluent macules with occasional itching), loss of taste, nausea, vomiting, and anorexia. It may inhibit pyridoxine, which should be supplemented during treatment (50 mg/d). Mercaptopropionylglycine (Thiola), 300–1200 mg in divided doses, with initial dosing matched with total quantitative cystine excretion (mg per mg) forms a soluble complex with cystine and can reduce stone formation and is the most commonly used sulfide-binding drug. Side effects and frequent dosing, however, decrease patient compliance.

Surgical treatment is similar to that for other stones except that most stones are recalcitrant to extracorporeal shock wave lithotripsy (SWL). One should have a low threshold to proceed with percutaneous stone extraction in symptomatic patients. Despite optimum medical therapy, a high stone recurrence rate frequently frustrates both patient and physician. Minimally invasive techniques and optimum medical therapy are paramount.

4. Xanthine—Xanthine stones are secondary to a congenital deficiency of xanthine dehydrogenase. This enzyme normally catalyzes the oxidation of hypoxanthine to xanthine and of xanthine to uric acid. It is of interest that allopurinol, used to treat hyperuricosuric calcium nephrolithiasis and uric acid lithiasis, produces iatrogenic xanthinuria. Blood and urine levels of uric acid are lowered, and hypoxanthine and xanthine levels are increased; however, there are no case reports of xanthine stone formation resulting from allopurinol treatment. It is unlikely that allopurinol completely inhibits xanthine dehydrogenase. Urinary stones develop in approximately 25% of patients with this enzymatic deficiency. The stones are radiolucent and are tannish yellow in color. Treatment should be directed by symptoms and evidence of renal obstruction. High fluid intake and urinary alkalinization are required for prophylaxis. If stones recur, a trial of allopurinol and a purine-restricted diet is appropriate.

5. Indinavir—Protease inhibitors are a popular and effective treatment in patients with acquired immunodeficiency syndrome. Indinavir is the most common protease inhibitor that results in radiolucent stones in up to 6% of patients who are prescribed this medication. Indinavir calculi are the only urinary stones to be radiolucent on noncontrast CT scans. They may be associated with calcium components and in these situations will be visible on noncontrast CT images. Temporary cessation of the medication with intravenous hydration frequently allows these stones to pass. The stones are tannish red and usually fall apart during basket extraction.

6. Rare—Silicate stones are very rare and are usually associated with long-term use of antacids containing silica. Surgical treatment is similar to that of other calculi.

Triamterene stones are radiolucent and have been identified with an increased frequency. They are associated with antihypertensive medications containing triamterene, such as Dyazide. Discontinuing the medication eliminates stone recurrences. Other medications that may become stone constituents include glafenine and antrafenine.

Rarely, patients arrive at an emergency room at an odd hour feigning signs and symptoms of passing a urinary stone in hopes of obtaining pain medications. They may add blood to their urine and give a believable story of a severe allergy to intravenous contrast medium. Occasionally, patients present a fake urinary stone, with specks of paint or other obvious curiosities. Such patients have Munchausen syndrome, and the diagnosis is difficult and made by exclusion.

▶ Symptoms and Signs at Presentation

Upper-tract urinary stones frequently cause pain when passing down the ureter. The character of the pain depends on the location. Calculi small enough to venture down the ureter usually have difficulty passing through the ureteropelvic junction, or entering the bladder at the ureterovesical junction (Figure 17–7). More than 60% of patients presenting with ureteral colic will have stones within 3 cm of the ureterovesical junction.

A. Pain

Renal colic and noncolicky renal pain are the two types of pain originating from the kidney. Renal colic usually is caused by stretching of the collecting system or ureter, whereas noncolicky renal pain is caused by distention of the renal capsule. These symptoms may overlap, making a clinical differentiation difficult or impossible. Urinary obstruction is the main mechanism responsible for renal colic. This may be mimicked by the pain a patient experiences when a retrograde ureteropyelogram is performed under local anesthesia, with excessive pressure resulting in overdistention of the collecting system. This pain is due to a direct increase in intraluminal pressure, stretching nerve endings.

Renal colic does not always wax and wane or come in waves like intestinal or biliary colic but may be relatively constant. Renal colic implies an intraluminal origin. Patients with renal calculi have pain primarily due to urinary obstruction.

Local mechanisms such as inflammation, edema, hyperperistalsis, and mucosal irritation may contribute to the perception of pain in patients with renal calculi. In the ureter, however, local pain is referred to the distribution of the ilioinguinal nerve and the genital branch of the genitofemoral nerve, whereas pain from obstruction is referred to the same areas as for collecting system calculi (flank and costovertebral angle), thereby allowing discrimination.

The vast majority of urinary stones present with the acute onset of pain due to acute obstruction and distention of the upper urinary tract. The severity and location of the pain can vary from patient to patient due to stone size, stone location, degree of obstruction, acuity of obstruction, and variation in individual anatomy (eg, intrarenal vs extrarenal pelvis). The stone burden does not correlate with the severity of the symptoms. Small ureteral stones frequently present with severe pain, whereas large staghorn configured calculi may present with a dull ache or flank discomfort.

The pain frequently is abrupt in onset and severe, and may awaken a patient from sleep. The severity of the pain is worsened by the unexpected nature of its onset. Patients frequently move constantly into unusual positions in an attempt to relieve the pain. This movement is in contrast to the lack of movement of someone with peritoneal signs; such a patient lies in a stationary position.

The symptoms of acute renal colic depend on the location of the calculus; several regions may be involved: renal calyx,

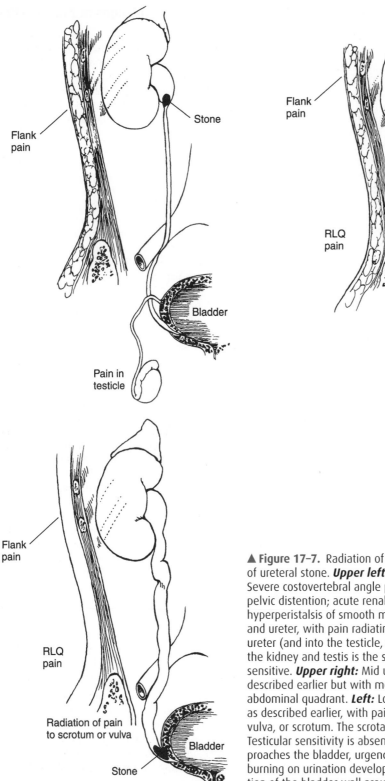

▲ **Figure 17–7.** Radiation of pain with various types of ureteral stone. ***Upper left:*** Ureteropelvic stone. Severe costovertebral angle pain from capsular and pelvic distention; acute renal and urethral pain from hyperperistalsis of smooth muscle of calyces, pelvis, and ureter, with pain radiating along the course of the ureter (and into the testicle, since the nerve supply to the kidney and testis is the same). The testis is hypersensitive. ***Upper right:*** Mid ureteral stone. Same as described earlier but with more pain in the lower abdominal quadrant. ***Left:*** Low ureteral stone. Same as described earlier, with pain radiating into bladder, vulva, or scrotum. The scrotal wall is hyperesthetic. Testicular sensitivity is absent. When the stone approaches the bladder, urgency and frequency with burning on urination develop as a result of inflammation of the bladder wall around the ureteral orifice.

renal pelvis, upper and mid ureter, and distal ureter. An orderly progression of symptoms as a stone moves down the urinary tract is the exception.

1. Renal calyx—Stones or other objects in calyces or caliceal diverticula may cause obstruction and renal colic. In general, nonobstructing stones cause pain only periodically, owing to intermittent obstruction. The pain is a deep, dull ache in the flank or back that can vary in intensity from severe to mild. The pain may be exacerbated after consumption of large amounts of fluid. Radiographic imaging may not reveal evidence of obstruction despite the patient's complaints of intermittent symptoms. It remains unclear how much of this pain is related to local mucosal irritation with activation of chemoreceptors. The presence of infection or inflammation in the calyx or diverticulum (eg, milk of calcium) in addition to obstruction may contribute to pain perception. Caliceal calculi occasionally result in spontaneous perforation with urinoma, fistula, or abscess formation.

Caliceal calculi are frequently small and numerous and appear to be able to pass spontaneously. Long-term retention against the flow of urine and against the forces of gravity and antegrade peristalsis suggests a significant element of obstruction. Effective long-term treatment requires stone extraction and elimination of the obstructive component.

Pain relief has been reported in many patients following SWL for small symptomatic caliceal calculi. Thus, if a patient continues to complain of pain in the face of a small caliceal calculus, SWL treatment may be justified for both diagnosis and treatment. Percutaneous, retrograde, and laparoscopic techniques have been successful in the management of calculi in calyces or caliceal diverticula.

2. Renal pelvis—Stones in the renal pelvis >1 cm in diameter commonly obstruct the ureteropelvic junction, generally causing severe pain in the costovertebral angle, just lateral to the sacrospinalis muscle and just below the 12th rib. This pain may vary from dull to excruciatingly sharp and is usually constant, boring, and difficult to ignore. It often radiates to the flank and also anteriorly to the upper ipsilateral abdominal quadrant. It may be confused with biliary colic or cholecystitis if on the right side and with gastritis, acute pancreatitis, or peptic ulcer disease if on the left, especially if the patient has associated anorexia, nausea, or emesis. Acquired or congenital ureteropelvic junction obstruction may cause a similar constellation of symptoms. Symptoms frequently occur on an intermittent basis following a drinking binge or consumption of large quantities of fluid.

Partial or complete staghorn configured calculi that are present in the renal pelvis are not necessarily obstructive. In the absence of obstruction, these patients often have surprisingly few symptoms such as flank or back pain. Recurrent urinary tract infections frequently culminate in radiographic evaluation with the discovery of a large calculus. If untreated, these "silent" staghorn calculi can often lead to significant morbidity, including renal deterioration, infectious complications, or both.

3. Upper and mid-ureter—Stones or other objects in the upper or mid ureter often cause severe, sharp back (costovertebral angle) or flank pain. The pain may be more severe and intermittent if the stone is progressing down the ureter and causing intermittent obstruction. A stone that becomes lodged at a particular site may cause less pain, especially if it is only partially obstructive. Stationary calculi that result in high-grade but constant obstruction may allow autoregulatory reflexes and pyelovenous and pyelolymphatic backflow to decompress the upper tract, with diminution in intraluminal pressure gradually easing the pain. Pain associated with ureteral calculi often projects to corresponding dermatomal and spinal nerve root innervation regions. The pain of upper ureteral stones thus radiates to the lumbar region and flank. Midureteral calculi tend to cause pain that radiates caudally and anteriorly toward the mid and lower abdomen in a curved, band-like fashion. This band initially parallels the lower costal margin but deviates caudad toward the bony pelvis and inguinal ligament. The pain may mimic acute appendicitis if on the right or acute diverticulitis if on the left side, especially if concurrent gastrointestinal symptoms are present.

4. Distal ureter—Calculi in the lower ureter often cause pain that radiates to the groin or testicle in males and the labia majora in females. This referred pain is often generated from the ilioinguinal or genital branch of the genitofemoral nerves. Diagnosis may be confused with testicular torsion or epididymitis. Stones in the intramural ureter may mimic cystitis, urethritis, or prostatitis by causing suprapubic pain, urinary frequency and urgency, dysuria, stranguria, or gross hematuria. Bowel symptoms are not uncommon. In women, the diagnosis may be confused with menstrual pain, pelvic inflammatory disease, and ruptured or twisted ovarian cysts. Strictures of the distal ureter from radiation, operative injury, or previous endoscopic procedures can present with similar symptoms. This pain pattern is likely due to the similar innervation of the intramural ureter and bladder.

B. Hematuria

A complete urinalysis helps to confirm the diagnosis of a urinary stone by assessing for hematuria and crystalluria and documenting urinary pH. Patients frequently admit to intermittent gross hematuria or occasional tea-colored urine (old blood). Most patients will have at least microhematuria. Rarely (in 10–15% of cases), complete ureteral obstruction presents without microhematuria.

C. Infection

Magnesium ammonium phosphate (struvite) stones are synonymous with infection stones. They are commonly associated with *Proteus, Pseudomonas, Providencia, Klebsiella,* and

Staphylococcus infections. They are rarely, if ever, associated with *E. coli* infections. Calcium phosphate stones are the second variety of stones associated with infections. Calcium phosphate stones with a urine pH <6.4 are frequently referred to as brushite stones, whereas infectious apatite stones have a urinary pH >6.4. Rarely, matrix stones with minimal crystalline components are associated with urinary tract infections. All stones, however, may be associated with infections secondary to obstruction and stasis proximal to the offending calculus. Culture-directed antibiotics should be administered before elective intervention.

Infection may be a contributing factor to pain perception. Uropathogenic bacteria may alter ureteral peristalsis by the production of exotoxins and endotoxins. Local inflammation from infection can lead to chemoreceptor activation and perception of local pain with its corresponding referral pattern.

1. Pyonephrosis—Obstructive calculi may culminate in the development of pyonephrosis. Unlike pyelonephritis, pyonephrosis implies gross purulent urine in an obstructed collecting system. It is an extreme form of infected hydronephrosis. Presentation is variable and may range from asymptomatic bacteriuria to florid urosepsis. Bladder urine cultures may be negative. Radiographic investigations are frequently nondiagnostic. Renal ultrasonography may be misguiding because of the nonspecific and variable appearance of pyonephrosis. Renal urine aspiration is the only way to make the definitive diagnosis. If the condition is noted at the time of a percutaneous nephrolithotomy, the procedure should be aborted to allow for adequate percutaneous drainage and treatment with appropriate intravenous antibiotics (Figure 17–8). If unrecognized and untreated, pyonephrosis may develop into a renocutaneous fistula.

2. Xanthogranulomatous pyelonephritis—Xanthogranulomatous pyelonephritis is associated with upper-tract obstruction and infection. Ultimately, this is a pathologic diagnosis with characteristic foamy macrophages. One-third of patients present with calculi; two-thirds present with flank pain, fever, and chills. Fifty percent of patients present with persistent bacteriuria. Urinalysis usually shows numerous red and white cells. This condition is a common imitator of other pathologic states of the kidney. It usually presents in a unilateral fashion. Laparoscopic or open surgical procedures, such as a simple nephrectomy for minimal or nonrenal function, can be challenging owing to marked and extensive reactive tissues.

D. Associated Fever

The association of urinary stones with fever is a relative medical emergency. Signs of clinical sepsis are variable and include fever, tachycardia, hypotension, and cutaneous vasodilation. Costovertebral angle tenderness may be marked with acute upper-tract obstruction; however, it cannot be relied upon to be present in instances of long-term obstruction. In such instances, a mass may be palpable resulting from a grossly hydronephrotic kidney. Fever associated with urinary tract obstruction requires prompt decompression. This may be accomplished with a retrograde catheter (double-J, or an externalized variety to serve as a port for selective urine collections, injection of contrast material, or both). If retrograde manipulations are unsuccessful, insertion of a percutaneous nephrostomy tube is required.

E. Nausea and Vomiting

Upper-tract obstruction is frequently associated with nausea and vomiting. Intravenous fluids are required to restore a euvolemic state. Intravenous fluids should not be used to force a diuresis in an attempt to push a ureteral stone down the ureter. Effective ureteral peristalsis requires coaptation of the ureteral walls and is most effective in a euvolemic state.

▶ Special Situations

A. Renal Transplantation

Urinary stones associated with renal transplantation are rare. Perirenal nerves are severed at the time of renal harvesting. Classic renal colic is not found in these patients. The patients usually are admitted with the presumptive diagnosis of graft rejection. Only after appropriate radiographic and ultrasonic evaluation, the correct diagnosis is made (Figure 17–9).

B. Pregnancy

Renal colic is the most common nonobstetric cause of acute abdominal pain during pregnancy (Figure 17–10). Despite marked hypercalciuria associated with pregnancy, calculi are relatively rare, with an incidence approximating 1:1500 pregnancies. Women with known urinary stone disease do not have an increased risk of stones during pregnancy. The

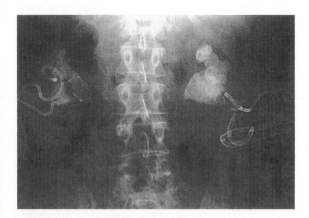

▲ **Figure 17–8.** Bilateral renal calculi seen on scout radiograph with numerous bilateral percutaneous nephrostomy tubes to drain severe bilateral pyonephrosis.

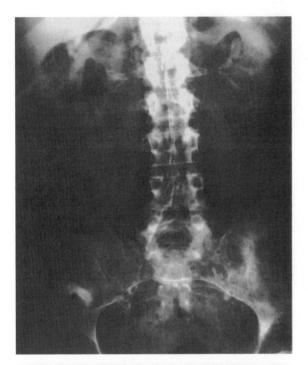

▲ **Figure 17–9.** Scout abdominal radiograph demonstrating renal calculus in a renal transplant in the right iliac fossa. Note native renal vasculature with marked calcifications secondary to malignant diabetes mellitus.

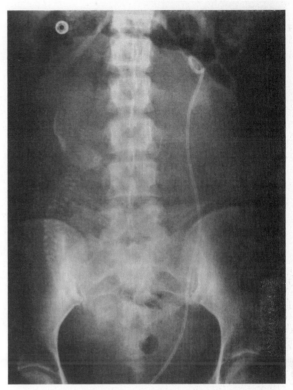

▲ **Figure 17–10.** Scout radiograph demonstrating left renal calculus with double-J ureteral stent in place. Skeletal fetal structures can be appreciated in this pregnant patient.

increased filtered load of calcium, uric acid, and sodium from the 25–50% increase in glomerular filtration rate associated with pregnancy has been thought to be a responsible factor in stone development.

The fetus demands special considerations regarding the potential dangers of radiation exposure (especially during the first trimester), medications, anesthesia, and surgical intervention. About 90% of symptomatic calculi present during the second and third trimesters. Initial investigations can be undertaken with renal ultrasonography and limited abdominal x-rays with appropriate shielding. Treatment requires balancing the safety of the fetus with the health of the mother. Temporizing measures to relieve upper-tract obstruction with a double-J ureteral stent or a percutaneous nephrostomy tube can be performed under local anesthesia. Treatment usually can be delayed until after delivery.

C. Dysmorphia

Patients with severe skeletal dysmorphia that is either congenital (spina bifida, myelomeningocele, cerebral palsy) or acquired (arthritis, traumatic spinal cord injuries) and concurrent urinary calculi represent a unique clinical situation requiring special considerations (Figure 17–11). These

skeletal abnormalities may preclude appropriate positioning for SWL or percutaneous approaches. Calculi on the concave side in a patient with severe scoliosis may eliminate percutaneous puncture access between the rib and the posterosuperior iliac spine. Retrograde manipulations may need to be performed with flexible endoscopes due to marked contractures, making conventional dorsal lithotomy positioning impossible. Many such patients have undergone supravesical urinary diversion so that retrograde access may be limited. Risks that need to be addressed include hypercalciuria associated with immobilization, relative dehydration due to patients' or attendants' attempts to reduce urinary output into external collecting devices, and the potential inability to drink without assistance. A full metabolic evaluation is even more important because these social and physical restrictions may be difficult or impossible to remedy.

D. Obesity

Obesity is a major risk factor for the development of urinary calculi. Surgical bypass procedures can cause hyperoxaluria. Massive weight gain or loss also may precipitate stone development. Obesity limits diagnostic and treatment options. A

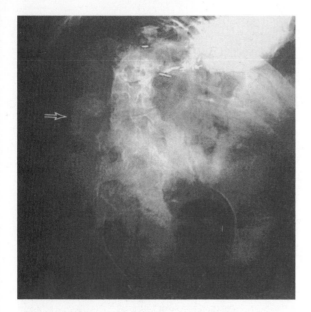

▲ **Figure 17-11.** Scout abdominal radiograph demonstrating a right renal calculus (*arrow*) in a patient with severe kyphoscoliosis. Respiratory compromise limited patient positioning for surgery.

large pannus may limit the physical examination and misguide incisions. Ultrasound examination is hindered by the attenuation of ultrasound beams. CT scan, magnetic resonance imaging, fluoroscopy tables, and lithotripters all have weight limitations, and patients weighing more than 300 pounds may be unsuited for diagnosis and treatment with these resources. Standard lithotripters have focal lengths <15 cm between the energy source and the F2 target, frequently making treatment of obese patients challenging. A large anterior pannus limits prone positioning on lithotripters. Standard Amplatz nephrostomy sheaths may not be long enough to enter the collecting system. Such sheaths may need to be advanced well below the skin or specialized long sheaths with long nephroscopes may be required. A preplaced heavy suture eases removal of such sheaths.

Risks of anesthesia are increased and special high-pressure respirators may be required if patients are placed in a prone position for a percutaneous procedure. Careful positioning for open procedures helps to reduce the likelihood of crush injuries and associated rhabdomyolysis. These patients are at increased risk of anesthetic complications. Postoperative prophylaxis for thromboembolic complications should be considered.

E. Medullary Sponge Kidney

Medullary sponge kidney is a common condition characterized by tubular ectasia associated with parenchymal cysts and clefts that predispose to nephrolithiasis in 50% of affected patients. It is most often an asymptomatic condition; however, it may present with renal colic, hematuria, or urinary tract infection. It is a radiographic diagnosis. The condition can involve select papillae or, more frequently, can be global. A full metabolic evaluation helps direct appropriate medical therapy.

F. Renal Tubular Acidosis

There are three main types of renal tubular acidosis: types I, II, and IV. Type I is associated with renal calculi.

Patients with type I renal tubular acidosis present with persistent acidemia with a low serum bicarbonate value unexplained by hyperventilation or known renal failure. The diagnosis should be suspected in those with a known family history, severe hypocitraturia, nephrocalcinosis, medullary sponge kidney, or a fasting urine pH >6.0 in the absence of infection. Patients usually present with nephrolithiasis (calcium phosphate), nephrocalcinosis, or osteomalacia (or a combination). This disease can be acquired as an adult or inherited with an autosomal dominant pattern. The diagnosis is confirmed by assessing the patient's response to an acid load. This is frequently produced by a rapid oral ammonium chloride load (0.1 g/kg over 1 hour). The dose can be given before bedtime in the evening; the patient is instructed to fast until a second morning voided urine sample and a serum bicarbonate level are obtained. A normal person responds by eliminating the acid load in the urine, resulting in a urinary pH <5.3. Those who do not respond in this fashion can be said to have type I renal tubular acidosis. In addition, the diagnosis should be challenged in those with normal citrate values. Treatment is centered on base replacement with potassium citrate or potassium bicarbonate solutions. Urinary citrate levels can be used to monitor effective treatment.

G. Associated Tumors

Squamous cell carcinoma of the upper urinary tract is uncommon but has been associated with calculi. Chronic irritation from calculi or infection may be contributory factors. Upper-tract calculi may predispose patients to transitional cell carcinoma.

H. Pediatric Patients

Urinary calculi are unusual in children. A full and thorough metabolic evaluation should be undertaken. Stone analysis is particularly helpful in directing these investigations. Children born prematurely and given furosemide while in the neonatal intensive care unit are at increased risk of developing urinary stone disease. Treatment may be limited by endoscope size. Preliminary data show no change in renal growth after SWL.

I. Caliceal Diverticula

Pyelocaliceal diverticula are cystic urine-containing eventrations of the upper tract lying within the renal parenchyma;

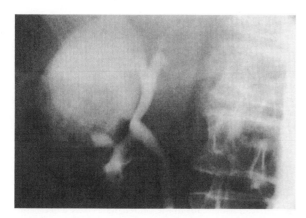

▲ **Figure 17–12.** Intravenous pyelogram demonstrating symptomatic right calyceal diverticula with numerous small calculi.

they communicate through a narrow channel into the main collecting system (Figure 17–12). These diverticula occur in approximately 0.2–0.5% of the population and are congenital in origin; up to 40% are associated with calculi. Type I diverticula are the most common and are closely related to minor calyces. Type II diverticula have a direct communication with the renal pelvis and tend to be larger and symptomatic. Caliceal diverticuli are usually asymptomatic, but patients may complain of flank pain or recurrent urinary tract infections. Frequently, many small calculi, rather than a solitary stone, are found in these obstructed cavities. When intervention was required in the past, treatment was with nephrectomy, heminephrectomy, or open surgical unroofing. Less invasive means are used today. Communications with the collecting system are commonly pinpoint and may be difficult to locate through a retrograde approach. Retrograde access into superior pole diverticula has been successful. Surprisingly, treatment may be successful with SWL if stone fragments are small enough to pass uneventfully. More commonly, percutaneous access and, more recently, laparoscopic means are used with success. Dilation of the caliceal neck, direct cauterization or sclerosis of the caliceal epithelium, or direct cauterization and sclerosis of the caliceal epithelium can help reduce stone recurrence rates.

J. Renal Malformations

Anatomic renal variants such as ectopic kidneys, including the horseshoe and pelvic kidney, predispose to renal calculi due to impaired urinary drainage. Pain symptoms appear to be no different from those reported in patients with normally positioned kidneys. Radiographic diagnosis may be difficult due to the unexpected location of the ureters and kidneys (Figure 17–13). If calculi can be targeted with SWL, most stone fragments pass surprisingly uneventfully. Large stone burdens should be approached percutaneously as in

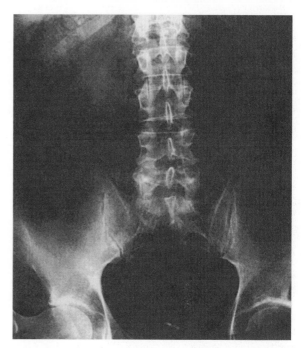

▲ **Figure 17–13.** Scout abdominal radiograph demonstrating horseshoe kidney with lateral ureteral deviation and double-J ureteral stent. Extraosseous calcifications are left lower calyceal stones.

normally positioned kidneys. Severe outlet obstruction should be corrected with laparoscopic or open surgery, and concurrent calculi can be removed at the same setting. Aberrant vasculature should be appreciated before percutaneous, laparoscopic, and open procedures are undertaken.

▶ Evaluation

A. Differential Diagnosis

Urinary stones can mimic other retroperitoneal and peritoneal pathologic states. A full differential diagnosis of the acute abdomen should be made, including acute appendicitis, ectopic and unrecognized pregnancies, ovarian pathologic conditions including twisted ovarian cysts, diverticular disease, bowel obstruction, biliary stones with and without obstruction, peptic ulcer disease, acute renal artery embolism, and abdominal aortic aneurysm—to mention a few. Peritoneal signs should be sought during physical examination.

B. History

A proper evaluation requires a thorough medical history. The nature of the pain should be evaluated, including its onset; character; potential radiation; activities that exacerbate or ease the pain; associated nausea, vomiting, or gross hematuria; and a history of similar pain. Patients with previous stones frequently have had similar types of pain in the past, but not always.

C. Risk Factors

1. Crystalluria—Crystalluria is a risk factor for stones. Stone formers, especially those with calcium oxalate stones, frequently excrete more calcium oxalate crystals, and those crystals are larger than normal (>12 μm). The rate of stone formation is proportional to the percentage of large crystals and crystal aggregates. Crystal production is determined by the saturation of each salt and the urinary concentration of inhibitors and promoters. Urine samples should be fresh; they should be centrifuged and examined immediately for optimum results. Cystine crystals are hexagonal; struvite stones appear as coffin lids; brushite ($CaHPO_4$) stones are splinter like and may aggregate with a spoke-like center; calcium apatite—$(Ca)_5(PO_4)_3(OH)$—and uric acid crystals appear as amorphous powder because the crystals are so small; calcium oxalate dihydrate stones are bipyramids; and calcium oxalate monohydrate stones are small biconcave ovals that may appear as a dumbbell. Cystine and struvite crystals are always abnormal and require further investigations. Other crystals are frequently found in normal urinalyses.

2. Socioeconomic factors—Renal stones are more common in affluent, industrialized countries. Immigrants from less industrialized nations gradually increase their stone incidence and eventually match that of the indigenous population. Use of soft water does not decrease the incidence of urinary stones.

3. Diet—Diet may have a significant impact on the incidence of urinary stones. As per capita income increases, the average diet changes, with an increase in saturated and unsaturated fatty acids; an increase in animal protein and sugar; and a decrease in dietary fiber, vegetable protein, and unrefined carbohydrates. A less energy-dense diet may decrease the incidence of stones. This fact has been documented during war years when diets containing minimal fat and protein resulted in a decreased incidence of stones. Vegetarians may have a decreased incidence of urinary stones. High sodium intake is associated with increased urinary sodium, calcium, and pH and a decreased excretion of citrate; this increases the likelihood of calcium salt crystallization because the urinary saturation of monosodium urate and calcium phosphate (brushite) is increased. Fluid intake and urine output may have an effect on urinary stone disease. The average daily urinary output in stone formers is 1.6 L/d.

4. Occupation—Occupation can have an impact on the incidence of urinary stones. Physicians and other white-collar workers have an increased incidence of stones compared with manual laborers. This finding may be related to differences in diet but also may be related to physical activity; physical activity may agitate urine and dislodge crystal aggregates. Individuals exposed to high temperatures may develop higher concentrations of solutes owing to dehydration, which may have an impact on the incidence of stones.

5. Climate—Individuals living in hot climates are prone to dehydration, which results in an increased incidence of urinary stones, especially uric acid calculi. Although heat may cause a higher fluid intake, sweat loss results in lowered voided volumes. Hot climates usually expose people to more ultraviolet light, increasing vitamin D_3 production. Increased calcium and oxalate excretion has been correlated with increased exposure time to sunlight. This factor has more impact on light-skinned people and may help explain why African Americans in the United States have a decreased stone incidence. Global warming may increase the incidence of urinary stone disease.

6. Family history—A family history of urinary stones is associated with an increased incidence of renal calculi. A patient with stones is twice as likely as a stone-free cohort to have at least one first-degree relative with renal stones (30% vs 15%). Those with a family history of stones have an increased incidence of multiple and early recurrences. Spouses of patients with calcium oxalate stones have an increased incidence of stones; this may be related to environmental or dietary factors. Large studies of identical twins have found that >50% of stones have a significant genetic component. New evidence is finding a significant association between urinary stones and cardiovascular disease.

7. Medications—A thorough history of medications taken may provide valuable insight into the cause of urinary calculi. The antihypertensive medication triamterene is found as a component of several medications, including Dyazide, and has been associated with urinary calculi with increasing frequency. Long-term use of antacids containing silica has been associated with the development of silicate stones. Carbonic anhydrase inhibitors may be associated with urinary stone disease (10–20% incidence). The long-term effect of sodium- and calcium-containing medications on the development of renal calculi is not known. Protease inhibitors in immunocompromised patients are associated with radiolucent calculi.

D. Physical Examination

A detailed physical examination is an essential component of the evaluation of any patient suspected of having a urinary calculus. The patient presenting with acute renal colic typically is in severe pain, often attempting to find relief in multiple, frequently bizarre, positions. This fact helps differentiate patients with this condition from those with peritonitis, who are afraid to move. Systemic components of renal colic may be obvious, with tachycardia, sweating, and nausea often prominent. Costovertebral angle tenderness may be apparent. An abdominal mass may be palpable in patients with long-standing obstructive urinary calculi and severe hydro-nephrosis.

Fever, hypotension, and cutaneous vasodilation may be apparent in patients with urosepsis. In such instances, there is an urgent need for decompression of the obstructed urinary tract, massive intravenous fluid resuscitation, and intravenous antibiotics. Occasionally, intensive care support is needed.

A thorough abdominal examination should exclude other causes of abdominal pain. Abdominal tumors, abdominal aortic aneurysms, herniated lumbar disks, and pregnancy may mimic renal colic. Referred pain may be similar owing to common afferent neural pathways. Intestinal ileus may be associated with renal colic or other intraperitoneal or retroperitoneal processes. Bladder palpation should be performed because urinary retention may present with pain similar to renal colic. Incarcerated inguinal hernias, epididymitis, orchitis, and female pelvic pathologic states may mimic urinary stone disease. A rectal examination helps exclude other pathologic conditions.

E. Radiologic Investigations

1. Computed tomography—Noncontrast spiral CT scans are now the imaging modality of choice in patients presenting with acute renal colic. It is rapid and is now less expensive than an intravenous pyelogram (IVP). It images other peritoneal and retroperitoneal structures and helps when the diagnosis is uncertain. It does not depend on an experienced radiologic technician to obtain appropriate oblique views when there is confusion with overlying bowel gas in a nonprepped abdomen. There is no need for intravenous contrast. Distal ureteral calculi can be confused with phleboliths. Prone positioning will help differentiate impacted ureterovesical junction calculi from stones that have already passed into the urinary bladder. Noncontrast images do not give anatomic details as seen on an IVP (eg, a bifid collecting system) that may be important in planning intervention. If intravenous contrast material is used during the study, a KUB film or three-dimensional reconstruction can give additional helpful information. Uric acid stones are visualized no differently from calcium oxalate stones. Matrix calculi have adequate amounts of calcium to be visualized easily by CT scan. HU can help predict stone type and hardness. Hard calcium oxalate monohydrate stones, for example, frequently have HU >1000, whereas uric acid stones frequently have HU <500. The increased use of CT scans has also increased the radiation exposure to stone patients, especially those with recurrent disease. CT scans should be used when the diagnosis is in doubt and should not be routinely utilized for diagnosis or surveillance.

2. Intravenous pyelography—An IVP can simultaneously document nephrolithiasis and upper-tract anatomy. It is rarely used today with the widespread availability of CT scan and ultrasound. Extraosseous calcifications on radiographs

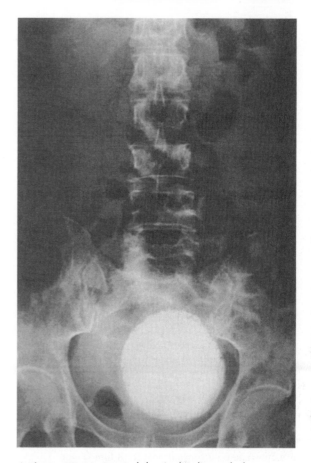

▲ **Figure 17–14.** Scout abdominal radiograph demonstrating large extraosseous calcification that represents a uterine fibroid. This easily could be confused with a large bladder calculus.

may be erroneously assumed to be urinary tract calculi (Figure 17–14). Oblique views easily differentiate gallstones from right renal calculi. Static hard-copy films can be interpreted by most clinicians. Anecdotally, small ureteral stones have passed spontaneously during such studies. An inadequate bowel preparation, associated ileus and swallowed air, and lack of available technicians may result in a less than ideal study when obtained during acute renal colic. A delayed, planned IVP may result in a superior study.

Acute forniceal rupture is not uncommonly associated with a highly obstructive ureteral calculus. It may result in dramatic radiographs but is of no clinical significance, and no specific intervention is required. The rupture may be precipitated by the osmotic diuresis of the intravenous contrast agent.

3. Tomography—Renal tomography is useful to identify calculi in the kidney when oblique views are not helpful.

It visualizes the kidney in a coronal plane at a set distance from the top of the x-ray table. Renal tomography may help identify poorly opacified calculi or stones difficult to appreciate secondary to overlying abdominal gas or morbid obesity when imaged with a traditional with a KUB.

4. KUB films and directed ultrasonography—A KUB film and renal ultrasound may be as effective as an IVP or CT scan in establishing a diagnosis. The ultrasound examination should be directed by notation of suspicious areas seen on a KUB film; it is, however, operator dependent. The distal ureter is easily visualized through the acoustic window of a full bladder. Edema and small calculi missed on an IVP can be appreciated with such studies. New studies comparing CT versus ultrasound for the acute diagnosis of urinary stones is underway.

5. Retrograde pyelography—Retrograde pyelography occasionally is required to delineate upper-tract anatomy and localize small or radiolucent offending calculi. Bulb ureterograms frequently leak contrast material back into the bladder, resulting in a suboptimal study. Advancing an angiographic exchange catheter with or without the aid of a guidewire 3–4 cm into the ureter is an alternative technique. Intermittent fluoroscopic images direct appropriate injection volumes and help reduce the likelihood of pyelolymphatic, pyelosinus, and pyelovenous reflux.

6. Magnetic resonance imaging—Magnetic resonance imaging is a poor study to document urinary stone disease.

7. Nuclear scintigraphy—Nuclear scintigraphic imaging of stones has recently been appreciated. Bisphosphonate markers can identify even small calculi that are difficult to appreciate on a conventional KUB film (Figure 17–15). Differential radioactive uptake dependent on stone composition appreciated during in vitro studies cannot be appreciated on in vivo studies. Nuclear scintigraphy cannot delineate upper-tract anatomy in sufficient detail to help direct a therapeutic plan.

▶ Intervention

A. Conservative Observation

Most ureteral calculi pass and do not require intervention. Spontaneous passage depends on stone size, shape, location, and associated ureteral edema (which is likely to depend on the length of time that a stone has not progressed). Ureteral calculi 4–5 mm in size have a 40–50% chance of spontaneous passage. In contrast, calculi >6 mm have a >15% chance of spontaneous passage. This does not mean that a 1-cm stone will not pass or that a 1- to 2-mm stone will always pass uneventfully.

Medical expulsive therapy (MET) helps facilitate spontaneous passage of ureteral stones. An alpha-blocker, nonsteroidal anti-inflammatory medications with or without low-dose steroids is now becoming standard care to optimize spontaneous ureteral stone passage. The vast majority of stones that pass do so within a 6-week period after the onset

of symptoms. Ureteral calculi discovered in the distal ureter at the time of presentation have a 50% chance of spontaneous passage, in contrast to a 25% and 10% chance in the mid and proximal ureter, respectively.

B. Dissolution Agents

The effectiveness of dissolution agents depends on stone surface area, stone type, volume of irrigant, and mode of delivery. Oral alkalinizing agents include sodium or potassium bicarbonate and potassium citrate. Extra care should be employed in patients susceptible to congestive heart failure or renal failure. Citrate is metabolized to bicarbonate and comes in a variety of preparations. Polycitra contains potassium and sodium citrate and citric acid. Bicitra contains only sodium citrate and citric acid. Food does not alter the effectiveness of these agents. Alternatively, orange juice alkalinizes urine. Intravenous alkalinization is effective with 1/6 molar sodium lactate.

Intrarenal alkalinization may be performed successfully under a low-pressure system (<25 cm water pressure). This may be achieved through a percutaneous nephrostomy tube or an externalized retrograde catheter. Agents include sodium bicarbonate, 2–4 ampules in 1 L of normal saline, producing a urinary pH between 7.5 and 9.0. Tromethamine-E and tromethamine can produce urinary pHs of 8.0–10.5 and are especially effective with pH-sensitive calculi as in uric acid and cystine lithiasis.

Cystine calculi can be dissolved with a variety of thiols, including D-penicillamine (0.5% solution), N-acetylcysteine (2–5% solution), and alpha-mercaptopropionylglycine (Thiola) (5% solution).

Struvite stone dissolution requires acidification and may be achieved successfully with Suby's G solution and hemiacidrin (Renacidin). Urinary pH may get down to 4.0. Hemiacidrin must be used with sterile urine, and careful monitoring of serum magnesium levels is required. The Food and Drug Administration has not approved hemiacidrin for upper-tract irrigations, and thus appropriate informed consent is required.

C. Relief of Obstruction

Urinary stone disease may result in significant morbidity and possible mortality in the presence of obstruction, especially with concurrent infection. A patient with obstructive urinary calculi with fever and infected urine requires emergent drainage. Retrograde pyelography to define upper-tract anatomy is logically followed by retrograde placement of a double-J ureteral stent. On occasion, such catheters are unable to bypass the offending calculus or may perforate the ureter. In such situations, one must be prepared to place a percutaneous nephrostomy tube.

D. Extracorporeal Shock Wave Lithotripsy

Extracorporeal SWL has revolutionized the treatment of urinary stones. The concept of using shock waves to fragment

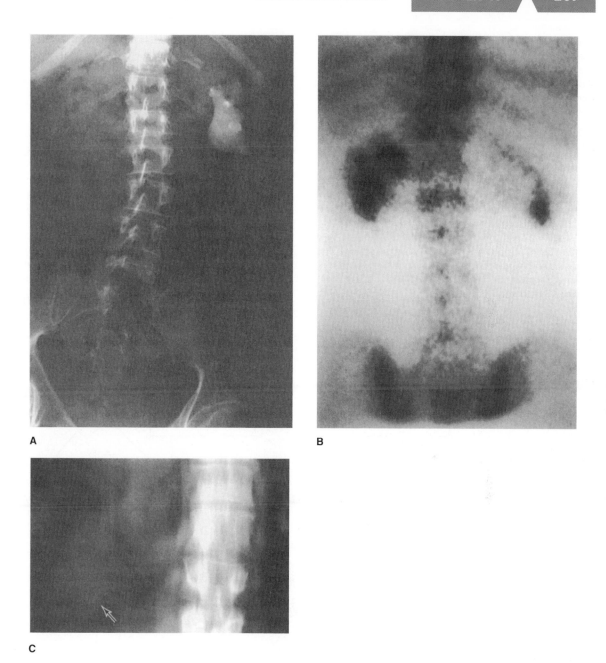

▲ Figure 17–15. A: Scout abdominal radiograph demonstrating large left staghorn renal calculus. **B:** Nuclear scinti-graphic evaluation of renal calculi. Posterior view demonstrating uptake on large left staghorn calculus after furosemide (Lasix) diuresis. Note right kidney with uptake in lower pole. **C:** Follow-up tomogram confirms calculus (*arrow*) in right lower pole missed on initial radiograph.

stones was noted in the 1950s in Russia. However, it was during the investigation of pitting on supersonic aircraft that Dornier, a German aircraft corporation, rediscovered that shock waves originating from passing debris in the atmosphere can crack something that is hard. It was the ingenious application of a model developed in hopes of understanding such shock waves that extracorporeal (outside the body) SWL emerged. The first clinical application with successful fragmentation of renal calculi was in 1980. The HM-1 (Human Model-1) lithotriptor underwent modifications in 1982 leading to the HM-2 and, finally, to the widespread application of the HM-3 in 1983 (Figure 17–16). Since then, thousands of lithotriptors have been put into use around the world, with millions of patients successfully treated.

All require an energy source to create the shock wave, a coupling mechanism to transfer the energy from outside to inside the body, and either fluoroscopic or ultrasonic modes, or both, to identify and position the calculi at a focus of converging shock waves. They differ in generated pain and anesthetic or anesthesiologist requirements, consumable components, size, mobility, cost, and durability. Focal peak pressures (400–1500 bar), focal dimensions (6 × 28 mm to 50 × 15 mm), modular design, varied distances (12–17.0 cm) between focus 1 (the shock wave source) and focus 2 (the target), and purchase price differentiate the various machines available today.

1. Shock wave physics—In contrast to the familiar ultrasonic wave with sinusoidal characteristics and longitudinal mechanical properties, acoustic shock waves are not harmonic and have nonlinear pressure characteristics. There is a steep rise in pressure amplitude that results in compressive forces (Figure 17–17). There are two basic types of shock wave sources, supersonic and finite amplitude emitters.

Supersonic emitters release energy in a confined space, thereby producing an expanding plasma and an acoustic shock wave. Such shock waves occur in nature—the familiar thunderstorm with lightning (an electrical discharge) followed by thunder (an acoustic sonic boom) is an analogous situation. Under controlled conditions, such an acoustic

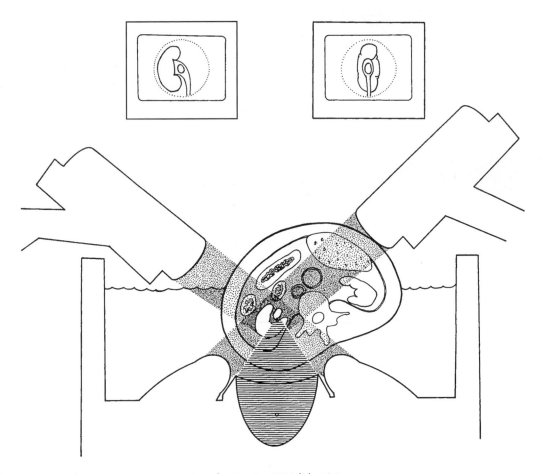

▲ **Figure 17–16.** Diagrammatic representation of a Dornier HM-3 lithotriptor.

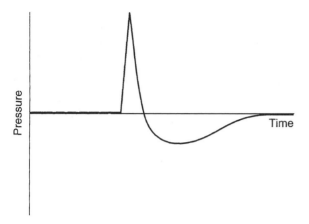

▲ **Figure 17-17.** Shock wave. Vertical axis represents pressure and horizontal axis represents time.

shock wave can successfully fragment calculi. The initial compression wave travels faster than the speed of sound in water and rapidly slows down to that speed. The traveling pressure wave is reduced in a nonlinear fashion. Medical applications have focused such waves to concentrate energy on a calculus (Figure 17–18).

Finite amplitude emitters, in contrast to point source energy systems, create pulsed acoustic shock waves by displacing a surface activated by electrical discharge. There are two major types of finite amplitude emitters, piezoceramic and electromagnetic. The piezoceramic variety results in a shock wave after an electrical discharge causes the ceramic component to elongate in such a manner that the surface is displaced and an acoustic pulse is generated. Thousands of such components placed on the concave side of a spheric surface directed toward a focus result in high stress, strain, and cavitation pressures (Figure 17–19). Electromagnetic systems are similar in concept to a stereo speaker system. An electrical discharge to a slab, adjacent to an insulating foil, creates an electric current that repulses a metal membrane, displacing it and generating an acoustic pulse into an adjacent medium. These waves need to be focused toward the offending stone.

All shock waves, despite their source, are capable of fragmenting stones when focused. Fragmentation is achieved by erosion and shattering (Figure 17–20). Cavitational forces result in erosion at the entry and exit sites of the shock wave. Shattering results from energy absorption with stress, strain, and shear forces. Surrounding biologic tissues are resilient because they are neither brittle nor are the shock waves focused on them.

2. Preoperative evaluation—Physical examination should be as thorough as in preparation for any other surgical

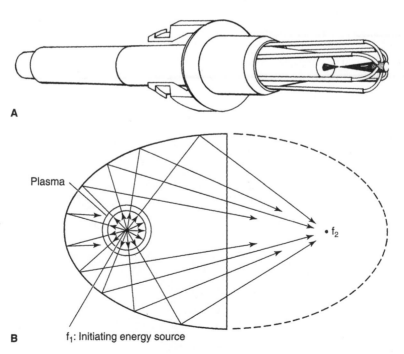

▲ **Figure 17-18.** **A:** Supersonic shock wave emission from a spark gap electrode. **B:** Reflecting the shock wave from focus 1 to focus 2 allows for stone fragmentation.

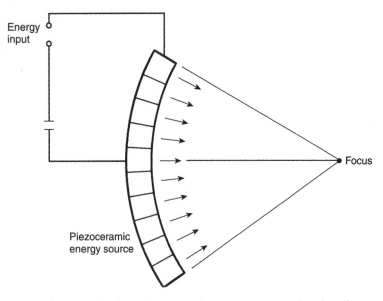

▲ **Figure 17–19.** Piezoceramic finite amplitude emitter. Ceramic components are placed on the concave surface of a sphere and each component is directed to an identified focus.

procedure. Vital signs including blood pressure should be noted. Body habitus including any gross skeletal abnormalities, contractures, or excessive weight (>300 lb) may severely limit or preclude SWL. Borderline individuals require simulation before treatment. Pregnant women and patients with large abdominal aortic aneurysms or uncorrectable bleeding disorders should not be treated with SWL. Individuals with cardiac pacemakers should be thoroughly evaluated by

a cardiologist. If SWL is contemplated, a cardiologist with thorough knowledge and with the ability to override the pacemaker should be present in the lithotripsy suite.

3. Intraoperative considerations

A. Stone localization—Proper patient positioning is a prerequisite for successful lithotripsy. Palpating the patient's ribs and pelvic bony girdle can approximate appropriate

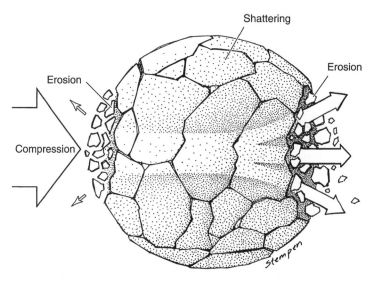

▲ **Figure 17–20.** Incoming shock waves result in fragmentation from erosion and shattering.

excess copper in the treatment of Wilson's disease, undergoes a thiol–disulfide exchange with cystine. This reduces the amount of urinary cystine that is relatively insoluble. Cystine solubility is pH dependent (pH 5.0: 150–300 mg/L; pH 7.0: 200–400 mg/L; pH 7.5: 220–500 mg/L). D-Penicillamine is associated with numerous and frequent side effects, including rashes and hematologic, renal, and hepatic abnormalities. An initial dosage of 250 mg daily in three to four divided doses may help reduce severe side effects. It may be increased gradually to 2 g/d. Dosage should be titrated with quantitative urinary cystine values. Penicillamine increases the requirement of pyridoxine (vitamin B_6), which should be supplemented with 25–50 mg/d.

Mercaptopropionylglycine (Thiola) is better tolerated by patients than is penicillamine. Mercaptopropionylglycine, a reducing agent, binds to the sulfide portion of cystine, forming a mixed disulfide (Thiola-cysteine) water-soluble compound. It may retard the rate of new stone formation. The dosage should be titrated with repeat 24-hour urinary cystine values. An initial dosage may be 200–300 mg three times daily, either 1 hour before or 2 hours after each meal. Side effects are not infrequent and may include drug fever; nausea, vomiting, and gastrointestinal upset; rash, wrinkling, or friable skin; lupus-like symptoms, decreased taste perception; and a variety of hematologic disorders.

BLADDER STONES

Bladder calculi usually are a manifestation of an underlying pathologic condition, including voiding dysfunction or a foreign body. Voiding dysfunction may be due to a urethral stricture, benign prostatic hyperplasia, bladder neck contracture, or flaccid or spastic neurogenic bladder, all of which result in static urine. Foreign bodies such as Foley catheters and forgotten double-J ureteral catheters can serve as nidi for stones (Figure 17–22). Most bladder calculi are seen in men. In developing countries, they are frequently found in prepubescent boys. Stone analysis frequently reveals ammonium urate, uric acid, or calcium oxalate stones. Bladder stones can be solitary or numerous (Figure 17–23). Patients present with irritative voiding symptoms, intermittent urinary stream, urinary tract infections, hematuria, or pelvic pain. Physical examination is unrevealing. A large percentage of bladder stones are radiolucent (uric acid). Ultrasound of the bladder identifies the stone with its characteristic postacoustic shadowing. The stone moves with changing body position.

Stones within a ureterocele do not move with body position (Figure 17–24) as seen on ultrasound examination. They frequently are nonobstructive. Endoscopic incision and stone removal rarely results in vesicoureteral reflux. The mode of

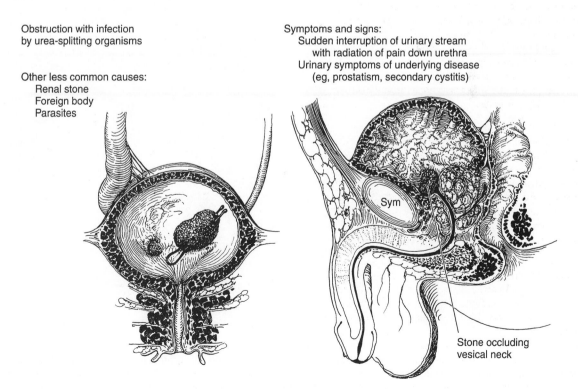

▲ **Figure 17–22.** Genesis and symptoms and signs of vesical calculus.

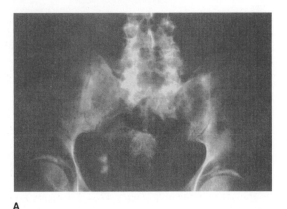

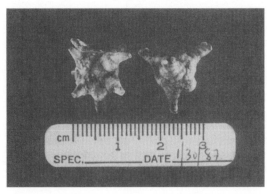

A   B

▲ **Figure 17–23.** *A:* Plain abdominal radiograph demonstrating two bladder calculi. *B:* Gross picture of removed bladder calculi. Note the characteristic shape of jackstones typically composed of uric acid.

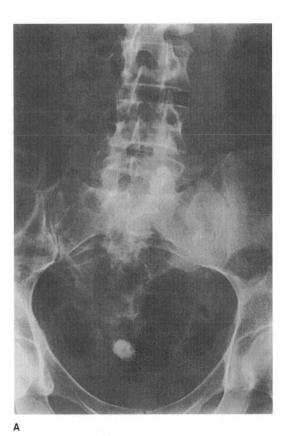

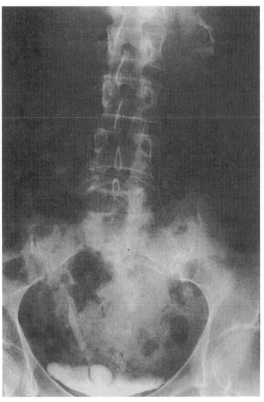

A   B

▲ **Figure 17–24.** *A:* Scout abdominal radiograph demonstrating extraosseous calcification in the region of the bladder. *B:* Intravenous pyelogram demonstrates stone to be within a ureterocele.

stone removal for other bladder stones should be directed by the underlying cause.

Early instruments used to remove bladder calculi were both clever and bizarre. Simple mechanical crushing devices are still used today. Mechanical lithotrites should be used with caution to prevent bladder injury when the jaws are closed. Ensuring a partially full bladder and endoscopic visualization of unrestricted lateral movement before forceful crushing of the stones helps reduce this troublesome complication. Cystolitholapaxy allows most stones to be broken and subsequently removed through a cystoscope. Electrohydraulic, ultrasonic, laser, and pneumatic lithotrites similar to those used through a nephroscope are effective. Cystolithotomy can be performed through a small abdominal incision.

PROSTATIC AND SEMINAL VESICLE STONES

Prostatic calculi are found within the prostate gland per se and are found uncommonly within the prostatic urethra. They are thought to represent calcified corpora amylacea and are rarely found in boys. Usually small and numerous, they are noted to be tannish gray in color during transurethral resection of the prostate. They are commonly located at the margin of the surgically resected adenoma and are composed of calcium phosphate. Although usually of no clinical significance, rarely they are associated with chronic prostatitis. Large prostatic calculi may be misinterpreted as a carcinoma. The prostate is usually mobile, however, and a radiograph or transrectal ultrasound helps to confirm the diagnosis.

Seminal vesicle stones are smooth and hard and are extremely rare. They may be associated with hematospermia. Physical examination reveals a stony hard gland, and when multiple stones are present, a crunching sensation may be noted. These stones occasionally are confused with tuberculosis of the seminal vesicle.

URETHRAL AND PREPUTIAL STONES

Urethral calculi usually originate from the bladder and rarely from the upper tracts. Most ureteral stones that pass spontaneously into the bladder can pass through the urethra unimpeded. Urethral stones may develop secondary to urinary stasis, secondary to a urethral diverticulum, near urethral strictures, or at sites of previous surgery. Most urethral stones in men present in the prostatic or bulbar regions and are solitary. Patients with recurrent pendulous urethral calculi without evidence of other pathologic conditions should be suspected of self-introduction of such stones in an attempt to obtain pain medications or for attention, as seen in Munchausen syndrome.

Females rarely develop urethral calculi owing to their short urethra and a lower incidence of bladder calculi. Most urethral stones found in women are associated with urethral diverticula.

Symptoms are similar to bladder calculi—intermittent urinary stream, terminal hematuria, and infection. The stones may present with dribbling or during acute urinary retention. Pain may be severe and, in men, may radiate to the tip of the penis. The diagnosis may be confirmed by palpation, endoscopic visualization, or radiographic study.

Treatment should be directed by the underlying cause. Stones associated with a dense urethral stricture or complex diverticula can be removed during definitive open surgical repair. Small stones may be grasped successfully and removed intact. More frequently, they need to be fragmented and removed. Long-standing, large impacted stones are best removed through a urethrotomy.

Preputial calculi are rare and usually occur in adults. They develop secondary to a severe obstructive phimosis. They may occur secondary to poor hygiene with inspissated smegma. Diagnosis is confirmed by palpation. Treating the underlying cause with a dorsal preputial slit or a formal circumcision prevents recurrent calculi.

BIBLIOGRAPHY

Urinary Ions
Calcium

Milosevic D et al: Determination of urine saturation with computer program EQUIL 2 as a method for estimation of the risk of urolithiasis. J Chem Inf Comput Sci 1998;38:646.

Moe OW, Bonny O: Genetic hypercalciuria. J Am Soc Nephrol 2005;16:729.

Traxer O et al: Effect of ascorbic acid consumption on urinary stone risk factors. J Urol 2003;170(2, Pt 1):397–401.

Wallace RB et al: Urinary tract stone occurrence in the Women's Health Initiative (WHI) randomized clinical trial of calcium and vitamin D supplements. Am J Clin Nutr 2011;94(1):270–277.

Oxalate

Knight J et al: Metabolism of fructose to oxalate and glycolate. Horm Metab Res 2010;42(12):868–873.

Thurgood LA et al: Comparison of the specific incorporation of intracrystalline proteins into urinary calcium oxalate monohydrate and dihydrate crystals. J Proteome Res 2010;9(9):4745–4757.

Tiselius HG: Standardized estimate of the ion activity product of calcium oxalate in urine from renal stone formers. Eur Urol 1989;16:48.

Uric Acid

Maalouf NM: Metabolic syndrome and the genesis of uric acid stones. J Ren Nutr 2011;21(1):128–131.

Marangella M: Uric acid elimination in the urine. Pathophysiological implications. Contrib Nephrol 2005;147:132.

Stoller ML: Gout and stones or stones and gout? J Urol 1995;154:1670.

Cystine

Pietrow PK et al: Durability of the medical management of cystinuria. J Urol 2003;169:68.

Purohit RS, Stoller ML: Stone clustering of patients with cystine urinary stone formation. Urology 2004;63:630.

Shekarriz B, Stoller ML: Cystinuria and other noncalcareous calculi. Endocrinol Metab Clin North Am 2002;31:951.

Xanthine

Gargah T et al: Xanthine urolithiasis. Saudi J Kidney Dis Transpl 2010;21(2):328–331.

Triamterene

Daudon M, Jungers P: Drug-induced renal calculi: Epidemiology, prevention and management. Drugs 2004;64(3):245–275.

Matrix Urinary Calculi

Shah HN et al: The management of renal matrix calculi: A single-centre experience over 5 years. BJU Int 2009;103(6):810–814.

Urinary Stone Inhibitors
Citrate

Seltzer MA et al: Dietary manipulation with lemonade to treat hypocitraturic calcium nephrolithiasis. J Urol 1996;156:907.

Shah O et al: Genetic and dietary factors in urinary citrate excretion. J Endourol 2005;19:177.

Spivacow FR et al: Long-term treatment of renal lithiasis with potassium citrate. Urology 2010;76(6):1346–1349.

Urinary Proteins

Selvam R, Kalaiselvi P: Oxalate binding proteins in calcium oxalate nephrolithiasis. Urol Res 2003;31:242.

Trace Elements

Schwartz BF et al: Rethinking the role of urinary magnesium in calcium urolithiasis. J Endourol 2001;15:233.

Renal Tubular Acidosis

Evan AP et al: Renal histopathology of stone-forming patients with distal renal tubular acidosis. Kidney Int 2007;71(8):795–801.

Water

Meschi T et al: Body weight, diet and water intake in preventing stone disease. Urol Int 2004;72(Suppl 1):29–33.

Urinary Stone Disease in Uncommon Situations
Spinal Cord Dysfunction

Ramsey S, McIlhenny C: Evidence-based management of upper tract urolithiasis in the spinal cord-injured patient. Spinal Cord 2011;49(9):948–954.

Pregnancy

Rosenberg E et al: Nephrolithiasis during pregnancy: Characteristics, complications, and pregnancy outcome. World J Urol 2011;29(6):743–747.

Renal Transplantation

Lu HF et al: Donor-gifted allograft urolithiasis: Early percutaneous management. Urology 2002;59:25.

Obesity

Nowfar S et al: The relationship of obesity and gender prevalence changes in United States inpatient nephrolithiasis. Urology 2011;78(5):1029–1033.

Taylor EN et al: Obesity, weight gain, and the risk of kidney stones. JAMA 2005;293:455.

Anatomic Renal Anomalies

Baskin LS et al: The horseshoe kidney: Therapeutic considerations with urolithiasis. J Endourol 1989;3:51.

Ganpule AP, Desai MR: Urolithiasis in kidneys with abnormal lie, rotation or form. Curr Opin Urol 2011;21(2):145–153.

Goumas-Kartalas I, Montanari E: Percutaneous nephrolithotomy in patients with spinal deformities. J Endourol 2010;24(7):1081–1089.

Pediatrics

Gürgöze MK, Sarı MY: Results of medical treatment and metabolic risk factors in children with urolithiasis. Pediatr Nephrol 2011;26(6):933–937.

Caliceal Diverticulae

Gross AJ, Herrmann TR: Management of stones in calyceal diverticulum. Curr Opin Urol 2007;17(2):136–140.

Tumors

Paonessa J et al: Squamous cell carcinoma of the renal pelvis associated with kidney stones: A case report. Med Oncol 2010;28(Suppl 1):S392–S394.

Medical Therapy

Berger AD et al: Patients with primary hyperparathyroidism—Why do some form stones? J Urol 2009;181(5):2141–2145.

Johri N et al: An update and practical guide to renal stone management. Nephron Clin Pract 2010;116(3):c159–c171.

Kenny JE, Goldfarb DS: Update on the pathophysiology and management of uric acid renal stones. Curr Rheumatol Rep 2010;12(2):125–129.

Pak CY et al: Adequacy of a single stone risk analysis in the medical evaluation of urolithiasis. J Urol 2001;165:378–381.

Surgical Therapy

Albala DM et al: Lower pole I: A prospective randomized trial of extracorporeal shock wave lithotripsy and percutaneous nephrostolithotomy for lower pole nephrolithiasis—Initial results. J Urol 2001;166:2072–2080.

Al-Kohlany KM et al: Treatment of complete staghorn stones: A prospective randomized comparison of open surgery versus percutaneous nephrolithotomy. J Urol 2005;173:469.

Extracorporeal Shock Wave Lithotripsy

Chaussy CG et al: First clinical experience with extracorporeally induced destruction of kidney stones by shock waves. J Urol 1982;127:417.

Drach GW et al: Report of the United States co-operative study of extracorporeal shock wave lithotripsy. J Urol 1986;135:1127.

Elbahnasy AM et al: Lower caliceal stone clearance after shock wave lithotripsy or ureteroscopy: The impact of lower pole radiographic anatomy. J Urol 1998;159:676.

Lingeman JE et al: Blood pressure changes following extracorporeal shock wave lithotripsy and other forms of treatment for nephrolithiasis. JAMA 1990;263:1789.

Percutaneous Nephrostolithotomy

Akman T et al: Factors affecting bleeding during percutaneous nephrolithotomy: Single surgeon experience. J Endourol 2011;25(2):327–333.

Cracco CM et al: New developments in percutaneous techniques for simple and complex branched renal stones. Curr Opin Urol 2011;21(2):154–160.

Irby PB et al: Percutaneous access techniques in renal surgery. Tech Urol 1999;5:29.

Ureteroscopy

Bagley DH: Removal of upper urinary tract calculi with flexible ureteropyeloscopy. Urology 1990;35:412.

Herrera-Gonzalez G et al: Effectiveness of single flexible ureteroscopy for multiple renal calculi. J Endourol 2011;25(3):431–435.

18

Injuries to the Genitourinary Tract

Jack W. McAninch, MD, FACS, FRCS(E)(Hon)

EMERGENCY DIAGNOSIS AND MANAGEMENT

About 10% of all injuries seen in the emergency room involve the genitourinary system to some extent. Many of them are subtle and difficult to define and require great diagnostic expertise. Early diagnosis is essential to prevent serious complications.

Initial assessment should include control of hemorrhage and shock along with resuscitation as required. Resuscitation may require intravenous lines and a urethral catheter in seriously injured patients. In men, before the catheter is inserted, the urethral meatus should be examined carefully for the presence of blood.

The history should include a detailed description of the accident. In cases involving gunshot wounds, the type and caliber of the weapon should be determined, since high-velocity projectiles cause much more extensive damage.

The abdomen and genitalia should be examined for evidence of contusions or subcutaneous hematomas, which might indicate deeper injuries to the retroperitoneum and pelvic structures. Fractures of the lower ribs are often associated with renal injuries, and pelvic fractures often accompany bladder and urethral injuries. Diffuse abdominal tenderness is consistent with perforated bowel, free intraperitoneal blood or urine, or retroperitoneal hematoma. Patients who do not have life-threatening injuries and whose blood pressure is stable can undergo more deliberate radiographic studies. This provides more definitive staging of the injury.

▶ Special Examinations (Figures 18–1 through 18–3)

When genitourinary tract injury is suspected on the basis of the history and physical examination, additional studies are required to establish its extent.

A. Catheterization and Assessment of Injury

Assessment of the injury should be done in an orderly fashion so that accurate and complete information is obtained. This process of defining the extent of injury is termed *staging*. The algorithms (Figures 18–1 through 18–3) outline the staging process for urogenital trauma.

1. Catheterization—Blood at the urethral meatus in men indicates urethral injury; catheterization should not be attempted if blood is present, but retrograde urethrography should be done immediately. If no blood is present at the meatus, a urethral catheter can be carefully passed to the bladder to recover urine; microscopic or gross hematuria indicates urinary system injury. If catheterization is traumatic despite the greatest care, the significance of hematuria cannot be determined, and other studies must be done to investigate the possibility of urinary system injury.

2. Computed tomography—Abdominal computed tomography (CT) with contrast media is the best imaging study to detect and stage renal and retroperitoneal injuries. It can define the size and extent of the retroperitoneal hematoma, renal lacerations, urinary extravasation, and renal arterial and venous injuries; additionally, it can detect intra-abdominal injuries (liver, spleen, pancreas, bowel). Spiral CT scanning, now common, is very rapid, but it may not detect urinary extravasation or ureteral and renal pelvic injuries. We recommend repeat scanning 10 minutes after the initial study to aid the diagnosis of these conditions.

3. Retrograde cystography—Filling of the bladder with contrast material is essential to establish whether bladder perforations exist. At least 300 mL of contrast medium should be instilled for full vesical distention. A film should be obtained with the bladder filled and a second one after the bladder has emptied itself by gravity drainage. These two films establish the degree of bladder injury as well as the size of the surrounding pelvic hematomas.

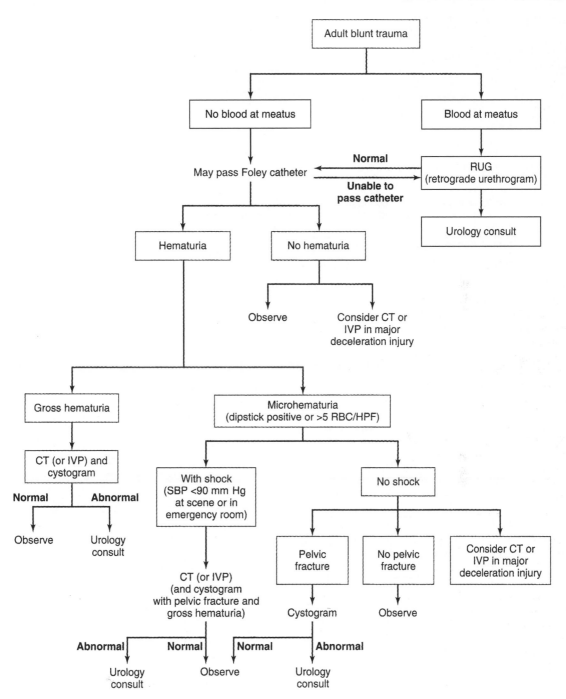

▲ **Figure 18–1.** Algorithm for staging blunt trauma in adults.

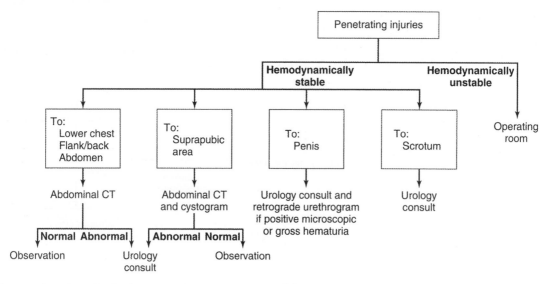

▲ **Figure 18–2.** Algorithm for staging penetrating trauma in adults.

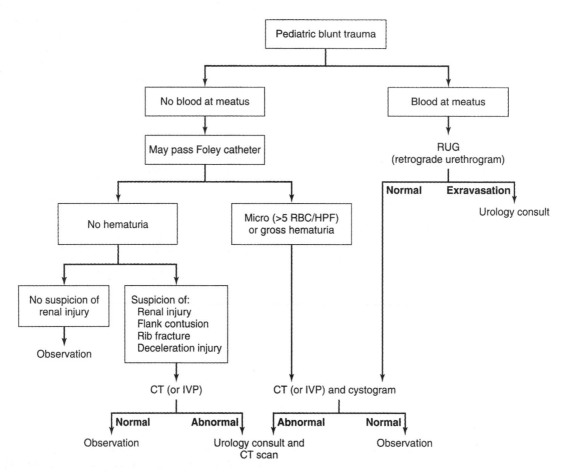

▲ **Figure 18–3.** Algorithm for staging blunt trauma in children

Cystography with CT scan is excellent for establishing bladder injury. At the time of scanning, this likewise must be done with retrograde filling of the bladder with 300 mL of contrast media to ensure adequate distention to detect injury.

4. Urethrography—A small (12F) catheter can be inserted into the urethral meatus and 3 mL of water placed in the balloon to hold the catheter in position. After retrograde injection of 20 mL of water-soluble contrast material, the urethra will be clearly outlined on film, and extravasation in the deep bulbar area in case of straddle injury—or free extravasation into the retropubic space in case of prostatomembranous disruption—will be visualized.

5. Arteriography—Arteriography may help define renal parenchymal and renal vascular injuries. It is also useful in the detection of persistent bleeding from pelvic fractures for purposes of embolization with Gelfoam or autologous clot.

6. Intravenous urography—Intravenous urography can be used to detect renal and ureteral injury. This is best done with high-dose bolus injection of contrast media (2.0 mL/kg) followed by appropriate films.

B. Cystoscopy and Retrograde Urography

Cystoscopy and retrograde urography may be useful to detect ureteral injury, but are seldom necessary, since information can be obtained by less invasive techniques.

C. Abdominal Sonography

Abdominal sonography has not been shown to add substantial information during initial evaluation of severe abdominal trauma.

INJURIES TO THE KIDNEY

Renal injuries are the most common injuries of the urinary system. The kidney is well protected by heavy lumbar muscles, vertebral bodies, ribs, and the viscera anteriorly. Fractured ribs and transverse vertebral processes may penetrate the renal parenchyma or vasculature. Most injuries occur from automobile accidents or sporting mishaps, chiefly in men and boys. Kidneys with existing pathologic conditions such as hydronephrosis or malignant tumors are more readily ruptured from mild trauma.

▶ Etiology (Figure 18–4)

Blunt trauma directly to the abdomen, flank, or back is the most common mechanism, accounting for 80–85% of all renal injuries. Trauma may result from motor vehicle accidents, fights, falls, and contact sports. Vehicle collisions at high speed may result in major renal trauma from rapid deceleration and cause major vascular injury. Gunshot and knife wounds cause most penetrating injuries to the kidney; any such wound in the flank area should be regarded as a

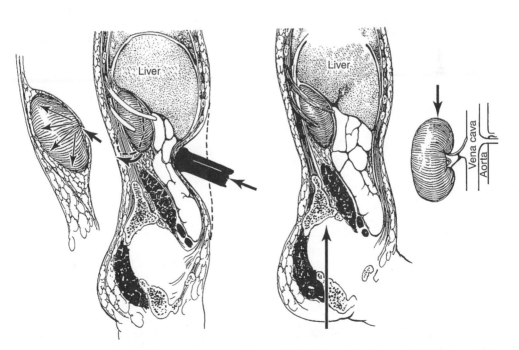

▲ **Figure 18–4.** Mechanisms of renal injury. **Left:** Direct blow to abdomen. Smaller drawing shows force of blow radiating from the renal hilum. **Right:** Falling on buttocks from a height (contrecoup of kidney). Smaller drawing shows direction of force exerted on the kidney from above. Tear of renal pedicle.

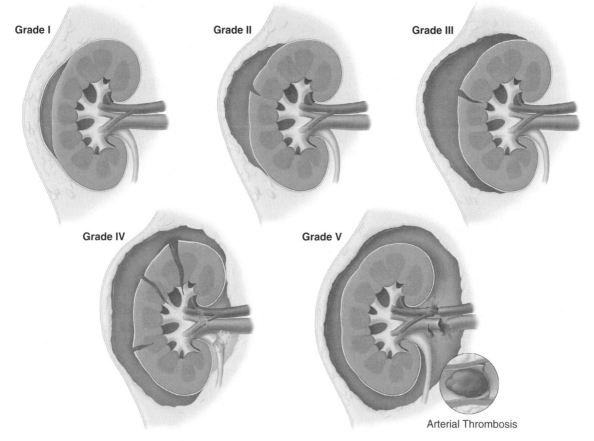

▲ **Figure 18–5.**

cause of renal injury until proved otherwise. Associated abdominal visceral injuries are present in 80% of renal penetrating wounds.

▶ Pathology and Classification (Figure 18–5)

A. Early Pathologic Findings

Lacerations from blunt trauma usually occur in the transverse plane of the kidney. The mechanism of injury is thought to be force transmitted from the center of the impact to the renal parenchyma. In injuries from rapid deceleration, the kidney moves upward or downward, causing sudden stretch on the renal pedicle and sometimes complete or partial avulsion. Acute thrombosis of the renal artery may be caused by an intimal tear from rapid deceleration injuries owing to the sudden stretch.

Pathologic classification of renal injuries is as follows:

Grade 1 (the most common)—Renal contusion or bruising of the renal parenchyma. Microscopic hematuria is common, but gross hematuria rarely occurs.

Grade 2—Renal parenchymal laceration into the renal cortex. Perirenal hematoma is usually small.

Grade 3—Renal parenchymal laceration extending through the cortex and into the renal medulla. Bleeding can be significant in the presence of large retroperitoneal hematoma.

Grade 4—Renal parenchymal laceration (single or multiple) extending into the renal collecting system; also main renal artery thrombosis from blunt trauma, segmental renal vein, or both; or artery injury with contained bleeding.

Grade 5—Multiple Grade 4 parenchymal lacerations, renal pedicle avulsion, or both; main renal vein or artery injury from penetrating trauma; main renal artery or vein thrombosis.

B. Late Pathologic Findings (Figure 18–6)

1. Urinoma—Deep lacerations that are not repaired may result in persistent urinary extravasation and late complications of a

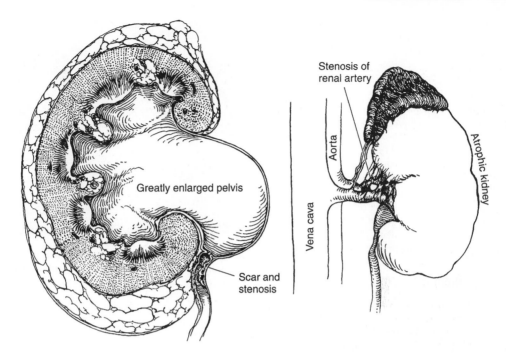

▲ **Figure 18-6.** Late pathologic findings in renal trauma. *Left:* Ureteropelvic stenosis with hydronephrosis secondary to fibrosis from extravasation of blood and urine. *Right:* Atrophy of kidney caused by injury (stenosis) of arterial blood supply.

large perinephric renal mass and, eventually, hydronephrosis and abscess formation.

2. Hydronephrosis—Large hematomas in the retroperitoneum and associated urinary extravasation may result in perinephric fibrosis engulfing the ureteropelvic junction, causing hydronephrosis. Follow-up excretory urography is indicated in all cases of major renal trauma.

3. Arteriovenous fistula—Arteriovenous fistulas may occur after penetrating injuries but are not common.

4. Renal vascular hypertension—The blood flow in tissue rendered nonviable by injury is compromised; this results in renal vascular hypertension in <1% of cases. Fibrosis from surrounding trauma has also been reported to constrict the renal artery and cause renal hypertension.

▶ Clinical Findings and Indications for Studies

Microscopic or gross hematuria following trauma to the abdomen indicates injury to the urinary tract. It bears repeating that stab or gunshot wounds to the flank area should alert the physician to possible renal injury whether or not hematuria is present. Some cases of renal vascular injury are not associated with hematuria. These cases are almost always due to rapid deceleration accidents and are an indication for imaging studies.

The degree of renal injury does not correspond to the degree of hematuria, since gross hematuria may occur in minor renal trauma and only mild hematuria in major trauma. However, not all adult patients sustaining blunt trauma require full imaging evaluation of the kidney (Figure 18–1). Miller and McAninch (1995) made the following recommendations based on findings in >1800 blunt renal trauma injuries: Patients with gross hematuria or microscopic hematuria with shock (systolic blood pressure <90 mm Hg) should undergo radiographic assessment; patients with microscopic hematuria without shock need not. However, should physical examination or associated injuries prompt reasonable suspicion of a renal injury, renal imaging should be undertaken. This is especially true of patients with rapid deceleration trauma, who may have renal injury without the presence of hematuria.

A. Symptoms

There is usually visible evidence of abdominal trauma. Pain may be localized to one flank area or over the abdomen. Associated injuries such as ruptured abdominal viscera or multiple pelvic fractures also cause acute abdominal pain and may obscure the presence of renal injury.

Catheterization usually reveals hematuria. Retroperitoneal bleeding may cause abdominal distention, ileus, and nausea and vomiting.

B. Signs

Initially, shock or signs of a large loss of blood from heavy retroperitoneal bleeding may be noted. Ecchymosis in the flank or upper quadrants of the abdomen is often noted. Lower rib fractures are frequently found. Diffuse abdominal tenderness may be found on palpation; an "acute abdomen" usually indicates free blood in the peritoneal cavity. A palpable mass may represent a large retroperitoneal hematoma or perhaps urinary extravasation. If the retroperitoneum has been torn, free blood may be noted in the peritoneal cavity but no palpable mass will be evident. The abdomen may be distended and bowel sounds absent.

C. Laboratory Findings

Microscopic or gross hematuria is usually present. The hematocrit may be normal initially, but a drop may be found when serial studies are done. This finding represents persistent retroperitoneal bleeding and development of a large retroperitoneal hematoma. Persistent bleeding may necessitate operation.

D. Staging and X-Ray Findings

Staging of renal injuries allows a systematic approach to these problems (Figures 18–1 through 18–3). Adequate studies help define the extent of injury and dictate appropriate management. For example, blunt trauma to the abdomen associated with gross hematuria and a normal urogram requires no additional renal studies; however, nonvisualization of the kidney requires immediate arteriography or CT scan to determine whether renal vascular injury exists. Ultrasonography and retrograde urography are of little use initially in the evaluation of renal injuries.

Staging begins with an abdominal CT scan, the most direct and effective means of staging renal injuries. This noninvasive technique clearly defines parenchymal lacerations and urinary extravasation; shows the extent of the retroperitoneal hematoma; identifies nonviable tissue; and outlines injuries to surrounding organs such as the pancreas, spleen, liver, and bowel (Figure 18–7). (If CT scan is not available, an intravenous pyelogram can be obtained [Figure 18–8].)

Arteriography defines major arterial and parenchymal injuries when previous studies have not fully done so. Arterial thrombosis and avulsion of the renal pedicle are best diagnosed by arteriography and are likely when the kidney is not visualized on imaging studies (Figure 18–9). The major causes of nonvisualization on an excretory urogram are total pedicle avulsion, arterial thrombosis, severe contusion caus-

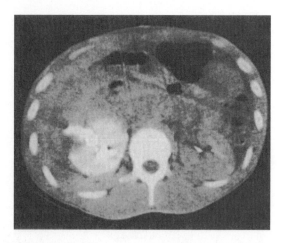

▲ **Figure 18–7.** Computed tomography scan of right kidney following knife stab wound. Laceration with urine extravasation is seen. Large right retroperitoneal hematoma is present.

ing vascular spasm, and absence of the kidney (either congenital or from operation).

Radionuclide renal scans have been used in staging renal trauma. However, in emergency management, this technique is less sensitive than arteriography or CT.

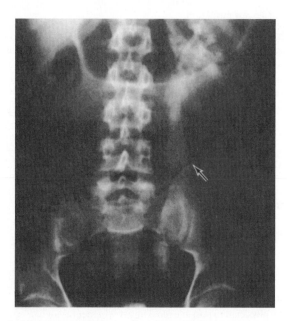

▲ **Figure 18–8.** Blunt renal trauma to left kidney demonstrating extravasation (at *arrow*) on intravenous urogram.

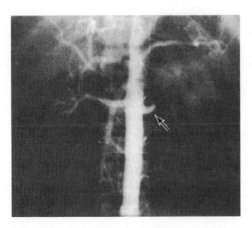

▲ **Figure 18–9.** Arteriogram following blunt abdominal trauma shows typical findings of acute renal artery thrombosis (*arrow*) of left kidney.

▷ Differential Diagnosis

Trauma to the abdomen and flank areas is not always associated with renal injury. In such cases, there is no hematuria, and the results of imaging studies are normal.

▷ Complications

A. Early Complications

Hemorrhage is perhaps the most important immediate complication of renal injury. Heavy retroperitoneal bleeding may result in rapid exsanguination. Patients must be observed closely, with careful monitoring of blood pressure and hematocrit. Complete staging must be done early (Figures 18–1 through 18–3). The size and expansion of palpable masses must be carefully monitored. Bleeding ceases spontaneously in 80–85% of cases. Persistent retroperitoneal bleeding or heavy gross hematuria may require early operation.

Urinary extravasation from renal fracture may show as an expanding mass (urinoma) in the retroperitoneum. These collections are prone to abscess formation and sepsis. A resolving retroperitoneal hematoma may cause slight fever (38.3°C [101°F]), but higher temperatures suggest infection. A perinephric abscess may form, resulting in abdominal tenderness and flank pain.

B. Late Complications

Hypertension, hydronephrosis, arteriovenous fistula, calculus formation, and pyelonephritis are important late complications. Careful monitoring of blood pressure for several months is necessary to watch for hypertension. At 3–6 months, a follow-up excretory urogram or CT scan should be obtained to be certain that perinephric scarring has not caused hydronephrosis or vascular compromise; renal

atrophy may occur from vascular compromise and is detected by follow-up urography. Heavy late bleeding may occur 1–4 weeks after injury.

▷ Treatment

A. Emergency Measures

The objectives of early management are prompt treatment of shock and hemorrhage, complete resuscitation, and evaluation of associated injuries.

B. Surgical Measures

1. Blunt injuries—Minor renal injuries from blunt trauma account for 85% of cases and do not usually require operation. Bleeding stops spontaneously with bed rest and hydration. Cases in which operation is indicated include those associated with persistent retroperitoneal bleeding, urinary extravasation, evidence of nonviable renal parenchyma, and renal pedicle injuries (<5% of all renal injuries). Aggressive preoperative staging allows complete definition of injury before operation.

2. Penetrating injuries—Penetrating injuries should be surgically explored. A rare exception to this rule is when staging has been complete and only minor parenchymal injury, with no urinary extravasation, is noted. In 80% of cases of penetrating injury, associated organ injury requires operation; thus, renal exploration is only an extension of this procedure.

C. Treatment of Complications

Retroperitoneal urinoma or perinephric abscess demands prompt surgical drainage. Malignant hypertension requires vascular repair or nephrectomy. Hydronephrosis may require surgical correction or nephrectomy.

Angioembolization done by interventional radiology provides excellent control of active bleeding from the kidney. This approach, in the trauma setting, is most often used when nonoperative management has been selected and renal parenchymal bleeding persists or develops after days or weeks of observation.

▷ Prognosis

With careful follow-up, most renal injuries have an excellent prognosis, with spontaneous healing and return of renal function. Follow-up CT and renal scan and monitoring of blood pressure ensure detection and appropriate management of late hydronephrosis and hypertension.

INJURIES TO THE URETER

Ureteral injury is rare but may occur, usually during the course of a difficult pelvic surgical procedure or as a result of stab or gunshot wounds. Rapid deceleration accidents may avulse the ureter from the renal pelvis. Endoscopic basket manipulation of ureteral calculi may result in injury.

▶ Etiology

Large pelvic masses (benign or malignant) may displace the ureter laterally and engulf it in reactive fibrosis. This may lead to ureteral injury during dissection, since the organ is anatomically malpositioned. Inflammatory pelvic disorders may involve the ureter in a similar way. Extensive carcinoma of the colon may invade areas outside the colon wall and directly involve the ureter; thus, resection of the ureter may be required along with resection of the tumor mass. Devascularization may occur with extensive pelvic lymph node dissections or after radiation therapy to the pelvis for pelvic cancer. In these situations, ureteral fibrosis and subsequent stricture formation may develop along with ureteral fistulas. Endoscopic manipulation of a ureteral calculus with a stone basket or ureteroscope may result in ureteral perforation or avulsion.

▶ Pathogenesis and Pathology

The ureter may be inadvertently ligated and cut during difficult pelvic surgery. In such cases, sepsis and severe renal damage usually occur postoperatively. If a partially divided ureter is unrecognized at operation, urinary extravasation and subsequent buildup of a large urinoma will ensue, which usually leads to ureterovaginal or ureterocutaneous fistula formation. Intraperitoneal extravasation of urine can also occur, causing ileus and peritonitis. After partial transection of the ureter, some degree of stenosis and reactive fibrosis develops, with concomitant mild-to-moderate hydronephrosis.

▶ Clinical Findings

A. Symptoms

If the ureter has been completely or partially ligated during operation, the postoperative course is usually marked by fever of 38.3°C–38.8°C (101°F–102°F) as well as flank and lower quadrant pain. Such patients often experience paralytic ileus with nausea and vomiting. If ureterovaginal or cutaneous fistula develops, it usually does so within the first 10 postoperative days.

Ureteral injuries from external violence should be suspected in patients who have sustained stab or gunshot wounds to the retroperitoneum. The midportion of the ureter seems to be the most common site of penetrating injury. There are usually associated vascular and other abdominal visceral injuries.

B. Signs

The acute hydronephrosis of a totally ligated ureter results in severe flank pain and abdominal pain with nausea and vomiting early in the postoperative course and with associated ileus.

Signs and symptoms of acute peritonitis may be present if there is urinary extravasation into the peritoneal cavity. Watery discharge from the wound or vagina may be identified as urine by determining the creatinine concentration of a small sample—urine has many times the creatinine concentration found in serum—and by intravenous injection of 10 mL of indigo carmine, which will appear in the urine as dark blue.

C. Laboratory Findings

Ureteral injury from external violence is manifested by microscopic hematuria in 90% of cases. Urinalysis and other laboratory studies are of little use in diagnosis when injury has occurred from other causes.

D. Imaging Findings

Diagnosis is by excretory urography or delayed abdominal spiral CT scan. A plain film of the abdomen may demonstrate a large area of increased density in the pelvis or in an area of retroperitoneum where injury is suspected. After injection of contrast material, delayed excretion is noted with hydronephrosis. Partial transection of the ureter results in more rapid excretion, but persistent hydronephrosis is usually present, and contrast extravasation at the site of injury is noted on delayed films (Figure 18–10).

In acute injury from external violence, the excretory urogram usually appears normal, with very mild fullness down to the point of extravasation at the ureteral transection.

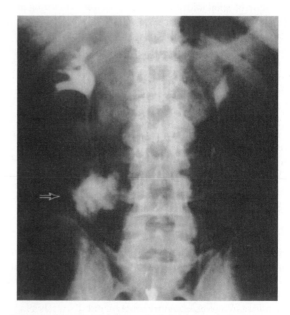

▲ **Figure 18–10.** Stab wound of right ureter shows extravasation (at *arrow*) on intravenous urogram.

Retrograde ureterography demonstrates the exact site of obstruction or extravasation.

E. Ultrasonography

Ultrasonography outlines hydroureter or urinary extravasation as it develops into a urinoma and is perhaps the best means of ruling out ureteral injury in the early postoperative period.

F. Radionuclide Scanning

Radionuclide scanning demonstrates delayed excretion on the injured side, with evidence of increasing counts owing to accumulation of urine in the renal pelvis. Its great benefit, however, is in the assessment of renal function after surgical correction.

▶ Differential Diagnosis

Postoperative bowel obstruction and peritonitis may cause symptoms similar to those of acute ureteral obstruction from injury. Fever, "acute abdomen," and associated nausea and vomiting following difficult pelvic surgery are definite indications for screening sonography or excretory urography to establish whether ureteral injury has occurred.

Deep wound infection must be considered postoperatively in patients with fever, ileus, and localized tenderness. The same findings are consistent with urinary extravasation and urinoma formation.

Acute pyelonephritis in the early postoperative period may also result in findings similar to those of ureteral injury. Sonography shows normal results, and urography shows no evidence of obstruction.

▶ Complications

Ureteral injury may be complicated by stricture formation with resulting hydronephrosis in the area of injury. Chronic urinary extravasation from unrecognized injury may lead to formation of a large retroperitoneal urinoma. Pyelonephritis from hydronephrosis and urinary infection may require prompt proximal drainage.

▶ Treatment

Prompt treatment of ureteral injuries is required. The best opportunity for successful repair is in the operating room when the injury occurs. If the injury is not recognized until 7–10 days after the event and no infection, abscess, or other complications exist, immediate reexploration and repair are indicated. Proximal urinary drainage by percutaneous nephrostomy or formal nephrostomy should be considered if the injury is recognized late or if the patient has significant complications that make immediate reconstruction unsatisfactory. The goals of ureteral repair are to achieve complete debridement, a tension-free spatulated anastomosis, water-tight closure, ureteral stenting (in selected cases), and retroperitoneal drainage.

A. Lower Ureteral Injuries

Injuries to the lower third of the ureter allow several options in management. The procedure of choice is reimplantation into the bladder combined with a psoas-hitch procedure to minimize tension on the ureteral anastomosis. An antireflux procedure should be done when possible. Primary ureteroureterostomy can be used in lower-third injuries when the ureter has been ligated without transection. The ureter is usually long enough for this type of anastomosis. A bladder tube flap can be used when the ureter is shorter.

Transureteroureterostomy may be used in lower-third injuries if extensive urinoma and pelvic infection have developed. This procedure allows anastomosis and reconstruction in an area away from the pathologic processes.

B. Midureteral Injuries

Midureteral injuries usually result from external violence and are best repaired by primary ureteroureterostomy or transureteroureterostomy.

C. Upper Ureteral Injuries

Injuries to the upper third of the ureter are best managed by primary ureteroureterostomy. If there is extensive loss of the ureter, autotransplantation of the kidney can be done as well as bowel replacement of the ureter.

D. Stenting

Most anastomoses after repair of ureteral injury should be stented. The preferred technique is to insert a silicone internal stent through the anastomosis before closure. These stents have a J memory curve on each end to prevent their migration in the postoperative period. After 3–4 weeks of healing, stents can be endoscopically removed from the bladder. The advantages of internal stenting are maintenance of a straight ureter with a constant caliber during early healing, the presence of a conduit for urine during healing, prevention of urinary extravasation, maintenance of urinary diversion, and easy removal.

▶ Prognosis

The prognosis for ureteral injury is excellent if the diagnosis is made early and prompt corrective surgery is done. Delay in diagnosis worsens the prognosis because of infection, hydronephrosis, abscess, and fistula formation.

INJURIES TO THE BLADDER

Bladder injuries occur most often from external force and are often associated with pelvic fractures. (About 15% of all

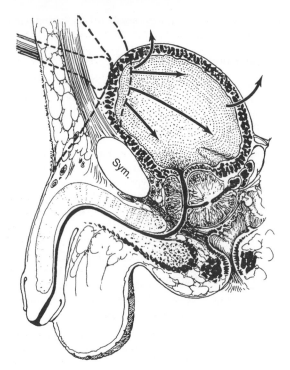

▲ **Figure 18–11.** Mechanism of vesical injury. A direct blow over the full bladder causes increased intravesical pressure. If the bladder ruptures, it will usually rupture into the peritoneal cavity.

pelvic fractures are associated with concomitant bladder or urethral injuries.) Iatrogenic injury may result from gynecologic and other extensive pelvic procedures as well as from hernia repairs and transurethral operations.

▶ Pathogenesis and Pathology (Figure 18–11)

The bony pelvis protects the urinary bladder very well. When the pelvis is fractured by blunt trauma, fragments from the fracture site may perforate the bladder. These perforations usually result in extraperitoneal rupture. If the urine is infected, extraperitoneal bladder perforations may result in deep pelvic abscess and severe pelvic inflammation.

When the bladder is filled to near capacity, a direct blow to the lower abdomen may result in bladder disruption. This type of disruption is ordinarily intraperitoneal. Since the reflection of the pelvic peritoneum covers the dome of the bladder, a linear laceration will allow urine to flow into the abdominal cavity. If the diagnosis is not established immediately and if the urine is sterile, no symptoms may be noted for several days. If the urine is infected, immediate peritonitis and acute abdomen will develop.

▶ Clinical Findings

Pelvic fracture accompanies bladder rupture in 90% of cases. The diagnosis of pelvic fracture can be made initially in the emergency room by lateral compression on the bony pelvis, since the fracture site will show crepitus and be painful to the touch.

A. Symptoms

There is usually a history of lower abdominal trauma. Blunt injury is the usual cause. Patients ordinarily are unable to urinate, but when spontaneous voiding occurs, gross hematuria is usually present. Most patients complain of pelvic or lower abdominal pain.

B. Signs

Heavy bleeding associated with pelvic fracture may result in hemorrhagic shock, usually from venous disruption of pelvic vessels. Evidence of external injury from a gunshot or stab wound in the lower abdomen should make one suspect bladder injury, manifested by marked tenderness of the suprapubic area and lower abdomen. An acute abdomen may occur with intraperitoneal bladder rupture. On rectal examination, landmarks may be indistinct because of a large pelvic hematoma.

C. Laboratory Findings

Catheterization usually is required in patients with pelvic trauma but not if bloody urethral discharge is noted. Bloody urethral discharge indicates urethral injury, and a urethrogram is necessary before catheterization (Figures 18–1 through 18–3). When catheterization is done, gross or, less commonly, microscopic hematuria is usually present. Urine taken from the bladder at the initial catheterization should be cultured to determine whether infection is present.

D. X-Ray Findings

A plain abdominal film generally demonstrates pelvic fractures. There may be haziness over the lower abdomen from blood and urine extravasation. A CT scan should be obtained to establish whether kidney and ureteral injuries are present.

Bladder disruption is shown on cystography. The bladder should be filled with 300 mL of contrast material and a plain film of the lower abdomen obtained. Contrast medium should be allowed to drain out completely, and a second film of the abdomen should be obtained. The drainage film is extremely important, because it demonstrates areas of extraperitoneal extravasation of blood and urine that may not appear on the filling film (Figure 18–12). With intraperitoneal extravasation, free contrast medium is visualized in the abdomen, highlighting bowel loops (Figure 18–13).

CT cystography is an excellent method for detecting bladder rupture; however, retrograde filling of the bladder with 300 mL of contrast medium is necessary to distend the bladder completely. Incomplete distention with consequent

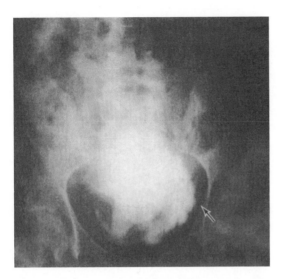

▲ **Figure 18–12.** Extraperitoneal bladder rupture. Extravasation (at *arrow*) seen outside the bladder in the pelvis on cystogram.

missed diagnosis of bladder rupture often occurs when the urethral catheter is clamped during standard abdominal CT scan with intravenous contrast injection.

▶ Complications

A pelvic abscess may develop from extraperitoneal bladder rupture; if the urine becomes infected, the pelvic hematoma

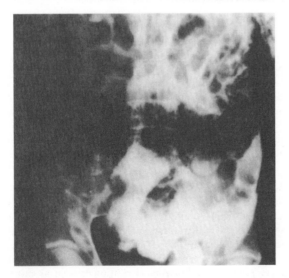

▲ **Figure 18–13.** Intraperitoneal bladder rupture. Cystogram shows contrast surrounding loops of bowel.

becomes infected too. Intraperitoneal bladder rupture with extravasation of urine into the abdominal cavity causes delayed peritonitis. Partial incontinence may result from bladder injury when the laceration extends into the bladder neck. Meticulous repair may ensure normal urinary control.

▶ Treatment

A. Emergency Measures

Shock and hemorrhage should be treated.

B. Surgical Measures

A lower midline abdominal incision should be made. As the bladder is approached in the midline, a pelvic hematoma, which is usually lateral, should be avoided. Entering the pelvic hematoma can result in increased bleeding from release of tamponade and in infection of the hematoma, with subsequent pelvic abscess. The bladder should be opened in the midline and carefully inspected. After repair, a suprapubic cystostomy tube is usually left in place to ensure complete urinary drainage and control of bleeding.

1. Extraperitoneal bladder rupture—Extraperitoneal bladder rupture can be successfully managed with urethral catheter drainage only. (Typically 10 days will provide adequate healing time.) Large blood clots in the bladder or injuries involving the bladder neck should be managed surgically.

As the bladder is opened in the midline, it should be carefully inspected and lacerations closed from within. Polyglycolic acid or chromic absorbable sutures should be used.

Extraperitoneal bladder lacerations occasionally extend into the bladder neck and should be repaired meticulously. Fine absorbable sutures should be used to ensure complete reconstruction so that the patient will have urinary control after injury. Such injuries are best managed with indwelling urethral catheterization and suprapubic diversion.

2. Intraperitoneal rupture—Intraperitoneal bladder ruptures should be repaired via a transperitoneal approach after careful transvesical inspection and closure of any other perforations. The peritoneum must be closed carefully over the area of injury. The bladder is then closed in separate layers by absorbable suture. All extravasated fluid from the peritoneal cavity should be removed before closure. At the time of closure, care should be taken that the suprapubic cystostomy is in the extraperitoneal position.

3. Pelvic fracture—Stable fracture of the pubic rami is usually present. In such cases, the patient can be ambulatory within 4–5 days without damage or difficulty. Unstable pelvic fractures requiring external fixation have a more protracted course.

4. Pelvic hematoma—There may be heavy uncontrolled bleeding from rupture of pelvic vessels even if the hematoma has not been entered at operation. At exploration and bladder repair, packing the pelvis with laparotomy tapes often controls the problem. If bleeding persists, it may be necessary to leave the tapes in place for 24 hours and operate again to remove them. Embolization of pelvic vessels with Gelfoam or skeletal muscle under angiographic control is useful in controlling persistent pelvic bleeding.

▶ Prognosis

With appropriate treatment, the prognosis is excellent. The suprapubic cystostomy tube can be removed within 10 days, and the patient can usually void normally. Patients with lacerations extending into the bladder neck area may be temporarily incontinent, but full control is usually regained. At the time of discharge, urine culture should be performed to determine whether catheter-associated infection requires further treatment.

INJURIES TO THE URETHRA

Urethral injuries are uncommon and occur most often in men, usually associated with pelvic fractures or straddle-type falls. They are rare in women. Various parts of the urethra may be lacerated, transected, or contused. Management varies according to the level of injury. The urethra can be separated into two broad anatomic divisions: the posterior urethra, consisting of the prostatic and membranous portions, and the anterior urethra, consisting of the bulbous and pendulous portions.

INJURIES TO THE POSTERIOR URETHRA

▶ Etiology (Figure 18–14)

The membranous urethra passes through the pelvic floor and voluntary urinary sphincter and is the portion of the posterior urethra most likely to be injured. When pelvic fractures occur from blunt trauma, the membranous urethra is sheared from the prostatic apex at the prostatomembranous junction. The urethra can be transected by the same mechanism at the interior surface of the membranous urethra.

▶ Clinical Findings

A. Symptoms

Patients usually complain of lower abdominal pain and inability to urinate. A history of crushing injury to the pelvis is usually obtained.

B. Signs

Blood at the urethral meatus is the single most important sign of urethral injury. The importance of this finding cannot be overemphasized, because an attempt to pass a urethral catheter may result in infection of the periprostatic

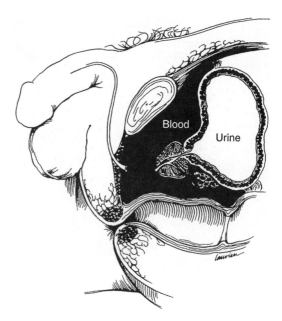

▲ **Figure 18–14.** Injury to the posterior (membranous) urethra. The prostate has been avulsed from the membranous urethra secondary to fracture of the pelvis. Extravasation occurs above the triangular ligament and is periprostatic and perivesical.

and perivesical hematoma and conversion of an incomplete laceration to a complete one. The presence of blood at the external urethral meatus indicates that immediate urethrography is necessary to establish the diagnosis.

Suprapubic tenderness and the presence of pelvic fracture are noted on physical examination. A large developing pelvic hematoma may be palpated. Perineal or suprapubic contusions are often noted. Rectal examination may reveal a large pelvic hematoma with the prostate displaced superiorly. Rectal examination can be misleading, however, because a tense pelvic hematoma may resemble the prostate on palpation. Superior displacement of the prostate does not occur if the puboprostatic ligaments remain intact. Partial disruption of the membranous urethra (currently 10% of cases) is not accompanied by prostatic displacement.

C. X-Ray Findings

Fractures of the bony pelvis are usually present. A urethrogram (using 20–30 mL of water-soluble contrast material) shows the site of extravasation at the prostatomembranous junction. Ordinarily, there is free extravasation of contrast material into the perivesical space (Figure 18–15). Incomplete prostatomembranous disruption is seen as minor extravasation, with a portion of contrast material passing into the prostatic urethra and bladder.

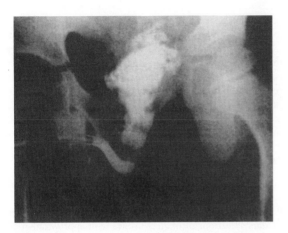

▲ **Figure 18–15.** Ruptured prostatomembranous urethra shows free extravasation on urethrogram. No contrast medium is seen entering the prostatic urethra.

D. Instrumental Examination

The only instrumentation involved should be for urethrography. Catheterization or urethroscopy should not be done, because these procedures pose an increased risk of hematoma, infection, and further damage to partial urethral disruptions.

▶ Differential Diagnosis

Bladder rupture may be associated with posterior urethral injuries in approximately 20% of cases. Cystography cannot be done preoperatively, since a urethral catheter should not be passed. Careful evaluation of the bladder at operation is necessary.

▶ Complications

Stricture, impotence, and incontinence as complications of prostatomembranous disruption are among the most severe and debilitating mishaps that result from trauma to the urinary system. Stricture following primary repair and anastomosis occurs in about 50% of cases. If the preferred suprapubic cystostomy approach with delayed repair is used, the incidence of stricture can be reduced to about 5%.

The incidence of impotence after primary repair is 30–80% (mean, about 50%). This figure can be reduced to 30–35% by suprapubic drainage with delayed urethral reconstruction.

Total urinary incontinence occurs in <2% of patients and is typically associated with severe sacral fracture and S2–4 nerve injury.

▶ Treatment

A. Emergency Measures

Shock and hemorrhage should be treated.

B. Surgical Measures

Urethral catheterization should be avoided.

1. Immediate management—Initial management should consist of suprapubic cystostomy to provide urinary drainage. A midline lower abdominal incision should be made, with care being taken to avoid the large pelvic hematoma. The bladder and prostate are usually elevated superiorly by large periprostatic and perivesical hematomas. The bladder often is distended by a large volume of urine accumulated during the period of resuscitation and operative preparation. The urine is often clear and free of blood, but gross hematuria may be present. The bladder should be opened in the midline and carefully inspected for lacerations. If a laceration is present, the bladder should be closed with absorbable suture material and a cystostomy tube inserted for urinary drainage. This approach involves no urethral instrumentation or manipulation. The suprapubic cystostomy is maintained in place for about 3 months. This allows resolution of the pelvic hematoma, and the prostate and bladder will slowly return to their anatomic positions.

Incomplete laceration of the posterior urethra heals spontaneously, and the suprapubic cystostomy can be removed within 2–3 weeks. The cystostomy tube should not be removed before voiding cystourethrography shows that no extravasation persists.

2. Delayed urethral reconstruction—Reconstruction of the urethra after prostatic disruption can be undertaken within 3 months, assuming there is no pelvic abscess or other evidence of persistent pelvic infection. Before reconstruction, a combined cystogram and urethrogram should be done to determine the exact length of the resulting urethral stricture. This stricture usually is 1–2 cm long and situated immediately posterior to the pubic bone. The preferred approach is a single-stage reconstruction of the urethral rupture defect with direct excision of the strictured area and anastomosis of the bulbous urethra directly to the apex of the prostate. A 16F silicone urethral catheter should be left in place along with a suprapubic cystostomy. Catheters are removed within a month, and the patient is then able to void (Figure 18–16).

3. Immediate urethral realignment—Some surgeons prefer to realign the urethra immediately. Persistent bleeding and surrounding hematoma create technical problems. The incidence of stricture, impotence, and incontinence appears to be higher than with immediate cystostomy and delayed reconstruction. However, several authors have reported success with immediate urethral realignment.

C. General Measures

After delayed reconstruction by a perineal approach, patients are allowed ambulation on the first postoperative day and usually can be discharged within 3 days.

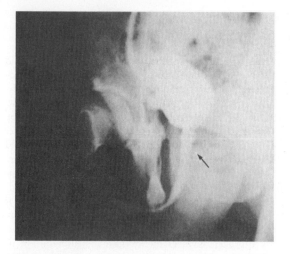

▲ **Figure 18–16.** Delayed repair of urethral injury. Normal voiding urethrogram after transpubic repair of stricture following prostatomembranous urethral disruption. *Arrow* indicates area of repair.

D. Treatment of Complications

Approximately 1 month after the delayed reconstruction, the urethral catheter can be removed and a voiding cystogram obtained through the suprapubic cystostomy tube. If the cystogram shows a patent area of reconstruction free of extravasation, the suprapubic catheter can be removed; if there is extravasation or stricture, suprapubic cystostomy should be maintained. A follow-up urethrogram should be obtained within 2 months to watch for stricture development.

Stricture, if present (<5%), is usually very short, and urethrotomy under direct vision offers easy and rapid cure. The patient may be impotent for several months after delayed repair. Impotence is permanent in about 10% of patients. Implantation of a penile prosthesis is indicated if impotence is still present 2 years after reconstruction (see Chapter 38). Incontinence after posterior urethral rupture and delayed repair is rare (<2%) and is usually related to the extent of injury rather than to the repair.

▶ Prognosis

If complications can be avoided, the prognosis is excellent. Urinary infections ultimately resolve with appropriate management.

INJURIES TO THE ANTERIOR URETHRA

▶ Etiology (Figure 18–17)

The anterior urethra is the portion distal to the urogenital diaphragm. Straddle injury may cause laceration or contusion of the urethra. Self-instrumentation or iatrogenic instrumentation may cause partial disruption.

▶ Pathogenesis and Pathology

A. Contusion

Contusion of the urethra is a sign of crush injury without urethral disruption. Perineal hematoma usually resolves without complications.

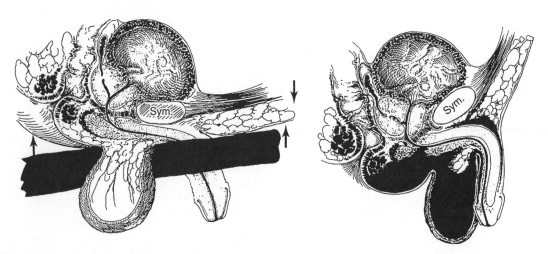

▲ **Figure 18–17.** Injury to the bulbous urethra. **Left:** Mechanism: usually a perineal blow or fall astride an object; crushing of urethra against inferior edge of pubic symphysis. **Right:** Extravasation of blood and urine enclosed within Colles' fascia (see Figures 18–1 through 18–9).

B. Laceration

A severe straddle injury may result in laceration of part of the urethral wall, allowing extravasation of urine. If the extravasation is unrecognized, it may extend into the scrotum, along the penile shaft, and up to the abdominal wall. It is limited only by Colles' fascia and often results in sepsis, infection, and serious morbidity.

▶ Clinical Findings

A. Symptoms

There is usually a history of a fall, and in some cases, a history of instrumentation. Bleeding from the urethra is usually present. There is local pain into the perineum and sometimes massive perineal hematoma. If voiding has occurred and extravasation is noted, sudden swelling in the area will be present. If diagnosis has been delayed, sepsis and severe infection may be present.

B. Signs

The perineum is very tender; a mass may be found, as may blood at the urethral meatus. Rectal examination reveals a normal prostate. The patient usually has a desire to void, but voiding should not be allowed until assessment of the urethra is complete. No attempt should be made to pass a urethral catheter, but if the patient's bladder is overdistended, percutaneous suprapubic cystostomy can be done as a temporary procedure.

When presentation of such injuries is delayed, there is massive urinary extravasation and infection in the perineum and the scrotum. The lower abdominal wall may also be involved. The skin is usually swollen and discolored.

C. Laboratory Findings

Blood loss is not usually excessive, particularly if secondary injury has occurred. The white count may be elevated with infection.

D. X-Ray Findings

A urethrogram, with instillation of 15–20 mL of water-soluble contrast material, demonstrates extravasation and the location of injury (Figure 18–18). A contused urethra shows no evidence of extravasation.

▶ Complications

Heavy bleeding from the corpus spongiosum injury may occur in the perineum as well as through the urethral meatus. Pressure applied to the perineum over the site of the injury usually controls bleeding. If hemorrhage cannot be controlled, immediate operation is required.

The complications of urinary extravasation are chiefly sepsis and infection. Aggressive debridement and drainage

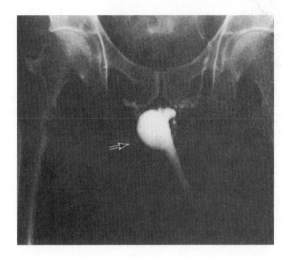

▲ **Figure 18–18.** Ruptured bulbar (anterior) urethra following straddle injury. Extravasation (at *arrow*) on urethrogram.

are required if there is infection. Stricture at the site of injury is a common complication, but surgical reconstruction may not be required unless the stricture significantly reduces urinary flow rates.

▶ Treatment

A. General Measures

Major blood loss usually does not occur from straddle injury. If heavy bleeding does occur, local pressure for control, followed by resuscitation, is required.

B. Specific Measures

1. Urethral contusion—The patient with urethral contusion shows no evidence of extravasation, and the urethra remains intact. After urethrography, the patient is allowed to void; and if the voiding occurs normally, without pain or bleeding, no additional treatment is necessary. If bleeding persists, urethral catheter drainage can be done.

2. Urethral lacerations—Instrumentation of the urethra following urethrography should be avoided. A small midline incision in the suprapubic area readily exposes the dome of the bladder so that a suprapubic cystostomy tube can be inserted, allowing complete urinary diversion while the urethral laceration heals. Percutaneous cystostomy may also be used in such injuries. If only minor extravasation is noted on the urethrogram, a voiding study can be performed within 7 days after suprapubic catheter drainage to search for extravasation. In more extensive injuries, one should wait 2–3 weeks before doing a voiding study through the suprapubic catheter. Healing at the site of injury may result in stricture formation. Most of these strictures are not severe and do not require surgical reconstruction. The suprapubic cystostomy catheter may be removed if no extravasation is documented. Follow-up with documentation of urinary flow rates will show whether there is urethral obstruction from stricture.

3. Urethral laceration with extensive urinary extravasation—After major laceration, urinary extravasation may involve the perineum, scrotum, and lower abdomen. Drainage of these areas is indicated. Suprapubic cystostomy for urinary diversion is required. Infection and abscess formation are common and require antibiotic therapy.

4. Immediate repair—Immediate repair of urethral lacerations can be performed, but the procedure is difficult and the incidence of associated stricture is high.

C. Treatment of Complications

Strictures at the site of injury may be extensive and require delayed reconstruction.

▶ Prognosis

Urethral stricture is a major complication but, in most cases, does not require surgical reconstruction. If, when stricture resolves, urinary flow rates are poor and urinary infection and urethral fistula are present, reconstruction is required.

INJURIES TO THE PENIS

Disruption of the tunica albuginea of the penis (penile fracture) can occur during sexual intercourse. At presentation, the patient has penile pain and hematoma. This injury should be surgically corrected.

Gangrene and urethral injury may be caused by obstructing rings placed around the base of the penis. These objects must be removed without causing further damage. Penile amputation is seen occasionally, and in a few patients, the penis can be surgically replaced successfully by microsurgical techniques.

Total avulsion of the penile skin occurs from machinery injuries. Immediate debridement and skin grafting are usually successful in salvage. Injuries to the penis should suggest possible urethral damage, which should be investigated by urethrography.

INJURIES TO THE SCROTUM

Superficial lacerations of the scrotum may be debrided and closed primarily. Blunt trauma may cause local hematoma and ecchymosis, but these injuries resolve without difficulty. One must be certain that testicular rupture has not occurred.

Total avulsion of the scrotal skin may be caused by machinery accidents or other major trauma. The testes and spermatic cords are usually intact. It is important to provide coverage for these structures: this is best done by immediate surgical debridement and by placing the testes and spermatic cords in the subcutaneous tissues of the upper thighs. Later reconstruction of the scrotum can be done with a skin graft or thigh flap.

INJURIES TO THE TESTIS

Blunt trauma to the testis causes severe pain and, often, nausea and vomiting. Lower abdominal tenderness may be present. A hematoma may surround the testis and make delineation of its margin difficult. Ultrasonography can be used as an aid to better define the organ. If rupture has occurred, the sonogram will delineate the injury, which should be surgically repaired.

BIBLIOGRAPHY

Emergency Diagnosis and Management

Brandes S et al: Consensus on genitourinary trauma. BJU Int 2004;94:277.

Demetriades D et al: Pelvic fractures: Epidemiology and predictors of associated abdominal injuries. J Am Coll Surg 2002;195(1):1.

Morey AF et al: Consensus on genitourinary trauma. BJU Int 2004;94:507.

Rosenstein D, McAninch JW: Urologic emergencies. Med Clin North Am 2004;88:495.

Tarman GJ et al: Lower genitourinary injury and pelvic fractures in pediatric patients. Urology 2002;59:123.

Titton RL et al: Urine leaks and urinomas: Diagnosis and imaging-guided intervention. Radiographics 2003;23:1133.

Yossepowitch O et al: Urological injuries during cesarean section: Intraoperative diagnosis and management. J Urol 2004;172:196.

Ziran BH et al: Delays and difficulties in the diagnosis of lower urologic injuries in the context of pelvic fractures. J Trauma 2005;58:533.

Injuries to the Kidney

Armenakas NA et al: Indications for nonoperative management of renal stab wounds. J Urol 1999;161:768.

Barsness KA et al: Renovascular injury: An argument for renal preservation. J Trauma 2004;57:310.

Buckley JC, McAninch JW: Pediatric renal injuries. J Urol 2004; 172:687.

Buckley JC, McAninch JW: Revision of current American Association for the Surgery of Trauma Renal Injury grading system. J Trauma 2011;70(1):35–37.

Elliott SP et al: Renal arterial injuries: Single center analysis of management strategies and outcomes. J Urol 2007;178(6):2451–2455.

Johnson B et al: A need for reevaluation of sports participation recommendations for children with a solitary kidney. J Urol 2005; 174:686.

Knudson MM et al: Outcome after major renovascular injuries: A Western Trauma Association multicenter report. J Trauma 2000;49:1116.

McAninch JW et al: Renal reconstruction after injury. J Urol 1991; 145:932.

Miller KS, McAninch JW: Radiographic assessment of renal trauma: Our 15-year experience. J Urol 1995;154:352.

Santucci RA et al: Evaluation and management of renal injuries: Consensus statement of renal trauma subcommittee. BJU Int 2004;93:937.

Santucci RA, Fisher MB: The literature increasingly supports expectant (conservative) management of renal trauma—A systematic review. J Trauma 2005;59:493.

Tasian GE et al: Evaluation of renal function after major renal injury: Correlation with the American Association for the Surgery of Trauma Injury Scale. J Urol 2010;183(1):196–200.

Voelzke BB, McAninch JW: The current management of renal trauma. Am Surg 2008;74(8):667–678.

Voelzke BB, McAninch JW: Renal gunshot wounds: Clinical management and outcome. J Trauma 2009;66(3):593–600.

Wessells H et al: Criteria for nonoperative treatment of significant penetrating renal lacerations. J Urol 1996;157:24.

Injuries to the Ureter

Elliott SP, McAninch JW: Ureteral injuries from external violence: The 25-year experience at San Francisco General Hospital. J Urol 2003;170:1213.

Injuries to the Bladder

Elliott SP, McAninch JW: Extraperitoneal bladder trauma: Delayed surgical management can lead to prolonged convalescence. J Trauma 2009;66(1):274–275.

Gomez RG et al: Consensus statement on bladder injuries. BJU Int 2004;94:27.

Power N et al: Computed tomographic cystography in bladder trauma: Pictorial essay. Can Assoc Radiol J 2004;55(5):304.

Injuries to the Urethra

Chapple C et al: Consensus statement on urethral trauma. BJU Int 2004;93:1195.

Koraitim MM: On the art of anastomotic posterior urethroplasty: A 27-year experience. J Urol 2005;173:135.

McAninch JW, Voelzke BB: Managing urethral trauma in children. US Pediatr 2008;4(1):85–88.

Myers JB, McAninch JW: Management of posterior urethral disruption injuries. Nat Clin Pract Urol 2009;6:154–163.

Park S, McAninch JW: Straddle injuries to the bulbar urethra: Management and outcomes in 78 patients. J Urol 2004;171(Suppl 2, Pt 1):722.

Yu NC et al: Fistulas of the genitourinary tract: A radiologic review. Radiographics 2004;24(5):1331.

Injuries to the Penis

Gomes CM et al: Genital trauma due to animal bites. J Urol 2001;165:80.

Mydlo JH: Surgeon experience with penile fracture. J Urol 2001;166:526.

Zargooshi J: Penile fracture in Kermanshah, Iran: Report of 172 cases. J Urol 2000;164:364.

Injuries to the Scrotum

Buckley JC, McAninch JW: Use of ultrasonography in diagnosis of testicular injuries in blunt scrotal trauma. J Urol 2006;175:175.

Mohr AM et al: Management of trauma to the male external genitalia: The usefulness of American Association for the Surgery of Trauma organ injury scales. J Urol 2003;170:2311.

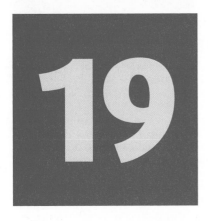

Immunology & Immunotherapy of Urologic Cancers

Eric J. Small, MD

Both experimental and naturally occurring tumors are capable of stimulating a specific antitumor immune response. This observation suggests that there are foreign proteins (antigens) on tumor cells that classically have been described as resulting in humoral and cellular immune responses. However, experimental models suggest that a T-cell (cell-mediated) response may be more important in the killing of tumor cells than a B-cell (humoral) response.

A detailed description of the components of the immune system is beyond the scope of this chapter, but certain features of the immune system as they pertain to diagnostic and therapeutic issues will be reviewed.

TUMOR ANTIGENS

Tumor antigens can be divided into tumor-specific antigens and tumor-associated antigens. Tumor-specific antigens are not found on normal tissue, and they permit the host to recognize a tumor as foreign. Tumor-specific antigens have been shown to exist in oncogenesis models utilizing chemical, physical, and viral carcinogens but appear to be less common in models of spontaneous tumor development.

The identification of tumor-specific antigens led to the theory of immune surveillance, which suggests that the immune system is continuously trolling for foreign (tumor-specific) antigens. This theory is supported by the observation that at least some cancers are more common in immune-suppressed patients such as transplant patients or human immunodeficiency virus–infected individuals. However, many cancers are not overrepresented in these patient populations. Furthermore, spontaneous tumor models, which more closely resemble human carcinogenesis, appear to have a less extensive repertoire of tumor-specific antigens but instead have been found to express many tumor-associated antigens.

Tumor-associated antigens are found in normal cells but either become less prevalent in normal tissue after embryogenesis (eg, alpha-fetoprotein [AFP]) or remain present in normal tissue but are overexpressed in cancer cells (eg, prostate-specific antigen [PSA]). In either case, the more ubiquitous nature of these antigens appears to cause reduced immune reactivity (also known as tolerance) to the specific antigen. The mechanisms of tolerance are complex and may be due in part to the absence of other required costimulatory molecules (such as B7, a molecule required for T-cell stimulation). Recent evidence has also implicated a number of immune checkpoints that result in downregulation of the cellular immune response. In particular, two molecules, CTLA-4 and PD-1, have been identified on activated lymphocytes that dampen the immune response, and therefore have been exploited as potential therapeutic targets.

The development of monoclonal technology has allowed the development of many antibodies against many tumor-associated antigens and has provided insight into the regulation and expression of these antigens. The reexpression or upregulation of these tumor-associated antigens during carcinogenesis may lead to immune response (or loss of tolerance). Many novel therapeutic approaches have sought to break this tolerance, and approaches to enhance a patient's immune response will be discussed.

▶ Humoral Immunity

A large number of monoclonal antibodies have been developed against a variety of tumor-associated antigens. Oncofetal antigens such as AFP and beta-human chorionic gonadotropin (β-hCG) are important markers in germ cell tumors. β-hCG is also expressed in a small percentage of patients with bladder carcinoma. Antibodies directed against specific targets such as vascular endothelial growth factor (VEGF) have been developed and have been tested for the treatment of advanced prostate cancer, renal cell carcinoma (RCC), and transitional cell carcinoma (TCC).

▶ Antibodies in Cancer Diagnosis and Detection

A. Prostate Cancer

Immunoassays are used to test both body fluids and tissues for the presence of tumor-associated antigens. In the urologic cancers, the most obvious example is the development of monoclonal antibodies against PSA. The utility and limitations of PSA are described elsewhere in this volume. Other antigens that have been tested in prostate cancer include prostatic acid phosphatase, which has largely been replaced by PSA in screening programs and in patients with low tumor burden. Prostatic acid phosphatase may be of some use in detecting or following bone metastases and as a predictive marker of response to therapy for metastatic disease. Antibodies to prostate-specific membrane antigen (PSMA) have been used, primarily for immunohistochemistry.

B. Renal Cell Carcinoma

Unfortunately, there are as yet no well-established antigens (or antibodies) that can be used to reliably evaluate and monitor RCC, although a variety of target antigens are being evaluated.

C. Bladder Cancer

Two oncofetal antigens, β-hCG and carcinoembryonic antigen, are expressed by a minority (≤20%) of TCCs. These markers are not routinely used, but in diagnostic dilemmas, measurement of serum levels of β-hCG or staining of tissue for this antigen may be useful.

D. Germ Cell Tumors

As described in Chapter 23, antibodies to hCG and AFP are routinely used to detect shed antigens from germ cell tumors in the bloodstream. These antigens can also be detected in tissue samples. While the use of serum markers in germ cell tumors is reviewed elsewhere, it is worth noting that the presence of the oncofetoprotein AFP, either in serum or in tissue specimens, is pathognomonic for a nonseminomatous germ cell tumor, regardless of results of routine pathologic evaluation. In addition to their diagnostic utility, AFP and hCG can be used as markers of response to therapy and as predictive factors of outcome. For example, the international germ cell tumor risk classification schema for patients with metastatic disease relies heavily on AFP and hCG levels as well as levels of a nonspecific marker, lactate dehydrogenase, to assign patients with nonseminomatous germ cell tumors to one of three risk levels (see Chapter 23).

E. Radioimmunodetection

Monoclonal antibodies to a specific antigen can be radiolabeled, and the preferential binding of the monoclonal antibody to tumor cells can be exploited. Theoretically, such an approach could be used for the presurgical evaluation of disease, postsurgical evaluation for minimal residual disease, confirmation of cancer identified by other imaging modalities, and detection of recurrent disease. There are several potential impediments to successful tumor radioimmunodetection. These include dilution of antibody in the bloodstream; metabolism of the antibody; nonspecific binding in liver, reticuloendothelial system, bone marrow, and elsewhere; binding of antibody by circulating or shed antigen; and the development of neutralizing human antimouse antibodies.

The only radioimmunodetection system for urologic cancers at this time is ^{111}In-capromab pendetide (Prostascint), a murine monoclonal antibody to PSMA. Its use has been hampered by a fairly laborious administration process, operator dependence in interpretation of scans, and a less than satisfactory positive predictive value. The use of ^{111}In-capromab pendetide is described in Chapter 10.

▶ Immunotherapy with Monoclonal Antibodies

Immunotherapy with monoclonal antibodies alone ("naked antibodies") has been fairly extensively evaluated. The use of monoclonal antibodies against tumor-associated antigens has met with only limited success in patients with solid tumors including prostate and kidney cancer. In lymphoproliferative disorders such as leukemia and lymphoma, some antibodies to tumor-associated surface antigens appear to result in tumor cell death. The mechanism for these effects is certainly multifactorial but may, in part, be mediated by resultant complement fixation.

Direct antiproliferative effects of antibodies on cancer cells can be achieved by antibodies against functionally important antigens. Thus, the inhibition of growth factors and growth factor receptors and the activation or inhibition of signal transducing molecules are attractive therapeutic targets. In urologic cancers, while no approved monoclonal antibody therapy exists, trials of antibodies against growth factors, VEGF (an angiogenic molecule), and signal transduction molecules are being undertaken. Kidney cancer is highly dependent on angiogenesis, and bevacizumab (an antibody agent against VEGF) has been shown to prolong time to progression (TTP) in metastatic disease. Two independent randomized phase 3 trials have demonstrated the superiority of alpha-interferon plus bevacizumab over alpha-interferon alone, with an improvement in TTP, leading to approval by the U.S. Food and Drug Administration (FDA) of bevacizumab for this indication. By contrast, in prostate cancer patients with progressive disease despite androgen deprivation therapy, the addition of bevacizumab to conventional chemotherapy with docetaxel failed to demonstrate a prolongation in overall survival, (although TTP was improved).

An alternative approach to naked antibodies is to conjugate any of a variety of cytotoxic agents to an antibody. The advantage of this approach is a "bystander effect," making it unnecessary to use an antibody that binds each and every cell. This can be achieved in a variety of ways. The most straightforward is to use the monoclonal antibody as a means of providing some targeting specificity for the cytotoxic agent used. Cytotoxic agents used include radioisotopes, chemotherapy, and toxins such as ricin. Other means of providing some specificity is to bind a prodrug (with an antibody) to the tumor site and then to activate the bound prodrug. Finally, targeting with bispecific antibodies (eg, to antigen and to an effector T cell, or to antigen and toxin) has been undertaken. These approaches have all been tested in prostate cancer, but all remain investigational at this point.

Cell-Mediated Immunity

There is considerable evidence, both clinical and preclinical, that tumor-associated antigens can elicit a cell-mediated immune response. In some models, when carcinogen-induced tumors in mice are resected and the mouse is reinoculated with tumor cells, the tumor fails to regrow, suggesting the development of immunity to specific antigens. Specific antigens that are rejected in immunized hosts are termed transplantation antigens. The specificity of tumor rejection has since been demonstrated to reside in T lymphocytes (at a minimum). Lymphocytes of cancer patients can sometimes be stimulated in vitro to recognize specific tumor-associated antigens and consequently demonstrate properties of cytolytic T lymphocytes. Unfortunately, the phenomenon of tumor rejection is by no means universal, either in the laboratory or clinically, and it is unusual to detect cytolytic T-lymphocyte activity against many tumor-associated antigens.

Nevertheless, there are several clinical scenarios that suggest that cell-mediated antitumor responses exist. These observations have promoted a broad search for the means of enhancing patients' immune responses to tumor-associated antigens. RCC is in many ways the prototypical immune-mediated tumor and, along with melanoma, has until recently been the primary target of immune manipulations.

Immunotherapy Involving Cell-Mediated Immunity

Evidence of cell-mediated immunity playing a role in tumor rejection lies in the results of a variety of immunotherapeutic interventions. Immunotherapy can be broadly classified as active or passive. This classification refers to the role the host's immune system plays. Thus, the passive transfer of preformed antibodies is contrasted to a vaccination program in which the host's immune system must be capable of mounting an immune response. Adoptive therapy refers to a middle ground in which efforts are made to reconstitute, modify, or bolster one of the effector cells involved ex vivo, followed by reinfusion into the patient, where the rest of the immune cascade must then be recruited.

Active Immunotherapy: Vaccination

Autologous vaccination programs (the vaccination of patients with their own tumor cells) have been extensively explored. The advantage of autologous vaccination is that the vaccine bears the antigens of the patient's tumor, although the distinct disadvantage is that not every patient has a tumor available for vaccine preparation, and the preparation of each vaccine is tremendously labor intensive. By contrast, allogeneic vaccines (the use of a generic vaccine or "off-the-shelf" antigen) have the benefit of mass production and ease of use, and the identification of specific tumor rejection antigens allows specific antigenic targeting. However, this approach runs the risk of a more narrow shared antigenic spectrum with the patient's tumor. Both autologous and allogeneic vaccination strategies have been evaluated in RCC and prostate cancer.

Several means exist to undertake vaccination. The simplest is to use intact but inactivated tumor cells. Inactivation can be achieved with ultraviolet radiation, external beam (photon) radiation, or freeze-thawing. Crude extracts of cells can also be used. The advantage of using cell extracts is that inactivation is not necessary and small particles and proteins that might be more easily phagocytosed are available. One can also enhance the immunogenicity of inoculated cells by growing the cells in cytokines, coinjecting with cytokines (nonspecific active immunotherapy, described later), or transfecting these cells with the genes for immune stimulatory cytokines or the costimulatory molecule B7. Clinical trials using prostate cancer cell lines transfected with the granulocyte-macrophage colony-stimulating factor (GM-CSF) gene (GVAX; Cell Genesys, South San Francisco, CA) for vaccination in patients with metastatic hormone refractory prostate cancer failed to show a therapeutic benefit. Purified protein or peptides represent a second potential vaccination schema. A trial of PSA in a vaccina and fowlpox (ProstaVax) vector demonstrated clinical activity, and confirmatory trials are underway. A third way of undertaking specific vaccination is to attempt to bypass the antigen-presenting function of the immune system and to directly stimulate professional antigen-presenting cells, such as dendritic cells, ex vivo. These cells can be stimulated by pulsing them with protein or peptides of interest or by transfecting them with a gene encoding the antigenic peptide of interest before reinfusion. Sipuleucel-T is an autologous dendritic cell product that has been shown to prolong life, and it is appropriate for patients with castration-resistant metastatic prostate cancer who do not have cancer-associated pain, visceral metastases, rapidly progressive disease, or the need for systemic steroids.

Nonspecific Active Immunotherapy: Cytokines and Biologic Response Modifiers

Bacillus Calmette-Guérin (BCG) is a live attenuated form of tubercle bacillus that appears to have local activity against some tumors but has been largely disappointing as systemic therapy. The utility of BCG in the treatment of superficial bladder cancer is well described and is beyond the scope of this chapter. The mechanism by which BCG can elicit a local immune response in the uroepithelium and thereby exhibit impressive anticancer activity is not well delineated. However, possible mechanisms of action include macrophage activation, lymphocyte activation, recruitment of dendritic cells, and natural killer cells. It is intriguing that this is strictly a local phenomenon and that BCG has no role in the treatment of muscle-invasive or metastatic disease.

Interleukin-2 (IL-2) is a naturally occurring cytokine that has multiple immunoregulatory properties. The observation that exogenously administered IL-2 could result in tumor regression in patients with RCC and melanoma was the first unequivocal indication that cancer regression could be mediated by immune manipulations. IL-2 stimulates lymphocyte proliferation, enhances cytolytic T-cell activity, induces natural killer cell activity, and induces gamma-interferon and tumor necrosis factor production. IL-2 has no direct cytotoxicity, but when administered exogenously will activate effector cells of the host immune system, including lymphocytes, natural killer cells, lymphokine-activated killer cells, and tumor-infiltrating lymphocytes. IL-2 has been administered in RCC in several different schemas, including high-dose intravenous bolus (IL-2 is FDA approved with this schedule), continuous intravenous infusion, and at lower doses subcutaneously. The high-dose regimens must be administered on an inpatient basis and are characterized by significant, albeit manageable, toxicities, including fever; malaise; vascular leak syndrome; hypotension; and cardiac, renal, and hepatic dysfunction. Subcutaneous IL-2 is self-administered by patients in the outpatient setting, and while clearly less toxic, still has associated malaise and constitutional symptoms. The optimal dosing regimen is not well established, and overall response proportions rarely exceed 20%. Durable complete responses of 5–8% have been reported with some of the high-dose regimens. IL-2 has also been combined with other active agents such as alpha-interferon and chemotherapy, although it is not clear if these combinations provide additional benefit. High-dose IL-2 is, to date, the only therapy of inducing durable complete remissions and potential cures. However, its toxicity profile makes this approach realistic for very carefully selected young patients with an excellent performance status, limited extent of metastases, and no significant comorbidities.

Alpha-interferon is a naturally occurring cytokine that has direct cytotoxic and possibly antiproliferative properties, but it also has immunoregulatory properties. It enhances major histocompatibility complex expression, thereby potentially increasing the efficiency of antigen processing and recognition. Alpha-interferon has anticancer activity in both RCC and superficial bladder cancer. Its primary toxicity is fever, malaise, and constitutional symptoms, although at higher doses, it can result in bone marrow toxicity, central nervous system toxicity, and hepatic toxicity. In RCC, as a single agent,

alpha-interferon can result in clinical responses in up to 20% of patients. In contradistinction to IL-2 as a single agent, durable complete responses are quite rare. Nevertheless, in randomized trials, alpha-interferon appears to confer a modest survival advantage over other agents now known to be largely inactive. As noted earlier, the addition of bevacizumab to alpha-interferon is superior to alpha-interferon alone. Alpha-interferon is also used as an intravesical treatment in superficial bladder cancer, where it has established activity, and is not infrequently used as second-line therapy after BCG. A recent trial of BCG plus interferon failed to demonstrate superiority over BCG alone in patients with superficial bladder cancer.

GM-CSF is perhaps the most important cytokine in eliciting cellular immune responses. Administered systemically as a subcutaneous injection, GM-CSF has been shown to reduce PSA in patients with both hormone-sensitive and hormone-resistant prostate cancer. However, the use of GM-CSF is neither proven to be of clinical benefit nor approved for this indication and must be considered investigational.

▶ Immunomodulation

A myriad of immunosuppressive factors exist within cancer patients that may serve to dampen antitumor immune responses. Some of these molecules represent natural pathways to inhibit autoimmunity, while some molecules may have been usurped by the tumor to evade immune recognition. Novel approaches are now being developed to target these pathways. For example, CTLA-4 is an inhibitory molecule that blocks activation of T cells. By preventing the action of CTLA-4, an anti-CTLA-4 antibody (ipilimumab) can augment and prolong T-cell immune responses. In animal models, ipilimumab can induce tumor rejection in immunogenic tumors and, in combination with antitumor vaccination, can induce rejection of minimally immunogenic tumors, including in the transgenic adenocarcinoma of mouse/prostate (TRAMP) prostate cancer model. Ipilimumab has been demonstrated to have modest anticancer activity as monotherapy in patients with metastatic CRPC, although it is not yet approved. The combination of CTLA-4 blockade with vaccination is of interest and is under investigation. The potential benefits of CTLA-4 blockade need to be balanced against not insignificant autoimmune toxicity, which can, rarely, result in colitis, dermatitis, hepatitis, and hypophysitis (panhypopituitarism).

▶ Adoptive Immunotherapy

Adoptive immunotherapy is the transfer of cellular products (effector cells) to the host or patient in an effort to develop an immune response. The use of adoptive immunotherapy was prompted by the observation that T cells derived from patients with melanoma or RCC had the ability to recognize antigens on the primary tumor. Thus, it was hoped that these cells could be harvested, activated ex vivo, and then reinfused into patients. Lymphokine-activated killer cells and tumor-infiltrating lymphocytes have been used to treat patients with metastatic RCC in the investigational setting, frequently along with IL-2. However, randomized trials comparing IL-2 alone with IL-2 plus cellular products have failed to demonstrate an improvement in response proportions or survival. Chapter 22 gives specific details of immunotherapy in RCC.

BIBLIOGRAPHY

Agarwala SS, Kirkwood JM: Interferons in the treatment of solid tumors. Oncology 1994;51:129.

Anichini A et al: Clonal analysis of the cytolytic T-cell response to human tumors. Immunol Today 1987;8:385.

Berd D et al: Induction of cell-mediated immunity to autologous melanoma cells and regression of metastases after treatment with a melanoma cell vaccine preceded by cyclophosphamide. Cancer Res 1986;46:2572.

Berd D et al: Treatment of metastatic melanoma with an autologous tumor-cell vaccine: Clinical and immunologic results in 64 patients. J Clin Oncol 1990;11:1858.

Berd D: Cancer vaccines: Reborn or just recycled? Semin Oncol 1998;25:605.

Bukowski RM: Natural history and therapy of metastatic renal cell carcinoma: The role of interleukin-2. Cancer 1997;80:1198.

Fyfe G et al: Results of treatment of 255 patients with metastatic RCC who received high-dose recombinant interleukin-2 therapy. J Clin Oncol 1995;13:688.

Gitlitz BJ et al: Immunotherapy and gene therapy. Semin Urol Oncol 1996;14:237.

Goedegebuure PS, Eberlen TJ: Vaccine trials for the clinician: Prospects for viral and non-viral vectors. Oncologist 1997;2:300.

Hewitt H et al: A critique of the evidence for active host defense against cancer based on personal studies of 27 murine tumors of spontaneous origin. Br J Cancer 1976;33:241.

Hoover HC Jr et al: Adjuvant active specific immunotherapy for human colorectal cancer: 6.5-year median follow-up of a phase III prospectively randomized trial. J Clin Oncol 1993;11:390.

Hsu FJ et al: Dendritic cells and their application in immunotherapeutic approaches to cancer therapy. PPO Updates 1997;11:1.

International Germ Cell Cancer Collaborative Group: International germ cell consensus classification: A prognostic factor-based staging system for metastatic germ cell cancers. J Clin Oncol 1997; 15:594.

Kantoff PW et al: Sipuleucel-T immunotherapy for castration resistant prostate cancer. N Engl J Med 2010;363:411–422.

Lamm DL: Long-term results of intravesical therapy for superficial bladder cancer. Urol Clin North Am 1992;19:573.

Morales A, Nickel JC: Immunotherapy for superficial bladder cancer. Urol Clin North Am 1992;19:549.

Morton DL et al: Prolongation of survival in metastatic after active specific immunotherapy with a new polyvalent melanoma vaccine. Ann Surg 1992;216:463.

Osanto S: Vaccine trials for the clinician: Prospects for tumor antigens. Oncologist 1997;2:284.

Rosenberg SA et al: Use of tumor-infiltrating lymphocytes and interleukin-2 in the immunotherapy of patients with metastatic melanoma. N Engl J Med 1988;319:1676.

Rosenberg SA et al: Treatment of 283 consecutive patients with metastatic melanoma or renal cell cancer using high-dose bolus interleukin-2. JAMA 1994;271:907.

Schlag P et al: Active specific immunotherapy with Newcastle-disease-virus-modified autologous tumor cells following resection of liver metastases in colorectal cancer. Cancer Immunol Immunother 1992;35:325.

Shepard HM et al: Monoclonal antibody therapy of human cancer: Taking the HER2 protooncogene to the clinic. J Clin Immunol 1991;11:117.

Simons JW, Mikhak B: Ex vivo gene therapy using cytokine-transduced tumor vaccines: Molecular and clinical pharmacology. Semin Oncol 1998;25:661.

Texter JH Jr, Neal CE: The role of monoclonal antibody in the management of prostate adenocarcinoma. J Urol 1998;160:2393.

Vanky F, Klein E: Specificity of auto-tumor cytotoxicity exerted by fresh, activated and propagated human T lymphocytes. Int J Cancer 1982;29:547.

Velders MP et al: Active immunization against cancer cells: Impediments and advances. Semin Oncol 1998;25:697.

Chemotherapy of Urologic Tumors

20

Eric J. Small, MD

The use of chemotherapy in the treatment of malignant tumors of the genitourinary system serves as a paradigm for a multidisciplinary approach to cancer. The careful integration of surgical and chemotherapeutic treatments has resulted in impressive advances in the management of urologic cancer. By definition, surgical interventions are directed at local management of urologic tumors, whereas chemotherapy and biologic therapy are systemic in nature. Although there is no question that there are times in the natural history of a genitourinary tumor when only one therapeutic method is required, a multidisciplinary approach is always called for. This chapter details the importance of a joint surgical–medical approach to patients with urologic cancer. A practicing urologist should collaborate closely with a medical oncologist and should feel comfortable speaking with patients about the uses, risks, and benefits of chemotherapy.

PRINCIPLES OF SYSTEMIC THERAPY

A. Clinical Uses of Chemotherapy

Systemic therapy is indicated in the treatment of disseminated cancer when either cure or palliation is the goal. In addition, chemotherapy may be used as part of a multimodality treatment plan in an effort to improve both local and distant control of the tumor. An understanding of the goals and limitations of systemic therapy in each of these settings is essential for its effective use.

1. Curative intent of metastatic disease—In considering the role of potentially curative chemotherapy in patients with metastatic disease, several factors must be taken into account. The first is the responsiveness of the tumor. Responsiveness is generally defined by the observed partial or complete responses that together constitute the overall objective response rate. The assessment of neoplasms with frequent bony metastases such as prostate cancer, renal cell carcinoma, and transitional cell carcinoma (TCC) is difficult, as a persistently abnormal bone scan does not necessarily

imply residual cancer. Patients in whom the only site of disease is bone generally must be considered nonassessable by conventional measures, and if available, intermediate markers of response (such as prostate-specific antigen [PSA]) are required. The transient worsening appearance of a bone scan with therapy but which represents healing bone is termed "bone scan flare," and can be indistinguishable from true disease progression. For this reason, assessment of all parameters including symptomatology, PSA in prostate cancer patients, CT and MRI is essential. For patients with metastatic prostate cancer in whom bone scan flare is suspected or possible, repeating scans several months later is essential.

If cure is the intent with systemic therapy, the relevant response criterion to consider is the percentage of patients achieving a complete response. This number is less than 10% in patients with metastatic renal cell carcinoma and hormone-refractory prostate cancer, 25% or less in patients with metastatic transitional cell carcinoma, and up to 80% in patients with metastatic germ cell malignancies. Under some circumstances, however (for example, in postchemotherapy residual masses in patients with germ cell carcinoma), an apparent partial response can be converted into a complete response with judicious resection (see Section A. 3).

The second feature to consider in treating patients with potentially curative systemic therapy is the anticipated toxicity of such therapy. In general, higher levels of toxicity are acceptable if a cure can be achieved, although care must be exercised to avoid a "cure worse than the disease." This is particularly true in the case of fairly toxic therapies such as interleukin-2 or bone marrow transplantation. These treatments can result in apparent cures of approximately 10% and 30%, respectively, of patients with metastatic renal cell carcinoma or refractory germ cell tumors (GCTs). Patients undergoing these rigorous therapies must be carefully selected and must be as fully informed as possible about potential toxicities.

2. Treatment of patients with incurable metastatic cancer—When the goal of systemic therapy is palliation of symptoms rather than cure, the toxicity of the treatment to be offered must be balanced against the cancer-related symptoms the patient is experiencing, and in general, more toxic therapies are not indicated. Nonetheless, an understanding of the potential capabilities of systemic therapy must be understood because even in otherwise incurable disease there may be a role for systemic therapy if there is a likelihood that the patient's life can be prolonged with its use. This is the case for docetaxel or cabazitaxel therapy in prostate cancer and combination cisplatinum based chemotherapy in bladder cancer. In addition, systemic chemotherapy can be associated with a control of pain, and an *improvement* in quality of life. This appears to be the case for both mitoxantrone and docetaxel in patients with metastatic hormone refractory prostate cancer.

3. Systemic therapy used in conjunction with surgery: adjuvant and neoadjuvant therapy—Systemic therapy administered after a patient has been rendered free of disease surgically is termed **adjuvant therapy**. Several important criteria must be met if adjuvant therapy is to be used outside of a research setting. First, an assessment must be undertaken of known risk factors predictive of relapse or development of distant metastases. Patients at low risk of relapse generally should not receive adjuvant therapy because they are unlikely to derive a benefit and will be unnecessarily exposed to the toxicity of therapy. Second, the proposed therapy must have been shown to decrease the rate of relapse and increase the disease-free interval (and, it is hoped, survival) in a randomized, phase III trial. Finally, because patients who are being treated with adjuvant therapy are free of disease and presumably asymptomatic, toxicity must be kept at a minimum. This opens the way to a tailored approach in which patients with high-risk disease, as determined by pathologic review of the surgical specimen, are treated in order to decrease the risk of micrometastatic disease.

By contrast, neoadjuvant therapy is administered before definitive surgical resection. Here, the potential advantages include early therapy of micrometastatic disease and tumor debulking to allow a more complete resection. Patients with known metastatic disease generally do not exhibit high enough response rates to systemic therapy to warrant local surgery following chemotherapy, with the clear exception of patients with GCT. Whether or not patients with metastatic renal cell carcinoma who exhibit a partial response to systemic therapy may benefit from resection of residual masses is not known. As with adjuvant therapy, the proposed therapy must have been demonstrated to impact favorably on rate of relapse, disease-free interval, and survival in a randomized phase III trial.

B. Chemotherapeutic Agents and Their Toxicity

The usefulness of antineoplastic agents lies in their therapeutic index or preferential toxicity to malignant cells over normal, nonmalignant cells. The mechanism of action of most chemotherapeutic drugs is based on their toxicity to rapidly dividing cells. Thus, in general, malignancies that have relatively rapid growth, such as GCT, are relatively chemosensitive, whereas slower growing neoplasms such as renal cell carcinoma are less sensitive. Toxicity from chemotherapeutic agents is seen primarily in normal, nonmalignant cells that are also rapidly dividing, such as hematopoietic cells in the bone marrow, gastrointestinal mucosa, and hair follicles, and is manifested in cytopenias, mucositis, and alopecia. Other common toxicities observed with agents frequently used in the treatment of genitourinary malignancies include nephrotoxicity, neurotoxicity, hemorrhagic cystitis, pulmonary fibrosis, and cardiotoxicity. Table 20–1 summarizes the spectrum of activity and primary toxicities of commonly used chemotherapeutic agents.

The development of chemotherapy drug resistance remains an important clinical problem in the field of oncology. Malignant cells develop resistance in a variety of ways, including the induction of transport pumps, which actively pump the drug out of the cell and through increased activity of enzymes necessary to inactivate the particular chemotherapeutic agent. Although there are several experimental methods of circumventing these mechanisms of drug resistance, one practical approach to this problem is the use of multiagent chemotherapy. Increased tumor cell killing is achieved by exposing neoplastic cells to multiple agents with different mechanisms of action. Furthermore, this approach allows the selection of agents with nonoverlapping toxicity profiles.

The use of increased dose intensity (higher doses of a drug administered over the same time period) as a means of overcoming drug resistance remains experimental in urologic malignancies with one clear exception. A subset of patients with otherwise incurable GCT appear to be curable with high-dose chemotherapy and autologous bone marrow transplant support (see the section Germ Cell Malignancies).

C. Unique Features of Genitourinary Malignancies

The systemic therapy of urologic malignancies offers unique challenges to the practitioner. Renal insufficiency due to obstructive uropathy from local extension of the tumor or postsurgical or postradiotherapy changes is not infrequent and may alter antineoplastic drug clearance. In patients with renal cell carcinoma, previous nephrectomy may also impact drug clearance. Furthermore, the common use of the nephrotoxic chemotherapeutic agent cisplatin in the treatment of urologic malignancies (most prominently, in bladder and testicular neoplasms) may further diminish renal function. Careful attention must be paid, therefore, to renal function throughout the course of systemic therapy, with appropriate dose adjustments made. Dosing adjustments also must be considered in patients who have undergone cystectomy because ileal conduits or neobladders have the capacity to resorb chemotherapeutic agents that are excreted in the urine in active form (most notably, methotrexate).

Table 20–1. Commonly used chemotherapeutic agents in urologic oncology, and their toxicity.

Agent	Activity	Common toxicities
Bleomycin	Germ cell tumors	Fever, chills, pulmonary fibrosis
Cabazitaxel	Prostate cancer	Myelosuppression
Capecitabine	Renal cell carcinoma	Mucositis, diarrhea, myelosuppression
Carboplatin	Bladder cancer, germ cell tumors	Myelosuppression
Cisplatin	Bladder cancer, germ cell tumors, prostate cancer	Renal insufficiency, peripheral neuropathy, auditory toxicity, myelosuppression
Docetaxel (Taxotere)	Bladder cancer, germ cell tumors, prostate cancer	Myelosuppression, neuropathy
Doxorubicin	Bladder cancer, prostate cancer	Myelosuppression, mucositis, cardiomyopathy
Etoposide (VP-16)	Germ cell tumors, prostate cancer[†]	Myelosuppression
Gemcitabine (Gemzar)	Bladder cancer, renal cell carcinoma	Myelosuppression
Ifosfamide	Germ cell tumors	Myelosuppression, neurologic (CNS) toxicity, cystitis
Methotrexate	Germ cell tumors, bladder cancer	Mucositis, myelosuppression, renal toxicity
Mitoxantrone	Prostate cancer	Myelosupression, cardiac
Paclitaxel (Taxol)	Bladder cancer, germ cell tumors	Myelosuppression, neuropathy
Vinblastine	Bladder cancer, germ cell tumors, prostate cancer[†]	Peripheral, autonomic neuropathy; myelosuppression

Frequent local extension in the pelvis presents additional unique problems. Patients with previous pelvic radiotherapy have markedly diminished bone marrow reserves, which may limit the use of myelosuppressive drugs. Furthermore, local pelvic relapses have the potential to be symptomatic and painful. Particularly in patients who have already received radiotherapy, systemic therapy may be important for palliation.

GERM CELL MALIGNANCIES

A. Overview

The evolution of therapy for GCT has been deliberate and thoughtful, and has resulted in cures of 80–85% of men with GCT, serving as a model for the treatment of curable cancers. Nonetheless, challenges in the management of GCT remain. Because of their young age, patients who have been cured are at risk of delayed, treatment-induced toxicity. Furthermore, an 80–85% cure rate also implies that 15–20% of patients with GCT will not be cured and ultimately will succumb to their disease. An understanding of staging and risk assessment is crucial if (1) patients with good risk features are not to be overtreated and exposed to undue toxic risks, and (2) patients with poor risk features are to receive adequate (curative) therapy.

The most common multiagent chemotherapy regimen for the treatment of GCT is a three-drug combination consisting of bleomycin, etoposide, and cisplatin (BEP). The treatment is repeated every 21 days. One cycle consists of cisplatin 20 mg/m^2 IV day 1–5, etoposide 100 mg/m^2 IV day 1–5, and bleomycin, 30 units IV, day 2, 9, and 16. Frequently the first 5 days of treatment require hospitalization. The deletion of bleomycin from this regimen results in the pulmonary embolus (PE) regimen. The substitution of ifosfamide for bleomycin yields the VIP regime (UP-16, ifosfamide, platinum).

B. Use of Chemotherapy for Patients with Stage I and II Disease

The standard of care for patients with stage I GCT remains orchiectomy followed by retroperitoneal lymphadenectomy or surveillance for nonseminoma patients. In seminoma patients, following orchiectomy, a single dose of carboplatin has been shown to be as effective as retroperitoneal radiation, and may be associated with a lower incidence of secondary malignancies, including contralateral testicular neoplasms. Surveillance is also an appropriate option for Stage I seminoma patients.

Patients with stage II nonseminomatous microscopic disease identified at lymphadenectomy (stage IIA) or patients with low-volume clinical stage II disease (stage IIB) who have undergone retroperitoneal lymphadenectomy may benefit from two cycles of adjuvant PE or cisplatin-etoposide-bleomycin (PEB) chemotherapy. The use of

Table 20–2. Commonly used chemotherapeutic regimens in urologic oncology.

Indication	Regimen name, if any	Components
Metastatic prostate cancer, castration resistant, front line	D/P M/P	Docetaxel + Prednisone Mitoxantrone + Prednisone
Metastatic prostate cancer, castration resistant, second line	—	Cabazitaxel + Prednisone
Bladder cancer metastatic second line	ITP	Ifosfamide, Paclitaxel, Cisplatinum
Germ cell tumors front line	BEP	Bleomycin, Etoposide, Cisplatinum, Etoposide, Cisplatinum
Germ cell tumors second line	VIP ITP	Etoposide, Ifosfamide, Cisplatinum Ifosfamide, Paclitaxel, Cisplatinum
Renal cell carcinoma (rarely)	Gem/cape	Gemcitabine, Capecitabine

adjuvant therapy results in a 96% long-term disease-free survival. While the relapse rate for patients who do not receive adjuvant therapy ranges from 20–40%, the vast majority of relapsing patients can also be cured with either three or four cycles of subsequent chemotherapy, yielding an identical long-term survival rate. The decision about adjuvant chemotherapy after lymphadenectomy must be individualized. Patients at high risk for relapse may choose to undergo two cycles of chemotherapy at that point in order to avoid the possibility of three to four cycles in the future.

C. Use of Chemotherapy in Patients with Advanced Disease

Patients with advanced GCT should be treated with systemic therapy after completion of their orchiectomy. This group includes some stage IIB nonseminomatous tumors and all stage IIC or higher tumors, both seminomas and nonseminomas. A variety of chemotherapy regimens will result in approximately 80% of patients with advanced GCT achieving a complete response and 70% achieving long-term apparent cures (good prognosis). By the same token, however, 20–30% of patients have a poor prognosis and will still ultimately die from their disease. Studies of pretreatment clinical characteristics have sought to identify prognostic features that can be prospectively used to segregate this diverse group of advanced GCT patients into poor- and good-prognostic subsets.

A common classification system has been developed by the International Germ Cell Cancer Collaborative Group (IGCCC). In this system, good-prognosis patients with nonseminomatous GCT have a testis or retroperitoneal primary tumor, no nonpulmonary visceral metastases, and low-serum tumor markers. Intermediate-prognosis patients are the same as good-prognosis patients but have intermediate serum tumor markers. Poor-prognosis patients have a mediastinal primary tumor or nonpulmonary visceral metastases

(liver, bone, brain) or high levels of serum tumor markers. Five-year overall survival for the good-, intermediate-, and poor-prognosis categories with current regimens is 92%, 80%, and 48%, respectively. By definition, seminomas are never in the poor-prognosis category. Seminomas are segregated into good-prognosis cases (any primary site, but no nonpulmonary visceral metastases), with an 86% 5-year survival, and intermediate-prognosis cases (any primary site but with the presence of nonpulmonary visceral metastases), with a 72% 5-year survival.

Because it is not likely that the extraordinarily high cure rate for good-prognosis patients can be improved upon, most efforts in the treatment of these patients have been aimed at optimizing treatment with less toxic regimens that will have equal efficacy. Trials evaluating (1) the elimination of bleomycin, (2) a reduction in the number of chemotherapy cycles administered, or (3) the substitution of carboplatin for cisplatin have been undertaken.

The outlook for poor-prognosis patients is not as good, with only approximately 30–60% of patients achieving a complete response. Thus, whereas the major concern in good-prognosis patients has been the reduction of toxicity, the major objective of clinical investigation in poor-prognosis patients has been to improve efficacy, with less concern for reducing toxicity. Clinical trials in poor-prognosis patients have by and large relied on one or both of two approaches. The first has been to exploit agents that have been demonstrated to be efficacious in the salvage setting, and the second has been to evaluate the role of dose escalation.

Currently acceptable regimens for good-prognosis patients are fairly well defined and include three cycles of PEB or four cycles of PE. By contrast, optimal therapy for poor-prognosis patients is not fully defined. Four cycles of PEB or four cycles of VIP are appropriate options. The use of high dose chemotherapy with peripheral stem cell transplant does not appear to improve outcomes over conventional high-risk therapy.

D. Adjunctive Surgery and "Salvage" Therapy

Postchemotherapy adjunctive surgery must be integrated into the treatment plan of patients with advanced GCT. Approximately 20% of patients with GCTs have residual masses after systemic therapy. The role of adjunctive surgery in patients with GCT with postchemotherapy residual masses has been reviewed. Except in rare circumstances, adjunctive surgery is not indicated in the presence of persistently elevated serum tumor markers. Adjunctive surgery usually can be undertaken safely within 1–2 months of completion of chemotherapy. It must be noted, however, that all patients who have received bleomycin, whether or not there is clinical evidence of pulmonary fibrosis, are at risk of development of oxygen-related pulmonary toxicity. The anesthesiologist must be made aware of the patient's previous exposure to bleomycin and every effort must be taken to maintain the FiO_2 as low as possible throughout the surgical procedure. Patients who are found to have active carcinoma in their resected specimens are frequently treated with further "salvage" chemotherapy, generally with a different regimen, although compelling evidence supporting this procedure is still forthcoming. Patients who appear to benefit from postsurgical chemotherapy are patients with incomplete resections, patients whose resected specimen contains more than 10% viable cancer cells, and patients who were in the IGCCC high-risk group prior to beginning frontline chemotherapy.

While approximately 80% of patients with GCT can currently be cured with platinum-based therapy, 20% ultimately die of their disease, either because a complete response is not achieved with induction therapy or because they relapse after becoming disease-free with primary therapy. Before the initiation of salvage therapy, the diagnosis of relapsed or primary, refractory GCT must be clearly established. In particular, falsely elevated human chorionic gonadotropin or alpha-fetoprotein values and false-positive radiographic studies of the chest due to previous bleomycin use must be ruled out. Persistent or slowly growing masses, particularly in the absence of serologic progression, may represent benign teratoma. Therapies based on ifosfamide, paclitaxel, or high-dose chemotherapy with autologous bone marrow transplant provide a salvage rate of approximately 25% in patients with relapsed or refractory GCT.

TRANSITIONAL CELL CARCINOMA OF THE UROEPITHELIUM

A. Nonmetastatic Disease

The development of effective chemotherapy regimens for the treatment of metastatic transitional cell carcinoma (TCC) has resulted in more widespread use of these regimens in combination with other modes for the treatment of locally advanced but nonmetastatic disease. In bulky inoperable invasive bladder tumors (T3b, T4, N_+), chemotherapy has been used as a means of cytoreduction in order to make surgery possible. Chemotherapy before surgery, termed **neoadjuvant therapy**, has also been used in muscle-invasive cancers that *are* resectable, in an effort to treat micrometastatic disease before cystectomy. It must be borne in mind that the pathologic complete response rate in the bladder after neoadjuvant chemotherapy is probably in the 20–40% range; therefore, definitive surgical resection after chemotherapy is usually required. A survival advantage has been demonstrated with neoadjuvant methotrexate, vinblastine, doxorubicin and cisplatin (MVAC) chemotherapy (compared with no chemotherapy, and this is therefore considered the standard of care for muscle invasive disease).

Adjuvant trials generally have been used to treat only patients found to have pathologic T3 and T4 lesions after radical cystectomy. Several small, randomized trials have shown a benefit to various adjuvant chemotherapy regimens; a large randomized multi-institution trial remains to be done.

Chemotherapy in combination with radiation therapy has been advocated by some as a bladder-preserving approach for muscle-invasive tumors. Patients are usually treated with two cycles of chemotherapy, followed by radiation therapy and concomitant cisplatin as a radiosensitizer. If follow-up cystoscopy reveals no cancer, consolidative multiagent systemic chemotherapy is administered. This approach appears to be particularly useful for smaller, lower-stage tumors. The presence of hydronephrosis or hydroureter is a contradiction to this approach, as these patients do less well with a bladder sparing approach. While longer follow-up is required, it appears that approximately 30–50% of patients can attain long-term disease-free status with a functional bladder with this approach.

B. Metastatic Disease

The development of successful therapy of metastatic bladder TCC has been based on the use of cisplatin. Until recently, two common cisplatin-based regimens are in wide use: (1) cisplatin, methotrexate, and vinblastine (CMV) and (2) the same drugs in a slightly different schedule and dose along with doxorubicin (Adriamycin), in a regimen known as MVAC. These regimens result in overall response rates of approximately 50–60% and complete remission rates in the 20–35% range. Median overall survival for patients with metastatic disease treated with these regimens is in the 8- to 14-month range. Despite early promise, however, long-term survival after MVAC or CMV remains in the single digits. Both CMV and MVAC are intensive regimens, with myelosuppression occurring commonly. The use of hematopoietic growth factors has made it easier to administer full doses on schedule, although this improvement in dose intensity does not appear to translate into a clinical benefit.

The combination of gemcitabine and cisplatin has been compared to MVAC, and has been shown to be less toxic and equivalent in efficacy to MVAC. As a consequence, gemcitabine/cisplatin can be considered the standard of care for the treatment of advanced TCC. However, it should be noted that the gemcitabine/cisplatin regime has been tested in a randomized study only in patients with metastatic disease, and its utility as an adjuvant or neoadjuvant has not been tested. For patients with impaired renal function, agents such as carboplatin and paclitaxel have been utilized.

RENAL CELL CARCINOMA

The treatment of metastatic renal cell carcinoma with chemotherapy remains largely unsatisfactory. The general lack of active agents and the excessive toxicity of many of the agents that exhibit some activity have contributed to the absence of adjuvant or neoadjuvant trials. Trials that used adjuvant interferon-alpha for patients considered at high risk for relapse after nephrectomy failed to show an advantage of the adjuvant therapy. A large adjuvant trial of the novel tyrosine kinase inhibitors, sorafenib and sunitinib, is underway.

Metastatic renal cell carcinoma is relatively resistant to chemotherapy. The fluoropyrimidines capecitabine has modest activity, as does gemcitabine, with response proportions of 10–15% reported. Renal cell carcinoma is one of very few neoplasms that clearly are responsive to biologic response modifiers. The utility of biologic response modifiers, antiangiogenic agents, tyrosine kinase inhibitors, and mammalian target of rapamycin (mTOR) inhibitors in renal cell carcinoma are discussed elsewhere in Chapter 20. These agents are used prior to using chemotherapy.

HORMONE-REFRACTORY PROSTATE CANCER

The systemic therapy of patients with metastatic prostate cancer in whom hormonal therapy has failed generally consists of secondary hormonal manipulations followed by chemotherapy. Approximately 15% of patients who have had progressive disease despite therapy with combined androgen blockade will have a fall in PSA when their antiandrogen is discontinued. This maneuver is mandated, therefore, before initiating other systemic therapy. Furthermore, second-line hormonal maneuvers such as adrenal androgen deprivation with ketoconazole, estrogens, or secondary anti-androgens such as nilutamide clearly have activity and, particularly in asymptomatic patients, should be considered. As noted previously, the evaluation of responses in patients with bone disease only is challenging. The use of the PSA in this setting has been fairly extensively evaluated, and it appears to be a reasonable intermediate endpoint. Thus, a decline in PSA of 30–50% appears to be predictive of longer survival for these patients.

Mitoxantrone is approved in combination with prednisone for the treatment of progressive, symptomatic hormone-refractory prostate cancer (HRPC). Twenty-nine percent of those treated with the combination experienced decreased pain, compared with 12% receiving prednisone alone. In addition, there were greater improvements in quality-of-life measures. The toxicity of the treatment was mild in both groups;

fewer than 2% of patients had infectious episodes. Median survival for both groups was approximately 1 year. Mitoxantrone has modest albeit definable activity in HRPC, although it probably does not significantly prolong survival.

Until recently, chemotherapy for prostate cancer was considered ineffective in prolonging survival. However, the results of two-phase III trials have established docetaxel-based chemotherapy as the standard-of-care for first-line treatment of metastatic HRPC. The every 3-week docetaxel regimens in each one of these trials demonstrated a modest but statistically significant (2 month) survival benefit over mitoxantrone/prednisone. The median survival with docetaxel was 18–19 months. Thus, every 3-week docetaxel/prednisone has emerged as the FDA-approved, first-line regimen for HRPC. Following therapy with docetaxel, patients who remain candidates for further chemotherapy can be treated with cabazitaxel, an agent shown to prolong life in this group of patients compared with mitoxantrone/prednisone. Zolendronic acid or Denosumab are indicated in castration-resistant prostate cancer (CRPC) patients with bone metastases, as each reduces the incidence of skeletal related events.

Many patients with advanced prostate cancer have bone pain or functional impairments that adversely affect quality of life, and provision of appropriate palliative care is an integral component of their management. In addition to the usual analgesics, glucocorticoids serve as anti-inflammatory agents and can alleviate bone pain. For patients with widespread bone metastases and pain not easily controlled with analgesics or local irradiation strontium 89 and samarium 153 can be administered intravenously; they are selectively concentrated in bone metastases and alleviate pain in 70% or more of treated patients.

BIBLIOGRAPHY

Bajorin DF, Bosl GJ: Bleomycin in germ cell tumor therapy: Not all regimens are created equal. J Clin Oncol 1997;15(5):1717–1719.

Beyer J et al: High-dose chemotherapy as salvage treatment in germ cell tumors: A multivariate analysis of prognostic factors. J Clin Oncol 1996;14:2638.

Beyer J et al: Long-term survival of patients with recurrent or refractory germ cell tumors after high dose chemotherapy. Cancer 1997;79:161.

Garrow GC, Johnson DH: Treatment of "good risk" metastatic testicular cancer. Semin Oncol 1992;19:159.

Harker WG et al: Cisplatin, methotrexate, and vinblastine (CMV): An effective chemotherapy regimen for metastatic transitional cell carcinoma of the urinary tract. A Northern California Oncology Group study. J Clin Oncol 1985;3:1463.

International Germ Cell Cancer Collaborative Group: International Germ Cell Consensus Classification: A prognostic factor-based staging system for metastatic germ cell cancers. J Clin Oncol 1997;15:594.

Kelly WK et al: Prostate-specific antigen as a measure of disease outcome in metastatic hormone-refractory prostate cancer. J Clin Oncol 1993;11:1566.

Oh WK, Kantoff PW: Management of hormone refractory prostate cancer: Current standards and future prospects. J Urol 1998; 160:1220.

Parkinson DR, Sznol M: High-dose interleukin-2 in the therapy of metastatic renal cell carcinoma. Semin Oncol 1995;22:61.

Petrylak DP et al: Docetaxel and estramustine compared with mitoxantrone and prednisone for advanced refractory prostate cancer. N Engl J Med 2004;351:1513.

Pont J et al: Adjuvant chemotherapy for high-risk clinical stage I nonseminomatous testicular germ cell cancer: Long-term results of a prospective trial. J Clin Oncol 1996;14:441.

Savarese D et al: Phase II Study of Docetaxel, Estramustine, and Low-Dose Hydrocortisone in Men with Hormone Refractory Prostate Cancer: A final report of CALGB 9780. J Clin Oncol 2002;19:2509.

Small EJ, Srinivas S: The antiandrogen withdrawal syndrome: Experience in a large cohort of unselected patients with advanced prostate cancer. Cancer 1995;76:1428.

Small EJ, Vogelzang NJ: Second-line hormonal therapy for advanced prostate cancer: A shifting paradigm. J Clin Oncol 1997;15:382.

Stadler WM, Vogelzang NJ: Low-dose interleukin-2 in the treatment of metastatic renal cell carcinoma. Semin Oncol 1995;22:67.

Sternberg SN et al: Methotrexate, vinblastine, doxorubicin, and cisplatin for advanced transitional cell carcinoma of the urothelium: Efficacy and patterns of response and relapse. Cancer 1989;64: 2448.

Tannock I et al: Chemotherapy with mitoxantrone plus prednisone or prednisone alone for symptomatic hormone-resistant prostate cancer: A Canadian randomized study with palliative end points. J Clin Oncol 1996;14:1756.

Tannock I et al: Docetaxel and prednisone or mitoxantrone and prednisone for advanced prostate cancer. N Engl J Med 2004;351:1502.

Vaughn DJ et al: Paclitaxel plus carboplatin in advanced carcinoma of the urothelium: An active and tolerable outpatient regimen. J Clin Oncol 1998;16:255.

von der Maase H et al: Gemcitabine and cisplatin versus methotrexate, vinblastine, doxorubicin and cisplatin in advanced or metastatic bladder cancer: Results of a large, randomized, multi-national, multi-center phase III study. J Clin Oncol 2000;17:3068.

Williams SD et al: Immediate adjuvant chemotherapy versus observation with treatment at relapse in pathologic stage II testicular cancer. N Engl J Med 1987;317:1433.

Williams SD et al: Treatment of disseminated germ cell tumors with cisplatin, bleomycin, and either vinblastine or etoposide. N Engl J Med 1987;316:1435.

Yagoda A et al: Chemotherapy for advanced renal cell carcinoma: 1983–1993. Semin Oncol 1995;22:42.

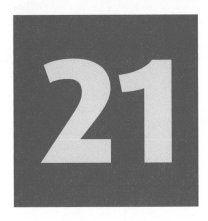

Urothelial Carcinoma: Cancers of the Bladder, Ureter, & Renal Pelvis

Badrinath R. Konety, MD, MBA, &
Peter R. Carroll, MD, MPH

BLADDER CARCINOMAS

▶ Incidence

Bladder cancer is the second most common cancer of the genitourinary tract. It accounts for 7% of new cancer cases in men and 2% of new cancer cases in women. The incidence is higher in whites than in African Americans, and there is a positive social class gradient for bladder cancer in both sexes. The average age at diagnosis is 65 years. At that time, approximately 75% of bladder cancers are localized to the bladder; 25% have spread to regional lymph nodes or distant sites.

▶ Risk Factors and Pathogenesis

Cigarette smoking accounts for 65% of cases in men and 20–30% in women. In general, smokers have approximately a two- to threefold increased risk of bladder cancer than nonsmokers, and the association appears to be dose related. The causative agents are thought to be alpha- and beta-naphthylamine, which are secreted into the urine of smokers. The risk of bladder appears to decrease after smoking cessation but may not reach the levels of never smokers.

Occupational exposure accounts for 15–35% of cases in men and 1–6% in women (Matanoski and Elliott, 1981). Workers in the chemical, dye, rubber, petroleum, leather, and printing industries are at increased risk. Specific occupational carcinogens include benzidine, beta-naphthylamine, and 4-aminobiphenyl, and the latency period between exposure and tumor development may be prolonged. Patients who have received cyclophosphamide (Cytoxan) for the management of various malignant diseases are also at increased risk (Fairchild et al, 1979). Ingestion of artificial sweeteners has been proposed to be a risk factor, but several studies have failed to confirm any association (Elcock and Morgan, 1993). Physical trauma to the urothelium induced by infection, instrumentation, and calculi increases the risk of malignancy (Hicks, 1982).

The exact genetic events leading to the development of bladder cancer are unknown, but they are likely to be multiple and may involve the activation of oncogenes and inactivation or loss of tumor suppressor genes (Olumi et al, 1990). Loss of genetic material on chromosome 9 appears to be a consistent finding in patients with both low-grade, low-stage and high-grade, high-stage disease (Miyao et al, 1993; Tsai et al, 1990), which suggests that this may be an early event in bladder cancer development. Loss of chromosome 9 in multiple tumors from an individual patient supports the concept that genetic changes in bladder cancer represent a "field defect" that may occur throughout the urothelium. More recent studies examining p53 tumor suppressor gene mutations in primary, recurrent, and upper-tract tumors suggest that these tumors can have a single clonal origin (Dalbagni et al, 2001; Sidransky et al, 1991). Additional genetic changes have been described that are specific for invasive bladder tumors. Chromosome 11p, which contains the c-Ha-ras proto-oncogene, is deleted in approximately 40% of bladder cancers (Olumi et al, 1990). Increased expression of the c-Ha-ras protein product, p21, has been detected in dysplastic and high-grade tumors but not in low-grade bladder cancers. Deletions of chromosome 17p have also been detected in over 60% of all invasive bladder cancers, but 17p deletions have not been described in superficial tumors. This finding is noteworthy because the p53 tumor suppressor gene maps to chromosome 17p. *TP53* alterations represent the most commonly identified genetic abnormality in human cancers, making deletion of this chromosome an important finding in carcinoma in situ (CIS) and muscle invasive bladder cancer. Mutations of the fibroblast growth factor receptor 3 (FGFr3) are found in >60% of papillomas and low-grade bladder tumors and hence it is considered an oncogene. Ras mutations are also found in both low- and high-grade or muscle invasive tumors but Ras and FGFr3 mutations appear to be mutually exclusive (Jebar et al, 2005) and both are involved in activation of the MAP Kinase pathway. p53 mutations are less common in low-grade tumors and loss of FGFr3 with increased expression of p53 has been associated with higher stage and grade (Knowles, 2007).

Staging

Currently, the most commonly used staging system allows for a precise and simultaneous description of the primary tumor stage (T stage), the status of lymph nodes (N stage), and metastatic sites (M stage) (American Joint Committee on Cancer, 1997). The T staging system is depicted in Figure 20–1. Nodal (N) stage is defined as Nx—cannot be assessed, N0—no nodal metastases, N1—single node <2 cm involved, N2—single node involved 2–5 cm in size or multiple nodes none >5 cm, N3—one or more nodes >5 cm in size involved.

Metastases (M) stage is defined as Mx—cannot be defined, M0—no distant metastases, M1—distant metastases present. Staging errors exist when one compares the clinical stage (that based on physical examination and imaging) with the pathologic stage (that based on removal of the bladder and regional lymph nodes). Overstaging is relatively uncommon, but clinical understaging may occur in up to 53% of patients (Dutta et al, 2001; Skinner, 1982).

Histopathology

Ninety-eight percent of all bladder cancers are epithelial malignancies, with the predominant majority being transitional cell carcinomas (TCCs). About 5% are adenocarcinomas or squamous cell carcinomas.

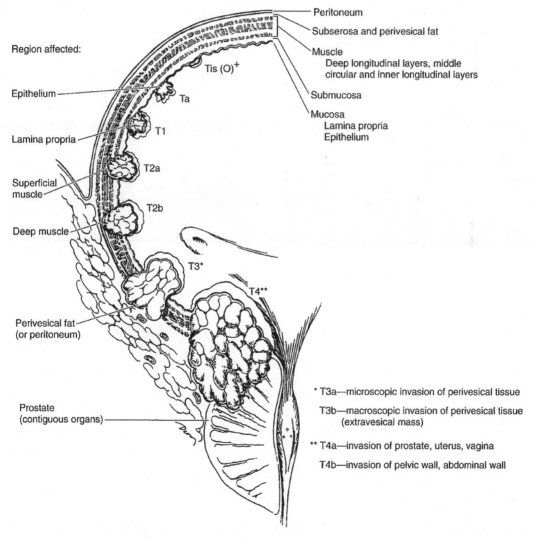

▲ **Figure 21–1.** Staging of bladder cancer.

A. Normal Urothelium

The normal urothelium is composed of 3–7 layers of transitional cell epithelium resting on a basement membrane composed of extracellular matrix (collagen, adhesive glycoproteins, glycosaminoglycans) (Figure 21–2A). The epithelial cells vary in appearance: The basal cells are actively proliferating cells resting on the basement membrane; the luminal cells, perhaps the most important feature of normal bladder epithelium, are larger umbrella-like cells that are bound together by tight junctions. Beyond the basement membrane is loose connective tissue, the lamina propria, in which occasionally smooth-muscle fibers can be identified. These fibers should be distinguished from deeper, more extensive muscle elements defining the true muscularis propria.

B. Papilloma/PUNLMP

The World Health Organization recognizes a papilloma as a papillary tumor with a fine fibrovascular stalk supporting an epithelial layer of transitional cells with normal thickness and cytology (Epstein et al, 1998). These are also termed papillary urothelial neoplasms of low malignant potential or PUNLMP. PUNLMPs are a rare benign condition that do not require aggressive therapy.

C. Transitional Cell Carcinoma

Approximately 90% of all bladder cancers are TCCs. These tumors most commonly appear as papillary, exophytic lesions (Figure 21–2B); less commonly, they may be sessile or ulcerated. Whereas the former group is usually superficial in nature, sessile growths are often invasive.

CIS is recognizable as flat, anaplastic epithelium. The urothelium lacks the normal cellular polarity, and cells contain large, irregular hyperchromatic nuclei with prominent nucleoli (Figure 21–2C).

D. Nontransitional Cell Carcinomas

1. Adenocarcinoma—Adenocarcinomas account for <2% of all bladder cancers. Primary adenocarcinomas of the bladder may be preceded by cystitis and metaplasia. Histologically, adenocarcinomas are mucus secreting and may have glandular, colloid, or signet-ring patterns. Whereas primary adenocarcinomas often arise along the floor of the bladder, adenocarcinomas arising from the urachus occur at the dome. Both tumor types are often localized at the time of diagnosis, but muscle invasion is usually present. Five-year survival is usually <40%, despite aggressive surgical management (Abenoza et al, 1987; Bernstein et al, 1988; Kramer et al, 1979).

2. Squamous cell carcinoma—Squamous cell carcinoma accounts for between 5% and 10% of all bladder cancers in the United States and is often associated here with a history of chronic infection, vesical calculi, or chronic catheter use. It

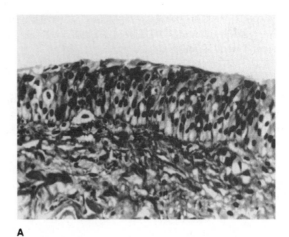

A

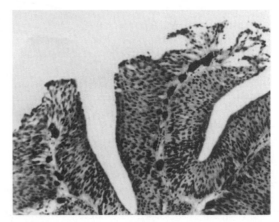

B

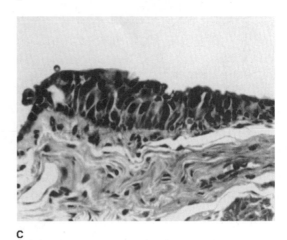

C

▲ **Figure 21-2. A:** Normal urothelium (125×). **B:** Moderately well differentiated, papillary bladder cancer (60×). **C:** Carcinoma in situ (200×).

may also be associated with bilharzial infection owing to *Schistosoma haematobium*, because squamous cell carcinoma accounts for approximately 60% of all bladder cancers in Egypt, parts of Africa, and the Middle East, where this infection is prevalent (El-Bolkainy et al, 1981). These tumors are often nodular and invasive at the time of diagnosis. Histologically they appear as poorly differentiated neoplasms composed of polygonal cells with characteristic intercellular bridges. Keratinizing epithelium is present, although often in small amounts.

3. Undifferentiated carcinomas—Undifferentiated bladder carcinomas, which are rare (accounting for <2%), have no mature epithelial elements. Very undifferentiated tumors with neuroendocrine features and small cell carcinomas tend to be aggressive and present with metastases (Choong et al, 2005; Quek et al, 2005).

4. Mixed carcinoma—Mixed carcinomas constitute 4–6% of all bladder cancers and are composed of a combination of transitional, glandular, squamous, or undifferentiated patterns. The most common type comprises transitional and squamous cell elements (Murphy, 1989). Most mixed carcinomas are large and infiltrating at the time of diagnosis.

E. Rare Epithelial and Nonepithelial Cancers

Rare epithelial carcinomas identified in the bladder include villous adenomas, carcinoid tumors, carcinosarcomas, and melanomas. Rare nonepithelial cancers of the urinary bladder include pheochromocytomas, lymphomas, choriocarcinomas, and various mesenchymal tumors (hemangioma, osteogenic sarcoma, and myosarcoma) (Murphy, 1989). Cancers of the prostate, cervix, and rectum may involve the bladder by direct extension. The most common tumors metastatic to the bladder include (in order of incidence) melanoma, lymphoma, stomach, breast, kidney, lung, and liver (Franks et al, 1999;Goldstein, 1967; Murphy, 1989).

▶ Clinical Findings

A. Symptoms

Hematuria is the presenting symptom in 85–90% of patients with bladder cancer. It may be gross or microscopic, intermittent rather than constant. In a smaller percentage of patients, it is accompanied by symptoms of vesical irritability: frequency, urgency, and dysuria. Irritative voiding symptoms seem to be more common in patients with diffuse CIS. Symptoms of advanced disease include bone pain from bone metastases or flank pain from retroperitoneal metastases or ureteral obstruction.

B. Signs

Patients with large-volume or invasive tumors may be found to have bladder wall thickening or a palpable mass—findings that may be detected on a careful bimanual examination

under anesthesia. If the bladder is not mobile, that suggests fixation of tumor to adjacent structures by direct invasion.

Hepatomegaly and supraclavicular lymphadenopathy are signs of metastatic disease. Lymphedema from occlusive pelvic lymphadenopathy may be seen occasionally. Patients may also present with back pain or pathologic fracture from bony metastases. On rare occasions, metastases can occur in unusual sites such as the skin presenting as painful nodules with ulceration (Block et al, 2006).

C. Laboratory Findings

1. Routine testing—The most common laboratory abnormality is hematuria. It may be accompanied by pyuria, which on occasion may result from concomitant urinary tract infection. Azotemia may be noted in patients with ureteral occlusion owing to the primary bladder tumor or lymphadenopathy. Anemia may be a presenting symptom owing to chronic blood loss, or replacement of the bone marrow with metastatic disease.

2. Urinary cytology—Exfoliated cells from both normal and neoplastic urothelium can be readily identified in voided urine. Larger quantities of cells can be obtained by gently irrigating the bladder with isotonic saline solution through a catheter or cystoscope (barbotage). Cytologic examination of exfoliated cells may be especially useful in detecting cancer in symptomatic patients and assessing response to treatment. Detection rates are high for tumors of high grade and stage as well as CIS but not as impressive for low-grade superficial tumors.

3. Other markers—Several new tests have been developed in order to overcome the shortcomings of urinary cytology such as the low sensitivity for low-grade superficial tumors and inter-observer variability. Commercially available tests include, the bladder tumor antigen (BTA) stat test (Bard Diagnostic Sciences, Inc, Redmond, WA), the BTA TRAK assay (Bard Diagnostic Sciences, Inc), NMP22 assay, and the NMP22 BladderChek test, ImmunoCyt and UroVysion. These tests can detect cancer specific proteins in urine (BTA/NMP22) or augment cytology by identifying cell surface or cytogenetic markers in the nucleus (UroVysion and ImmunoCyt). Other tests under investigation include identification of the Lewis X antigen on exfoliated urothelial cells, and the determination of telomerase activity in exfoliated cells. Several studies have examined the performance of these voided urinary markers for the detection and follow-up of patients with bladder cancer (Grossfeld et al, 2001; Konety and Getzenberg, 2001) (Table 21–1).

These tests have been demonstrated to enhance detection of bladder cancer when used either individually or in combination with cytology. They have been used to detect both new index tumors as well as recurrent tumors. Some of the protein markers lack the specificity of cytology thereby hampering their widespread use. Studies are currently evaluating the precise role of these urinary markers in bladder cancer

Table 21–1. Exfoliated markers for the detection of bladder cancer.

Marker	Sensitivity (%)	Specificity (%)	PPV (%)	NPV (%)
Cytology	35–61	93–100	—	—
NMP22	49–68	86–88	29–65	60–100
BTA stat	57–83	68–85	20–56	70–95
BTA TRAK	54–91	28–84	62	73
Telomerase	62–80	60–99	84	89
UroVysion	30–72	63–95	45–92	31–88
ImmunoCyt	76–85	63–75	29–63	81–96
Cytokeratin 20	91	85	95	76

PPV, positive predictive value; NPV, negative predictive value.

and their optimal role in the diagnosis and surveillance of bladder cancer is still being determined.

D. Imaging

Although bladder cancers may be detected by various imaging techniques, their presence is confirmed by cystoscopy and biopsy. Imaging is therefore used to evaluate the upper urinary tract and, when infiltrating bladder tumors are detected, to assess the depth of muscle wall infiltration and the presence of regional or distant metastases. Intravenous urography used to be one of the most common imaging tests for the evaluation of hematuria. However, it has virtually been replaced by computed tomography (CT) urography, which is more accurate, for evaluation of the entire abdominal cavity, renal parenchyma, and ureters in patients with hematuria (Gray Sears et al, 2002). Bladder tumors may be recognized as pedunculated, radiolucent filling defects projecting into the lumen (Figure 21–3); nonpapillary, infiltrating tumors may result in fixation or flattening of the bladder wall. Hydronephrosis from ureteral obstruction is usually associated with deeply infiltrating lesions and poor outcome after treatment (Haleblian et al, 1998).

Superficial (Ta, Tis) bladder cancers staged with a properly performed TUR and examination under anesthesia do not require additional imaging of the bladder or pelvic organs. However, higher stage lesions are often understaged, and the addition of imaging may be useful. Both CT and magnetic resonance imaging (MRI) (Figure 20–4) have been used to characterize the extent of bladder wall invasion and detect enlarged pelvic lymph nodes, with overall staging accuracy ranging from 40% to 85% for CT and from 50% to 90% for MRI (Fisher et al, 1985; Wood et al, 1988). Both techniques rely on size criteria for the detection of lymphadenopathy: lymph nodes >1 cm are thought to be suggestive of metastases; unfortunately, small-volume pelvic lymph node

metastases are often missed. Because invasive bladder cancers may metastasize to the lung or bones, staging of advanced lesions is completed with chest x-ray and radionuclide bone scan. Bone scans can be avoided if the serum alkaline phosphatase is normal (Berger, 1981). More recently positron emission tomography (PET) CT scans have been utilized to assess metastases from bladder cancer. Early data suggests that PET CT may be able to detect microscopic metastases in lymph nodes that otherwise appear normal with a sensitivity of 70% and specificity of 94% (Kibel et al, 2009). However it is still unclear if such information does lead to significant change in management.

E. Cystourethroscopy and Tumor Resection

The diagnosis and initial staging of bladder cancer is made by cystoscopy and transurethral resection (TUR). Cystoscopy can be done with either flexible or rigid instruments, although the former is associated with less discomfort and only requires local anesthesia. Superficial, low-grade tumors usually appear as single or multiple papillary lesions. Higher-grade lesions are larger and sessile. CIS may appear as flat areas of erythema and mucosal irregularity. Use of fluorescent cystoscopy with blue light can enhance the ability to detect lesions by as much as 20% (Jocham et al, 2005). In this procedure, hematoporphyrin derivatives that accumulate preferentially in cancer cells are instilled into the bladder and fluorescence incited using a blue light. Cancer cells with accumulated porphyrin such as 5-aminolevulinic acid or hexaminolevulinate (HAL) are detected as glowing red under the fluorescent light (Loidl et al, 2005). This technology can be particularly useful in the detection of CIS.

Once a tumor is visualized or suspected, the patient is scheduled for examination under anesthesia and TUR or biopsy of the suspicious lesion. The objectives are tumor diagnosis, assessment of the degree of bladder wall invasion

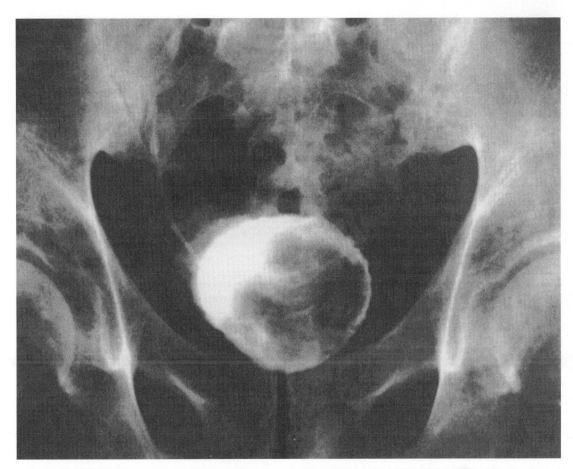

▲ **Figure 21–3.** Image of the urinary bladder obtained on an intravenous urogram. The filling defect represents a papillary bladder cancer.

(staging), and complete excision of the low-stage lesions amenable to such treatment. The American Urologic Associations' best practice guidelines for bladder cancer state that as a standard, all patients undergo as complete a resection as possible of all visible tumors (Hall et al, 2007).

Patients are placed in the lithotomy position. A careful bimanual examination is performed. The presence of any palpable mass and mobility of the bladder are noted along with any degree of fixation to contiguous structures. Cystoscopy is repeated with one or more lenses (30° and 70°) that permit complete visualization of the entire bladder surface. A resectoscope is then placed into the bladder, and visible tumors are removed by electrocautery. Suspicious areas may be biopsied with cup biopsy forceps and the areas may be cauterized with an electrode. Some clinicians routinely perform random bladder biopsies of normal-appearing urothelium both close to and remote from the tumor. The value of random bladder biopsies is controversial. Detection of CIS on these biopsies can alter treatment though more recent studies suggest that only 1.5% of low-risk and 3.5% of high-risk patients may have tumor detected on such biopsies (van der Meijden et al, 1999; May et al, 2003). Findings of the random biopsy can alter treatment in up to 7% of patients (May et al, 2003). Using fluorescent cystoscopy may allow for more precise assessment of the completeness of tumor resection, thereby reducing the risk of leaving behind unresected tumor.

▶ Natural History and Selection of Treatment

A. Standard Histopathological Assessment

The natural history of bladder cancers is defined by two separate but related processes: tumor recurrence and progression. Progression, including metastasis, represents the greater

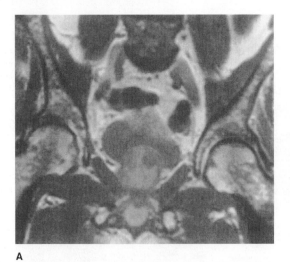
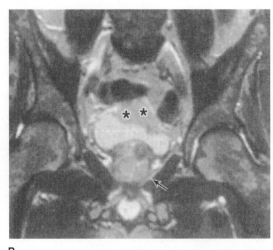

A   **B**

▲ **Figure 21–4.** MRI scan of invasive bladder carcinoma: **A:** T1-weighted image; **B:** T2-weighted image. Bladder wall invasion is best assessed on T2-weighted images because of heightened contrast between tumor (*asterisks*) and detrusor muscle along with ability to detect interruption of the thin high-intensity line representing normal bladder wall. The heterogeneous appearance of the prostate (*arrow*) on the T2-weighted image owes to benign prostatic hypertrophy, confirmed at cystectomy. MRI, magnetic resonance imaging.

biologic risk. However, recurrence, even without progression, represents substantial patient morbidity in that it requires periodic reevaluation (cytology, cystoscopy, etc), repeat endoscopic ablation, and often intravesical chemotherapy (which may be costly, uncomfortable, and associated with complications). Treatment decisions are based on tumor stage and grade. Staging is performed using the tumor, node, metastasis (TNM) staging system (Figure 20–1; Table 20–2) while grading has changed from the Ash-Broder system (I–III or I–IV). The new WHO-ISUP system segregates tumors into papillary urothelial neoplasm of low malignant potential (PUNLMP), low grade or high grade.

At initial presentation, 74% of bladder tumors are superficial or nonmuscle invasive—stage Tis, Ta, or T1 (David et al, 2009). Invasion into the muscle wall and beyond is identified in a smaller number of patients, approximately 26; regional or distant metastases are found in approximately 25%. Unfortunately, 80% of patients with invasive or metastatic disease have no previous history of bladder cancer (Kaye and Lange, 1982). About 47% of the tumors are high grade and 53% are low grade at diagnosis (David et al, 2009). A majority of patients with T1 disease can be further subclassified into groups based on the level of lamina propria invasion. The depth of lamina propria invasion is predictive of the likelihood of recurrence and progression (Orsola et al 2005). There are strong correlations between tumor grade and stage

Table 21–2. Initial treatment options for bladder cancers.

Cancer stage	Initial treatment options
Tis	Complete TUR followed by intravesical BCG
Ta (single, low-to-moderate grade, not recurrent)	Complete TUR
Ta (large, multiple, high grade, or recurrent)	Complete TUR followed by intravesical chemo- or immunotherapy
T1	Complete TUR followed by intravesical chemo- or immunotherapy or radical cystectomy
T2–T4	Radical cystectomy Neoadjuvant chemotherapy followed by radical cystectomy Radical cystectomy followed by adjuvant chemotherapy Concomitant chemotherapy and irradiation
Any T, N+, M+	Systemic chemotherapy followed by selective surgery or irradiation

TUR, transurethral resection.

and tumor recurrence, progression, and survival (Frazier et al, 1993). Patients with low-stage, low-grade disease have a low risk (<5%) of progression to invasive disease, while as many as 40% of patients with low-stage but high-grade disease will progress with extended follow-up (Herr, 2000). Disease-free survival is excellent for patients with pathologically confirmed superficial disease (pT0, pT1, pTIS, 80–88%). However, it falls for patients with pT2 (53–80%), pT3 (39–68%), and pT4 (25–40%) tumors (Frazier et al, 1993; Stein et al, 2001; Thrasher et al, 1994)—owing to the greater likelihood of metastasis in tumors of higher stage. Although lymph node metastases are uncommon (5%) in tumors of low stage, they are increasingly more common in higher stage tumors: 10–30% for pT3A, 31–46% for pT3B, and 35–64% for pT4 (Frazier et al, 1993; Stein et al, 2001). In patients with organ-confined disease, the presence of pelvic lymph node metastases appears to be the most important prognostic factor (Vieweg et al, 1999). The presence of lymphovascular invasion even in those with node-negative disease may portend a worse prognosis (Lotan et al, 2005).

Although metastasis is less common with superficial bladder cancers, such tumors may progress; most recur and require additional treatment. Tumor progression occurs in <6% of patients with Ta disease, but in up to 53% of those with T1 disease, with or without concomitant CIS (Cookson et al, 1997; Heney et al, 1983). Tumor progression occurs in 10–20% of patients with grade I tumors, 19–37% with grade II tumors, and 33–64% with grade III tumors (Lutzeyer et al, 1982; Torti et al, 1987). Using the more recent grading system, progression is observed in 5% of those with low-grade tumors, 15–40% with high-grade tumors, while PUNLMPs almost never demonstrate any risk of progression (Epstein et al, 1998).

Tumor recurrence is related to history of disease and grade, number, and size of the tumor. It is more common in the first 12–24 months after diagnosis (but can become manifest many years later), and patients with one recurrence are more likely to have another. Patients with T1, multiple (>4), large (>3), or high-grade tumors are at greater risk, as are those with either CIS or severe dysplasia in normal-appearing urothelium remote from the tumor site (Heney et al, 1983; Wolf et al, 1985). Tumors can be stratified into low-, intermediate- and high-risk categories based on these criteria and this can be used to guide management decisions.

B. Molecular Markers

Conventional histopathologic analysis of bladder tumors, including determination of tumor grade and stage, may not reliably predict the behavior of many bladder cancers. Assessment of molecular markers of disease, with immunohistochemical methods, in biopsy specimens or cystectomy specimens can yield useful prognostic information.

Tumor growth and metastasis require the growth of new blood vessels, through angiogenesis. Angiogenic stimulators, such as the fibroblastic growth factors and vascular endothelial growth factor, and angiogenic inhibitors, such as thrombospondin-1 and angiostatin regulate angiogenesis. Immunohistochemical quantification of angiogenesis in a given tumor by measuring microvessel density is a useful prognostic indicator for a variety of human malignancies, including bladder cancer. In bladder cancer, microvessel density has been associated with lymph node metastases, disease progression, and overall survival of patients with invasive bladder cancer treated with radical cystectomy (Bochner et al, 1997; Dickinson et al, 1994; Jaeger et al, 1995). The p53 gene is a tumor suppressor gene that plays a key role in the regulation of the cell cycle. When deoxyribonucleic acid (DNA) damage occurs, the level of p53 protein increases, causing cell cycle arrest and repair of DNA. Mutations in the p53 gene result in the production of an abnormal protein product, allowing cells with damaged DNA to continue through the cell cycle. The altered p53 protein has a prolonged half-life compared with the wild-type protein, allowing for its detection by immunohistochemical techniques. Patients with altered p53 expression (indicating possible mutation of the p53 gene) appear to have an increased risk for disease recurrence and a decreased overall survival when compared with patients with normal p53 expression (Esrig et al, 1995). Cancers that are p53 positive are associated with recurrence rates of 62% for pT1, 56% for pT2, and 80% for pT3a, compared with 7%, 12%, and 11%, respectively, for cancers without p53 reactivity.

Alteration of the retinoblastoma (Rb) gene, a tumor suppressor gene, is associated with high-grade, high-stage bladder cancers. In addition, Rb alteration appears to be significantly associated with decreased overall survival in such patients (Cordon-Cardo et al, 1992; Logothetis et al, 1992). Studies in which both p53 and Rb have been examined in patients with invasive bladder cancer suggest that bladder tumors with alterations in both genes have a poorer prognosis and decreased overall survival when compared with tumors with wild-type p53 and Rb.

Assessment of other markers that may correlate with outcome in patients with bladder cancer includes that of tumor growth fraction (proliferative index) and cellular adhesion molecule expression (E-cadherin) (Lipponen and Eskelinen, 1995; Okamura et al, 1990).

C. Treatment Selection

Patients with superficial bladder cancers can be treated with TUR followed by selective intravesical chemotherapy or immunotherapy. Patients with initial low-grade small tumors are at low risk of progression and may be treated by TUR alone followed by surveillance or intravesical chemotherapy. In some patients with recurrent, low-grade tumors, fulguration of such tumors using electrocautery in an office setting under local anesthesia is also an acceptable alternative. Recent data suggest that some low-grade tumors can be observed at least for a period of time without significant increased risk of progression or metastases (Soloway et al, 2003). Patients with T1, high-grade, multiple, large, recurrent tumors or those associated with CIS on bladder biopsies are at a higher risk of progression and recurrence and should be considered candidates for intravesical chemotherapy or immunotherapy after complete and careful TUR. A second resection of the same area may be required to accurately stage disease and determine treatment (Herr et al, 1999; Grimm et al, 2003). Repeat resections may also enhance response to intravesical therapy (Herr, 2005). Management of T1 tumors is somewhat controversial; some clinicians advise radical cystectomy, especially for high-grade lesions, which are associated with a high rate of progression. However, progression rates can be reduced by intravesical immunotherapy (Cookson and Sarosdy, 1992; Herr et al, 1989). Recurrence of T1 disease after a trial of intravesical therapy warrants more aggressive therapy such as cystectomy (Herr, 1991; Herr and Sogani, 2001).

Patients with more invasive, but still localized, tumors (T2, T3) are candidates for more aggressive local treatment, including partial or radical cystectomy, or a combination of radiation and systemic chemotherapy. Radical TUR alone may be a viable option in select patients with T2 disease, particularly if no tumor is found on repeat resection since 10-year survival rates as high as 83% can be achieved (Herr, 2001). However, this approach must be used with caution since there is a substantial risk of leaving residual disease behind (Solsona et al, 1998). Superficial ductal or acinar in situ carcinoma of the prostatic urethra, not invading the basement membrane or prostatic stroma, may be treated with TUR and intravesical chemotherapy or immunotherapy rather than cystectomy. However, patients with more extensive involvement of the prostatic urethra by TCC, or recurrence after conservative therapy, require more aggressive therapy. Patients with unresectable local tumors (T4B) are candidates for systemic chemotherapy, followed by surgery (or possibly irradiation). Patients with either local or distant metastases should receive systemic chemotherapy followed by the selective use of either irradiation or surgery, depending on the response.

▶ Treatment

A. Intravesical Chemotherapy

Immunotherapeutic or chemotherapeutic agents can be instilled into the bladder directly via catheter, thereby avoiding the morbidity of systemic administration in most cases. Intravesical therapy can have a prophylactic or therapeutic objective, either to reduce recurrence in patients whose tumors have been completely resected. Intravesical chemotherapy is used in two settings. When instilled immediately following TUR, it acts prophylactically to reduce tumor cell implantation (Solsona et al, 1999). It can also be used therapeutically to reduce risk of recurrence and progression particularly for low-risk superficial tumors. Therefore,

Table 23–3. Delivery of intravesical chemotherapy or immunotherapy.

Use	Timing	Goal
Adjunctive	At TUR	Prevent implantation
Prophylactic	After complete TUR	Prevent or delay recurrence or progression
Therapeutic	After incomplete TUR	Cure residual disease

TUR, transurethral resection.

intravesical chemotherapy or immunotherapy may be delivered in three different fashions to achieve individual goals (Table 20–3). Considerable experience has been gained, but comparison of different agents is difficult owing to the paucity of randomized trials and variations in dose, contact time, patient population, and intervals between treatments. Most agents are administered weekly for 6 weeks except when being used prophylactically where a single dose is administered immediately following TUR. Maintenance therapy (ie, monthly or bimonthly intravesical therapy) may decrease recurrence rates further. Although local toxicity is relatively common—primarily irritative voiding symptoms—systemic toxicity is rare because of the limited absorption of drugs across the lumen of the bladder. Severe systemic complications can be avoided by not administering intravesical chemotherapy in patients with gross hematuria. Efficacy may be improved by increasing contact time and drug concentration (ie, by restricting fluid intake before administration, asking the patient to lie in different positions during treatment, avoiding instillation of air during drug administration, and requiring the patient to avoid urinating for 1–2 hours thereafter). The most common agents in the United States are mitomycin C, thiotepa, and Bacillus Calmette-Guérin (BCG). Patients in whom treatment with one agent fails may respond to another.

1. Mitomycin C—Mitomycin C is an antitumor, antibiotic, alkylating agent that inhibits DNA synthesis. With a molecular weight of 329, systemic absorption is minimal. The usual dose is 40 mg in 40 cc of sterile water or saline given once a week for 6 weeks. The same dose is utilized for a single prophylactic instillation. Between 39% and 78% of patients with residual tumor experience, a complete response to intravesical mitomycin C (Kowalkowski and Lamm, 1988) and recurrence is reduced in 2–33% after complete TUR (Herr et al, 1987). Side effects are noted in 10–43% of patients and consist largely of irritative voiding symptoms including urinary frequency, urgency, and dysuria. Unique to this drug is the appearance of a rash on the palms and genitalia in approximately 6% of patients, but this effect can be alleviated if patients wash their hands and genitalia at the time of voiding after intravesical administration. Instillation of Mitomycin C into the bladder immediately post-TUR has been shown to decrease recurrences and prolong the interval to recurrence (Sylvester et al, 2004). Hence it is now considered standard of care to instill one dose of 40 mg of Mitomycin C into the bladder immediately post-TUR to reduce risk of recurrence (Hall et al, 2007). The efficacy of Mitomycin C can be enhanced by administering it in a more concentrated solution of 40 mg in 20 cc of sterile water after alkalinizing the urine and with reduced fluid intake (Au et al, 2001).

2. Thiotepa—Thiotepa is an alkylating agent with a molecular weight of 189. Although various doses have been used, 30 mg weekly seems to be sufficient. Up to 55% of patients respond completely. Most series show significantly lower recurrence rates in patients taking thiotepa than in those taking a placebo (Herr et al, 1987; Kowalkowski and Lamm, 1988). Cystitis is not uncommon after instillation but is usually mild and self-limited. Myelosuppression manifested as leukopenia and thrombocytopenia occurs in up to 9% of patients owing to systemic absorption. A complete blood count should be obtained in all patients before successive instillations.

3. BCG—BCG is an attenuated strain of *Mycobacterium bovis*. Many different strains of BCG exist, and the marketed preparations vary in the number, pathogenicity, viability, and immunogenicity of organisms (Catalona and Ratliff, 1990). The exact mechanism by which BCG exerts its antitumor effect is unknown, but it seems to be immunologically mediated. Mucosal ulceration and granuloma formation are commonly seen after intravesical instillation. Activated helper T lymphocytes can be identified in the granulomas, and interleukin-2 reportedly can be detected in the urine of treated patients (Haaf et al, 1986). BCG has been shown to be very effective both therapeutically and prophylactically. It appears to be the most efficacious intravesical agent for the management of CIS. Complete responses are recorded in 36–71% of patients with residual carcinoma (Catalona and Ratliff, 1990; Herr et al, 1987). Recurrence rates are reduced substantially in patients treated after endoscopic resection (11–27% versus a 70% recurrence after endoscopic resection alone) (Catalona and Ratliff, 1990; Herr et al, 1985; Herr et al, 1987; Lamm, 1985). BCG has been shown to be superior to intravesical chemotherapy in preventing recurrence in patients with high-risk superficial bladder cancer (Lamm et al, 1991). Although BCG appears to be effective in delaying progression of high-risk superficial bladder cancer, 40–50% of these patients will experience disease progression with extended follow-up and many patients will ultimately require cystectomy (Cookson et al, 1997; Davis et al, 2002; Herr et al, 1995). The most commonly recommended induction regimen for BCG is weekly for 6 weeks followed by a period of 6 weeks where no BCG is given. Maintenance therapy should be considered in high-risk patients (Lamm et al, 2000). The optimal regimen for maintenance therapy is unclear. Published regimens involve three instillations once a week at 3- to 6-month intervals for 3 years following TUR. Only a small proportion (16–32%) of patients received all the treatments in prior studies, which highlights the difficulty of administering maintenance therapy and its side effects (van der Meijden et al, 2003; Lamm et al, 2000). Maintenance BCG appears to be more effective than intravesical chemotherapy with mitomycin C for intermediate- and high-risk superficial bladder cancer (Bohle, 2003). BCG is more effective than chemotherapy in preventing progression of superficial cancers (Sylvester et al, 2005). Side effects of intravesical BCG administration are relatively common, although severe complications are uncommon. Most patients experience some degree of urinary frequency and urgency. Hemorrhagic cystitis occurs in approximately 7% of patients, and evidence of distant infection is found in <2%. Patients with mild systemic or moderate local symptoms should be treated with isoniazid (300 mg daily) and pyridoxine (vita-min B_6 50 mg/day), and the dosage of BCG should be reduced. Isoniazid is continued while symptoms persist and stopped 1 day before the next instillation.

Patients with severe systemic symptoms should have instillations stopped. Patients with prolonged high fever (>103°F), symptomatic granulomatous prostatitis, or evidence of systemic infection require treatment with isoniazid and rifampin (600 mg daily). Patients with signs and symptoms of BCG sepsis (eg, high fever, chills, confusion, hypotension, respiratory failure, jaundice) should be treated with isoniazid, rifampin, and ethambutol (1200 mg). The addition of cycloserine (500 mg twice daily) or prednisolone (40 mg daily) increases survival rates (Lamm, 1992).

4. New intravesical agents and approaches—The rate of metachronous tumor recurrence is high compared with that of low-grade cancers occurring in other organs (eg, nasopharynx, colon). Recurrence of superficial bladder cancer is related to cancer stage, grade and number of tumors, associated dysplasia, and DNA content. Recurrent tumors may be due to regrowth of previously resected cancers, growth of new cancers at remote sites, or implantation and subsequent proliferation of cells released into the bladder at the time of endoscopic treatment of the original tumor. Several investigators have studied the efficacy of single-dose therapy delivered at the time of complete TUR (Oosterlinck et al, 1993; Tolley et al, 1988). Such therapy has been shown to decrease recurrence rates, probably by decreasing the risk of tumor cell implantation at the time of initial cancer resection. Studies of interferon-alpha and valrubicin (an anthracycline derivative) suggest that these agents, either alone or perhaps in combination with other agents, may be effective in either high-risk patients or those who fail to respond to first-line therapy (Belldegrun et al, 1998; Sarosdy et al, 1998; Steinberg et al, 2000). Preliminary studies suggest that low-dose BCG, in combination with interferon, may be successful in preventing recurrences up to 24 months in 57% of patients who are BCG naïve and in 42% of those who have failed prior

BCG therapy (O'Donnell et al, 2004). Other agents that have been tested in the context of salvage intravesical therapy following BCG failure have been Gemcitabine as well as Docetaxel. Gemcitabine showed promise in an early, phase I study but subsequent studies have not demonstrated similar efficacy in this setting (Dalbagni et al, 2006). Docetaxel also demonstrated a good response in an initial phase I study but subsequent follow-up revealed that the response was not durable unless further induction and maintenance doses were administered (Barlow et al, 2009).

B. Surgery

1. TUR—TUR is the initial form of treatment for all bladder cancers. It allows a reasonably accurate estimate of tumor stage and grade and the need for additional treatment. Patients with single, low-grade, noninvasive tumors may be treated with TUR alone; those with superficial disease but high-risk features should be treated with TUR followed by selective use of intravesical therapy, as described above. TUR alone has rarely been used in the management of patients with invasive bladder cancer because of a high likelihood of recurrence and progression. Such an approach has been used infrequently for carefully selected patients with comorbid medical conditions and either no residual disease or minimal disease only at restaging TUR of bladder tumor (Herr et al, 1987; Solsona et al, 1998). Careful follow-up of patients with superficial bladder cancers is mandatory because disease will recur in 30–80% of patients, depending on cancer grade, tumor stage, and number of tumors. Disease status at 3 months after initial resection is an important predictor of the risk of subsequent recurrence and progression (Holmang and Johansson, 2002; Solsona et al, 2000). For patients who presented initially with solitary, low-grade lesions and who are free of recurrence at 3 months, repeat cystoscopy at 1 year is suggested. Patients who presented initially with multiple or higher grade lesions (or both) and those who have recurrences at 3 months require more careful surveillance. In such patients, cystoscopy at 3-month intervals is necessary. Although periodic cystoscopy is suggested for all patients with a history of bladder cancer, the risk of recurrence decreases as the tumor-free interval increases. After 5 years without recurrence, the risk of recurrence has been estimated to be 22%; the rate is 2% for 10 years (Morris et al, 1995).

2. Partial cystectomy—Patients with solitary, infiltrating tumors (T1–T3) localized along the posterior lateral wall or dome of the bladder are candidates for partial cystectomy, as are patients with cancers in a diverticulum. Disease remote from the primary tumor must be excluded by random bladder biopsies preoperatively. To minimize tumor implantation resulting from contamination of the wound with cancer cells at the time of surgery, short-course, limited-dose (1000–1600 cGy) irradiation can be used, and an intravesical chemotherapeutic agent can be instilled preoperatively (Ojeda and Johnson, 1983). Although survival rates of well-selected

patients may approach those for patients with similar stage tumors treated by radical cystectomy, local recurrences are common (Sweeney et al, 1992; Whitmore, 1983). Patients with concomitant CIS and those with lymph node metastases do not respond well to partial cystectomy (Holzbeierlein et al, 2004). Given current techniques of bladder replacement surgery, partial cystectomy is uncommonly indicated in the management of patients with invasive bladder cancer.

3. Radical cystectomy—Radical cystectomy implies removal of the anterior pelvic organs: in men, the bladder with its surrounding fat and peritoneal attachments, the prostate, and the seminal vesicles; in women, the bladder and surrounding fat and peritoneal attachments, cervix, uterus, anterior vaginal vault, urethra, and ovaries. This remains the "gold standard" of treatment for patients with muscle invasive bladder cancer. However, in select female patients, the vaginal vault and urethra can be spared along with the uterus, fallopian tubes, and ovaries, particularly in those who are premenopausal. Sparing of the urethra allows for construction of a neobladder that can be anastomosed to the urethral remnant. Disease-free survival 5 years after surgery is based on tumor stage: 88% for patients with PT0, PTa, or PTIS disease; 80% for patients with PT1 disease; 81% for patients with PT2 disease; 68% for patients with PT3a and 47% for those with PT3b disease; and 44% for patients with PT4a disease (Stein et al, 2001). Recurrences after surgery usually occur within the first 3 years. Local pelvic recurrence rates are low (7–10%); most patients who fail therapy have distant disease recurrence.

The risk of urethral tumor occurrence or recurrence in men who undergo radical cystectomy is 6.1–10.6%. Risk factors for urethral tumor involvement in men include infiltration of the prostatic stroma or prostatic urethra with cancer or CIS. Patients with these risk factors are candidates for urethrectomy either at the time of radical cystectomy or as a separate procedure (Zabbo and Montie, 1984). Although prostatic urethral disease is a risk factor for urethral recurrence, recent evidence suggests that urethrectomy may be omitted and orthotopic urinary diversion performed safely in men with only proximal prostatic urethral involvement and a negative urethral margin at radical cystectomy (Iselin et al, 1997).

Urethrectomy was once routinely performed in all women undergoing radical cystectomy. However, recent clinical experience suggests that bladder replacement is an acceptable procedure in women as well as men. Women with bladder cancer who have an uninvolved urethral margin at the time of cystectomy and whose tumor was not located at the bladder neck are candidates for this procedure. Approximately 66% of women undergoing radical cystectomy for the management of bladder cancer fall into this group (Stein et al, 1995; Stein et al, 1998; Stenzl et al, 1995).

In such women, even the uterus, substantial portion of the vaginal vault, fallopian tubes, and ovaries can be spared. A bilateral pelvic lymph node dissection is usually performed simultaneously with radical cystectomy. Lymph node metastases are identified in approximately 20–35% of patients (Stein et al, 2001)—an incidence that reflects the inability of any imaging mode to identify consistently small-volume lymph node metastases preoperatively. Patients with lymph node metastases have a poorer prognosis. However, some patients (10–33%) with limited disease in regional lymph nodes may be cured by radical cystectomy and lymphadenectomy (Lerner et al, 1993; Stein et al, 2001; Vieweg et al, 1999). Even patients with pathologically negative nodes appear to benefit from an extensive lymphadenectomy (Konety, 2003). Patients with fewer than five positive lymph nodes and organ-confined disease in the primary tumor tend to have a better prognosis than patients with more extensive disease. These patients may also benefit from adjuvant chemotherapy (see Section Chemotherapy).

Urinary diversion may be accomplished using a variety of techniques. Methods have been developed that allow construction of reservoirs that are continent and do not require the patient to wear an external appliance for collection of urine (see Chapter 25).

C. Radiotherapy

External beam irradiation (5000–7000 cGy), delivered in fractions over a 5- to 8-week period, is an alternative to radical cystectomy in well-selected patients with deeply infiltrating bladder cancers. Treatment is generally well tolerated, but approximately 15% of patients may have significant bowel, bladder, or rectal complications. Five-year survival rates for stages T2 and T3 disease range from 18% to 41% (Goffinet et al, 1975; Quilty and Duncan, 1986; Woon et al, 1985). Unfortunately, local recurrence is common, occurring in approximately 33–68% of patients. Consequently, radiation as monotherapy is usually offered only to those patients who are poor surgical candidates due to advanced age or significant comorbid medical problems.

D. Chemotherapy

Approximately 15% of patients who present with bladder cancer are found to have regional or distant metastases; approximately 30–40% of patients with invasive disease develop distant metastases despite radical cystectomy or definitive radiotherapy. Without treatment, survival is limited. Early results with single chemotherapeutic agents and, subsequently, combinations of drugs have shown that a significant number of patients with metastatic bladder cancer respond partially or completely (Scher and Sternberg, 1985). The single most active agent is cisplatin, which, when used alone, produces responses in approximately 30% of patients (Yagoda, 1983). Other effective agents include methotrexate, doxorubicin, vinblastine, cyclophosphamide, gemcitabine, and 5-fluorouracil. Response rates improve when active agents are combined. The regimen of methotrexate, vinblastine, doxorubicin (Adriamycin), and cisplatin (MVAC) has

been the most commonly used for patients with advanced bladder cancer (Sternberg et al, 1988; Tannock et al, 1989). Approximately 13–35% of patients receiving such regimens attain a complete response. However, the median survival time is approximately 1 year, and the sustained survival rate is 20–25%. Treatment with MVAC is associated with substantial toxicity, including a toxic death rate of 3–4%.

Other newer agents demonstrating activity in this disease include ifosfamide, gemcitabine, paclitaxel, and gallium nitrate (Fagbemi and Stadler, 1998). A study demonstrated similar overall survival, time to treatment failure, and response rate for patients treated with MVAC and those treated with the combination of gemcitabine and cisplatin (von der Maase et al, 2000). The advantage of gemcitabine and cisplatin over MVAC is significantly lower toxicity and improved tolerability.

E. Combination Therapy

Once it became apparent that patients with metastatic bladder cancer could benefit from combination chemotherapy, investigators began treating patients with locally invasive (T2–T4), but not metastatic, cancer similarly. Chemotherapy can be given before planned radical cystectomy (neoadjuvant) in an attempt to decrease recurrence rates and, in selected cases, allow for bladder preservation. Approximately 22–43% of patients achieve a complete response to chemotherapy alone (Scher et al, 1988; Scher, 1990). However, additional treatment is still indicated because a substantial number of patients who believed to be free of tumors after chemotherapy alone are found to have infiltrating disease at the time of surgery (Scher et al, 1989). Results from a recent randomized trial suggest that neoadjuvant chemotherapy followed by surgery improve duration of survival when compared with surgery alone for patients with invasive disease. Patients who undergo neoadjuvant chemotherapy are more likely to have no residual tumor in the bladder at cystectomy and this portends a better long-term survival (Grossman et al, 2003). Alternatively, adjuvant chemotherapy may be offered to selected patients after radical cystectomy because of an increased risk of recurrence due to the presence of locally advanced disease (ie, P3, P4, or N_+) (Freiha et al, 1996; Logothetis et al, 1988; Scher, 1990; Skinner et al, 1991; Stockle et al, 1992; Stockle et al, 1995). These studies suggest that patients initially managed with radical cystectomy who are found to be at an increased risk of systemic relapse due to the presence of lymph node metastases or regionally advanced disease are candidates for adjuvant chemotherapy.

Owing to high local and systemic failure rates after definitive irradiation, several investigators have explored the possibility of combining irradiation with systemic chemotherapy to decrease recurrence rates, improve patient survival, and allow bladder preservation. Trials of single-agent chemotherapy and irradiation have shown better local response rates than are found in historical series of irradiation alone (Jakse et al, 1985; Pearson and Raghaven, 1985; Shipley et al, 1984).

More recently, investigators have treated patients with invasive bladder cancer with complete TUR followed by concomitant chemotherapy and radiation (Cervek et al, 1998; Chauvet et al, 1996; Given et al, 1995; Kachnic et al, 1997; Serretta et al, 1998; Shipley et al, 1997; Tester et al, 1996; Zietman et al, 1997; Zeitman et al, 2001). Cisplatin and Gemcitabine have been the chemotherapeutic agents with the best radiosensitizing activity in these regimens (Oh et al, 2009). Early cystectomy is offered to those who do not tolerate chemotherapy, radiation, or both owing to toxicity and those whose cancers fail to respond to such therapy. Complete response rates to chemoradiation may be as high as 50–70% initially, with 5-year overall survival rates approaching 50–60%. However, local recurrence is common, exceeding 50% in many of these studies. Studies with longer median follow-up of almost 7 years suggest that the occurrence of late failure with superficial disease recurrence may be around 26% (Zeitman et al, 2001). However patients who develop superficial disease recurrence (most commonly CIS) are more likely to require salvage cystectomy with only 34% being alive with a preserved bladder at 8 years compared to 61% of those who do not have such disease recurrence. Owing to invasive local recurrences, only 18– 44% of patients may be alive with an intact bladder 5 years after chemoradiation. Local disease stage and completeness of initial TUR are predictive of response and survival while delivery of radiation therapy by itself is not (Rodel et al, 2002). Predictors of poor outcome after combined chemoradiation for invasive bladder cancer include hydronephrosis at presentation, advanced clinical tumor stage, inability to complete the entire treatment protocol, and poor performance status. A recent study has suggested that chemoradiation may also be inappropriate for patients with bladder tumors that are p53-positive (Herr et al, 1999). Combined chemotherapy and radiation has also been used successfully to treat high-grade superficially invasive tumors (T1) (Akcetin et al, 2005).

Systemic adjuvant chemotherapy for locally invasive, but not metastatic, bladder cancer should not yet be considered standard therapy. The durability of the response, ultimate survival rates, and optimal candidates for the treatment regimens described will be determined only after completion of randomized studies.

URETERAL AND RENAL PELVIC CANCERS

▶ Incidence

Carcinomas of the renal pelvis and ureter are rare, accounting for only 4% of all urothelial cancers. The ratio of bladder–renal pelvic–ureteral carcinomas is approximately 51:3:1 (Williams and Mitchell, 1973). The mean age at diagnosis is 65 years, and the male–female ratio is 2–4:1 (Babaian and Johnson, 1980). Urothelial cancer often presents as a widespread urothelial abnormality: Patients with a single upper-tract carcinoma are at risk of developing bladder carcinomas

(30–50%) and contralateral upper-tract carcinoma (2–4%). Conversely, patients with primary bladder cancer are at low risk (<2%) of developing upper urinary tract cancers (Oldbring et al, 1989). However, patients with multiple, recurrent superficial and in situ bladder cancers that are successfully treated by TUR and BCG are at a substantial lifelong risk of development of upper-tract cancers (Herr, 1998). The cumulative risks of such cancers have been estimated to be 10% at 5 years of follow-up, 26% at 5–10 years, and 34% at >10 years.

▶ Etiology

As with bladder carcinoma, smoking and exposure to certain industrial dyes or solvents are associated with an increased risk of upper urinary tract TCCs. However, these tumors also occur with increased frequency in patients with a long history of excessive analgesic intake, those with Balkan nephropathy, and those exposed to Thorotrast, a contrast agent previously used for retrograde pyelography. Patients with carcinomas associated with analgesic abuse are more likely to be women, have higher stage disease, and be younger than others (Mahoney et al, 1977). All the major constituents of the analgesic compounds consumed (acetaminophen, aspirin, caffeine, and phenacetin) may be associated with an increased risk of upper urinary tract cancer (Jensen et al, 1989; Ross et al, 1989). Balkan nephropathy is an interstitial inflammatory disease of the kidneys that affects Yugoslavians, Rumanians, Bulgarians, and Greeks (Markovic, 1972); associated upper-tract carcinomas are generally superficial and more likely to be bilateral. The exact mechanism of tumor induction in these patients remains unknown.

▶ Pathology

The mucosal lining of the renal pelvis and ureter is similar to that of the urinary bladder, being composed of transitional cell epithelium. Thus, most renal pelvic and ureteral cancers (90% and 97%, respectively) are TCCs. Grading is similar to that for bladder carcinomas. Papillomas account for approximately 15–20% of cases (Grabstald et al, 1971). They are isolated in just over 50% of patients and multiple in the rest, and in approximately 25% of patients with isolated papillomas and 50% of patients with multiple papillomas, carcinomas eventually develop. Among patients with carcinomas of the ureter, multicentricity approaches 50%. There is a relationship between tumor grade and the likelihood of urothelial abnormalities elsewhere: Low-grade cancers are associated with a low incidence of urothelial atypia or CIS in remote sites; however, these abnormalities are common with high-grade neoplasms (McCarron et al, 1982). Most upper urinary tract TCCs are localized at the time of diagnosis; the most common metastatic sites include regional lymph nodes, bone, and lung.

Squamous carcinomas account for approximately 10% of renal pelvic cancers and are much rare in the ureter. Most carcinomas are usually sessile and infiltrating at the time of diagnosis. Such tumors are commonly identified in patients with a history of chronic inflammation from infection or calculous disease. Adenocarcinomas are very rare tumors of the upper urinary tract and, like squamous carcinomas, tend to be far advanced at the time of diagnosis.

Mesodermal tumors of the renal pelvis and ureter are quite rare. Benign tumors include fibroepithelial polyps (the most common), leiomyomas, and angiomas. Fibroepithelial polyps occur most commonly in young adults and are characterized radiographically by a long, slender, and polyploid filling defect within the collecting system. The most common malignant mesodermal tumors are leiomyosarcomas. The ureter and renal pelvis may be invaded by cancers of contiguous structures, such as primary renal, ovarian, or cervical carcinomas. True metastases to the ureter are rare. The most common metastatic tumors include those of stomach, prostate, kidney, and breast as well as lymphomas.

▶ Staging and Natural History

Staging of both renal pelvic and ureteral carcinomas (Table 21–4) is based on an accurate assessment of the degree of tumor infiltration and parallels the staging system developed for bladder cancer (Grabstald et al, 1971; American Joint Committee on Cancer, 1997). Tumor stage and grade correlate with survival (Reitelman et al, 1987). Low-grade and low-stage cancers of the renal pelvis and ureter are associated with survival rates between 60% and 90%, compared with 0% and 33% for tumors of higher grade or those that have penetrated deep into or through the renal pelvic or ureteral wall (Hall et al, 1998). The latter figures reflect a high likelihood of regional or distant metastases—40% and 75% in patients with stages T2–T4 cancers, respectively. Upper urinary tract cancers are associated with a high rate of recurrent bladder cancer with as many as 40% of patients experiencing recurrent bladder tumors (Bagley and Grasso, 2010).

Table 21–4. Staging of ureteral and renal pelvic carcinoma.

	TNM[†]
Confined to mucosa	Ta, Tis
Invasion of lamina propria	T1
Invasion of muscularis	T2
Extension through muscularis into fat or renal parenchyma	T3
Spread to adjacent organs	T4
Lymph node metastases	N+
Metastases	M+

[†]Tumor, Node, Metastasis.
Drawn from American Joint Committee on Cancer, 1997.

▶ Clinical Findings

A. Symptoms and Signs

Gross hematuria is noted in 70–90% of patients. Flank pain, present in 8–50%, is the result of ureteral obstruction from blood clots or tumor fragments, renal pelvic or ureteral obstruction by the tumor itself, or regional invasion by the tumor. Irritative voiding symptoms are present in approximately 5–10% of patients. Constitutional symptoms of anorexia, weight loss, and lethargy are uncommon and are usually associated with metastatic disease. A flank mass owing to hydronephrosis or a large tumor is detected in approximately 10–20% (Geerdsen, 1979), and flank tenderness may be elicited as well. Supraclavicular or inguinal adenopathy or hepatomegaly may be identified in a small percentage of patients with metastatic disease.

B. Laboratory Findings

Hematuria is identified in most patients but may be intermittent. Elevated liver function levels due to liver metastases are noted in a few patients. Pyuria and bacteriuria may be identified in patients with concomitant urinary tract infection from obstruction and urinary stasis.

As with bladder cancers, upper urinary tract cancers may be identified by examining exfoliated cells in the urinary sediment. In addition, specimens may be obtained directly with a ureteral catheter or by passing a small brush through the lumen of an open-ended catheter (Dodd et al, 1997; Gill et al, 1973). Detection depends on the grade of the tumor and the adequacy of the specimen obtained: 20–30% of low-grade cancers may be detected by cytologic testing compared with >60% of higher grade lesions (McCarron et al, 1983); using barbotage or a ureteral brush increases diagnostic accuracy. The utility of the newer voided markers, such as the UroVysion have been found to have better sensitivity and specificity relative to cytology of upper-tract washings for the diagnosis of renal pelvis and ureteric tumors (Akkad et al, 2007).

C. Imaging

Findings on intravenous or CT urography in patients with upper urinary tract cancers are usually abnormal. The most common abnormalities identified include an intraluminal filling defect, unilateral nonvisualization of the collecting system, and hydronephrosis (Almgard et al, 1973; Williams and Mitchell, 1973). Ureteral and renal pelvic tumors must be differentiated from nonopaque calculi, blood clots, papillary necrosis, and inflammatory lesions such as ureteritis cystica, fungus infections, or tuberculosis. The urography is often indeterminate, requiring retrograde pyelography for more accurate visualization of collecting-system abnormalities and simultaneous collection of cytologic specimens. CT urography is being increasingly used as the test of choice for evaluating the upper tract. During retrograde pyelography, contrast material is injected into the ureteral orifice with a

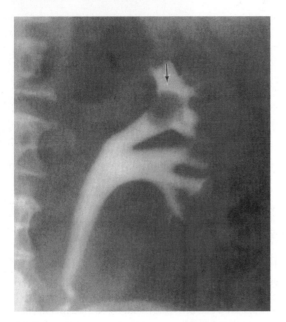

▲ **Figure 21–5.** Filling defect representing a transitional cell carcinoma (*arrow*) on retrograde pyelography.

bulb or acorn-tip catheter. Intraluminal filling defects may then be identified in the ureter or renal pelvis (Figure 21–5). Ureteral tumors are often characterized by dilation of the ureter distal to the lesion, creating the appearance of a "goblet." Nonopaque ureteral calculi appear as a narrowing of the ureter distal to the calculus. A ureteral catheter passed up the ureter may coil distal to a ureteral tumor (Bergman's sign)

(Bergman et al, 1961). Ultrasonography, CT, and MRI frequently identify soft-tissue abnormalities of the renal pelvis but may fail to identify ureteral filling defects directly, although they may show hydronephrosis (Figure 21–6). All three imaging techniques differentiate blood clot and tumor from nonopaque calculi. In addition, CT and MRI allow simultaneous examination of abdominal and retroperitoneal structures for signs of regional (lymph node) or more distant metastases.

D. Ureteropyeloscopy

The use of rigid and flexible ureteropyeloscopes has allowed direct visualization of upper urinary tract abnormalities. These instruments are passed transurethrally through the ureteral orifice; in addition, they (and the similarly constructed but larger nephroscopes) can be passed percutaneously into renal calyces and the pelvis directly. The latter instrument carries with it the theoretic possibility of tumor spillage along the percutaneous tract. Indications for ureteroscopy include evaluation of filling defects within the upper urinary tract and after positive results on cytologic study or after noting unilateral gross hematuria in the absence of a filling defect. Ureteroscopy is also performed as a surveillance procedure in patients who have undergone conservative surgery for removal of a ureteral or renal pelvic tumor. Visualization, biopsy, and, on occasion, complete tumor resection, fulguration, or laser vaporization of the tumor are possible endoscopically. Performance of ureteroscopy with biopsy to establish the diagnosis in a patient with positive urine cytology and an upper-tract filling defect may not always be necessary as these patients are presumed to have upper-tract TCC for which nephroureterectomy may be

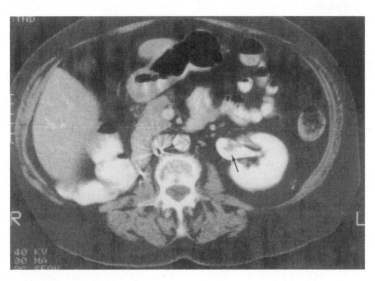

▲ **Figure 21–6.** Computed tomography scan showing the presence of a renal pelvic tumor (*arrow*).

considered. However, any delay that may ensue from first performing a ureteroscopy with biopsy does not appear to jeopardize subsequent patient survival (Boorjian et al, 2005). Ureteroscopic visualization with biopsy is accurate and can identify cancer in a majority of patients. A diagnosis of cancer can be obtained >90% of the time with grade determination possible in >80% of cases (Keeley et al, 1997). It is harder to obtain lamina propria or muscle in ureteroscopic cup biopsy specimens, which limits evaluation for stage of disease. Correlation of grade determined by tumor biopsy to that of the nephroureterectomy specimen is observed in 78% of cases. Biopsies tend to underestimate tumor grade in 22% of patients and stage in 45% of Ta tumors (Guarnizo et al, 2000). Multiple biopsies and biopsy of tumors in the proximal ureter tend to be more reliable in accurately determining stage and grade of ureteric tumors (Guarnizo et al, 2000).

▶ Treatment

Treatment of renal pelvic and ureteral tumors should be based primarily on grade, stage, position, and multiplicity. Renal function and anatomy should be assessed. The standard therapy for both tumor types has been nephroureterectomy with excision of a bladder cuff owing to the possibility of multifocal disease within the ipsilateral collecting system. This procedure may be performed using either an open or laparoscopic approach (Jarrett et al, 2001; Landman et al, 2002). When the operation is performed for proximal ureteral or renal pelvic cancers, the entire distal ureter with a small cuff of bladder needs to be removed to avoid recurrence within this segment (Reitelman et al, 1987; Strong et al, 1976). Tumors of the distal ureter may be treated with distal ureterectomy and ureteral reimplantation into the bladder if no proximal defects suggestive of cancer have been noted (Babaian and Johnson, 1980).

Indications for more conservative surgery, including open or endoscopic excision, are not well defined. Absolute indications for renal-sparing procedures include tumor within the collecting system of a single kidney and bilateral urothelial tumors of the upper urinary tract or in patients with two kidneys but marginal renal function. In patients with two functioning kidneys, endoscopic excision alone should be considered only for low-grade and noninvasive tumors. One must realize that endoscopic examination may fail to detect the degree of infiltration adequately and therefore may understage some tumors. Limited experience with endoscopic resection, fulguration, or vaporization suggests that the procedure is safe in properly selected patients (Blute et al, 1989). However, recurrences have been noted in 15–80% of patients treated with open or endoscopic excision (Blute et al, 1989; Keeley et al, 1997; Maier et al, 1990; Orihuela and Smith, 1988; Stoller et al, 1997). Recurrence may be avoided by treating with instillation of immunotherapeutic or chemotherapeutic agents such as BCG or mitomycin C (Keeley and Bagley, 1997; Orihuela and Smith, 1988; Studer et al,

1989). These agents can be delivered to the upper urinary tract through single or double-J ureteral catheters (Patel and Fuchs, 1998). If patients are treated conservatively, it has been suggested that routine follow-up should include routine endoscopic surveillance because imaging alone may be inadequate for detecting recurrence (Chen et al, 2000).

Radiotherapy plays a limited role in upper urinary tract cancers. Although controversial, postoperative irradiation is believed by some investigators to decrease recurrence rates and improve survival in patients with deeply infiltrating cancers. Patients with metastatic, transitional cell cancers of the upper urinary tract should receive cisplatin-based chemotherapeutic regimens as described for patients with metastatic bladder cancers. There is recent evidence suggesting that neoadjuvant chemotherapy in those with invasive upper-tract tumors may be better tolerated and yield higher response rates as it is delivered in the setting of more normal renal function (Lane et al, 2010). Adjuvant chemotherapy does not appear to improve survival significantly in patients with upper urinary tract neoplasms.

BIBLIOGRAPHY

Bladder Carcinomas

Abenoza P et al: Primary adenocarcinoma of urinary bladder. Urology 1987;29:2.

Akcetin Z et al: Radiochemotherapy after transurethral resection is an effective treatment method in T1G3 bladder cancer. Anticancer Res 2005;25:1623.

American Joint Committee on Cancer: Cancer Staging Manual. Lippincott, 1997.

Au J et al: Methods to Improve Efficacy of Intravesical Mitomycin C: Results of a Randomized Phase III Trial. J Natl Cancer Inst 2001; 93:597.

Barlow L et al: A single-institution experience with induction and maintenance intravesical docetaxel in the management of non-muscle-invasive bladder cancer refractory to bacille Calmette-Guérin therapy. BJU Int 2009;104:1098

Belldegrun A et al: Superficial bladder cancer: The role of interferon-alpha. J Urol 1998;159:1793.

Berger GL et al: Lack of value of routine preoperative bone and liver scans in cystectomy candidates. J Urol 1981;125:637.

Bernstein SA et al: Primary signet-ring cell carcinoma of urinary bladder. Urology 1988;31:432.

Block CE et al: Cutaneous metastases from transitional cell carcinoma of the bladder. Urology 2006;67:846.

Bochner BH et al: Relationship of tumor angiogenesis and nuclear p53 accumulation in invasive bladder cancer. Clin Cancer Res 1997;3:1615.

Bohle A et al: Intravesical bacillus Calmette-Guerin versus mitomycin C for superficial bladder cancer: A formal meta-analysis of comparative studies on recurrence and toxicity. J Urol 2003;169:90.

Catalona WJ, Ratliff TL: Bacillus Calmette-Guérin and superficial bladder cancer. Surg Annu 1990;22:363.

Cervek J et al: Invasive bladder cancer: Our experience with bladder sparing approach. Int J Radiat Oncol Biol Phys 1998;41:273.

Chauvet B et al: Concurrent cisplatin and radiotherapy for patients with muscle invasive bladder cancer who are not candidates for radical cystectomy. J Urol 1996;156:1258.

Choong NW et al: Small cell carcinoma of the urinary bladder. The Mayo Clinic experience. Cancer 2005;103:1172.

Cookson MS, Sarosdy M: Management of stage T1 bladder cancer with intravesical bacillus Calmette-Guérin therapy. J Urol 1992; 148:797.

Cookson MS et al: The treated natural history of high-risk superficial bladder cancer: 15-year outcome. J Urol 1997;158:62.

Cordon-Cardo C et al: Altered expression of the retinoblastoma gene product: Prognostic indicator in bladder cancer. J Natl Cancer Inst 1992;84:1251.

Dalbagni G et al: Genetic alterations in tp53 in recurrent urothelial cancer: A longitudinal study. Clin Cancer Res 2001;7:2797.

Dalbagni G et al: Phase II trial of intravesical gemcitabine in bacilli Calmette-Guérin refractory transitional cell carcinoma of the bladder. J Clin Oncol 2006;24:2729

David KA et al: Surveillance of urothelial carcinoma: Stage and grade migration, 1993–2005 and survival trends, 1993–2000. Cancer 2009;115:1435.

Davis JW et al: Superficial bladder carcinoma treated with Bacillus Calmette-Guerin: Progression-free and disease specific survival with minimum 10 year followup. J Urol 2002;167:494.

Dickinson AJ et al: Quantification of angiogenesis as an independent predictor of prognosis in invasive bladder carcinomas. Br J Urol 1994;74:762.

Dutta SC et al: Clinical under staging of high risk nonmuscle invasive urothelial carcinoma treated with radical cystectomy. J Urol 2001;166:490.

El-Bolkainy MN et al: The impact of schistosomiasis on the pathology of bladder carcinoma. Cancer 1981;48:2643.

Elcock M, Morgan RW: Update on artificial sweeteners and bladder cancer. Regul Toxicol Pharmacol 1993;17:35.

Epstein JI et al: The World Health Organization/International Society of Urological Pathology consensus classification of urothelial (transitional cell) neoplasms of the urinary bladder. Am J Surg Pathol 1998;22:1435.

Esrig D et al: Prognostic importance of p53 and Rb alterations in transitional cell carcinoma of the bladder. J Urol 1995;153(Pt 2):362A.

Fagbemi S, Stadler W: New chemotherapy regimens for advanced bladder cancer. Semin Urol Oncol 1998;16:23.

Fairchild WV et al: The incidence of bladder cancer after cyclophosphamide therapy. J Urol 1979;122:163.

Fisher MR et al: Urinary bladder MR imaging. 2. Neoplasm. Radiology 1985;157:471.

Franks ME et al: Hepatocellular carcinoma metastatic to the bladder after liver transplantation. J Urol 1999;162:799.

Frazier HA et al: The value of pathologic factors in predicting cancer-specific survival among patients treated with radical cystectomy for transitional cell carcinoma of the bladder and prostate. Cancer 1993;71:3993.

Freiha F et al: A randomized trial of radical cystectomy versus radical cystectomy plus cisplatin, vinblastine, and methotrexate chemotherapy for muscle invasive bladder cancer. J Urol 1996;155:495.

Given RW et al: Bladder-sparing multimodality treatment of muscle-invasive bladder cancer: A five-year follow-up. Urology 1995;46:499.

Goffinet DR et al: Bladder cancer: Results of radiation therapy in 384 patients. Radiology 1975;117:149.

Goldstein AG: Metastatic carcinoma to the bladder. J Urol 1967; 98:209.

Gray Sears CL et al: Prospective comparison of computerized tomography and excretory urography in the initial evaluation of asymptomatic microhematuria. J Urol 2002;168:2457.

Grimm MO et al: Effect of routine repeat transurethral resection for superficial bladder cancer: A long-term observational study. J Urol 2003;170:433.

Grossfeld GD et al: Evaluation of asymptomatic microscopic hematuria in adults (Part II): American Urological Association Best Practice Policy. Urology 2001;57:604.

Grossman HB et al: Neoadjuvant chemotherapy plus cystectomy compared with cystectomy alone for locally advanced bladder cancer. N Engl J Med 2003;349:859.

Haaf EO et al: Detection of interleukin 2 in urine of patients with superficial bladder tumors after treatment with intravesical BCG. J Urol 1986;136:970.

Haleblian GE et al: Hydronephrosis as a prognostic indicator in bladder cancer patients. J Urol 1998;160:2011.

Hall CG et al: Guideline for the management of nonmuscle invasive bladder cancer (Stage Ta, T1, and Tis): 2007 update. J Urol 2007;178:2314.

Heney NM et al: Superficial bladder cancer: Progression and recurrence. J Urol 1983;130:1083.

Herr HW: Progression of stage T1 bladder tumors after intravesical bacillus Calmette-Guérin. J Urol 1991;145:40.

Herr HW: The value of a second transurethral resection in evaluating patients with bladder tumors. J Urol 1999;162:74.

Herr HW: Tumor progression and survival of patients with high grade, noninvasive papillary (TaG3) bladder tumors: 15-year outcome. J Urol 2000;163:60.

Herr HW: Transurethral resection of muscle-invasive bladder cancer: 10-year outcome. J Clin Oncol 2001;19:89.

Herr HW: Restaging transurethral resection of high risk superficial bladder cancer improves the initial response to bacillus Calmette-Guerin therapy. J Urol 2005;174:2134.

Herr HW, Sogani PC: Does early cystectomy improve the survival of patients with high risk superficial bladder tumors? J Urol 2001;166:1296.

Herr HW et al: Experience with intravesical bacillus Calmette-Guérin therapy of superficial bladder tumors. Urology 1985; 25:119.

Herr HW et al: An overview of intravesical therapy for superficial bladder tumors. J Urol 1987;138:1363.

Herr HW et al: Superficial bladder cancer treated with bacillus Calmette-Guérin: A multivariate analysis of factors affecting tumor progression. J Urol 1989;141:22.

Herr HW et al: Intravesical bacillus Calmette-Guerin therapy prevents tumor progression and death from superficial bladder cancer: Ten-year follow-up of a prospective randomized trial. J Clin Oncol 1995;13:1404.

Herr HW et al: Can p53 help select patients with invasive bladder cancer for bladder preservation? J Urol 1999;161:20.

Hicks RM: Promotion in bladder cancer. Carcinogenesis 1982;7:139.

Holmang S, Johansson SL: Stage Ta–T1 bladder cancer: The relationship between findings at first followup cystoscopy and subsequent recurrence and progression. J Urol 2002;167:1634.

Holzbeierlein J et al: Partial cystectomy: A contemporary review of the Memorial Sloan-Kettering Cancer Center experience and recommendations for patient selection. J Urol 2004;172:878.

Iselin C et al: Does prostate transitional cell carcinoma preclude orthotopic bladder reconstruction after radical cystoprostatectomy for bladder cancer? J Urol 1997;158:2123.

Jaeger TM et al: Tumor angiogenesis correlates with lymph node metastases in invasive bladder cancer. J Urol 1995;154:69.

Jakse G et al: Combination of chemotherapy and irradiation for non-resectable bladder carcinoma. World J Urol 1985;3:121.

Jebar AH et al: FGFR3 and Ras gene mutations are mutually exclusive genetic events in urothelial cell carcinoma. Oncogene 2005;24:5218.

Jocham D et al: Improved detection and treatment of bladder cancer using hexaminolevulinate imaging: A prospective, phase III multicenter study. J Urol 2005;174:862.

Kachnic LA et al: Bladder preservation by combined modality therapy for invasive bladder cancer. J Clin Oncol 1997;15:1022.

Kaye KW, Lange PH: Mode of presentation of invasive bladder cancer: Reassessment of the problem. J Urol 1982;128:31.

Kibel AS et al: Prospective study of [18F]fluorodeoxyglucose positron emission tomography/computed tomography for staging of muscle-invasive bladder carcinoma. J Clin Oncol 2009;27:4314.

Knowles MA: Role of FGFR3 in urothelial carcinoma: Biomarker and potential therapeutic target. World J Urol 2007;25:581.

Konety BR, Getzenberg RH: Urine based markers of urological malignancy. J Urol 2001;165:600.

Kowalkowski TS, Lamm DL: Intravesical chemotherapy of superficial bladder cancer. In: Resnick M (ed) Current Trends in Urology. Williams & Wilkins, Philadelphia, PA, 1988.

Kramer SA et al: Primary non-urachal adenocarcinoma of the bladder. J Urol 1979;121:278.

Lamm DL: Bacillus Calmette-Guérin immunotherapy for bladder cancer. J Urol 1985;134:40.

Lamm DL: Complications of bacillus Calmette-Guérin immunotherapy. Urol Clin North Am 1992;19:565.

Lamm DL et al: A randomized trial of intravesical doxorubicin and immunotherapy with bacillus Calmette-Guérin for transitional cell carcinoma of the bladder. N Engl J Med 1991;325:1205.

Lamm DL et al: Maintenance bacillus Calmette-Guérin immunotherapy for recurrent Ta, T1 and carcinoma in situ transitional cell carcinoma of the bladder: A randomized Southwest Oncology Group study. J Urol 2000;163:1124.

Lerner SP et al: The rationale for en bloc pelvic lymph node dissection for bladder cancer patients with nodal metastases: Long-term results. J Urol 1993;149:758.

Lipponen PK, Eskelinen MJ: Reduced expression of E-cadherin is related to invasive disease and frequent recurrence in bladder cancer. J Cancer Res Clin Oncol 1995;121:303.

Logothetis CJ et al: Adjuvant cyclophosphamide, doxorubicin, and cisplatin chemotherapy for bladder cancer: An update. J Clin Oncol 1988;6:1590.

Logothetis CJ et al: Altered expression of retinoblastoma protein and known prognostic variables in locally advanced bladder cancer. J Natl Cancer Inst 1992;84:1256.

Loidl W et al: Flexible cystoscopy assisted by hexaminolevulinate induced fluorescence: A new approach for bladder cancer detection and surveillance? Eur Urol 2005;47:323.

Lotan Y et al: Lymphovascular invasion is independently associated with overall survival, cause-specific survival, and local and distant recurrence in patients with negative lymph nodes at radical cystectomy. J Clin Oncol 2005;23:6533.

Lutzeyer W et al: Prognostic parameters in superficial bladder cancer: An analysis of 315 cases. J Urol 1982;127:250.

Matanoski GM, Elliott EA: Bladder cancer epidemiology. Epidemiol Rev 1981;3:203.

May F et al: Significance of random bladder biopsies in superficial bladder cancer. Eur Urol 2003;44:47.

Miyao N et al: Role of chromosome 9 in human bladder cancer. Cancer Res 1993;53:4066.

Morris S et al: Superficial bladder cancer: How long should a tumor-free patient have check cystoscopies? Br J Urol 1995;75:193.

Murphy WM: Diseases of the urinary bladder, urethra, ureters, and renal pelvis. In: Murphy WM (ed) Urological Pathology. Saunders, Philadelphia, 1989.

O'Donnell MA et al: Interim results from a national multicenter phase II trial of combination bacillus Calmette-Guerin plus interferon alfa-2b for superficial bladder cancer. J Urol 2004;172:888.

Oh KS et al: Combined-modality therapy with gemcitabine and radiation therapy as a bladder preservation strategy: Long-term results of a phase I trial. Int J Radiat Oncol Biol Phys 2009;74:511.

Ojeda L, Johnson DE: Partial cystectomy: Can it be incorporated into an integrated therapy program? Urology 1983;22:115.

Okamura K et al: Growth fractions of transitional cell carcinomas of the bladder defined by the monoclonal antibody Ki-67. J Urol 1990;144:875.

Olumi AF et al: Molecular analysis of human bladder cancer. Semin Urol 1990;8:270.

Oosterlinck W et al: A prospective European Organization for Research and Treatment of Cancer Genitourinary Group Randomized trial comparing transurethral resection followed by a single intravesical instillation of epirubicin or water in single stage Ta, T1 papillary carcinoma of the bladder. J Urol 1993;149:749.

Orsola A et al: Initial high-grade T1 urothelial cell carcinoma: Feasibility and prognostic significance of lamina propria invasion microstaging (T1a/b/c) in BCG-treated and BCG-non-treated patients. Eur Urol 2005;48:231

Pearson BS, Raghaven D: First line intravenous cisplatin for deeply invasive bladder cancer: Update on 70 cases. Br J Urol 1985;57:690.

Quek ML et al: Radical cystectomy for primary neuroendocrine tumors of the bladder: The university of southern California experience. J Urol 2005;174:93.

Quilty PM, Duncan W: Primary radical radiotherapy for T3 transitional cell cancer of the bladder: Analysis of survival and control. Int J Radiat Oncol Biol Phys 1986;12:853.

Rodel C et al: Combined-modality treatment and selective organ preservation in invasive bladder cancer: Long-term results. J Clin Oncol 2002;20:3061.

Sarosdy M et al: Oral bropirimine immunotherapy of bladder carcinoma in situ after prior intravesical bacille Calmette-Guérin. Urology 1998;51:226.

Scher HI: Neoadjuvant therapy of invasive bladder tumors. In: Williams R, Carroll PR (eds) Treatment Perspectives in Urologic Oncology. Pergamon Press, New York, 1990.

Scher HI, Sternberg CN: Chemotherapy of urologic malignancies. Semin Urol 1985;3:239.

Scher HI et al: Neoadjuvant M-VAC (methotrexate, vinblastine, doxorubicin and cisplatin) effect on the primary bladder lesion. J Urol 1988;139:470.

Scher HI et al: Neoadjuvant chemotherapy for invasive bladder cancer: Experience with the M-VAC regimen. Br J Urol 1989;64:250.

Serretta V et al: Urinary NMP22 for the detection of recurrence after transurethral resection of transitional cell carcinoma of the bladder: Experience in 137 patients. Urology 1998;52:793.

Shipley WU et al: Cisplatin and full dose irradiation for patients with invasive bladder carcinoma: A preliminary report of tolerance and local response. J Urol 1984;132:899.

Shipley WU et al: Invasive bladder cancer: Treatment strategies using transurethral surgery, chemotherapy and radiation therapy with selection for bladder conservation. Int J Radiat Oncol Biol Phys 1997;39:937.

Sidransky D et al: Identification of p53 gene mutations in bladder cancers and urine samples. Science 1991;252:706.

Silverman DT et al: Bladder cancer. In: Schottenfeld D, Fraumeni JF Jr (eds) Cancer Epidemiology and Prevention. Oxford University Press, New York, NY, 2006. pp. 1101–1127.

Skinner DG: Management of invasive bladder cancer: A meticulous lymph node dissection can make a difference. J Urol 1982;128:34.

Skinner DG et al: The role of adjuvant chemotherapy following cystectomy for invasive bladder cancer: A prospective comparative trial. J Urol 1991;145:459.

Soloway MS et al: Expectant management of small, recurrent, non-invasive papillary bladder tumors. J Urol 2003;170:438

Solsona E et al: Feasibility of transurethral resection for muscle infiltrating carcinoma of the bladder: Long-term followup of a prospective study. J Urol 1998;159:95.

Solsona E et al: Effectiveness of a single immediate mitomycin C instillation in patients with low risk superficial bladder cancer: Short and long-term followup. J Urol 1999;161:1120.

Solsona E et al: The 3-month clinical response to intravesical therapy as a predictive factor for progression in patients with high risk superficial bladder cancer. J Urol 2000;164:685.

Stein JP et al: Indications for lower urinary tract reconstruction in women after cystectomy for bladder cancer: A pathological review of female cystectomy specimens. J Urol 1995;154:1329.

Stein JP et al: Prospective pathologic analysis of female cystectomy specimens: Risk factors for orthotopic diversion in women. Urology 1998;51:951.

Stein JP et al: Radical cystectomy in the treatment of invasive bladder cancer: Long-term results in 1,054 patients. J Clin Oncol 2001; 19:666.

Steinberg G et al: Efficacy and safety of Valrubicin for the treatment of bacillus Calmette-Guérin refractory carcinoma in situ of the bladder. J Urol 2000;163:761.

Stenzl A et al: The risk of urethral tumors in female bladder cancer: Can the urethra be used for orthotopic reconstruction of the lower urinary tract? J Urol 1995;153(3 Pt 2):950.

Sternberg CN et al: M-VAC (methotrexate vinblastine doxorubicin and cisplatin) for advanced transitional cell carcinoma of the urothelium. J Urol 1988;139:461.

Stockle M et al: Adjuvant polychemotherapy of nonorgan-confined bladder cancer after radical cystectomy revisited: Long-term results of a controlled prospective study and further clinical experience. J Urol 1995;153:47.

Stockle M et al: Advanced bladder cancer (stages pT3b, pT4a, pN1 and pN2): Improved survival after radical cystectomy and 3 adjuvant cycles of chemotherapy. Results of a controlled prospective trial. J Urol 1992;148:302.

Sweeney P et al: Partial cystectomy. Urol Clin North Am 1992;19:701.

Sylvester RJ et al: A single immediate postoperativeinstillation of chemotherapy decreases the risk of recurrence in patients with stage Ta T1bladder cancer: A meta-analysis of published results of randomized clinical trials. J Urol 2004;171:2186.

Sylvester RJ et al: Bacillus Calmette-Guérin versus chemotherapy for the intravesical treatment of patients with carcinoma in situ of the bladder: A meta-analysis of the published results of randomized clinical trials. J Urol 2005;174:86.

Tannock I et al: M-VAC (methotrexate vinblastine doxorubicin and cisplatin) chemotherapy for transitional cell carcinoma: The Princess Margaret Hospital experience. J Urol 1989;142:289.

Tester W et al: Neoadjuvant combined modality program with selective organ preservation for invasive bladder cancer: Results of Radiation Therapy Oncology Group phase II trial 8802. J Clin Oncol 1996;14:119.

Tolley D et al: Effect of mitomycin C on recurrence of newly diagnosed superficial bladder cancer: Interim report from the Medical Research Council Subgroup on Superficial Bladder Cancer. Br Med J 1988;296:1759.

Torti FM et al: Superficial bladder cancer: The primacy of grade in the development of invasive disease. J Clin Oncol 1987;5:125.

Trasher JB et al: Clinical variables which serve as predictors of cancer-specific survival among patients treated with radical cystectomy for transitional cell carcinoma of the bladder and prostate. Cancer 1994;73:1708.

Tsai YC et al: Allelic losses of chromosomes 9, 11, and 17 in human bladder cancer. Cancer Res 1990;50:44.

van der Meijden A et al: Significance of bladder biopsies in Ta, T1 bladder tumors: A report from the EORTC Genito-Urinary Tract Cancer Cooperative Group. EORTC-GU Group Superficial Bladder Committee. Eur Urol 1999;35:267.

van der Meijden A et al: Maintenance Bacillus Calmette-Guerin for Ta T1 bladder tumors is not associated with increased toxicity: Results from a European Organisation for Research and Treatment of Cancer Genito-Urinary Group Phase III Trial. Eur Urol 2003;44:429.

Vieweg J et al: Impact of primary stage on survival in patients with lymph node positive bladder cancer. J Urol 1999;161:72.

von der Maase H et al: Gemcitabine and cisplatin versus methotrexate, vinblastine, doxorubicin and cisplatin in advanced or metastatic bladder cancer: Results of a large, randomized, multinational, multicenter phase III study. J Clin Oncol 2000;17:3068.

Whitmore WF: Management of invasive bladder neoplasms. Semin Urol 1983;1:34.

Wolf H et al: Urothelial dysplasia concomitant with bladder tumours: A determinant for future new occurrences in patients treated by full course radiotherapy. Lancet 1985;I:1005.

Wood DP et al: The role of magnetic resonance imaging in the staging of bladder carcinoma. J Urol 1988;140:741.

Woon SY et al: Bladder carcinoma: Experience with radical and preoperative radiotherapy in 421 patients. Cancer 1985;56:1293.

Yagoda A: Chemotherapy for advanced urothelial cancer. Semin Urol 1983;1:60.

Zabbo A, Montie JE: Management of the urethra in men undergoing radical cystectomy for bladder cancer. J Urol 1984;131:267.

Zietman A et al: The case for radiotherapy with or without chemotherapy in high-risk superficial and muscle-invading bladder cancer. Semin Urol Oncol 1997;15:161.

Zietman AL et al: Selective bladder conservation using transurethral re-section, chemotherapy, and radiation: Management and consequences of Ta, T1, and Tis recurrence within the retained bladder. Urology 2001;58:380.

Ureteral and Renal Pelvic Cancers

Akkad T et al: Fluorescence in situ hybridization for detecting upper urinary tract tumors–a preliminary report. Urology 2007;70:753.

Almgard LE et al: Carcinoma of the ureter with special reference to malignancy grading and prognosis. Scand J Urol Nephrol 1973;7:165.

American Joint Committee on Cancer: Cancer Staging Manual. Lippincott-Raven, Philadelphia, 1997.

Babaian RJ, Johnson DE: Primary carcinoma of the ureter. J Urol 1980;123:357.

Bagley DH, Grasso M: Uretersocopic laser treatment of upper urinary tract neoplasms. World J Urol 2010;28:143.

Bergman H et al: New roentgenologic signs of carcinoma of the ureter. Am J Roentgenol 1961;86:707.

Blute ML et al: Impact of endourology on diagnosis and management of upper urinary tract urothelial cancer. J Urol 1989;141:1298.

Boorjian S et al: Impact of delay to nephroureterectomy for patients undergoing ureteroscopic biopsy and laser tumor ablation of upper tract transitional cell carcinoma. Urology 2005;66:283.

Chen GL et al: Surveillance of upper tract transitional cell carcinoma: The role of ureteroscopy, retrograde pyelography, cytology and urinalysis. J Urol 2000;164:1901.

Dodd L et al: Endoscopic brush cytology of the upper urinary tract: Evaluation of its efficacy and potential limitations in diagnosis. Acta Cytol 1997;41:377.

Geerdsen J: Tumours of the renal pelvis and ureter: Symptomatology, diagnosis, treatment, and prognosis. Scand J Urol Nephrol 1979; 13:287.

Gill WB et al: Retrograde brushing: A new technique for obtaining histologic and cytologic material from ureteral renal pelvic and renal caliceal lesions. J Urol 1973;109:573.

Grabstald H et al: Renal pelvic tumors. JAMA 1971;218:845.

Guarnizo E et al: Ureteroscopic biopsy of upper tract urothelial carcinoma improved diagnostic accuracy and histopathological considerations using a multi-biopsy approach. J Urol 2000;163:52.

Hall M et al: Prognostic factors, recurrence, and survival in transitional cell carcinoma of the upper urinary tract: A 30-year experience in 252 patients. Urology 1998;52:594.

Herr H: Long-term results of BCG therapy: Concern about upper tract tumors. Semin Urol Oncol 1998;16:13.

Jarrett TW et al: Laparoscopic nephroureterectomy for the treatment of transitional cell carcinoma of the upper urinary tract. Urology 2001;57:448.

Jensen OM et al: The Copenhagen case-control study of renal pelvis and ureter cancer: Role of analgesics. Int J Cancer 1989;44:965.

Keeley F et al: Ureteroscopic treatment and surveillance of upper urinary tract transitional cell carcinoma. J Urol 1997;157:1560.

Keeley FX, Bagley DH: Adjuvant mitomycin C following endoscopic treatment of upper tract transitional cell carcinoma. J Urol 1997;158:2074.

Keeley FX et al: Diagnostic accuracy of ureteroscopic biopsy in upper tract transitional cell carcinoma. J Urol 1997;157:33.

Landman J et al: Comparison of hand assisted and standard laparoscopic radical nephroureterectomy for the management of localized transitional cell carcinoma. J Urol 2002;167:2387.

Lane BR et al: Chronic kidney disease after nephroureterectomy for upper tract urothelial carcinoma and implications for the administration of perioperative chemotherapy. Cancer 2010;116:2967.

Mahoney JF et al: Analgesic abuse renal parenchymal disease and carcinoma of the kidney or ureter. Aust N Z J Med 1977;7:463.

Maier U et al: Organ-preserving surgery in patients with urothelial tumors of the upper urinary tract. Eur Urol 1990;18:197.

Markovic B: Endemic nephritis and urinary tract cancer in Yugoslavia, Bulgaria and Romania. J Urol 1972;107:212.

McCarron JP et al: Systematic mapping of nephroureterectomy specimens removed for urothelial cancer: Pathological findings and clinical correlations. J Urol 1982;128:243.

McCarron JP et al: Tumors of the renal pelvis and ureter: Current concepts and management. Semin Urol 1983;1:75.

Oldbring J et al: Carcinoma of the renal pelvis and ureter following bladder carcinoma: Frequency risk factors and clinicopathological findings. J Urol 1989;141:1311.

Orihuela E, Smith AD: Percutaneous treatment of transitional cell carcinoma of the upper urinary tract. Urol Clin North Am 1988;15:425.

Patel A, Fuchs G: New techniques for the administration of topical adjuvant therapy after endoscopic ablation of upper urinary tract transitional cell carcinoma. J Urol 1998;159:71.

Reitelman C et al: Prognostic variables in patients with transitional cell carcinoma of the renal pelvis and proximal ureter. J Urol 1987; 138:1144.

Ross RK et al: Analgesics, cigarette smoking, and other risk factors for cancer of the renal pelvis and ureter. Cancer Res 1989;49:1045.

Stoller M et al: Endoscopic management of upper tract urothelial tumors. Tech Urol 1997;3:152.

Strong DW et al: The ureteral stump after nephroureterectomy. J Urol 1976;115:654.

Studer UE et al: Percutaneous bacillus Calmette-Guérin perfusion of the upper urinary tract for carcinoma in situ. J Urol 1989;142: 975.

Williams CB, Mitchell JP: Carcinoma of the ureter: A review of 54 cases. Br J Urol 1973;45:377.

Zimmerman R et al: Utility of the Bard BTA test in detecting upper urinary tract transitional cell carcinoma. Urology 1998;51:956.

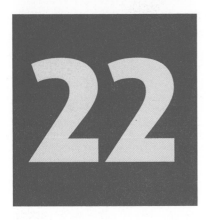

Renal Parenchymal Neoplasms

Badrinath R. Konety, MD, MBA, Daniel A. Vaena, MD, & Richard D. Williams, MD

BENIGN TUMORS

With the liberal use of computed tomography (CT) scans and magnetic resonance imaging (MRI), benign renal masses are being detected more frequently. Benign renal tumors include, oncocytoma, angiomyolipoma, leiomyoma, lipoma, hemangioma, and juxtaglomerular tumors.

▶ Renal Oncocytoma

Renal oncocytoma has a spectrum of behavior ranging from benign to malignant. Composed of large epithelial cells with finely granular eosinophilic cytoplasm (oncocytes), oncocytomas occur in various organs and organ systems including adrenal, salivary, thyroid, and parathyroid glands as well as the kidney. An estimated 3–5% of renal tumors are oncocytomas (Romis et al, 2004). Men are affected more often than women.

Renal oncocytomas generally occur and are contained within a well-defined fibrous capsule. Metastasis is extremely rare though invasion of the lymphovascular spaces has been observed. On cut section, the surface of the tumor is usually tan or light brown with a central stellate scar, but necrosis typical of renal adenocarcinoma is absent. The tumors are usually solitary and unilateral, although several bilateral cases and multiple oncocytomas occurring simultaneously (**oncocytomatosis**) have been reported (Tickoo et al, 1999).

Oncocytomas can also be associated with benign tumors of hair follicles (**fibrofolliculomas**), colon polyps/tumors, and pulmonary cysts as part of the Birt–Hogg–Dubé syndrome (Toro et al, 1999). The familial renal oncocytoma syndrome has also been described (Philips et al, 2001). These patients may have a characteristic genetic abnormality involving a gene located on 17p encoding a protein named **folliculin** (Nickerson et al, 2002) Histologically, well-differentiated oncocytomas are made up of large, uniform cells containing an intensely eosinophilic cytoplasm, which on ultrastructural studies is found to be packed with mitochondria. Mitotic

activity is absent, and nuclear pleomorphism is uncommon (Figure 22–1). Consistent chromosomal alterations such as loss of chromosome 1 or Y and translocations in the short arm of chromosome 11 have been described in oncocytomas (Lindgren et al, 2004; Philips et al, 2001). The cellular origin of renal oncocytes has not been fully elucidated, although some early evidence suggested that oncocytes resemble proximal convoluted tubular cells (Merino and Librelsi, 1982). Other findings suggest that their origin may be a precursor stem cell (Cohen et al, 1988) or the intercalated cells of the collecting ducts (Storkel et al, 1989).

The diagnosis of oncocytoma is predominantly pathologic because there are no reliable distinguishing clinical characteristics. Gross hematuria and flank pain occur in <20% of patients. No characteristic features of the tumors appear on CT, ultrasound (US), intravenous urography (IVU), or MRI. Angiographic features of oncocytomas include the "spoke-wheel" appearance of tumor arterioles, the "lucent rim sign" of the capsule, and a homogeneous capillary nephrogram phase. Unfortunately, these findings are not invariable, and similar findings have been reported in patients with renal cell carcinoma (RCC).

High-grade oncocytomas may be intermixed with elements of RCC and can be found as coexisting lesions within the same or opposite kidney (Licht et al, 1993). The role of fine-needle aspiration in the preoperative diagnosis of oncocytomas remains controversial and limited due to a lack of characteristic features that distinguish oncocytoma from RCC.

▶ Angiomyolipoma (Renal Hamartoma)

Angiomyolipoma is a rare benign tumor of the kidney seen in two distinct clinical populations. Angiomyolipomas are found in approximately 45–80% of patients with tuberous sclerosis and are typically bilateral and asymptomatic. Tuberous sclerosis is a familial inherited disorder comprising adenoma sebaceum, mental retardation, and epilepsy. In patients without tuberous sclerosis, renal angiomyolipomas can be

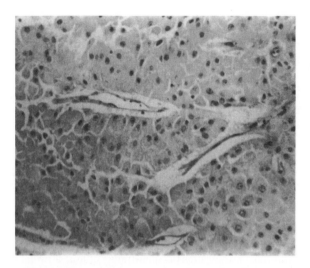

▲ **Figure 22–1.** Histologic section of a grade I (benign renal oncocytoma (original magnification, ×100).

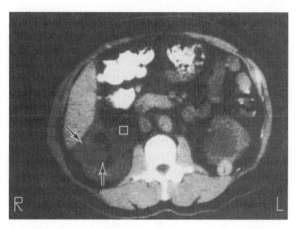

▲ **Figure 22–2.** Computed tomogram of an angiomyolipoma (*arrows*).

unilateral and tend to be larger than those associated with tuberous sclerosis (Anderson and Hatcher, 1990). There is no known histologic difference between the lesions seen in these two populations. As many as 25% of cases can present with spontaneous rupture and subsequent hemorrhage into the retroperitoneum (Wong et al, 1981).

Angiomyolipomas are unencapsulated yellow to gray lesions, typically round to oval, that elevate the renal capsule, producing a bulging smooth or irregular mass. They are characterized by three major histologic components: mature fat cells, smooth muscle, and blood vessels. Renal hamartomas may extend to perirenal or renal sinus fat and involve regional lymphatics and other visceral organs (Ditonno et al, 1992). The presence of renal hamartomas in extrarenal sites is a manifestation of multicentricity rather than metastatic potential, because only one well-documented case of malignant transformation of angiomyolipoma has been reported (Lowe et al, 1992).

Female patients with a rare condition termed **lymphangioleiomyomatosis** may have multiple renal and hepatic angiomyolipomata, multiple pulmonary cysts, enlarged abdominal lymph nodes, and lymphangiomyomas (Avila et al, 2000; Urban et al, 1999). The diagnosis of renal angiomyolipoma has evolved with the widespread use of US and CT. Ultrasonography and CT are frequently diagnostic in lesions with high fat content. Fat visualized on US appears as very high intensity echoes. Fat imaged by CT has a negative density, −20 to −80 Hounsfield units, which is pathognomonic for angiomyolipomas when observed in the kidney (Figure 22–2) (Pitts et al, 1980). MRI can also be utilized to identify fat within the lesion and confirm a diagnosis of angiomyolipoma. MRI is particularly useful in distinguishing lipid poor angiomyolipoma which have much lower fat content

compared to routine angiomyolipomas, from other solid renal lesions (Kim et al, 2006).

The management of angiomyolipomas historically has been correlated with symptoms. Steiner and colleagues (1993) reported a long-term follow-up study of 35 patients with angiomyolipomas. They proposed that patients with isolated lesions <4 cm be followed up with yearly CT or US. Patients with asymptomatic or mildly symptomatic lesions >4 cm should be followed up with semiannual US. Patients with lesions >4 cm with moderate or severe symptoms (bleeding or pain) should undergo renal-sparing surgery or renal arterial embolization. Recent data indicate that even larger angiomyolipoma's (AML's) upto 8 cm can be observed and treated as dictated by symptoms. Approximately 25–30% of patients who are observed will ultimately require treatment in the form of embolization, surgery or radio frequency ablation (Sooriakumaran, 2010). However the long-term efficacy of selective embolization remains suboptimal and the long-term efficacy of radiofrequency ablation is yet to be determined. More recent data also suggests that immunosuppressive agents such as sirolimus (an inhibitor of mammalian target of rapamycin or mTOR) may also be effective in treating AML arising in patients with tuberous sclerosis (Bissler et al, 2008).

▶ Other Rare Benign Renal Tumors

Several other benign renal tumors are quite rare, including leiomyomas, hemangiomas, lipomas, and juxtaglomerular cell tumors. With the exception of juxtaglomerular tumors, there are no features that unequivocally establish the diagnosis before surgery; therefore, the pathologist most often provides the diagnosis after nephrectomy.

Leiomyomas are rare small tumors typically found in smooth-muscle-containing areas of the kidney including the renal capsule and renal pelvis. Two groups of renal leiomyomas have been described (Steiner et al, 1990). The more common group comprises cortical tumors that are <2 cm and may be multiple. These tumors are typically found at autopsy and are not clinically significant. A larger, commonly solitary leiomyoma has been described, which may cause symptoms and is confirmed pathologically after nephrectomy.

Hemangiomas are small vascular tumors occurring in the kidney with a frequency second only to that in the liver among visceral organs. Multiple lesions in one kidney occur in approximately 12% of cases; however, they are rarely bilateral. They can occasionally be the elusive source of hematuria in an otherwise well-evaluated patient. The diagnosis may be determined by CT angiography, MR angiography, or by direct visualization by endoscopy (Ekelund and Gothlin, 1975).

Renal lipomas are very uncommon deposits of mature adipose cells without evident mitosis that arise from the renal capsule or perirenal tissue. They are seen primarily in middle-aged females and, owing to the characteristic CT differentiation of fat, are best detected radiographically on CT scanning.

The **juxtaglomerular cell tumor** is the most clinically significant member of this subgroup of rare benign tumors because it causes significant hypertension that can be cured by surgical treatment. It is a very rare lesion, with <100 reported cases and may have characteristic chromosomal alterations (Brandal et al, 2005). The tumors occur more commonly in young adults, more often females in their 20s and 30s and are rarely malignant. The tumors originate from the pericytes of afferent arterioles in the juxtaglomerular apparatus and can be shown to contain renin secretory granules. They are typically encapsulated and located in the cortical area. Symptoms of the "typical" tumors include hypertension, hypokalemia, hyperaldosteronism, and high renin (Dong et al, 2010). Some atypical cases may demonstrate just hypertension with normal potassium levels or may even be non functional. The diagnosis is confirmed by selected renal vein sampling for renin. Although complete nephrectomy was advocated in the past, several recent reports indicate that partial nephrectomy can be equally effective (Haab et al, 1995).

ADENOCARCINOMA OF THE KIDNEY (RCC)

In the United States in 2010, an estimated 58,240 new cases of adenocarcinoma of the kidney were expected to be diagnosed, and 13,040 deaths were expected to occur from this disease (Jemal et al, 2010). RCC accounts for roughly 2.8% of adult cancers and constitutes approximately 85% of all primary malignant renal tumors. There appears to be an increase in the incidence of all stages of RCC over the past few decades (Hock et al, 2002; Mindrup et al, 2005). RCC occurs most commonly in the fifth to sixth decade and has a male–female ratio of 2:1. The incidence of renal cancer may vary based on race, with black men demonstrating a higher incidence than in men of all other races. Black men may also have a higher likelihood of a subsequent RCC in the contralateral kidney (Rabbani et al, 2002). Asians appear to have the lowest incidence of RCC (Miller, 1996).

▶ Etiology

The cause of renal adenocarcinoma is unknown. Occupational exposures, chromosomal aberrations, and tumor suppressor genes have been implicated. Cigarette smoking is the only risk factor consistently linked to RCC by both epidemiologic case-control and cohort studies (La Vecchia et al, 1990), with most investigations demonstrating at least a twofold increase in risk for the development of RCC in smokers (Yu et al, 1986). Exposure to asbestos, solvents, and cadmium has also been associated with an increased incidence of RCC (Mandel et al, 1995).

RCC occurs in two forms, inherited and sporadic. In 1979, Cohen and colleagues described a pedigree with hereditary RCC in which the pattern of inheritance was consistent with an autosomal dominant gene with a balanced reciprocal translocation between the short arm of chromosome 3 and the long arm of chromosome 8. Subsequent work has documented that both the hereditary and sporadic forms of RCC are associated with structural changes in chromosome 3p (Erlandsson, 1998; Kovacs et al, 1988; Noordzij and Mickisch, 2004).

Other hereditary forms of RCC have been described. **Von Hippel-Lindau disease** is a familial cancer syndrome in which affected individuals have a mutation of chromosome 3p predisposition to develop tumors in multiple organs, including cerebellar hemangioblastoma, retinal angiomata, and bilateral clear cell RCC. In 1993, Latif and colleagues identified the von Hippel–Lindau gene, leading to the detection of a germ line mutation in approximately 75% of families affected by von Hippel–Lindau disease (Chen et al, 1995). It has also been recognized that at least 50% of cases of sporadic clear cell RCC has mutations in the Von Hippel–Lindau (VHL) gene (Gnarra et al, 1994).

Hereditary papillary renal carcinoma was described in 1994 and is characterized by a predisposition to develop multiple bilateral renal tumors with a papillary histologic appearance (Zbar et al, 1994). In contrast to von Hippel–Lindau patients, the major neoplastic manifestations appear to be confined to the kidney.

Acquired cystic disease of the kidneys is a well-recognized entity of multiple bilateral cysts in the native kidneys of uremic patients (Reichard et al, 1998). The risk of developing RCC has been estimated to be >30 times higher in patients receiving dialysis who have cystic changes in their kidney than in the general population (Brennan et al, 1991). Several series reported in the literature suggest that RCC occurs in 3–9% of patients with acquired cystic disease of the kidneys (Gulanikar et al, 1998). Most RCC cases have been described in patients undergoing hemodialysis, but RCC has been reported in association with peritoneal dialysis (Smith et al, 1987) and successful renal transplants (Vaziri et al, 1984) and in patients with long-term renal insufficiency not requiring dialysis (Bretan et al, 1986; Fallon and Williams, 1989).

Pathology

RCC originates from the proximal renal tubular epithelium, as evidenced by electron microscopy (Makay et al, 1987) and immunohistochemical analysis (Holthöfer, 1990). These tumors occur with equal frequency in either kidney and are randomly distributed in the upper and lower poles. RCCs originate in the cortex and tend to grow out into perinephric tissue, causing the characteristic bulge or mass effect that aids in their detection by diagnostic imaging studies. Grossly, the tumor is characteristically yellow to orange because of the abundance of lipids, particularly in the clear cell type. RCCs do not have true capsules but may have a pseudocapsule of compressed renal parenchyma, fibrous tissue, and inflammatory cells.

Histologically, RCC is most often a mixed adenocarcinoma containing clear cells, granular cells, and, occasionally, sarcomatoid-appearing cells. The classifications of the subtypes of RCC are based on morphology and cytogenetic characteristics. Most RCCs are classified into one of the following histologic subtypes: conventional clear cell, papillary (chromophilic), chromophobe, collecting duct, neuroendocrine, and unclassified (Mostofi and Davis, 1998). Benign renal tumors are papillary adenoma, renal oncocytoma, and metanephric adenoma. Clear cells are rounded or polygonal with abundant cytoplasm, which contains cholesterol, triglycerides, glycogen, and lipids (Figure 22–3).

The cells present in the papillary (chromophilic) type contain less glycogen and lipids, and electron microscopy reveals that the granular cytoplasm contains many mitochondria and cytosomes. Chromophobe-type carcinomas contain large polygonal cells with distinct cell borders and reticulated cytoplasm, which can stain diffusely with Hale's colloidal iron (Theones et al, 1988). Oncocytic RCC or oncocytomas tend to have cytoplasm packed with mitochondria, giving it a granular appearance. Collecting duct tumors tend to have irregular borders and a basophilic cytoplasm with extensive anaplasia and are likely to invade blood vessels and cause infarction of tissue. Sarcomatoid cells are spindle shaped and form sheets or bundles. This later cell type rarely occurs as a pure form and is most commonly a

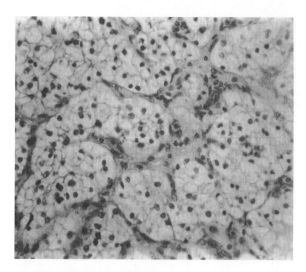

▲ **Figure 22–3.** Photomicrograph of clear cell renal adenocarcinoma (original magnification, ×125).

small component of either the clear cell or papillary cell type (or both).

Pathogenesis

RCCs are vascular tumors that tend to spread either by direct invasion through the renal capsule into perinephric fat and adjacent visceral structures or by direct extension into the renal vein. Approximately 25–30% of patients have evidence of metastatic disease at presentation. The most common site of distant metastases is the lung. However, liver, bone (osteolytic), ipsilateral adjacent lymph nodes and adrenal gland, brain, the opposite kidney, and subcutaneous tissue are frequent sites of disease spread.

Tumor Staging and Grading

A. Tumor Staging

The ultimate goal of staging is to select appropriate therapy and obtain prognostic information. Appropriate studies for a complete clinical staging evaluation include history and physical examination, complete blood count, serum chemistries (renal and hepatic function), urinalysis, chest x-ray (chest CT scan for an equivocal exam), CT scan of abdomen and pelvis, and a radionuclide bone scan (with x-rays of abnormal areas).

The original staging system described by Robson (1963) is easy to use, but it does not relate directly to prognosis and hence is no longer commonly used. The tumor-node-metastasis (TNM) system more accurately classifies the

Table 22–1. TNM classification system for renal cell carcinoma.[a]

Classification	Definition
T—Primary tumor	
TX	Primary tumor cannot be assessed
T0	No evidence of primary tumor
T1	Tumor 7.0 cm or less in greatest dimension, limited to the kidney
T1a	Tumor less than 4.0 cm in greatest dimension, limited to the kidney
T1b	Tumor 4.0-7.0 cm in greatest dimension, limited to the kidney
T2	Tumor more than 7.0 cm in greatest dimension, limited to the kidney
T2a	Tumor >7 cm but ≤10 cm in greatest dimension, limited to kidney
T2b	Tumor >10 cm in greatest dimension, limited to kidney
T3	Tumor extends into major veins or perinephric tissues but not into ipsilateral adrenal gland or beyond Gerota's fascia
T3a	Tumor invades renal vein or its segmental branches or perirenal fat or renal sinus fat but not beyond Gerota's fascia
T3b	Tumor grossly extends into vena cava below the diaphragm
T3c	Tumor grossly extends into vena cava above diaphragm or into the wall of the vena cava
T4	Tumor invades beyond Gerota's fascia including contiguous extension into ipsilateral adrenal gland
N—Regional lymph nodes	
NX	Regional lymph nodes cannot be assessed
N0	No regional lymph node metastasis
N1	Metastasis in regional lymph nodes
M—Distant metastases	
MX	Distant metastasis cannot be assessed
M0	No distant metastasis
M1	Distant metastasis

[a]All sizes measured in greatest dimension.

extent of tumor involvement and is currently most often used. The TNM classification system for RCC has undergone multiple revisions with the most recent edition being the 2010 version (Table 22–1). In the most recent American Joint Committee on Cancer TNM staging, stage T1 disease is further divided into T1a (tumor size <4 cm) and T1b (size 4–7 cm) as there is a difference in long-term survival between stage T1a and T1b (Ficarra et al, 2005).

B. Tumor Grading

Fuhrman grading has become commonly used by pathologists in North America (Fuhrman et al, 1982; Goldstein, 1997). The system uses four grades based on nuclear size and irregularity and nucleolar prominence. The system is most effective in predicting metastasis (50% of high-grade tumors within 5 years). When high-grade, predominantly granular tumors are corrected for grade and stage, there is no apparent difference between clear cell and granular cell tumor prognosis (McNichols et al, 1981). However, patients presenting with advanced disease do poorly irrespective of tumor grade.

▶ Clinical Findings

A. Symptoms and Signs

The classically described triad of gross hematuria, flank pain, and a palpable mass occurs in only 7–10% of patients and is frequently a manifestation of advanced disease. Patients may also present with hematuria, dyspnea, cough, and bone pain that are typically symptoms secondary to metastases. With the routine use of CT scanning for evaluation of nonspecific findings, asymptomatic renal tumors are increasingly detected incidentally (>50%).

B. Paraneoplastic Syndromes

RCC is associated with a wide spectrum of paraneoplastic syndromes including erythrocytosis, hypercalcemia, hypertension, and nonmetastatic hepatic dysfunction. Overall, these manifestations can occur in 10–40% of patients with RCC.

RCC is the most common cause of paraneoplastic erythrocytosis, which is reported to occur in 3–10% of patients with this tumor (Sufrin et al, 1989). In patients with RCC, the elevated erythrocyte mass is physiologically inappropriate and may result either from enhanced production of erythropoietin from the tumor or as a consequence of regional renal hypoxia promoting erythropoietin production from nonneoplastic renal tissue (Hocking, 1987).

Hypercalcemia has been reported to occur in up to 20% of patients with RCC (Muggia, 1990). Hypercalcemia may be due to production of a parathyroid hormone-related peptide that mimics the function of parathyroid hormone (Strewler et al, 1987) or other humoral factors such as osteoclast-activating factor, tumor necrosis factor, and transforming growth factor-alpha (Muggia, 1990).

Hypertension associated with RCC has been reported in up to 40% of patients (Sufrin et al, 1989), and renin production by the neoplasm has been documented in 37%. The excess renin and hypertension associated with RCC are typically refractory to antihypertensive therapy but may respond after nephrectomy (Gold et al, 1996).

In 1961, Stauffer described a reversible syndrome of hepatic dysfunction in the absence of hepatic metastases associated with RCC. Hepatic function abnormalities include elevation of alkaline phosphatase and bilirubin, hypoalbuminemia, prolonged prothrombin time, and hypergammaglobulinemia. Stauffer's syndrome tends to occur in association with fever, fatigue, and weight loss and typically resolves after nephrectomy. The reported incidence of Stauffer's syndrome varies from 3% to 20% (Gold et al, 1996). It may be due to overproduction of granulocyte-macrophage colony stimulating factor by the tumor (Chang et al, 1992).

RCC is known to produce a multitude of other biologically active products that result in clinically significant syndromes, including adrenocorticotropic hormone (Cushing's syndrome), enteroglucagon (protein enteropathy), prolactin (galactorrhea), insulin (hypoglycemia), and gonadotropins (gynecomastia and decreased libido; or hirsutism, amenorrhea, and male pattern balding) (Sufrin et al, 1986).

A paraneoplastic syndrome present at the time of disease diagnosis does not, in and of itself, confer a poor prognosis. However, patients whose paraneoplastic metabolic disturbances fail to normalize after nephrectomy (suggesting the presence of clinically undetectable metastatic disease) have very poor prognoses (Hanash, 1982).

C. Laboratory Findings

In addition to the laboratory abnormalities associated with the various RCC paraneoplastic syndromes, anemia, hematuria, and an elevated sedimentation rate are frequently observed.

Anemia occurs in about 30% of RCC patients. The anemia typically is not secondary to blood loss or hemolysis and is commonly normochromic. The serum iron and total iron-binding capacity are usually low, as in the anemia of chronic disease. Iron therapy is usually ineffective; however, surgical removal of early-stage tumors usually leads to physiologic correction of the anemia. The potential role of recombinant erythropoietin for patients with unresectable disease represents a potential, but untested, option.

Gross or microscopic hematuria can be seen in up to 60% of patients presenting with RCC. An elevated erythrocyte sedimentation rate is also commonly seen, with a reported incidence as high as 75%. These findings are nonspecific, and normal findings do not rule out a diagnosis of RCC.

D. X-Ray Findings

Although many radiologic techniques are available to aid in the detection and diagnosis of renal masses, CT scanning remains the primary technique with which others must be compared. Other radiologic techniques used include US and MRI.

E. Ultrasonography

US examination is a noninvasive, relatively inexpensive technique able to further delineate a renal mass. It is approximately 98% accurate in distinguishing simple cysts from solid lesions. Strict ultrasonographic criteria for a simple cyst include through transmission, a well-circumscribed mass without internal echoes, and adequate visualization of a strong posterior wall (Figure 22–4).

F. CT Scanning

CT scanning is more sensitive than US for detection of renal masses. A typical finding of RCC on CT is a mass that becomes enhanced with the use of intravenous contrast media. In general, RCC exhibits an overall decreased density in Hounsfield units compared with normal renal parenchyma but shows either a homogeneous or heterogeneous pattern of enhancement (increase in density of >10 Hounsfield units) following contrast administration (Figure 22–5). In addition to defining the primary lesion, CT scanning is also the method of choice in staging the patient by visualizing the renal hilum, perinephric space, renal vein and vena cava, adrenals, regional lymphatics, and adjacent organs. In patients with equivocal chest x-ray findings, a CT scan of the chest is indicated. Patients who present with symptoms consistent with brain metastases should be evaluated with either head CT or MRI. Spiral CT with 3-dimensional reconstruction has become useful for evaluating tumors before nephron-sparing surgery to delineate the 3-dimensional extent of the tumor and precisely outline the vasculature, which can aid the surgeon in preventing positive surgical margins (Holmes et al, 1997). Intraoperative ultrasonography is also often used to confirm the extent and number of masses in the kidney at the time of performing a partial nephrectomy.

G. Renal Angiography

With the widespread availability of CT scanners, the role of renal angiography in the diagnostic evaluation of RCC has markedly diminished and is now very limited. There remain a very few specific clinical situations in which angiography may be useful; for example, guiding the operative approach in a patient with an RCC in a solitary kidney when attempting to perform a partial nephrectomy may be indicated (Figure 22–6). However, CT angiography or MR angiography can give better information with less risk to the patient.

H. Radionuclide Imaging

Determination of metastases to bones is most accurate by radionuclide bone scan, although the study is nonspecific and requires confirmation with bone x-rays of identified abnormalities to verify the presence of the typical osteolytic lesions. There is evidence that patients without bone pain

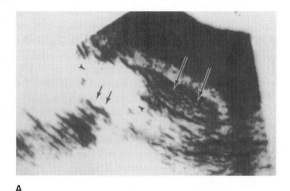

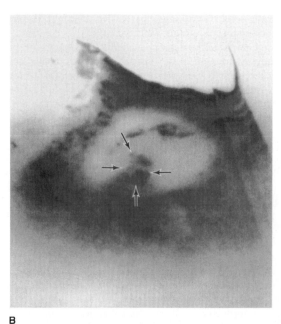

A   B

▲ **Figure 22–4.** ***A:*** Ultrasound image of a simple renal cyst showing renal parenchyma (*long arrows*), cyst wall (*arrowheads*), and a strong posterior wall (*short arrows*). ***B:*** Ultrasound image of a solid renal mass (*arrows*).

and with a normal alkaline phosphatase level have a very low incidence of bone metastases (Henriksson et al, 1992), and thus a routine bone scan is not necessary in such patients.

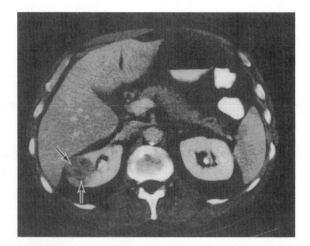

▲ **Figure 22–5.** Computed tomogram (contrast enhancement) of a renal cell carcinoma (*arrows*).

I. Magnetic Resonance Imaging

MRI is equivalent to CT for staging of RCC (Hricak et al, 1988). Its primary advantage is in the evaluation of patients with suspected vascular extension (Figure 22–7). Prospective trials have demonstrated that MRI is superior to CT in assessing inferior vena caval involvement (Kabala et al, 1991) and is at least as accurate as venacavography (Horan et al, 1989). In contrast to both CT and cavography, MRI evaluation does not require either iodinated contrast material or ionizing radiation. Recent studies using MRI angiography with gadolinium or CT angiography have improved vascular evaluation of renal neoplasms (Bluemke and Chambers, 1995). MR angiography can also be used to delineate the vascular supply before planned nephron-sparing surgery.

J. Positron Emission Tomography (PET) and Targeted Imaging

This technique allows the measurement of systemically administered biochemical agents such as 18-fluoro-2-deoxyglucose (FDG), which can accumulate in the kidney. Although FDG-PET scanning can yield false-positive results in some patients with RCC (Bachor et al, 1996), it may be useful in monitoring response to systemic therapy in those with metastatic disease (Hoh et al, 1998). FDG-PET may also be more accurate than routine CT scanning in detecting

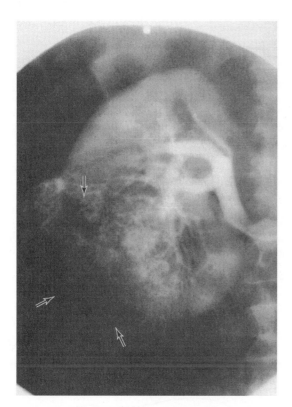

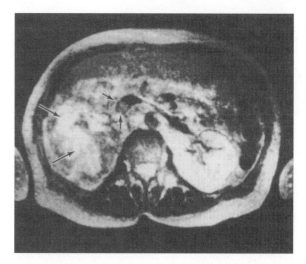

▲ **Figure 22–7.** Transaxial magnetic resonance image (T2) of a renal cell carcinoma (*long arrows*) with vena caval tumor thrombus (*short arrows*).

▲ **Figure 22–6.** Right renal angiogram showing typical neovascularity (*arrows*) in a large lower pole renal cell cancer.

disease recurrence or progression, which may alter treatment decisions in up to 50% of cases (Ramdave et al, 2001). However, most recent studies suggest that FDG-PET is of insufficient sensitivity to be useful for staging RCC.

The enzyme carbonic anhydrase IX (CA IX) is expressed at high levels in clear cell RCC. CA IX is regulated by the VHL gene through HIF1α and with loss of the VHL tumor suppressor gene being very common in clear cell RCC, there is loss of regulation of CA IX expression which is significantly increased. It is expressed at low levels in the gastrointestinal, mucosa, and biliary tract but not in other normal tissues. This characteristic can be exploited to detect clear cell RCC using a radiolabeled monoclonal antibody scan using the antibody G250 which targets carbonic anhydrase IX (Stillebroer et al, 2010). Up to 80% of clear cell RCC are found to express G250 antigen and in nearly imaging studies (Oosterwijnk et al, 1993). Other renal tumors such as chromophobe and papillary RCC demonstrate very little CA IX expression. More recently an immuno-PET approach has been used combining the monoclonal antibody to CA IX and a PET scan to better visualize renal lesions. In early studies,

94% of renal tumors were correctly identified using this approach (Divgi et al, 2007).

K. Fine-Needle Aspiration

Fine-needle aspiration of renal lesions is the diagnostic approach of choice in those patients with clinically apparent metastatic disease who may be candidates for nonsurgical therapy. Other settings in which fine-needle aspiration may be appropriate include establishing a diagnosis in patients who are not surgical candidates, differentiating a primary RCC from a renal metastasis in patients with known primary cancers of nonrenal origin, and evaluating some radiographically indeterminate lesions. Fine needle aspiration is being increasingly used to confirm the diagnosis of a neoplasm particularly in patients who may undergo observation or percutaneous ablative therapy (Shah et al, 2005). While core needle biopsies may be able to accurately diagnose malignancy in up to 100% of cases >4 cm and 95% of cases <4 cm, this may require multiple cores for accuracy (Wunderlich et al, 2005). Rare reports of seeding of the needle tract have been reported but the risk of seeding is reported to be <0.01% (Volpe et al, 2007). Recently, core biopsies of the primary renal mass have been more commonly utilized in patients with metastatic disease (when biopsying a metastatic site is not feasible), in order to guide appropriate targeted systemic therapy (prior to or instead of cytoreductive nephrectomy), since the choice of systemic therapy can be influenced by the specific RCC histology. The accuracy of needle core biopsies is reported to be >90% with sensitivity ranging between 70–100% and specificity of 100% (Volpe et al, 2007). The accuracy of fine needle aspiration cytology of renal masses is reported to be slightly lower mainly because of lower sensitivity. Specificity can still be high and close to 100%.

L. Instrumental and Cytologic Examination

Patients presenting with hematuria should also be evaluated with cystoscopy. Blood effluxing from the ureteral orifice identifies the origin of bleeding from the upper tract. Most renal pelvis tumors can be distinguished radiographically from RCC; however, endoscopic evaluation of the bladder, ureters, and renal pelvis is occasionally helpful in making a diagnosis. In addition, although urine cytologic study is rarely helpful in the diagnosis of RCC, cytologic study of urine with renal pelvis washing is frequently diagnostic in renal pelvis tumors.

▶ Differential Diagnosis

When a patient presents with clinical findings consistent with metastatic disease and is found to have a renal mass, a diagnosis of RCC can be straightforward. Most patients present with a renal mass discovered after an evaluation of hematuria or pain or as an incidental finding during an imaging workup of an unrelated problem. The differential diagnosis of RCC includes other solid renal lesions. The great majority of renal masses are simple cysts. Once the diagnosis of a cyst is confirmed by US, no additional evaluation is required if the patient is asymptomatic. Equivocal findings or the presence of calcification within the mass warrant further evaluation by CT. A wide variety of pathologic entities appear as solid masses on CT scans, and differentiation of benign from malignant lesions is frequently difficult. Findings on CT scan that suggest malignancy include amputation of a portion of the collecting system, presence of calcification, a poorly defined interface between the renal parenchyma and the lesion, invasion into perinephric fat or adjacent structures, and the presence of abnormal periaortic adenopathy or distant metastatic disease. The frequency of benign lesions among renal masses <7 cm in size is as high as 16–20% (Duchene et al, 2003; Snyder et al, 2006). Masses >7 cm are rarely benign.

Some characteristic lesions can be defined using CT criteria in combination with clinical findings. Angiomyolipomas (with large fat components) can easily be identified by the low-attenuation areas classically produced by substantial fat content. A renal abscess may be strongly suspected in a patient presenting with fever, flank pain, pyuria, and leukocytosis, and an early needle aspiration and culture should be performed. Other benign renal masses (in addition to those previously described) include granulomas and arteriovenous malformations. Renal lymphoma (both Hodgkin's disease and non-Hodgkin's disease), transitional cell carcinoma of the renal pelvis, adrenal cancer, and metastatic disease (most commonly from a lung or breast cancer primary) are additional diagnostic possibilities that may be suspected based on CT and clinical findings.

▶ Treatment

A. Specific Measures

1. Localized disease—Surgical removal of the early-stage lesion remains the only potentially curative therapy available for RCC patients. Appropriate therapy depends almost entirely on the stage of tumor at presentation and therefore requires a thorough staging evaluation. The prognoses of patients with stages T1–T3a disease are similar following radical nephrectomy.

Radical or partial nephrectomies are the primary treatments for localized RCC. The goal is to achieve the removal of tumor and to take a wide margin of normal tissue. Radical nephrectomy entails en bloc removal of the kidney and its enveloping fascia (Gerota's) including the ipsilateral adrenal, proximal one-half of the ureter, and lymph nodes up to the area of transection of the renal vessels (Figure 22–8).

Various open incisions provide optimal access for the radical nephrectomy, including an anterior subcostal (unilateral chevron) or thoracoabdominal incision, and, occasionally, a midline incision or the classic flank incision.

The likelihood of local recurrence after radical nephrectomy is 2–3% (Itano et al, 2000). Repeat resection of isolated local recurrence can be curative and yield a survival benefit

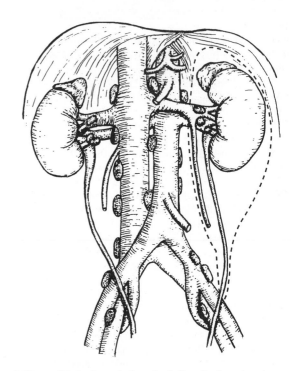

▲ **Figure 22–8.** Boundaries of a left radical nephrectomy. Dotted line represents both the surgical margin and Gerota's fascia.

(Itano et al, 2000; Tanguay et al, 1996). The role of regional lymphadenectomy in RCC remains controversial. Between 18% and 33% of patients undergoing radical nephrectomy with lymph node dissection for RCC have metastatic disease identified (Skinner et al, 1988). Although several retrospective studies (Thrasher and Paulson, 1993) and a prospective, nonrandomized study (Herrlinger et al, 1991) suggest that regional lymphadenectomy can improve survival in patients with T1–T2 RCC. More recent studies including a randomized prospective study as well as a population-based study failed to show any survival benefit that could be obtained by routinely performing regional lymphadenectomy especially in patients with organ-confined disease (Blom et al, 1999; Joslyn et al, 2005). Removal of the adrenal is unnecessary if the tumor is not in the upper pole, because adrenal involvement is uncommon in this instance.

Preoperative renal artery embolization (angioinfarction) has been used in the past as a surgical adjunct to facilitate radical nephrectomy, but because there is no conclusive evidence that preoperative embolization actually decreases blood loss or facilitates surgery, its use should be limited to patients with very large tumors in which the renal artery may be difficult to reach early in the procedure. In addition, this technique may be useful to palliate patients with nonresectable tumors and significant symptoms such as hemorrhage, flank pain, or paraneoplastic syndromes.

Radiation therapy has been advocated as a neoadjuvant (preoperative) or adjuvant method to radical nephrectomy, but there is no evidence that postsurgical radiation therapy to the renal bed, whether or not residual tumor is present, contributes to prolonged survival.

RCC may invade renal vascular spaces and produce tumor thrombi extending into renal veins, inferior vena cava, hepatic veins, and, occasionally, the right atrium. Between 5% and 10% of patients presenting with RCC have some degree of vena caval involvement (Figure 22–9) (Skinner et al, 1988). Patients presenting with involvement of the vena cava below the hepatic veins (T3bN0M0) but without evidence of regional or distant metastases have a prognosis similar to patients with stage T2 disease when treated by radical excision. The surgical approach to the removal of caval thrombi depends entirely on the level of cephalad extension. In general, these thrombi do not invade the wall of the cava and therefore can be removed without resection of the caval wall. For tumor thrombi that have reached the level of the right atrium, the use of cardiopulmonary bypass is typically required.

Laparoscopic or robotic radical nephrectomy and partial nephrectomy can also be accomplished successfully and safely. Laparoscopic/robotic radical nephrectomy is being used increasingly for patients with localized renal tumors. This approach results in quicker recovery with efficacy comparable to that of open radical nephrectomy and is now the approach of choice in appropriate patients with <10 cm tumors and without local extension or a renal vein or caval thrombus (Gill et al, 2001; Portis et al, 2002).

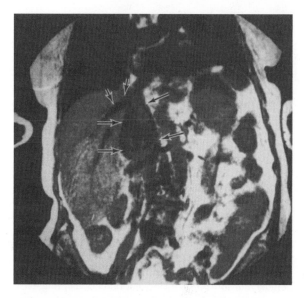

▲ **Figure 22–9.** Coronal magnetic image (T1) of a large vena caval tumor thrombus (*long arrows*) in a patient with renal cell carcinoma. Thrombus extends just to entrance of hepatic veins (*short arrows*).

The approach to the patient with either bilateral RCC or disease in a solitary kidney differs from the standard approach of radical nephrectomy. Bilateral RCC occurs with a frequency as high as 3% (Smith, 1986). Radical nephrectomy in these patients or in those with solitary kidneys obviously commits patients to long-term dialysis or renal transplantation and the morbidities of these conditions. Staging these patients is essentially the same as previously outlined, with the notable exception that either MR or CT angiography is often used to assess the extent of tumor within the kidney and the renal artery anatomy. Surgical alternatives to radical nephrectomy include open or laparoscopic/robotic partial nephrectomy, ex vivo partial nephrectomy (bench surgery followed by autotransplantation) (Novick et al, 1980), and enucleation of multiple lesions (Marshall et al, 1986). Given the lack of curative adjuvant therapy, the risk of inadequate excision, and subsequent recurrence from various renal-sparing approaches, partial nephrectomy with an adequate parenchymal margin remains the preferred treatment.

Partial nephrectomy and wedge resection with an adequate margin of normal parenchyma is considered standard primary surgical therapy for patients with tumors <4 cm in size, even in the presence of a normal contralateral kidney. Local recurrence of tumor in the same kidney ranges from 0% to 10%, and it is between 0% and 3% for tumors <4 cm in size (Hafez et al, 1997; Morgan and Zincke, 1990; Uzzo and Novick, 2001). In patients with multiple small tumors, such as those with von Hippel–Lindau disease, enucleation of the tumor(s) is also an acceptable approach. Long-term follow-up demonstrates that partial nephrectomy has a similar outcome as radical nephrectomy (Herr, 1999). Laparoscopic or robotic partial nephrectomy for these small tumors is recently gaining in use. The main advantages of the laparoscopic/robotic approach to partial nephrectomy are lower blood loss, less pain, and faster recovery.

Additional therapeutic approaches being increasingly applied for the treatment of small, incidentally discovered renal lesions include the use of cryoablation, high-intensity focused US, and radiofrequency ablation (Murphy and Gill, 2001). Cryoablation with liquid nitrogen or argon gas, either percutaneously using MRI guidance or via laparoscopic probes, has proved to be feasible and effective in selected patients (Gill et al, 2000; Shingleton and Sewell, 2002). Radiofrequency ablation has also been accomplished via the percutaneous approach with minimal morbidity in small groups of patients (Pavlovich et al, 2002). These approaches are particularly attractive in patients with single or multiple small lesions or older individuals with many comorbidities. The long-term effectiveness of both radiofrequency ablation as well as cryoablation appears to be acceptable (Kimura et al, 2010). It appears that cryoablation is superior to radiofrequency ablation in terms of long-term cancer control. Bleeding, scarring of renal pelvis, and urine leak are among the commonly reported complications with the ablative therapies.

Observation as treatment can also be considered an acceptable management approach for small (<3.0 cm) lesions, particularly in elderly patients. One recent study noted a growth rate of 0–1.3 cm/year in 40 patients followed up for a mean of 3.5 years (Bosniak, 1995), indicating that with careful follow-up, watchful waiting may be appropriate in selected patients. Only one-third of small (<4 cm) renal masses are observed to increase in size over 2 years with none experiencing disease progression (Volpe et al, 2004). This further suggests that at least initially observation is a reasonable option particularly for older patients with comorbidities who may not be amenable to surgery.

2. Disseminated disease—Approximately 30% of patients with RCC will present with advanced disease. Metastatic RCC has a variable natural history, with 5-year survival rates typically <10% (Motzer et al, 1996). Infrequently, the disease may have a more protracted course. The biological diversity of RCC is illustrated by the 6.6% response rate (including 3% complete responders) in the placebo arm of a phase III trial of interferon-gamma (IFN-γ) in advanced RCC (Gleave et al, 1998).

Role of stratification factors: The experience with IFN has led to the understanding that patients can be grouped into three different risk categories, which predicts their overall survival from metastatic RCC. The so-called Motzer criteria, or Memorial Sloan-Kettering Cancer Center risk group, stratify patients into good, intermediate and poor risk based on performance status, prior nephrectomy, hemoglobin, lac-

tate dehydrogenase (LDH), and calcium level (Motzer et al, 1999). Importantly, even though IFN is currently no longer used in the treatment of RCC, these risk groups were utilized to select different patient populations in the development of currently available targeted therapies (below).

A. SURGERY—The role of radical nephrectomy in the management of patients with advanced disease has been reevaluated based on the results of randomized clinical trials. Historically, radical nephrectomy was primarily used as a palliative procedure in the setting of metastatic disease for managing patients with severe hemorrhage or unremitting pain. Over the past 20 years, retrospective observations of the potential for nephrectomy to improve the outcome of patients receiving biologic response modifier therapy prompted a prospective evaluation of this effect. The Southwest Oncology Group performed a randomized phase III trial, randomizing patients with advanced RCC to nephrectomy followed by interferon-alpha (IFN-α) 2b versus interferon alone. The median survival of patients undergoing nephrectomy followed by interferon was 3 months longer compared to those receiving only interferon (Flanigan et al, 2001). A similar, smaller, randomized trial conducted in Europe demonstrated similar findings (Mickisch et al, 2001). These two studies have prompted a shift in the standard of care for patients with metastatic RCC and good performance status who desire systemic therapy to include a nephrectomy prior to systemic therapy. Nephrectomy in the presence of metastatic disease (cytoreductive nephrectomy) can be performed via the open approach or laparoscopically. Patients who undergo the nephrectomy laparoscopically may have shorter hospital stay, less blood loss, and obtain adjuvant therapy earlier (Rabets et al, 2004)

The continued role of cytoreductive nephrectomy prior to systemic therapy has undergone considerable scrutiny after 2004, with the availability of new targeted systemic therapy (anti-vascular endothelial growth factor (anti-VEGF) tyrosine kinase inhibitors (TKIs) and mTOR inhibitors). While a majority of patients who received these drugs in clinical trials (and in current medical practice in 2010) have had prior cytoreductive nephrectomy, no randomized comparison regarding the role of cytoreductive nephrectomy in prolonging survival in the targeted therapy era is yet available. An ongoing clinical trial in Europe is examining this question. Trials are also examining the role of neoadjuvant-targeted therapy prior to cytoreductive nephrectomy.

Patients presenting with a solitary metastatic site particularly in the lung that is amenable to surgical resection may be candidates for combined nephrectomy and removal of the metastatic foci (Hoffman et al, 2005). This approach can result in 5-year survival rates of 30–40% with patients developing metachronous solitary lung metastases having a better prognosis (Hoffman et al, 2005). In patients who are destined to receive adjuvant therapy, even limited resection of metastases can yield improved survival further emphasizing the potential benefit of tumor debulking (Vogl et al, 2006).

The important role of surgical resection of solitary brain metastases has been highlighted by several randomized trials demonstrating an improvement in survival in patients with solitary brain metastases who undergo both surgical resection and whole-brain radiotherapy compared with patients who receive only radiation therapy (Patchell et al, 1990; Vecht et al, 1993).

B. RADIATION THERAPY—Radiation therapy is an important method in the palliation of patients with metastatic RCC. Despite the belief that RCC is a relatively radioresistant tumor, effective palliation of metastatic disease to the brain, bone, and lungs is reported in up to two-thirds of patients (Fossa et al, 1982; Onufrey and Mohiuddin, 1985).

C. BIOLOGIC RESPONSE MODIFIERS—The use of metastatic RCC as a model for the investigation of various biologic response modifiers was a consequence of both the lack of effective chemotherapy and the long-recognized biologic "eccentricities" of this tumor. Spontaneous regression of metastatic RCC is a well-recognized, albeit rare, event (Kavoussi et al, 1986; Vogelzang et al, 1992). Although no specific evidence exists, many believe this phenomenon to be immunologically mediated.

Studies using partially purified human leukocyte interferon in renal cancer were first reported in 1983, with subsequent studies using human lymphoblastoid interferon and, subsequently, recombinant interferon-alpha (r-IFN-α). Various doses and schedules of r-IFN-α have demonstrated reproducible overall response rates of 10–15% in advanced renal cancer (Pastore et al, 2001). A modest impact on survival has been demonstrated in some randomized trials of IFN-α. The Medical Research Council compared IFN-α to medroxyprogesterone acetate and demonstrated a 2.5-month median survival improvement favoring the IFN-α arm (Medical Research Council Renal Cancer Collaborators, 1999). Other large randomized studies have failed to demonstrate a survival advantage of IFN-α compared to other biologic response modifiers (Motzer et al, 2000; Negrier et al, 1998). IFN-α is commonly administered 3–5 days/week as a subcutaneous injection. Patients most likely to have a clinical benefit from interferon therapy are those who have minimal tumor burden (ie, primary kidney tumor removed), lung or nodal metastases only, and an excellent performance status. Given the modest activity of interferon in patients with advanced disease, trials of interferon administered in the adjuvant setting to patients at high risk of recurrence have been conducted but have not demonstrated clinical benefit (Pizzocaro et al, 2001; Trump et al, 1996). The experience with beta and gamma interferons has been less extensive. In 1989, Aulitzky and colleagues reported a 30% response rate in a trial of low-dose IFN-γ (Aulitzky et al, 1989). Unfortunately, subsequent trials, including a phase III trial, have demonstrated response rates of <10% (Gleave et al, 1998).

Interleukin-2 (IL-2), a T-cell growth factor, was first identified in 1976. Recombinant IL-2 was for a long time the only agent approved by the US Food and Drug Administration for patients with advanced renal carcinoma. The approval was based on several nonrandomized trials showing overall response rates for high-dose IL-2 in the 15% range and a complete response rate of 5%, resulting in some long-term survivors being seen with this treatment. The wide variability in response rates to IL-2 is likely a function of patient selection. Fyfe and colleagues (1995) reported a retrospective evaluation of 255 patients treated with high-dose IL-2 and found that an Eastern Cooperative Oncology Group performance score of 0 was a significant predictor of clinical response. More recently, the Cytokine Working Group presented the results of the SELECT trial, which was designed to prospectively evaluate predictive factors for response to high-dose IL-2. This trial showed that in optimally selected patients, response rates could be as high as 30%, with optimal criteria being clear cell histology and good or intermediate UCLA SANI score (which takes into account number of metastatic sites, thyroid function, lymph node status, constitutional symptoms, and histology). (Mc Dermott et al, 2001).

Randomized trials comparing IFN-α, IL-2, and IL-2 plus INF-α have demonstrated higher objective response rates to the combination therapy, with no difference in survival and significantly higher toxicity associated with the combination (Negrier et al, 1998). Biochemotherapy regimens have been evaluated with a phase III trial demonstrating no advantage to the combination of IL-2, IFN-α, and fluorouracil versus IL-2 and IFN (Negrier et al, 2000).

With the advent of the targeted therapy era for RCC (forthcoming section), and given the low response rates to IFN, and the significant toxicities of high-dose IL-2 (despite it being the only treatment to date with potential for durable responses), immunotherapy treatments are currently offered to a minority of carefully selected patients and in centers with expertise.

D. TARGETED THERAPY—There has been significant progress in the development of several antiangiogenic agents and inhibitors of tyrosine kinase and other cell cycle activators in RCC, with currently six drugs having FDA approval for treatment of metastatic RCC in different settings and routinely used in clinical practice. Both inherited and sporadic RCCs appear to have mutations of the VHL gene resulting in loss of the gene product. This causes increased levels of hypoxia-inducible factor-alpha that in turn promotes increased expression of VEGF and promotes angiogenesis.

Bevacizumab is a monoclonal antibody that binds and inactivates VEGF A. It has shown the ability to yield partial responses, delay disease progression, and improve survival in patients with advanced renal cancer (Yang et al, 2003). Randomized trials comparing IFN with the IFN and bevacizumab combination have shown the superiority of the combination in terms of progression-free survival (Escudier et al, 2010; Rini et al, 2010).

Anti-VEGF TKIs are small molecules that are orally bioavailable. Currently FDA approved are sorafenib, sunitinib, and pazopanib. Sunitinib and pazopanib were shown to have significant activity in the first-line setting with higher response rates and longer progression-free survival compared to IFN or placebo (Motzer et al, 2007; Sternberg et al, 2010). Sorafenib was shown to have activity in patients who had previously received cytokine immunotherapy. (Escudier et al, 2009). Anti-VEGF TKI administration requires significant expertise in managing toxicities, which for instance include hypertension, diarrhea, rash, hand-foot skin reactions, cardiac abnormalities, and many others. Not all drugs in this class exhibit the same toxicities or frequency thereof. Most patients who entered clinical trials with TKIs had clear cell histology and prior cytoreductive nephrectomy.

mTOR inhibitors are another important class of agents with activity against RCC. The mTOR pathway interacts with the VEGF pathway at the molecular level and is another contributor of angiogenesis in RCC. Temsirolimus was the first mTOR inhibitor to be FDA approved and has been demonstrated to prolong survival in patients with advanced renal cancer who present with poor risk or multiple sites of metastases (Hudes et al, 2007). The phase III trial that demonstrated the efficacy of temsirolimus also notably included several patients with nonclear cell histology, a rare finding in the trials of TKIs. Everolimus was subsequently FDA-approved based on its ability to prolong progression-free survival as second-line therapy for patients with metastatic clear-cell RCC (Motzer et al, 2010). mTOR inhibitors can cause mouth sores, fatigue, pneumonitis, and hypertriglyceridemia among other side effects.

Given all the drugs available for metastatic RCC in 2010, there are many challenges ahead of us in understanding what is the best sequence of therapies to treat patients suffering from advanced RCC today. The sequential nature of the treatments also makes it difficult to prove overall survival benefits with each individually used drug in a clinical trial. The current belief is that the overall survival of patients with metastatic RCC has increased over time, approaching a median overall survival of 2 years (as opposed to 1 year in the interferon era). It is also to be highlighted that much of the clinical benefit seen with the targeted agents is not evidenced by tumor shrinkage (response rates, which are generally modest), but instead from increased duration of tumor control (progression-free survival and projected overall survival) benefits. Finally, in making decisions about which systemic therapy to use for a specific patient, many factors are taken into consideration including performance status, histology, sites and number of metastases, mode of administration, anticipated tolerance to each individual drug, line of therapy, and socioeconomic and clinical trial considerations.

B. Follow-up Care

There is no universal agreement on the frequency or studies required in the follow-up care of patients with RCC. A stage-specific follow-up schedule is recommended for patients who have undergone radical or partial nephrectomy (Levy et al, 1998; Hafez et al, 1997). Patients with stage T1 disease need less stringent follow-up with yearly chest x-rays and liver and renal function tests. Those with stage T2 or T3 disease require more frequent follow-up of at least 3-month or 6-month intervals in the early postoperative period. Repeat CT scans of the abdomen should also be obtained, especially in those who have undergone partial nephrectomy, to rule out local recurrence. Patients with metastatic disease who are not undergoing therapy need continued follow-up to provide appropriate supportive care.

▶ Prognosis

The prognosis of patients is most clearly related to the stage of disease at presentation. Recent studies report 5-year survival rates for patients with stage T1–T2 disease in the 80–100% range, with stage T3 in the 50–60% range. Patients presenting with metastatic disease have a poorer prognosis, with only a 16–32% 5-year survival rate.

NEPHROBLASTOMA (WILMS TUMOR)

Nephroblastoma, also known as Wilms tumor, is the most common solid renal tumor of childhood, accounting for roughly 5% of childhood cancers. Approximately 650 new cases are reported annually. The peak age for presentation is during the third year of life, and there is no sex predilection. The disease is seen worldwide with a similar age of onset and sex distribution. Tumors are commonly unicentric, but they occur in either kidney with equal frequency. In 5% of cases the tumors are bilateral.

Wilms tumor occurs in familial and nonfamilial forms. The National Wilms Tumor Study (NWTS) group documented the occurrence of a familial Wilms tumor in approximately 1% of cases (Breslow and Beckwith, 1982). Although a relatively rare neoplasm, Wilms tumor has become a very important model for the study of tumorigenesis and has become a prototypical neoplasm for collaborative clinical trials, with approximately 85% of all new cases diagnosed in North America enrolled in NWTS group protocols (Beckwith, 1997). Approximately 10% of patients with Wilms tumors have recognized congenital malformations. Among the more common disorders associated with Wilms tumor are the WAGR syndrome (Wilms, aniridia, genitourinary malformation, mental retardation), overgrowth syndromes, such as Beckwith–Wiedemann syndrome and isolated hemihypertrophy, and nonovergrowth disorders, such as isolated aniridia and trisomy 18 (Weiner et al, 1998). Genitourinary abnormalities such as hypospadias, cryptorchidism, and renal fusion are found in 4.5–7.5% of patients with unilateral Wilms tumor and in up to 13.4% of those with bilateral disease (Breslow et al, 1993). Some of these genetic syndromes are associated with alterations in the WT1 gene but other genes such as the IGF1, H19, and p57 genes can also be implicated (Beckwith–Wiedemann).

Etiology

In 1972 Knudson and Strong proposed a two-hit hypothesis to explain the earlier age of onset and bilateral presentation in children with a familial history of Wilms tumor. In this hypothesis, the pathogenesis of the sporadic form of Wilms tumor results from two postzygotic mutations in a single cell. In contrast, the familial form of the disease arises after one prezygotic mutation and a subsequent postzygotic event. Karyotypic analyses of Wilms tumor patients with various congenital malformations and loss of heterozygosity studies helped identify a region on the short arm of chromosome 11 (11p13) (Huff, 1994; Riccardi et al, 1978). This work ultimately led to the identification of a gene associated with Wilms tumor development (WT1), which maps to chromosome 11p13 (Coppes et al, 1994). Although alterations in this gene have been associated with Wilms tumor and genitourinary abnormalities, only 5–10% of sporadic Wilms tumors have been demonstrated to have WT1 mutations (Varanasi et al, 1994). Genetic linkage studies of families with an inherited susceptibility to Wilms tumors suggest that other Wilms tumor genes exist (Weiner et al, 1998).

Pathogenesis and Pathology

In 1990 Beckwith and colleagues proposed a simplified nomenclature and classification of Wilms tumor precursor lesions known as nephrogenic rests (NR). Two distinct categories of NR were identified and designated as perilobar NR and intralobar NR. One concept of Wilms tumor development proposed that some NR remain dormant for many years, with some undergoing involution and sclerosis and others giving rise to Wilms tumors (Beckwith, 1997; Beckwith et al, 1990). The typical Wilms tumor consists of blastemal, epithelial, and stromal elements in varying proportions (Figure 22–10). Tumors composed of blastema and stroma or blastema alone have been described. Pure tubular and papillary forms that are very similar to papillary RCC have also been described.

The NWTS correlated pathologic specimens with clinical outcome and divided various histologic features into favorable and unfavorable prognostic groups. The unfavorable subgroup includes tumors that contain focal or diffuse elements of anaplastic cells or two other neoplastic entities considered not to be Wilms tumor variants, clear cell sarcoma of the kidney, and rhabdoid tumor of the kidney (Beckwith, 1997; Beckwith and Palmer, 1978). Favorable histology tumors comprise all Wilms tumors without anaplasia. Anaplastic tumors are characterized by extreme nuclear atypia, hyperdiploidy, and numerous complex translocations. Anaplasia occurs in 5% of Wilms tumors and incidence increases with age. It is more common in African-American children and is linked to p53 mutations (Bardesey et al, 1994). Presence of diffuse anaplasia indicates a worse prognosis compared to focal anaplasia.

Grossly, Wilms tumors are generally large, multilobulated, and gray or tan in color with focal areas of hemorrhage and

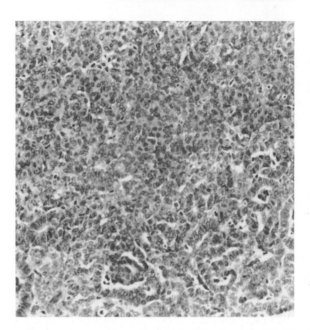

▲ **Figure 22–10.** Wilms tumor with characteristic tubular/glomeruloid structures and blastema (original magnification ×40).

necrosis. A fibrous pseudocapsule is occasionally seen. Tumor dissemination can occur by direct extension through the renal capsule, hematogenously via the renal vein and vena cava, or via lymphatic spread. Metastatic disease is present at diagnosis in 10–15% of patients, with the lungs (85–95%) and liver (10–15%) the most common sites of involvement. Regional lymphatics are involved in as many as 25% of patients. Metastases to liver, bone, and brain are uncommon.

Tumor Staging

The NWTS staging system is most widely used and is based on surgical and pathologic findings. The original classification was used in the first and second NWTS trials and was modified for NWTS III (D'Angio et al, 1989). Further modifications have been introduced to the staging in the NWTS V study.

Stage I—Tumor limited to kidney and completely excised. No penetration of renal capsule or involvement of renal sinus vessels. Tumor was not ruptured before or during removal. There is no residual tumor apparent beyond the margins of resection.

Stage II—Tumor extends beyond the kidney but is completely removed. There is either penetration through the outer surface of the renal capsule, invasion of renal sinus vessels, biopsy of tumor before removal, or spillage of tumor locally during removal. There is no residual tumor apparent at or beyond the margins of excision and no lymph node involvement.

Stage III—Residual nonhematogenous tumor confined to abdomen. Any one or more of the following occur: (a) regional lymph node involvement; (b) diffuse peritoneal contamination by tumor, such as spillage of tumor beyond the flank before or during surgery, or by tumor growth that has penetrated through the peritoneal surface; (c) implants are found on the peritoneal surfaces; (d) the tumor extends beyond the surgical margins either microscopically or grossly; (e) the tumor is not completely resectable because of local infiltration into vital structures; (f) tumor spill not confined to the flank occurred either before or during surgery; (g) transected tumor thrombus.

Stage IV—Hematogenous metastases to lung, liver, bone, and brain.

Stage V—Bilateral renal involvement at diagnosis. An attempt should be made to stage each side according to the previously given criteria on the basis of extent of disease before biopsy.

▶ Clinical Findings

A. Symptoms and Signs

The diagnosis of Wilms tumor is most commonly made after the discovery of an asymptomatic mass by a family member or a physician during a routine physical examination. Common symptoms at presentation include abdominal pain and distention, anorexia, nausea and vomiting, fever, and hematuria. The most common sign is an abdominal mass. Hypertension is seen in 25–60% of cases and is caused by elevated renin levels (D'Angio et al, 1982; Pizzo et al, 1989). Up to 30% of patients demonstrate hematuria and coagulopathy can occur in 10%.

B. Laboratory Analysis

Urinalysis may show evidence of hematuria, and anemia may be present, particularly in patients with evidence of subcapsular hemorrhage. Patients with liver metastases may have abnormal serum chemistries.

C. X-Ray Imaging

Abdominal US and CT scanning are performed initially to evaluate the mass. CT of the abdomen is performed with suspected Wilms tumor and can be useful in providing information regarding tumor extension, the status of the contralateral kidney, and the presence of regional adenopathy. CT scanning remains an imperfect technique with a relatively high false-positive rate for hepatic invasion in right-sided tumors, and 7% of cases of surgically confirmed synchronous bilateral Wilms tumors were missed by preoperative CT imaging in the NWTS IV (Ritchey et al, 1995).

Abdominal MRI can sometimes be useful to distinguish between NR and Wilms tumor but is otherwise not routinely indicated. MRI can also provide important information in defining the extent of tumor into the inferior vena cava, including those with intracardiac extension. MRI is limited in that there is no bowel contrast agent, and its use in children requires sedation (Babyn et al, 1995).

Chest x-ray remains the initial examination of choice to evaluate for the presence of lung metastases. The role of a chest CT scan is controversial, and it is probably not indicated for routine use in low-risk patients; however, when done concomitantly with an abdominal CT, chest CT may provide clinically useful information in high-risk patients. If pulmonary metastases are seen on chest x-ray, CT of the chest will not alter current therapy. However, the need for chest CT imaging in patients with negative results of chest x-ray remains controversial, because it is not clear whether those lesions detected by CT alone require more aggressive treatment (Weiner et al, 1998).

D. Needle Biopsy

Preoperative biopsy is indicated routinely only in tumors deemed too large for safe primary surgical resection and for which preoperative chemotherapy or radiation therapy is planned.

▶ Differential Diagnosis

The differential diagnosis of a flank mass in a child includes hydronephrosis, cystic kidneys, intrarenal neuroblastoma, mesoblastic nephroma, and various very rare sarcomas.

Ultrasonography can confirm the presence of hydronephrosis and evaluate for the presence of cystic kidneys. Neuroblastoma, while pathologically distinct from Wilms tumor, frequently presents in the abdomen as a mass arising from the adrenal glands or paraspinal ganglion. Neuroblastomas are radiographically indistinguishable from Wilms tumors, but there are several features that may aid in the differentiation. In contrast to Wilms tumors, which are typically confined to one side of the abdomen, neuroblastomas usually cross the midline. Wilms tumors are intrarenal masses and rarely cause a change in the axis of the kidney, while neuroblastomas may cause an outward and downward displacement of the kidney (drooping lily). Children with neuroblastomas are more likely to present with metastatic disease, and these tumors have a higher frequency of calcification observed radiographically. In addition, neuroblastomas may produce various tumor markers including vanillylmandelic acid and other catecholamines that are not seen in patients with Wilms tumor (Pizzo et al, 1989).

Mesoblastic nephromas are benign hamartomas and cannot be preoperatively distinguished from Wilms tumors. They are most commonly seen in the neonatal period and are typically identified by surgical pathology after nephrectomy. The tumor can occur in adults (Truong et al, 1998).

▶ Treatment

The goal of therapy is to provide the highest possible cure rate with the lowest treatment-related morbidity. Significant improvements in survival rates for children with Wilms tumor have been achieved by an improved understanding of the disease and a multimodality approach to therapy, advocated by the National Wilms Tumor Registry (NWTS), which incorporates surgery, radiation therapy, and chemotherapy.

A. Surgical Measures

For patients with unilateral kidney involvement whose tumors are deemed surgically resectable (tumors not crossing the midline or involving adjacent visceral organs), radical nephrectomy via a transabdominal incision is the procedure of choice.

Retroperitoneal lymph node dissection is not of proven value and is not recommended. However, biopsy of regional lymphatics (renal hilum and para-aortic nodes) and careful examination of the opposite kidney and the remainder of the abdomen provide crucial data for staging and prognosis. Tumor extending into the vena cava should be removed unless there is evidence of total obstruction. Excision of tumor extending into adjacent organs can be attempted if feasible. Complete excision of all tumors would allow downstaging and decrease the amount of additional chemotherapy. A major point of emphasis during surgical extirpation is to avoid spillage because there is evidence that this increases abdominal recurrence of disease (Ross and Kay, 1999; Shamberger et al, 1999).

A child with bilateral Wilms tumor, like an adult with bilateral RCC, requires an individualized approach. Patients with favorable histology tumors can frequently be managed with preoperative chemotherapy followed by renal-sparing surgery (Kumar et al, 1998). In patients for whom preoperative chemotherapy is planned, a biopsy for diagnosis and staging is indicated (Blute et al, 1987). In some centers, needle aspiration biopsy has proved to be a reliable diagnostic tool when evaluated by experienced pathologists (Hanash, 1989). In patients with unfavorable histology tumors, the therapeutic approach consists of aggressive surgery followed by chemotherapy and radiation therapy.

B. Chemotherapy

Wilms tumor has been long recognized as a chemosensitive neoplasm. Consecutive multicenter randomized trials conducted by the National Wilms' Tumor Study Group (NWTSG), starting in the 1960s, have carefully explored various treatment strategies to determine the role of various antineoplastics and the integration of surgery and radiotherapy, with the goal of optimizing response rates and cure while minimizing the toxicity of therapy. Current studies are focused on continued efforts to minimize toxicity (primarily by decreasing chemotherapy treatment duration and removing radiotherapy) in those favorable subgroups with impressive cure rates, and modifying efforts in poor-risk subgroups to improve response and survival.

Patients with stage I favorable or anaplastic histology and stage II favorable histology tumors undergo surgical resection and have adjuvant chemotherapy with vincristine and dactinomycin combinations without radiotherapy. Patients with stage III and IV favorable histology tumors undergo surgical resection and have adjuvant therapy with vincristine, dactinomycin, and doxorubicin, with adjuvant radiotherapy. Patients with stage II–IV focally anaplastic histology tumors receive therapy similar to that for advanced-stage favorable histology tumors. In the NWTS V, patients with stage II–IV anaplastic tumors are receiving vincristine, doxorubicin, cyclophosphamide, and etoposide (Kalapurakal et al, 2004). Salvage chemotherapy regimens include agents such as cyclophosphamide, ifosfamide, carboplatin, and etoposide. For stage V or bilateral Wilms tumors, diagnosis is established by bilateral biopsies followed by chemotherapy. Second-look surgery may be necessary to reassess response 6–8 weeks after chemotherapy. Renal sparing procedures can be attempted but the rate of renal failure is high.

C. Radiation Therapy

Wilms tumor has long been recognized as a radiosensitive tumor. Despite the proven efficacy of radiation therapy in children, its use is complicated by its potential for growth disturbances and recognized cardiac, pulmonary, and hepatic toxicities. The development of effective chemotherapy combinations has practically replaced radiation therapy in the preoperative setting. The first and second NWTS trials demonstrated that postoperative radiotherapy was not required for patients with favorable histology stage I disease. NWTS III failed to show an advantage for postoperative radiotherapy in patients with favorable stage II disease and demonstrated that the relapse rate of patients with stage III disease was no different for patients receiving 1000 cGy compared with the traditional 2000 cGy (D'Angio et al, 1989). Postoperative radiation is recommended for patients with stage III or IV disease with favorable histology, stages II–IV with focal anaplasia and clear cell sarcoma, and all stages of rhabdoid tumor of the kidney (Weiner et al, 1998).

▶ Prognosis

The multimodality approach to the treatment of children with Wilms tumors has significantly improved outcomes. The 4-year survival of patients with favorable histology Wilms tumor now approaches 90% (Weiner et al, 1998). The most important negative prognostic factors remain the unfavorable histologic subtypes (clear cell sarcoma, rhabdoid, and anaplastic tumors). Although the addition of doxorubicin in NWTS III significantly improved the 2-year survival rate for patients with clear cell sarcomas (61.5–90.3%), it did not affect the survival of children with rhabdoid tumors. Analysis of patients with bilateral Wilms tumors registered with NWTS II and III revealed a 3-year survival rate of 82% (Blute et al, 1987).

Future challenges include improvements in therapy for patients with anaplastic tumors (stages II–IV), clear cell sarcoma, and rhabdoid tumors, and efforts to improve outcomes in favorable histology tumors while decreasing both short-term and late toxicities. Long-term toxicity in these patients include renal failure, cardiac toxicity with congestive heart failure due to chemotherapy, and lung radiation as well as a higher risk for secondary malignancies.

SECONDARY RENAL TUMORS

The kidney is a frequent site for metastatic spread of both solid and hematologic tumors. Wagle et al (1975) surveyed 4413 autopsies at a major cancer center and found 81 (18%) cases of secondary carcinoma of the kidney (hematologic tumors were excluded). The most frequent primary site of cancer was lung (20%), followed by breast (12%), stomach (11%), and renal (9%). The authors noted that metastases to the renal parenchyma typically demonstrated capsular and stromal invasion with sparing of the renal pelvis and that bilateral secondary renal involvement was found in approximately 50% of cases.

Albuminuria and hematuria are relatively common findings in patients with secondary renal metastases; however, pain and renal insufficiency are rare (Olsson et al, 1971; Wagle et al, 1975). Secondary metastatic disease to the kidneys tends to be a late event, frequently in the setting of widely disseminated disease, which typically portends a poor prognosis. Therapy is dictated by the responsiveness of the primary neoplasm; that is, patients with breast and ovarian cancers for which there is effective therapy are more likely to respond than patients with primary lung or gastric cancers.

Autopsy series have reported clinically evident renal invasion by lymphoma to be 0.5–7%, with the rates of Hodgkin's and non-Hodgkin's lymphoma distributed equally (Goffinet et al, 1977; Weimar et al, 1981). Renal involvement is usually in the form of bilateral, multiple, discrete tumor nodules. Renal involvement by non-Hodgkin's lymphoma is typically characterized by diffuse, aggressive histologic findings (ie, diffuse large cell) in the setting of extensive disease. Therapy typically consists of combination chemotherapy, with the prognosis of patients similar to that of patients without renal involvement but with widely disseminated, aggressive lymphomas (Geffen et al, 1985).

BIBLIOGRAPHY

Anderson EE, Hatcher PA: Renal angiomyolipoma. Probl Urol 1990;4:230.

Aulitzky W et al: Successful treatment of metastatic renal cell carcinoma with a biologically active dose of recombinant interferon-gamma. J Clin Oncol 1989;7:1875.

Avila NA et al: Lymphangioleiomyomatosis: Abdominopelvic CT and US findings. Radiology 2000;216:147.

Babyn P et al: Imaging patients with Wilms' tumor. Hematol Oncol Clin North Am 1995;9:1217.

Bachor R et al: Positron emission tomography in the diagnosis of renal cell carcinoma. Urologe A 1996;35:146.

Bardesey N et al: Anaplastic Wilms tumor: A subtype displaying poor prognosis harbors p53 gene mutations. Nat Genet 1994;7:91.

Beckwith JB: New developments in the pathology of Wilms' tumor. Cancer Invest 1997;15:153.

Beckwith JB, Palmer NF: Histopathology and prognosis of Wilms' tumor: Results from the first National Wilms' Tumor Study. Cancer 1978;41:1937.

Beckwith JB et al: Nephrogenic rests, nephroblastomatosis, and the pathogenesis of Wilms' tumor. Pediatr Pathol 1990;10:1.

Bissler JJ et al: Sirolimus for angiomyolipoma in tuberous sclerosis complex or lymphangioleiomyomatosis. N Engl J Med 2008;358:140.

Blom JHM et al: Radical nephrectomy with and without lymph node dissection: Preliminary results of the EORTC randomized phase III protocol 30881. Eur Urol 1999;36:570.

Bluemke DA, Chambers TP: Spiral CT angiography: An alternative to conventional angiography. Radiology 1995;195:317.

Blute ML et al: Bilateral Wilms' tumor. J Urol 1987;138:968.

Bonsib SM et al: Sarcomatoid renal tumors: Clinicopathologic correlation of three cases. Cancer 1987;59:527.

Bosniak MA: Observation of small incidentally detected renal masses. Semin Urol Oncol 1995;13:267.

Brandal P et al: Chromosomal abnormalities in juxtaglomerular cell tumors. Cancer 2005;104:504.

Brennan JF et al: Acquired renal cystic disease: Implications for the urologist. Br J Urol 1991;67:342.

Breslow N et al: Epidemiology of Wilms' tumor. Med Pediatr Oncol 1993;21:172.

Breslow NE, Beckwith JB: Epidemiological features of Wilms' tumor: Results of the National Wilms' Tumor Study. J Natl Cancer Inst 1982;68:429.

Bretan PN Jr et al: Chronic renal failure: A significant risk factor in the development of acquired renal cysts and renal cell carcinoma: Case reports and a review of the literature. Cancer 1986;57:1971.

Chang SY et al: Inhibitory effects of suramin on a human renal cell carcinoma line causing hepatic dysfunction. J Urol 1992;147:1147.

Chen F et al: Germline mutations in the von Hippel-Lindau disease tumor suppressor gene: Correlation with phenotype. Hum Mutat 1995;5:66.

Cohen AJ et al: Hereditary renal-cell carcinoma associated with a chromosomal translocation. N Engl J Med 1979;301:592.

Cohen C et al: Histogenesis of renal cell carcinoma and renal oncocytoma: An immunohistochemical study. Cancer 1988;62:1946.

Coppes MJ et al: Genetic events in the development of Wilms' tumor. N Engl J Med 1994;331:586.

D'Angio GJ et al: Wilms' tumor: Genetic aspects and etiology: A report of the National Wilms' Tumor Study (NWTS) Committee of the NWTS Group. In: Kuss R et al (eds) Renal Tumors: Proceedings of the First International Symposium on Kidney Tumors. Alan R. Liss, New York, NY, 1982.

D'Angio GJ et al: Treatment of Wilms' tumor: Results of the Third National Wilms' Tumor Study. Cancer 1989;64:349.

Ditonno P et al: Extrarenal angiomyolipomas of the perinephric space. J Urol 1992;147:447.

Divgi CR et al: Preoperative characterization of clear-cell renal carcinoma using iodine-124-labelled antibody chimeric G250 (124I-cG250) and PET in patients with renal masses: A phase I trial. Lancet Oncol 2007;8:304.

Dong D et al: Juxtaglomerular cell tumor of the kidney: A new classification scheme. Urol Oncol 2010;28:34.

Duchene DA et al: Histopathology of surgically managed renal tumors: Analysis of a contemporary series. Urology 2003;62:827.

Ekelund L, Gothlin J: Renal hemangiomas: An analysis of 13 cases diagnosed by angiography. Am J Roentgenol Radium Ther Nucl Med 1975;125:788.

Erlandsson R: Molecular genetics of renal cell carcinoma. Cancer Genet Cytogenet 1998;104:1.

Escudier B et al: Sorafenib in advanced renal cell carcinoma. N Engl J Med 2007;356:125.

Escudier B et al: Sorafenib for treatment of renal cell carcinoma: Final efficacy and safety results of the phase III treatment approaches in renal cancer global evaluation trial. J Clin Oncol 2009;27(20):3312.

Escudier et al: Phase III Trial of Bevacizumab Plus Interferon Alfa-2a in Patients With Metastatic Renal Cell Carcinoma (AVOREN): Final Analysis of Overall Survival. J Clin Oncol 2010;28(13):2144

Fallon B, Williams RD: Renal cancer associated with acquired cystic disease of the kidney and chronic renal failure. Semin Urol 1989;4:228.

Ficarra V et al: Multiinstitutional European validation of the 2002 TNM staging system in conventional and papillary localized renal cell carcinoma. Cancer 2005;104:968.

Flanigan RC et al: Nephrectomy followed by interferon alfa-2b compared with interferon alfa-2b alone for metastatic renal cell cancer. N Engl J Med 2001;345:1655.

Fossa SD et al: Radiotherapy of metastasis from renal cancer. Eur Urol 1982;8:340.

Fuhrman SA et al: Prognostic significance of morphologic parameters in renal cell carcinoma. Am J Surg Pathol 1982;6:655.

Fyfe G et al: Results of treatment of 255 patients with metastatic renal cell carcinoma who received high-dose recombinant interleukin-2 therapy. J Clin Oncol 1995;13:688.

Geffen DB et al: Renal involvement in diffuse aggressive lymphomas: Results of treatment with combination chemotherapy. J Clin Oncol 1985;3:646.

Gill IS et al: Laparoscopic renal cryoablation in 32 patients. Urology 2000;56:748.

Gill IS et al: Laparoscopic radical nephrectomy in 100 patients. Cancer 2001;92:1843.

Gitlitz BJ et al: Treatment of metastatic renal cell carcinoma with high-dose bolus interleukin-2 in a non-intensive care unit: An analysis of 124 consecutively treated patients. Cancer J 2001;7:112.

Gleave ME et al: Interferon gamma-1b compared with placebo in metastatic renal cell carcinoma. N Engl J Med 1998;338:1265.

Gnarra JR et al: Mutations in of the VHL tumor suppressor gene in renal cell carcinoma. Nat Genet 1994;7(1):85–90

Goffinet DR et al: Clinical and surgical (laparotomy) evaluation of patients with non-Hodgkin's lymphomas. Cancer Treat Rep 1977;61:981.

Gold PJ et al: Paraneoplastic manifestations of renal cell carcinoma. Semin Urol Oncol 1996;14:216.

Goldstein NS: The current state of renal cell carcinoma grading. Cancer 1997;80:977.

Greene FL et al (ed): AJCC Cancer Staging Manual, 6th edn. Springer-Verlag, New York, 2002.

Gulanikar AC et al: Prospective pretransplant ultrasound screening in 206 patients for acquired renal cysts and renal cell carcinoma. Transplantation 1998;66:1669.

Haab F et al: Renin secreting tumors: Diagnosis, conservative surgical approach and long-term results. J Urol 1995;153:1781.

Hafez KS et al: Patterns of tumor recurrence and guidelines for followup following nephron-sparing surgery for sporadic renal cell carcinoma. J Urol 1997;157:2067.

Hanash KA: The nonmetastatic hepatic dysfunction syndrome associated with renal cell carcinoma (hypernephroma): Stauffer's syndrome. Prog Clin Biol Res 1982;100:301.

Hanash KA: Recent advances in the surgical treatment of bilateral Wilms' tumor. In: Murphy GP, Khoury S (eds) Therapeutic Progress in Urological Cancers. Alan R. Liss, New York, NY, 1989.

Henriksson C et al: Skeletal metastases in 102 patients evaluated before surgery for renal cell carcinoma. Scand J Urol Nephrol 1992;26:363.

Herr HW: Partial nephrectomy for unilateral renal carcinoma and a normal contralateral kidney: 10-year followup. J Urol 1999;161:33.

Herrlinger A et al: What are the benefits of extended dissection of the regional lymph nodes in the therapy of renal cell carcinoma? J Urol 1991;146:1224.

Hock LM et al: Increasing incidence of all stages of kidney cancer in the last 2 decades in the United States: An analysis of Surveillance, Epidemiology and End Results Program data. J Urol 2002;167:57.

Hocking WG: Hematologic abnormalities in patients with renal diseases. Hematol Oncol Clin North Am 1987;1:229.

Hoffman H-S et al: Prognostic factors and survival after resection of metastatic renal cell carcinoma. Eur Urol 2005;48:77.

Hoh CK et al: Positron emission tomography in urologic oncology. J Urol 1998;159:347.

Holmes NM et al: Renal imaging with spiral CT scan: Clinical applications. Tech Urol 1997;3:202.

Holthöfer H: Immunohistology of renal cell carcinoma. Eur Urol 1990;18(suppl):15.

Horan JJ et al: The detection of renal cell carcinoma extension into the renal vein and inferior vena cava: A prospective comparison of venacavography and MRI. J Urol 1989;142:943.

Hricak H et al: Detection and staging of renal neoplasms: A reassessment of MR imaging. Radiology 1988;166:643.

Hudes et al: Temsirolimus, interferon alfa, or both for advanced renal cell carcinoma. N Engl J Med2007;356(22):2271

Huff V: Inheritance and functionality of Wilms' tumor genes. Cancer Bull 1994;46:254.

Itano NB et al: Outcome of isolated renal cell carcinoma fossa recurrence after nephrectomy. J Urol 2000;164:322.

Jemal A et al: Cancer statistics, 2010. CA Cancer J Clin 2010;60:277.

Joslyn SA et al: Impact of lymphadenectomy and nodal burden in renal cell carcinoma: Retrospective analysis of the National Surveillance, Epidemiology, and End Results database. Urology 2005;65:675.

Kabala JE et al: Magnetic resonance imaging in the staging of renal cell carcinoma. Br J Radiol 1991;64:683.

Kalapurakal JA et al: Management of Wilms tumor: Current practice and future goals. Lancet Oncol 2004;5:37.

Kavoussi LR et al: Regression of metastatic renal cell carcinoma: A case report and literature review. J Urol 1986;125:1005.

Kim JK et al: Renal angiomyolipoma with minimal fat: Differentiation from other neoplasm at double-echo chemical shift FLASH MR imaging. Radiology 2006;239:174.

Kimura M et al: Minimally invasive surgery using ablative modalities for the localized renal mass. Int J Urol 2010;17:215

Kovacs G et al: Consistent chromosome 3p deletion and loss of heterozygosity in renal cell carcinoma. Proc Natl Acad Sci USA 1988;85:1571.

Kumar R et al: Conservative surgical management of bilateral Wilms' tumor: Results of the United Kingdom Children's Cancer Study Group. J Urol 1998;160:1450.

Latif F et al: Identification of the von Hippel-Lindau disease tumor suppressor gene. Science 1993;260:1317.

La Vecchia C et al: Smoking and renal cell carcinoma. Cancer Res 1990;50:5231.

Levy DA et al: Stage specific guidelines for surveillance after radical nephrectomy for local renal cell carcinoma. J Urol 1998;159:1163.

Licht MR et al: Renal oncocytoma: Clinical and biological correlates. J Urol 1993;150:1380.

Lindgren V et al: Cytogenetic analysis of a series of 13 renal oncocytomas: J Urol 2004;171:602.

Lowe BA et al: Malignant transformation of angiomyolipoma. J Urol 1992;147:1356.

Makay B et al: The ultrastructure and immunocytochemistry of renal cell carcinoma. Ultrastruct Pathol 1987;11:483.

Mandel JS et al: International renal cell cancer study. IV. Occupation. Int J Cancer 1995;61:601.

Marshall FF et al: The feasibility of surgical enucleation for renal cell carcinoma. J Urol 1986;135:231.

McDermott D et al: A randomized phase III trial of high-dose interleukin-2 versus subcutaneous IL2/interferon in patients with metastatic renal cell carcinoma. Proc Am Soc Clin Oncol 2001;20(abst 685):172a.

McNichols DW et al: Renal cell carcinoma: Long-term survival and late recurrence. J Urol 1981;126:17.

Medical Research Council Renal Cancer Collaborators: Interferon-α and survival in metastatic renal carcinoma: Early results of a randomised controlled trial. Lancet 1999;353:14.

Merino MJ, Librelsi VA: Oncocytomas of the kidney. Cancer 1982;50:1952.

Mickisch G et al: P-170 glycoprotein glutathione and associated enzymes in relation to chemoresistance of primary human renal cell carcinomas. Urol Int 1990;45:170.

Mickisch G et al: Radical nephrectomy plus interferon-alfa-based immunotherapy compared with interferon-alfa alone in metastatic renal-cell carcinoma: A randomised trial. Lancet 2001;358:966.

Miller BA: Racial/Ethnic Patterns of Cancer in the United States, 1988–1992. NIH Pub. No. 96–4104. National Cancer Institute, Bethesda, MD, 1996.

Morgan WR, Zincke H: Progression and survival after renal-conserving surgery for renal cell carcinoma: Experience in 104 patients and extended followup. J Urol 1990;144:852.

Mindrup SR et al: The prevalence of renal cell carcinoma diagnosed at autopsy. BJU Int 2005;95:31.

Mostofi FK, Davis CJ Jr: Histologic Typing of Kidney Tumors. Springer-Verlag, Berlin, 1998.

Motzer RJ et al: Renal-cell carcinoma. N Engl J Med 1996;335:865.

Motzer et al: Survival and prognostic stratification of 670 patients with advanced renal cell carcinoma. J Clin Oncol 1999;17(8):2530–2540.

Motzer RJ et al: Phase III trial of interferon alfa-2a with or without 13-cis-retinoic acid for patients with advanced renal cell carcinoma. J Clin Oncol 2000;18:2972.

Motzer RJ et al: Sunitinib in patients with renal cell carcinoma. JAMA 2006;295:2516.

Motzer RJ et al: Sunitinib versus interferon alpha in metastatic renal cell carcinoma. N Engl J Med 2007;356:115.

Motzer RJ et al: Phase 3 trial of everolimus for metastatic renal cell carcinoma: Final results and analysis of prognostic factors. Cancer 2010;116:4256

Muggia FM: Overview of cancer-related hypercalcemia: Epidemiology and etiology. Semin Oncol 1990;17:3.

Murphy DP, Gill IS: Energy based renal tumor ablation: A review. Semin Urol Oncol 2001;19:133.

Negrier S et al: Recombinant human interleukin-2, recombinant human interferon alfa-2a, or both in metastatic renal cell carcinoma. N Engl J Med 1998;338:1272.

Negrier S et al: Treatment of patients with metastatic renal carcinoma with a combination of subcutaneous interleukin-2 and interferon alfa with or without fluorouracil. J Clin Oncol 2000;18:4009.

Nickerson ML et al: Mutations in a novel gene lead to kidney tumors, lung wall defects, and benign tumors of the hair follicle in patients with the Birt–Hogg–Dube syndrome. Cancer Cell 2002;2:157.

Noordzij MA, Mickisch GH: The genetic make-up of renal tumors. Urol Res 2004;32:251.

Novick AC et al: Extracorporeal renal surgery and autotransplantation: Indications, techniques and results. J Urol 1980;123:806.

Olsson CA et al: Pulmonary cancer metastatic to the kidneys: A common renal neoplasm. J Urol 1971;105:492.

Onufrey V, Mohiuddin M: Radiation therapy in the treatment of metastatic renal cell carcinoma. Int J Radiat Oncol Biol Phys 1985;11:2007.

Oosterwijk E et al: Antibody localization in human renal cell carcinoma: A phase I study of monoclonal antibody G250. J Clin Oncol 1993;11(4):738.

Pastore RD et al: Renal cell carcinoma and interferon at the millennium. Cancer Invest 2001;19:281.

Patchell RA et al: A randomized trial of surgery in the treatment of single metastases to the brain. N Engl J Med 1990;322:494.

Pavlovich CP et al: Percutaneous radio frequency ablation of small renal tumors: Initial results. J Urol 2002;167:10.

Philips JL et al: The genetic basis of renal epithelial tumors: Advances in research and its impact on prognosis and therapy. Curr Opin Urol 2001;11:463.

Pitts WR et al: Ultrasonography, computed tomography and pathology of angiomyolipoma of the kidney: Solution to a diagnostic dilemma. J Urol 1980;124:907.

Pizzo PA et al: Solid tumors of childhood. In: de Vita VT Jr et al: (eds) Cancer Principles and Practice of Oncology. Lippincott, Philadelphia, 1989.

Pizzocaro G et al: Interferon adjuvant to radical nephrectomy in Robson stages II and III renal cell carcinoma: A multicentric randomized study. J Clin Oncol 2001;9:425.

Portis AJ et al: Long-term followup after laparoscopic radical nephrectomy. J Urol 2002;167:1257.

Rabbani F et al: Temporal change in risk of metachronous contralateral renal cell carcinoma: Influence of tumor characteristics and demographic factors. J Clin Oncol 2002;20:2370.

Rabets JC et al: Laparoscopic versus open cytoreductive nephrectomy for metastatic renal cell carcinoma. Urology 2004;64:930.

Ramdave S et al: Clinical role of F-18-fluorodeoxyglucose positron emission tomography for detection and management of renal cell carcinoma. J Urol 2001;166:825.

Reichard EAP et al: Renal neoplasms in patients with renal cystic disease. Abdom Imaging 1998;23:237.

Riccardi VM et al: Chromosomal imbalance in the Aniridia–Wilms' tumor association: 11p interstitial deletion. Pediatrics 1978;61:604.

Rini BI et al: Phase III trial of bevacizumab plus interferon alfa versus interferon alfa monotherapy in patients with metastatic renal cell carcinoma: Final results of CALGB 90206. J Clin Oncol 2010;28(13):2137

Ritchey ML et al: Accuracy of current imaging modalities in the diagnosis of synchronous bilateral Wilms tumor: A report from the National Wilms' Tumor Study Group. Cancer 1995;75:600.

Robson CJ: Radial nephrectomy for renal cell carcinoma. J Urol 1963;89:37.

Romis L et al: Frequency, clinical presentation and evolution of renal oncocytomas: Multicentric experience from a European database. Eur Urol 2004;45:53.

Ross JH, Kay R: Surgical considerations for patients with Wilms' tumor. Semin Urol Oncol 1999;17:33.

Shah RB et al: Image guided biopsy in the evaluation of renal mass lesions in contemporary urological practice: Indications, adequacy, clinical impact and limitations of the pathological diagnosis. Hum Pathol 2005;36:1309.

Shamberger RC et al: Surgery-related factors and local recurrence of Wilms' tumor in National Wilms' Tumor Study 4. Ann Surg 1999; 229:292.

Shingleton WB, Sewell PE: Percutaneous renal cryoablation of renal tumors in patients with Von-Hippel-Lindau disease. J Urol 2002;167:1268.

Skinner DG et al: Technique of radical nephrectomy. In: Skinner DG, Lieskovsky G (eds) Genitourinary Cancer. Saunders, Philadelphia, 1988.

Smith RB: The treatment of bilateral renal cell carcinoma or renal cell carcinoma in the solitary kidney. In: deKernion JB, Pavone-Macaluso M (eds) Tumors of the Kidney. Williams & Wilkins, Baltimore, MD, 1986.

Smith JW et al: Acquired renal cystic disease: Two cases of associated adenocarcinoma and a renal ultrasound survey of a peritoneal dialysis population. Am J Kidney Dis 1987;10:41.

Snyder ME et al: Incidence of benign lesions for clinically localized renal masses smaller than 7 cm in radiological diameter: Influence of sex. J Urol 2006;176:2391.

Sooriakumaran P et al: Angiomyolipomata: Challenges, solutions, and future prospects based on over 100 cases treated. BJU Int 2010;105:106.

Stauffer MH: Nephrogenic hepatosplenomegaly. (Abstract.) Gastroenterology 1961;40:694.

Steiner MS et al: Leiomyoma of the kidney: Presentation of 4 new cases and the role of computerized tomography. J Urol 1990;143:994.

Steiner MS et al: The natural history of renal angiomyolipoma. J Urol 1993;150:1782.

Sternberg CN et al: Pazopanib in locally advanced or metastatic renal cell carcinoma: Results of a phase III trial. J Clin Oncol 2010 28:1061

Stillebroer AB et al: Carbonic anhydrase IX in renal cell carcinoma: Implications for prognosis, diagnosis and therapy. Eur Urol 2010;58:75.

Storkel S et al: The human chromophobe cell renal carcinoma: Its probable relation to intercalated cells of the collecting duct. Virchows Arch B Cell Pathol Incl Mol Pathol 1989;56:237.

Strewler GJ et al: Parathyroid hormone-like protein from human renal carcinoma cells: Structural and functional homology with parathyroid hormone. J Clin Invest 1987;80:1803.

Sufrin G et al: Serologic markers, paraneoplastic syndromes, and ectopic hormone production in renal adenocarcinoma. In: de Kernion JB, Pavone-Macaluso M (eds) Tumors of the Kidney. Williams & Wilkins, Baltimore, MD, 1986.

Sufrin G et al: Paraneoplastic and serologic syndromes of renal adeno-carcinoma. Semin Urol 1989;7:158.

Tanguay S et al: Therapy of locally recurrent renal cell carcinoma after nephrectomy. J Urol 1996;155:26.

Theones W et al: Chromophobe cell carcinoma and its variants: A report on 32 cases. J Pathol 1988;155:277.

Thrasher JB, Paulson DF: Prognostic factors in renal cancer. Urol Clin North Am 1993;20:247.

Tickoo SK et al: Renal oncocytosis: A morphologic study of fourteen cases. Am J Surg Pathol 1999;23:1094.

Toro JR et al: Birt–Hogg–Dubé syndrome: A novel marker of kidney neoplasia. Arch Dermatol 1999;135:1195.

Trump DL et al: Randomized controlled trial of adjuvant therapy with lymphoblastoid interferon in resected, high-risk renal cell carcinoma. (Abstract.) Proc Am Soc Clin Oncol 1996;15:648.

Truong LD et al: Adult mesoblastic nephroma: Expansion of the morphologic spectrum and review of literature. Am J Surg Pathol 1998;22:827.

Uhlenbrock D et al: Angiomyolipoma of the kidney: Comparison between magnetic resonance imaging, computed tomography, and ultrasonography for diagnosis. Acta Radiol 1988;29:523.

Urban T et al: Pulmonary lymphangioleiomyomatosis: A study of 69 patients. Medicine 1999;78:321.

Uzzo RG, Novick AC: Nephron sparing surgery for renal tumors: Indications, techniques and outcomes. J Urol 2001;161:6.

Varanasi R et al: Fine structure analysis of the WT1 gene in sporadic Wilms' tumors. Proc Natl Acad Sci U S A 1994;91:3554.

Vaziri ND et al: Acquired renal cystic disease in renal transplant recipients. Nephron 1984;37:203.

Vecht CJ et al: Treatment of single brain metastases: Radiotherapy alone or combined with neurosurgery? Ann Neurol 1993;33:583.

Vogelzang NJ et al: Spontaneous regression of histologically proved pulmonary metastases from renal cell carcinoma: A case with 5-year followup. J Urol 1992;148:1247.

Vogl UM et al: Prognostic factors in metastatic renal cell carcinoma: Metastasectomy as independent prognostic variable. Br J Cancer 2006;95:691.

Volpe A et al: The natural history of incidentally detected small renal masses. Cancer 2004;100:738.

Volpe A et al: Techniques, safety and accuracy of sampling of renal tumors by fine needle aspiration and core biopsy. J Urol 2007;178:379.

Wagle DG et al: Secondary carcinomas of the kidney. J Urol 1975;114:30.

Weimar G et al: Urogenital involvement by malignant lymphomas. J Urol 1981;125:230.

Weiner JS et al: Current concepts in the biology and management of Wilms' tumor. J Urol 1998;159:1316.

Wong AL et al: Renal angiomyolipoma: A review of the literature and a report of 4 cases. Br J Urol 1981;53:406.

Wunderlich H et al: The accuracy of 250 fine needle biopsies of renal tumors. J Urol 2005;174:2422.

Yagoda A et al: Chemotherapy for advanced renal cell carcinoma: 1983–1993. Semin Oncol 1995;22:42.

Yang JC et al: A randomized trial of bevacizumab, an anti-vascular endothelial growth factor antibody for metastatic renal cancer. N Engl J Med 2003;349:427.

Yu MC et al: Cigarette smoking, obesity, diuretic use and coffee consumption as risk factors for renal cell carcinoma. J Natl Cancer Inst 1986;77:351.

Zbar B et al: Hereditary papillary renal cell carcinoma. J Urol 1994;151:561.

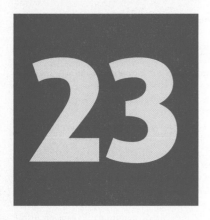

23

Neoplasms of the Prostate Gland

Matthew R. Cooperberg, MD, MPH, Joseph C. Presti Jr., MD,
Katsuto Shinohara, MD, & Peter R. Carroll, MD, MPH

The prostate gland is the male organ most commonly afflicted with either benign or malignant neoplasms. McNeal et al (1988) popularized the concept of zonal anatomy of the prostate. Three distinct zones have been identified (Figure 23–1). The peripheral zone accounts for 70% of the volume of the young adult prostate, the central zone accounts for 25%, and the transition zone accounts for 5%. These anatomic zones have distinct ductal systems but, more important, are differentially afflicted with neoplastic processes. Sixty to seventy percent of carcinomas of the prostate (CaP) originate in the peripheral zone, 10–20% in the transition zone, and 5–10% in the central zone (McNeal et al, 1988). Benign prostatic hyperplasia (BPH) uniformly originates in the transition zone (Figure 23–2).

BENIGN PROSTATIC HYPERPLASIA

Incidence and Epidemiology

BPH is the most common benign tumor in men, and its incidence is age related. The prevalence of histologic BPH in autopsy studies rises from approximately 20% in men aged 41–50, to 50% in men aged 51–60, and to >90% in men older than 80 years. Although clinical evidence of disease occurs less commonly, symptoms of prostatic obstruction are also age related. At age 55, approximately 25% of men report obstructive voiding symptoms. At age 75, 50% of men complain of a decrease in the force and caliber of their urinary stream.

Risk factors for the development of BPH are poorly understood. Some studies have suggested a genetic predisposition, and some have noted racial differences. Approximately 50% of men younger than 60 years who undergo surgery for BPH may have a heritable form of the disease. This form is most likely an autosomal dominant trait, and first-degree male relatives of such patients carry an increased relative risk of approximately fourfold.

Etiology

The etiology of BPH is not completely understood, but it seems to be multifactorial and endocrine controlled. The prostate is composed of both stromal and epithelial elements, and each, either alone or in combination, can give rise to hyperplastic nodules and the symptoms associated with BPH. Each element may be targeted in medical management schemes.

Observations and clinical studies in men have clearly demonstrated that BPH is under endocrine control. Castration results in the regression of established BPH and improvement in urinary symptoms. Additional investigations have demonstrated a positive correlation between levels of free testosterone and estrogen and the volume of BPH. The latter may suggest that the association between aging and BPH might result from the increased estrogen levels of aging causing induction of the androgen receptor, which thereby sensitizes the prostate to free testosterone. There is evidence that estrogens acting through stromal and epithelial estrogen receptors may contribute, in part, to diseases of the prostate. Genetic or environmental factors that influence 5α-reductase appear to be important in the development of BPH as well (Alan et al, 2008; Gail et al, 2008).

Pathology

As discussed earlier, BPH develops in the transition zone. It is truly a hyperplastic process resulting from an increase in cell number. Microscopic evaluation reveals a nodular growth pattern that is composed of varying amounts of stroma and epithelium. Stroma is composed of varying amounts of collagen and smooth muscle. The differential representation of the histologic components of BPH explains, in part, the potential responsiveness to medical therapy. Thus, α-blocker therapy may result in excellent responses in patients with BPH that has a significant component of

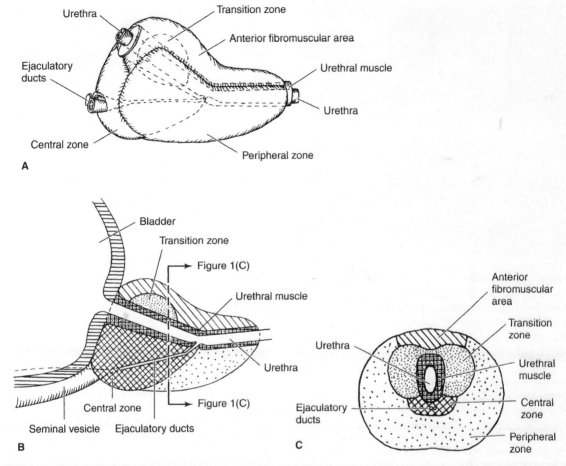

▲ **Figure 23–1. A:** Schematic lateral view of the prostate. **B:** Cut section of the same. **C:** Transverse view of area shown in B.

smooth muscle, while those with BPH predominantly composed of epithelium might respond better to 5α-reductase inhibitors. Patients with significant components of collagen in the stroma may not respond to either form of medical therapy. Unfortunately, one cannot reliably predict responsiveness to a specific therapy (see later).

As BPH nodules in the transition zone enlarge, they compress the outer zones of the prostate, resulting in the formation of a so-called surgical capsule. This boundary separates the transition zone from the peripheral zone and serves as a cleavage plane for open enucleation of the prostate during open simple prostatectomies performed for BPH.

▶ Pathophysiology

One can relate the symptoms of BPH to either the obstructive component of the prostate or the secondary response of the bladder to the outlet resistance. The obstructive component can be subdivided into the mechanical and the dynamic obstruction.

As prostatic enlargement occurs, mechanical obstruction may result from intrusion into the urethral lumen or bladder neck, leading to a higher bladder outlet resistance. Prior to the zonal classification of the prostate, urologists often referred to the "three lobes" of the prostate, namely, the median and the two lateral lobes. Prostatic size on digital rectal examination (DRE) correlates poorly with symptoms, in part, because the median lobe is not readily palpable.

The dynamic component of prostatic obstruction explains the variable nature of the symptoms experienced by patients. The prostatic stroma, composed of smooth muscle and collagen, is rich in adrenergic nerve supply. The level of autonomic stimulation thus sets a tone to the prostatic urethra. Use of α-blocker therapy decreases this tone, resulting in a decrease in outlet resistance.

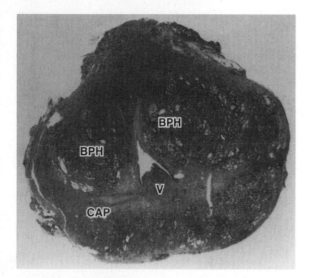

▲ **Figure 23–2.** Whole mount of prostate at level of midprostatic urethra. Note verumontanum (V) and areas of prostate cancer (CAP) in peripheral zone and areas of benign prostatic hyperplasia (BPH) in transition zone.

The irritative voiding complaints (see later) of BPH result from the secondary response of the bladder to the increased outlet resistance. Bladder outlet obstruction leads to detrusor muscle hypertrophy and hyperplasia as well as collagen deposition. Although the latter is most likely responsible for a decrease in bladder compliance, detrusor instability is also a factor. On gross inspection, thickened detrusor muscle bundles are seen as trabeculation on cystoscopic examination. If left unchecked, mucosal herniation between detrusor muscle bundles ensues, causing diverticula formation (so-called false diverticula composed of only mucosa and serosa).

▶ Clinical Findings

A. Symptoms

The symptoms of BPH can be divided into obstructive and irritative complaints. Obstructive symptoms include hesitancy, decreased force and caliber of stream, sensation of incomplete bladder emptying, double voiding (urinating a second time within 2 hours of the previous void), straining to urinate, and postvoid dribbling. Irritative symptoms include urgency, frequency, and nocturia.

The self-administered questionnaire originally developed by the American Urological Association (AUA) is both valid and reliable in identifying the need to treat patients and in monitoring their response to therapy. The AUA Symptom Score Questionnaire has been extensively validated and translated, and it is now more commonly called the International Prostate Symptom Score (IPSS) (Table 23–1). The

IPSS is perhaps the single most important tool used in the evaluation of patients with BPH and is recommended for all patients before the initiation of therapy. This assessment focuses on seven items that ask patients to quantify the severity of their obstructive or irritative complaints on a scale of 0–5. Thus, the score can range from 0 to 35. An IPSS of 0–7 is considered mild, 8–19 is considered moderate, and 20–35 is considered severe. The relative distribution of scores for BPH patients and control subjects is, respectively, 20% and 83% in those with mild scores, 57% and 15% in those with moderate scores, and 23% and 2% in those with severe scores (McConnell et al, 1994). As with other quality-of-life surveys, a reasonable degree of both literacy and numeracy is necessary for valid results. A multimedia version of the IPSS has been proposed which is more reliable among low-education populations (Bryant et al, 2009).

A detailed history focusing on the urinary tract excludes other possible causes of symptoms that may not result from the prostate, such as urinary tract infection, neurogenic bladder, urethral stricture, or prostate cancer.

B. Signs

A physical examination, DRE, and focused neurologic examination are performed on all patients. The size and consistency of the prostate is noted, even though prostate size, as determined by DRE, does not correlate with severity of symptoms or degree of obstruction. BPH usually results in a smooth, firm, elastic enlargement of the prostate. Induration, if detected, must alert the physician to the possibility of cancer and the need for further evaluation (ie, prostate-specific antigen [PSA], transrectal ultrasound [TRUS], and biopsy).

C. Laboratory Findings

A urinalysis to exclude infection or hematuria and serum creatinine measurement to assess renal function are required. Renal insufficiency may be observed in 10% of patients with prostatism and warrants upper-tract imaging. Patients with renal insufficiency are at an increased risk of developing postoperative complications following surgical intervention for BPH. Serum PSA is considered optional, but most physicians will include it in the initial evaluation. PSA, compared with DRE alone, certainly increases the ability to detect CaP, but because there is much overlap between levels seen in BPH and CaP, its use remains controversial (see Section "Prostate Cancer Screening and Chemoprevention").

D. Imaging

Upper-tract imaging (renal ultrasound or computed tomography [CT] urogram) is recommended only in the presence of concomitant urinary tract disease or complications from BPH (eg, hematuria, urinary tract infection, renal insufficiency, history of stone disease). TRUS is useful to determine prostate size for men planning to undergo prostate surgery who are suspected to have severe prostate enlargement based on DRE.

Table 23–1. Questionnaire for international prostate symptom score.

Urinary symptoms (symptom score criteria)	AUA Score					
	Not at all	Less than 1 time in 5	Less than half the time	About half the time	More than half the time	Almost always
1. Incomplete emptying Over the past month, how often have you had a sensation of not emptying your bladder completely after you finished urinating?	0	1	2	3	4	5
2. Frequency Over the past month, how often have you had to urinate again less than 2 hours after you finished urinating?	0	1	2	3	4	5
3. Intermittency Over the past month, how often have you found you stopped and started again several times when you urinate?	0	1	2	3	4	5
4. Urgency Over the past month, how often have you found it difficult to postpone urination?	0	1	2	3	4	5
5. Weak stream Over the past month, how often have you had a weak urinary stream?	0	1	2	3	4	5
6. Straining Over the past month, how often have you had to push or strain to begin urination?	0	1	2	3	4	5
	None	1 time	2 times	3 times	4 times	5 or more times
7. Nocturia Over the past month, how many times did you most typically get up to urinate from the time you went to bed at night until the time you got up in the morning?	0	1	2	3	4	5

International Prostate Symptom Score (IPSS) = sum of questions A1 to A7

Quality of life due to urinary problems

	Delighted	Pleased	Mostly satisfied	Mixed—about equally satisfied and unsatisfied	Mostly dissatisfied	Unhappy	Terrible
If you were to spend the rest of your life with your urinary condition just the way it is now, how would you feel about that?	0	1	2	3	4	5	6

Source: McConnell JD: *Benign Prostatic Hyperplasia; Diagnosis and Treatment.* Clinical Practice Guideline No. 8. AHCPR Publication No. 94–0582. Agency for Health Care Policy and Research, Public Health Service, US Department of Health and Human Services, Rockville, MD, 1994.

E. Cystoscopy

Cystoscopy is not routinely recommended to determine the need for treatment but may assist in choosing the surgical approach in patients opting for invasive therapy. When marked obstructive symptoms exist in the setting of relative minimal prostate enlargement, cystoscopy may be useful to identify a high bladder neck, urethral stricture, or other pathology. If BPH is associated with hematuria, then cystoscopy is mandatory to rule out other bladder pathology.

F. Additional Tests

Measurement of flow rate, determination of postvoid residual urine, and pressure-flow studies are considered optional. Cystometrograms and urodynamic profiles are reserved for patients with suspected neurologic disease or those who have failed prostate surgery.

▶ Differential Diagnosis

Other obstructive conditions of the lower urinary tract, such as urethral stricture, bladder neck contracture, bladder stone, or CaP, must be entertained when evaluating men with presumptive BPH. A history of previous urethral instrumentation, urethritis, or trauma should be elucidated to exclude urethral stricture or bladder neck contracture. Hematuria and pain are commonly associated with bladder stones. CaP may be detected by abnormalities on the DRE or an elevated PSA (see later).

A urinary tract infection, which can mimic the irritative symptoms of BPH, can be readily identified by urinalysis and culture; however, a urinary tract infection can also be a complication of BPH. Although irritative voiding complaints are also associated with carcinoma of the bladder, especially carcinoma in situ, the urinalysis usually shows evidence of hematuria. Likewise, patients with neurogenic bladder disorders may have many of the signs and symptoms of BPH, but a history of neurologic disease, stroke, diabetes mellitus, or back injury may be present as well. In addition, examination may show diminished perineal or lower extremity sensation or alterations in rectal sphincter tone or the bulbocavernosus reflex. Simultaneous alterations in bowel function (constipation) might also alert one to the possibility of a neurologic origin.

▶ Treatment

After patients have been evaluated, they should be informed of the various therapeutic options for BPH. It is advisable for patients to consult with their physicians to make an educated decision on the basis of the relative efficacy and side effects of the treatment options.

Specific treatment recommendations can be offered for certain groups of patients. For those with mild symptoms (IPSS score, 0–7), watchful waiting is generally advised. On the other end of the therapeutic spectrum, absolute surgical indications include urinary retention refractory to medical management and attempts at catheter removal, recurrent urinary tract infection, recurrent gross hematuria, bladder stones, renal insufficiency, or large bladder diverticula.

A. Watchful Waiting

Very few studies on the natural history of BPH have been reported. The risk of progression or complications is uncertain. However, in men with symptomatic BPH, it is clear that progression is not inevitable and that some men undergo spontaneous improvement or resolution of their symptoms.

Retrospective studies on the natural history of BPH are inherently subject to bias, related to patient selection and the type and extent of follow-up. Very few prospective studies addressing the natural history of BPH have been reported. A large randomized study compared finasteride with placebo in men with moderately to severely symptomatic BPH and enlarged prostates on DRE (McConnell et al, 1998). Patients in the placebo arm of the study had a 7% risk of developing urinary retention over 4 years.

As mentioned earlier, watchful waiting is the appropriate management of men with mild symptom scores (0–7). Men with moderate or severe symptoms can also be managed in this fashion if they so choose. Neither the optimal interval for follow-up nor specific end points for intervention have been defined.

B. Medical Therapy

1. α-Blockers—The human prostate and bladder base contains α_1-adrenoreceptors, and the prostate shows a contractile response to corresponding agonists. The contractile properties of the prostate and bladder neck seem to be mediated primarily by the subtype α_{1a}-receptors. α-Blockade has been shown to result in both objective and subjective degrees of improvement in the symptoms and signs of BPH in some patients. α-Blockers can be classified according to their receptor selectivity as well as their half-life (Table 23–2).

Phenoxybenzamine and prazosin are the prototypical nonselective and selective α-blockers, but today, they are primarily of historical interest.

Long-acting α_1-blockers make once-a-day dosing possible, but dose titration is still necessary. Terazosin is initiated at 1 mg daily for 3 days and increased to 2 mg daily for 11 days and then to 5 mg/d. Dosage can be escalated to 10 mg daily if necessary. Therapy with doxazosin is started at 1 mg daily for 7 days and increased to 2 mg daily for 7 days, and then to 4 mg daily. Dosage can be escalated to 8 mg daily if necessary. Possible side effects include orthostatic hypotension, dizziness, tiredness, retrograde ejaculation, rhinitis, and headache.

Selective blockade of the α_{1a}-receptors, which are localized in the prostate and bladder neck, results in fewer systemic

Table 23–2. Classification of medical therapy and recommended dosage in BPH.

Classification	Oral dosage
α-Blockers	
Nonselective	
Phenoxybenzamine	10 mg twice a day
α1, short acting	
Prazosin	2 mg twice a day
α1, long acting	
Terazosin	5 or 10 mg daily
Doxazosin	4 or 8 mg daily
α_{1a}-Selective	
Tamsulosin	0.4 or 0.8 mg daily
Alfuzosin	10 mg daily
Silodosin	8 mg daily
5α-Reductase inhibitors	
Finasteride	5 mg daily
Dutasteride	0.5 mg daily

(particularly cardiovascular) side effects, thus obviating the need for dose titration with these agents (tamsulosin, alfuzosin, and silodosin). Other side effects such as retrograde ejaculation still can occur.

Several randomized, double-blind, placebo-controlled trials, individually comparing α-blockers with placebo, have demonstrated the safety and efficacy of all of these agents.

2. 5α-Reductase inhibitors—Finasteride is a 5α-reductase inhibitor that blocks the conversion of testosterone to dihydrotestosterone (DHT). This drug affects the epithelial component of the prostate, resulting in a reduction in the size of the gland and improvement in symptoms. Six-month therapy is required to see the maximum effects on prostate size (20% reduction) and symptomatic improvement.

Several randomized, double-blind, placebo-controlled trials have compared finasteride with placebo. Efficacy, safety, and durability are well established. However, symptomatic improvement is seen only in men with enlarged prostates (>40 cm^3). Side effects are uncommon and include decreased libido, decreased ejaculate volume, and impotence. Serum PSA is reduced by approximately 50% in patients being treated with finasteride, but individual values may vary.

Dutasteride differs from finasteride as it inhibits both isoenzymes of 5α-reductase. Similar to finasteride, it reduces serum PSA and total prostate volume. Randomized, placebo-controlled trials have shown the efficacy of dutasteride in symptomatic relief, symptoms scores, peak urinary flow rate, and reduced risk of acute urinary retention and the need for surgery. Side effects are relatively uncommon and include erectile dysfunction, decreased libido, gynecomastia, and ejaculation disorders. Few studies comparing finasteride and

dutasteride head-to-head. One retrospective analysis of >5000 men older than 65 years treated with 5α-reductase inhibitors in the mid-2000s found small but statistically significantly differences, with rates of urinary retention of 12% and 14.7% for dutasteride and finasteride, respectively ($p = 0.0042$), and rates of prostate surgery of 3.9% and 5.1%, respectively ($p = 0.03$) (Fenter et al, 2008).

3. Combination therapy—The first randomized, double-blind, placebo-controlled study investigating combination α-blocker and 5α-reductase inhibitor therapy was a four-arm Veterans Administration Cooperative Trial comparing placebo, finasteride alone, terazosin alone, and combination finasteride and terazosin (Lepor et al, 1996). More than 1200 patients participated, and significant decreases in IPSS and increases in urinary flow rates were seen only in the arms containing terazosin. However, one must note that enlarged prostates were not an entry criterion; in fact, prostate size in this study was much smaller than that in previous controlled trials using finasteride (32 vs 52 cm^3). McConnell and colleagues conducted a long-term, double-blind trial involving 3047 men to compare the effects of placebo, doxazosin, finasteride, and combination therapy on measures of the clinical progression of BPH (McConnell et al, 2003). The risk of overall clinical progression—defined as an increase above baseline of at least four points in the IPSS, acute urinary retention, urinary incontinence, renal insufficiency, or recurrent urinary tract infection—was significantly reduced by doxazosin (39% risk reduction) and finasteride (34% risk reduction), as compared with placebo. The reduction in risk associated with combination therapy (66% risk reduction) was significantly greater than that associated with doxazosin or finasteride alone. Patients most likely to benefit from combination therapy are those in whom baseline risk of progression is very high, generally patients with larger glands and higher PSA values.

4. Phytotherapy—Phytotherapy refers to the use of plants or plant extracts for medicinal purposes. The use of phytotherapy in BPH has been popular in Europe for years, and its use in the United States is growing as a result of patient-driven enthusiasm. Several plant extracts have been popularized, including the saw palmetto berry (*Serenoa repens*), the bark of *Pygeum africanum*, the roots of *Echinacea purpurea* and *Hypoxis rooperi*, pollen extract, and the leaves of the trembling poplar. *S. repens* has been the most well-studied agent, usually at 320 mg/day. Given the poor regulation of the nutritional supplement industry, actual tablet content may vary extremely from the dose noted on the product label (Feifer et al, 2002). A prospective, randomized clinical trial of saw palmetto showed no benefit beyond placebo for either IPSS improvement or urinary flow rate (Bent et al, 2006). An updated systematic review including this and other trials confirmed no improvement over placebo for this approach (Wilt et al, 2009).

C. Surgical Therapy

1. Transurethral resection of the prostate—The vast majority of subtotal prostatectomies undertaken for BPH can be completed endoscopically. Most of these procedures involve the use of a spinal or general anesthetic and usually require an overnight hospital stay. Magnitude and durability of IPSS and flow rate improvement with transurethral resection of the prostate (TURP) is superior to that of any minimally invasive therapy. However, the length of hospital stay of patients undergoing TURP is greater. Risks of TURP include retrograde ejaculation (75%), impotence (5–10%), and incontinence (<1%). Complications include bleeding; urethral stricture or bladder neck contracture; perforation of the prostate capsule with extravasation; and, if severe, transurethral resection (TUR) syndrome resulting from a hypervolemic, hyponatremic state due to absorption of the hypotonic irrigating solution.

Clinical manifestations of the TUR syndrome include nausea, vomiting, confusion, hypertension, bradycardia, and visual disturbances. The risk of the TUR syndrome increases with resection times >90 minutes and is usually seen in older men. Treatment includes diuresis and, in severe cases, hypertonic saline administration. TURP can now be performed with a bipolar electrode, allowing resection to be performed under saline irrigation. This approach eliminates the hyponatremia responsible for TUR syndrome, though significant fluid volume absorption can still occur with prolonged resection.

2. Transurethral incision of the prostate—Men with moderate to severe symptoms and a small prostate often have posterior commissure hyperplasia (elevated bladder neck). These patients will often benefit from an incision of the prostate. This procedure is more rapid and less morbid than TURP. Outcomes in well-selected patients are comparable, although a lower rate of retrograde ejaculation with transurethral incision has been reported (25%). The technique involves two incisions using the Collins knife at the 5- and 7-o'clock positions. The incisions are started just distal to the ureteral orifices and are extended outward to the verumontanum.

3. Transurethral vaporization of the prostate (TUVP)—Increasingly popular in recent years, ablative techniques use photo- or electroevaporation to ablate obstructing prostate tissue. The two most commonly used devices for these procedures are the neodymium-doped yttrium-aluminum-garnet (Nd:YAG) KTP "GreenLight" laser, which is preferentially absorbed by hemoglobin, and the plasma vaporization "Button" electrode. The latter works with a standard contemporary bipolar generator used for bipolar TURP.

As with modern TURP, these procedures are performed under saline irrigation. The goal of the procedure in either case is to produce a central prostate defect comparable with what would be expected after a traditional TURP, but with less bleeding and lower risk of perforation. The potential downsides are greater irritative voiding symptoms in the short term after the procedure and less durability of the result than a standard TURP. Also, as tissue is destroyed rather than resected, no specimen is sent to pathology for review.

4. Holmium laser enucleation of the prostate (HoLEP)—Rather than progressive resection or ablation of tissue from the urethra outward as with TURP and its derivatives, HoLEP denotes an anatomic dissection in the plane between the central and peripheral zones of the prostate. This approach is felt to provide the largest defect and perhaps the longest durability, but entails a longer learning curve than TURP or TUVP.

5. Simple (subtotal) prostatectomy—When the prostate is too large to be removed endoscopically, an open enucleation is necessary. What constitutes "too large" is subjective and will vary depending upon the surgeon's experience with TURP. Glands >100 g are usually considered for open enucleation. Open prostatectomy may also be initiated when concomitant bladder diverticulum or a large bladder stone is present or if dorsal lithotomy positioning is not possible.

Open prostatectomies can be done with either a suprapubic or retropubic approach. A *simple suprapubic prostatectomy* is performed transvesically and is the operation of choice in dealing with concomitant bladder pathology. After the bladder is opened, a semicircular incision is made in the bladder mucosa, distal to the trigone. The dissection plane is initiated sharply, and then blunt dissection with the finger is performed to remove the adenoma. The apical dissection should be done sharply to avoid injury to the distal sphincteric mechanism. After the adenoma is removed, hemostasis is attained with suture ligatures, and both a urethral and a suprapubic catheter are inserted before closure. In a *simple retropubic prostatectomy*, the bladder is not entered. Rather, a transverse incision is made in the surgical capsule of the prostate, and the adenoma is enucleated as described earlier. Only a urethral catheter is needed at the end of the procedure. *Robot-assisted simple prostatectomy* has been reported in recent small series (Sutherland et al, 2011).

6. Transurethral microwave thermotherapy—Microwave hyperthermia is most commonly delivered with a transurethral catheter. Some devices cool the urethral mucosa to decrease the risk of injury. However, if temperatures are not >45°C, cooling is unnecessary. Improvement in IPSS and flow rate has been documented, but as these procedures are done in the office with no visual verification of tissue ablation, results have been mixed. Strong financial incentives, however, have driven frequent utilization in certain clinical contexts.

Very sparse prospective data are available to fairly compare any of the above procedures with TURP or with each other. A recent meta-analysis found few differences, but the component studies tended to be small and with limited follow-up (Ahyai et al, 2010). All of the newer procedures are more expensive than TURP, and comparative cost-effectiveness studies are sorely needed.

CARCINOMA OF THE PROSTATE

▶ Incidence and Epidemiology

Prostate cancer is the most common noncutaneous cancer detected among American men. More than 200,000 cases are detected annually (Jemal et al, 2010). Approximately 30,000 men die of the disease annually—more than any other tumor type except lung cancer. However, prostate cancer mortality at the population level has declined by roughly 40% since the mid-1990s, during a time in which men have been living longer and therefore have been more likely to reach the older ages at which prostate cancer mortality would be expected to increase. There are no known dietary or other environmental trends that can explain this decline in mortality rates. The explanation is controversial but is likely multifactorial, reflecting a combination of screening programs and improvements in treatment.

These improvements in prostate cancer mortality have come at the cost of significant rates of overdiagnosis and overtreatment. The number of prostate cancer deaths annually is far outweighed by the number of diagnoses, and most men diagnosed ultimately die of other causes, most often cardiovascular disease. Of all cancers, the prevalence of CaP increases the most rapidly with age. However, unlike most cancers, which have a peak age of incidence, the incidence of CaP continues to increase with advancing age. The lifetime risk of a 50-year-old man for latent CaP (ie, detected as an incidental finding at autopsy, not related to the cause of death) is 40%; for lifetime diagnosis of CaP, 15%; and for death from CaP, 2.9%. Thus, many prostate cancers are indolent and inconsequential to the patient while others are virulent, and if detected too late or left untreated, they result in a patient's death. This broad spectrum of biological activity can make decision making for individual patients difficult, and highlight the critical need for risk stratification of prostate cancers, which will be discussed in further detail later.

Several risk factors for prostate cancer have been identified. As discussed earlier, increasing age heightens the risk for CaP. Which of the factors associated with the aging process are responsible for this observation is unknown. The probability of CaP diagnosis in a man younger than 40 years is 1 in 10,000; for men 40–59 years old, it is 1 in 103; and for men 60–79 years old, it is 1 in 8. African Americans are at a higher risk for CaP than whites. In addition, African American men tend to present with higher disease risk than whites. Controversial data have been reported suggesting that mortality from this disease may also be higher for African Americans. A positive family history of CaP also increases the relative risk for CaP. The age of disease onset in the family member with the diagnosis of CaP affects a patient's relative risk. If the age of onset is 70, the relative risk is increased fourfold; if the age of onset is 60, the relative risk is increased fivefold; and if the age of onset is 50, the relative risk is increased sevenfold.

Although diagnostic biases due to varying penetrance of PSA screening exist across countries, differences in the incidence of prostate cancer are real. These differences may be related, in part, to differences in diet (Chan et al, 2005). Epidemiologic studies have shown that the incidence of clinically significant prostate cancer is much lower in parts of the world where people eat a predominantly low fat, plant-based diet. In addition, migrant studies demonstrate that when men from a low-risk country move to the United States and begin eating a westernized diet, their rates of prostate cancer increase severalfold and approach that of the host country. Total fat intake, animal fat intake, and red meat intake are associated with an increased risk of prostate cancer, whereas intake of fish is associated with a decreased risk. There is considerable controversy on the impact of obesity on prostate cancer. Some studies suggest that obesity is associated with an increased risk of more advanced disease and a higher recurrence rate after treatment. In addition, lycopene, selenium, omega-3 fatty acids (fish), and vitamin E intake have been shown to be protective, whereas vitamin D and calcium increase risk. No dietary supplementation study has yet shown a tangible benefit in terms of reducing risk of diagnosis or mortality. Previous vasectomy has been suggested as a factor that heightens the risk for CaP, but this association has not been validated in larger studies (Cox et al, 2002).

▶ Pathology

More than 95% of the prostate cancers are adenocarcinomas. The histology of the remaining 5% of prostate cancer is heterogeneous, arising from stromal, epithelial, or ectopic cells. Nonadenocarcinoma variants can be categorized into two groups based on the cellular origin: epithelial and nonepithelial. Epithelial variants consist of endometrioid, mucinous, signet-ring, adenoid cystic, adenosquamous, squamous cell, transitional cell, neuroendocrine, and comedocarcinoma. Nonepithelial variants include rhabdomyosarcoma, leiomyosarcoma, osteosarcoma, angiosarcoma, carcinosarcoma, malignant lymphoma, and metastatic neoplasms among others.

The remainder of this discussion will focus on adenocarcinoma. However, it is increasingly evident that neuroendocrine ("small cell") differentiation may occur in response to prolonged androgen deprivation. This can be recognized by staining such tissue for neuroendocrine markers (chromogranin A, neuron-specific enolase) and/or by measuring such markers in serum.

The cytologic characteristics of CaP include hyperchromatic, enlarged nuclei with prominent nucleoli (Figure 23–3). Cytoplasm is often abundant; thus, nuclear-to-cytoplasmic ratios are not often helpful in making a diagnosis of CaP, unlike their usefulness in diagnosing many other neoplasms. Cytoplasm is often slightly blue tinged or basophilic, which may assist in the diagnosis. The diagnosis of CaP is truly an

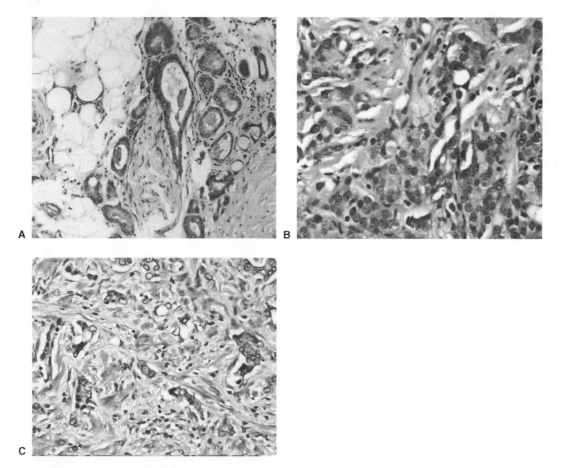

▲ **Figure 23–3.** Gleason primary grade 3 (**A**), grade 4 (**B**), and grade 5 (**C**) cancer (200×). **A:** Glands are well developed with variation in contour and morphology. The glands grow in an infiltrative pattern. Nuclear features of malignancy include mild nuclear enlargement, granular chromatin, and nucleoli. **B:** Malignant cells have trabecular, glandular, and infiltrative growth pattern forming small solid nests and abortive, fused glandular lumens. Malignant nuclear features include marked nuclear enlargement and macronucleoli. **C:** Highly infiltrative growth pattern with single cells and small nests of malignant epithelial cells. Cytologic features include marked nuclear pleomorphism and anisonucleosis with irregular contours, coarse irregular chromatin distribution, and macronucleoli.

architectural one. The basal cell layer is absent in CaP, whereas it is present in normal glands, BPH glands, and the precursor lesions of CaP. If the diagnosis of CaP is in question, high-molecular-weight keratin immunohistochemical staining is useful, as it preferentially stains basal cells. Absence of staining is thus consistent with CaP. Those biopsies that remain equivocal could be stained with new markers such as AMACR or EPCA, which appear to identify those with the disease, but who have equivocal or negative biopsies based on standard tissue staining.

Prostatic intraepithelial neoplasia (PIN) and atypical small acinar proliferation (ASAP) are thought to be precursor lesions. However, the risk of prostate cancer appears to

be higher in those with the latter histology. Men found to have either lesion may be at an increased risk of prostate cancer and warrant repeat biopsy, particularly if an extended-core biopsy was not performed initially. High-grade PIN (HGPIN) is characterized by cellular proliferations within preexisting ducts and glands, with nuclear and nucleolar enlargement similar to prostate cancer. However, unlike cancer, HGPIN retains a basal cell layer identifiable by immunohistochemistry.

Approximately 60–70% of cases of CaP originate in the peripheral zone, 10–20% originate in the transition zone, and 5–10% in the central zone. Although prostate cancer is frequently multifocal, the use of widespread screening and extended biopsy techniques has resulted in the increasing detection of unifocal and smaller cancers.

Penetration of the prostatic capsule by cancer is a common event and often occurs along perineural spaces. Seminal vesicle invasion is associated with a high likelihood of regional or distant disease. Locally advanced CaP may invade the bladder trigone, resulting in ureteral obstruction. Rectal involvement is rare as Denonvilliers' fascia represents a strong barrier. (Of note, this barrier is largely one way, as rectal cancer may invade the prostate relatively commonly.) Lymphatic metastases are most often identified in the obturator, external iliac, and internal lymph node chains. Other sites of nodal involvement include the common iliac, presacral, and periaortic lymph nodes.

The axial skeleton is the most usual site of distant metastases, with the lumbar spine being most frequently implicated (Figure 23–4). The next most common sites in decreasing order are proximal femur, pelvis, thoracic spine, ribs, sternum, skull, and humerus. The bone lesions of metastatic CaP are typically osteoblastic. Involvement of long bones can lead to pathologic fractures. Vertebral body involvement with significant tumor masses extending into the epidural space can result in cord compression. Visceral metastases most commonly involve the lung, liver, and adrenal gland. Central nervous system involvement is usually a result of direct extension from skull metastasis.

▶ Molecular Genetics and Pathobiology

Molecular profiling of human tissues has identified differential expression of specific genes and proteins in the progression from normal precursor tissue to preneoplastic lesions to cancer (both androgen dependent and independent). In doing so, diagnostic, prognostic, and therapeutic markers have been discovered.

Chromosomal rearrangements or copy number abnormalities at 8p, 10q, 11q, 13q, 16q, 17p, and 18q have been described in prostate cancers. Some of these such as specific loss at 8p23.2 and/or gain at 11q13.1 are predictive of prostate cancer progression.

The entire prostate microenvironment, not just the epithelial compartment, is important for both normal and neoplastic growth as significant epithelial–mesenchymal/stromal interactions occur (Chung et al, 2005). Molecular events may not always be spontaneous, but the product of environmental influences. For instance, both epidemiologic and molecular data suggest that inflammation may be related to prostate cancer development (Nelson et al, 2004). RNASEL, encoding an interferon-inducible ribonuclease, and MSR1, encoding subunits of the macrophage scavenger receptor, are candidate-inherited susceptibility genes for prostate cancer, including familial cancer. Proliferative inflammatory atrophy lesions containing activated inflammatory cells and proliferating epithelial cells appear likely to be precursors to PIN lesions and prostatic carcinomas.

Using a novel bioinformatics approach, Tomlins and colleagues identified two transcription factors ERG and EtV1 that were overexpressed in prostate cancer tissue. Furthermore, TMPRSS2 was fused to these genes suggesting that fusion accounted for overexpression. This genetic rearrangement appears to be the most common identified in prostate cancer. The TMPRSS2:ERG fusion has been identified in approximately 50% of prostate tumors and likely represents an early molecular event in carcinogenesis. Furthermore, this fusion may yield a distinct phenotype with a more aggressive natural history, independent of Gleason grade (Narod et al, 2008).

Some overexpressed genes or combinations of genes may be important biomarkers capable of not only identifying cancer in equivocal biopsy samples (alpha-methylacyl coenzyme A racemase [AMACR] and early prostate cancer antigen [EPCA]) but also in predicting response to treatment and progression (Rubin, 2004). Multiple research efforts have identified other promising multiparametric models to improve risk stratification and prediction (Cuzick et al, 2011; Mucci et al,

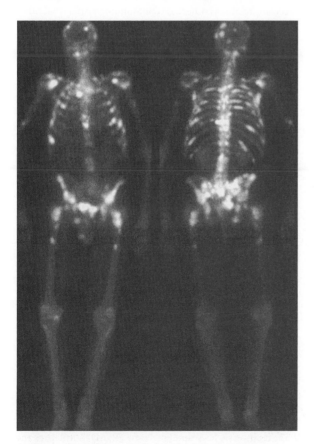

▲ **Figure 23–4.** Whole body bone scintigram showing multiple bone metastases.

2008; Paris et al, 2010; Penney et al, 2011), though none of these has yet been well validated or reached clinical practice. Beyond genetic analyses, parallel advances in proteomics and metabolomics likewise are yielding novel insights into both the pathophysiology of prostate cancer and improved risk stratification of the disease (Sreekumar et al, 2009).

The number of prostate cancers attributable to heritable factors may be greater than once thought (Lichtenstein et al, 2000). Although the loci 8q, 3p, 7p/q, 9q, 10q, 11q, 17q, and 22q have been identified as harboring potential predisposition genes in those with a family history of prostate cancer, a multigene model may best explain familial clustering of this disease. In addition, men with a family history of breast and/or ovarian cancer may be offered a predictive genetic test to determine whether or not they carry the family specific BRCA1/2 mutations as they are at increased risk of breast and prostate cancers.

▶ Clinical Findings

A. Symptoms

The large majority of patients with early-stage CaP are asymptomatic. The presence of symptoms often suggests locally advanced or metastatic disease. Obstructive or irritative voiding complaints can result from local growth of the tumor into the urethra or bladder neck or from its direct extension into the trigone of the bladder. Much more commonly, however, such symptoms are attributable to coexisting BPH. Metastatic disease to the bones may cause bone pain. Metastatic disease to the vertebral column with impingement on the spinal cord may be associated with symptoms of cord compression, including paresthesias and weakness of the lower extremities and urinary or fecal incontinence.

B. Signs

A physical examination, including a DRE, is needed. Induration or nodularity, if detected, must alert the physician to the possibility of cancer and the need for further evaluation (ie, PSA, TRUS, and biopsy). Locally advanced disease with bulky regional lymphadenopathy may lead to lymphedema of the lower extremities. Specific signs of cord compression relate to the level of the compression and may include weakness or spasticity of the lower extremities and a hyperreflexic bulbocavernosus reflex.

C. General Laboratory Findings

Azotemia can result from bilateral ureteral obstruction either from direct extension into the trigone or from retroperitoneal adenopathy. Anemia may be present in metastatic disease. Alkaline phosphatase may be elevated in the presence of bone metastases. Serum acid phosphatase may be elevated with disease outside the confines of the prostate.

D. Prostate-Specific Antigen and Other Tumor Markers

PSA is a serine protease in the human kallikrein (hK) family produced by benign and malignant prostate tissues. It circulates in the serum as uncomplexed (free or unbound) or complexed (bound) forms. PSA is used both as a diagnostic (screening) tool and as a means of risk-stratifying known prostate cancers. In both contexts, its use is complicated by the fact that PSA is *prostate* specific, not *prostate cancer* specific. Other prevalent conditions such as BPH and prostatitis—as well as urethral instrumentation and perineal insults such as prolonged bike ride—can elevate the PSA, producing false-positive results.

A "normal" PSA has traditionally been defined as ≤4 ng/mL, and the positive predictive value of a serum PSA between 4 and 10 ng/mL is approximately 20–30%. For levels in excess of 10 ng/mL, the positive predictive value increases from 42% to 71.4%. In light of variation with age and ethnicity, age- and race-specific reference ranges have been proposed (Oesterling et al, 1993). More importantly, the results of the Prostate Cancer Prevention Trial (PCPT) study, which included biopsy regardless of PSA level—thus avoiding the ascertainment bias otherwise confounding virtually all other studies of PSA—demonstrated that there is no level of PSA below which prostate cancer risk falls to zero. PSA is rather indicative of a continuum of risk—the higher the level, the higher the risk (Thompson et al, 2004).

Current prostate cancer screening and detection strategies therefore include with PSA other risk factors such as family history, race, age, and others (Greene et al, 2009). Online risk calculators integrating these variables have been made generated to determine risk of prostate cancer and risk of high-grade prostate cancer. A calculator based on the PCPT data, for example, is available at http://tinyurl.com/caprisk.

Use of medications such as 5α-reductase inhibitors (including the 1 mg finasteride formulation marked for alopecia as Propecia) must be ascertained, as these medications can artificially lower the PSA by approximately 50%. Interestingly, serum PSA levels have also been noted to be decreased in men with high body mass indexes compared with normal weight men, likely as a result of hemodilution (Banez et al, 2007).

Numerous strategies to refine PSA for cancer detection have been explored. Their common goal in general has been to decrease the number of false-positive test results, thus increasing the specificity and positive predictive value of the test and lead to fewer unnecessary biopsies, lower costs, and reduced morbidity of cancer detection. Attempts at refining PSA have included PSA velocity (PSAV) (change of PSA over time), PSA kinetics (standardizing levels in relation to the size of the prostate), and PSA isoforms (free vs protein-bound molecular forms of PSA).

1. PSA kinetics—PSAV refers to the rate of change of serum PSA; its inverse, PSA doubling time (PSADT) indicates the amount of time required for the PSA to double. A retrospective study has shown that men with prostate cancer have a more rapidly rising serum PSA in the years before diagnosis than do men without prostate cancer. Patients whose serum PSA increases by 0.75 ng/mL per year appear to be at an increased risk of harboring cancer. However, PSAV must be interpreted with caution. An elevated PSAV should be considered significant only when several serum PSA assays are carried out by the same laboratory over a period of at least 18 months. Very rapid PSA increases may be indicative of prostatitis (symptomatic or otherwise) rather than cancer. Recent studies have questioned whether PSA kinetics in fact add significantly to the absolute PSA level in the prediagnosis setting (Vickers et al, 2011), and the optimal use of PSA kinetics remains controversial.

2. PSA density—PSA levels are elevated on average approximately 0.12 ng/mL per gram of BPH tissue. Thus, patients with enlarged glands due to BPH may have elevated PSA levels. The ratio of PSA to gland volume is termed the PSA density. Some investigators advocate prostate biopsy only if the PSA density exceeds 0.1 or 0.15, while others have not found PSA density to be useful. Problems with this approach include the facts that (1) epithelial–stromal ratios vary from gland to gland and only the epithelium produces PSA and (2) errors in calculating prostatic volume based on TRUS may approach 25%. The positive predictive value of PSA density is slightly higher than the use of a PSA level >4 ng/mL in several series (30–40% vs 20–30%). The other major problem with PSA doubling (PSAD) is that it still requires TRUS, which, while a lower risk procedure than biopsy, is still invasive and uncomfortable. Thus, PSAD may be most useful in settings in which the prostate volume is already known (ie, PSA rising after a negative prior biopsy).

Instead of adjusting the PSA to total prostate volume, some have advocated adjusting it to transition zone volume (PSA transition zone density, PSAT [Djavan et al, 2002]). However, like PSA density, such calculations are subject to error, require TRUS, and do not seem to be superior to the use of PSA in most patients.

3. Molecular forms of PSA—Various molecular isoforms of PSA have been identified and studied. Approximately 90% of the serum PSA is bound to α_1-antichymotrypsin (ACT), and lesser amounts are free or are bound to α_2-macroglobulins. In the latter form, no epitopes to the antibodies used in the current assays are available, while PSA bound ACT may have three of its five epitopes masked. Early studies suggest that prostate cancer patients demonstrate a lower percentage of free PSA than do patients with benign disease. A large multicenter study has reported that in men with a normal DRE and a total PSA level between 4 and 10 ng/mL, a 25% free PSA cutoff would detect 95% of cancers while avoiding 20% of unnecessary biopsies. The cancers associated with >25% free PSA were more prevalent in older patients and generally were less threatening in terms of tumor grade and volume (Catalona et al, 1998). The predictive utility of percentage of free PSA in subsequent studies, however, has been mixed.

More recent studies have focused on other PSA subtypes. A serum panel adding free PSA, intact PSA, and hK2 to total PSA has been shown to improve predictive accuracy for prostate cancer diagnosis among men with a PSA >3 (Vickers et al, JCO 2010) and is currently undergoing validation studies. A truncated form of PSA designated −2proPSA has also shown promise in this setting and is likewise undergoing validation studies (Catalona et al, 2011; Mikolajczyk et al, 2004).

4. PCA3—Prostate cancer antigen 3 (PCA3) is a noncoding, prostate-specific mRNA, which is overexpressed in the majority of prostate cancers, with a median 66-fold upregulation compared with adjacent noncancer tissue (Hessels et al, 2007). PCA3 predicts the presence of cancer in a biopsy setting with an accuracy of 74.6% (Groskopf et al, 2006). PCA3 may be particularly useful in the evaluation of men with a negative prior biopsy and a rising PSA (Haese et al, 2008).

▶ Diagnosis and Evaluation

A. Prostate Biopsy

Prostate biopsy should be considered in men with an elevated serum PSA, abnormal DRE, or a combination of the two, depending additionally on the patient's overall health, comorbidities, life expectancy, levels of anxiety and of risk aversion, and information preferences. Prostate biopsy is performed under TRUS guidance using a spring-loaded biopsy device coupled to the imaging probe. Biopsies are taken throughout the peripheral zone of the prostate, with optional additional sampling of any abnormal areas on DRE and/or TRUS. Traditionally, six (sextant) biopsies were taken along a parasagittal line between the lateral edge and the midline of the prostate at the apex, midgland, and base bilaterally. However, several investigators have shown that increasing the number (≥10) and performing more laterally directed biopsies of the peripheral zone will increase detection rates 14–20% over the more traditional sextant technique. Although a small number of prostate cancers will originate in the transition zone, specific transition zone biopsies add little to overall cancer detection rates when an extended-pattern biopsy is performed. Some practitioners do add biopsies of the anterior commissure, a relatively frequent site of initially missed cancers found on second or subsequent biopsy. There is ongoing interest in the use of even more extended biopsy schemes ("saturation biopsy") or use of a transperineal approach to improve cancer detection, usually in those who have had a negative biopsy, but are thought to be at an increased risk of prostate cancer based on a persistently abnormal serum PSA.

Prostate biopsy is usually performed using local anesthesia and preprocedure antibiotic prophylaxis (usually a fluoroquinolone). The use of local anesthesia, either applied topically along the anterior rectal wall, injected into or adjacent to the prostate, or a combination of the two, decreases pain associated with the procedure. Hematospermia, hematochezia, and hematuria are common occurring in approximately 40–50% of patients. With rising prevalence of antibiotic-resistant bacteria, rates of sepsis despite standard prophylaxis have been growing (Lange et al, 2009). These can be life threatening even in otherwise-healthy men, and patients are counseled to return immediately to the emergency department for any high fevers after the procedure.

Saturation schemes consist of 20 or more cores that emphasize sampling of the peripheral zone. One of the more common saturation schemes involves taking two cores from the lateral base, three cores from the lateral mid, three cores from the apex (including anterior apex), and one core from the parasagittal mid and one core from the parasagittal base. While initial saturation schemes included two cores at both the parasagittal mid and parasagittal base, unique identification of cancer in these areas is rare and thus it has been recommended to only obtain one care for each of these areas. Investigators have demonstrated that saturation biopsies can be performed in the office using a periprostatic block. They observed no improved yield by using a saturation biopsy as the initial biopsy scheme or the first repeat biopsy scheme but rather advocate it as a second repeat biopsy strategy (Jones et al, 2002).

The Reduction by Dutasteride of Prostate Cancer Events (REDUCE) trial allows us to prospectively look at both cancer detection rates and quality of cancers in a repeat biopsy situation. Recall that entry criteria for this trial mandated a prior negative biopsy (minimum of a negative sextant biopsy) within 6 months of enrollment. In the placebo arm, 3346 patients underwent a repeat biopsy within 1–2 years of enrollment and 17.2% were found to have cancer of which 30% were high grade (Gleason score >7). At the repeat biopsy between years 3 and 4, 11.7% of 2343 patients were found to have cancer of which 21% were high grade. Considering only patients with primary Gleason pattern 4 or 5, 8.7% and 2.6% of the cancers were high grade at the 2- and 4-year biopsy, respectively. This study also compared the relative merit of PCA3 and F/T PSA in the repeat biopsy population. No significant difference was seen between these two markers for predicting cancer (Andriole et al, 2010).

B. Grading and Staging

The Gleason system is the most commonly employed grading system. The system relies on the low-power appearance of the glandular architecture under the microscope. In assigning a grade to a given tumor, pathologists assign a primary grade to the pattern of cancer that is most commonly observed and a secondary grade to the second most commonly observed pattern in the specimen. Grades range from 1 to 5 (Figure 23–3). If the entire specimen has only one pattern present, then both the primary and secondary grade are reported as the same grade (eg, 3 + 3). The *Gleason score* or *Gleason sum*

is obtained by adding the primary and secondary grades together.

Traditionally, Gleason grades ranged from 1 to 5, and Gleason scores thus ranged from 2 to 10. Gleason scores of 2–4, 5–7, and 8–10 corresponded to well-, moderately, and poorly differentiated tumors, respectively. However, pathology grading practices have changed over time, and this grouping is largely outdated (though it is still sometimes reported in the literature). In contemporary pathology practice, Gleason patterns 1 and 2 are rarely assigned, so *Gleason pattern 3* corresponds with low-grade disease (variable-sized glands that percolate through normal stroma and between normal glands), *Gleason pattern 4* corresponds with intermediate-grade disease (incompletely formed glands with variable amounts of fusion and more infiltrative growth pattern), and *Gleason pattern 5* corresponds with high-grade disease (single infiltrating cells with no gland formation). Variations in growth such as cribriform patterns and comedocarcinoma are also observed.

A Gleason score 6 (3 + 3) tumor is uniformly low grade. In differentiating intermediate- and high-grade tumors, the primary Gleason pattern is the most important determinant of biologic risk. Thus, among Gleason score 7 tumors, those assigned 4 + 3 are more aggressive than those read as 3 + 4. Many clinical series have failed to distinguish between these two populations and, therefore, caution must be exercised in reviewing these series.

The 2010 AJCC TNM staging system for CaP is presented in Table 23–3. Note that with respect to the primary tumor categorization (T stage), the clinical staging system uses results of the DRE and TRUS, but not the results of the biopsy. Some examples to illustrate this staging system are as follows. If a patient has a palpable abnormality on one side of the prostate, even though biopsies demonstrate bilateral disease, his clinical stage remains T2a. If a patient has a normal DRE, with TRUS demonstrating a lesion on one side and a biopsy confirming cancer, his clinical stage is also T2a (using results of DRE and TRUS). A T1c cancer must have *both* a normal DRE and a normal TRUS. It should be noted that compared with risk factors such as Gleason score and PSA levels, clinical T stage in prostate cancer is a relatively weak prognostic factor. Partly due to the subjectivity of DRE and TRUS interpretation, and given adjustment for more objective measures of tumor volume such as percent of biopsy cores involved, T stage often drops out of multivariable models of prostate cancer prognosis, at least among T1 and T2 tumors which account for the vast majority of tumors diagnosed in contemporary practice (Reese et al, 2011)

C. Imaging

1. TRUS—As described earlier, TRUS is useful in helping guide prostatic biopsies and other prostate-directed interventions. TRUS also provides useful local staging information if cancer is detected, usually with greater accuracy than

Table 23–3. TNM staging system for prostate cancer.

T—Primary tumor	
Tx	Cannot be assessed
T0	No evidence of primary tumor
Tis	Carcinoma in situ (PIN)
T1a	≤5% of tissue in resection for benign disease has cancer, normal DRE
T1b	>5% of tissue in resection for benign disease has cancer, normal DRE
T1c	Detected from elevated PSA alone, normal DRE and imaging
T2a	Tumor palpable by DRE or visible by imaging, involving less than half of one lobe of the prostate
T2b	Tumor palpable by DRE or visible by imaging, involving more than half of one lobe of the prostate
T2c	Tumor palpable by DRE or visible by imaging, involving both lobes of the prostate
T3a	Extracapsular extension on one or both sides
T3b	Seminal vesicle involvement on one or both sides
T4	Tumor directly extends into bladder neck, sphincter, rectum, levator muscles, or into pelvic sidewall
N—Regional lymph nodes (obturator, internal iliac, external iliac, presacral lymph nodes)	
Nx	Cannot be assessed
N0	No regional lymph node metastasis
N1	Metastasis in a regional lymph node or nodes
M—Distant metastasis	
Mx	Cannot be assessed
M0	No distant metastasis
M1a	Distant metastasis in nonregional lymph nodes
M1b	Distant metastasis to bone
M1c	Distant metastasis to other sites

DRE, digital rectal examination; PIN, prostatic intraepithelial neoplasia; PSA, prostate-specific antigen; TRUS, transrectal ultrasound.

Source: American Joint Committee on Cancer: *Cancer Staging Manual*, 7th ed. Lippincott-Raven, 2010.

DRE. If visible, CaP tends to appear as a hypoechoic lesion in the peripheral zone and/or hypervascularity seen on power Doppler examination. The sonographic criteria for extracapsular extension are bulging of the prostate contour or angulated appearance of the lateral margin. The criteria for seminal vesicle invasion are a posterior bulge at the base of the seminal vesicle or asymmetry in echogenicity of the seminal vesicle associated with hypoechoic areas at the base of the prostate. In some protocols under development, 3D TRUS permits a three-dimensional image to be constructed from a series of 2D images by a computer algorithm. Use of an intravenous microbubbles may also improve visualization of tumor microvasculature, and targeted microbubbles under development may further improve this emerging modality (Sanna et al, 2011). Elastography—an imaging modality based on differential compressibility of benign and malignant tissue—may also emerge as a useful adjunct to standard TRUS (Mahdavi et al, 2011).

2. Endorectal magnetic resonance imaging (MRI)—Use of an endorectal coil improves cancer detection and staging compared with the use of a standard body coil. While rendering high image quality, the use of an endorectal coil appears to be operator dependent, requiring education and expertise. Routine use of this technology may not alter treatment decisions compared with the information gained by assessment of more standard clinicopathologic information. Use of magnetic resonance spectroscopy (MRS) in conjunction with MRI may improve the accuracy of imaging. Prostate cancer is associated with proportionately lower levels of citrate and higher levels of choline and creatine compared with BPH or normal prostate tissue. The combined metabolic and anatomic information provided by a multiparametric MRI exam and MRS may allow for a more accurate assessment of cancer location and stage. The reported staging accuracy of endorectal MRI varies from 51% to 92%. It appears to add novel information to the assessment of some patients over the use of nomograms alone, but it may be best utilized in high-risk patients where it is most accurate and helpful (Afnan et al, 2010; Verma et al, 2010).

3. Axial imaging (CT, MRI)—Cross-sectional imaging of the pelvis in patients with CaP is selectively performed to exclude lymph node metastases in high-risk patients who are thought to be candidates for definitive local therapy, whether it be surgery or irradiation. Both CT and body coil-based MRI are used for this purpose. Neither modality is particularly accurate for local T staging. Patients identified as having lymphadenopathy on imaging may occasionally undergo CT-guided fine-needle aspiration if the diagnosis is equivocal. If lymph node metastases are confirmed, such patients may be candidates for alternative treatment regimens. However, the incidence of lymph node metastases in contemporary radical prostatectomy (RP) series is low (<10%). In addition, imaging is costly and its sensitivity is limited (30–40%). Various criteria can be used to identify patients for axial imaging, including negative bone scans and either T3 cancers or a PSA >20 ng/mL and primary Gleason grade 4 or 5 cancers. Like bone scan, cross-sectional imaging—CT in particular—is widely overused for staging of low-risk tumors which are very unlikely to be associated with lymph node metastases.

Intravenous administration of superparamagnetic nanoparticles, which gain access to lymph nodes by means of interstitial-lymphatic fluid transport, at the time of high-resolution MRI, appears to improve visualization of small nodal metastases, but this agent is not yet approved for use in the United States.

4. Bone scan—When prostate cancer metastasizes, it most commonly does so to the bone (Figure 23–4). Soft tissue metastases (eg, lung and liver) are rare at the time of initial presentation. Although a bone scan has been considered a standard part of the initial evaluation of men with newly diagnosed prostate cancer, good evidence has been accumulated that it can be excluded in most of these men on the basis of serum PSA. Several investigators have shown that bone scans can be omitted in patients with newly diagnosed, untreated prostate cancer who are asymptomatic, have T1 and T2 disease, and have serum PSA concentrations <20 ng/mL. These recommendations in fact are incorporated into clinical guidelines for the management of clinically localized prostate cancer, but bone scan remains widely overused among men with low-risk disease, as confirmed in a number of recent studies (Palvolgi et al, 2011).

5. Antibody imaging—ProstaScint is a murine monoclonal antibody to prostate-specific membrane antigen (PSMA), which is conjugated to [111]indium. After infusion of the antibody, single photon emission computed tomography (SPECT) images are usually obtained at 30 minutes to access vasculature and at 72–120 hours. It has been studied—and is Food and Drug Administration (FDA) approved—for initial staging and workup of recurrent disease. However, the antibody recognizes an intracellular epitope of PSMA; only soft tissues are imaged and the test may suffer from both false-positive and -negative results in both clinical situations described earlier. Use of new antibodies, which recognize the extracellular domain of PSMA, appear to allow for recognition of both bone and soft tissue metastases and could be used as agents for therapy, not only improved imaging (Bander et al, 2006).

D. Multivariable Risk Assessment

As discussed elsewhere in this chapter, contemporary treatment patterns for prostate cancer are marked by both overtreatment of low-risk disease and undertreatment of high-risk disease. A key approach to mitigating this problem is better and more consistent risk stratification intended to help identify the best timing and intensity of treatment for a given patient. The critical variables for optimal risk stratification have been detailed earlier: the PSA level, the Gleason score, and some measure of tumor volume—clinical T stage and/or extent of biopsy core involvement (eg, percent of cores positive or percent of all biopsy tissue positive). More than 100 risk formulae, lookup tables, nomograms, and other instruments have been published to help with this task (Cooperberg, 2008; Shariat et al, 2008). Some key instruments are described as follows.

1. Risk groups—One of the first widely adopted approaches to risk stratification is a three-level risk group classification published by D'Amico et al and formally adopted by the AUA's practice guideline for localized prostate cancer treatment (D'Amico et al, 1998; Thompson, 2007). In this classification, men are assigned to one of three groups as follows:

Low risk: PSA ≤10, Gleason ≤6, and clinical stage T1 or T2a.

Intermediate risk: PSA 10–20, Gleason 7, or clinical stage T2b.

High risk: PSA >20, Gleason 8–10, or clinical stage T2c or T3a.

The major advantage to this system is its simplicity, and it is used very commonly. However, it has significant drawbacks. First, it overweights T stage which, as noted earlier, is not an accurate measure of tumor extent within the T2 category. Second, it does not distinguish between Gleason 3 + 4 and 4 + 3 tumors, which (again, as noted earlier) behave very differently within the Gleason 7 category. Finally, and most importantly, it is not a true multivariable instrument in that it does not account for information from the various risk variables. Both a PSA 19.8, Gleason 4 + 3, stage T2b tumor and a PSA 4.2, Gleason 3 + 4, stage T1c tumor are "intermediate risk" in this classification, but would be expected to behave quite differently.

2. Lookup tables and nomograms—Most risk instruments are based on multivariable logistic regression or Cox proportional hazards models depending on the outcome of interest. For example, the well-validated lookup tables first published by Partin et al predict pathologic outcomes such as extracapsular extension and seminal vesicle invasion (Makarov et al, 2007).

A nomogram is a graphical representation of a regression model. First popularized in urology by Kattan et al (2003), nomograms are alternatives to lookup tables (see Figure 23–5). To use a nomogram, a patient is assigned a number of points for each risk factor; these are then summed to yield a prediction for the outcome (eg, 5-year biochemical recurrence-free survival), usually with a ±10% margin of error.

Many other nomograms have been published since, intended to predict pathologic outcomes, biochemical outcomes after surgery or radiation therapy, or longer-term outcomes such as metastasis or mortality. Two important caveats should be noted. First, a given nomogram is developed based on data from a specific cohort of men, usually treated in one or a few academic centers in which a small number of highly trained surgeons or radiation oncologists treat large volumes of patients. A great deal of caution must be exercised in calculating specific risks of recurrence for patients treated in other settings by different clinicians, and ideally nomograms should be formally validated in a given setting before they are used routinely in that setting (Greene, 2004).

Second, with computer software, it is very easy to calculate multiple nomogram scores simultaneously, creating a temptation to use the nomogram scores to compare treatment options such as surgery or radiation. Nomograms cannot be used this way—the cohorts of patients used to develop each are very different, as are the definitions of the outcomes reported. In particular, with few exceptions, nomograms predict likelihood of PSA recurrence after treatment, which is defined very differently after radiation than after surgery. Thus, nomograms may be useful to give a patient undergoing a specific treatment a sense of the likely outcomes, but should not help guide treatment decisions.

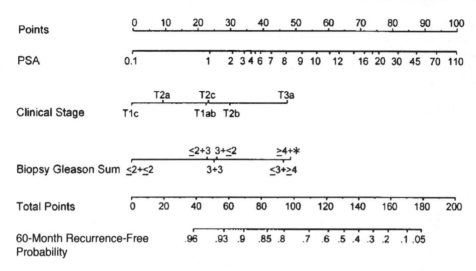

▲ Figure 23–5.

3. CAPRA score—Because of these limitations—and the fact that nomograms are difficult to calculate for hundreds or thousands of patients in research settings and cannot be used to consistently identify low- or high-risk cohorts—the UCSF Cancer of the Prostate Risk Assessment (CAPRA) score was developed, intended to combine the accuracy of nomograms with the ease of calculation of a risk grouping system (Cooperberg et al, 2005). To calculate the CAPRA score, points are assigned based primarily on the PSA and Gleason score, with lesser weights given to T stage, percent of biopsy cores positive, and patient age (Figure 23–6):

Points are added to yield a 0–10 score. Overall, every 2-point increase in score (eg, from 2 to 4 or from 5 to 7)

indicates roughly a doubling of risk. CAPRA scores in the 0–2 range indicate relatively low-risk disease, CAPRA 3–5 tumors are intermediate risk, and CAPRA 6–10 tumors are high risk. The CAPRA score has been widely validated in the United States and Europe in multiple contexts. It was recently found to offer better accuracy than competing instruments in an independent head-to-head comparison study (Lugghezani, Eur Urol 2009). Moreover, it has been shown to predict metastasis and mortality as well as biochemical outcomes—after surgery, radiation therapy, and hormonal therapy (Cooperberg et al, 2009). A postoperative version incorporating pathologic data has also been published recently, but it has not yet been externally validated (Cooperberg et al, Cancer 2011).

Variable	Level	Points	Variable	Level	Points
PSA	≤6	0	T-stage	T1/T2	0
	6.1-10	1		T3a	1
	10.1-20	2			
	20.1-30	3	% of biopsy cores positive	<34%	0
	>30	4		≥34%	1
Gleason (primary/secondary)	1-3/1-3	0			
	1-3/4-5	1	Age	<50	0
	4-5/1-5	3		≥50	1

▲ Figure 23–6.

It is important to note that the CAPRA score is primarily meant to indicate *relative* rather than absolute risk. Thus, a tumor with a CAPRA score of 4 has an intermediate risk of recurrence or progression after surgery or radiation. This tumor will be *more likely* to progress than one with a score of 2, and *less likely* than one with a score of 6, regardless of treatment approach or setting. The *specific* risk (eg, likelihood of being free of disease at 5 years after treatment), while roughly consistent across different cohorts, will depend at least in part on factors such as surgeon skill and experience, pathology grading practices, etc.

▶ Prostate Cancer Screening and Chemoprevention

Prostate cancer screening is a subject of substantial ongoing controversy in the United States and elsewhere. Some organizations, such as the AUA, generally support at least offering screening to men with good life expectancy (at least 10 years), whereas others are neutral and some, such as the US Preventive Services Task Force (2008), are relatively hostile to screening (Greene et al, 2009).

The case for CaP screening is supported by the following: the disease is burdensome in this country; PSA improves detection of clinically important tumors without significantly increasing the detection of unimportant tumors; most PSA-detected tumors are curable; prostate cancer mortality is declining in regions where screening occurs; and curative treatments are available. If screening is undertaken, it appears that the use of both DRE and serum PSA is preferable to either one used alone. Although most guidelines recommend that screening be undertaken at age 50, some have advocated for earlier screening starting at age 40, based on (1) less confounding of PSA assessment by BPH at earlier ages and (2) the fact that a small but significant number of men already have high-risk or advanced prostate cancer by the age of 50. There is broader consensus that screening should start earlier for men with risk factors such as family history and/or African American ethnicity. Although annual screening is most often recommend in the United States, some feel that men with very low serum PSA level (eg, ≤1 ng/mL) may be able to be screened at less frequent intervals (every 2 or 3 years). Determining an optimal interval for screening is another rationale for establishing a baseline PSA level at age 40. Similarly, if the PSA level remains <1 ng/mL by the age of 60, then the likelihood of death from prostate cancer by the age of 85 falls to <1% (Vickers et al, BMJ 2010).

Two large randomized screening trials were reported in 2009, which, if anything, only fueled the controversy surrounding screening. The Prostate, Lung, Colorectal and Ovarian (PLCO) Cancer Screening Trial randomized 76,693 men in the United States to annual PSA screening or usual care. The risk of prostate cancer death with 7 to 10 years follow-up was very low both in screened and unscreened men and did not differ significantly between them. However, the duration of follow-up was too short to observe a difference given the long natural of prostate cancer. Moreover, a very high proportion of men in the "control" arm of the study, in fact, were screened with PSA before the start of the study and/or during the study. Finally, the rate of prostate biopsy among men who crossed the predefined PSA threshold of 4.0 ng/mL was quite low. These limitations limit the ability of this study to fairly test the hypothesis, even as longer follow-up accumulates in the future (Andriole et al, 2009). Despite these limitations, a recent subset analysis found a substantial decrease in prostate cancer–specific mortality for men undergoing screening with no major comorbidity, while those with comorbid disease demonstrated a trend toward *increased* mortality in the screening arm (Crawford et al, 2011).

The European Randomized Study of Screening for Prostate Cancer (ERSPC) randomized 162,387 men in seven countries to PSA screening at 2- or 4-year intervals, with biopsy thresholds ranging from 2.5 to 4.0 ng/mL. This was a larger study than PLCO, with longer follow-up and much less contamination among control patients. The study demonstrated that screening was associated with a 20% relative reduction in prostate cancer–specific mortality at 9 years median follow-up. A follow-up analysis found that with adjustment for compliance with screening, the reduction in mortality rose to 31%. The hazard curves in the ERSPC study only began to diverge approximately 7 years into the trial; thus, with longer follow-up, the observed benefit to screening will likely be further magnified (Schroder, 2009). In a subanalysis of patients from one of the ERSPC study centers with particularly high compliance and long (14 years) follow-up, the mortality reduction was nearly 50% (Hugosson, 2010).

The primary argument against screening is that many cancers identified through screening efforts would never result in clinically significant disease in the patient if left untreated, a phenomenon called overdetection. Some have estimated that between 29% and 48% of cancers detected by an aggressive screening program are such cancers (Draisma et al, 2003; Etzioni et al, 2002). This underscores the importance of informed consent before screening is undertaken and the need to discuss all treatment options, including active surveillance, in those found to have the disease. Indeed, overdetection is primarily a problem to the extent that it leads to overtreatment, which in fact is a pervasive problem in the United States and elsewhere (Cooperberg, JCO 2010). It is hoped that properly risk-adapted management strategies, including greater use of active surveillance for men with lower risk disease, may ultimately ameliorate the controversy surrounding screening, at least to an extent.

▶ Chemoprevention

There is much interest in prostate cancer prevention due to the disease's high prevalence, slowly progressive nature, long latency period, and high absolute mortality. The ideal therapeutic intervention would arrest disease progression during the latency period and decrease the incidence of clinical disease. The ideal agent should be nontoxic and of low cost and the ideal patient would be one at high risk of the disease. To date, several promising chemopreventive agents have been identified and are under laboratory and clinical investigation.

In the PCPT, 18,882 men aged 55 or older with normal DRE and PSA level <3 ng/mL were randomized to either placebo or the 5α-reductase inhibitor, finasteride (5 mg/day) (Thompson et al, 2003). Prostate cancer was detected in 18.4% of those on finasteride and 24.4% on placebo, for a 24.8% reduction in prevalence. Cancers of Gleason grades 7, 8, 9, or 10 were more common in the finasteride group than in the placebo group (37.0% vs 22.2%). This apparent increase in the risk of high-grade cancers may be artifactual for several reasons, related most importantly to downsizing of benign prostate tissue by the medication and resulting improvement in the receiver operating characteristic curve of prostate biopsy for the *detection* of high-grade cancer (by analogy, one is more likely to find a given needle in a smaller haystack than in a larger haystack). However, this question—whether the higher incidence of high-grade disease is attributable to detection bias—remains controversial, and the FDA decided recently not only to decline an expanded label for chemoprevention for 5α-reductase inhibitors but also to add an explicit warning to the labels regarding risk of high-grade prostate cancer (Theoret et al, 2011). Sexual side effects were more common in those receiving finasteride, whereas urinary symptoms were more common in those receiving placebo.

Another recently reported placebo-controlled, randomized trial (the REDUCE study) found a similar 22.8% reduction in incidence of prostate cancer among men 50–75 years of age, with PSA levels 2.5–10 ng/mL and a prior negative biopsy, who were treated with dutasteride rather than placebo. As in the PCPT, urinary symptoms were significantly ameliorated on the treatment arm, at the expense of sexual side effects among some participants (Andriole et al, 2010).

Uptake of prostate cancer chemoprevention with 5α-reductase inhibitors has been slow since the PCPT was first reported, but a guideline from the AUA and American Society of Clinical Oncology advises that men at risk be informed of chemoprevention as an option (Kramer et al, 2009). Other chemoprevention studies are ongoing, but no other agents have yet been found to be as promising as finasteride and dutasteride. In one notable negative study (the SELECT study), a randomized, placebo-controlled trial of >35,000 men, selenium and vitamin E were shown to be of no benefit for prostate cancer chemoprevention (Lippman et al, 2009).

▶ **Treatment**

A. Localized Disease

1. General considerations—The optimal form of therapy for all stages of CaP remains a subject of great debate.

Treatment dilemmas persist in the management of localized disease (T1 and T2) because of the uncertainty surrounding the relative efficacy of various modalities, including RP, radiation therapy, and surveillance. Currently, treatment decisions are based on the grade and stage of the tumor, the life expectancy of the patient, the ability of each therapy to ensure disease-free survival, its associated morbidity, and patient and physician preferences. Until recently, there was little information to be sure that treatment of early stage disease had an important impact on overall and cancer-specific survival. A well-conducted randomized trial of RP versus surveillance in men with early stage prostate cancer generally diagnosed before the PSA era was conducted in Scandinavia (Bill-Axelson et al, 2011). With 13 years follow-up, men who underwent RP were less likely to die of prostate cancer (relative risk, 0.62). The advantage to surgery was most apparent in younger patients (<65 years old at diagnosis).

No randomized controlled trials comparing active local therapies (eg, surgery and radiation therapy) have been published. Studies of nonrandomized but prospectively accrued cohorts with high quality data have recently shown, after extensive risk adjustment and various controls for confounding, a consistent mortality benefit for surgery relative to external beam radiation therapy or hormonal therapy, and for any local therapy (surgery or radiation) relative to hormonal therapy alone (Cooperberg, Cancer 2010; Zelefsky, 2010). The differences seem to be greatest for men with relatively high-risk tumors. Other similar studies are ongoing. Despite the ongoing controversies, what is clear is that many men with low-risk disease are candidates for active surveillance; those with low- to intermediate-risk disease should receive local monotherapy (surgery or radiation), and those with higher-risk disease usually need multimodal therapy, either radiation with hormonal therapy or surgery followed selectively by radiation depending on the pathology and early PSA outcomes. These strategies are described in further detail later.

2. Watchful waiting and active surveillance—Although local cancer progression may occur, with watchful waiting for early stage prostate cancer, disease-specific mortality at 10 years is low varying generally between 4% and 15%. However, in further follow-up from 15 to 20 years, a substantial increase in the risk of local and systemic progression and death from prostate cancer may be seen (Johansson, Andren et al, 2004). The risk of progression is related significantly to cancer grade. The risk of progression is low in those with Gleason grades 2–6 (no pattern 4 or 5), but increases significantly for those with high-grade disease, even among men diagnosed at relatively advanced age (Lu-Yao, 2009). Most of the men, in these previously reported series of men managed with watchful waiting, had palpable disease and, therefore, larger, more significant cancer than most of those detected currently based on serum PSA. In addition, most men were not followed carefully with periodic clinical, radiographic, and laboratory (PSA) reevaluation. They were treated, usually with androgen deprivation, when symptomatic metastatic disease was detected.

A more modern concept of watchful waiting is better termed "**active surveillance.**" In surveillance, men with very well-characterized, early-stage, and low- to intermediate-grade cancer are followed very carefully with serial DRE and PSA assessments, and follow-up TRUS-guided biopsies to ensure stability of the tumor. Cancers are usually treated at the first sign of subclinical progression (Cooperberg et al, 2011a, 2011b; Dall'Era, Cancer 2008; Klotz, 2010). Although between 20% and 41% of men on such regimens may require treatment at 3–5 years of follow-up, treatment at progression appears to be as effective as it would have been if delivered at the time of diagnosis for most men. Optimal surveillance strategies, end points for intervention, and exact risks of surveillance have not been well defined, as yet. There is little question, however, that given the trends toward diagnosis of low-risk, often indolent tumors, active surveillance remains underused as an initial management strategy and likely will play a greater role in the coming years.

3. Radical prostatectomy—The first radical perineal prostatectomy was performed by Hugh Hampton Young in 1904, and Terence Millin first described the radical retropubic approach in 1945. However, the procedure remained unpopular because of frequent complications of incontinence and impotence. The rebirth of RP has resulted from a better understanding of the surgical anatomy of the pelvis. Description of the anatomy of the dorsal vein complex and prostate apex anatomy resulted in modifications in the surgical technique leading to reduced operative blood loss. In addition, improved visualization made possible a more precise apical dissection, allowing better sparing of the external urethral sphincter and resulting improved continence. Description of the course of the cavernous nerves enabled further modifications of the surgical technique—so-called nerve-sparing techniques—in appropriate cases, resulting in better long-term preservation of erection function.

Lymph node dissection, once done routinely, may be performed only in those at significant risk of lymph node metastases. Such men can be identified with use of probability tables and nomograms as described earlier. Previously, only limited node dissections were performed harvesting lymph nodes from the obturator fossa. However, results from extended dissections showed that more than half of lymph node metastases are found outside this region. Therefore, a more extended and meticulous dissection is advised. Some feel that this may not only have diagnostic value but also could have a therapeutic impact in those with limited nodal disease (Allaf et al, 2004; Bader et al, 2003).

Considerable experience has been gained recently using a laparoscopic approach to RP. This can be performed through an extra- or transperitoneal approach. The advent of the DaVinci surgical robot has transformed laparoscopic

prostatectomy and has been adopted very rapidly in the United States. Laparoscopy reduces blood loss substantially, shortens the overall recovery time, and in some series reduces hospitalization time. Whether robot-assisted or unassisted laparoscopic surgery results in better or worse results in terms of the critical outcomes of cancer control, preservation of continence, and preservation of erectile function, however, remains unclear (Ficcara, Eur Urol 2009). Randomized trails were not performed, and even high-quality comparative cohort data remain fairly sparse, though this situation is gradually starting to change. The best evidence to date suggests that outcomes after robot-assisted surgery are probably comparable with—and are certainly not worse than—those obtained with the open approach (Barocas, 2010). However, the robot and associated disposable equipment are expensive, so the cost–benefit relationships remain unclear. It should be noted, however, that unlike some other novel technologies in prostate cancer care, Medicare and other payors do not offer any additional reimbursement for robot-assisted surgery. These costs in most cases are absorbed by the hospitals.

The prognosis of patients treated by RP correlates with the pathologic grade and stage of the specimen, and by the PSA response. PSA should fall to undetectable levels within 6 weeks of surgery in most cases. Distant metastases occur in about 85% of patients with positive lymph nodes; some men with limited micrometastatic nodal involvement may be cured by RP and lymphadenectomy, but all men with node involvement should be offered adjuvant androgen deprivation therapy. A high percentage of patients with seminal vesical involvement at RP, and a smaller proportion of those with extracapsular extension, are likewise destined to distant failure. There are several nomograms and other scoring systems available to help determine prognosis after surgery, similar to those discussed earlier for risk assessment prior to treatment (Cooperberg et al, Cancer 2011; Stephenson et al, 2005).

Patients with organ-confined cancer have 10-year disease-free survival ranging from 70% to 85% in several series. Those with focal extracapsular extension demonstrate 85% and 75% disease-free survival at 5 and 10 years, respectively. Patients with more extensive extracapsular extension demonstrate 70% and 40% disease-free survival at 5 and 10 years, respectively. High-grade tumors (Gleason sum >7) have a higher risk of progression than do low-grade tumors. Disease-free survival at 10 years for patients with Gleason sum 2–6 tumors is in excess of 70%; for Gleason sum 7, 50%; and for Gleason sum >8, 15%. The impact of positive surgical margins is controversial, and may relate to the extent, location, and grade of tumor at the margin. Neoadjuvant androgen deprivation, studied by several investigators, reduces the risk of positive surgical margins, but it does not appear to impact long-term biochemical relapse-free survival.

The management of patients with adverse pathologic features (positive surgical margins, extracapsular extension, and/or seminal vesicle invasion) at RP remains controversial. A large multicenter trial sponsored by the Southwest

Oncology Group found a nearly 30% relative reduction in metastasis and cancer-specific mortality with 12 years follow-up for those given adjuvant radiation therapy compared with those observed. However, if all men with these disease features were given adjuvant radiation, many would be overtreated. The problem is that of the men in the control group, fewer than one-third ever received radiation, even after PSA relapse, and radiation was given relatively late in these cases (Thompson et al, 2009). Retrospective studies have shown that administering salvage radiation at relatively low PSA levels results in improved outcomes, with stratification down to a PSA of 0.5 ng/mL. What is unknown is whether there is a benefit to true *adjuvant* radiation—that is, radiation given to a man with adverse pathology but an undetectable PSA—compared with *early salvage*—that is, deferring treatment among those with undetectable PSAs but administering radiation at the first sign of a rising PSA identified with an ultrasensitive assay (ie, with a PSA >0.01 but <0.1 ng/mL). Relatively good evidence supports earlier rather than later salvage radiation—that is, treating at as low a detectable PSA level as possible (Stephenson, 2007).

Morbidity associated with RP can be significant and is in part related to the experience of the surgeon. Immediate intraoperative complications include blood loss, rectal injury, and ureteral injury. Blood loss is more common with the retropubic approach than with the perineal approach because in the former, the dorsal venous complex must be divided. As noted earlier, laparoscopic approaches decrease such bleeding. Rectal injury is rare with the retropubic approach and more common with the perineal approach but usually can be immediately repaired without long-term sequelae. Ureteral injury is rare with any technique. Laparoscopic approaches carry the additional risks of laparoscopic access and insufflation, as well as risks related to transperitoneal access when this approach is used.

Perioperative complications include deep venous thrombosis, pulmonary embolism, lymphocele formation, and wound infection. Late complications include urinary incontinence and impotence. Reported rates of incontinence vary widely depending on the series, how continence is defined and reported, how long after surgery continence is assessed, and other factors. Age, urethral length, and surgeon experience are predictive of continence recovery. The return of continence after surgery may be gradual: many men regain continence by 2–3 months, but recovery can continue up to 1 year. Most academic series report long-term continence rates of 80–95%; rates from population-based studies are lower.

Preservation of potency varies as a function of age, preoperative sexual function, and preservation of one or both neurovascular bundles. However, the nerve-sparing procedure should be used selectively, for extracapsular extension may be a common finding in patients with presumed localized CaP. If extracapsular extension is present, preservation of the neurovascular bundle may increase the likelihood that the tumor will recur. However, it should also be noted that nerve sparing

is not a binary decision: the cavernosal nerve is not a single, well-defined structure, but rather it is a network of small nerve fibers running among the fascial layers surrounding the prostate. On each side, those tissues may be completely spared, partially spared, or widely excised depending on the preoperative findings. Like continence, reported rates of potency preservation vary very widely—from 40% to 82% in men younger than 60 years when both nerves are preserved and drops to 20–60% when only one nerve is preserved. For men between the ages of 60 and 69 years, comparable rates are 25–75% with bilateral nerve sparing and 10–50% with unilateral nerve sparing. As with continence, these figures are derived for the most part of academic series and may not be achieved in all practices. Recovery of sexual function generally occurs within 6–24 months following surgery. Potency can be improved with early use of PDE-5 inhibitors and other, more aggressive approaches to "penile rehabilitation." (See Chapter 38 for more information on impotence.)

4. Radiation therapy—external beam therapy—Traditional external beam radiotherapy (XRT) techniques allow the safe delivery of 6500–7000 cGy to the prostate. Standard XRT techniques depend upon bony landmarks to define treatment borders or a single CT slice to define the target volume. These standard XRT techniques generally involve the use of open square or rectangular fields with minimal to no blocking and are characterized by the use of relatively small boost fields. Often, these XRT techniques fail to provide adequate coverage of the target volume in as many as 20–41% of patients with CaP irradiated.

Improved imaging and use of novel treatment planning (three-dimensional, conformal radiation therapy [3DCRT] and intensity-modulated radiation therapy [IMRT]) allow for better targeting, conforming, or shaping radiation volume more closely around the prostate, and the use of higher doses without exceeding tolerance of surrounding normal tissues. Such radiotherapy has resulted in dramatic reductions in acute and late toxicity of radiation treatment and improved tumor control compared with conventional dose radiotherapy. Doses ≥72 cGy appear to result in improved biochemical outcomes compared with lower doses. Day-to-day variations in patient/prostate position can be accounted for by the use of daily online CT scanning, transabdominal ultrasound imaging, and insertion of an endorectal balloon or imaging of radiopaque fiducial markers placed before treatment. Whole pelvic radiation, including regional lymph nodes, especially when combined with androgen deprivation, has demonstrated improved outcomes in those with intermediate and high-risk prostate cancer, though not all radiation oncologists agree with these findings.

In addition to the use of dose escalation and improved tumor targeting, several investigators have shown that the results of radiation therapy may be improved with the use of neoadjuvant, concurrent, and adjuvant androgen deprivation. On the basis of numerous randomized trials, androgen deprivation improves the outcome of radiation in those with intermediate- or high-risk disease. The use of short-term (3–4 months) neoadjuvant and concurrent androgen deprivation is recommended for those with intermediate-risk disease, whereas those with high-risk disease should receive neoadjuvant, concurrent, and long-term adjuvant (24 months) androgen deprivation (Bolla et al, 2002; Horwitz et al, 2008; Roach, 2003).

As with RP, men who receive radiation may experience side effects especially those related to urinary, bowel, and sexual function. Most such side effects are limited in extent. Although men who undergo surgery are more likely to suffer incontinence, men who undergo radiation are more likely to suffer obstructive or irritative voiding or bowel symptoms (urgency, frequency, diarrhea, hematuria, rectal bleeding, and tenesmus). Although the impact of surgery on sexual function occurs early and may improve with time, the impact of radiation on sexual function may not be seen for 18–24 months. Sexual side effects may be exacerbated with the concurrent use of androgen deprivation, especially if used long term (Wu et al, 2008). Long-term risks, such as urethral stricture, rectourinary fistula, and radiation cystitis, are uncommon but can be quite challenging to manage. There is a doubling of the risk of rectal cancer and bladder cancer starting 10 years after prostate radiation, though the absolute risks of these uncommon tumors remains low (Bhojani et al, 2010).

Novel radiation approaches include stereotactic radiation (eg, CyberKnife) and proton-beam radiation. As with robot-assisted surgery, these technologies are heavily marketed in some areas but have not yet been shown to offer any clear benefit with respect to cancer control or quality-of-life preservation. Unlike robot-assisted surgery, however, in which hospitals absorb the costs of the technology, costs for novel radiation modalities—including IMRT—are borne by payors, and generally much higher than those associated with surgery or brachytherapy.

Readers are referred to Chapter 25 for a more detailed discussion of radiation therapy in CaP.

5. Radiation therapy—brachytherapy—A resurgence in the interest in brachytherapy has occurred because of the technologic developments making it possible to place radioactive seeds under TRUS guidance. Previously, free-hand seed placement techniques were used; however, very high failure rates were observed and the technique was virtually abandoned. Currently, with the use of computer software, one can preplan a precise dose of radiotherapy to be delivered by TRUS guidance. Implants can be permanent (iodine 125 or palladium 103) in that the seeds are placed in the prostate, and the radiation dose is delivered over time or temporary in that the seeds are loaded into hollow-core catheters and both the seeds (iridium 192) and catheters are removed after a short period of hospitalization and radiation exposure. Permanent implants have a lower dose rate, but a higher total dose delivered compared to temporary implants which have a higher dose rate, but deliver a lower total dose. External beam radiation can be given to those with intermediate- and high-risk cancers, who receive permanent brachytherapy, and is routinely given to most who undergo temporary or high dose rate brachytherapy. Some clinicians are determining whether men with low-risk disease can be treated effectively with high dose rate brachytherapy alone without the use of neo- or adjuvant external beam radiation.

As opposed to external beam radiation, androgen deprivation does not appear to improve the outcomes of men with intermediate disease who are treated with brachytherapy. Androgen deprivation is often used to shrink the prostate prior to brachytherapy to facilitate seed placement, though this does come at the price of additional side effects (Potters et al, 2001). Men with high-risk disease who choose brachytherapy receive external beam radiation and adjuvant androgen deprivation as described for those managed with eternal beam techniques alone.

Readers are referred to Chapter 25 for a more detailed discussion of brachytherapy in CaP.

6. Cryosurgery—There has been a resurgence of interest in cryosurgery as a treatment for localized CaP in the past several years. This is due to an increased interest in less invasive forms of therapy for localized CaP as well as several recent technical innovations, including improved percutaneous techniques, expertise in TRUS, improved cryotechnology, and better understanding of cryobiology.

Freezing of the prostate is carried out by using a multi-probe cryosurgical device. Multiple hollow-core probes are placed percutaneously under TRUS guidance. Most surgeons routinely perform two freeze–thaw cycles in all patients, and if the iceball does not adequately extend to the apex of the prostate, the cryoprobes are pulled backward into the apex and additional freeze–thaw cycles are undertaken. The temperature at the edge of the iceball is 0°C to −2°C, while actual cell destruction requires −25°C to −50°C. Therefore, actual tissue destruction occurs a few millimeters inside the iceball edge and cannot be monitored precisely by ultrasound imaging. Double freezing creates a larger tissue destruction area and theoretically brings the iceball edge and destruction zone edge closer together. An intraurethral warming device minimizes urethral freezing and subsequent sloughing, thus minimizing risk of severe urinary symptoms and/or retention.

With modern (third generation) cryoablation systems, severe complications such as rectourethral fistulas are much less common than they once were. However, erectile dysfunction is very common after cryotherapy, more so than after nerve-sparing surgery or radiation therapy, and cryotherapy has not been widely adopted for primary treatment. However, it is frequently effective for men with biopsy-confirmed locally persistent/recurrent disease after radiation.

7. Focal therapy—Prostate cancer tends to be an infiltrative disease, with cancerous glands interspersed with normal ones, and is frequently multifocal. Therefore, focal therapy—treating only the tumor while sparing the normal prostate and surrounding structures—is more challenging than for tumors that grow as discrete lesions. Multiple modalities are under investigation for this purpose—including limited cryotherapy, high-intensity focused ultrasound (HIFU), interstitial laser therapy, and others. There are several challenges to these approaches, chief among which is that PSA is not a reliable indicator of cancer status after focal ablation, so repeat biopsies after treatment are generally indicated. Ultimately, widespread adoption of focal therapy awaits validation of better imaging modalities currently under development that will identify—and ideally grade–prostate lesions with greater accuracy.

B. Recurrent Disease

1. Overview—A substantial number of men who are treated with either surgery or radiation for presumed clinically localized prostate cancer will relapse based on evidence of a detectable or rising serum PSA after treatment, respectively. Although a persistently detectable serum PSA after surgery is considered a failure, what constitutes biochemical failure after radiation is a matter of some debate. By one count, 152 different definitions have been proposed: 53 after surgery and 99 after radiation therapy. The AUA endorsed the common surgical definition of PSA ≥0.2 ng/mL with a confirmatory value >0.2 ng/mL (Cookson, 2007). The American Society for Therapeutic Radiology and Oncology (ASTRO) adopted the definition of three consecutive rises in serum PSA above nadir. However, this has since been modified to improve its specificity by defining failure as a rise of at least 2 ng/mL greater than the nadir level. It must be recognized that these definitions are neither intended nor able to allow comparisons between surgery and radiation patients, because the surgical definition will identify recurrence about 5 years earlier than the radiation definition (Nielsen et al, 2008). Biochemical failure may have a variable natural history after any kind of initial treatment and may signify localized disease, systemic disease, or a combination of the two. After either form of treatment, an interval to PSA failure <3–6 years and a posttreatment PSADT <3 months place a man at increased risk for metastases and subsequent prostate cancer–specific mortality.

2. Following radical prostatectomy—The likelihood of recurrence following RP is related to cancer grade, pathologic stage, and the extent of extracapsular extension. Cancer recurrence is more common in those with positive surgical margins, established extracapsular extension, seminal vesicle invasion, and high-grade disease. For those patients in whom a detectable PSA level develops after RP, the site of recurrence (local vs distant) can be established with reasonable certainty based on the interval from surgery to the detectable PSA concentration, PSADT, and selective use of imaging studies. Indeed, the likelihood of ultimate prostate cancer–specific mortality following PSA recurrence after RP ranges from 1% to 99%, depending on the Gleason score, time to recurrence, and PSADT (Freedland et al, 2005). Patients at low risk (eg, long interval to recurrence, slow PSA kinetics) and/or those with limited life expectancy may be observed, those with suspected local recurrence (particularly in the setting of positive margins) may benefit from salvage radiation therapy, and those with probable or documented distant disease should receive systemic therapy with androgen deprivation.

3. Following radiation therapy—A rising PSA level following definitive radiotherapy is indicative of cancer recurrence. For those who undergo radiation and experience biochemical failure as defined earlier, the site of recurrence may be identified using PSA kinetics, time to failure as noted earlier, prostate biopsies, and selective use of imaging. Up to one-third of patients will experience a "PSA bounce" following radiation (especially brachytherapy), which is defined by a rise in serum PSA followed by a decline. Such patients are not at an increased risk of cancer recurrence and repeat prostate biopsy should be deferred in such patients. Most patients who fail radiation therapy, irrespective of the site of recurrence, currently are managed with androgen deprivation. Those with documented local recurrence may be candidates for salvage prostatectomy, cryosurgery, or additional radiation. However, morbidity can be high with these forms of treatment, as is subsequent relapse.

C. Metastatic Disease

1. Initial endocrine therapy—Since death due to CaP is almost invariably a result of failure to control metastatic disease, a great deal of research has concentrated on efforts to improve control of distant disease. It is well known that most prostatic carcinomas are hormone dependent and that the large majority of men with metastatic CaP respond initially to various forms of androgen deprivation. Testosterone, the major circulating androgen, is produced by the Leydig cells in the testes (95%), with a smaller amount being produced by peripheral conversion of other steroids. Free testosterone enters prostate cells and is converted to DHT, the major intracellular androgen. DHT binds to a cytoplasmic receptor protein and the complex moves to the cell nucleus, where it modulates transcription. Androgen deprivation may be induced at several levels along the pituitary–gonadal axis using a variety of methods or agents (Table 23–4).

Use of a class of drugs (LHRH agonists) has allowed induction of androgen deprivation without orchiectomy or administration of diethylstilbestrol. There are four LHRH agonists currently approved by the FDA for the treatment of prostate cancer: goserelin acetate, triptorelin pamoate, histrelin acetate, and leuprolide acetate. These can be delivered by injection monthly or as depot preparations lasting

Table 23–4. Androgen ablation therapy for prostate cancer.

Level	Agent	Dose route	Dose (mg)	Frequency
Pituitary				
	Diethylstilbestrol	Oral	1–3	Daily
	Goserelin	Subcutaneous	10.8	Every 3 months
	Goserelin	Subcutaneous	3.6	Every month
	Leuprolide	Intramuscular	22.5–30	Every 3–4 months
	Leuprolide	Intramuscular	7.5	Every month
	Histrelin	Subcutaneous	50	Annual
	Triptorelin	Intramuscular	11.25–22.5	Every 3–6 months
	Degarelix	Intramuscular	80	Every month
Adrenal				
	Ketoconazole	Oral	400	Daily
	Aminoglutethimide	Oral	250	Four times a day
	Abiraterone	Oral	1000	Daily
Testicle				
	Orchiectomy			
Prostate cell				
	Bicalutamide	Oral	50	Daily
	Flutamide	Oral	250	Three times a day
	Nilutamide	Oral	150	Daily

3–6 months. A subcutaneous implant that releases leuprolide acetate at a constant rate for 1 year is also available. A second-generation LHRH antagonist (degarelix) was recently released. LHRH antagonists avoid the "flare" phenomenon associated with LHRH agonists, in which serum testosterone concentrations increase before falling. Such an increase could cause symptoms in those with advanced cancer. Currently, administration of LHRH agonists is the most common form of primary androgen blockade used in the United States. Orchiectomy, once common, is much less commonly performed today. Like LHRH agonists, estrogens achieve castration by feedback inhibition of the hypothalamic–pituitary axis and, perhaps, by a direct cytotoxic effect. Although effective, their use is limited due to an increased risk of negative cardiovascular effects. Transdermal preparations are under investigation.

Because of its rapid onset of action, ketoconazole should be considered in patients with advanced prostate cancer who present with spinal cord compression or disseminated intravascular coagulation. Although testosterone is the major circulating androgen, the adrenal gland secretes the androgens dehydroepiandrosterone, dehydroepiandrosterone sulfate, and androstenedione. Prostate cancer cells have also been identified to synthesize androgen directly in the setting of LHRH agonist therapy, thus escaping castration via autocrine pathways. Ketoconazole and the novel agent abiraterone inhibit androgen biosynthesis throughout the body—in the testes and adrenals and within the tumor cells (De Bono et al, 2011).

Some investigators believe that suppressing both testicular and adrenal androgens (combined androgen blockade) allows for a better initial and a longer response compared with those methods that inhibit production of only testicular androgens. Complete androgen blockade can be achieved by combining an androgen receptor antagonist (flutamide, bicalutamide, or nilutamide) with the use of an LHRH agonist or orchiectomy. When patients with metastatic prostate cancer are stratified with regard to extent of disease and performance status, those patients with limited disease and a good performance status who are treated with combined androgen blockade (an LHRH agonist and antiandrogen agent) seem to survive longer than those treated with an LHRH agonist alone (Crawford et al, 1989). However, another study comparing the use of an antiandrogen with and without an orchiectomy failed to demonstrate a survival difference between the two arms (Eisenberger et al, 1998). A meta-analysis of monotherapy and complete androgen blockade for the treatment of men with advanced prostate carcinoma suggested that there might be a small survival advantage to complete androgen blockade. This advantage must be balanced against an increased risk of side effects and costs among those on combined therapy (Samson, 2002), often for a number of years.

Ongoing trials are studying the use of intermittent androgen deprivation to determine whether this might result in a delay in the appearance of the hormone-refractory state. Intermittent therapy, compared with continuous therapy, may be associated with improved quality of life as serum testosterone levels may normalize during periods off therapy. High-dose antiandrogen monotherapy (bicalutamide 150 mg/day) is an alternative to castration both in patients with locally advanced and metastatic disease who are interested in maintaining libido and erectile function. In those with locally advanced disease, no significant difference in overall survival has been demonstrated between bicalutamide monotherapy and castration. However, in those with metastatic disease, castration is associated with better survival, and antiandrogen monotherapy is not commonly used in the United States.

The timing of initial endocrine therapy in CaP has been an area of great debate for many years. Data from the Veterans Administration Cooperative Studies from the 1960s did not demonstrate a clear survival advantage for early intervention with androgen ablation therapy in patients with advanced CaP. However, a randomized study from the Medical Research Council comparing early with delayed endocrine therapy in patients with advanced CaP demonstrated improved survival as well as lower complication rates (cord compression, ureteric obstruction, bladder outlet obstruction, and pathologic fractures) in patients treated with early endocrine therapy (Medical Research Council, 1997).

In patients who undergo RP and are found to have microscopic lymph node involvement, early endocrine therapy has also resulted in a survival advantage (Messing et al, 2006). Most would agree that androgen deprivation should be instituted in all those with metastatic disease, whether symptomatic or not. In addition, there may be an advantage to early therapy in those without radiographic evidence of cancer, but who relapse after initial therapy and are found to have rapid PSADTs as such patients are at great risk of developing metastatic disease early and dying of their disease. Androgen deprivation is not without side effects including hot flashes, anemia, loss of libido and sexual function, loss of bone mineral density, increased weight and body fat, and cognitive changes. In addition, increases in total cholesterol, low- and high-density lipoproteins, and serum triglycerides have been reported. Men on androgen deprivation should be monitored for such side effects as treatment for most is readily available. Many men diagnosed with prostate cancer suffer from low bone mineral density, which can be exacerbated with androgen deprivation therapy. Many agents may prevent generalized and localized bone loss, including calcium and vitamin D supplements and, if significant, bisphosphonates. Anemia is usually mild, but may be managed with recombinant erythropoietin. Although there are a number of treatments for men with hot flashes that are especially troublesome, medroxyprogesterone acetate (300–400 mg IM monthly) is an effective treatment with limited side effects.

Ultimately, most prostate cancers will adapt to survive without androgens, at which point they are denoted "hormone refractory" or "castrate resistant." The armamentarium available for treatment of advanced prostate cancer in this health state is evolving very rapidly. Briefly, interventions now available include the following:

- Cessation of antiandrogen therapy if the patient has been on combined androgen blockade.
- Secondary hormonal therapy aimed at the androgen biosynthesis pathway (ketoconazole, abiraterone).

- Immunotherapy via administration of autologous dendritic cells primed for recognition of prostatic acid phosphatase (sipuleucel-T).
- Receptor activator of NFκB (RANK) ligand antibody therapy to slow development and progression of bone metastases (denosumab).
- Taxane-based chemotherapy (docetaxel, cabazitaxel).

Other drugs currently in late-stage development include MDV3100, a novel antiandrogen, and XL184, a multityrosine kinase inhibitor.

These agents all have nonoverlapping mechanisms of action, and there is no a priori reason an individual patient could not receive all of them. However, no data exist to guide optimal sequencing of these strategies. Moreover, the costs of expensive novel treatments accumulate very quickly, and there is a clear need for much better personalization of treatment based on biomarkers and other predictors of response currently in development.

Readers are referred to Chapter 19 for a detailed discussion of the therapy for hormone-refractory prostate cancer.

BIBLIOGRAPHY

Prostate Gland Anatomy

McNeal JEet al: Zonal distribution of prostatic adenocarcinoma: Correlation with histologic pattern and direction of spread. Am J Surg Pathol 1988;12(12):897–906.

Benign Prostatic Hyperplasia

Ahyai SA et al: Meta-analysis of functional outcomes and complications following transurethral procedures for lower urinary tract symptoms resulting from benign prostatic enlargement. Eur Urol 2010;58:384.

Alan R et al: Serum steroid and sex hormone-binding globulin concentrations and the risk of incident benign prostatic hyperplasia: Results from the prostate cancer prevention trial. Am J Epidemiol 2008;168(12):1416–1424.

Andriole G et al: The effects of 5alpha-reductase inhibitors on the natural history, detection and grading of prostate cancer: Current state of knowledge. J Urol 2005;174(6):2098–3104.

Bent S et al: Saw Palmetto for benign prostatic hyperplasia. N Engl J Med 2006;354:557.

Boyle P et al: Updated meta-analysis of clinical trials of *Serenoa repens* extract in the treatment of symptomatic benign prostatic hyperplasia. BJU Int 2004;93(6):751–756.

Bryant MD et al: Multimedia version of a standard medical questionnaire improves patient understanding across all literacy levels. J Urol 2009;182:1120.

Elzayat EA et al: Holmium laser enucleation of the prostate: A size-independent new "gold standard". Urology 2005;66(5, Suppl):108–113.

Feifer AH et al: Analytical accuracy and reliability of commonly used nutritional supplements in prostate disease. J Urol 2002;168:150. PMID 12050511.

Gail S et al: The role of estrogens and estrogen receptors in normal prostate growth and disease. Steroids 2008;73(3):233–244.

Gravas S et al: Critical review of lasers in benign prostatic hyperplasia (BPH). BJU Int 2011;107:1030.

Hoffman RM et al: Transurethral microwave thermotherapy vs transurethral resection for treating benign prostatic hyperplasia: A systematic review. BJU Int 2004;94(7):1031–1036.

Lepor H et al: The efficacy of terazosin, finasteride, or both in benign prostatic hyperplasia. Veterans Affairs Cooperative Studies Benign Prostatic Hyperplasia Study Group. N Engl J Med 1996;335(8):533–539.

McConnell JD et al: Benign prostatic hyperplasia: Diagnosis and treatment. Agency for Health Care Policy and Research. Clin Pract Guidel Quick Ref Guide Clin 1994;8:1–17.

McConnell JD et al: The effect of finasteride on the risk of acute urinary retention and the need for surgical treatment among men with benign prostatic hyperplasia. Finasteride Long-Term Efficacy and Safety Study Group. N Engl J Med 1998;338(9):557–563.

McConnell JD et al: The long-term effect of doxazosin, finasteride, and combination therapy on the clinical progression of benign prostatic hyperplasia. N Engl J Med 2003;349(25):2387–2398.

Roehrborn CG et al: Long-term sustained improvement in symptoms of benign prostatic hyperplasia with the dual 5alpha-reductase inhibitor dutasteride: Results of 4-year studies. BJU Int 2005;96(4):572–577.

Roehrborn CG , Schwinn DA : Alpha1-adrenergic receptors and their inhibitors in lower urinary tract symptoms and benign prostatic hyperplasia. J Urol 2004;171(3):1029–1035.

Sutherland DE et al: Robot-assisted simple prostatectomy for severe benign prostatic hyperplasia. J Endourol 2011;25(4):641.

Wei JT et al: Urologic diseases in America project: Benign prostatic hyperplasia. J Urol 2008;173:1256.

Wilt TA et al: *Serenoa repens* for benign prostatic hyperplasia. Cochrane Database Syst Rev 2009;2:CD001423.

Prostate Cancer

Epidemiology and Guidelines

Barqawi AB et al: Observed effect of age and body mass index on total and complexed PSA: Analysis from a national screening program. Urology 2005;65(4):708–712.

Chan JM et al: The relative impact and future burden of prostate cancer in the United States. J Urol 2004;172(5, Pt 2):S13–S16; discussion S17.

Cooperberg MR et al: Time trends and local variation in primary treatment of localized prostate cancer. J Clin Oncol 2010; 28(7):1117.

Cox B et al: Vasectomy and risk of prostate cancer. JAMA 2002; 287(23):3110–3115.

Jemal A et al: Cancer statistics, 2010. CA Cancer J Clin 2010;60: 277.

Penson DF , Chan JM: Urologic diseases in America project: Prostate cancer. J Urol 2007;177:2020.

Thompson IM et al: Guideline for the management of clinically localized prostate cancer: 2007 update. J Urol 2007;177:2106.

Genetics, Pathobiology, and Pathology

Baillargeon J et al: The association of body mass index and prostate-specific antigen in a population-based study. Cancer 2005;103(5):1092–1095.

Chan JM et al: Role of diet in prostate cancer development and progression. J Clin Oncol 2005;23(32):8152–8160.

Chang BL et al: Two-locus genome-wide linkage scan for prostate cancer susceptibility genes with an interaction effect. Hum Genet 2005:1–9.

Chung LW et al: Molecular insights into prostate cancer progression: The missing link of tumor microenvironment. J Urol 2005; 173(1):10–20.

Cuzick J et al: Prognostic value of an RNA expression signature derived from cell cycle proliferation genes in patients with prostate cancer: A retrospective study. Lancet Oncol 2011;12:245.

Dong JT: Prevalent mutations in prostate cancer. J Cell Biochem 2006;97(3):433–447.

Hughes C et al: Molecular pathology of prostate cancer. J Clin Pathol 2005;58(7):673–684.

Jiang Z et al: Discovery and clinical application of a novel prostate cancer marker: Alpha-methylacyl CoA racemase (P504S). Am J Clin Pathol 2004;122(2):275–289.

Lichtenstein P et al: Environmental and heritable factors in the causation of cancer: Analyses of cohorts of twins from Sweden, Denmark, and Finland. N Engl J Med 2000;343(2):78–85.

Moore CK et al: Prognostic significance of high grade prostatic intraepithelial neoplasia and atypical small acinar proliferation in the contemporary era. J Urol 2005;173(1):70–72.

Mucci LA et al: Testing a multigene signature of prostate cancer death in the Swedish Watchful Waiting Cohort. Cancer Epidemiol Biomarkers Prev 2008;17:1682.

Narod SA et al: Fusion in the ETS gene family and prostate cancer. Br J Cancer 2008;99:847–851.

Nelson WG et al: The role of inflammation in the pathogenesis of prostate cancer. J Urol 2004;172(5, Pt 2):S6–S11; discussion S11–S12.

Paris PL et al: A group of genome-based biomarkers that add to a Kattan nomogram for predicting progression in men with high-risk prostate cancer. Clin Cancer Res 2010;16:195.

Penney KL et al: mRNA expression signature of Gleason grade predicts lethal prostate cancer. J Clin Oncol 2011;29:2391.

Rubin MA et al: Decreased alpha-methylacyl CoA racemase expression in localized prostate cancer is associated with an increased rate of biochemical recurrence and cancer-specific death. Cancer Epidemiol Biomarkers Prev 2005;14(6):1424–1432.

Schalken JA et al: Molecular prostate cancer pathology: Current issues and achievements. Scand J Urol Nephrol Suppl 2005;216:82–93.

Sreekumar A et al: Metabolomic profiles delineate potential role for sarcosine in prostate cancer progression. Nature 2009;457:910.

Taplin ME et al: Prognostic significance of plasma chromogranin a levels in patients with hormone-refractory prostate cancer treated in Cancer and Leukemia Group B 9480 study. Urology 2005;66(2):386–391.

Tomlins SA et al: Recurrent fusion of TMPRSS2 and ETS transcription factor genes in prostate cancer. Science 2005;310(5748):644–648.

Varambally S et al: Integrative genomic and proteomic analysis of prostate cancer reveals signatures of metastatic progression. Cancer Cell 2005;8(5):393–406.

Wang X et al: Autoantibody signatures in prostate cancer. N Engl J Med 2005;353(12):1224–1235.

Screening and Chemoprevention, and Biopsy

Andriole GL et al: Mortality results from a randomized prostate-cancer screening trial. N Engl J Med 2009;360(13):1310–1319.

Andriole GL et al: Effect of dutasteride on the risk of prostate cancer. N Engl J Med 2010;362(13):1192–1202.

Carroll PR et al: Serum prostate-specific antigen for the early detection of prostate cancer: Always, never, or only sometimes? J Clin Oncol 2011;29:345.

Crawford ED et al: Comorbidity and mortality results from a randomized prostate cancer screening trial. Clin Oncol 2011;29(4):355–361.

Draisma G et al: Lead time and overdiagnosis in prostate-specific antigen screening: Importance of methods and context. J Natl Cancer Inst 2009;101:374–383.

Greene KL et al: Prostate specific antigen best practice statement: 2009 update. J Urol 2009;182(5):2232–2241.

Harris RE et al: Aspirin, ibuprofen, and other non-steroidal anti-inflammatory drugs in cancer prevention: A critical review of non-selective COX-2 blockade (review). Oncol Rep 2005;13(4):559–583.

Hugosson J et al: Mortality results from the Göteborg randomised population-based prostate-cancer screening trial. Lancet Oncol 2010;11(8):725–732.

Jones JS et al: Saturation biopsy with periprostatic block can be performed in the office. J Urol 2002;168:2108.

Kramer BS et al: Use of 5-α-reductase inhibitors for prostate cancer chemoprevention: American Society of Clinical Oncology/American Urological Association 2008 clinical practice guideline. J Clin Oncol 2009;27:1502–1516.

Lippman SM et al: Effect of selenium and vitamin E on risk of prostate cancer and other cancers: the Selenium and Vitamin E Cancer Prevention Trial (SELECT). JAMA 2009;301:39.

Nelson WG : Agents in development for prostate cancer prevention. Expert Opin Investig Drugs 2004;13(12):1541–1554.

Parnes HL et al: Prevention of hormone-related cancers: Prostate cancer. J Clin Oncol 2005;23(2):368–377.

Schröder FH et al: Screening and prostate-cancer mortality in a randomized European study. N Engl J Med 2009;360(13):1320–1328.

Theoret MR et al: The Risks and Benefits of 5α-Reductase Inhibitors for Prostate-Cancer Prevention. N Engl J Med 2011;365(2):97–99.

Thompson IM et al: The influence of finasteride on the development of prostate cancer. N Engl J Med 2003;349(3):215–224.

Thompson IM et al: Prevalence of prostate cancer among men with a prostate-specific antigen level < or =4.0 ng per milliliter. N Engl J Med 2004;350(22):2239–2246.

Unger JM et al: Estimated impact of the Prostate Cancer Prevention Trial on population mortality. Cancer 2005;103(7):1375–1380.

U.S. Preventive Services Task Force: Screening for prostate cancer. Ann Intern Med 2008;149:185–191.

Vickers AJ et al: Prostate specific antigen concentration at age 60 and death or metastasis from prostate cancer: Case-control study. BMJ 2010;341:c4521.

Serum Tumor Markers

Banez LL et al: Obesity-related plasma hemodilution and PSA concentration among men with prostate cancer. JAMA 2007;298:2275.

Catalona WJ et al: Use of the percentage of free prostate-specific antigen to enhance differentiation of prostate cancer from benign prostatic disease: A prospective multicenter clinical trial. JAMA 1998;279(19):1542–1547.

Catalona WJ et al: Serum pro-prostate specific antigen preferentially detects aggressive prostate cancers in men with 2 to 4 ng/ml prostate specific antigen. J Urol 2004;171(6, Pt 1):2239–2244.

Catalona WJ et al: A multicenter study of [-2]pro-prostate specific antigen combined with prostate specific antigen and free prostate specific antigen for prostate cancer detection in the 2.0 to 10.0 ng/ml prostate specific antigen range. J Urol 2011;185:1650.

Cooney KA et al: Age-specific distribution of serum prostate-specific antigen in a community-based study of African-American men. Urology 2001;57(1):91–96.

D'Amico AV et al: Preoperative PSA velocity and the risk of death from prostate cancer after radical prostatectomy. N Engl J Med 2004;351(2):125–135.

D'Amico AV et al: Prostate specific antigen doubling time as a surrogate end point for prostate cancer specific mortality following radical prostatectomy or radiation therapy. J Urol 2004;172(5, Pt 2):S42–S46; discussion S46–S47.

Djavan B et al: Complexed prostate-specific antigen, complexed prostate-specific antigen density of total and transition zone, complexed/total prostate-specific antigen ratio, free-to-total prostate-specific antigen ratio, density of total and transition zone prostate-specific antigen: Results of the prospective multicenter European trial. Urology 2002;60(4, Suppl 1):4–9.

Eggener SE et al: Predictors of subsequent prostate cancer in men with a prostate specific antigen of 2.6 to 4.0 ng/ml and an initially negative biopsy. J Urol 2005;174(2):500–504.

Etzioni R et al: Prostate-specific antigen and free prostate-specific antigen in the early detection of prostate cancer: Do combination tests improve detection? Cancer Epidemiol Biomarkers Prev 2004;13(10):1640–1645.

Groskopf J et al: APTIMA PCA3 molecular urine test: Development of a method to aid in the diagnosis of prostate cancer. Clin Chem 2006;52:1089.

Haese A et al: Clinical utility of the PCA3 urine assay in European men scheduled for repeat biopsy. Eur Urol 2008;54:1081.

Hessels D et al: Detection of TMPRSS2-ERG fusion transcripts and prostate cancer antigen 3 in urinary sediments may improve diagnosis of prostate cancer. Clin Cancer Res 2007;13:5103.

Lein M et al: A multicenter clinical trial on the use of (-5, -7) pro prostate specific antigen. J Urol 2005;174(6):2150–2153.

Mikolajczyk SD et al: Proenzyme forms of prostate-specific antigen in serum improve the detection of prostate cancer. Clin Chem 2004;50(6):1017–1025.

Oesterling JE et al: Serum prostate-specific antigen in a community-based population of healthy men. Establishment of age-specific reference ranges. JAMA 1993;270(7):860–864.

Pan CC et al: The association between presentation PSA and race in two sequential time periods in prostate cancer patients seen at a university hospital and its community affiliates. Int J Radiat Oncol Biol Phys 2003;57(5):1292–1296.

Patel DA et al: Preoperative PSA velocity is an independent prognostic factor for relapse after radical prostatectomy. J Clin Oncol 2005;23(25):6157–6162.

Paul B et al: Detection of prostate cancer with a blood-based assay for early prostate cancer antigen. Cancer Res 2005;65(10):4097–5100.

Roddam AW et al: Use of prostate-specific antigen (PSA) isoforms for the detection of prostate cancer in men with a PSA level of 2–10 ng/ml: Systematic review and meta-analysis. Eur Urol 2005;48(3):386–399; discussion 398–399.

Tewari A et al: Racial differences in serum prostate-specific antigen (PSA) doubling time, histopathological variables and long-term PSA recurrence between African-American and white American men undergoing radical prostatectomy for clinically localized prostate cancer. BJU Int 2005;96(1):29–33.

Thompson IM et al: Operating characteristics of prostate-specific antigen in men with an initial PSA level of 3.0 ng/ml or lower. JAMA 2005;294(1):66–70.

Vickers AJ et al: Reducing unnecessary biopsy during prostate cancer screening using a four-kallikrein panel: An independent replication. J Clin Oncol 2010;28:2493.

Vickers AJ et al: An empirical evaluation of guidelines on prostate-specific antigen velocity in prostate cancer detection. J Natl Cancer Inst 2011;103:462.

Staging and Risk Assessment

Cooperberg MR et al: The University of California, San Francisco Cancer of the Prostate Risk Assessment score: A straightforward and reliable preoperative predictor of disease recurrence after radical prostatectomy. J Urol 2005;173(6):1938–1942.

Cooperberg MR . Prostate cancer risk assessment: choosing the sharpest tool in the shed. Cancer 2008;113(11):3062–3066.

Cooperberg MR et al: Risk assessment for prostate cancer metastasis and mortality at the time of diagnosis. J Natl Cancer Inst 2009; 101(12):878–887.

D'Amico AV et al: Biochemical outcomes after radical prostatectomy, external beam radiation therapy, or interstitial radiation therapy for clinically localized prostate cancer. JAMA 1998;280:969.

Lughezzani G et al: Head-to-head comparison of the three most commonly used preoperative models for prediction of biochemical recurrence after radical prostatectomy. Eur Urol 2010;57:562.

Makarov DV et al: Updated nomogram to predict pathologic stage of prostate cancer given prostate-specific antigen level, clinical stage, and biopsy Gleason score (Partin tables) based on cases from 2000 to 2005. Urology 2007;69:1095.

Porten SP et al: The independent value of tumour volume in a contemporary cohort of men treated with radical prostatectomy for clinically localized disease. BJU Int 105:472, 2010.

Reese AC et al: Inaccuracies in assignment of clinical stage for localized prostate cancer. Cancer 117:283, 2011.

Shariat SF et al: An updated catalog of prostate cancer predictive tools. Cancer 2008;113:3075–3099.

Zhou P et al: Predictors of prostate cancer-specific mortality after radical prostatectomy or radiation therapy. J Clin Oncol 2005;23(28):6992–6998.

Imaging

Afnan J et al: Update on prostate imaging. Urol Clin North Am 2010;37:23.

Bander NH : Technology insight: monoclonal antibody imaging of prostate cancer. Nat Clin Pract Urol 2006;3:216.

Halpern EJ et al: Prostate: High-frequency Doppler US imaging for cancer detection. Radiology 2002;225(1):71–77.

Harisinghani MG et al: Noninvasive detection of clinically occult lymph-node metastases in prostate cancer. N Engl J Med 2003;348(25):2491–2499.

Kizu H et al: Fusion of SPECT and multidetector CT images for accurate localization of pelvic sentinel lymph nodes in prostate cancer patients. J Nucl Med Technol 2005;33(2):78–82.

Mahdavi SS et al: Evaluation of visualization of the prostate gland in vibro-elastography images. Med Image Anal 2011;15(4):589–600.

Palvolgi R et al: Bone scan overuse in staging of prostate cancer: An analysis of a Veterans Affairs Cohort. Urology 2011;77:1330–1337.

Ponsky LE et al: Evaluation of preoperative ProstaScint scans in the prediction of nodal disease. Prostate Cancer Prostatic Dis 2002;5(2):132–135.

Sanna V et al: Development of polymeric microbubbles targeted to prostate-specific membrane antigen as prototype of novel ultrasound contrast agents. Mol Pharm 2011;8(3):748–757.

Thomas CT et al: Indium-111-capromab pendetide radioimmunoscintigraphy and prognosis for durable biochemical response to salvage radiation therapy in men after failed prostatectomy. J Clin Oncol 2003;21(9):1715–1721.

Verma S et al: Prostate MRI and 3D MR spectroscopy: how we do it. Am J Roentgenol 2010;194(6):1414–1426.

Prostate Biopsy

Epstein JI et al: Utility of saturation biopsy to predict insignificant cancer at radical prostatectomy. Urology 2005;66(2):356–360.

Karakiewicz PI et al: Development and validation of a nomogram predicting the outcome of prostate biopsy based on patient age, digital rectal examination and serum prostate specific antigen. J Urol 2005;173(6):1930–1934.

Lange D et al: Bacterial sepsis after prostate biopsy–A new perspective. Urology 2009;74:1200.

Obek C et al: Comparison of 3 different methods of anesthesia before transrectal prostate biopsy: A prospective randomized trial. J Urol 2004;172(2):502–505.

Pelzer AE et al: Are transition zone biopsies still necessary to improve prostate cancer detection? Results from the Tyrol screening project. Eur Urol 2005;48(6):916–921; discussion 921.

Pinkstaff DM et al: Systematic transperineal ultrasound-guided template biopsy of the prostate: Three-year experience. Urology 2005; 65(4):735–739.

Presti JC Jr et al: The optimal systematic prostate biopsy scheme should include 8 rather than 6 biopsies: Results of a prospective clinical trial. J Urol 2000;163(1):163–166; discussion 166–167.

Rabets JC et al: Prostate cancer detection with office based saturation biopsy in a repeat biopsy population. J Urol 2004;172(1):94–97.

Remzi M et al: The Vienna nomogram: Validation of a novel biopsy strategy defining the optimal number of cores based on patient age and total prostate volume. J Urol 2005;174(4, Pt 1):1256–1260; discussion 1260–1261; author reply 1261.

Sheikh M et al: Patients' tolerance and early complications of transrectal sonographically guided prostate biopsy: Prospective study of 300 patients. J Clin Ultrasound 2005;33(9):452–456.

Radical Prostatectomy

Allaf ME et al: Anatomical extent of lymph node dissection: Impact on men with clinically localized prostate cancer. J Urol 2004;172(5, Pt 1):1840–1844.

Bader P et al: Disease progression and survival of patients with positive lymph nodes after radical prostatectomy. Is there a chance of cure? J Urol 2003;169(3):849–854.

Barocas DA et al: Robotic assisted laparoscopic prostatectomy versus radical retropubic prostatectomy for clinically localized prostate cancer: Comparison of short-term biochemical recurrence-free survival. J Urol 2010;183:990.

Bhatta-Dhar N et al: No difference in six-year biochemical failure rates with or without pelvic lymph node dissection during radical prostatectomy in low-risk patients with localized prostate cancer. Urology 2004;63(3):528–531.

Bill-Axelson A et al: Radical prostatectomy versus watchful waiting in early prostate cancer. N Engl J Med 2011;364:1708–1717.

Bolla M et al: Postoperative radiotherapy after radical prostatectomy: A randomised controlled trial (EORTC trial 22911). Lancet 2005;366(9485):572–578.

Cooperberg MR et al: Comparative risk-adjusted mortality outcomes after primary surgery, radiotherapy, or androgen-deprivation therapy for localized prostate cancer. Cancer 2010;116:5226.

Cooperberg MR et al: The CAPRA-S score: A straightforward tool for improved prediction of outcomes after radical prostatectomy. Cancer 2011;117(22):5039–5046.

Dotan ZA et al: Pattern of prostate-specific antigen (PSA) failure dictates the probability of a positive bone scan in patients with an increasing PSA after radical prostatectomy. J Clin Oncol 2005;23(9):1962–1968.

Ficarra V et al: Retropubic, laparoscopic, and robot-assisted radical prostatectomy: A systematic review and cumulative analysis of comparative studies. Eur Urol 2009 55:1037–1063.

Guillonneau B et al: Laparoscopic radical prostatectomy: Oncological evaluation after 1,000 cases a Montsouris Institute. J Urol 2003;169(4):1261–1266.

Karakiewicz PI et al: Prognostic impact of positive surgical margins in surgically treated prostate cancer: Multi-institutional assessment of 5831 patients. Urology 2005;66(6):1245–1250.

Lunacek A et al: Anatomical radical retropubic prostatectomy: "Curtain dissection" of the neurovascular bundle. BJU Int 2005;95(9):1226–1231.

Messing EM et al: Immediate versus deferred androgen deprivation treatment in patients with node-positive prostate cancer after radical prostatectomy and pelvic lymphadenectomy. Lancet Oncol 2006;7:472–479.

Patel DA et al: Preoperative PSA velocity is an independent prognostic factor for relapse after radical prostatectomy. J Clin Oncol 2005;23(25):6157–6162.

Rogers CG et al: Natural history of disease progression in patients who fail to achieve an undetectable prostate-specific antigen level after undergoing radical prostatectomy. Cancer 2004;101(11):2549–2556.

Stephenson AJ et al: Postoperative nomogram predicting the 10-year probability of prostate cancer recurrence after radical prostatectomy. J Clin Oncol 2005;23(28):7005–7012.

Stephenson AJ et al: Predicting the outcome of salvage radiation therapy for recurrent prostate cancer after radical prostatectomy. J Clin Oncol 2007;25:2035.

Stephenson AJ et al: Prostate cancer–specific mortality after radical prostatectomy for patients treated in the prostate-specific antigen era. J Clin Oncol 2009;27:4300.

Swindle P et al: Do margins matter? The prognostic significance of positive surgical margins in radical prostatectomy specimens. J Urol 2005;174(3):903–907.

Thompson IM et al: Adjuvant radiotherapy for pathological T3N0M0 prostate cancer significantly reduces risk of metastases and improves survival: Long-term followup of a randomized clinical trial. J Urol 2009;181:956.

Zelefsky MJ et al: Metastasis after radical prostatectomy or external beam radiotherapy for patients with clinically localized prostate cancer: A comparison of clinical cohorts Adjusted for case mix. J Clin Oncol 2010;28:1508.

Radiation

Ashman JB et al: Whole pelvic radiotherapy for prostate cancer using 3D conformal and intensity-modulated radiotherapy. Int J Radiat Oncol Biol Phys 2005;63(3):765–771.

Ataman F et al: Late toxicity following conventional radiotherapy for prostate cancer: Analysis of the EORTC trial 22863. Eur J Cancer 2004;40(11):1674–1681.

Bhojani N et al: The rate of secondary malignancies after radical prostatectomy versus external beam radiation therapy for localized prostate cancer: A population-based study on 17,845 patients. Int J Radiat Oncol Biol Phys 2010;76(2):342–348.

Bolla M et al: Long-term results with immediate androgen suppression and external irradiation in patients with locally advanced prostate cancer (an EORTC study): A phase III randomised trial. Lancet 2002;360(9327):103–106.

Buyyounouski MK et al: Defining biochemical failure after radiotherapy with and without androgen deprivation for prostate cancer. Int J Radiat Oncol Biol Phys 2005;63(5):1455–1462.

Ciezki JP et al: A retrospective comparison of androgen deprivation (AD) vs. no AD among low-risk and intermediate-risk prostate cancer patients treated with brachytherapy, external beam radiotherapy, or radical prostatectomy. Int J Radiat Oncol Biol Phys 2004;60(5):1347–1350.

D'Amico AV et al: 6-month androgen suppression plus radiation therapy vs radiation therapy alone for patients with clinically localized prostate cancer: A randomized controlled trial. JAMA 2004;292(7):821–827.

Hanks GE et al: Phase III trial of long-term adjuvant androgen deprivation after neoadjuvant hormonal cytoreduction and radiotherapy in locally advanced carcinoma of the prostate: The Radiation Therapy Oncology Group Protocol 92–02. J Clin Oncol 2003;21(21):3972–3978.

Horwitz EM et al: Ten-year follow-up of radiation therapy oncology group protocol 92–02: A phase III trial of the duration of elective androgen deprivation in locally advanced prostate cancer. J Clin Oncol 2008;26:2497–2504.

Konski A et al: Is proton beam therapy cost effective in the treatment of adenocarcinoma of the prostate. J Clin Oncol 2007;25:3603.

Lawton CA et al: Androgen suppression plus radiation versus radiation alone for patients with stage D1/pathologic node-positive adenocarcinoma of the prostate: Updated results based on national prospective randomized trial Radiation Therapy Oncology Group 85–31. J Clin Oncol 2005;23(4):800–807.

Lee CT et al: Comparison of treatment volumes and techniques in prostate cancer radiation therapy. Am J Clin Oncol 2005;28(6):618–625.

Merrick GS et al: Impact of supplemental external beam radiotherapy and/or androgen deprivation therapy on biochemical outcome after permanent prostate brachytherapy. Int J Radiat Oncol Biol Phys 2005;61(1):32–43.

Potters L et al: Potency after permanent prostate brachytherapy for localized prostate cancer. Int J Radiat Oncol Biol Phys 2001;50:1235.

Roach M III et al: Phase III trial comparing whole-pelvic versus prostate-only radiotherapy and neoadjuvant versus adjuvant combined androgen suppression: Radiation Therapy Oncology Group 9413. J Clin Oncol 2003;21(10):1904–1911.

Vargas CE et al: Lack of benefit of pelvic radiation in prostate cancer patients with a high risk of positive pelvic lymph nodes treated with high-dose radiation. Int J Radiat Oncol Biol Phys 2005; 63(5):1474–1482.

Zietman AL et al: Comparison of conventional-dose vs high-dose conformal radiation therapy in clinically localized adenocarcinoma of the prostate: A randomized controlled trial. JAMA 2005;294(10):1233–1239.

Zietman AL et al: PSA bounces after neoadjuvant androgen deprivation and external beam radiation: Impact on definitions of failure. Int J Radiat Oncol Biol Phys 2005;62(3):714–718.

Active Surveillance

Albertsen PC et al: Impact of comorbidity on survival among men with localized prostate cancer. J Clin Oncol 2011;29:1335.

Cooperberg MR et al: Outcomes of active surveillance for men with intermediate-risk prostate cancer. J Clin Oncol 2011a;29:228–234.

Cooperberg MR et al: Active surveillance for prostate cancer: Progress and promise. J Clin Oncol 2011b;29(27):3669–3676. Review.

Harlan SR et al: Time trends and characteristics of men choosing watchful waiting for initial treatment of localized prostate cancer: Results from CapSure. J Urol 2003;170(5):1804–1807.

Hayes JH et al: Active surveillance compared with initial treatment for men with low-risk prostate cancer: A decision analysis. JAMA 2010;304(21):2373–2380.

Kattan MW et al: Counseling men with prostate cancer: a nomogram for predicting the presence of small, moderately differentiated, confined tumors. J Urol 2003;170(5):1792–1797.

Klotz L et al: Clinical results of long-term follow-up of a large, active surveillance cohort with localized prostate cancer. J Clin Oncol 2009;28:126–131.

Lu-Yao GL et al: Outcomes of localized prostate cancer following conservative management. JAMA 2009;302(11):1202–1209.

Porten S et al: Changes in prostate cancer grade on serial biopsy in men undergoing active surveillance. J Clin Oncol 2011;29:795–800.

Ross AE et al: Prostate-specific antigen kinetics during follow-up are an unreliable trigger for intervention in a prostate cancer surveillance program. J Clin Oncol 2010;28:2810.

Tosoian JJ et al: Active surveillance program for prostate cancer: An update of the Johns Hopkins experience. J Clin Oncol 2011;29:2185.

Cryotherapy and HIFU

Colombel M , Gelet A : Principles and results of high-intensity focused ultrasound for localized prostate cancer. Prostate Cancer Prostatic Dis 2004;7(4):289–294.

Donnelly BJ et al: Role of transrectal ultrasound guided salvage cryosurgery for recurrent prostate carcinoma after radiotherapy. Prostate Cancer Prostatic Dis 2005;8(3):235–242.

Onik G : The male lumpectomy: Rationale for a cancer targeted approach for prostate cryoablation. A review. Technol Cancer Res Treat 2004;3(4):365–370.

Shinohara K : Prostate cancer: Cryotherapy. Urol Clin North Am 2003;30(4):725–736, viii.

Quality of Life

Miller DC et al: Long-term outcomes among localized prostate cancer survivors: Health-related quality-of-life changes after radical prostatectomy, external radiation, and brachytherapy. J Clin Oncol 2005;23(12):2772–2780.

Pardo Y et al: Quality-of-life impact of primary treatments for localized prostate cancer in patients without hormonal treatment. J Clin Oncol 2010;28:4687.

Sanda MG et al: Quality of life and satisfaction with outcome among prostate-cancer survivors. N Engl J Med 2008;358:1250–1261.

Sonn GA et al: Differing perceptions of quality of life in patients with prostate cancer and their doctors. J Urol 2009;182:2296.

Speight JL et al: Longitudinal assessment of changes in sexual function and bother in patients treated with external beam radiotherapy or brachytherapy, with and without neoadjuvant androgen ablation: Data from CapSure. Int J Radiat Oncol Biol Phys 2004; 60(4):1066–1075.

Steineck G et al: Quality of life after radical prostatectomy or watchful waiting. N Engl J Med 2002;347(11):790–796.

Wei JT et al: Comprehensive comparison of health-related quality of life after contemporary therapies for localized prostate cancer. J Clin Oncol 2002;20:557–566.

Wu AK et al: Health related quality of life in patients treated with multimodal therapy for prostate cancer. J Urol 2008;180:2415.

Relapse and Androgen Deprivation

Chaudhary UB et al: Secondary hormonal manipulations in the management of advanced prostate cancer. Can J Urol 2005;12(3): 2666–2676.

Chen CD et al: Molecular determinants of resistance to antiandrogen therapy. Nat Med 2004;10(1):33–39.

Cookson MS : Variation in the definition of biochemical recurrence in patients treated for localized prostate cancer: The American Urological Association prostate guidelines for localized prostate cancer update panel report and recommendations for a standard in the reporting of surgical outcomes. J Urol 2007; 177:540.

Crawford ED et al: A controlled trial of leuprolide with and without flutamide in prostatic carcinoma. N Engl J Med 1989;321(7): 419–424.

De La Taille A et al: Intermittent androgen suppression in patients with prostate cancer. BJU Int 2003;91(1):18–22.

Eisenberger MA et al: Bilateral orchiectomy with or without flutamide for metastatic prostate cancer. N Engl J Med 1998;339(15): 1036–1042.

Freedland SJ et al: Risk of prostate cancer–specific mortality following biochemical recurrence after radical prostatectomy. JAMA 2005;294:433–439.

Kumar RJ et al: Preventing and treating the complications of hormone therapy. Curr Urol Rep 2005;6(3):217–223.

Lee AK , D'Amico AV : Utility of prostate-specific antigen kinetics in addition to clinical factors in the selection of patients for salvage local therapy. J Clin Oncol 2005;23(32):8192–8197.

Moul JW et al: Early versus delayed hormonal therapy for prostate specific antigen only recurrence of prostate cancer after radical prostatectomy. J Urol 2004;171(3):1141–1147.

Nielsen ME et al: Is it possible to compare PSA recurrence-free survival after surgery and radiotherapy using revised ASTRO Criterion— "Nadir+2"? Urology 2008;72:389.

Schroder FH et al: Early versus delayed endocrine treatment of pN1–3 M0 prostate cancer without local treatment of the primary tumor: Results of European Organisation for the Research and Treatment of Cancer 30846—A phase III study. J Urol 2004; 172(3):923–927.

Studer UE et al: Immediate versus deferred hormonal treatment for patients with prostate cancer who are not suitable for curative local treatment: Results of the randomized trial SAKK 08/88. J Clin Oncol 2004;22(20):4109–4118.

Secondary Therapy and Chemotherapy

Beltran H et al: New therapies for castration-resistant prostate cancer: Efficacy and safety. Eur Urol 2011;60(2):279–290.

D'Amico AV et al: Surrogate end point for prostate cancer specific mortality in patients with nonmetastatic hormone refractory prostate cancer. J Urol 2005;173(5):1572–1576.

De Bono JS et al: Abiraterone and increased survival in metastatic prostate cancer. N Engl J Med 2011;364(21):1995–2005.

Fizazi K et al: Denosumab versus zoledronic acid for treatment of bone metastases in men with castration-resistant prostate cancer: A randomised, double-blind study. Lancet 2011;377:813.

Goodin S et al: Effect of docetaxel in patients with hormone-dependent prostate-specific antigen progression after local therapy for prostate cancer. J Clin Oncol 2005;23(15):3352–3357.

Kantoff PW et al: Sipuleucel-T immunotherapy for castration-resistant prostate cancer. N Engl J Med 2010:363:411.

Rozhansky F et al: Prostate-specific antigen velocity and survival for patients with hormone-refractory metastatic prostate carcinoma. Cancer 2005;106(1):63–67.

Tannock IF et al: Docetaxel plus prednisone or mitoxantrone plus prednisone for advanced prostate cancer. N Engl J Med 2004; 351(15): 1502–1512.

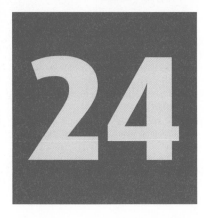

Genital Tumors

Joseph C. Presti, Jr., MD

TUMORS OF THE TESTIS

GERM CELL TUMORS OF THE TESTIS

▶ Epidemiology and Risk Factors

Malignant tumors of the testis are rare, with approximately 9 new cases per 100,000 males reported in the United States each year. Of all primary testicular tumors, 90–95% are germ cell tumors (seminoma and nonseminoma), while the remainders are nongerminal neoplasms (Leydig cell, Sertoli cell, gonadoblastoma). The lifetime probability of developing testicular cancer is 0.2% for a white male in the United States. Survival of patients with testicular cancer has improved dramatically in recent years, reflecting the development and refinement of effective combination chemotherapy. Of the 8480 new cases of testicular cancer in the United States in 2010, only 350 deaths are expected.

The incidence of testicular cancer shows marked variation among different countries, races, and socioeconomic classes. Scandinavian countries report up to 6.7 new cases per 100,000 males annually; Japan reports 0.8 per 100,000 males. In the United States, the incidence of testicular cancer in blacks is approximately one-fourth that in whites. Within a given race, individuals in the higher socioeconomic classes have approximately twice the incidence of those in the lower classes.

Testicular cancer is slightly more common on the right side than on the left, which parallels the increased incidence of cryptorchidism on the right side. Of primary testicular tumors, 1–2% are bilateral, and about 50% of these tumors occur in men with a history of unilateral or bilateral cryptorchidism. Primary bilateral tumors of the testis may happen synchronously or asynchronously but tend to be of the same histologic type. Seminoma is the most common germ cell tumor in bilateral *primary* testicular tumors, while malignant lymphoma is the most common bilateral tumor of the testis.

Although the cause of testicular cancer is unknown, both congenital and acquired factors have been associated with

tumor development. The strongest association has been with the cryptorchid testis. Approximately 7–10% of testicular tumors develop in patients who have a history of cryptorchidism; seminoma is the most common form of tumor these patients have. However, 5–10% of testicular tumors occur in the contralateral, normally descended testis. The relative risk of malignancy is highest for the intra-abdominal testis (1 in 20) and is significantly lower for the inguinal testis (1 in 80). Placement of the cryptorchid testis into the scrotum (orchiopexy) lowers the risk of malignancy if it is performed prior to the age of 13 (Pettersson et al, 2007).

Exogenous estrogen administration to the mother during pregnancy has been associated with an increased relative risk for testicular tumors in the fetus, ranging from 2.8 to 5.3 over the expected incidence. Other acquired factors such as trauma and infection-related testicular atrophy have been associated with testicular tumors; however, a causal relationship has not been established.

▶ Classification

Numerous classification systems have been proposed for germ cell tumors of the testis. Classification by histologic type proves to be the most useful with respect to treatment. The two major divisions are seminoma and nonseminomatous germ cell tumors (NSGCTs), which include embryonal, teratoma, choriocarcinoma, and mixed tumors.

▶ Tumorigenic Hypothesis for Germ Cell Tumor Development

During embryonal development, the totipotential germ cells can travel down normal differentiation pathways and become spermatocytes. However, if these totipotential germ cells travel down abnormal developmental pathways, seminoma or embryonal carcinomas (totipotential tumor cells) develop. If the embryonal cells undergo further differentiation along intraembryonic pathways, teratoma will result. If the embryonal cells undergo further differentiation

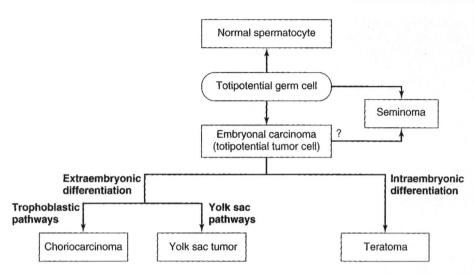

▲ **Figure 24–1.** Tumorigenic model for germ cell tumors of the testis.

along extraembryonic pathways, either choriocarcinoma or yolk sac tumors are formed (Figure 24–1). This model helps to explain why specific histologic patterns of testicular tumors produce certain tumor markers. Note that yolk sac tumors produce alpha-fetoprotein (AFP) just as the yolk sac produces AFP in normal development. Likewise, choriocarcinoma produces human chorionic gonadotropin (hCG) just as the normal placenta produces hCG.

▶ Pathology

A. Seminoma (35%)

Three histologic subtypes of pure seminoma have been described. However, stage for stage, there is no prognostic significance to any of these subtypes. Classic seminoma accounts for 85% of all seminomas and is most common in the fourth decade of life. Grossly, coalescing gray nodules are observed. Microscopically, monotonous sheets of large cells with clear cytoplasm and densely staining nuclei are seen. It is noteworthy that syncytiotrophoblastic elements are seen in approximately 10–15% of cases, an incidence that corresponds approximately to the incidence of hCG production in seminomas.

Anaplastic seminoma accounts for 5–10% of all seminomas. Diagnosis requires the presence of three or more mitoses per high-power field, and the cells demonstrate a higher degree of nuclear pleomorphism than the classic types. Anaplastic seminoma tends to present at a higher stage than the classic variety. When stage is taken into consideration, however, this subtype does not convey a worse prognosis.

Spermatocytic seminoma accounts for 5–10% of all seminomas. Microscopically, cells vary in size and are characterized

by densely staining cytoplasm and round nuclei that contain condensed chromatin. More than half of the patients with spermatocytic seminoma are older than 50 years.

B. Embryonal Cell Carcinoma (20%)

Two variants of embryonal cell carcinoma are common: the adult type and the infantile type or yolk sac tumor (also called endodermal sinus tumor). Histologic structure of the adult variant demonstrates marked pleomorphism and indistinct cellular borders. Mitotic figures and giant cells are common. Cells may be arranged in sheets, cords, glands, or papillary structures. Extensive hemorrhage and necrosis may be observed grossly.

The infantile variant, or yolk sac tumor, is the most common testicular tumor of infants and children. When seen in adults, it usually occurs in mixed histologic types and possibly is responsible for AFP production in these tumors. Microscopically, cells demonstrate vacuolated cytoplasm secondary to fat and glycogen deposition and are arranged in a loose network with large intervening cystic spaces. Embryoid bodies are commonly seen and resemble 1- to 2-week-old embryos consisting of a cavity surrounded by syncytio- and cytotrophoblasts.

C. Teratoma (5%)

Teratomas may be seen in both children and adults. They contain more than one germ cell layer in various stages of maturation and differentiation. Grossly, the tumor appears lobulated and contains variable-sized cysts filled with gelatinous or mucinous material. Mature teratoma may have elements resembling benign structures derived from ectoderm, mesoderm, and endoderm, while immature teratoma consists of undifferentiated primitive tissue. In contrast to its ovarian counterpart, the mature teratoma of the testis does not attain the same degree of differentiation as teratoma of the ovary. Microscopically, ectoderm may be represented by squamous epithelium or neural tissue; endoderm may be represented by intestinal, pancreatic, or respiratory tissue; and mesoderm may be represented by smooth or skeletal muscle, cartilage, or bone.

D. Choriocarcinoma (<1%)

Pure choriocarcinoma is rare. Lesions tend to be small within the testis and usually demonstrate central hemorrhage on gross inspection. Microscopically, syncytio- and cytotrophoblasts must be visualized. The syncytial elements are typically large, multinucleated cells with vacuolated, eosinophilic cytoplasm; the nuclei are large, hyperchromatic, and irregular. Cytotrophoblasts are uniform cells with distinct cell borders, clear cytoplasm, and a single nucleus.

Clinically, choriocarcinomas behave in an aggressive fashion characterized by early hematogenous spread. Paradoxically, small intratesticular lesions can be associated with widespread metastatic disease.

E. Mixed Cell Type (40%)

Within the category of mixed cell types, most (up to 25% of all testicular tumors) are teratocarcinomas, which are a combination of teratoma and embryonal cell carcinoma. Up to 6% of all testicular tumors are of mixed cell type, with seminoma being one of the components. Treatment for these mixtures of seminoma and NSGCT is similar to that of NSGCT alone.

F. Carcinoma In Situ

In a series of 250 patients with unilateral testicular cancer, Berthelsen et al (1982) demonstrated the presence of carcinoma in situ (CIS) in 13 (5.2%) of the contralateral testes. This is approximately twice the overall incidence of bilateral testicular cancer. The presence of contralateral atrophy or ultrasonographic microlithiasis in patients with testicular tumors warrants contralateral biopsy. If diagnosed, CIS is usually treated by external beam radiation therapy.

▶ Patterns of Metastatic Spread

With the exception of choriocarcinoma, which demonstrates early hematogenous spread, germ cell tumors of the testis typically spread in a stepwise lymphatic fashion. Lymph nodes of the testis extend from T1 to L4 but are concentrated at the level of the renal hilum because of their common embryologic origin with the kidney. The primary landing site for the right testis is the interaortocaval area at the level of the right renal hilum. Stepwise spread, in order, is to the precaval, preaortic, paracaval, right common iliac, and right external iliac lymph nodes. The primary landing site for the left testis is the para-aortic area at the level of the left renal hilum. Stepwise spread, in order, is to the preaortic, left common iliac, and left external iliac lymph nodes. In the absence of disease on the left side, no crossover metastases to the right side have ever been identified. However, right-to-left crossover metastases are common. These observations have resulted in modified surgical dissections to preserve ejaculation in selected patients (see Section "Treatment").

Certain factors may alter the primary drainage of a testis neoplasm. Invasion of the epididymis or spermatic cord may allow spread to the distal external iliac and obturator lymph nodes. Scrotal violation or invasion of the tunica albuginea may result in inguinal metastases. Although the retroperitoneum is the most commonly involved site in metastatic disease, visceral metastases may be seen in advanced disease. The sites involved in decreasing frequency include lung, liver, brain, bone, kidney, adrenal, gastrointestinal tract, and spleen. As mentioned previously, choriocarcinoma is the exception to the rule and is characterized by early hematogenous spread, especially to the lung. Choriocarcinoma has also a predilection for unusual sites of metastasis such as the spleen.

▶ Clinical Staging

Many clinical staging systems have been proposed for testicular cancer. However, most are variations of the original system proposed by Boden and Gibb (1951). In this system, a stage A lesion was confined to the testis, stage B demonstrated regional lymph node spread, and stage C was spread beyond retroperitoneal lymph nodes. Numerous clinical staging systems have also been suggested for seminoma. A stage I lesion is confined to the testis. Stage II has retroperitoneal nodal involvement (IIA is <2 cm, IIB is >2 cm). Stage III has supradiaphragmatic nodal involvement or visceral involvement. The TNM classification of American Joint Committee (2010) has attempted to standardize clinical stages as in Table 24–1.

▶ Clinical Findings

A. Symptoms

The most common symptom of testicular cancer is a painless enlargement of the testis. Enlargement is usually gradual, and a sensation of testicular heaviness is not unusual. The typical delay in treatment from initial recognition of the lesion by the patient to definitive therapy (orchiectomy) ranges from 3 to 6 months. The length of delay correlates with the incidence of metastases. The importance of patient awareness and self-examination is apparent. Acute testicular pain is seen in approximately 10% of cases and may be the result of intratesticular hemorrhage or infarction.

Approximately 10% of patients present with symptoms related to metastatic disease. Back pain (retroperitoneal

Table 24–1. TNM classification of tumors of the testis.

T—Primary tumor

TX:	Cannot be assessed
T0:	No evidence of primary tumor
Tis:	Intratubular cancer (CIS)
T1:	Limited to testis and epididymis, no vascular invasion
T2:	Invades beyond tunica albuginea and into tunica vaginalis or has vascular invasion
T3:	Invades spermatic cord
T4:	Invades scrotum

N—Regional lymph nodes

NX:	Cannot be assessed
N0:	No regional lymph node metastasis
N1:	Lymph node metastasis ≤2 cm, or multiple nodes, none >2 cm and <6 nodes positive
N2:	Nodal mass >2 cm and ≤5 cm or ≥6 nodes positive
N3:	Nodal mass >5 cm

M—Distant metastasis

MX:	Cannot be assessed
M0:	No distant metastasis
M1a:	Distant metastasis present in nonregional lymph nodes or lungs
M1b:	Nonpulmonary visceral metastases

S—Serum tumor markers

SX:	Markers not available
S0:	Marker levels within normal limits
S1:	Lactic acid dehydrogenase (LDH) <1.5 × normal and hCG <5000 mIU/mL and AFP <1000 ng/mL
S2:	LDH 1.5–10 × normal or hCG 5000–50,000 mIU/mL or AFP 1000–10,000 ng/mL
S3:	LDH >10 × normal or hCG >50,000 mIU/mL or AFP >10,000 ng/mL

Source: American Joint Committee on Cancer: Cancer Staging Manual, 7th ed. Springer-Verlag, New York, 2010.

metastases involving nerve roots) is the most common symptom. Other symptoms include cough or dyspnea (pulmonary metastases); anorexia, nausea, or vomiting (retroduodenal metastases); bone pain (skeletal metastases); and lower extremity swelling (vena caval obstruction).

Approximately 10% of patients are asymptomatic at presentation, and the tumor may be detected incidentally following trauma, or it may be detected by the patient's sexual partner.

B. Signs

A testicular mass or diffuse enlargement is found in most cases. The mass is typically firm and nontender and the epididymis should be easily separable from it. A hydrocele may accompany the testicular tumor and help to camouflage it. Transillumination of the scrotum can help to distinguish between these entities.

Palpation of the abdomen may reveal bulky retroperitoneal disease; assessment of supraclavicular, scalene, and inguinal nodes should be performed. Gynecomastia is present in 5% of all germ cell tumors but may be present in 30–50% of Sertoli and Leydig cell tumors. Its cause seems to be related to multiple complex hormonal interactions involving testosterone, estrone, estradiol, prolactin, and hCG. Hemoptysis may be seen in advanced pulmonary disease.

C. Laboratory Findings and Tumor Markers

Anemia may be detected in advanced disease. Liver function tests may be elevated in the presence of hepatic metastases. Renal function may be diminished (elevated serum creatinine) if ureteral obstruction secondary to bulky retroperitoneal disease is present. The assessment of renal function (creatinine clearance) is mandatory in patients with advanced disease who require chemotherapy.

Several biochemical markers are of importance in the diagnosis and management of testicular carcinoma, including AFP, hCG, and lactic acid dehydrogenase (LDH). AFP is a glycoprotein with a molecular mass of 70,000 daltons and a half-life of 4–6 days. Although present in fetal serum in high levels, beyond the age of 1 year, it is present only in trace amounts. While present to varying degrees in many NSGCTs (Table 24–2), it is never found in seminomas.

hCG is a glycoprotein with a molecular mass of 38,000 daltons and a half-life of 24 hours. It is composed of two subunits: alpha and beta. The alpha subunit is similar to the alpha subunits of luteinizing hormone (LH), follicle-stimulating hormone (FSH), and thyroid-stimulating hormone (TSH). The beta subunit conveys the activity to each of these hormones and allows for a highly sensitive and specific radioimmunoassay in the determination of hCG levels. A normal man should not have significant levels of beta-hCG. While more commonly elevated in NSGCTs, hCG levels may be elevated in up to 7% of seminomas.

LDH is a cellular enzyme with a molecular mass of 134,000 daltons that has five isoenzymes; it is normally found in muscle (smooth, cardiac, skeletal), liver, kidney, and brain.

Table 24–2. Incidence of elevated tumor markers by histologic type in testis cancer.

	hCG (%)	AFP (%)
Seminoma	7	0
Teratoma	25	38
Teratocarcinoma	57	64
Embryonal	60	70
Choriocarcinoma	100	0

AFP, alpha-fetoprotein; hCG, human chorionic gonadotropin.

Elevation of total serum LDH and in particular isoenzyme-I was shown to correlate with tumor burden in NSGCTs. LDH may also be elevated in seminoma.

Other markers have been described for testis cancer, including placental alkaline phosphatase (PLAP) and gamma-glutamyl transpeptidase (GGT). These markers, however, have not contributed as much to the management of patients as those mentioned previously.

D. Imaging

The primary testicular tumor can be rapidly and accurately assessed by scrotal ultrasonography. This technique can determine whether the mass is truly intratesticular, can be used to distinguish the tumor from epididymal pathology, and may also facilitate testicular examination in the presence of a hydrocele.

Once the diagnosis of testicular cancer has been established by inguinal orchiectomy, careful clinical staging of disease is mandatory. Chest radiographs (posteroanterior and lateral) and computed tomography (CT scan) of the abdomen and pelvis are used to assess the two most common sites of metastatic spread, namely, the lungs and retroperitoneum. The role of CT scanning of the chest remains controversial because of its decreased specificity. Of note is the fact that routine chest x-rays (CXR) detect 85–90% of pulmonary metastases. Pedal lymphangiography (LAG) is rarely used owing to its invasiveness as well as low specificity, although it may be warranted in patients undergoing a surveillance protocol (see Section "Treatment").

▶ Differential Diagnosis

An incorrect diagnosis is made at the initial examination in up to 25% of patients with testicular tumors and may result in delay in treatment or a suboptimal surgical approach (scrotal incision) for exploration. Epididymitis or epididymoorchitis is the most common misdiagnosis in patients with testis cancer. Early epididymitis should reveal an enlarged, tender epididymis that is clearly separable from the testis. In advanced stages, the inflammation may spread to the testis and result in an enlarged, tender, and indurated testis and epididymis. A history of acute onset of symptoms including fever, urethral discharge, and irritative voiding symptoms may make the diagnosis of epididymitis more likely. Ultrasonography may identify the enlarged epididymis as the cause of the scrotal mass.

Hydrocele is the second most common misdiagnosis. Transillumination of the scrotum may readily distinguish between a translucent, fluid-filled hydrocele, and a solid testicular tumor. Since 5–10% of testicular tumors may be associated with hydroceles, if the testis cannot be adequately examined, a scrotal ultrasound examination is mandatory. Aspiration of the hydrocele should be avoided because positive cytologic results have been reported in hydroceles associated with testicular tumors.

Other diagnoses to be considered include spermatocele, a cystic mass most commonly found extending from the head of the epididymis; hematocele associated with trauma; granulomatous orchitis, most commonly resulting from tuberculosis and associated with beading of the vas deferens; and varicocele, which is engorgement of the pampiniform plexus of veins in the spermatic cord and should disappear when the patient is in the supine position.

Although most intratesticular masses are malignant, one benign lesion, an epidermoid cyst, may be seen on rare occasions. Usually, these cysts are very small benign nodules located just underneath the tunica albuginea; however, on occasion, they can be large. The diagnosis is usually made following inguinal orchiectomy; as frozen sections, the larger lesions are often difficult to distinguish from teratoma.

▶ Treatment

Inguinal exploration with cross-clamping of the spermatic cord vasculature and delivery of the testis into the field is the mainstay of exploration for a possible testis tumor. If cancer cannot be excluded by examination of the testis, radical orchiectomy is warranted. Scrotal approaches and open testicular biopsies should be avoided. Further therapy depends on the histologic characteristics of the tumor as well as the clinical stage.

A. Low-Stage Seminoma

Seminoma is exquisitely radiosensitive. About 95% of all stage I seminomas are cured with radical orchiectomy and retroperitoneal irradiation (usually 2500–3000 cGy). This low dose of radiation is usually well tolerated, with minimal gastrointestinal side effects. Because radiation therapy is associated with some morbidity and secondary malignancy risk, there is an increasing interest in surveillance in stage I seminoma. Because of the slow growth rate of seminoma, surveillance must be performed for up to 10 years and typically consists of a history and physical exam and tumor markers every 3–4 months for years 1–3, every 6 months for years 4–7, and then annually up to 10 years. Imaging while on surveillance includes abdominal and pelvic CT at each visit and CXR at alternate visits. Alternatively, single-agent carboplatin has been used in low-stage seminoma (NCCN, 2010).

Low-volume retroperitoneal disease can also be treated effectively with retroperitoneal irradiation with an average 5-year survival rate of 87%. Prophylactic mediastinal radiation is no longer employed because this may cause considerable myelosuppression and thus compromise the patient's ability to receive chemotherapy if required. Chemotherapy should be used as salvage therapy for patients who relapse following irradiation.

B. High-Stage Seminoma

Patients with bulky seminoma and any seminoma associated with an elevated AFP should receive primary chemotherapy. Seminomas are also sensitive to platinum-based regimens, as are their NSGCT counterparts. Good-risk patients (see later) receive four cycles of etoposide and cisplatin (EP) or three cycles of cisplatin, etoposide, and bleomycin (PEB). Intermediate-risk patients receive four cycles of PEB.

Ninety percent of patients with advanced disease achieve a complete response with chemotherapy. Residual retroperitoneal masses following chemotherapy are often fibrosis (90%) unless the mass is well circumscribed and in excess of 3 cm, under which circumstances approximately 40% of patients harbor residual seminoma. A positron emission tomography (PET scan) should be performed in patients with a residual mass and if positive, surgical resection is warranted. In such cases, surgical excision is warranted.

C. Low-Stage Nonseminomatous Germ Cell Tumors

Standard treatment for stage I disease in the United States has included retroperitoneal lymph node dissection (RPLND). However, because three-fourths of patients with clinical stage I disease are cured by orchiectomy alone and the morbidity of RPLND is not negligible, other alternatives have been explored. These options include surveillance and open nerve-sparing RPLND.

Surveillance in stage I NSGCT was proposed because, as mentioned previously, 75% of patients with clinical stage I disease have, in fact, pathologic stage I disease. In addition, infertility related to disruption of sympathetic nerve fibers is common following RPLND. Clinical staging has been markedly improved in the presence of CT scanning and LAG. And finally, effective chemotherapy regimens have been developed for relapse. Patients are considered candidates for surveillance if the tumor is an NSGCT confined within the tunica albuginea, the tumor does not demonstrate vascular invasion, tumor markers normalize after orchiectomy, radiographic imaging shows no evidence of disease (CXR, CT), and the patient is considered reliable.

Surveillance should be considered an active process on the part of both the physician and the patient. Patients are followed every 1–2 months for the first 2 years, every 3 months in year 3, every 4 months in year 4, and every 6 months in year 5. Tumor markers and CXR are obtained at each visit, and CT scans are obtained every 2–3 months in year 1, every 3–4 months in year 2, every 4 months in year 3, every 6 months in year 4, and once a year in year 5. Most relapses occur, however, within the first 8–10 months. With rare exceptions, patients who relapse can be cured by chemotherapy or surgery, or both.

Retroperitoneal lymph node dissection has been the preferred treatment of low-stage NSGCTs in the United States until recently. A thoracoabdominal or midline transabdominal approach may be used, and all nodal tissue between the ureters from the renal vessels to the bifurcation of the common iliac vessels is removed. Patients with negative nodes or N1 disease do not require adjuvant therapy, whereas the

recommendation for those with N2 disease is to receive two cycles of chemotherapy because their relapse rate approaches 50%.

While effective in surgically staging and potentially curing a subset of patients, RPLND is associated with significant morbidity, especially with respect to fertility in young men. With a standard RPLND, sympathetic nerve fibers are disrupted, resulting in loss of seminal emission. Currently, a modified RPLND can be performed that preserves ejaculation in up to 90% of patients. By modifying the dissection below the level of the inferior mesenteric artery to include only the nodal tissue ipsilateral to the tumor, important sympathetic fibers from the contralateral side are preserved, thus maintaining emission.

An alternative approach to patients with clinical stage I disease and vascular invasion in the primary is two cycles of chemotherapy. While obviating the need for surgery, such an approach is associated with neurotoxicity and fertility issues for these young patients.

D. High-Stage Nonseminomatous Germ Cell Tumors

Patients with bulky retroperitoneal disease (>3-cm nodes or three or more 1-cm cuts on CT scan) or metastatic NSGCT are treated with primary platinum-based combination chemotherapy following orchiectomy. Good-risk patients are treated with either four cycles of EP or three cycles of PEB. Intermediate- and poor-risk patients receive four cycles of PEB. If tumor markers normalize and a residual mass is apparent on imaging studies, resection of that mass is mandatory, because 20% of the time it will harbor residual cancer, 40% of the time it will be teratoma, and 40% of the time it will be fibrosis (Figure 24–2). In patients with residual cancer in the resected tissue, the histologic picture is usually embryonal cell carcinoma, but malignant teratoma is seen in <5% of cases. Malignant teratoma is unresponsive to chemotherapy, and only 15% of patients survive following surgical resection. If tumor markers fail to normalize following primary chemotherapy, salvage chemotherapy is required (cisplatin, etoposide, bleomycin, ifosfamide). Even if patients attain a complete response after chemotherapy (normal tumor markers, no mass on CT scan or CXR), some investigators advocate an RPLND because viable germ cell tumor may be seen in up to 10% of cases.

Although the treatment plan described cures up to 70% of patients with high-volume disease, there are patients who fail to respond. Also, the potential complications from chemotherapy including sepsis, neuropathy, renal toxicity, and death must be considered. It is thus apparent that it is important to be able to discriminate between patients who are likely to respond to standard chemotherapy (good risk) and those who may require more aggressive regimens (intermediate or high risk). Table 24–3 stratifies patients with advanced testicular cancer into risk groups based upon the primary tumor

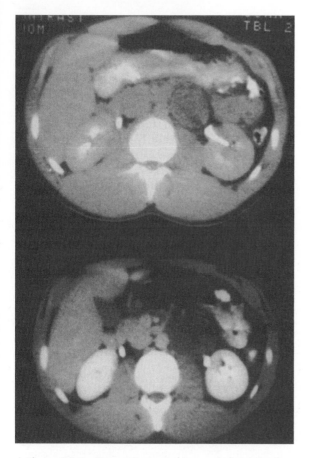

▲ **Figure 24–2.** **Upper:** Computed tomography scan of patient with bulky retroperitoneal mass after radical orchiectomy for embryonal carcinoma. **Lower:** Residual cystic mass after chemotherapy; it was resected and found to be teratoma.

site, location of metastases, and serum tumor markers. The rate of decline of serum tumor markers during chemotherapy has also been used to predict response in patients with advanced disease.

▶ Follow-up Care

All patients with testicular cancer require regular follow-up care. As discussed previously, patients on a surveillance protocol require vigorous follow-up. For those who have undergone surgery (RPLND) or radiotherapy, in general, they are followed at 3-month intervals for the first 2 years, then every 6 months until 5 years, and then yearly. Follow-up visits should include careful examination of the remaining testis, the abdomen, and the lymph node areas. Laboratory investigation should include AFP, hCG, and LDH levels. A CXR and an abdominal film (if an LAG was performed) should also be included at each visit. Abdominal CT scans are used less frequently as risk of relapse in the retroperitoneum is low following RPLND.

▶ Prognosis

Survival in testicular cancer has improved dramatically over the past several years, reflecting the continuing improvement and refinement in combination chemotherapy. For seminoma treated by orchiectomy and radiotherapy, the 5-year disease-free survival rate is 98% for stage I and 92–94% for stage II-A in several recent series. Higher stage disease treated by orchiectomy and primary chemotherapy has a 5-year disease-free survival rate of 35–75%, yet the lower value comes from older series in which more crude chemotherapy regimens were employed.

Survival in patients with NSGCTs treated by orchiectomy and RPLND for stage I disease ranges from 96% to 100%. For low-volume stage II disease treated with chemotherapy plus surgery, >90% 5-year disease-free survival rates are attainable. Patients with bulky retroperitoneal or disseminated

Table 24–3. Risk classification for testicular cancer.

Risk status	Nonseminoma	Seminoma
Good risk	Testicular or retroperitoneal primary No nonpulmonary visceral metastases Postorchiectomy markers S1 level	Any primary site No nonpulmonary visceral metastases Normal AFP, any hCG, any LDH
Intermediate risk	Testicular or retroperitoneal primary No nonpulmonary visceral metastases Postorchiectomy markers S2 level	Any primary site No nonpulmonary visceral metastases Normal AFP, any hCG, any LDH
Poor risk	Mediastinal primary tumor Nonpulmonary visceral metastases Postorchiectomy markers S3 level	None

AFP, alpha-fetoprotein; hCG, human chorionic gonadotropin; LDH, lactic acid dehydrogenase.

disease treated with primary chemotherapy followed by surgery have a 5-year disease-free survival rate of 55–80%.

NON–GERM CELL TUMORS OF THE TESTIS

Approximately 5–6% of all testis tumors are non–germ cell tumors of the testis. Three types will be considered, namely, Leydig cell tumors, Sertoli cell tumors, and gonadoblastomas.

LEYDIG CELL TUMORS

▶ Epidemiology and Pathology

Leydig cell tumors are the most common non–germ cell tumors of the testis and account for 1–3% of all testicular tumors. They follow a bimodal age distribution: the 5- to 9-year-old and the 25- to 35-year-old age groups. Twenty-five percent of these tumors occur in childhood. Bilaterality is seen in 5–10% of cases. The cause of these tumors is unknown; unlike germ cell tumors, there is no association with cryptorchidism.

Pathologic examination reveals a small, yellow, well-circumscribed lesion devoid of hemorrhage or necrosis. Microscopically, hexagonally shaped cells with granular, eosinophilic cytoplasm containing lipid vacuoles are seen. Reinke crystals are fusiform-shaped cytoplasmic inclusions that are pathognomonic for Leydig cells.

▶ Clinical Findings

Prepubertal children usually present with virilization, and tumors are benign. Adults are usually asymptomatic, although gynecomastia may be present in 20–25%. Ten percent of tumors in adults are malignant. Laboratory findings include elevated serum and urinary 17-ketosteroids as well as estrogens.

▶ Treatment and Prognosis

Radical orchiectomy is the initial treatment for Leydig cell tumors. Clinical staging is similar to that for germ cell tumors, and levels of the 17-ketosteroids can be helpful in distinguishing between benign and malignant lesions. Elevations of 10–30 times normal are typical of malignancy. RPLND is recommended for malignant lesions. Because of the rarity of these lesions, the role of chemotherapy remains to be defined. Prognosis is excellent for benign lesions, while it remains poor for patients with disseminated disease.

SERTOLI CELL TUMORS

▶ Epidemiology and Pathology

Sertoli cell tumors are exceedingly rare, composing <1% of all testicular tumors. A bimodal age distribution is seen: 1-year old or younger and the 20- to 45-year-old age group. Approximately 10% of the lesions are malignant. Gross examination reveals a yellow or gray-white lesion with cystic components. Benign lesions are well circumscribed, while malignant lesions show ill-defined borders. Microscopically, tumors appear heterogeneous with mixed amounts of epithelial and stromal components. Sertoli cells are columnar or hexagonal cells with a large nucleus and solitary nucleolus and contain vacuolated cytoplasm.

▶ Clinical Findings

A testicular mass is the most common presentation. Virilization is often seen in children, and gynecomastia may be present in 30% of adults. Because of the rarity of these tumors, minimal endocrine data are available on these patients.

▶ Treatment

Radical orchiectomy is the initial procedure of choice. In cases of malignancy, RPLND is indicated; however, the roles of chemotherapy and radiotherapy remain unclear.

GONADOBLASTOMAS

▶ Epidemiology and Pathology

Gonadoblastomas comprise 0.5% of all testicular tumors and are almost exclusively seen in patients with some form of gonadal dysgenesis. Most of these tumors occur in patients younger than 30 years, although the age distribution ranges from infancy to >70 years. Gross examination reveals a yellow or gray-white lesion that can vary in size from microscopic to >20 cm and may exhibit calcifications. Microscopically, three cell types are seen: Sertoli cells, interstitial cells, and germ cells.

▶ Clinical Findings

The clinical manifestations are predominantly related to the underlying gonadal dysgenesis and are discussed elsewhere in this book. It is noteworthy that four-fifths of patients with gonadoblastomas are phenotypic females. Males typically have cryptorchidism or hypospadias.

▶ Treatment and Prognosis

Radical orchiectomy is the primary treatment of choice. In the presence of gonadal dysgenesis, a contralateral gonadectomy is recommended because the tumor tends to be bilateral in 50% of cases in this setting. Prognosis is excellent.

SECONDARY TUMORS OF THE TESTIS

Secondary tumors of the testis are rare. Three categories are considered: lymphoma, leukemia, and metastatic tumors.

LYMPHOMA

▶ Epidemiology and Pathology

Lymphoma is the most common testicular tumor in a patient older than 50 years and is the most common secondary neoplasm of the testis, accounting for 5% of all testicular tumors. It may be seen in three clinical settings: (1) late manifestation of widespread lymphoma; (2) initial presentation of clinically occult disease; and (3) primary extranodal disease. Gross examination reveals a bulging, gray or pink lesion with ill-defined margins. Hemorrhage and necrosis are common. Microscopically, diffuse histiocytic lymphoma is the most common type.

▶ Clinical Findings

Painless enlargement of the testis is common. Generalized constitutional symptoms occur in one-fourth of patients. Bilateral testis involvement occurs in 50% of patients, usually asynchronously.

▶ Treatment and Prognosis

Fine needle aspiration should be considered in patients with a known or suspected diagnosis of lymphoma while radical orchiectomy is reserved for those with suspected primary lymphoma of the testicle. Further staging and treatment should be handled in conjunction with the medical oncologist. Prognosis is related to the stage of disease. Some reports support adjuvant chemotherapy for primary testicular lymphoma, with improved survival rates of up to 93% after 44 months of follow-up.

LEUKEMIC INFILTRATION OF THE TESTIS

The testis is a common site of relapse for children with acute lymphocytic leukemia. Bilateral involvement may be present in one-half of cases. Testis biopsy rather than orchiectomy is the diagnostic procedure of choice. Bilateral testicular irradiation with 20 Gy and reinstitution of adjuvant chemotherapy constitute the treatment of choice. Prognosis remains guarded.

METASTATIC TUMORS

Metastasis to the testis is rare. These lesions are typically incidental findings at autopsy. The most common primary site is the prostate, followed by the lung, gastrointestinal tract, melanoma, and kidney. The typical pathologic finding is neoplastic cells in the interstitium with relative sparing of the seminiferous tubules.

EXTRAGONADAL GERM CELL TUMORS

▶ Epidemiology and Pathology

Extragonadal germ cell tumors are rare, accounting for approximately 3% of all germ cell tumors. Debate continues over whether these lesions originate from "burned-out" testicular primaries or originate de novo. Most retroperitoneal tumors have their origin from a testicular primary, whereas mediastinal germ cell tumors are truly ectopic.

The most common sites of origin in decreasing order are mediastinum, retroperitoneum, sacrococcygeal area, and pineal gland. All germ cell types may be observed. Seminoma composes more than half of the retroperitoneal and mediastinal tumors.

▶ Clinical Findings

Clinical presentation depends on the site and volume of disease. Mediastinal lesions may present with pulmonary complaints. Retroperitoneal lesions may present with abdominal or back pain and a palpable mass. Sacrococcygeal tumors are most commonly seen in neonates and may present with a palpable mass and bowel or urinary obstruction. Pineal tumors may present with headache, visual or auditory complaints, or hypopituitarism.

Metastatic spread is to regional lymph nodes, lung, liver, bone, and brain. Metastatic workup is similar, therefore, to that of testicular germ cell tumors. A careful testicular examination is mandatory along with ultrasonography to exclude an occult testicular primary.

▶ Treatment and Prognosis

Treatment of extragonadal germ cell tumors parallels that of testicular tumors. Low-volume seminoma can be managed with radiotherapy. High-volume seminoma should receive primary chemotherapy. Prognosis parallels that of testicular seminoma. Primary chemotherapy should be employed for nonseminomatous elements with surgical excision of residual masses; however, prognosis remains poor for these patients.

TUMORS OF THE EPIDIDYMIS, PARATESTICULAR TISSUES, AND SPERMATIC CORD

Primary tumors of the epididymis are rare and are most commonly benign. Adenomatoid tumors of the epididymis are the most common and typically occur in the third and fourth decade of life. They are typically asymptomatic, solid lesions that arise from any portion of the epididymis.

Leiomyomas are the second most common tumor of the epididymis. These lesions tend to be painful and are often associated with a hydrocele. Cystadenomas are benign lesions of the epididymis that are bilateral in 30% of cases and are frequently seen in association with von Hippel–Lindau disease. Histologically, these lesions are difficult to distinguish from renal cell carcinoma. Malignant lesions of the epididymis are extremely rare. In general, an inguinal approach should be used, and if frozen section confirms a benign lesion, epididymectomy should be performed. If a malignant tumor is diagnosed, radical orchiectomy must be performed.

Tumors of the spermatic cord are typically benign. Lipomas of the cord account for most of these lesions. Of the malignant lesions, rhabdomyosarcoma is the most common, followed by leiomyosarcoma, fibrosarcoma, and liposarcoma.

Clinical diagnosis of tumors of the spermatic cord can be difficult. Differentiating between a hernia and a spermatic cord tumor may be possible only at exploration. In general, these lesions should be approached through an inguinal incision. The cord should be occluded at the internal ring and frozen sections obtained. If malignancy is diagnosed, attention should be directed toward performing wide local excision to avoid local recurrence. Staging of disease is similar to that of testicular tumors. For rhabdomyosarcoma, RPLND should be performed with adjuvant radiotherapy and chemotherapy. The value of RPLND for the other malignant spermatic cord tumors remains to be determined. Prognosis relates to the histologic status, stage, and site of disease.

TUMORS OF THE PENIS

▶ Epidemiology and Risk Factors

Carcinoma of the penis accounts for <1% of cancers among males in the United States, with approximately one to two new cases being reported per 100,000 men. There is marked variation in incidence with geographic location. In areas such as Africa and regions of South America, penile carcinoma may compose 10–20% of all malignant lesions. Penile carcinoma occurs most commonly in the sixth decade of life, although rare case reports have included children.

The one etiologic factor most commonly associated with penile carcinoma is poor hygiene. The disease is virtually unheard of in males circumcised near birth. One theory postulates that smegma accumulation under the phimotic foreskin results in chronic inflammation leading to carcinoma. A viral cause has also been suggested as a result of the association of this tumor with cervical carcinoma.

▶ Pathology

A. Precancerous Dermatologic Lesions

Leukoplakia is a rare condition that most commonly occurs in diabetic patients. A white plaque typically involving the meatus is seen. Histologic examination reveals acanthosis, hyperkeratosis, and parakeratosis. This lesion may precede or occur simultaneously with penile carcinoma.

Balanitis xerotica obliterans is a white patch originating on the prepuce or glans and usually involving the meatus. The condition is most commonly observed in middle-aged diabetic patients. Microscopic examination reveals atrophic epidermis and abnormalities in collagen deposition.

Giant condylomata acuminata are cauliflower-like lesions arising from the prepuce or glans. The cause is believed to be viral (human papillomavirus). These lesions may be difficult to distinguish from well-differentiated squamous cell carcinoma.

B. Carcinoma In Situ (Bowen Disease, Erythroplasia of Queyrat)

Bowen disease is a squamous cell carcinoma in situ typically involving the penile shaft. The lesion appears as a red plaque with encrustations.

Erythroplasia of Queyrat is a velvety, red lesion with ulcerations that usually involve the glans. Microscopic examination shows typical, hyperplastic cells in a disordered array with vacuolated cytoplasm and mitotic figures.

C. Invasive Carcinoma of the Penis

Squamous cell carcinoma composes most penile cancers. It most commonly originates on the glans, with the next most common sites, in order, being the prepuce and shaft. The appearance may be papillary or ulcerative.

Verrucous carcinoma is a variant of squamous cell carcinoma composing 5–16% of penile carcinomas. This lesion is papillary in appearance, and on histologic examination, it is noted to have a well-demarcated deep margin unlike the infiltrating margin of the typical squamous cell carcinoma.

▶ Patterns of Spread

Invasive carcinoma of the penis begins as an ulcerative or papillary lesion, which may gradually grow to involve the entire glans or shaft of the penis. Buck's fascia represents a barrier to corporal invasion and hematogenous spread. Primary dissemination is via lymphatic channels to the femoral and iliac nodes. The prepuce and shaft skin drain into the superficial inguinal nodes (superficial to fascia lata), while the glans and corporal bodies drain to both superficial and deep inguinal nodes (deep to fascia lata). There are many cross-communications so that penile lymphatic drainage is bilateral to both inguinal areas. Drainage from the inguinal nodes is to the pelvic nodes. Involvement of the femoral nodes may result in skin necrosis and infection or femoral vessel erosion and hemorrhage. Distant metastases are clinically apparent in <10% of cases and may involve lung, liver, bone, or brain.

▶ Tumor Staging

The staging system used most commonly in the United States was proposed by Jackson (1966), and the stages are as follows: In stage I, the tumor is confined to the glans or prepuce. Stage II involves the penile shaft. Stage III has operable inguinal node metastasis. In stage IV, the tumor extends beyond the penile shaft, with inoperable inguinal or distant metastases. The TNM classification of the American Joint Committee (1996) is given in Table 24–4.

Table 24–4. TNM classification of tumors of the penis.

T—Primary tumor	
TX:	Cannot be assessed
T0:	No evidence of primary tumor
Tis:	Carcinoma in situ
Ta:	Noninvasive verrucous carcinoma
T1:	Invades subepithelial connective tissue
T2:	Invades corpus spongiosum or cavernosum
T3:	Invades urethra or prostate
T4:	Invades other adjacent structures
N—Regional lymph nodes	
NX:	Cannot be assessed
N0:	No regional lymph node metastasis
N1:	Metastasis in single superficial inguinal node
N2:	Metastasis in multiple or bilateral superficial inguinal nodes
N3:	Metastasis in deep inguinal or pelvic nodes
M—Distant metastasis	
MX:	Cannot be assessed
M0:	No distant metastasis
M1:	Distant metastasis present

Source: American Joint Committee on Cancer: *TNM Classification—Genitourinary Sites,* 2010.

Clinical Findings

A. Symptoms

The most common complaint at presentation is the lesion itself. It may appear as an area of induration or erythema, an ulceration, a small nodule, or an exophytic growth. Phimosis may obscure the lesion and result in a delay in seeking medical attention. In fact, 15–50% of patients delay for at least 1 year in seeking medical attention. Other symptoms include pain, discharge, irritative voiding symptoms, and bleeding.

B. Signs

Lesions are typically confined to the penis at presentation. The primary lesion should be characterized with respect to size, location, and potential corporal body involvement. Careful palpation of the inguinal area is mandatory because >50% of patients present with enlarged inguinal nodes. This enlargement may be secondary to inflammation or metastatic spread.

C. Laboratory Findings

Laboratory evaluation is typically normal. Anemia and leukocytosis may be present in patients with long-standing disease or extensive local infection. Hypercalcemia in the absence of osseous metastases may be seen in 20% of patients and appears to correlate with volume of disease.

D. Imaging

Metastatic workup should include CXR, bone scan, and CT scan of the abdomen and pelvis. Disseminated disease is present in <10% of patients at presentation.

Differential Diagnosis

In addition to the dermatologic lesions discussed previously, carcinoma of the penis must be differentiated from several infectious lesions. Syphilitic chancre may present as a painless ulceration. Serologic and dark field examination should establish the diagnosis. Chancroid typically appears as a painful ulceration of the penis. Selective cultures for *Haemophilus ducreyi* should identify the cause. Condylomata acuminata appear as exophytic, soft, "grape cluster" lesions anywhere on the penile shaft or glans. Biopsy can distinguish this lesion from carcinoma if any doubt exists.

Treatment

A. Primary Lesion

Biopsy of the primary lesion is mandatory to establish the diagnosis of malignancy. Treatment varies depending on the pathology as well as the location of the lesion. CIS may be treated conservatively in reliable patients. Fluorouracil cream application or neodymium:YAG laser treatment is effective for CIS and is preserving of the penis. Patients must come for frequent follow-up examinations to monitor response.

The goal of treatment in invasive penile carcinoma is complete excision with adequate margins. For lesions involving the prepuce, this may be accomplished by simple circumcision. For lesions involving the glans or distal shaft, partial penectomy with a 2-cm margin to decrease local recurrence has traditionally been suggested. Less aggressive surgical resections such as Mohs micrographic surgery and local excisions directed at penile preservation yet attaining a negative surgical margin have gained popularity. For lesions involving the proximal shaft or when partial penectomy results in a penile stump of insufficient length for sexual function or directing the urinary stream, total penectomy with perineal urethrostomy has been recommended.

B. Regional Lymph Nodes

As discussed previously, penile carcinoma spreads primarily to the inguinal lymph nodes. However, enlargement of inguinal nodes at presentation does not necessarily imply metastatic disease. In fact, up to 50% of the time this enlargement is caused by inflammation. Thus, patients who present with enlarged inguinal nodes should undergo treatment of the primary lesion followed by a 4- to 6-week

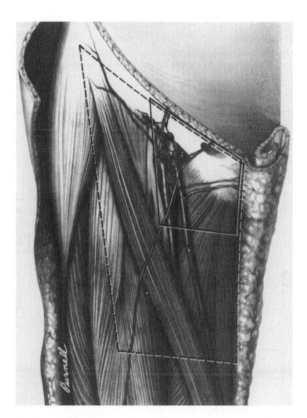

▲ **Figure 24–3.** Comparison of limits of dissection of complete (dashed line) versus limited (solid line) inguinal lymphadenectomy.

course of oral broad-spectrum antibiotics. Persistent adenopathy following antibiotic treatment should be considered to be metastatic disease, and sequential bilateral ilioinguinal node dissections should be performed. If lymphadenopathy resolves with antibiotics, observation in low-stage primary tumors (Tis, T1) is warranted. However, if lymphadenopathy resolves in higher stage tumors, more limited lymph node samplings should be considered, such as the sentinel node biopsy described by Cabanas (1977) or a modified (limited) dissection as suggested by Catalona (1988) (Figure 24–3). If positive nodes are encountered, bilateral ilioinguinal node dissection should be performed. A decision tree for penile carcinoma is presented in Figure 24–4. Patients who initially have clinically negative nodes but in whom clinically palpable nodes later develop should undergo a unilateral ilioinguinal node dissection.

Patients who have inoperable disease and bulky inguinal metastases are treated with chemotherapy (cisplatin and 5-fluorouracil). In some cases, regional radiotherapy can provide significant palliation by delaying ulceration and infectious complications and alleviating pain.

C. Systemic Disease

Four chemotherapeutic agents demonstrate activity against penile carcinoma: bleomycin, methotrexate, cisplatin, and 5-fluorouracil. However, no long term responders have been reported.

▶ Prognosis

Survival in penile carcinoma correlates with the presence or absence of nodal disease. Five-year survival rates for patients with node-negative disease range from 65% to 90%. For patients with positive inguinal nodes, this rate decreases to 30–50% and with positive iliac nodes decreases to <20%. In the presence of soft tissue or bony metastases, no 5-year survivors have been reported.

▶ Other Penile Tumors

Squamous cell carcinoma accounts for 98% of penile cancers. Sporadic cases of melanoma, basal cell carcinoma, and Paget disease have been reported. The incidence of Kaposi sarcoma of the penis is increasing with the increasing prevalence of the human immunodeficiency virus. It appears as a painful papule on the glans or shaft with bluish-purple discoloration. These lesions tend to be radiosensitive.

TUMORS OF THE SCROTUM

Tumors of the scrotal skin are rare. The most common benign lesion is a sebaceous cyst. Squamous cell carcinoma is the most common malignant tumor of the scrotum, although rare cases of melanoma, basal cell carcinoma, and Kaposi sarcoma have been reported. In the past, squamous cell carcinoma of the scrotum most commonly resulted from exposure to environmental carcinogens including chimney soot, tars, paraffin, and some petroleum products. Today, most cases result from poor hygiene and chronic inflammation.

Biopsy of the scrotal lesion must be performed to establish a histologic diagnosis. Wide excision with a 2-cm margin should be performed for malignant tumors. Surrounding subcutaneous tissue should be excised with the primary tumor; however, resection of the scrotal contents is rarely necessary. Primary closure using the redundant scrotal skin is usually possible. The management of inguinal nodes should be similar to that of penile cancer.

Prognosis correlates with the presence or absence of nodal involvement. In the presence of inguinal node metastasis, the 5-year survival rate is approximately 25%; there are virtually no survivors if iliac nodes are involved.

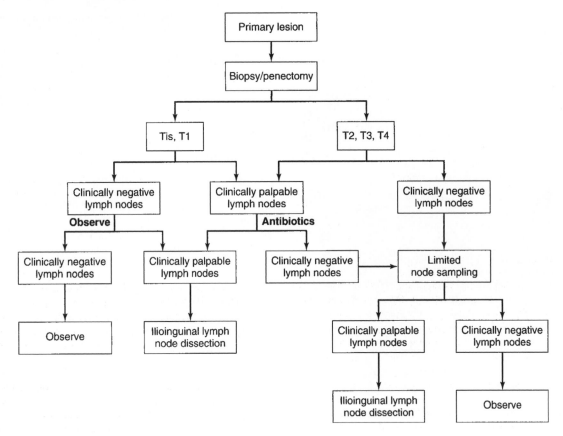

▲ **Figure 24–4.** Management of penile carcinoma.

BIBLIOGRAPHY

Tumors of the Testis

American Joint Committee on Cancer: Cancer Staging Manual, 7th ed. Springer-Verlag, New York, 2010.

Berthelsen JG et al: Screening for carcinoma in situ of the contra-lateral testis in patients with germinal testicular cancer. Br Med J 1982;285:1683.

Boden G, Gibb R: Radiotherapy and testicular neoplasms. Lancet 1951;2:1195.

National Comprehensive Cancer Network Clinical Practice Guide-lines in Oncology: Testicular Cancer, 2010. Available at: http://www.nccn.org/professionals/physician_gls/f_guidelines.asp

Pettersson A et al: Age at surgery for undescended testis and risk of testicular cancer. N Engl J Med 2007;356:1835.

Tumors of the Penis

Cabanas RM: An approach for the treatment of penile carcinoma. Cancer 1977;39:456.

Catalona WJ: Modified inguinal lymphadenectomy for carcinoma of the penis with preservation of saphenous veins: Technique and preliminary results. J Urol 1988;140:306.

Jackson SM: The treatment of carcinoma of the penis. Br J Surg 1966;53:33.

Carroll PR, Presti JC Jr: Testis cancer. Urol Clin North Am 1998;25(3): entire issue.

Urinary Diversion & Bladder Substitutions

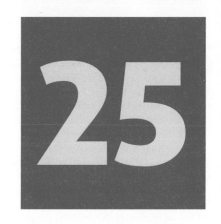

Badrinath R. Konety, MD, MBA,

Susan Barbour, RN, MS, WOCN, & Peter R. Carroll, MD, MPH

Selected patients with lower urinary tract cancers or severe functional or anatomic abnormalities of the bladder may require urinary diversion. Although this can be accomplished by establishing direct contact between the urinary tract and the skin surface, it is most often performed by incorporating various intestinal segments into the urinary tract. Virtually every segment of the gastrointestinal tract has been used to create urinary reservoirs or conduits. No single technique is ideal for all patients and clinical situations. A decision is based on a patient's underlying disease and its method of treatment as well as on renal function, individual anatomy, and personal preference. An ideal method of urinary diversion would most closely approximate the normal bladder: it would be nonrefluxing, low pressure, continent, and nonabsorptive.

Individual methods of urinary diversion can be categorized in various ways, such as (1) by the segment of intestine used and (2) by whether the method provides complete continence or simply acts as a conduit carrying urine from the renal pelvis or ureter to the skin, where the urine is collected in an appliance attached to the skin surface. Continent forms of urinary diversion can be categorized further according to whether they are attached to the urethra (ie, as a bladder substitute) or are placed in the abdomen and rely on another mechanism for continence (continent urinary reservoir).

PREOPERATIVE COUNSELING AND PREPARATION

All candidates for urinary diversion or bladder substitution should undergo careful preoperative counseling and preparation, including a detailed discussion of the objectives and potential complications of each method. Any potential impact of a procedure on sexual function, body image, and lifestyle should be discussed. Overall satisfaction of most patients undergoing urinary diversion appears to be high (Allareddy et al, 2006; Dutta et al, 2002; Fujisawa et al, 2000a;

Hara et al, 2002). However, because they allow freedom from an external appliance, continent forms of urinary diversion, especially bladder substitution, may be of great psychological and functional benefit to well-selected patients (Bjerre, 1995; Okada et al, 1997). More recent data suggest that the differences in quality of life between continent and noncontinent diversion may not be as significant as previously expected (Gilbert et al, 2007).

A careful history taken from the patient should note any previous abdominal or pelvic surgery, irradiation, or systemic disease. A history of intestinal resection or irradiation, renal failure, diverticulitis, regional enteritis, or ulcerative colitis would be especially important to consider when selecting a method of urinary diversion or bladder substitution. A complete blood count and measurement of serum electrolytes, urea nitrogen, and creatinine should be performed. The upper urinary tract should be imaged with intravenous urography, ultrasound, or computed tomography to determine whether hydronephrosis, renal parenchymal scarring, or calculous disease exists. Contrast imaging of the small or large bowel or colonoscopy should be considered preoperatively for patients with a history of significant intestinal irradiation, occult bleeding, or other gastrointestinal diseases. Patients with benign bladder diseases—such as a reduced bladder capacity due to neurologic disorders or irradiation, bladder fistulas, or interstitial cystitis—are occasionally considered candidates for urinary diversion or bladder substitution to manage urinary incontinence; however, with such patients, careful evaluation of bladder function and anatomy is required, as adequate urinary function can often be restored by urinary tract reconstruction, pharmacologic manipulation, or intermittent catheterization.

Patients undergo a standard mechanical and oral antibiotic bowel cleansing program beginning 1 or 2 days before surgery. Recent data suggest that mechanical bowel preparation can be avoided in colon and rectal surgery without increased risk of postoperative infectious complications. It may actually contribute to postoperative ileus. Hence use of clear liquid diet without mechanical bowel preparation prior to surgery may be adequate (Slim et al, 2009). Administration of combined oral and intravenous antibiotics prior to bowel surgery is advised as it appears to reduce the risk of wound infections by as much as 75% (Nelson et al, 2009). Much of patients' dissatisfaction with urinary diversion can be attributed to poor stomal construction or siting (Fitzgerald et al, 1997). The patient should be preoperatively evaluated in the lying, sitting, and standing positions with their clothes on. The stoma should preferably be located above or below the belt line. The most common site for stoma placement is through the rectus abdominis muscle sheath to avoid the later development of a parastomal hernia. The ideal location is free of creases, folds, previous incisions, and in a location visible to the patient to ensure ability to care for stoma. In obese patients or patients with a short mesentery, the stoma should be placed closer to the level of the umbilicus or in the right upper quadrant.

INTESTINAL CONDUIT URINARY DIVERSION

▶ Ileal Conduit

Ureteroileal urinary diversion is the most common method of urinary diversion in the United States. The conduit is constructed using a segment of ileum 18–20 cm long and located approximately 15–20 cm proximal to the ileocecal valve (Figure 25–1). Longer conduits may be required in obese patients, but a short segment minimizes the absorptive surface of the bowel in contact with urine. Once the appropriate length of bowel is selected and isolated, the mesentery is divided proximally and distally and individual mesenteric blood vessels are ligated. The bowel is divided, thus isolating the segment selected for conduit construction. The continuity of the small intestine is reestablished, with the anastomoses being above the plane of the conduit allowing for normal bowel function. The conduit is usually positioned in the right lower quadrant of the abdomen in an isoperistaltic direction. The posterior closed end of the conduit can be sewn with an absorbable suture to exclude the staple line and fixed to the posterior peritoneum or the sacral promontory to prevent volvulus of the conduit. The ureters are reimplanted individually in an end-to-side fashion or joined together (Wallace technique) and anastomosed in an end-to-end fashion, creating a refluxing ureteroileal anastomosis. Ureteral stents (7–8F, single-J, Silastic) are usually placed through the ureteral anastomosis and conduit and into the renal pelvis to facilitate urinary drainage while the anastomosis is healing.

The preselected stoma site is identified and a small circle of skin and underlying fat excised. The fascia is incised in a cruciate fashion. The end of the conduit is brought through the rectus abdominis muscle and anchored to the fascia, and the stoma is then formed. The stoma should protrude,

without tension, approximately 1–1.5 in above the skin surface.

▶ Jejunal Conduit

Jejunal conduit urinary diversion is used rarely and mainly in cases where other segments cannot be used due to significant ileal and colonic disease caused by previous irradiation or inflammatory bowel disease. Electrolyte disturbances are more common when the jejunum is used for conduit construction and hence this bowel segment is used only if none of the other intestinal segments can be used to fashion a conduit.

▶ Colon Conduit

There are several advantages to using the large bowel in construction of urinary conduits: nonrefluxing ureterointestinal anastomoses are easily performed, possibly abrogating the deleterious effects of reflux on the upper urinary tracts (Richie and Skinner, 1975); stomal stenosis is uncommon because of the wide diameter of the large bowel; limited absorption of electrolytes occurs; and the blood supply to the transverse and sigmoid colon is abundant. Either the transverse or the sigmoid colon can be used, allowing for placement of the conduit high or low in the abdomen, depending on the integrity and condition of the ureters. Use of the transverse colon for conduit construction is especially well suited for patients who have received extensive pelvic irradiation or when the middle and distal ureters are absent.

The blood supply of the transverse colon is based on the middle colic artery. The greater omentum is separated from the superior surface of the transverse colon, and a segment of bowel, usually 15 cm in length, is selected for the conduit (Figure 25–2). Short mesenteric incisions are made, and the colon is divided proximally and distally. Once the conduit is isolated, bowel continuity is reestablished. The proximal end of the conduit is closed and fixed in the midline posteriorly. The ureters are brought through small incisions in the posterior peritoneum and reimplanted into the base of the conduit. The stoma may be positioned on either the patient's right or left side.

A sigmoid conduit is constructed in a similar manner. Great care should be taken to preserve the blood supply by carefully selecting a segment with a good blood supply and by making short mesenteric incisions. The conduit is positioned lateral to the reapproximated sigmoid colon. Ureteral reimplantation and stoma construction are completed.

The ureters can be reimplanted into the large intestine either in a nonrefluxing submucosal tunnel or in a refluxing end-to-side manner. A submucosal tunnel can be created by incising the tenia up to the mucosa of the large bowel for a distance of 3–4 cm. A "button" of mucosa is removed, and the ureter is anastomosed to the mucosa of the bowel. The muscularis

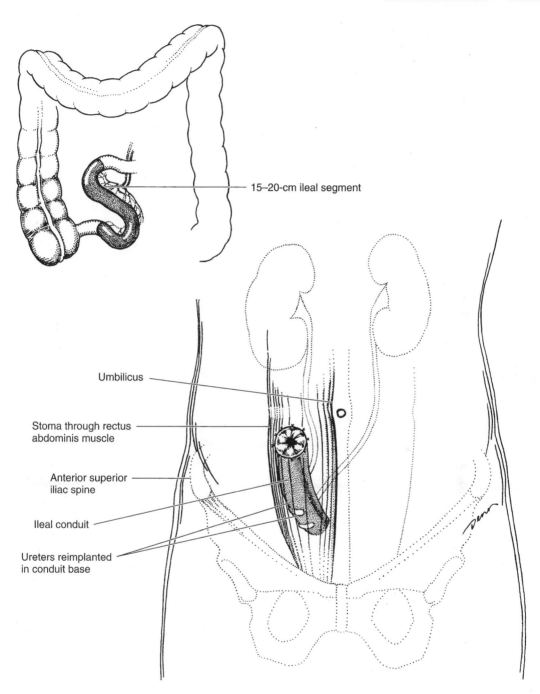

15–20-cm ileal segment

Umbilicus

Stoma through rectus
abdominis muscle

Anterior superior
iliac spine

Ileal conduit

Ureters reimplanted
in conduit base

▲ **Figure 25–1.** Ileal conduit.

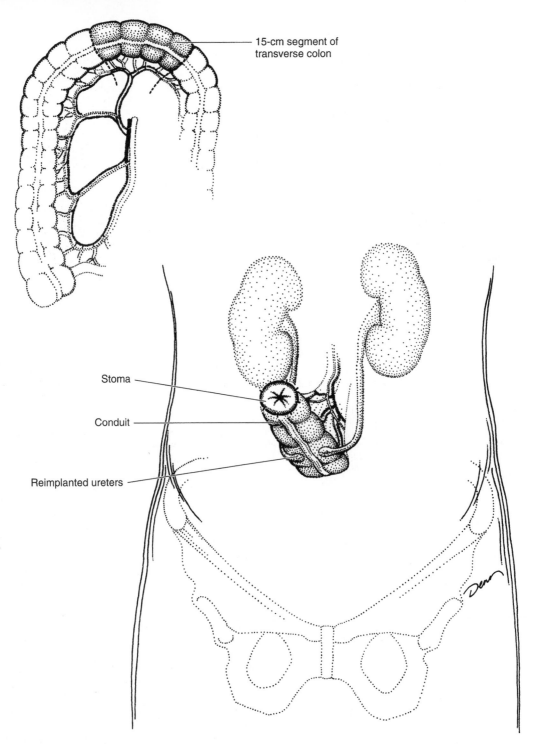

15-cm segment of transverse colon

Stoma

Conduit

Reimplanted ureters

▲ **Figure 25–2.** Transverse colon conduit.

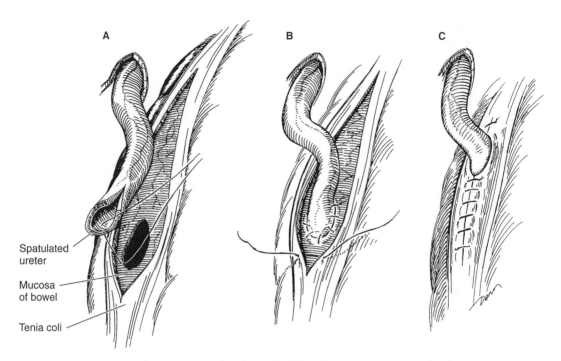

Spatulated
ureter

Mucosa
of bowel

Tenia coli

▲ **Figure 25–3.** Creation of a submucosal tunnel in the wall of the colon to prevent ureteral reflux of urine. **A:** Incision in the tenia coli. **B:** Anastomosis of distal ureter to large intestine mucosa. **C:** Muscularis (tenia) approximated over ureter.

of the tenia is reapproximated over the ureter to complete the tunnel (Figure 25–3).

CONTINENT URINARY DIVERSION AND BLADDER SUBSTITUTION

▶ General Considerations

Various procedures have been developed for construction of bladder substitutes or continent urinary reservoirs that preclude the need for an external urine collection appliance. Such reservoirs or bladder substitutes are composed of three segments: ureterointestinal (afferent limb) anastomosis, the reservoir itself, and the conduit carrying the urine from the reservoir to the surface (efferent continence mechanism). Bladder substitutes rely on the intact urethra and sphincter to provide outlet resistance and carry urine to the urethral meatus. In men and women whose urethrae are involved by cancer or are not functional owing to benign diseases, an efferent continence mechanism can be constructed with the appendix or short segments of tapered, intussuscepted, or reimplanted intestine.

The decision to proceed with bladder replacement is dependent on the risk of urethral recurrence and the continence of the patient. Both men and women who have low risk of urethral recurrence and those who have intact external urinary sphincters should be considered for bladder replacement rather than construction of a continent urinary reservoir. The risk of urethral occurrence or recurrence in men who undergo radical cystectomy is 6.1–10.6%. Carcinoma in situ and tumor multifocality appear to be risk factors for prostatic urethral tumor involvement in men with bladder cancer (Nixon et al, 2002). Although prostatic urethral disease is a risk factor for urethral recurrence, recent evidence suggests that orthotopic diversion may be considered in those with only proximal prostatic urethral involvement and negative urethral margins at cystectomy (Iselin et al, 1997). Although orthotopic bladder replacement was once reserved for men, it is now commonly performed in women as well (Stein et al, 1997). Women with bladder cancer whose tumors are not located at the bladder neck and have a clear urethral margin at the time of cystectomy are candidates for this procedure. Approximately 66% of women undergoing radical cystectomy for the management of bladder cancer fall into this group (Stein et al, 1995, 1998a; Stenzl et al, 1995). Intraoperative inspection and frozen section assessment of the bladder neck limits the risk of urethral recurrence.

The bowel segments should be opened and refashioned (detubularized) to interrupt the normal high-pressure contractions of the intact intestine (Hinman, 1988). A large radius is preferred, as this results in a reservoir with a larger geometric capacity and lower pressure. Continent reservoirs and bladder substitutes may be made of small intestine, large intestine, or a combination of both. Even though bladder substitution is perceived by some as a more complex procedure, prior studies have demonstrated complication and reoperation rates similar to those of ileal conduit urinary diversion in the hands of experienced surgeons (Gburek et al, 1998; Parekh et al, 2000). Long-term results of bladder replacement demonstrate excellent functional outcomes (Abol-Enein and Ghoneim, 2001; Elmajian et al, 1996; Hautmann et al, 1999; Stein et al, 1997; Stenzl et al, 2001; Steven and Poulsen, 2000). Daytime continence can be expected in 87–100% of men and 82–100% of women. Nighttime continence is achieved in 86–94% of men and 72–82% of women. Nearly all men are able to void to completion, while approximately 25–50% of women require intermittent catheterization to completely empty the neobladder. It is beyond the scope of this chapter to review all techniques and minor modifications; instead, the most common techniques and the general principles of continent diversion are reviewed.

▶ Ureterosigmoidostomy

The first direct anastomosis of the ureters into the intact colon was performed by Smith in 1878 (Smith, 1879). Peritonitis (from fecal spillage) and pyelonephritis (resulting from ascending infection and stricturing of the ureteral anastomosis) led initially to very high surgical mortality rates. Recognizing that ascending infection from the rectum into the kidney was a major problem, surgeons developed techniques to reimplant the ureters into the colon in an antirefluxing fashion. Since patients will retain large amounts of urine and fecal material simultaneously in the rectum, assurance of adequate rectal sphincter function is important preoperatively. Since ammonia may be absorbed across the bowel surface, patients with liver disease who may be at an increased risk of hyperammonemic encephalopathy should not undergo this procedure. Patients who have primary diseases of the colon or have received extensive pelvic irradiation should undergo alternative forms of diversion.

The ureters are identified at or below the common iliac arteries. The overlying peritoneum is incised and the ureters are mobilized carefully to preserve their blood supply. A site low in the sigmoid is selected for ureteral reimplantation. The ureters are reimplanted separately into the respective ipsilateral tenia coli, using the antirefluxing techniques described earlier. The peritoneum is sutured over the completed ureteral anastomosis (Figure 25–4).

One particularly worrisome complication of ureterosigmoidostomy is development of adenocarcinoma at the site where the ureters have been reimplanted into the large intestine. The incidence of anastomosis site adenocarcinoma is uncertain, but there seems to be a several thousandfold

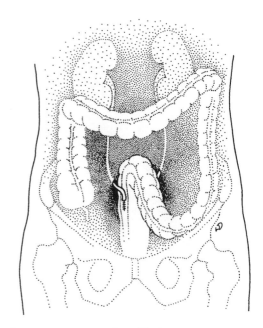

▲ **Figure 25–4.** Ureterosigmoidostomy.

increase in its incidence in patients who have undergone ureterosigmoidostomy over individuals who have not undergone this type of surgery. The induction period varies but may be approximately 20 years; thus, the risk is especially high in young patients. Experimental studies have shown that the development of adenocarcinoma seems dependent on the presence of urine, feces, urothelium, and colonic epithelium in close approximation. All those who undergo ureterosigmoidostomy should be counseled to undergo yearly sigmoidoscopy starting 5 years after the procedure and at any time occult or gross gastrointestinal bleeding or a major change in bowel habits is noted.

▶ Reservoirs Constructed of Small Intestine

Nils Kock was responsible for the early and ongoing development of a continent urinary reservoir fashioned entirely of small intestine (Kock et al, 1982; Nieh, 1997). This reservoir includes the construction of nipple valves as the proximal and distal ends of the reservoir to prevent ureteric reflux (proximally) and incontinence (distally). The Koch reservoir is no longer commonly used due to a high incidence of complications related to the nipple valves.

In an attempt to decrease the complication rate associated with the afferent intussuscepted antireflux nipple of the Kock ileal neobladder, Stein and colleagues (1998b) have described an innovative antireflux technique (Figure 25–5). This new reservoir, the T pouch, has several important advantages over the Kock ileal neobladder: (1) It requires a smaller segment of ileum to create the antireflux technique, (2) the serosal-lined

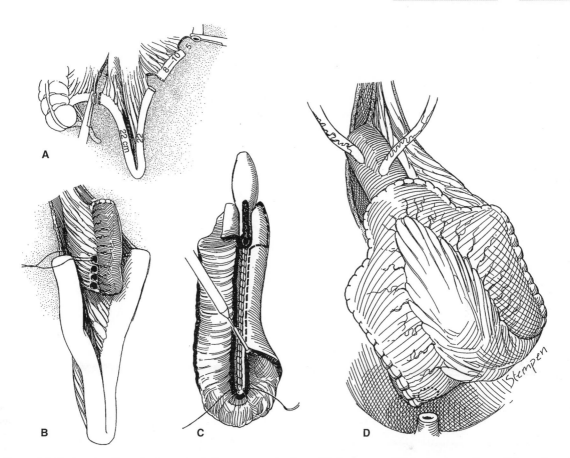

▲ **Figure 25–5.** Construction of a T pouch. **A:** Two segments of small intestine are isolated; one portion will form the reservoir, and the smaller, more proximal portion will form the antireflux segment. **B:** The longer reservoir portion of the segments is folded into a V. The smaller, antireflux segment is fixed to the serosa of the reservoir portion. **C:** The antireflux segment has been opened and tapered with a stapling device. The ileal segments selected for the reservoir portion of the pouch are joined anteriorly and then opened, exposing the mucosa. As the opening reaches the ostium of the antireflux segment, the incisions are carried laterally and create wide flaps that can then be closed over the ostium to cover the tapered antireflux segment. **D:** The reservoir portion is closed.

antireflux mechanism eliminates the need for intussusception, (3) blood supply is better preserved, and (4) urine is not in contact with the implanted portion of the ileum.

Camey described a technique of bladder substitution whereby an intact segment of ileum was anastomosed directly to the urethra (Lilien and Camey, 1984). A 40-cm segment of ileum was isolated from the gastrointestinal tract, and its midpoint was anastomosed, without tension, directly to the urethra. The ureters were reimplanted into either end of the ileal segment in an antirefluxing fashion. However, failure to detubularize the ileal segment led to a high incidence of urinary incontinence compared with substitutes fashioned from detubularized small-bowel segments (Hautmann et al, 1999; Studer and Zingg, 1997). Forty- to sixty-centimeter segments of ileum can be detubularized and

folded into U-, S-, or W-shaped reservoirs, which can be connected directly to the urethra (Figure 25–6). The ureters are reimplanted directly into a short segment of ileum at the proximal end of the bowel segment, isolated to fashion the diversion, which is not detubularized. End-to-side ureteric anastomosis into this isoperistaltic segment of ileum prevents reflux. With the Hautmann type of ileal neobladder (W configuration), nondetubularized segments of ileum can be left intact at either end of the W and the ureters individually implanted into each of these segments. This would make it easier to dissect the ureter if a nephroureterectomy is required at a later date for upper-tract tumor recurrence. The larger diameter and lower pressure of these reservoirs compared with those of nondetubularized bowel have led to better continence rates.

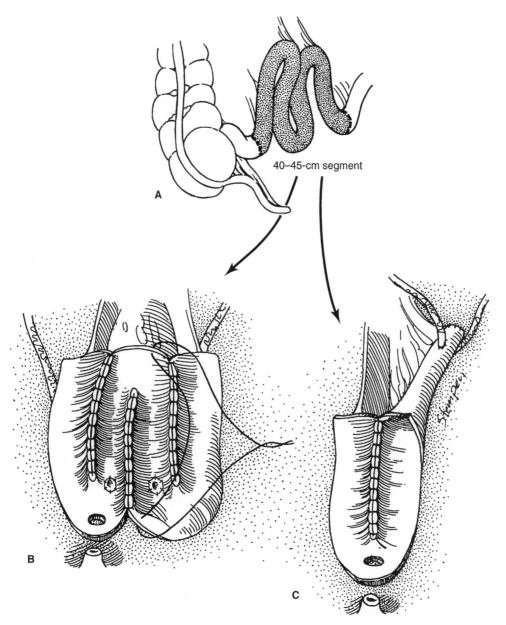

▲ **Figure 25–6.** Bladder substitutes constructed entirely of small intestine. **A:** Forty to forty-five centimeters of small intestine is selected. **B:** Small intestine is opened and fashioned into a W. The ureters are reimplanted into the second and third limbs of the reservoir, and the reservoir is attached to the urethra. **C:** Small intestine is folded into a J with the most proximal portion of the segment not opened. The ureters are reimplanted into the intact ileal segment of the reservoir, and the reservoir is attached to the urethra.

▶ Reservoirs Constructed of Large Intestine

Various investigators have described using segments of the large intestine alone or combinations of large- and small-bowel segments to fashion urinary reservoirs (Bihrle, 1997;

Lampel et al, 1996). Bladder substitutes have been constructed using detubularized bowel segments from the ileo-cecal region or sigmoid colon. Use of the ascending colon and terminal ileum to construct continent urinary reservoirs has gained great popularity. Cecum and ascending colon are

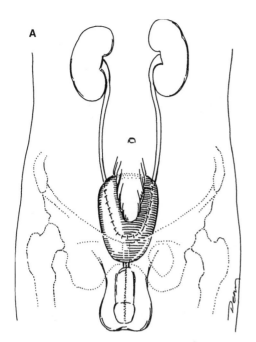
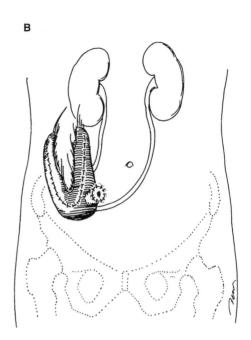

▲ **Figure 25–7.** Use of the ileocecal segment to construct (**A**) a bladder substitute attached to the urethra or (**B**) a continent urinary reservoir placed in the abdomen using plicated terminal ileum as a stoma.

detubularized and refashioned or augmented with the small intestine to provide for a spherical reservoir. The ureters are reimplanted in a nonrefluxing fashion (Figure 25–7). The reservoir can be anastomosed directly to the urethra. In women or in men who require a urethrectomy, a continent, catheterizable stoma can be fashioned of appendix or tapered terminal ileum (Figure 25–8).

▶ Postoperative Care

Postoperative care varies depending on the method of urinary diversion or bladder substitution. As with all patients who have undergone major abdominal surgery, early ambulation, use of intermittent compression stockings, and incentive spirometry may be used to prevent pulmonary emboli or respiratory complications. Nasogastric tubes are optional and can be used in patients with abdominal distension, nausea, and emesis. Serum electrolytes and creatinine should be monitored postoperatively for the development of metabolic abnormalities. If single J ureteral stents have been placed, they are usually removed sometime after postoperative day 5; double J stents may stay in place for up to 3 weeks in patients undergoing neobladders. Continent urinary reservoirs and bladder substitutes produce mucus. They should be irrigated regularly in the early postoperative period to prevent mucus accumulation. Mucus production decreases over time, and irrigation ultimately

becomes unnecessary. Upper urinary tract surveillance for hydronephrosis should be performed on a regular basis using ultrasound or computed tomography. An initial assessment of the upper urinary tract is made in the early postoperative period; if upper urinary tract dilation is not found, the patient undergoes repeat imaging on a yearly basis or as dictated by surveillance protocols for the stage of bladder cancer.

COMPLICATIONS

Complications occurring after urinary diversion, bladder substitution, or continent urinary diversion are generally a product of surgical technique, the underlying disease process and its treatment, the age of the patient, and the length of follow-up (Carlin et al, 1997; Gburek et al, 1998). Early complications, which are uncommon (occurring in approximately 10–20% of patients), include excessive bleeding, intestinal obstruction/ileus, urinary extravasation, and infection. Late complications (10–20% of patients) include metabolic disorders, stomal problems (stenosis or hernia), pyelonephritis, and calculi. Rarely, spontaneous neobladder rupture may occur presumably due to overdistention or blunt abdominal trauma (Nippgen et al, 2001). Such patients usually present with peritonitis and acute abdominal pain. Perforation of continent cutaneous diversions can occur and can be related to vigorous catheterization.

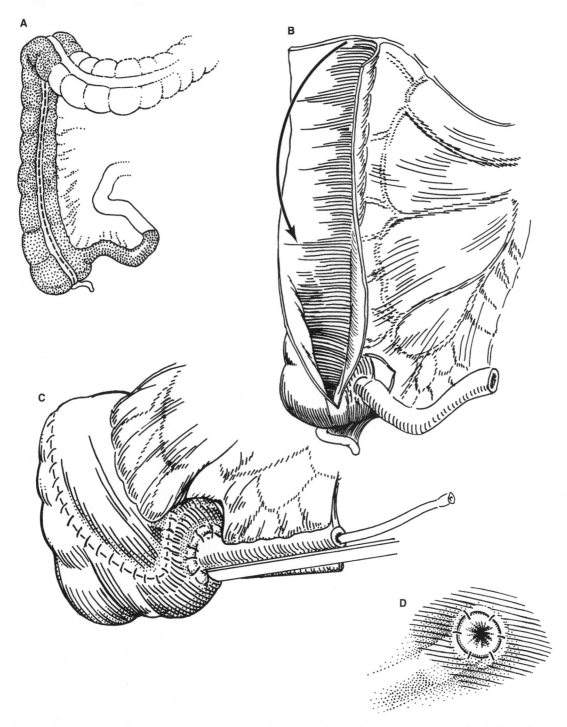

▲ **Figure 25–8.** **A:** Continent urinary reservoir constructed from the ileocecal segment. **B:** Bowel detubularized. **C:** Stoma constructed by tapering the terminal ileum with intestinal stapling instrument or sutures. **D:** Completed stoma.

Metabolic and Nutritional Disorders

Fluid, electrolyte, nutrient, and waste product excretion or absorption normally occurs across the intestinal wall. Metabolic abnormalities may occur when intestinal segments are interposed into the urinary tract. As pointed out previously, use of the jejunum may result in hyponatremic, hypochloremic, hyperkalemic metabolic acidosis in up to 40% of patients. The jejunum is unable to maintain large solute gradients, so large amounts of water and solute pass through the jejunal wall. Sodium and chloride are rapidly excreted into the conduit, and potassium is passively absorbed. Aldosterone is produced, resulting in reabsorption of hydrogen and excretion of potassium into the distal tubule of the kidney and consequent acidosis and movement of potassium from the body's intracellular stores. As water is lost into the conduit, extracellular fluid volume is reduced, as is the glomerular filtration rate. The renin–angiotensin system is activated which further stimulates aldosterone secretion. Urea may be absorbed from the jejunal lumen, which (with dehydration) contributes to azotemia. This syndrome is often characterized clinically by nausea, vomiting, anorexia, and muscle weakness.

The pathogenesis and nature of metabolic abnormalities occurring after incorporation of the ileum or colon into the urinary tract differ from those associated with jejunal conduits. When such segments are used, sodium and chloride are absorbed across the bowel surface. Chloride is absorbed in slight excess of sodium, resulting in a net loss of bicarbonate into the bowel lumen. Preexisting renal failure contributes to the development and severity of the disorder, as does a large bowel surface area and long contact time. Hyperchloremic acidosis is more common in patients who undergo ureterosigmoidostomy than in patients who undergo simple conduit construction using either the ileum or the colon, because of the larger surface area and longer contact time with urine associated with ureterosigmoidostomies. Hyperchloremic metabolic acidosis may manifest clinically as weakness, anorexia, vomiting, Kussmaul breathing, and coma. One potential long-term complication of chronic acidosis may be decreased bone calcium content and osteomalacia (Kawakita et al, 1996; McDougal et al, 1988).

Bile salts are important for fat digestion and uptake of vitamins A and D. Bile salt metabolism may be altered after ileal resection (Olofsson et al, 1998). Resection of small segments of the ileum may be associated with mild malabsorption and steatorrhea owing to increased concentrations of bile salts delivered to the colon. The increased concentration of such salts leads to decreased colonic absorption of water and electrolytes. Resection of large segments of ileum may reduce bile salt reabsorption to very low levels, leading to severe fat malabsorption. Bowel transit time may be reduced further by resection of the ileocecal valve. Cholestyramine may be used to treat secretory bile salt diarrhea. If diarrhea persists, addition of agents such as loperamide that decrease bowel motility and increase transit time may be effective. Cholelithiasis may be more common after ileal resections as well.

Vitamin B_{12} deficiency may occur as a result of either gastric or ileal resection (Fujisawa et al, 2000b; Terai et al, 1997). Because B_{12} stores are likely to last for years, its deficiency may not become apparent for several years after intestinal surgery. B_{12} deficiency results in megaloblastic anemia and peripheral nerve paresthesias. The levels of this vitamin can be assessed in patients after ileal or gastric resection. Alternatively, yearly replacement by injection of Vitamin B_{12} is adequate in those in whom deficiency is noted.

Stoma

A good deal of patients' dissatisfaction with urinary diversion can be attributed to stomal complications. Stoma construction is especially important in procedures in which a pouch must be worn. Careful stomal construction as outlined earlier is essential (Fitzgerald et al, 1997). Most peristomal skin problems can be avoided with adequate siting, good surgical technique coupled with regular follow-up with a nurse specialized in ostomy care and follow-up (Enterostomal Therapy Nurse; wound, ostomy, and continence nurse [WOCN]). Complications related to the stoma can be separated into (1) stomal complications: necrosis, stenosis, hernia, retraction, or prolapse and (2) peristomal complications: dermatitis related to fungal infections, contact allergic reactions, mechanical trauma, and contact dermatitis leading to alkaline encrustations from urine on the skin over time. They are often related, as a stenotic stoma may be difficult to pouch leading to chronic skin irritation. External stomal and peristomal complications rates range from 15% to 65% (Szymanski, 2010). The likelihood of stomal stenosis increases with time. Stomal stenosis can lead to conduit elongation and upper-tract obstruction. This condition can be diagnosed relatively easily by catheterizing the stoma and measuring the residual urine volume. It is corrected by revision of the stoma. Parastomal herniation tends to occur as a delayed complication in 5–28% of patients (Franks and Hrebinko, 2001; Symanski et al, 2010). One cause for this is the location of the stoma lateral to the rectus muscle, which eliminates the circumferential support provided by the muscle cuff around the stoma. The hernia typically tends to occur around the superolateral aspect of the stoma. Placing the stoma such that the conduit is traversing the rectus muscle may not always decrease the likelihood of parastomal hernia (Gray, 2005). Some degree of stomal bulge without a hernia is commonly noted in most patients with conduits. Repair of a stomal hernia requires reinforcing the rectus fascia with mesh, either intraperitoneally through the previous midline incision or through an incision lateral to the stoma. In some cases, it may be necessary to move the stoma to a new site, preferably to the contralateral side of the abdominal wall. Recurrence rates following hernia repair were high previously but have declined considerably to 0–7% in recent series (Franks and Hrebinko, 2001; Ho and Fawcett, 2004).

Skin irritation or infections are most common in procedures in which an appliance is worn and there is prolonged contact of the skin with urine. Some patients' skin may be sensitive to adhesive agents.

Stomal or skin problems are minimized by selecting an appropriate pouching system. Extended wear pouches provide better skin protection because of better adhesion and delayed moisture absorption (Colwell, 2005). The treatment of parastomal conditions is summarized in Table 25–1.

The most troublesome stomal complication of external urinary appliances is unexpected pouch leakage. This is often a result of improper application of the pouch but may be caused by poor stomal construction. With a properly constructed and located stoma, the choice of the pouch is relatively simple and is often determined by patient preference. Factors that must be taken into account when selecting a pouch include patient dexterity and preference, available resources, and stomal construction. Pouches have an adhesive skin barrier that attaches to the skin and a bag that collects urine. An opening is made in the middle of the skin barrier; this opening should be of a diameter just larger than the stoma to avoid erosion of the stoma or prolonged contact of the skin with urine, typically one-eighth of an inch on each side unless the stoma is retracted or at skin level then the

Table 25–1. Common peristomal skin problems and their management.

Problem/Description	Cause	Management
Fungal infections/yeast dermatitis • Usually confluent circumferential rash (fine papules and pustules) with satellite lesions. May be pruritic	• Yeast overgrowth on skin exposed to excess moisture (barrier opening too large, pouch leakage)	• Antifungal powder (Nystatin) or systemic therapy with fluconazole (Diflucan)
Allergic contact dermatitis • Area of erythema, pruritus, and/or blistering that corresponds to allergen	• Allergic reaction in sensitive patient • Once allergic reaction is chronic, it is more difficult to treat and identify irritant	• Identify irritant (skin patch test) and discontinue product • Apply hydrocortisone cream for short period to reduce skin reaction • Topical antihistamines (diphenhydramine gel) • Avoid solvents and soaps under pouch
Mechanical trauma • Denuded peristomal skin without rash or pruritus	• Frequent or excessive pouch changing leading to skin stripping • Pressure trauma from belt or convexity • Overuse of tape around the barrier	• Minimize pouch changes • Encourage gentle skin care or use of protective sealant • Consider nonadhesive pouches (used with belt)
Pseudoverrucous skin lesions • Warty raised macerated lesions around the stoma. May cause bleeding and pain • Late complication	• Urine contact with peristomal skin over extended period • As the lesions develop, patients often keep making the opening larger, compounding the problem	• Ensure correct opening in pouch • Patient will need to cover lesions initially for resolution, and they will need to change their pouch more frequently until the lesions have resolved

Peristomal hernia
• Reducible bulge under or around stoma
	• Not clear at this time—may be related to abdominal aperture size created at the time of surgery
	  • May be avoided by placing stoma within rectus abdominis sheath
		• Flexible pouching system
		  • Surgical repair with mesh or re-siting (tends to recur)
		• Hernia support belt applied while hernia is reduced (Nu-Hope)

Alkaline encrustation	• Crystal deposits on exposed peristomal skin	• Increase oral fluid intake • Acidify urine with 1 g ascorbic acid daily • 20-minute vinegar soaks at the time of pouch change

Note: The patient should see a wound, ostomy, and continence nurse (WOCN), if available.

opening may be more secure if there is one-fourth-inch clearance on each side to avoid undermining (Doughty, 2005).

Most patients favor using disposable urinary collection pouches. Disposable, one-piece pouches are single use. Two-piece systems allow the patient to remove the pouch, leaving the skin barrier intact. A larger collection device is often attached to the pouch at night.

▶ Continence and Urinary Function

One of the common late complications of continent urinary diversion is urinary incontinence that can occur following both cutaneous diversion and in neobladders. Nighttime incontinence is particularly a problem with neobladders and can occur in about 20–50% of all patients (Lee et al, 2003; Meyer et al, 2004). Daytime incontinence is significantly lower and ranges from <10% to 33%. Reported continence rates are higher with the T pouch at around 87% (daytime) and 72% (nighttime) (Stein, 2004). The wide variations in reported continence rates stem from varying definitions of continence. Improvement in continence is observed with time and increasing neobladder capacity reaching 92% for daytime and 80% at nighttime by 2 years (Studer, 1996). Bladder capacity increases gradually and stabilizes to reach >450 cc and continence also improves over time in these patients (Permenis, 2004). Incomplete emptying can occur in a small percentage of patients requiring long-term self-catheterization. Women who undergo neobladder construction are especially at risk for hypercontinence, which can occur in 12% to as high as 60% of patients and must be counseled preoperatively in this regard (Stein et al, 2009; Stenzl et al, 2001). Day- and nighttime continence rates appear to be similar between male and female patients and the most common types of neobladders reconstruction (Studer vs Hautmann) (Lee et al, 2003; Stenzl et al, 2001). Sphincteric damage and low urethral resting pressures are believed to be the reasons for incontinence while urethral denervation, poor pouch contractility, and/or exaggerated acute angulation of the neobladder urethral junction are believed to be the reasons for hypercontinence and retention. Frequent bladder emptying, urethral collagen injection, artificial urinary sphincter placements, and urethral slings are all potential treatment options for incontinence while catheterization is the main therapy for urinary retention.

▶ Pyelonephritis and Renal Deterioration

Pyelonephritis occurs in approximately 10% of patients who have undergone urinary diversion. Treatment is based on a properly collected urine sample for culture. A urine sample should not be collected from the pouch; rather, the pouch should be removed, the stoma cleansed with an antiseptic, and a catheter advanced gently through the stoma. If infection has occurred in a patient with a simple conduit, the volume of residual urine within the conduit should be recorded. Obstruction and stasis of urine within the reconstructed urinary tract are risk factors for the development of infection.

Although many patients with preexisting dilation of the upper urinary tract show improvement or resolution of the dilation after urinary diversion or bladder substitution, progressive renal deterioration as manifested by hydronephrosis or an increasing serum creatinine level (or both) occurs in some patients who undergo these procedures. The incidence of either complication increases after 10 years. The presence of hydronephrosis, particularly in patients with a conduit diversion, may indicate the presence of ureteric reflux or obstruction at the ureterovesical junction. A loopogram will help demonstrate if there is retrograde flow of contrast from conduit to the ureter and renal pelvis. In some situations, it may be necessary to obtain a radionuclide renal scan (MAG3) to determine if there is antegrade flow of urine from the kidney through the ureters. Pyelographic evidence of upper urinary tract deterioration has been noted in up to 50% of patients who have undergone urinary diversion at an early age. Recurrent upper urinary tract infection and high-pressure ureteral reflux and obstruction, usually in combination, contribute to the likelihood of renal deterioration. Upper-tract deterioration is less likely following ileal continent diversion. While a majority of kidneys will demonstrate mild dilation, 97% of patients show no change in renal parenchymal size and 100% show no change in serum creatinine 10–15 years following the Studer type of ileal neobladder (Perimenis, 2004).

▶ Calculi

Calculi occur in approximately 8% of patients who undergo urinary diversion or bladder substitution (Cohen and Streem, 1994; Terai et al, 1996). Such patients have several risk factors for the development of various calculi. Nonabsorbable staples, mesh, or suture material used to construct conduits or reservoirs may act as a nidus for stone formation. Colonization in either conduits or reservoirs is common, whereas symptomatic infection is much rare. Certain bacteria can contribute to stone formation; some bacteria commonly found in the urinary tract, including *Proteus*, *Klebsiella*, and *Pseudomonas* species, produce urease, a urea-splitting enzyme that contributes to the formation of ammonia and carbon dioxide. Hydrolysis of these products results in an alkaline urine supersaturated with magnesium ammonium phosphate, calcium phosphate, and carbonate apatite crystals. Management of such infection-related stones requires stone removal, resolution of infection, and, often, use of adjunctive agents to complete stone dissolution.

The likelihood of stone formation is increased by the development of systemic acidosis. Prolonged contact of the urine with the intestinal surface facilitates the exchange of chloride for bicarbonate. Bicarbonate loss results in systemic acidosis and hypercalciuria. The combination of hypercalciuria and alkaline urine predisposes a patient to the development of calcium calculi. In addition, the terminal ileum is responsible for bile salt absorption; if this portion of the intestine is used for conduit or bladder reservoir construction, excess bile salts in the intestine may bind calcium and result in increased absorption of oxalate, which may lead to the development of oxalate-containing calculi. Hypocitraturia may also be a risk factor for stone disease in patients undergoing bladder replacement (Osther et al, 2000). Excess conduit length, urine stasis, and dehydration make the development of calculi more likely.

BIBLIOGRAPHY

General

Allareddy V et al: Quality of life in long term bladder cancer survivors. Cancer 2006;106:2355.

Bjerre BD et al: Health-related quality of life after cystectomy: Bladder substitution compared with ileal conduit diversion. A questionnaire survey. Br J Urol 1995;75:200.

Carlin BI et al: Comparison of the ileal conduit to the continent cutaneous diversion and orthotopic neobladder in patients undergoing cystectomy: A critical analysis and review of the literature. Semin Urol Oncol 1997;15:189.

Dutta SC et al: Health-related quality of life assessment after radical cystectomy: Comparison of ileal conduit with continent orthotopic neobladder. J Urol 2002;168:164.

Fitzgerald J et al: Stomal construction, complications, and reconstruction. Urol Clin North Am 1997;24:729.

Fujisawa M et al: Health-related quality of life with orthotopic neobladder versus ileal conduit according to the SF-36 survey. Urology 2000a;55:862.

Hara I et al: Health-related quality of life after radical cystectomy for bladder cancer: A comparison of ileal conduit and orthotopic bladder replacement. BJU Int 2002;89:10.

Okada Y et al: Quality of life survey of urinary diversion patients: Comparison of continent urinary diversion versus ileal conduit. Int J Urol 1997;4:26.

Colon Conduit

Richie JP: Sigmoid conduit urinary diversion. Urol Clin North Am 1986;13:225.

Continent Urinary Diversion and Bladder Substitution

Abol-Enein H, Ghoneim MA: Functional results of orthotopic ileal neobladder with serous-lined extramural ureteral reimplantation: Experience with 450 patients. J Urol 2001;165:1427.

Bihrle R: The Indiana Pouch continent urinary reservoir. Urol Clin North Am 1997;24:773.

Gburek BM et al: Comparison of the Studer ileal neobladder and ileal conduit urinary diversion with respect to perioperative outcome and late complications. J Urol 1998;160:721.

Gilbert SM et al: Measuring health-related quality of life outcomes in bladder cancer patients using the Bladder Cancer Index (BCI). Cancer 2007;109:1756–1762.

Hautmann R et al: The ileal neobladder: Complications and functional results in 363 patients after 11 years of followup. J Urol 1999;161:422.

Iselin C et al: Does prostate transitional cell carcinoma preclude orthotopic bladder reconstruction after radical cystoprostatectomy for bladder cancer? J Urol 1997;158:2123.

Kock NG et al: Urinary diversion via a continent ileal reservoir: Clinical results in 12 patients. J Urol 1982;128:469.

Lampel A et al: Continent diversion with the Mainz pouch. World J Urol 1996;14:85.

Lilien OM, Camey M: 25-year experience with replacement of the human bladder (Camey procedure). J Urol 1984;132:886.

Nelson RL et al: Antimicrobial prophylaxis for colorectal surgery. Cochrane Database Syst Rev 2009;21(1):CD001181.

Nieh P: The Kock Pouch urinary reservoir. Urol Clin North Am 1997;24:755.

Nixon RG et al: Carcinoma in situ and tumor multifocality predict the risk of prostatic urethral involvement at radical cystectomy in men with transitional cell carcinoma of the bladder. J Urol 2002;167:502.

Parekh DJ et al: Continent urinary reconstruction versus ileal conduit: A contemporary single-institution comparison of perioperative morbidity and mortality. Urology 2000;55:852.

Slim K et al: Updated systematic review and meta-analysis of randomized clinical trials on the role of mechanical bowel preparation before colorectal surgery. Ann Surg 2009;249:203–209.

Stein JP et al: Indications for lower urinary tract reconstruction in women after cystectomy for bladder cancer: A pathological review of female cystectomy specimens [see comments]. J Urol 1995; 154:1329.

Stein J et al: Orthotopic lower urinary tract reconstruction in women using the Kock ileal neobladder: Updated experience in 34 patients. J Urol 1997;158:400.

Stein J et al: Prospective pathologic analysis of female cystectomy specimens: Risk factors for orthotopic diversion in women. Urology 1998a;51:951.

Stein J et al: The T Pouch: An orthotopic ileal neobladder incorporating a serosal lined ileal antireflux technique. J Urol 1998b;159:1836.

Stein JP et al: The orthotopic T pouch ileal neobladder: Experience with 209 patients. J Urol 2004;172:584.

Stenzl A et al: The risk of urethral tumors in female bladder cancer: Can the urethra be used for orthotopic reconstruction of the lower urinary tract? J Urol 1995;153(3 Pt 2):950.

Stenzl A et al: Urethra-sparing cystectomy and orthotopic urinary diversion in women with malignant pelvic tumors. Cancer 2001; 92:1864.

Steven K, Poulsen AL: The orthotopic Kock ileal neobladder: Functional results, urodynamic features, complications, and survival in 166 men. J Urol 2000;164:288.

Studer U, Zingg E: Ileal orthotopic bladder substitutes. Urol Clin North Am 1997;24:781.

Ureterosigmoidostomy

Smith T: An account of an unsuccessful attempt to treat extroversion of the bladder by a new operation. St Barth Hosp Rep 1879;15:29.

Complications

Carlin BI et al: Comparison of the ileal conduit to the continent cutaneous diversion and orthotopic neobladder in patients undergoing cystectomy: A critical analysis and review of the literature. Semin Urol Oncol 1997;15:189.

Cohen T, Streem S: Minimally invasive endourologic management of calculi in continent urinary reservoirs. Urology 1994;43:865.

Franks ME, Hrebinko RL Jr: Technique of parastomal hernia repair using synthetic mesh. Urology 2001;57:551.

Fujisawa M et al: Long-term assessment of serum vitamin B_{12} concentrations in patients with various types of orthotopic intestinal neobladder. Urology 2000b;56:236.

Gburek B et al: Comparison of Studer ileal neobladder and ileal conduit urinary diversion with respect to perioperative outcome and late complications. J Urol 1998;160:721.

Ho KM, Fawcett DP: Parastomal hernia repair using the lateral approach. BJU Int 2004;94:598.

Kawakita M et al: Bone demineralization following urinary intestinal diversion assessed by urinary Pyridium cross-links and dual energy x-ray absorptiometry. J Urol 1996;156:355.

Lee KS et al: Hautmann and Studer orthotopic neobladders: A contemporary experience. J Urol. 2003;169:2188.

McDougal WS et al: Boney demineralization following intestinal diversion. J Urol 1988;140:853.

Meyer JP et al: A three-centre experience of orthotopic neobladder reconstruction after radical cystectomy: Initial results. BJU Int 2004;94:1317.

Nippgen JBW et al: Spontaneous late rupture of orthotopic detubularized ileal neobladders: Report of five cases. Urology 2001; 58:43.

Olofsson G et al: Bile acid malabsorption after continent urinary diversion with an ileal reservoir. J Urol 1998;160:724.

Osther PJ et al: Stone risk after bladder substitution with the ileal-urethral Kock reservoir. Scand J Urol Nephrol 2000;34:257.

Perimenis P et al: Ileal orthotopic bladder substitute combined with an afferent tubular segment: Long-term upper urinary tract changes and voiding pattern. Eur Urol 2004;46:604.

Stein R et al: Long-term metabolic effects in patients with urinary diversion. World J Urol 1998;16:292.

Stein JP et al: Long term oncological outcome in women undergoing radical cystectomy and orthotopic diversion for bladder cancer. J Urol 2009;181:2052–2059.

Stenzl A et al: Urethra-sparing cystectomy and orthotopic urinary diversion in women with malignant pelvic tumors. Cancer 2001;92:1864.

Studer UE et al: Summary of 10 years' experience with an ileal low-pressure bladder substitute combined with an afferent tubular isoperistaltic segment. World J Urol 1996;14:29.

Terai A et al: Urinary calculi as a late complication of the Indiana continent urinary diversion: Comparison with the Kock pouch procedure. J Urol 1996;155:66.

Ostomy Care

Bass EM et al: Does preoperative stoma marking and education by the enterostomal therapist affect outcomes? Dis Colon Rectum 1997;40:440.

Colwell JC: Dealing with ostomies: Good care, good devices, good quality of life. J Support Oncol 2005;3:72.

Colwell JC, Fichera A: Care of the obese patient with an ostomy. J Wound Ostomy Continence Nurs 2005;32:378.

Doughty D: Principles of ostomy management in the oncology patient. J Support Oncol 2005;3:59.

Fitzgerald J et al: Stomal construction, complications, and reconstruction. Urol Clin North Am 1997;24:729.

Gray M et al: What treatments are effective for the management of peristomal hernia? J Wound Ostomy Continence Nurs 2005;32:87.

Szymanski KM et al: External stoma and peristomal complications following radical cystectomy and ileal conduit diversion: A systematic review. Ostomy Wound Management 2010;1:28.

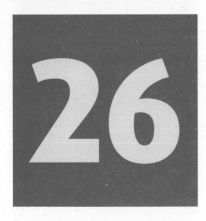

Radiotherapy of Urologic Tumors

Alexander R. Gottschalk, MD, PhD,

Joycelyn L. Speight, MD, PhD, & Mack Roach III, MD

The primary management of genitourologic malignant diseases has been tied to the use of radiation for more than 100 years. In 1895, Roentgen described x-rays; by 1899, a patient with skin cancer was cured with radiation; and within 10 years, radiation was used to treat prostate cancer (Pasteau and Degrais, 1914). Radiotherapy became a mainstay of treatment for bladder and testicular cancers and later prostate cancer as supervoltage sources became available. Although chemotherapy and aggressive surgery have supplanted some of the uses of radiotherapy, radiation continues to play a major role in the management of carcinomas of the penis, urethra, prostate, and bladder. In this chapter, we review general principles and the indications for using radiation as a component in the primary management of urologic malignant diseases. The role of radiation as an agent of palliation has been well documented elsewhere and is excluded from this chapter.

GENERAL PRINCIPLES OF RADIOTHERAPY

Mechanisms of Cytotoxicity

The effects of radiation on tumor and surrounding normal tissues are thought to be mediated primarily through the induction of unrepaired double-strand breaks in DNA. Excited electron species generated in the presence of oxygen form peroxide radicals, which fix chemical lesions and result in the generation of either repairable or nonrepairable DNA double-strand breaks. High linear energy transfer radiation (including neutrons and heavy-charged particles) is associated with less repairable DNA damage. Classically, the expression of radiation damage is not seen until the target cells enter mitosis. Differentiated normal tissues with low mitotic activity, such as the heart and spinal cord, tend to express the effects of radiation much later than cells from more kinetically active tissues, such as the epithelial cells lining the rectum, bladder, or urethra. However, differentiated normal tissues with low mitotic activity are more sensitive to the use of high dose per fraction or high linear energy transfer radiotherapy. In organs

in which the functional stromal cells are postmitotic, such as muscle cells and neurons, the damage is expressed by slowly dividing support cells such as endothelial cells.

In addition to the classic mechanism described earlier, radiation has been shown to induce programed cell death (apoptosis). Androgen-independent human prostate cancer cells activate a genetic program of apoptotic cell death in response to exposure to ionizing radiation, in a dose-dependent fashion (Sklar, 1993). Results from animal models suggest that it is better to achieve maximal androgen suppression before starting radiation treatment however, in humans this may be sequence and volume dependent as well (Roach M, 2012; Zietman, 2000).

Radiation Sensitivity and Tolerance

Radiation tolerance levels have been determined for nearby normal tissues that are likely to be affected during conventional fractionated radiotherapy treatment of tumors arising from the urinary tract. The term *conventional fractionation* generally refers to the delivery of a single daily dose of 180 cGy (1.8 Gy) to 200 cGy (2.0 Gy). When used alone, cumulative doses of at least 65 Gy are necessary for local control of gross disease (adenocarcinomas, transitional cell carcinomas [TCCs], and squamous cell carcinomas) arising from the prostate, bladder, urethra, or ureters. When used prophylactically for presumed microscopic disease (lymph nodes) or postoperatively, doses of 45–50 Gy are generally sufficient. For testicular seminomas, doses of 25 Gy are usually adequate.

Total dose, dose per fraction, and volume of normal tissue irradiated are the major risk factors for radiation-induced complications. The presence of several comorbid conditions such as previous surgery, diabetes, inflammatory bowel diseases, or old age is also associated with an increased risk of radiation-induced complications. Accurate estimates of the "true tolerance" of surrounding normal tissues have been hampered until recently by our inability to reconstruct the actual relationship between normal tissue doses and volumes in three dimensions. Early reports assumed that organ movement and day-to-day treatment setup error had an insignificant impact on the doses of radiation delivered to surrounding normal tissues. Studies have demonstrated that these assumptions are inaccurate and probably result in an underestimate of the true tolerance of surrounding normal tissues to radiation (Langen and Jones, 2001).

▶ Dose Per Fraction Considerations

Dose per fraction, the total dose, volume, and overall treatment time are all critical determinants of chronic genitourinary toxicity. The linear quadratic equation (L-Q equation) has been adopted by many clinical investigators as the most useful model for comparing various doses and fractionation schemes (Fowler et al, 2001). This equation can be written as follows:

$$\text{Effect (E)} = n\,(\alpha d + \beta d)$$

where

d = Dose per fraction
α = Nonrepairable effects
β = Repairable effects
n = Number of identical fractions

For comparing two different fractionation schemes, assuming a similar overall treatment time, the L-Q equation also can be written as follows:

$$D_2/D_1 = (1 + d_1\beta/\alpha)/(1 + d_2\beta/\alpha)$$

where

D = Total dose and $D_1 = n_1 d_1$
d = Dose per fraction

For most clinical circumstances, it is assumed that the α/β ratio for late-reacting normal tissues such as the bladder or rectum is 3. For early-responding normal tissues and for tumor, it is assumed that the α/β ratio is 10.

▶ Altered Fractionation Schedules

Radiobiologic modeling using the α/β ratios as described previously has been used to develop "altered fractionation schedules" to improve the therapeutic ratio between efficacy and toxicity. *Accelerated hyperfractionation* was until recently the most frequently used altered fractionation schedule. With accelerated hyperfractionation, more than one treatment is given per day with a minimum of 6 hours between treatments, using a decreased dose per fraction. Since most radiation-induced damage is repaired within 6 hours, the use of multiple treatments per day in theory should allow greater doses of radiation to be given over a shorter period of time, reducing the opportunity for tumor repopulation. Using α/β modeling, the late effects predicted using 1.2 Gy fractions twice daily (separated by 6 hours) to 69.6 Gy would be expected to be equivalent

to those using conventional fractionation to 58 Gy. In contrast, early-responding tissues such as the epithelium of the bladder would be expected to respond as though they had been treated with a dose of 65 Gy using conventional fractionation. This model predicts an increase in acute effects, including tumor response, but a decrease in late effects, such as fibrosis.

Hypofractionation involves the use of larger than conventional fraction sizes. Such an approach results in nearly a 10% reduction in the total dose to the tumor without sparing late complications (assuming that the values chosen for the α/β ratio are correct for normal tissues and for tumors) (Fowler et al, 2001). Several recent investigators have argued that the α/β ratio for prostate cancer is much lower than previously thought and that this formed a strong rationale for the use of high dose rate (HDR) to treat prostate cancer (Brenner and Hall, 1999; Fowler et al, 2001; King and Fowler, 2001). For patients being treated with external-beam radiotherapy (EBRT), a growing number of investigators are studying the use of hypofractionated radiotherapy in an attempt to shorten overall time and cost, but to date, only one randomized trial suggests that cancer control rates might be better (Arcangeli et al, 2010, 2011; Lee, 2009; McCammon et al, 2009; Ritter et al, 2009). Some studies show no advantages, while others suggest there may be advantages to the use of hypofractionation (Arcangeli et al, 2010, 2011; Miles, 2008; Speight, 2005). Because of day-to-day setup variation, some type of online monitoring is advisable to ensure that this can be carried out safely.

▶ Brachytherapy

The term *brachytherapy* refers to a treatment technique that places radioactive sources in close proximity to or directly into the tumor. Brachytherapy can be classified as either interstitial or intracavity. Interstitial brachytherapy involves the placement of radioactive needles, afterloaded needles or catheters, or radioactive seeds directly into the prostate, bladder, penis, or periurethral soft tissues. Intracavitary brachytherapy includes placement of radioactive catheters into a lumen or orifice, such as in the urethra, to treat urethral and penile tumors. Permanent implants involve the use of radioactive seeds that are left in the patient. Nowadays, temporary implants generally involve the use of needles or catheters that act as conduits for delivering radiation from high-activity seeds attached to a long wire. Most modern temporary implants are delivered using HDR brachytherapy systems to deliver moderately high doses of radiation over a relatively short period of time (minutes). HDR brachytherapy is usually delivered over two or more treatment sessions to reduce the risk of late complications. Low dose rate brachytherapy is usually delivered in a continuous fashion over days to weeks via temporary or permanent implants, respectively. Figure 26–1 depicts an example of a transrectal ultrasound–based iodine-125 permanent interstitial implant of the prostate. Figure 26–2 shows an example of intracavitary brachytherapy for a urethral tumor in a female patient.

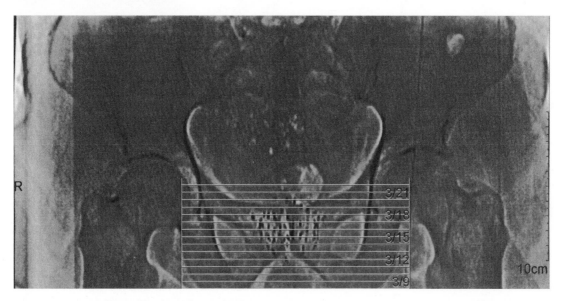

▲ **Figure 26–1.** Brachytherapy: Example of an ultrasound-guided permanent interstitial implant of the prostate.

SPECIFIC UROLOGIC SITES

▶ Prostate Cancer

Few urologists are aware that radiotherapy was first used to successfully treat prostate cancer 100 years ago and that it was not until 1949 that Memmelaar first reported the successful

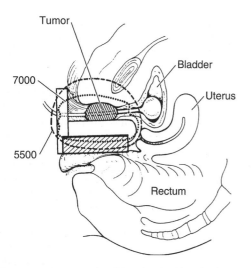

▲ **Figure 26–2.** Example of intraluminal brachytherapy for urethral cancer. (Reproduced with permission from Sailer SL, Shipley WU, Wang CC: Carcinoma of the female urethra: A review of results with radiation therapy. J Urol 1988;140:1.)

use of the retropubic approach—the radical RRP—for treatment of prostate cancer (Memmelaar, 1949). In the 1950s and 1960s, it was believed that radiotherapy provided comparable results with less morbidity. However, in 1979, Walsh and Donker demonstrated the potential value of the RRP to preserve nerves (Elder, 1982). Radical perineal prostatectomies became less fashionable in the 1980s after Walsh and others reported improvements in the RRP that promised to reduce blood loss, minimize the risk of incontinence, and preserve potency (Reiner, 1979). The comparative effectiveness of RRP compared with radiotherapy is very controversial in part because of major selection biases toward more favorable patients undergoing surgery and major advances in the accuracy and doses of radiation that can now be delivered (Giordano et al, 2008; Roach et al, 2008; Speight, 2007). Although some retrospective studies suggest better outcomes with surgery, inherent biases shed doubt on the validity of these conclusions (Roach et al, 2008).

For example, Giordano et al set to systematically evaluate the effect of selection biases in observational studies of treatment effectiveness in men with localized prostate cancer (Giordano et al, 2008). They identified men from the Medicare-linked database—Surveillance, Epidemiology, and End Results. They noted that controlling for comorbidity, extent of disease, and other characteristics by multivariate analyses or by propensity analyses had remarkably small impact on these improbable results. They concluded that observational studies of treatment outcomes should be viewed with caution. As is shown in Figure 26–3, they noted that men treated by radical prostatectomy had a better adjusted survival rate than men without prostate cancer suggesting selection

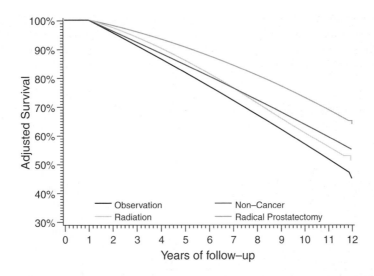

▲ **Figure 26-3.** As is shown, men treated by radical prostatectomy had a better adjusted survival rate than men without prostate cancer suggesting selection biases for favorable outcomes for these men compared with those treated with radiotherapy. (From Giordano SH et al: Limits of observational data in determining outcomes from cancer therapy. Cancer 2008;112:2456–2466.)

biases for favorable outcomes for these men compared with those treated with radiotherapy. Prostate-specific antigen (PSA) control rates appear to be very similar between contemporary high dose radiation and surgical series (Jabbari et al, 2010; Kupelian, 2004; Stone et al, 2009).

A. Conventional Treatment

1. "Conventional," three-dimensional, and intensity-modulated radiation therapy—Conventional external beam radiation therapy (EBRT) has been used in the United States for treating prostate cancer since the late 1960s through the late 1980s (Bagshaw et al, 1988). The placement of the treatment fields was based on bony anatomic landmarks. It is now known that this technique resulted in inadequate coverage of the target volume in nearly one-third of patients. Computed tomography has improved our ability to localize and reconstruct pelvic anatomy, allowing more accurate design of treatment portals.

Based on these studies, the local control rate following EBRT has been estimated to be between 70% and 90%. The end points of these studies were based primarily on a clinical assessment of "local control." These end points are now known to underestimate the true incidence of local failures because of the presence of occult cancer in clinically controlled patients. Many patients whose disease was once thought to be controlled locally, based on physical examination, do in fact have persistent disease when assessed by PSA or biopsy, or both (Crook et al, 2000). Although the posttreatment PSA is more sensitive, it is a less specific end point for treatment failure than is biopsy, because distant failures can contribute to a rising level. PSA has been long recognized as an acceptable end point for the assessment of disease status, but over the last few years, its value and limitations after radiotherapy have become much cleared (Roach et al, 2003, 2006a, 2006b, 2007; Rodrigues et al, 2011).

The standard or so-called Phoenix Definition for a recurrence is reached when a patient's PSA rises by more than 2 ng/mL above the nadir (lowest) posttreatment value (Abramowitz et al, 2008). Despite its use to determine biochemical failure, PSA is not the most important predictor of survival being less important than Gleason score or T-stage even if very elevated to an ultra-high levels (eg, ≥50 ng/mL). In contrast, the importance of GS and stage has been well demonstrated by the long-term results of Phase III randomized trials conducted by the Radiation Therapy Oncology Group (RTOG) (Roach et al, 2000). In a multivariate analysis, Gleason score, clinical stage, and pathologic node status were correlated with overall and cause-specific survival. The use of this type of risk stratification system to predict overall survival has been validated using contemporary patients (Roach et al, 2007). A benefit of the RTOG risk groups is their use in defining for whom and how long hormonal therapy should be used. Numerous other risk stratification schemes are currently in popular use by radiation oncologists in the management of prostate cancer, but the greatest degree of consensus is probably the groupings recommended by the National Comprehensive Cancer Network (NCCN) (Mohler et al, 2010).

2. Three-dimensional conformal radiotherapy (3-DCRT) and intensity-modulated radiotherapy (IMRT)—Many of the technical challenges with delivering accurate and high dose radiation have been addressed by the incorporation of (1) computed tomography–assisted localization and reconstruction of the pelvic anatomy in the early 1990s resulting in 3-DCRT; (2) computer optimization algorithms to improve dose conformality in the mid-1990s to create IMRT; (3) online imaging to create so-called image-guided IMRT or IGRT as the new standard of care for treating clinically localized prostate cancer (Boyer et al, 2001).

The most common type of IGRT used involves the use of intraprostatic markers (usually by urologist) that can be used to adjust for setup (positioning) errors and organ displacement immediately prior to each treatment (Shinohara, 2008). More sophisticated technologies have been developed but have not been proven to render better results and are more expensive (Langen et al, 2003; Willoughby et al, 2006). Because IGRT allows more accurate administration of radiation to the target, less normal tissue receives radiation, and, therefore, less side effects are observed (Millender et al, 2004). This may in turn permit increased doses of radiation to be given and theoretically lead to improved local control.

▶ Dose Escalation Radiotherapy

Following the early Phase I–II studies conducted by the RTOG (9406), higher doses (>70 Gy) became widely accepted as standard among radiation oncologist (Michalski et al, 2009). To date, however, the use of higher doses has resulted only in improved rates of freedom from PSA failure (Dearnaley et al, 2005; Kuban et al, 2008; Peeters et al, 2006; Zietman et al, 2005). In contrast, the evidence for the use of androgen deprivation therapy (ADT) in conjunction with EBRT appears to be more compelling (Roach, 2007). RTOG 0815 is an ongoing Phase III trial attempting to determine whether ADT can be omitted when high doses of radiation are used. An earlier study conducted by the Medical Research Council (MRC) suggests that the use of ADT did not obviate the need for modest dose escalation (Dearnaley et al, 2007) (Table 26–1).

A. Brachytherapy

Alternative forms of radiation for the treatment of prostate cancer grew in popularity in the late 1990s but plateaued with the development of IGRT and proton beam radiotherapy. The most common of these alternative forms of radiation is brachytherapy. The major theoretic advantages with this form of radiation are the ability to deliver a very high dose of radiation to a localized area with a decreased number of treatment visits. The use of modern-era imaging techniques for visualizing the placement of radioactive seeds has obviated the need for open surgical procedures. Transrectal ultrasound–guided closed techniques are currently the standard. *Permanent implants* involve the use of low dose rate (LDR) radiation delivered to a very higher total dose (eg, >100 Gy). *Temporary implants* generally involve a lower total dose but at a higher dose rate, hence the term "high dose rate" brachytherapy. An example of an ultrasound-based iodine-125 permanent seed implant of the prostate, performed at our institution, is shown in Figure 26–1.

The failure rates reported in several older studies (done in the late 1960s and 1970s) suggested that the permanent implants are less effective than EBRT. More recent series suggest that the results of permanent implants may be equal to or better than other treatments (Jabbari et al, 2010; Pickles et al, 2010).

At most centers, intermediate- and high-risk patients are treated with a combination of EBRT and interstitial implant with or without hormonal therapy. Some clinicians routinely add EBRT for all patients undergoing permanent seed implants (Critz et al, 2000). However, most brachytherapists agree that low-risk patients can be equally well treated without the additional cost or morbidity of EBRT, while patients with intermediate-risk disease usually receive EBRT (Frank et al, 2007; Merrick et al, 2006; Nag et al, 1999). Although proponents of prostate brachytherapy commonly believe that the morbidity associated with interstitial brachytherapy is less than that associated with 3-DCRT, prospective studies using validated quality-of-life instruments suggest that acute morbidity is greater with permanent implants, whereas long-term morbidity tends to be similar (Sanda et al, 2008).

Temporary implants have the advantage of decreasing radiation exposure to hospital personnel and greater flexibility because of the ability to compensate for less than optimal needle placement. Temporary implants tend to be used for patients with more advanced disease in part because they are usually combined with EBRT and because HDR can be used to cover disease that is thought to be outside the gland. Iridium-192 is the only widely used isotope for temporary prostate implants. Based on the available data, in the hands of experts, it appears that HDR represents an excellent treatment option.

B. Neutrons, Protons, and Heavy-Charged Particles

Particle beam radiation is an alternative form of EBRT. This class of radiation involves the use of heavy particles (eg, neutrons), charged particles (eg, protons), or heavy-charged particles (eg, carbon). The theoretic advantage of proton-based radiotherapy is the potential for a more conformal dose distribution. Two prospective randomized trials have been completed to date. The first showed a significant improvement in

Table 26–1. Major Phase III randomized trials addressing the issue of dose of radiation.

First author (year) source	Trial design	5 y estimated control low vs high dose arm	T-Stages and PSA (Median)[a]	Impact of higher doses of radiation
Pollack et al (2002) MD Anderson	70 vs 78 Gy	60/90%	T1–3 7.8 ng/mL	Improved PSA control rates and trend for reduced DM
Sathya et al (2005) Ontario and Hamilton	66 Gy EBRT vs 40 Gy EBRT + 35 Gy iridium 192 boost	~40/70%	T2 and T3 19 ng/mL	Better outcomes with iridium implant (higher biologic dose)
Lukka et al (2005) NCI Canada	66 Gy in 33 fractions vs 52.5 Gy in 20 fractions	53/60%	T1c to T2c 10.5 ng/mL	Patients receiving lower doses did worse
Zietman et al (2005) Proton Radiation Oncology Group	70 Gy vs 79 GyE (protons)	60/82%	T1–2, PSA 6.3 ng/mL	Improved PSA control rates, no difference in OS, CSS, DM
Peeters et al (2006) The Netherlands	68 vs 78 Gy	64/74%	T1–4 10–20 ng/mL	Improved PSA control rates (not by Phoenix definition) no difference in OS, CSS, DM
Dearnaley et al (2007) MRC RT01	64[b] vs 74 Gy[b]	60/71%	T1–3 12.8 ng/mL	Improved PSA control rates, no difference in OS, CSS, DM

OS, overall survival, CSS, cause-specific survival, DM, distant metastasis.
[a]Estimated from papers.
[b]Neoadjuvant androgen deprivation therapy used on each arm.

local control in patients with high-grade tumors but no improvement in disease-free, relapse-free, or overall survival (Shipley et al, 1995). There was no benefit to other subsets of patients, and the 5-year actuarial rates of rectal bleeding were significantly higher ($p = 0.002$) with mixed beam treatment. The second trial essentially confirmed the dose response findings of earlier x-ray–based dose escalation trials with better PSA control for men treated to 79 Gy than those treated to 70 Gy (Zietman et al, 2005).

The attractiveness of heavy particles such as neutron (or carbon) based radiotherapy relates to the relative lack of oxygen dependence. Heavy-charged particles (such as carbon) are thought to have the advantages of both neutrons and protons. Early studies using this technology have been encouraging, but the series are small, follow-up is relatively short, and this equipment has limited availability (Tsuji et al, 2005). Longer follow-up studies will be required to assess the impact of these alternative types of radiation on long-term survival.

▶ Hormonal Therapy and Radiotherapy

Regarding *hormonal therapy and radiotherapy*, there currently exists no uniform consensus as to who should receive hormonal therapy and how long it should last. However, the best evidence suggests that low-risk patients do not benefit, intermediate-risk patients benefit from short-term hormonal therapy, and high-risk patients benefit from long-term hormonal therapy (Roach et al, 2010). The standard for "short-term" hormonal therapy consists of combined androgen blockade using a luteinizing hormone-releasing hormone agent and an antiandrogen 2 months before (neoadjuvant)

and 2 months during radiotherapy with or without 2 additional months of ADT for a total of 4–6 months of combined ADT. Patients receiving hormonal therapy appear to benefit with or without whole-pelvic radiotherapy. Most patients with high-risk disease (T3 GS = 7–10 or GS = 8–10) should also receive long-term adjuvant ADT with a luteinizing hormone-releasing hormone agonist for 2–3 years or longer in selected patients (Roach et al, 2010). Tables 26–2 and 26–3 summarize the major Phase III trials including short- and long-term ADT and EBRT, respectively. ADT alone is not as effective as ADT combined with EBRT (Mason et al, 2010; Widmark et al, 2009).

A. Postoperative Radiotherapy and Salvage Brachytherapy

The objectives of local regional postoperative radiotherapy may include attempting to eliminate microscopic residual tumor in the surgical bed, regional periprostatic tissues, and regional lymph nodes. As such, there are several potential indications for the use of adjuvant radiation, including (1) positive surgical margins, (2) seminal vesicle involvement, (3) lymph node involvement, (4) extracapsular extension, (5) increasing PSA, and (6) biopsy-proven recurrence. The presence of any of these variables is associated with a higher incidence of local recurrence. Radiotherapy may be administered prior to evidence of a recurrence or so-called adjuvant treatment or after documented failure (usually based on a detectable or rising PSA) or so-called salvage treatment. Adjuvant EBRT reduces the incidence of local recurrence in patients with postsurgical microscopic residual tumor after radical

Table 26–2. External beam radiotherapy +/– short-term neoadjuvant ADT.

First author (year) source	Pts	Arms	Benefit
Roach et al (2008) RTOG 8610	456 pts, T2-4	44 WP –> 66–70 Gy +/– 4 mo NHT (2 mo before and 2 mo concurrent)	Improved 10-y CSS, reduced DM: 47 –> 35%
D'Amico et al (2004) Dana Farber	206 pts	45 Gy to P& SV –> boost P to 70 Gy +/– 6 mo ADT (2 mo before, during, and after)	8-yr OS: 61 –> 74% for all pts, mainly those with no or minimal comorbidities 5-y: bF: 45 –> 21% CSS: 94 –> 100% FF salvage HT: 57 –> 82%
Denham et al (2005) TTROG	818 pts, T2b-T4	66 Gy to prostate & SV 0 vs 3 mo vs 6 mo NHT (2 & 5 mos before RT)	Compared 0 vs 3 vs 6 mo ADT: bFFS: 38 vs 52 vs 56% 6 vs 0 mo improved DM and PCSS
Crook et al (2004) Princess Margret	378 pts, T1c-T4	66–67 Gy to prostate (+WP 45–46 Gy if risk of LN >15%) 3 mo vs 8 mo nADT	No difference in 5-y FFF or OS. For high-risk pts only, DFS improved in the 8-month arm (71% vs 42%, $p = 0.01$)
Laverdiere (2004) Quebec	481 pts, T2-3N0	64 Gy to prostate-only: Study 1: 0 vs 3 mo ADT vs 10 mo ADT Study 2: 5 mo ADT vs 10 mo ADT	7 y bPFS: 42 –> 67% with 3–10 mo HT vs no HT No diff in bPFS with 5 vs 10 mo ADT in 2nd study

ADT, androgen deprivation therapy; NHT, neoadjuvant hormonal therapy; AHT, adjuvant hormonal therapy; bFFS, biochemical freedom from failure; OS, overall survival; CSS, cause-specific survival.

prostatectomy. The major Phase III trials have consistently shown a delay in the risk of biochemical and clinical failure and the trial with the longest follow-up shows a reduction in the mortality associated with adjuvant EBRT compared with delayed treatment (Bolla et al, 2002; Thompson et al, 2009; Wiegel et al, 2009). There is a common impression among some urologists that the risk of complications outweighs the benefits of adjuvant radiotherapy, but this impression is probably due to the consequence of older treatment techniques. More contemporary series suggest that, with modern equipment and 3-D planning, the incidence of complications is relatively low (Moinpour et al, 2008; Pinkawa et al, 2008; Thompson, 2009).

The findings from these trials are consistent with those of retrospective studies that suggest that patients who are treated before clinically manifesting a local recurrence appear to have improved disease-free survival, time to distant metastasis, and freedom from biochemical relapse compared with patients undergoing salvage treatment (Nudell et al, 1999; Valicenti et al, 1999). Only 50% of such patients are successfully treated for biopsy-proven recurrence at 3 years (Rogers et al, 1998). Salvage radiotherapy, however, is the only curative option in men experiencing PSA failure after surgery. A nomogram reported by Stephenson et al provides a reasonable estimate of the overall effectiveness of men undergoing salvage EBRT for most patients (Stephenson et al, 2007). Overall only 25%

Table 26–3. External beam radiotherapy +/– long-term adjuvant +/– neoadjuvant ADT.

Study	Pts	Arms	Benefit
RTOG 8531 (Pilepich et al, 2005)	945 pts, cT3, pT3, or LN+	65–70 Gy +/– indefinite AHT the last week of RT	Improved 10 y OS
Bolla et al (2002) EORTC 22863	415 pts, T3–4 or T1–2 G ≥ 7	70 Gy +/– 3 y AHT starting on first day of RT	Improved 10 y OS and CSS
Hanks et al (2003) RTOG 9202	1554 pts, T2c-T4 PSA <150 ng/mL	65–70 Gy + 4 mo NHT +/– 2 y AHT	10 y OS: 52 –> 54% overall survival advantage for GS 8–10: 32 –> 45% CSS and DM advantage
Bolla et al (2009) EORTC 22961	970 pts, T2c-T4N0/+ or T1c-2bN+	70 Gy; 6 mo ADT vs 3 y AHT	3 y LHRH improved 5 y OS; prostate cancer mortality: 4.7% vs 3.2%, no difference in fatal cardiac events (3–4%)

ADT, androgen deprivation therapy; NHT, neoadjuvant hormonal therapy; AHT, adjuvant hormonal therapy; OS, overall survival; CSS, cause-specific survival.

are long-term disease free with some subsets doing substantially better. For example, those with a pre-EBRT PSA <0.5 ng/mL, a long doubling time (>6 years), and positive margins but negative seminal vesicles and lymph nodes may achieve progression free rate of up to 80% at 6 years when treated with conventional dose radiation and ADT.

Although definitive proof from a prospective randomized trial is lacking, it seems reasonable to assume that patients who have no other disease away from the pelvis would benefit from adjuvant treatment. Retrospective studies suggest that pelvic lymph nodal treatment may improve outcomes compared with ADT alone (Da Pozzo et al, 2009; Spiotto et al, 2007). The RTOG is currently conducting a Phase III trial addressing this question (RTOG 0534).

Patients experiencing local recurrences after EBRT or brachytherapy may be candidates for salvage radiotherapy (Aaronson et al, 2009; Lee et al, 2007). Unfortunately, the complication rate is quite high in some series (Nguyen et al, 2009). The RTOG is conducting a Phase I–II trial (RTOG 0526) of brachytherapy salvage of EBRT failures as well.

B. Complications of Radiotherapy for Prostate Cancer

Most patients experience urinary frequency and dysuria during the course of their treatment. In patients receiving whole-pelvic irradiation, mild diarrhea may develop, but moderate to severe late complications are similar (Pinkawa et al, 2008; Pinkawa et al, 2011). Mild, self-limited rectal bleeding occurs in approximately 10% of patients and is dose and volume related. Urinary incontinence is usually associated with a history of a prior transurethral resection of the prostate. Hematuria and ureteral strictures occur in <2–10% of patients and are usually mild and self-limited. Following conventional EBRT Fecal incontinence was uncommon, but rectal urgency due to reduction in rectal dispensability occurred in 10% of patients (Lukka et al, 2005). Loss of erectile function is the most worrisome, the most common, long-term complication of radiotherapy. Impotence is reported in 35–40% of patients who were potent before treatment and maybe critically dependent on the dose of radiation received by the bulb of the penis (Roach et al, 2010). One rather large prospective study concluded that sexual dysfunction may be slightly lower after EBRT than after brachytherapy, but both had a lower impact on function than radical prostatectomy or cryosurgery (Sanda et al, 2008). However, most patients experience a decrease in the frequency and quality of intercourse, and most note a decrease in the volume of ejaculate. Potency diminishes further with time owing to aging and late radiation–induced normal tissue injury.

Acute urinary toxicity associated with brachytherapy is more common and longer lasting than that seen with 3-DCRT. The incidence of strictures is also higher. Acute obstruction occurs in 2–20% of patients. Although incontinence is quite uncommon following radiotherapy, it can occur in up to 50% of patients if they have had a previous transurethral resection of the prostate. The frequency of rectal toxicity following brachytherapy is generally believed to be less than that with 3DCRT (Sanda et al, 2008).

NONPROSTATE GENITOURINARY CANCERS

▶ Urinary Tract Tumors

Urothelial cancers (UCs) can occur along the entirety of the urinary tract, from the kidney to the urethra. Most occur in the bladder, though up to 5% of UC occur in the upper urinary tract. The majority of these involve the renal pelvis (Munoz, 2000). The role for radiation therapy in the management of UC varies by site, ranging from a palliative and up-and-coming role, as in the management of renal cell cancers, to an established and joint role with surgery and chemotherapy, as in organ-sparing approaches for the management of muscle-invasive bladder cancer, to a primary role, as can be considered for the management of penile cancer. This section will review the common uses of EBRT and brachytherapy in the management of urinary tract malignancies.

▶ Bladder Cancer

In the absence of durable local control, the natural history of bladder cancer is that of progressive growth and invasion with the eventual development of distant metastases. At diagnosis, the majority of patients (85%) with TCC of the bladder have superficial mucosal lesions (Ta, T1); however, 70% of patients recur locally following transurethral resection of the bladder tumor (TURBT). About 50–65% of these patients will progress to muscle-invasive disease (Brake, 2000). The presence of TCC in situ is associated with a more aggressive natural history, with higher probability of recurrence and progression to muscle invasive disease (Wolf, 1994). The addition of intravesicle immunotherapy (Bacille Calmette-Guerin, BCG) or chemotherapy decreases the overall recurrence rate by approximately 30% compared with TURBT alone. Nonetheless, within the first 5 years, tumor progression is noted in 20–40% of patients despite this additional treatment (Smith, 1999; Soloway, 2002). The development of muscle invasion (T2–T4) is accompanied by a significant increase in the incidence of metastatic spread and cause-specific death. Unfortunately, more than half of the patients diagnosed with muscle-invasive TCC have disseminated disease, often occult, at diagnosis. Five-year survival rates of up to 60% are reported for early invasive lesions (T1/T2a, N0); however, rates fall to ≤40% for more advanced tumors (T2b/T4, N+). Late systemic disease recurrence, most frequently pulmonary metastases, with or without local recurrence accounts for the decline in survival (Stein, 2001; Dalbagni et al, 2001), emphasizing the importance of adjuvant cytotoxic chemotherapy in the management of TCC. Following decades of unsuccessful single and bimodality treatments, contemporary management utilizes combinations of cyto-toxic chemotherapy, radiotherapy, and/or surgery in an attempt to improve survival and, if possible, achieve organ preservation.

A. EBRT Management of Bladder Cancer

EBRT has had no role in the management of in situ (Tis) or superficial (T1) bladder cancer. Investigators at the University of Erlangen, Germany, proposed a role for post-TURBT EBRT or EBRT with chemotherapy (EBRT/CT; cisplatin or carboplatin with 5-fluorouracil) for high-risk (T1G3, T1G1–2 associated with Tis, multifocality or tumor diameter >5 cm) or multiple recurrent superficial bladder cancers (Weiss, 2006). Eighty-eight percent of (121/137) patients treated with EBRT or EBRT/CT 4–6 weeks after initial TURBT were found to have a complete response (CR) at restaging TURBT. Patients not achieving a CR (16/137; 12%) were managed with immediate cystectomy. Five- and 10-year DSS and OS rates for patients with CR were 89% and 75% and 79% and 53%, respectively. When the evaluation was limited to patients with T1G3 tumors, 5- and 10-year DSS and OS rates were 80% and 64% and 71% and 47%, respectively. These rates are comparable with those seen in primary cystectomy series in T1 bladder cancer (Amling, 1994; Freeman, 1995; Malkowicz, 1990). Of note, patients receiving EBRT/CT had significantly higher 5-year DSS rates than patients treated with EBRT only. These findings are provocative; however, a randomized trial comparing EBRT or EBRT/CT with BCG will be necessary to fully investigate the utility of this organ-sparing approach. A Phase III randomized trial by Harland et al reported that adjuvant EBRT provided no benefit over observation alone for time to progression, progression-free survival, or OS for T1G3 bladder tumors (Harland et al, 2007).

The primary use of EBRT has been in muscle-invasive TCC; however, many oncologists have felt that the role for radiotherapy in the management of TCC has been limited. Surgical and medical oncologists typically recommend EBRT only for those patients who are medically unfit for or refuse cystectomy, or as palliation for locally advanced, unresectable tumors. Radical cystectomy remains the "gold standard" for the management of recurrent superficial and primary muscle-invasive TCC in the United States, despite the absence of robust evidence supporting its superiority. In fact, the "optimum" management approach remains undetermined.

In earlier studies, neither radiotherapy monotherapy nor precystectomy radiotherapy has shown DSS or OS benefits versus radical cystectomy (Huncharek, 1998). However, most of these studies had small sample sizes, compared pathologically and clinically staged patients, and used inadequate radiotherapy techniques by current standards. Radiotherapy monotherapy yields poorer local control rates but comparable 5-year survival rates to radical cystectomy. For muscle-invasive TCC, three of four randomized trials comparing EBRT (≤50 Gy) plus immediate cystectomy versus primary EBRT (60 Gy) and delayed (salvage) cystectomy demonstrated equivalent long-term survival rates with either treatment; only one trial demonstrated a significant benefit associated with immediate cystectomy (Bloom, 1982; Miller, 1977; Sell, 1991). In addition, no significant difference in 5- and 10-year survival rates or rates of development of distant metastases is seen with delayed or salvage cystectomy (Horowich, 1995; Petrovich, 2001). The use of combined modality treatments to achieve organ preservation without compromising treatment outcome has become a management approach of choice for many malignancies, including breast, esophageal, laryngeal, and anorectal cancers. Demonstration of equivalent outcomes with salvage surgery has made organ preservation a reasonable and appropriate treatment choice for some patients with muscle-invasive TCC.

B. Combined Modality Management of Muscle-Invasive Bladder Cancer (Transurethral Bladder Resection, Chemotherapy, and EBRT) and Organ Preservation

Several prospective randomized trials evaluating combined modality therapy for bladder preservation have been completed. In general, each of the trials has followed a common bladder-preservation algorithm including maximal TURBT, followed by induction chemoradiation, and an assessment of treatment response. Individuals with clinically CR continued with bladder-sparing therapy; all others were recommended for extirpative surgery. Completeness of TURBT (visibly complete vs not visibly complete) is associated with significantly lower salvage cystectomy rates.

The key features of the contemporary bladder-sparing trials are summarized in Table 26–4.

As a body of work, more than 1000 patients have been enrolled on these trials. Various cytotoxic agents have been evaluated for efficacy and safety when administered with EBRT. The timing of chemotherapy delivery has also been addressed. Concurrent chemoradiation schedules offer higher CR rates compared with sequential administration (Shipley, 1998, 2005). Combinations of cisplatin-based chemotherapy with 5-fluorouracil (5-FU), paclitaxel, or gemcitabine appear well suited for multimodality treatment for tolerability, radiosensitizing, and complementary cell-killing effects (Kaufman, 2000; von der Maase, 2005). Cisplatinum-based chemotherapy regimens administered concurrently with EBRT were well tolerated and resulted in a significant increase in freedom from distant metastases and OS. However, additional cycles of neoadjuvant chemotherapy were found not beneficial with regard to CR rates, metastasis-free survival, or overall survival, and were associated with higher morbidity and mortality (Tester, 1993; Shipley, 1998). Gemcitabine and the taxanes have also demonstrated significant single-agent activity against TCC. Assessment of concurrent cisplatin and paclitaxel with EBRT followed by adjuvant

Table 26–4. Contemporary combined modality bladder preservation trials.

Series (y)	Induction treatment[a]	CR Rate[b]	5-y OS
Shipley: RTOG 85-12 (1987)	CDDP + EBRT	66%	52%
Tester: RTOG 88-02 (1993) (Tester, 1993)	MCV + CDDP + EBRT	75%	51%
Sauer et al (1998)	CDDP/Carbo + EBRT	71%	56%
Shipley: RTOG 89-03 (1998) (Shipley, 1998)	+/– neoadj MCV then CDDP + EBRT	59%	49%
Kaufman: RTOG 95-06 (2000) (Kaufman, 2000)	5FU + CDDP + EBRT	67%	
Arias (2000)	Neoadj MVAC then CDDP + EBRT	68%	48%
Hussain: SWOG (2001) (Hussain, 2001)	CDDP + 5FU + EBRT		45%
Rodel: Erlangen (2002) (Rodel, 2002)	CDDP/Carbo + EBRT	72%	50%
Hagan: RTOG 97-06 (2003) (Hagan, 2003)	CDDP + bid EBRT	74%	
Kaufman: RTOG 99-06 (2009)	TAX + CDDP + bid EBRT	81%	56%
RTOG 0223	TAX + CDDP + bid EBRT vs 5FU + CDDP + bid EBRT	N/A	N/A
RTOG 0524	PAX + TMaB + EBRT vs PAX + EBRT	N/A	N/A

[a]All patients underwent TURBT before induction treatment.
[b]Complete response rate at the time of postinduction cystoscopy.

CR rate, complete response rate; OS, overall survival; RTOG, Radiation Therapy Oncology Group; CDDP, cisplatin; EBRT, external beam radiotherapy; neoadj, neoadjuvant; MCV, methotrexate, cisplatin, vinblastine; 5FU, 5-fluorouracil; TAX, Taxotere; bid EBRT, twice daily EBRT; GEM, gemcitabine; MVAC, methotrexate, vinblastine, Adriamycin, cisplatin; Carbo, carboplatin; Pax, paclitaxel; TMaB, trastuzumab.

gemcitabine and cisplatin has yielded acceptable toxicity and shown a promising 81% CR rate (Kaufman, 2009). For patients not medically fit for cisplatin chemotherapy, a recent abstract has shown promising results using 5FU and mitomycin C concurrently with radiotherapy suggests the superiority of combined chemoradiation to radiation alone (James, 2010).

For patients achieving a CR to the induction phase of treatment, this approach, followed by consolidation chemotherapy, yields long-term, disease-free, overall, and metastases-free survival rates equivalent to those achieved with radical cystectomy. Five-year survival rates range from 50% to 62%, with nearly two-thirds of the surviving patients maintaining a well-functioning bladder. The incidence of cystectomy performed for palliation of treatment-related morbidity is low (Zeitman, 2001). Overall survival and metastases-free survival rates realized from these organ-preserving strategies approximate those achieved with primary radical cystectomy (Nichols et al, 2000; Stein, 2001; Zeitman, 2000), suggesting that overall survival is driven by the presence or absence of occult distant disease at diagnosis. Limited overall survival, driven by high rates of distant metastases, highlights the need to optimize systemic therapy and better select for patients who are likely to benefit from local treatment.

Several studies have evaluated epidermal growth factor receptor (EGFR) and Her-2/neu expression in bladder cancer. Immunohistochemical staining has revealed Her-2/neu over expression in 40–80% of tumors. Data regarding the relationship between expression and treatment response and outcome are conflicting. One report evaluated the use of EGFR and/or Her-2 with chemotherapy and radiotherapy resistance and treatment outcomes (Chakravarti et al, 2005). EGFR expression appears to be a favorable prognostic factor for muscle-invasive TCC and correlates with significantly higher absolute and disease-specific survival ($p = 0.044$ and $p = 0.42$, respectively). A trend toward decreased incidence of distant metastases was also associated with EGFR expression. Her-2 expression was significantly correlated with reduced response rates to chemoradiation. Unlike other studies, p53, p16 had no prognostic significance (del Muro, 2004). In vitro, a synergistic effect between EGFR and ionizing radiation has been shown to increase apoptosis when compared with EGFR alone (Maddineni et al, 2005). The potential diagnostic and therapeutic implications of these findings remain to be clarified.

Following chemoradiation, residual tumor will be found in 20–30% of patients at restaging cystoscopy and TURBT. In addition, 20–30% of patients who achieve a CR develop a new or recurrent TCC. Typically, half of these tumors are superficial and half are muscle invasive. Persistent and superficial recurrences of TCC are successfully managed with TURBT with or without intravesical chemotherapy. Treatment outcomes for patients with superficial recurrences are comparable with those for patients who achieve a CR. Invasive recurrences are managed with prompt cystectomy. Salvage surgery is not associated with compromised in overall survival (Rodel, 2002; Dunst et al, 2001; Zeitman, 2001). Although no difference in overall survival is seen in patients who subsequently develop a superficial disease relapse, the 5-year survival rate is less for patients with a native bladder than for patients who do not develop a recurrence.

C. Improving Treatment Outcomes

It appears that an EBRT dose–response relationship exists for TCC. The ability to deliver higher radiotherapy doses requires sophisticated treatment planning and delivery techniques that can spare the small bowel and rectum. Anatomy-based, image-guided EBRT has multiple goals including accurate tumor targeting, the ability to safely deliver higher radiation doses, and minimizing normal tissue toxicity. The importance of image-guided conformal EBRT has been discussed in the section on prostate cancer. Here again, treatment precision including accommodation for organ motion and patient positioning is particularly important. As with prostate and other pelvic malignancies, external pressure from surrounding bowel and rectum, as well as changes in the volume of urine within the bladder, leads to considerable variation in the position of the bladder (Pos et al, 2003; Langen, 2001). Fiducial marker placement and real-time imaging has been used and appears promising (Shimizu, 2000). For bladder-sparing treatment of TCC, this also preserves the option for later creation of continent diversions for patients who have an incomplete response to induction chemoradiation.

Other approaches to dose intensification include brachytherapy and *altered fractionation* regimens. Select European centers have used interstitial brachytherapy, usually in addition to EBRT, to treat TCC with reported local control rates of 70–90%, excellent preservation of bladder function, and low treatment-related toxicity. However, in the absence of randomized prospective trials comparing treatment outcome and toxicity, interstitial brachytherapy cannot be considered a standard of care for TCC. As discussed in Section "General Principles of Radiotherapy, dose escalation via altered fractionation schedules (Housset et al, 1993; Hagan, 2003; Sangar et al, 2005; Kaufman, 2000) enhances the therapeutic ratio by delivering a higher effective radiotherapy dose. Aggressive dose-intensified regimens yield higher CR rates though at the cost of moderately severe toxicity. Longer follow-up data are needed to comprehensively assess efficacy and safety.

Bladder preservation therapy provides an alternative treatment option for select patients with invasive TCC, without compromised survival. Patient selection for bladder-sparing approaches is of prime importance. Only those patients that would be suitable primary surgical candidates should be considered for this approach, since salvage cystectomy may be indicated. The optimal regimen of combined radiotherapy and chemotherapy remains to be determined.

D. Toxicity of Radiotherapy Treatment for Bladder Cancer

Treatment-related toxicities during and after chemoradiation primarily affect the bladder, rectum, and small bowel. Acute enteritis and cystitis are frequent complaints occurring in the majority of patients. These are usually mild and are managed symptomatically. Severe marrow-related toxicity is reported in ≤10% of organ-preservation patients. Rates of chronic bladder dysfunction of up to 10% have been reported, but symptomatic reduction in the bladder capacity is rare. Chronic, moderately severe rectal and small-bowel injuries are reported in 3–4% and 1–2%, respectively. Mortality rates are ≤1% (Chao, 1995). With wider use of conformal radiotherapy techniques, continued declines in toxicity may be anticipated.

▶ Cancers of the Kidney, Renal Pelvis, and Ureter

In the past, EBRT has had limited use in the management of primary renal cell carcinoma (RCC). There is new data using advanced techniques that make radiation therapy and up-and-coming modality in the treatment of RCC. *In vivo* and *in vitro* experiments have demonstrated variable though low radiosensitivity to conventionally fractionated EBRT (Ning et al, 1997). Randomized trials have failed to show a survival or relapse-free survival benefit from preoperative or postoperative radiotherapy (van der werf Messing, 1981; van der werf Messing, 1973; Juusela et al, 1977; Finney, 1973; Kjaer, 1987). More contemporary retrospective studies with better patient selection and using contemporary EBRT techniques have suggested a benefit of postoperative EBRT in select patients with a high-risk of local-regional failure (T3a and T3c) (Makarewicz, 1998; Kao et al, 1994; Stein, 1992). Stereotactic body radiotherapy (SBRT) is capable of delivering high-dose per fraction to kidney tumors and appears to overcome any potential radioresistance of RCC. Initial studies using SBRT on primary RCC tumors in nonsurgical patients have shown a reasonable rate of local control (Beitler, 2004; Svedman, 2008; Wersall, 2005).

Similarly, scant data exist supporting a benefit from EBRT for renal pelvis or ureteral carcinoma. Some studies have shown a local control benefit from postnephroureterectomy irradiation in T3-T4, N0, or node-positive patients (Maulard-Durdux et al, 1996; Cozad, 1992, 1995).

A role exists for palliative EBRT for metastatic renal cell renal pelvis and ureteral carcinomas. Palliative radiotherapy is effective at relieving pain from bone metastases, palliation of neurologic sequelae from brain metastases, spinal cord and nerve root compression, or invasion (Sheehan et al, 2003; Huguenin et al, 1998; Onufrey and Mohiuddin, 1985; Wronski et al, 1997). SBRT has also been used with a high degree of success in the palliation of spinal metastases from RCC (Nguyen, 2010).

URETHRAL CANCERS

Primary urethral cancers are very rare in both men and women. The National Cancer Institute Surveillance, Epidemiology and End Results (SEER) database in the United States identified only 1615 cases in the time period between 1973 and 2002 (www.seer.cancer.gov). As a result, knowledge regarding risk factors is extremely limited and no consensus exists regarding optimal management. Squamous cell histologies appear to be the most common followed by adenocarcinoma and TCC. Distal or anterior lesions appear to have a more favorable prognosis than proximal or posterior lesions.

▶ Cancer of the Female Urethra

Urethral adenocarcinoma comprises <0.003% of urogenital tract cancers in women (Meis, 1987). The treatment strategy for each patient is largely based upon tumor size and location; however, prognosis remains relatively poor, regardless of treatment approach.

Surgical excision has been used for small lesions of the distal urethra with limited success (Bracken, 1976). Both EBRT and brachytherapy are alternatives to surgical resection of early-stage urethral cancers <1 cm in size. For larger lesions, or lesions that extend into surrounding structures, preoperative EBRT radiation to the inguinal, external iliac, and hypogastric nodes is recommended (Grigsby, 1998b). Doses of 45–50 Gy are delivered to clinically uninvolved nodes, with an additional 10–15 Gy boost to any involved nodes. A total dose of 60–70 Gy is delivered to the tumor through reduced fields.

Tumors involving the posterior urethra often involve the bladder and have a high incidence of nodal involvement. Locally advanced tumors may be managed with preoperative radiotherapy and exenteration. If feasible, early lesions may be treated with surgical resection and postoperative EBRT or EBRT alone. Local control rates of 20–30% and correspondingly low 5-year survival rates are noted (Grigsby, 1998b). Preoperative EBRT doses are typically in the range of 45–50 Gy. Definitive and postoperative doses deliver 45–50 Gy to the pelvis and clinically uninvolved nodes, with an additional 10–15 Gy boost to involved nodes. A total dose of 60 Gy is delivered to the entire surface of the vaginal mucosa and brachytherapy is employed to deliver a final dose of 70–80 Gy (Grigsby, 1998a) to the primary tumor.

Urethral strictures are the most frequently reported complication of radiotherapy treatment. Urinary incontinence, cystitis, and vaginal atrophy and stenosis may also occur. Fistulas and small-bowel obstruction due to radiation or tumor necrosis are uncommon.

▶ Cancer of the Penis and Male Urethra

Surgery has been the primary management choice for penile cancer. Although quite effective, neither a partial nor a total penectomy is a desirable therapeutic choice. Because of the rarity of penile cancer, no randomized trials comparing various treatment options has been or is likely to be completed. High success rates achievable with surgical salvage have made possible attempts at organ preservation with the use of radiation alone. Similarly, the relative paucity of cases has precluded the development of standardized radiotherapy management; a minimum dose of 60–65 Gy is needed for control of the primary tumor. Careful patient selection is important, with optimal candidates described as having distal, well to moderately well-differentiated tumors that are ≤4 cm in diameter.

Both EBRT and interstitial brachytherapy may be used to treat penile lesions. If not previously performed, circumcision is required prior to radiotherapy treatment. Small superficial lesions of the glans and distal shaft may be treated with orthovoltage or low-energy electron beams. Larger, invasive lesions of the penis, penile urethra, and bulbous urethra are managed with EBRT alone or EBRT followed by an interstitial brachytherapy boost. Brachytherapy is required to achieve doses to the primary >65 Gy. Prophylactic irradiation of the bilateral inguinal and pelvic lymph nodes to 45–50 Gy accompanies management of all but the most superficial primary lesions. Palpable and clinically suspicious nodes receive 65–70 Gy. Local failure rates of 15–37% have been reported (Sarin et al, 1997; Rozan, 1995). Lesions of the prostatic urethra are managed in a manner similar to that of prostate cancer.

The high risk of systemic failure associated with urethral tumors results in 5-year survival rates of 55% and 15% for distal and proximal urethral tumors, respectively (Heysek et al, 1985). Neoadjuvant chemotherapy and radiotherapy, with surgery reserved for salvage, is one strategy for more advanced lesions (Eisenberger, 1992; Husein et al, 1990). Similar to the strategy used for organ preservation in other sites, concurrent chemoradiotherapy (Cohen, 2008) has been used for advance lesions.

Regarding *treatment toxicity*, acute, transient sequelae include brisk, moist desquamation of the skin of the penis, urinary frequency, urgency, dysuria, nocturia, and intermittent diarrhea. The risk of soft tissue necrosis, fibrosis, and phimosis are dose-limiting sequelae for penile irradiation. Urethral or meatal stricture or both are the most common complication of penile and urethral irradiation and are dose and technique dependent. Symptomatic strictures are managed with urethral dilation, with urethrotomy reserved for severe cases. Although sexual activity is almost uniformly interrupted during the course of treatment, most patients maintain full or slightly diminished potency after radiotherapy (Opjordsmoen and Fossa, 1994).

▶ Testicle Tumors

Testicular cancer is the most common malignancy in men aged 15–34 years. For unknown reasons, the incidence of testicular carcinoma has been increasing worldwide, with the greatest increases seen in seminoma. Testicular cancer remains one of the most curable cancers with 5-year relative survival rates of 96–99% for nonmetastatic cases. EBRT has played a primary role in the management of pure seminoma germ cell tumors (GCTs) of the testicles, but predominantly an adjuvant or palliative role in management of *nonseminomatous GCT (NSGCT)*. Furthermore, EBRT has a limited role as palliative therapy in disseminated NSGCT, since patients with brain metastases may still be cured with chemotherapy.

▶ Germ Cell Tumors

Seminoma accounts for 40% of testicular GCTs and occurs in slightly older men (median age, 33 years) than does nonseminoma testicular GCT. Nonseminoma GCTs (embryonal carcinoma, teratoma, choriocarcinoma, yolk sac tumor, and mixed GCT) comprise the remaining 60% of testicular tumors, peak at a slightly younger age (median age, 27 years), and are associated with elevations in β-hCG or α-fetoprotein or both in 80% of cases. Radical inguinal orchiectomy with high ligation of the spermatic cord remains the therapeutic mainstay for pure *seminomatous GCT*, followed by surveillance, radiotherapy, or chemotherapy.

Adjuvant radiotherapy has been used to reduce the risk of local and regional recurrence in ipsilateral pelvic and para-aortic lymph nodes. Figure 26–4 shows the incidence and location of nodal metastases in early-stage, left- and right-sided testicular tumors. The classic prophylactic postorchiectomy EBRT portals used to reduce the incidence of ipsilateral pelvic and para-aortic nodal recurrences is shown in Figure 26–5A and B. The exquisite radiosensitivity of pure seminoma has permitted progressive reduction in the radiotherapy dose used to treat seminoma, without a reduction relapse-free survival rates (Jones et al, 2005; Gurkaynak et al, 2003; Niewald et al, 1995). The role for EBRT in the management of pure seminoma has changed greatly over the past 10 years. Since equivalent disease-specific and overall survival rates may be achieved with adjuvant EBRT or surveillance for stage I seminoma (pT1–3, N0, M0, S0), in addition to the absence of treatment-related sequelae and the risk of secondary malignancy (Chao, 1995; Huyge, 2004; Travis, 1997; Zagars, 2004), surveillance has become a preferred approach for many centers (Choo et al, 2005; Miki et al, 1998; Warde, 1995, 2002, 1997).

Investigators at Princess Margaret Hospital (PMH) noted 80–85% 5-year relapse-free rate (RFR) for stage I patients participating in an active surveillance protocol, compared with those undergoing adjuvant EBRT (95–99%) (Warde, 2005). Comparable 5-year cause-specific survival rates were achieved with EBRT salvage following surveillance and postorchiectomy EBRT, 99.8% and 100%, respectively. The 10-year actuarial risk of requiring chemotherapy salvage was not significantly increased with surveillance.

The primary site of relapse in the surveillance population was determined to be isolated para-aortic lymph nodes (89%). Only 10% of relapses involved pelvic nodal regions. Seventy percent of relapses following prophylactic para-aortic and pelvic nodal EBRT were also in supra-diaphragmatic locations. These findings prompted their conclusion that surveillance should be the standard of care in stage I seminoma (Warde, 2005). However, until recently, surveillance had not been widely accepted as a management standard. A pattern of care study evaluating treatment practices at hospital centers in Canada and the United States showed significant variations in practice patterns (Choo et al, 2002). In addition, not all patients choose postorchiectomy observation, nor are all patients suitable candidates for surveillance protocols. Patients who are not compliant and patients with pathologic features, who are associated with significantly higher recurrence rates including tumors >4 cm, rete testis invasion, lymphovascular space invasion, and age ≤33 years may not be ideal candidates for surveillance (Parker et al, 2002; Richie, 2003; Warde, 1997, 2002). Additional considerations are the long-term side effects of frequent radiographic examinations over several years and the cost associated with surveillance. A summary of surveillance guidelines for stage I testicular seminoma is shown in Table 26–5.

The pattern of recurrence following surveillance and prophylactic EBRT spurred investigations of use of smaller treatment fields, targeting the para-aortic nodes and omitting treatment of the pelvic nodes (limited-field irradiation; Figure 26–5A), including a randomized trial by the MRC. Relapse-free survival rates using limited-field EBRT were equivalent to those seen with classic "dog-leg" irradiation, and hematologic, gastrointestinal, and gonadal toxicity were reduced. Pelvic nodal recurrences, however, were higher with limited-field EBRT (Fossa et al, 1999; Kiricuta et al, 1996; Logue et al, 2003; Niazi et al, 2005; Rowland et al, 2005; Sultanem, 1998). Patients who elect limited-field EBRT should probably have pelvic surveillance for a minimum of 10 years as a component of their treatment plan. Pelvic nodal recurrences are readily salvaged with EBRT or chemotherapy (Power et al, 2005). In

Table 26–5. Surveillance guidelines for stage I testicular seminoma.

Every 3–4 months, years 1–3[a]
History and physical
Serum AFP, β-hCG, LDH
Every 3–4 months, years 1–10
Abdominal/pelvic CT scan
Every 6 months, years 1–10
Chest x-ray

[a]After year 3, the frequency changes to every 6 months until year 7 and then annually.

AFP, α-fetoprotein; hCG, human chorionic gonadotrophin; LDH, lactate dehydrogenase.

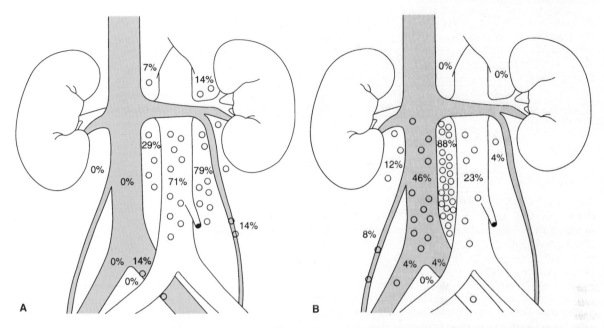

▲ **Figure 26–4. A:** Incidence and location of lymph nodes at risk for an early-stage left-sided testicular seminoma. **B:** Incidence and location of lymph nodes at risk for an early-stage right-sided testicular seminoma. (Adapted from Donohue JP et al: Distribution of nodal nets in nonseminomatous testis cancer. J Urol 1982;126:315.)

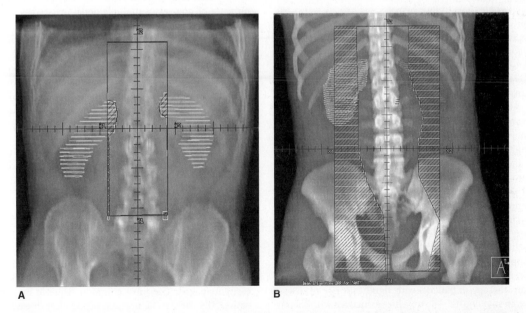

▲ **Figure 26–5. A:** Para-aortic treatment field ("limited-field") for prophylactic nodal irradiation for stage I testicular seminoma. **B:** Pelvic and para-aortic treatment field ("hockey stick or dog-leg") for prophylactic nodal irradiation for stage I testicular seminoma.

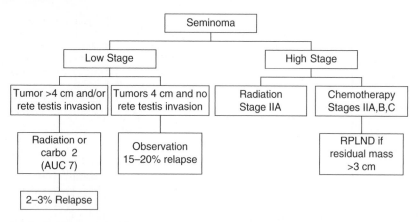

▲ **Figure 26–6.** Risk-adapted strategy for the management of stage I seminoma.

addition to the benefit of reduced treatment portals, it is reasonable to assume that increased use of IMRT will lead to further reductions in acute EBRT-related toxicity but the long term impact on the risk of second cancers is uncertain.

The greatest change in the management of stage I seminoma has been the use single agent carboplatin. Five Phase II trials conducted in Europe assessed relapse-free survival rates with two cycles of postorchiectomy, adjuvant carboplatin. With follow-up ranging from 14 to 74 months, relapse rates were <1% and grade three to four hematologic toxicity were <5%. The MRC conducted a prospective Phase III trial that randomized men with stage I seminoma to 20–30 Gy limited-field (para-aortic nodal) or large-field (pelvis and para-aortic nodal irradiation) EBRT or one cycle of adjuvant carboplatin (AUCx7) (Oliver et al, 2004; Oliver et al, 2005; Reiter et al, 2001; Dieckmann et al, 2000; Krege et al, 1997; Germa-Lluch et al, 2002). At 4 years median follow-up, the results indicated that single-cycle carboplatin was noninferior to prophylactic nodal irradiation; relapse-free survival rates were equivalent, patients receiving carboplatin were less likely to take time off from work, and significantly fewer secondary tumors were reported.

With an absence of consensus regarding treatment for stage I seminoma, the Spanish Germ Cell Cooperative group developed a risk-adapted management strategy (Figure 26–6) (Aparicio et al, 2005). In 2010, the NCCN published new practice guidelines for the management of testicular seminoma (http://www.nccn.org) incorporating the data from the contemporary seminoma trials. The impetus for these treatment recommendations appears to be the judicious use of adjuvant therapy in patients with significant risk of disease relapse. In so doing, the late toxicities associated with chemotherapy and radiotherapy may be reduced or avoided.

The use for adjuvant postorchiectomy EBRT in *stage II seminoma* (*pT1–3, N1–3, M0, S0–1*) is determined by the bulk of the retroperitoneal lymphadenopathy. Stage IIA (single or multiple nodes all ≤2 cm) and IIB (single or multiple nodes

2–5 cm) patients are successfully treated with EBRT directed to the para-aortic and ipsilateral pelvic lymph nodes, using the so-called hockey stick or dog-leg fields (Figure 26–5B). Doses of 20–30 Gy to the pelvis and para-aortic nodes followed by a 5–10-Gy boost to bulky nodes yield 5-year and 10-year relapse-free, cause-specific, and overall survival rates of 85%, 94%, and 93%, respectively (Chung et al, 2004; Classen et al, 2003; Rowland et al, 2005; Warde, 1998). Heterogeneity within clinical stages IIA and IIB seminoma due to the presence of one versus multiple nodal masses has led to the suggested use of single agent carboplatin with EBRT, particularly for stage IIB (Patterson et al, 2001). Patients with bulky retroperitoneal nodal disease (≥5 cm, IIC) have high rates of distant relapse. Standard of care is three cycles of cisplatin-etoposide and bleomycin (PEB) or four cycles of etoposide and cisplatinum, followed by surveillance. Residual disease <3 cm may be closely observed, treated with radiotherapy, or surgically resected. Masses ≥3 cm should be resected. Prophylactic mediastinal irradiation for stage II seminoma has long been abandoned. Supradiaphragmatic recurrence rates approximate 3% and may be successfully salvaged with multiagent chemotherapy. EBRT has no role in the primary management of stages IIC, III, and IV seminoma.

A. Toxicity from Radiotherapy Treatment of Testicular Seminoma

Treatment-related toxicity associated with pelvic and para-aortic EBRT is primarily gastrointestinal in nature and can be easily managed. The most common sequelae may include nausea, diarrhea, rectal urgency, peptic ulcer disease, gastroesophageal reflux disease (GERD), and transient reduction in spermatogenesis (Garcia-Serra et al, 2005; Joos et al, 1997). It has been estimated that 50% or more of the men diagnosed with testicular cancer have impaired spermatogenesis at the time of diagnosis, complicating precise characterization of

EBRT effects on fertility (Fossa et al, 1986; Gordon et al, 1997; Pasquolotto, 2003). The severity and duration of oligospermia appears to be dose related and testicular scatter doses are thought to be responsible for fertility disturbances. Radiation-related disturbances in spermatogenesis can be minimized by maintaining scatter doses to <20 cGy and the use of smaller treatment fields (Joos et al, 1997; Melchior et al, 2001). This is readily achieved with contemporary treatment approaches. Patients treated with postorchiectomy EBRT have >50% chance of regaining normal spermatogenesis and all patients regain at least some spermatogenesis, usually within 1–2 years after treatment completion (Gordon et al, 1997; Nalesnik et al, 2004). The existence of severe disturbances in spermatogenesis late in the post-EBRT course probably results from impaired pretreatment sperm cell production and less so the impact of scatter radiation on the remaining testicle.

A small but measurable increase in the risk of second malignancies after a 10–20-year latent period has been reported (Hughes et al, 2003; Travis, 1997; Zagars, 2004). In some reports, however, the overall observed incidence of second nonseminomatous malignancy was not significantly increased when compared with the expected incidence (Chao, 1995; Travis, 1997).

SUMMARY

Therapeutic radiation has an extensive history in the management of genitourinary (GU) malignancies. Major advances have been made in its use, particularly for prostate cancer, muscle-invasive TCC of the bladder and testicular seminoma, and a continued role for radiation therapy in the multidisciplinary management of genitourinary malignancies seems certain. Overall treatment outcomes continue to improve, accompanied by diminishing rates of toxicity. With continued technologic development, including the use of adaptive radiotherapy, the discovery and application of novel treatment agents, and the combined efforts of each discipline within urologic oncology, patients with GU tumors have greater opportunities to become and remain disease free.

BIBLIOGRAPHY

General Principles of Radiobiology, and Prostate Cancer

Aaronson DS et al: Salvage permanent perineal radioactive-seed implantation for treating recurrence of localized prostate adenocarcinoma after external beam radiotherapy. BJU Int 2009;104: 600–604.

Abramowitz MC et al: The Phoenix definition of biochemical failure predicts for overall survival in patients with prostate cancer. Cancer 2008;112:55–60.

Arcangeli G et al: Acute and late toxicity in a randomized trial of conventional versus hypofractionated three-dimensional conformal radiotherapy for prostate cancer. Int J Radiat Oncol Biol Phys 2011;79(4):1013–1021.

Arcangeli G et al: A prospective phase III randomized trial of hypofractionation versus conventional fractionation in patients with high-risk prostate cancer. Int J Radiat Oncol Biol Phys 2010; 78:11–18.

Bagshaw MA et al: Status of prostate cancer at Stanford University. NCI Monogr. 1988;7:47–60.

Bolla M et al: Long-term results with immediate androgen suppression and external irradiation in patients with locally advanced prostate cancer (an EORTC study): A phase III randomised trial. Lancet 2002;360:103–106.

Bolla M et al: Duration of androgen suppression in the treatment of prostate cancer. N Engl J Med 2009;360:2516–2527.

Boyer A et al: Intensity-modulated radiotherapy: Current status and issues of interest. Int J Radiat Oncol Biol Phys 2001;51:880–914.

Brenner DJ, Hall EJ: Fractionation and protraction for radiotherapy of prostate carcinoma. Int J Radiat Oncol Biol Phys 1999;43: 1095–1101.

Critz FA et al: Simultaneous irradiation for prostate cancer: Intermediate results with modern techniques. J Urol 2000;164:738–741; discussion 741–733.

Crook J et al: Report of a multicenter Canadian phase III randomized trial of 3 months vs. 8 months neoadjuvant androgen deprivation before standard-dose radiotherapy for clinically localized prostate cancer. Int J Radiat Oncol Biol Phys 2004;60:15–23.

Crook J et al: Postradiotherapy prostate biopsies: What do they really mean? Results for 498 patients. Int J Radiat Oncol Biol Phys 2000;48:355–367.

D'Amico AV et al: 6-month androgen suppression plus radiation therapy vs radiation therapy alone for patients with clinically localized prostate cancer: A randomized controlled trial. JAMA 2004;292:821–827.

Da Pozzo LF et al: Long-term follow-up of patients with prostate cancer and nodal metastases treated by pelvic lymphadenectomy and radical prostatectomy: The positive impact of adjuvant radiotherapy. Eur Urol 2009 55(5):1003–1011.

Dearnaley DP et al: Phase III pilot study of dose escalation using conformal radiotherapy in prostate cancer: PSA control and side effects. Br J Cancer 2005;92:488–498.

Dearnaley DP et al: Escalated-dose versus standard-dose conformal radiotherapy in prostate cancer: First results from the MRC RT01 randomised controlled trial. Lancet Oncol 2007;8:475–487.

Denham JW et al: Short-term androgen deprivation and radiotherapy for locally advanced prostate cancer: Results from the Trans-Tasman Radiation Oncology Group 96.01 randomised controlled trial. Lancet Oncol 2005;6:841–850.

Elder JS et al: Radical perineal prostatectomy for clinical stage B2 carcinoma of the prostate. J Urol 1982;127:704–706.

Fowler J et al: Is alpha/beta for prostate tumors really low? Int J Radiat Oncol Biol Phys 2001;50:1021–1031.

Frank SJ et al: Interstitial implant alone or in combination with external beam radiation therapy for intermediate-risk prostate cancer: A survey of practice patterns in the United States. Brachytherapy. 2007;6:2–8.

Giordano SH et al: Limits of observational data in determining outcomes from cancer therapy. Cancer 2008;112:2456–2466.

Hanks GE et al: Phase III trial of long-term adjuvant androgen deprivation after neoadjuvant hormonal cytoreduction and radiotherapy in locally advanced carcinoma of the prostate: The Radiation Therapy Oncology Group Protocol 92–02. J Clin Oncol 2003;21: 3972–3978.

Jabbari S et al: Equivalent biochemical control and improved prostate-specific antigen nadir after permanent prostate seed implant brachytherapy versus high-dose three-dimensional conformal radiotherapy and high-dose conformal proton beam radiotherapy boost. Int J Radiat Oncol Biol Phys 2010;76:36–42.

King CR, Fowler JF: A simple analytic derivation suggests that prostate cancer alpha/beta ratio is low. [Comment In: Int J Radiat Oncol Biol Phys. 2001 Sep 1;51(1):1–3 UI: 21407940]. Int J Radiat Oncol Biol Phys 2001;51:213–214.

Kuban DA et al: Long-term results of the M. D. Anderson randomized dose-escalation trial for prostate cancer. Int J Radiat Oncol Biol Phys 2008;70:67–74.

Kupelian PA et al: Radical prostatectomy, external beam radiotherapy <72 Gy, external beam radiotherapy > or = 72 Gy, permanent seed implantation, or combined seeds/external beam radiotherapy for stage T1-T2 prostate cancer. Int J Radiat Oncol Biol Phys 2004;58:25–33.

Langen KM, Jones DT: Organ motion and its management. Int J Radiat Oncol Biol Phys 2001;50:265–278.

Langen KM et al: Evaluation of ultrasound-based prostate localization for image-guided radiotherapy. Int J Radiat Oncol Biol Phys 2003;57:635–644.

Laverdiere J et al: The efficacy and sequencing of a short course of androgen suppression on freedom from biochemical failure when administered with radiation therapy for T2-T3 prostate cancer. J Urol 2004;171:1137–1140.

Lee B et al: Feasibility of high-dose-rate brachytherapy salvage for local prostate cancer recurrence after radiotherapy: The University of California-San Francisco experience. Int J Radiat Oncol Biol Phys 2007;67:1106–1112.

Lee WR: Extreme hypofractionation for prostate cancer. Expert Rev Anticancer Ther 2009;9:61–65.

Litwin M: Measuring health related quality of life in men with prostate cancer. J Urol 1994;152:1882–1887.

Lukka H et al: Randomized trial comparing two fractionation schedules for patients with localized prostate cancer. J Clin Oncol 2005;23:6132–6138.

Mason MD et al: Intergroup randomized phase 3 study of androgen deprivation therapy (ADT) + radiation therapy (RT) in locally advanced prostate cancer (CaP) (NCIC-CTG, SWOG, MRC-UK, and INT: T94–0110; NCT00002633). In: Cox, ed. Proceedings of the American Society for Radiation Oncology 52nd Annual Meeting, San Diego: Elsevier; 2010:S2.

McCammon R et al: Toxicity assessment of pelvic intensity-modulated radiotherapy with hypofractionated simultaneous integrated boost to prostate for intermediate- and high-risk prostate cancer. Int J adiat Oncol Biol Phys 2009;75(2):413–420.

Memmelaar J: Total prostatovesiculectomy; retropubic approach. J Urol 1949;62:340–348.

Merrick GS et al: Permanent prostate brachytherapy: Is supplemental external-beam radiation therapy necessary? Oncology (Williston Park) 2006;20:514–522; discussion 522–515.

Michalski JM et al: Long-term toxicity following 3D conformal radiation therapy for prostate cancer from the RTOG 9406 Phase I/II Dose Escalation Study. Int J Radiat Oncol Biol Phys 2009;76(1):14–22.

Miles EF, Lee WR: Hypofractionation for prostate cancer: A critical review. Semin Radiat Oncol 2008;18:41–47.

Millender LE et al: Daily electronic portal imaging for morbidly obese men undergoing radiotherapy for localized prostate cancer. Int J Radiat Oncol Biol Phys 2004;59:6–10.

Mohler J et al: NCCN clinical practice guidelines in oncology: Prostate cancer. J Natl Compr Canc Netw 2010;8:162–200.

Moinpour CM et al: Health-related quality of life results in pathologic stage C prostate cancer from a Southwest Oncology Group trial comparing radical prostatectomy alone with radical prostatectomy plus radiation therapy. J Clin Oncol 2008;26:112–120.

Nag S et al: American Brachytherapy Society (ABS) recommendations for transperineal permanent brachytherapy of prostate cancer. Int J Radiat Oncol Biol Phys 1999;44:789–799.

Nguyen PL et al: Patient-reported quality of life after salvage brachytherapy for radio-recurrent prostate cancer: A prospective Phase II study. Brachytherapy 2009;8:345–352.

Nudell DM et al: Radiotherapy after radical prostatectomy: Treatment outcomes and failure patterns. Urology 1999;54:1049–1057.

Pasteau O, Degrais P: The radium treatment of cancer of prostate. Arch Roentgen Ray 1914;18:396–410.

Peeters ST et al: Dose-response in radiotherapy for localized prostate cancer: Results of the Dutch multicenter randomized phase III trial comparing 68 Gy of radiotherapy with 78 Gy. J Clin Oncol 2006;24:1990–1996.

Pickles T et al: Brachytherapy or conformal external radiotherapy for prostate cancer: A single-institution matched-pair analysis. Int J Radiat Oncol Biol Phys 2010;76:43–49.

Pilepich MV, Winter K, Lawton CA, et al: Androgen suppression adjuvant to definitive radiotherapy in prostate carcinoma—long-term results of phase III RTOG 85-31. Int J Radiat Oncol Biol Phys 2005;61:1285–1290.

Pinkawa M et al: Health-related quality of life after adjuvant and salvage postoperative radiotherapy for prostate cancer—A prospective analysis. Radiother Oncol 2008;88:135–139.

Pinkawa M et al: Quality of life after whole pelvic versus prostate-only external beam radiotherapy for prostate cancer: A matched-pair comparison. Int J Radiat Oncol Biol Phys 2011;81(1):23–28.

Pollack A et al: Prostate cancer radiation dose response: Results of the M. D. Anderson phase III randomized trial. Int J Radiat Oncol Biol Phys 2002;53:1097–1105.

Reiner WB, Walsh PC: An anatomical approach to the surgical management of the dorsal vein and Santorini's plexus during radical retropubic surgery. J Urol. 1979;121:198.

Ritter M et al: Hypofractionation for prostate cancer. Cancer J 2009;15:1–6.

Roach M III et al: Predicting long-term survival, and the need for hormonal therapy: A meta-analysis of RTOG prostate cancer trials. Int J Radiat Oncol Biol Phys 2000;47:617–627.

Roach M III et al: Serum prostate-specific antigen and survival after external beam radiotherapy for carcinoma of the prostate. Urology 2003;61:730–735.

Roach M III et al: Defining biochemical failure following radiotherapy with or without hormonal therapy in men with clinically localized prostate cancer: Recommendations of the RTOG-ASTRO Phoenix Consensus Conference. Int J Radiat Oncol Biol Phys 2006a;65:965–974.

Roach M III et al: Defining high risk prostate cancer with risk groups and nomograms: Implications for designing clinical trials. J Urol 2006b;176:S16–S20.

Roach M III: Dose escalated external beam radiotherapy versus neoadjuvant androgen deprivation therapy and conventional dose external beam radiotherapy for clinically localized prostate cancer: Do we need both? Strahlenther Onkol 2007;183(Spec No 2):26–28.

Roach M III et al: Staging for prostate cancer: Time to incorporate pretreatment prostate-specific antigen and Gleason score? Cancer 2007;109:213–220.

Roach M III: "Short- and long-term mortality with localized prostate cancer": Errors and omissions? Arch Intern Med 2008;168:1351; author reply 1353.

Roach M III et al: Short-term neoadjuvant androgen deprivation therapy and external-beam radiotherapy for locally advanced prostate cancer: Long-term results of RTOG 8610. J Clin Oncol 2008;26:585–591.

Roach MWK et al: Prostate cancer. In: Hoppe P, Phillips and Roach M (eds.). Textbook of Radiation Oncology, 3rd ed. Elsevier, Philadelphia, PA, 2010:925–986.

Roach M III et al: Radiation dose-volume effects and the penile bulb. Int J Radiat Oncol Biol Phys 2010;76:S130–S134.

Roach M et al: Radiation Therapy Oncology Group (RTOG) 9413: Randomized trial comparing whole pelvic radiotherapy (WPRT) to prostate only (PORT) and neoadjuvant hormone therapy (NHT) to adjuvant hormone therapy (AHT). 2012 ASCO Genitourinary Symposium. San Francisco, California, 2012.

Rodrigues G et al: Impact of ultrahigh baseline PSA levels on biochemical and clinical outcomes in two Radiation Therapy Oncology Group Prostate Clinical Trials. Int J Radiat Oncol Biol Phys 2011;80(2):445–452.

Rogers R et al: Radiation therapy for the management of biopsy-proven, local recurrence following radical prostatectomy. J Urol 1998;160:1748–1753.

Sanda MG et al: Quality of life and satisfaction with outcome among prostate-cancer survivors. N Engl J Med 2008;358:1250–1261.

Sathya JR et al: Randomized trial comparing iridium implant plus external-beam radiation therapy with external-beam radiation therapy alone in node-negative locally advanced cancer of the prostate. J Clin Oncol 2005;23:1192–1199.

Shinohara K, Roach M III: Technique for implantation of fiducial markers in the prostate. Urology 2008;71:196–200.

Shipley WU et al: Advanced prostate cancer: The results of a randomized comparative trial of high dose irradiation boosting with conformal protons compared with conventional dose irradiation using photons alone. Int J Radiat Oncol Biol Phys 1995;32:3–12.

Sklar G: Combined antitumor effect of suramin plus irradiation in human prostate cancer cells: The role of apoptosis. J Urol 1993;150: 1526–1532.

Speight JL, Roach M III. Advances in the treatment of localized prostate cancer: The role of anatomic and functional imaging in men managed with radiotherapy. J Clin Oncol 2007;25:987–995.

Speight JL, Roach M III: Radiotherapy in the management of clinically localized prostate cancer: Evolving standards, consensus, controversies and new directions. J Clin Oncol 2005;23:8176–8185.

Spiotto MT et al: Radiotherapy after prostatectomy: Improved biochemical relapse-free survival with whole pelvic compared with prostate bed only for high-risk patients. Int J Radiat Oncol Biol Phys 2007;69:54–61.

Stephenson AJ et al: Predicting the outcome of salvage radiation therapy for recurrent prostate cancer after radical prostatectomy. J Clin Oncol 2007;25:2035–2041.

Stone NN et al: Multicenter analysis of effect of high biologic effective dose on biochemical failure and survival outcomes in patients with Gleason score 7–10 prostate cancer treated with permanent prostate brachytherapy. Int J Radiat Oncol Biol Phys 2009;73: 341–346.

Thompson IM et al: Adjuvant radiotherapy for pathological T3N0M0 prostate cancer significantly reduces risk of metastases and improves survival: Long-term followup of a randomized clinical trial. J Urol 2009;181:956–962.

Tsuji H et al: Hypofractionated radiotherapy with carbon ion beams for prostate cancer. Int J Radiat Oncol Biol Phys 2005;63:1153–1160.

Valicenti RK et al: The efficacy of early adjuvant radiation therapy for pT3N0 prostate cancer: A matched-pair analysis. Int J Radiat Oncol Biol Phys 1999;45:53–58.

Widmark A et al: Endocrine treatment, with or without radiotherapy, in locally advanced prostate cancer (SPCG-7/SFUO-3): An open randomised phase III trial. Lancet 2009;373:301–308.

Wiegel T et al: Phase III postoperative adjuvant radiotherapy after radical prostatectomy compared with radical prostatectomy alone in pT3 prostate cancer with postoperative undetectable prostate-specific antigen: ARO 96–02/AUO AP 09/95. J Clin Oncol 2009;27:2924–2930.

Willoughby T et al: Target localization and real-time tracking using the Calypso 4D Localization System in patients with localized prostate cancer. Int J Rad Bio Phys 2006;65:528–534.

Zietman AL: The case for neoadjuvant androgen suppression before radiation therapy. Mol Urol 2000;4:203–208; discussion 215.

Zietman AL et al: Comparison of conventional-dose vs high-dose conformal radiation therapy in clinically localized adenocarcinoma of the prostate: A randomized controlled trial. JAMA 2005;294:1233–1239.

Urinary Track Tumors

Munoz JJ: Upper tract urothelial neoplasms: Incidence and survival during the last 2 decades. J Urol 2000;164(5):1523–1525.

Bladder Cancer

Amling et al: Radical cystectomy for stages Ta, Tis and T1 transitional cell carcinoma of the bladder. J Urol 1994;151:31–35.

Bloom HJ et al: Treatment of T3 bladder cancer: Controlled trial of pre-operative radiotherapy and radical cystectomy versus radical radiotherapy. Br J Urol 1982;54(2):136–151.

Brake M et al: Recurrence and progression of stage T1, grade 3 transitional cell carcinoma of the bladder following intravesical immunotherapy with Bacillus Calmette-Guerin. J Urol 2000;163(6):1697–1701.

Chakravarti A et al: Expression of the epidermal growth factor receptor and Her-2 are predictors of favorable outcome and reduced complete response rates, respectively, in patients with muscle-invading bladder cancers treated by concurrent radiation and cisplatin-based chemotherapy: A report from the Radiation Therapy Oncology Group. Int J Radiat Oncol Biol Phys 2005; 62(2):309–317.

Dalbagni G et al: Cystectomy for bladder cancer: A contemporary series. J Urol 2001;165:1111.

del Muro et al: p53 and p21 expression levels predict organ preservation and survival in invasive bladder carcinoma treated with a combined-modality approach. Cancer 2004;100:1859.

Dunst J et al: Bladder preservation in muscle-invasive bladder cancer by conservative surgery and radiochemotherapy. Semin Surg Oncol 2001;20(1):24–31.

Freeman JA et al: Radical cystectomy for high risk patients with superficial bladder cancer in the era of orthotopic urinary reconstruction. Cancer 1995;76(5):833–839.

Hagan MP et al: RTOG 97–06: Initial report of a phase I-II trial of selective bladder conservation using TURBT, twice-daily accelerated irradiation sensitized with cisplatin, and adjuvant MCV combination chemotherapy. Int J Radiat Oncol Biol Phys 2003;57(3):665–672.

Harland SJ et al: A randomized trial of radical radiotherapy for the management of pT1G3 NXM0 transitional cell carcinoma of the bladder. J Urol 2007;178(3, Pt 1):807–813.

Horowich A: Organ conservation in bladder cancer. Eur J Cancer 1995;31(Suppl):208.

Housset M et al: Combined radiation and chemotherapy for invasive transitional-cell carcinoma of the bladder: A prospective study. J Clin Oncol 1993;11(11):2157–2157.

Huncharek M et al: Planned preoperative radiation therapy in muscle invasive bladder cancer: Results of a meta-analysis. Anticancer Res 1998;18(3B):1931–1934.

Hussain MH et al: Combination cisplatin, 5-fluorouracil and radiation therapy for locally advanced unresectable or medically unfit bladder cancer cases: A Southwest Oncology Group Study. J Urol 2001;165(1):56–60.

James N et al: Results of a 2 × 2 phase III randomized trial of synchronous chemo-radiotherapy compared to radiotherapy alone and standard vs. reduced high volume RT in muscle invasive bladder cancer (BC2001 CRUK/01/004). Int J Radiat Oncol Biol Phys 2010;78(3):S2–S3.

Kaufman DS et al: Phase I-II study (RTOG 99–06) of patients with muscle-invasive bladder cancer undergoing selective bladder-conservation employing TURBT transurethral surgery, paclitaxel, cisplatin and twice-daily radiotherapy followed by selective bladder preservation or radical cystectomy and adjuvant chemotherapy. Urology 2009;73(4):833–837.

Kaufman DS et al: The initial results in muscle-invading bladder cancer of RTOG 95–06: Phase I/II trial of transurethral surgery plus radiation therapy with concurrent cisplatin and 5-fluorouracil followed by selective bladder preservation or cystectomy depending on the initial response. Oncologist 2000;5(6):471–476.

Langen KM, Jones DT: Organ motion and its management. Int J Radiat Oncol Biol Phys 2001;50(1):265–278.

Maddineni SB et al: Differential radiosensitisation by ZD1839 (Iressa), a highly selective epidermal growth factor receptor tyrosine kinase inhibitor in two related bladder cancer cell lines. Br J Urol 2005;92(1):125–130.

Malkowicz et al: The role of radical cystectomy in the management of high grade superficial bladder cancer (PA, P1, PIS, and P2). J Urol 1990;144(3):641–645.

Miller LS: Bladder cancer: Superiority of preoperative irradiation and cystectomy in clinical stages B2 and C. Cancer 1977;39(2, Suppl): 973–980.

Nichols RC et al: Radiation therapy and concomitant paclitaxel/carboplatin chemotherapy for muscle-invasive transitional cell carcinoma of the bladder: A well tolerated combination. Int J Cancer 2000;90:281.

Onufrey V, Mohiuddin M: Radiation therapy in the treatment of metastatic renal cell carcinoma. Int J Radiat Oncol Biol Phys 1985;11(11):2007–2009.

Petrovich Z: Radiotherapy for carcinoma of the bladder. Am J Clin Oncol 2001;24:1–9.

Pos FJ et al: Concomitant boost radiotherapy for muscle invasive bladder cancer. Radiother Oncol 2003;68(1):75–80.

Rodel C et al: Organ preservation in patients with invasive bladder cancer: Initial results of an intensified protocol of transurethral

surgery and radiation therapy plus concurrent cisplatin and 5-fluorouracil. Int J Radiat Oncol Biol Phys 2002;52(5):1303–1309.

Sangar VK et al: Phase I study of conformal radiotherapy with concurrent gemcitabine in locally advanced bladder cancer. Int J Radiat Oncol Biol Phys 2005;61(2):420–425.

Sauer R et al: Efficacy of radiochemotherapy with platin derivatives compared to radiotherapy alone in organ-sparing treatment of bladder cancer. Int J Radiat Oncol Biol Phys 1998;40:121.

Sell A et al: Treatment of advanced bladder cancer category T2 T3 and T4a. A randomized multicenter study of preoperative irradiation and cystectomy versus radical irradiation and early salvage cystectomy for residual tumor. DAVECA protocol 8201. Danish Vesical Cancer Group. Scand J Urol Nephrol Suppl 1991;138:193–201.

Shimizu S et al: Use of an implanted marker and real-time tracking of the marker for the positioning of prostate and bladder cancers. Int J Radiat Oncol Biol Phys 2000;48(5):1591.

Shipley WU et al: Treatment of invasive bladder cancer by cisplatin and radiation in patients unsuitable for surgery. JAMA 1987; 258:93.

Shipley WU et al: Phase III trial of neoadjuvant chemotherapy in patients with invasive bladder cancer treated with selective bladder preservation by combined radiation therapy and chemotherapy: Initial results of Radiation Therapy Oncology Group 89–03. J Clin Oncol 1998;16(11):3576–3583.

Shipley WU et al: Selective bladder preservation by trimodality therapy for patients with muscularis propria-invasive bladder cancer and who are cystectomy candidates—The Massachusetts General Hospital and Radiation Therapy Oncology Group experiences. Semin Radiat Oncol 2005;15(1):36–41.

Smith JA Jr et al: Bladder cancer clinical guidelines panel summary report on the management of non-muscle invasive bladder cancer (stages Ta, T1 and TIS). Am Urol Assoc J Urol 1999;162:(5): 1697–1701.

Soloway MS et al: Contemporary management of stage T1 transitional cell carcinoma of the bladder. J Urol 2002;167(4):1573–1583.

Stein JP et al: Radical cystectomy in the treatment of invasive bladder cancer: Long-term results in 1,054 patients. J Clin Oncol 2001; 19(3):666–675.

Tester W et al: Combined modality program with possible organ preservation for invasive bladder carcinoma: Results of RTOG protocol 85–12. Int J Radiat Oncol Biol Phys 1993;25(5):783–790.

von der Maase H et al: Long-term survival results of a randomized trial comparing gemcitabine plus cisplatin, with Methotrexate, Vinblastine, Doxorubicin, plus cisplatin in patients with bladder cancer. J Clin Oncol 2005;23(21):4602–4608.

Wolf H et al: Natural history of carcinoma in situ of the urinary bladder. Scand J Urol Nephrol Suppl 1994;157:147–151.

Zeitman AL et al: Selective bladder conservation using transurethral resection, chemotherapy, and radiation: Management and consequences of Ta, T1, and Tis recurrence within the retained bladder. Urology 2001;58(3):380–385.

Zeitman AL, Shipley WU: Organ-conserving approaches to muscle invading bladder cancer: Alternatives to the radical cystectomy in the new century. Ann Intern Med 2000;32:34.

Cancers of the Kidney, Renal Pelvis, and Ureter

Beitler JJ et al: Definitive, high-dose-per-fraction, conformal, stereotactic external radiation for renal cell carcinoma. Am J Clin Oncol 2004;27:646–648.

Cozad SC et al: Adjuvant radiotherapy in high stage transitional cell carcinoma of the renal pelvis and ureter. Int J Radiat Oncol Biol Phys 1992;24(4):743–745.

Cozad SC et al: Transitional cell carcinoma of the renal pelvis or ureter: Patterns of failure. Urology 1995;46(6):796–800.

Finney R: An evaluation of postoperative radiotherapy in hypernephroma treatment—A clinical trial. Cancer 1973;32:1332–1340.

Huguenin PU et al: Radiotherapy for metastatic carcinomas of the kidney or melanomas: An analysis using palliative end points. Int J Radiat Oncol Biol Phys 1998;41(2):401–405.

Juusela H et al: Pre-operative irradiation in the treatment of renal adenocarcinoma. Scand J Urol Nephrol 1977;11:277–281.

Kao GD et al: Locally advanced renal cell carcinoma: Low complication rate and efficacy of postnephrectomy radiation therapy planned with CT. Radiology 1994;193(3):725–730.

Kjaer M et al: Postoperative radiotherapy in stage II and III renal adenocarcinoma. A randomized trial by the Copenhagen Renal Cancer Study Group. Int J Rad Oncol Biol Phys 1987;13(5):665–672.

Makarewicz R et al: The value of postoperative radiotherapy in advanced renal cell cancer. Neoplasma 1998;45(6):380–383.

Maulard-Durdux C et al: Postoperative radiation therapy in 26 patients with invasive transitional cell carcinoma of the upper urinary tract: No impact on survival? J Urol 1996;155(1):115–117.

Nguyen QN et al: Management of spinal metastases from renal cell carcinoma using stereotactic body radiotherapy. Int J Radiat Oncol Biol Phys 2010;76(4):1185–1192.

Ning S et al: Radiobiologic studies of radioimmunotherapy and external beam radiotherapy in vitro and in vivo in human renal cell carcinoma xenografts. Cancer 1997;15(80):2519–2518.

Sheehan JP et al: Radiosurgery in patients with renal cell carcinoma metastasis to the brain: Long-term outcomes and prognostic factors influencing survival and local tumor control. J Neurosurg 2003;98(2):342–349.

Stein M et al: The value of postoperative irradiation in renal cell carcinoma. Radiother Oncol 1992;24:41–44.

Svedman et al: Stereotactic body radiotherapy of primary and metastatic renal lesions for patients with only one functioning kidney. Acta Oncol 2008;47:1578–1583.

van der Werf-Messing B et al: Renal cell carcinoma trial. Strahlentherapie 1981;76:169–175.

van der Werf-Messing B: Proceedings: Cancer of the kidney. Cancer 1973;32(5):1056–1061.

Wersall PJ et al: Extracranial stereotactic radiotherapy for primary and metastatic renal cell carcinoma. Radiother Oncol 2005;77:88–95.

Wronski M et al: External radiation of brain metastases from renal carcinoma: A retrospective study of 119 patients from the M. D. Anderson Cancer Center. Int J Radiat Oncol Biol Phys 1997;37(4):753–759.

Cancer of the Female Urethra

Bracken RB et al: Primary carcinoma of the female urethra. J Urol 1976;116(2):188–192.

Grigsby PW: Carcinoma of the urethra in women. Int J Radiat Oncol Biol Phys 1998a;41:535.

Grigsby PW: Female urethra. In: Perez CA, Brady LW, eds. Principles and Practice of Radiation Oncology. 3rd ed. Lippincott–Raven, Philadelphia, 1998b.

Meis JM et al: Adenocarcinoma of the urethra in women. A clinicopathologic study. Cancer 1987;60(5):1038–1052.

Cancer of the Penis and Male Urethra

Cohen MS et al: Coordinated chemoradiation therapy with genital preservation for the treatment of primary invasive carcinoma of the male urethra. J Urol 2008;179(2):536–541.

Eisenberger MA: Chemotherapy for carcinomas of the penis and urethra. Urol Clin North Am 1992;2:333.

Heysek RV et al: Carcinoma of the male urethra. J Urol 1985;134:753.

Husein AM et al: Chemotherapy with cisplatin and 5-fluorouracil for penile and urethral squamous cell carcinomas. Cancer 1990; 65:433.

Opjordsmoen S, Fossa SD: Quality of life in patients treated for penile cancer: A follow-up study. Br J Urol 1994;74(5):652.

Rozan R et al: Interstitial brachytherapy for penile carcinoma: A multicentric survey (259 patients). Radiother Oncol 1995;36(2): 83–93.

Sarin R et al: Treatment results and prognostic factors in 101 men treated for squamous cell carcinoma of the penis. Int J Radiat Oncol Biol Phys 1997;38(4):713.

Testicle Tumors

Aparicio J et al: Risk-adapted management for patients with clinical stage I seminoma: The Second Spanish Germ Cell Cancer Cooperative Group study. J Clin Oncol 2005;23(34):8717–8723.

Chao CK et al: Secondary malignancy among seminoma patients treated with adjuvant radiation therapy. Int J Radiat Oncol Biol Phys 1995;33:831.

Choo R et al: Survey of radiation oncologists: Practice patterns of the management of stage I seminoma of testis in Canada and a selected group in the United States. Can J Urol 2002;9(2):1479–1485.

Choo R et al: Long-term outcome of postorchiectomy surveillance for Stage I testicular seminoma. Int J Radiat Oncol Biol Phys 2005;61(3):736–740.

Chung PW et al: Stage II testicular seminoma: Patterns of recurrence and outcome of treatment. Eur Urol 2004;45(6):754–759; discussion 759–760.

Classen J et al: Radiotherapy for stages IIA/B testicular seminoma: Final report of a prospective multi-center clinical trial. J Clin Oncol 2003;21(6):1101–1106.

Dieckmann KP et al: Adjuvant treatment of clinical stage I seminoma is a single course of carboplatin sufficient? Urology 2000; 55(1):102.

Fossa SD et al: Optimal planning target volume for stage I testicular seminoma: A Medical Research Council randomized trial. J Clin Oncol 1999;17:1146.

Fossa SD et al: Post-treatment fertility in patients with testicular cancer. III. Influence of radiotherapy in seminoma patients. Br J Urol 1986;58(3):315–319.

Garcia-Serra AM et al: Long-term results of radiotherapy for early-stage testicular seminoma. Am J Clin Oncol 2005;28(2):119–124.

Germa-Lluch JR et al: Clinical pattern and therapeutic results achieved in 1490 patients with germ-cell tumours of the testis: The experience of the Spanish Germ-Cell Cancer Group (GG). Eur Urol 2002;42(6):553–562; discussion 562–563.

Gordon W Jr et al: A study of reproductive function in patients with seminomas treated with radiotherapy and orchidectomy: (SWOG-8711) Southwest Oncology Group. Int J Radiat Oncol Biol Phys 1997;38(1):83–04.

Gurkaynak M et al: Stage I testicular seminoma: Para-aortic and iliac irradiation with reduced dose after orchiectomy. Urol Int 2003; 71(4):385–388.

Hughes MA et al: Two secondary malignancies after radiotherapy for seminoma: Case report and review of the literature. Urology 2003; 62(4):748.

Huyghe E et al: Fertility after testicular cancer treatments: Results of a large multicenter study. Cancer 2004;100(4):732–737.

Jones WG et al: Randomized trial of 30 versus 20 Gy in the adjuvant treatment of stage I testicular seminoma: A report on Medical Research Council Trial TE18, European Organisation for the Research and Treatment of Cancer Trial 30942 (ISRCTN18525328). J Clin Oncol 2005;23(6):1200–1208.

Joos H et al: Endocrine profiles after radio-therapy in stage I seminoma: Impact of two different radiation treatment modalities. Radiother Oncol 1997;43(2):159–162.

Kiricuta IC et al: Omission of the pelvic irradiation in stage I testicular seminoma: A study of post–orchiectomy para-aortic radiotherapy. Int J Radiat Oncol Biol Phys 1996;35:293.

Krege S et al: Phase II study: Adjuvant single-agent carboplatin therapy for clinical stage I seminoma. Eur Urol 1997;31(4): 405–407.

Logue JP et al: Short course para-aortic radiation for stage I seminoma of the testis. Int J Radiat Oncol Biol Phys 2003;57(5): 1304–1309.

Melchior D et al: Long term results and morbidity of paraaortic compared with paraaortic and iliac adjuvant radiation in clinical stage I seminoma. Anticancer Res 2001;21(4B):2989–2993.

Miki T et al: Long-term results of adjuvant irradiation or surveillance for stage I testicular seminoma. Int J Urol 1998;5:357.

Nalesnik JG et al: Fertility in men after treatment for stage 1 and 2A seminoma. Am J Clin Oncol 2004;27(6):584–588.

Niazi TM et al: Long-term results of paraaortic irradiation for patients with stage I seminoma of the testis. Int J Radiat Oncol Biol Phys 2005;61(3):741–744.

Niewald M et al: Low-dose radiotherapy for stage I seminoma: Early results. Radiother Oncol 1995;37(2):164–166.

Oliver RT et al: A randomised comparison of single agent carboplatin with radiotherapy in the adjuvant treatment of stage I seminoma of the testis, following orchidectomy: MRC TE19/EORTC 30982. J Clin Oncol 2004 ASCO Annual Meeting Proceedings (Post-Meeting Edition) 2004;22(14S):4517.

Oliver RT et al: Radiotherapy versus single-dose carboplatin in adjuvant treatment of stage I seminoma: A randomised trial. Lancet 2005;366(9482):293–300.

Parker C et al: The prognostic significance of the tumour infiltrating lymphocyte count in stage I testicular seminoma managed by surveillance. Eur J Cancer 2002;38(15):2014–2019.

Pasqualotto FF et al: Detection of testicular cancer in men presenting with infertility. Rev Hosp Clin Fac Med Sao Paulo 2003;58(2):75–80.

Patterson H et al: Combination carboplatin and radiotherapy in the management of stage II testicular seminoma: Comparison with radiotherapy treatment alone. Radiother Oncol 2001;59(1):5–11.

Power RE et al: Pelvic recurrence in stage I seminoma: A new phenomenon that questions modern protocols for radiotherapy and follow-up. Int J Urol 2005;12(4):378–382.

Reiter WJ et al: Twelve-year experience with two courses of adjuvant single-agent carboplatin therapy for clinical stage I seminoma. J Clin Oncol 2001;19(1):101–104.

Richie JP: Prognostic factors for relapse in stage I seminoma managed by surveillance: A pooled analysis. J Urol 2003;170(3):1041.

Rowland RG et al: Para-aortic irradiation for stage I testicular seminoma: Results of a prospective study in 675 patients. A trial of the German testicular cancer study group (GTCSG). Urol Oncol 2005;23(2):141.

Sultanem K et al: Para-aortic irradiation only appears to be adequate treatment for patients with stage I seminoma of the testis. Int J Radiat Oncol Biol Phys 1998;40:455.

Travis LB et al: Risk of second malignant neoplasms among long-term survivors of testicular cancer. J Natl Cancer Inst 1997;89(19):1429.

Warde P et al: Prognostic factors for relapse in stage I testicular seminoma treated with surveillance. J Urol 1997;157:1705.

Warde P et al: Should surveillance be considered the standard of care in stage I seminoma? J Clin Oncol ASCO Annual Meet Proc 2005a; 23:4520.

Warde P, Gospodarowicz M: Adjuvant carboplatin in stage I seminoma. Lancet 2005b;366(9482):267–268.

Warde P, Gospodarowicz M: Management of stage II seminoma. J Clin Oncol 1998;16:290.

Warde P et al: Stage I testicular seminoma: Results of adjuvant irradiation and surveillance. J Clin Oncol 1995;13(9):2255–2262.

Warde P et al: Prognostic factors for relapse in stage I seminoma managed by surveillance: A pooled analysis. J Clin Oncol 2002; 20(22):4448–4452.

Zagars GK et al: Mortality after cure of testicular seminoma. J Clin Oncol 2004;22(4):640–647.

Neurophysiology & Pharmacology of the Lower Urinary Tract

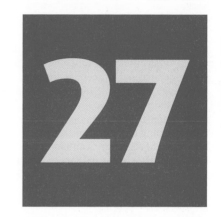

Karl-Erik Andersson, MD, PhD

INTRODUCTION

The bladder, in concert with the urethra and the pelvic floor, is responsible for storage and periodic expulsion of urine. The integrated function of these components of the lower urinary tract (LUT) is dependent on a complex control system in the brain, spinal cord and peripheral ganglia, and on local regulatory factors (de Groat, 2006). Dysfunction of the central nervous control systems or of the components of the LUT can produce insufficient voiding and retention of urine, or different types of urinary incontinence (mainly urgency and stress incontinence), or the symptom complex of the "overactive bladder" (OAB), characterized by urgency, frequency with or without urgency incontinence, often with nocturia (Abrams et al, 2002).

Pharmacologic treatment of urinary incontinence and LUT symptoms (LUTSs) including OAB is the main option, and several drugs with different modes and sites of action have been tried (Andersson 2007; Andersson and Wein, 2004; Andersson et al, 2009a, 2009b; Ouslander, 2004; Zinner et al, 2004). However, to be able to optimize treatment, knowledge about the mechanisms of micturition and of the targets for treatment is necessary. Theoretically, failure to store urine can be improved by agents that decrease detrusor activity and increase bladder capacity, and/or increase outlet resistance.

In this chapter, a brief review is given of the normal nervous control of the LUT and of some therapeutic principles used in the treatment of urinary incontinence.

NEURAL CIRCUITS CONTROLLING STORAGE AND EXPULSION OF URINE

Normal micturition occurs in response to afferent signals from the LUT (Birder et al, 2010; de Groat, 2006; Fowler et al, 2008). Both bladder filling and voiding are controlled by neural circuits in the brain, spinal cord, and peripheral ganglia. These circuits coordinate the activity of the smooth muscle in the detrusor and urethra with that of the striated muscles in the urethral sphincter and pelvic floor. Suprapontine influences are believed to act as on–off switches to shift the LUT between the two modes of operation: storage and elimination. In adults, urine storage and voiding are under voluntary control and depend upon learned behavior. In infants, however, these switching mechanisms function in a reflex manner to produce involuntary voiding. In adults, injuries or diseases of the central nervous system (CNS) can disrupt the voluntary control of micturition and cause the reemergence of reflex micturition, resulting in OAB and detrusor overactivity (DO). Because of the complexity of the CNS control of the LUT, OAB and DO can occur as a result of a variety of neurological disorders as well as changes in the peripheral innervation and smooth and skeletal muscle components (Andersson and Arner 2004; Andersson and Wein, 2004).

Filling of the bladder and voiding involve a complex pattern of afferent and efferent signaling in *parasympathetic (pelvic nerves), sympathetic (hypogastric nerves)*, and *somatic (pudendal nerves)* pathways. These pathways constitute reflexes, which either keep the bladder in a relaxed state, enabling urine storage at low intravesical pressure, or which initiate bladder emptying by relaxing the outflow region and contracting detrusor. Integration of the autonomic and somatic efferents result in that contraction of the detrusor muscle is preceded by a relaxation of the outlet region, thereby facilitating bladder emptying. On the contrary, during the storage phase, the detrusor muscle is relaxed and the outlet region is contracted to maintain continence.

PARASYMPATHETIC PATHWAYS

The sacral parasympathetic pathways m diate contraction of the detrusor smooth muscle and relaxation of the outflow region. The preganglionic *parasympathetic* neurons are located to the sacral parasympathetic nucleus (SPN) in the spinal cord at the level of S2–S4. The axons pass through the pelvic nerves and synapse with the postganglionic nerves either in the pelvic plexus, in ganglia on the surface of the bladder (vesical ganglia), or within the walls of the bladder and urethra (intramural ganglia). The ganglionic neurotransmission is predominantly mediated by acetylcholine acting on nicotinic receptors, although the transmission can be modulated by adrenergic, muscarinic, purinergic, and peptidergic presynaptic receptors. The postganglionic neurons in the pelvic nerve mediate the excitatory input to the normal human detrusor smooth muscle by releasing acetylcholine acting on muscarinic receptors (see later). However, an atropine-resistant (nonadrenergic, noncholinergic [NANC]) contractile component is regularly found in the bladders of most animal species. Such a component can also be demonstrated in functionally and morphologically altered human bladder tissue (O'Reilly et al, 2002), but contributes only to a few percent to normal detrusor contraction (Andersson and Wein, 2004). Adenosine triphosphate (ATP) is the most important mediator of the NANC contraction, although the involvement of other transmitters cannot be ruled out (Andersson and Wein, 2004). The pelvic nerve also conveys parasympathetic nerves to the outflow region and the urethra. These nerves exert an inhibitory effect on the smooth muscle, by releasing nitric oxide and other transmitters (Andersson and Wein, 2004).

SYMPATHETIC PATHWAYS

The *sympathetic* innervation of the bladder and urethra originates from the intermediolateral nuclei in the thoracolumbar region (T10–L2) of the spinal cord. The axons leave the spinal cord via the splanchnic nerves and travel either through the inferior mesenteric ganglia (IMF) and the hypogastric nerve or pass through the paravertebral chain to the lumbosacral sympathetic chain ganglia and enter the pelvic nerve. Thus, sympathetic signals are conveyed in both the hypogastric nerve and the pelvic nerve. The ganglionic sympathetic transmission is, like the parasympathetic preganglionic transmission, predominantly mediated by acetylcholine acting on nicotinic receptors. Some preganglionic terminals synapse with the postganglionic cells in the paravertebral ganglia or in the IMF, while other synapse closer to the pelvic organs and short postganglionic neurons innervate the target organs. Thus, the hypogastric and pelvic nerves contain both pre- and postganglionic fiber. The predominant effect of the sympathetic innervation is to contract the bladder base and the urethra. In addition, the sympathetic innervation inhibits the parasympathetic pathways at spinal and ganglionic levels. In the human bladder, electrical field stimulation in vitro causes nerve release of noradrenaline, which in the normal detrusor causes relaxation. However, the importance of the sympathetic innervation for relaxation of the human detrusor has never been established. In contrast, in several animal species, the adrenergic innervation has been demonstrated to mediate relaxation of the detrusor during filling (Andersson and Arner, 2004).

SOMATIC PATHWAYS

The *somatic* innervation of the urethral rhabdosphincter and of some perineal muscles (eg, compressor urethrae and urethrovaginal sphincter) is provided by the pudendal nerve. These fibers originate from sphincter motor neurons located in the ventral horn of the sacral spinal cord (levels S2–S4) in a region called Onuf's (Onufrowicz's) nucleus (Thor and de Groat, 2010; Thor and Donatucci, 2004).

AFFERENT PATHWAYS

The *afferent* nerves to the bladder and urethra originate in the dorsal root ganglia at the lumbosacral level of the spinal cord and travel via the pelvic nerve to the periphery (de Groat and Yoshimura, 2010; Kanai and Andersson, 2010). Some afferents originate in dorsal root ganglia at the thoracolumbar level and travel peripherally in the hypogastric nerve. The afferent nerves to the striated muscle of the external urethral sphincter travel in the pudendal nerve to the sacral region of the spinal cord. The most important afferents for the micturition process are myelinated $A\delta$-fibers and unmyelinated C-fibers traveling in the pelvic nerve to the sacral spinal cord, conveying information from receptors in the bladder wall. The $A\delta$-fibers respond to passive distension and active contraction, thus conveying information about bladder filling. The activation threshold for $A\delta$-fibers is 5–15 mm H_2O. This is the intravesical pressure at which humans report the first sensation of bladder filling. C-fibers have a high mechanical threshold and respond primarily to chemical irritation of the bladder urothelium/suburothelium or to cold. Following chemical irritation, the C-fiber afferents exhibit spontaneous firing when the bladder is empty and increased firing during bladder distension. These fibers are normally inactive and are therefore termed "silent fibers." Afferent information about the amount of urine in the bladder is continuously conveyed to the mesencephalic periaqueductal gray (PAG), and from there to the pontine micturition center (PMC), also called Barrington's nucleus (Holstege, 2005; Kuipers et al, 2006).

AFFERENT SIGNALING FROM THE UROTHELIUM/SUBUROTHELIUM

Recent evidence suggests that the urothelium/suburothelium may serve not only as a passive barrier but also as a specialized sensory and signaling unit, which, by producing nitric oxide, ATP, and other mediators, can control the activity in afferent nerves, and thereby the initiation of the micturition reflex (Andersson, 2002; Birder, 2010; Birder and de Groat, 2007; de Groat, 2004). The urothelium has been shown to express, for example, nicotinic, muscarinic, tachykinin, adrenergic, bradykinin, and transient receptor potential (TRP) receptors (Birder, 2010; Birder and de Groat, 2007). Low pH, high K^+, increased osmolality, and low temperatures can all influence afferent nerves, possibly via effects on the vanilloid receptor (capsaicin- [CAP] gated ion channel, TRPV1), which is expressed both in afferent nerve terminals and in the urothelial cells (Birder et al, 2001; Birder et al, 2002). A network of interstitial cells, extensively linked by Cx43-containing gap junctions, was found to be located beneath the urothelium in the human bladder (Brading and McCloskey, 2005; McCloskey, 2010; Sui et al, 2002; Sui et al, 2004). This interstitial cellular network was suggested to operate as a functional syncytium, integrating signals and responses in the bladder wall. The firing of suburothelial afferent nerves, conveying sensations and regulating the threshold for bladder activation, may be modified by both inhibitory (eg, nitric oxide) and stimulatory (eg, ATP, tachykinins, prostanoids) mediators. ATP, generated by the urothelium, has been suggested as an important mediator of urothelial signaling (Andersson, 2002). Supporting such a view, intravesical ATP induces DO in conscious rats (Pandita and Andersson, 2002). Furthermore, mice lacking the P2X$_3$ receptor were shown to have hypoactive bladders (Cockayne et al, 2000; Vlaskovska et al, 2001). Interstitial cells can also be demonstrated within the detrusor muscle (Brading and McCloskey, 2005; McCloskey, 2010). They may be involved in impulse transmission, but their role has not been clarified.

There seem to be other, thus far unidentified, factors in the urothelium that could influence bladder function (Andersson and Wein, 2004). Even if these mechanisms can be involved in, for example, the pathophysiology of OAB, their functional importance remains to be established.

NEURAL CONTROL OF BLADDER FILLING

During the storage phase, the bladder has to relax in order to maintain a low intravesical pressure. Urine storage is regulated by two separate storage reflexes, of which one is sympathetic (autonomic) and the other is somatic (Thor and Donatucci, 2004). The *sympathetic storage reflex* (pelvic-to-hypogastric reflex) is initiated as the bladder distends (myelinated Aδ-fibers) and the generated afferent activity travels in the pelvic nerves to the spinal cord. Within the spinal cord, sympathetic firing from the lumbar region (L1–L3) is initiated, which, by effects at the ganglionic level, decreases excitatory parasympathetic inputs to the bladder. Postganglionic neurons release noradrenaline, which facilitates urine storage by stimulating β$_3$-adrenoceptors (ARs) in the detrusor smooth muscle (see later). As mentioned previously, there is little evidence for a functionally important sympathetic innervation of the human detrusor, which is in contrast to what has been found in several animal species. The sympathetic innervation of the human bladder is found mainly in the outlet region, where it mediates contraction. During micturition, this sympathetic reflex pathway is markedly inhibited via supraspinal mechanisms to allow the bladder to contract and the urethra to relax. Thus, the Aδ afferents and the sympathetic efferent fibers constitute a vesico-spinal-vesical storage reflex, which maintains the bladder in a relaxed mode while the proximal urethra and bladder neck are contracted.

In response to a sudden increase in intra-abdominal pressure, such as during a cough, laugh, or sneeze, a more rapid *somatic storage reflex* (pelvic-to-pudendal reflex), also called the guarding or continence reflex, is initiated. The evoked afferent activity travels along myelinated Aδ afferent nerve fibers in the pelvic nerve to the sacral spinal cord, where efferent somatic urethral motor neurons, located in the nucleus of Onuf, are activated. Afferent information is also conveyed to the PAG and from there to the PMC (the L region). From this center, impulses are conveyed to the motor neurons in the nucleus of Onuf. Axons from these neurons travel in the pudendal nerve and release acetylcholine, which activates nicotinic cholinergic receptors on the rhabdosphincter, which contracts. This pathway is tonically active during urine storage. During sudden abdominal pressure increases, however, it becomes dynamically active to contract the rhabdosphincter. During micturition, this reflex is strongly inhibited via spinal and supraspinal mechanisms to allow the rhabdosphincter to relax and permit urine passage through the urethra. In addition to this spinal somatic storage reflex, there is also supraspinal input from the pons, which projects directly to the nucleus of Onuf and is of importance for voluntary control of the rhabdosphincter (Blok et al, 1997; Holstege, 2005; Sugaya et al, 2005).

NEURAL CONTROL OF BLADDER EMPTYING

▶ Vesico-Bulbo-Vesical Micturition Reflex

Electrophysiological experiments in cats and rats provide evidence for a voiding reflex mediated through a vesico-bulbo-vesical pathway involving neural circuits in the pons, which constitute the PMC. Other regions in the brain, important for micturition, include the hypothalamus and cerebral cortex (Fowler et al, 2008; Griffiths, 2004; Griffiths et al, 2005; Holstege, 2005). Bladder filling leads to increased activation of tension receptors within the bladder wall and thus to increased afferent activity in Aδ-fibers. These fibers project on spinal tract neurons mediating increased sympathetic firing to maintain continence as discussed earlier (storage reflex). In addition, the spinal tract neurons convey the afferent activity to more rostral areas of the spinal cord and the brain. As mentioned previously, one important receiver of the afferent information from the bladder is the PAG in the rostral brain stem (Fowler et al, 2008; Holstege, 2005; Kuipers et al, 2006). The PAG receives information both from afferent neurons in the bladder and from more rostral areas in the brain, that is, cerebral cortex and hypothalamus. This information is integrated in the PAG and the medial part of the PMC (the M region), which also control the descending pathways in the micturition reflex. Thus, PMC can be seen as a switch in the micturition reflex, inhibiting parasympathetic activity in the descending pathways when there is low activity in the afferent fibers and activating the parasympathetic pathways when the afferent activity reaches a certain threshold. The threshold is believed to be set by the inputs from more rostral regions in the brain. In cats, lesioning of regions above the inferior colliculus usually facilitates micturition by elimination of inhibitory inputs from more rostral areas of the brain. On the other hand, transections at a lower level inhibit micturition. Thus, the PMC seems to be under a tonic inhibitory control. A variation of the inhibitory input to PMC results in a variation of bladder capacity. Experiments on rats have shown that the micturition threshold is regulated by, for example, gamma-aminobutyric acid (GABA)-ergic inhibitory mechanisms in the PMC neurons.

▶ Vesico-Spinal-Vesical Micturition Reflex

Spinal lesions rostral to the lumbosacral level interrupt the vesico-bulbo-vesical pathway and abolish the supraspinal and voluntary control of micturition (Anderson and Wein, 2004). This results initially in an areflexic bladder accompanied by urinary retention. An automatic vesico-spinal-vesical micturition reflex develops slowly, although voiding is generally insufficient due to bladder-sphincter dyssynergia, that is, simultaneous contraction of bladder and urethra. It has been demonstrated in chronic spinal cats that the afferent limb of this reflex is conveyed through unmyelinated C-fibers, which usually do not respond to bladder distension, suggesting changed properties of the afferent receptors in the bladder. Accordingly, the micturition reflex in chronic spinal cats is blocked by CAP, which blocks C-fiber–mediated neurotransmission.

TARGETS FOR PHARMACOLOGIC INTERVENTION

CENTRAL NERVOUS SYSTEM TARGETS

Anatomically, several CNS regions may be involved in micturition control: supraspinal structures, such as the cortex and diencephalon, midbrain, and medulla, and also spinal structures (Fowler et al, 2008; Fowler and Griffiths, 2010; Griffiths, 2004; Griffiths et al, 2005; Holstege, 2005; Sugaya et al, 2005). Several transmitters are involved in the micturition reflex pathways described earlier and may be targets for drugs aimed for control of micturition (de Groat and Yoshimura, 2001). However, few drugs with a CNS site of action have been developed (Andersson and Pehrson, 2003).

▶ Opioid Receptors

Endogenous opioid peptides and corresponding receptors are widely distributed in many regions in the CNS of importance for micturition control (de Groat and Yoshimura, 2001). It has been well established that morphine, given by various routes of administration to animals and humans, can increase bladder capacity or block bladder contractions.

Furthermore, given intrathecally to anesthetized rats and intravenously to humans, the mu-opioid receptor antagonist, naloxone, has been shown to stimulate micturition, suggesting that a tonic activation of mu-opioid receptors has a depressant effect on the micturition reflex. However, intrathecal naloxone was not effective in stimulating micturition in conscious rats at doses blocking the effects of intrathecal morphine (Andersson and Wein, 2004).

Morphine given intrathecally was effective in patients with DO due to spinal cord lesions, but it was associated with side effects, such as nausea and pruritus. Further side effects of opioid receptor agonists comprise respiratory depression, constipation, and abuse (Andersson and Wein, 2004). Attempts have been made to reduce these side effects by increasing selectivity toward one of the different opioid receptor types. At least three different opioid receptors—μ, δ, and κ—bind stereospecifically with morphine and have been shown to interfere with voiding mechanisms. Theoretically, selective receptor actions, or modifications of effects mediated by specific opioid receptors, may have useful therapeutic effects for micturition control.

Tramadol is a well-known analgesic drug. By itself, it is a weak mu-receptor agonist, but it is metabolized to several different compounds, some of them almost as effective as morphine at the mu-receptor. However, the drug also inhibits serotonin (5-HT) and noradrenaline reuptake (Raffa and Friderichs, 1996). This profile is of particular interest, since both mu-receptor agonism and amine reuptake inhibition may be useful principles for treatment of DO/OAB.

When tramadol is given to a normal, awake rat, the most conspicuous changes in the cystometrogram are increases in threshold pressure and bladder capacity. Naloxone can more or less completely inhibit these effects (Pandita et al, 2003). However, there are differences between the effects of tramadol and morphine. Morphine has a very narrow range between the doses causing inhibition of micturition and those increasing bladder capacity and evoking urinary retention. Tramadol has effects over a much wider range of doses, which means that it could be therapeutically more useful for micturition control. It may be speculated that the difference is dependent on the simultaneous influence of the 5-HT and noradrenaline uptake inhibition (Pandita et al, 2003).

In rats, tramadol abolished experimentally induced DO caused by cerebral infarction (Pehrson et al, 2003). Tramadol also inhibited DO induced by apomorphine in rats (Pehrson and Andersson, 2003)—a model of bladder dysfunction in Parkinson's disease. Whether or not tramadol may have a clinically useful effect on DO/OAB remains to be studied in randomized controlled clinical trials (RCTs).

Safarinejad and Hosseini (2006) evaluated in a double-blind, placebo-controlled, randomized study the efficacy and safety of tramadol in patients with idiopathic DO. A total of 76 patients 18 years or older were given 100 mg tramadol sustained release every 12 hours for 12 weeks. Clinical evaluation was performed at baseline and every 2 weeks during treatment. Tramadol significantly reduced the number of incontinence periods and induced significant improvements in urodynamic parameters. The main adverse event was nausea. It was concluded that in patients with nonneurogenic DO, tramadol provided beneficial clinical and urodynamic effects. Even if tramadol may not be the best suitable drug for treatment of LUTS/OAB, the study proofs the principle of modulating micturition via the mu-receptor.

▶ Serotonin (5-HT) Mechanisms

Lumbosacral autonomic, as well as somatic, motor nuclei (Onuf's nuclei) receive a dense serotonergic input from the raphe nuclei, and multiple 5-HT receptors have been found at sites where afferent and efferent impulses from and to the LUT are processed (Ramage, 2006). The main receptors shown to be implicated in the control of micturition are the 5-HT_{1A}, 5-HT_2, and 5-HT_7 receptors (Ramage, 2006). There is some evidence in the rats for serotonergic facilitation of voiding; however, the descending pathway is essentially an inhibitory circuit, with 5-HT as a key neurotransmitter.

It has been speculated that selective serotonin reuptake inhibitors (SSRIs) may be useful for treatment of DO/OAB. On the other hand, there are reports suggesting that the SSRIs in patients without incontinence actually can cause incontinence, particularly in the elderly, and one of the drugs (sertraline) seemed to be more prone to produce urinary incontinence than the others (Movig et al, 2002). Patients exposed to serotonin uptake inhibitors had an increased risk (15 out of 1000 patients) for developing urinary incontinence. So far, there are no RCTs demonstrating the value of SSRIs in the treatment of DO/OAB.

Duloxetine is a combined noradrenaline and serotonin reuptake inhibitor, which has been shown to significantly increase sphincteric muscle activity during the filling/storage phase of micturition in the cat acetic acid model of irritated bladder function (Katofiasc et al, 2002; Thor et al, 1995). Bladder capacity was also increased in this model, both effects mediated centrally through both motor efferent and sensory afferent modulation. The effects of duloxetine was studied in a placebo-controlled study comprising women with OAB (Steers et al, 2007) and was, compared with placebo, shown to cause significant improvements or decreases in voiding and incontinence episodes, for increases in the daytime voiding intervals, and for improvements in quality-of-life (I-QoL) scores. Urodynamic studies showed no significant increases in maximum cystometric capacity or in the volume threshold for DO.

▶ GABA Mechanisms

Both in the brain and the spinal cord, GABA has been identified as a main inhibitory transmitter (de Groat and Yoshimura, 2001). GABA functions appear to be triggered by binding of GABA to its inotropic receptors, $GABA_A$ and

$GABA_C$, which are ligand-gated chloride channels, and its metabotropic receptor, $GABA_B$ (Chebib and Johnston, 1999). Since blockade of $GABA_A$ and $GABA_B$ receptors in the spinal cord and brain (Pehrson and Andersson, 2002) stimulated rat micturition, an endogenous activation of $GABA_{A+B}$ receptors may be responsible for continuous inhibition of the micturition reflex within the CNS. In the spinal cord, $GABA_A$ receptors are more numerous than $GABA_B$ receptors, except for the dorsal horn where $GABA_B$ receptors predominate.

Experiments using conscious and anesthetized rats demonstrated that exogenous GABA, muscimol ($GABA_A$ receptor agonist), and baclofen ($GABA_B$ receptor agonist) given intravenously, intrathecally, or intracerebroventricularly inhibit micturition (Pehrson et al, 2002). Baclofen given intrathecally attenuated oxyhemoglobin-induced DO, suggesting that the inhibitory actions of $GABA_B$ receptor agonists in the spinal cord may be useful for controlling micturition disorders caused by C-fiber activation in the urothelium and/or suburothelium (Pehrson et al, 2002).

Stimulation of the PMC results in an immediate relaxation of the external striated sphincter and a contraction of the detrusor muscle of the bladder demonstrated in cats a direct pathway from the PMC to the dorsal gray commissure of the sacral cord (Blok et al, 1997). It was suggested that the pathway produced relaxation of the external striated sphincter during micturition via inhibitory modulation by GABA neurons of the motoneurons in the sphincter of Onuf (Blok et al, 1997). In rats, intrathecal baclofen and muscimol ultimately produced dribbling urinary incontinence (Pehrson et al, 2002).

Thus, normal relaxation of the striated urethral sphincter is probably mediated via $GABA_A$ receptors (Pehrson et al, 2002; Pehrson and Andersson, 2002), $GABA_B$ receptors having a minor influence on motoneuron excitability (Rekling et al, 2000).

Gabapentin was originally designed as an anticonvulsant GABA mimetic capable of crossing the blood–brain barrier (Maneuf et al, 2003). The effects of gabapentin, however, do not appear to be mediated through interaction with GABA receptors, and its mechanism of action remains controversial (Maneuf et al, 2003), even if it has been suggested that it acts by binding to a subunit of the $\alpha_2\delta$ unit of voltage-dependent calcium channels. Gabapentin is also widely used not only for seizures and neuropathic pain but also for many other indications, such as anxiety and sleep disorders, because of its apparent lack of toxicity.

In a pilot study, Carbone et al (2003) reported on the effect of gabapentin on neurogenic DO. These investigators found a positive effect on symptoms and significant improvement in urodynamic parameters after treatment with gabapentin, and suggested that the effects of the drug should be explored in further controlled studies in both neurogenic and nonneurogenic DO. Kim et al (2004) studied the effects of gabapentin in patients with OAB and nocturia not responding to antimuscarinics. They found that 14 out of 31 patients improved with oral gabapentin. The drug was generally well tolerated, and the authors suggested that it can be considered in selective patients when conventional modalities have failed. It is possible that gabapentin and other $\alpha_2\delta$ ligands (eg, pregabalin and analogs) will offer new therapeutic alternatives.

Noradrenaline Mechanisms

Noradrenergic neurons in the brainstem project to the sympathetic, parasympathetic, and somatic nuclei in the lumbosacral spinal. Bladder activation through these bulbospinal noradrenergic pathways may involve excitatory α_1-ARs, which can be blocked by α_1-AR antagonists (Yoshiyama et al, 2000). In rats undergoing continuous cystometry, doxazosin, given intrathecally, decreased micturition pressure, both in normal rats and in animals with postobstruction bladder hypertrophy. The effect was much more pronounced in the animals with hypertrophied OABs. Doxazosin given intrathecally, but not intra-arterially, to spontaneously hypertensive rats exhibiting bladder overactivity, normalized bladder activity (Persson et al, 1998). It was suggested that doxazosin has a site of action at the level of the spinal cord and ganglia.

A central site of action for α_1-AR antagonists has been discussed as an explanation for the beneficial effects of these drugs in LUTS (especially storage symptoms) associated with benign prostatic hyperplasia (BPH) (Andersson and Gratzke, 2007; Andersson and Wein, 2004).

Dopamine Mechanisms

Patients with Parkinson's disease may have neurogenic DO, possibly as a consequence of nigrostriatal dopamine depletion and failure to activate inhibitory D1 receptors (Andersson, 2004). However, other dopaminergic systems may activate D2 receptors, facilitating the micturition reflex. Apomorphine, which activates both D1 and D2 receptors, induced bladder overactivity in anesthetized rats via stimulation of central dopaminergic receptors. The effects were abolished by infracollicular transection of the brain and by prior intraperitoneal administration of the centrally acting dopamine receptor blocker, spiroperidol. It has been shown that the DO induced by apomorphine in anesthetized rats resulted from synchronous stimulation of the micturition centers in the brainstem and spinal cord, and that the response was elicited by stimulation of both dopamine D1 and D2 receptors. Blockade of central dopamine receptors may be expected to influence voiding; however, the therapeutic potential of drugs having this action has not been established (Andersson and Wein, 2004).

NK-1 Receptor Mechanisms

The main endogenous tachykinins, substance P, neurokinin A (NKA), and neurokinin B (NKB), and their preferred receptors, NK1, NK2, and NK3, respectively, have been demonstrated in various CNS regions, including those involved in micturition control (Covenas et al, 2003; Lecci and Maggi, 2001; Saffroy et al, 2003).

Aprepitant, an NK-1 receptor antagonist used for treatment of chemotherapy-induced nausea and vomiting (Massaro and Lenz, 2005), significantly improved symptoms of OAB in postmenopausal women with a history of urgency incontinence or mixed incontinence, as shown in a well-designed pilot RCT (Green et al, 2006). Aprepitant was generally well tolerated and the incidence of side effects, including dry mouth, was low. Another NK-1 receptor antagonist, *serlopitant*, significantly decreased daily micturitions but did not offer advantages in efficacy compared with tolterodine (Frenkl et al, 2010). The results of these studies suggest that NK-1 receptor antagonism holds promise as a potential treatment approach for OAB, but so far, the drugs available have not been very effective.

PERIPHERAL TARGETS

There are many possible peripheral targets for pharmacologic control of bladder function (Andersson and Arner, 2004). Although many effective drugs are available targeting these systems, most of them are less useful in the clinical situation due to the lack of selectivity for LUT, which may result in intolerable side effects.

Muscarinic Receptors

Muscarinic receptors comprise five subtypes, M_1–M_5, encoded by five distinct genes, and in both animal and human bladders, the mRNAs for all muscarinic receptor subtypes have been demonstrated, with a predominance of mRNAs encoding M_2 and M_3 receptors. These receptors are also functionally coupled to G proteins, but the signal transduction systems vary (Andersson and Arner, 2004; Giglio and Tobin, 2009).

Detrusor smooth muscle contains muscarinic receptors mainly of the M_2 and M_3 subtypes. The M_3 receptors in the human bladder are the most important for detrusor contraction (Andersson and Wein, 2004). In the human detrusor, Schneider et al (2004) confirmed that the muscarinic receptor subtype mediating carbachol-induced contraction was the M_3 receptor, and they also demonstrated that the L-type calcium channel blocker, nifedipine, almost completely inhibited carbachol-induced detrusor contraction, whereas an inhibitor of store-operated Ca^{2+} channels caused little inhibition. The Rho-kinase inhibitor, Y-27632, produced a concentration-dependent attenuation of the carbachol-induced contractile responses. Schneider et al (2004) concluded that carbachol-induced contraction of human detrusor is mediated via M_3 receptors, and furthermore, largely depends on transmembrane Ca^{2+}-flux through nifedipine-sensitive calcium channels as well as activation of the Rho-kinase pathway. These conclusions were supported by Takahashi et al (2004) who found that in human detrusor muscle, carbachol induces contraction, not only by increasing $[Ca^{2+}]$ but also by increasing the Ca^{2+} sensitivity of the contractile apparatus in a Rho-kinase and protein kinase C-dependent manner.

It has been suggested that M_2 receptors may oppose sympathetically mediated smooth muscle relaxation, mediated by β-ARs (Hegde, 1997). M_2 receptor stimulation may also activate nonspecific cation channels and inhibit K_{ATP} channels through activation of protein kinase C. However, the functional role for the M_2 receptors in the normal bladder has not been clarified, but in certain disease states, M_2 receptors may contribute to contraction of the bladder. Thus, in the denervated rat bladder, M_2 receptors, or a combination of M_2 and M_3 receptors mediate contractile responses. Both types of receptor seemed to act in a facilitatory manner to mediate contraction (Braverman et al, 2002). In obstructed, hypertrophied rat bladders, there was an increase in total M_2 receptor density but a reduction in M_3 receptor density (Braverman and Ruggieri, 2003). The functional significance of this change for voiding function has not been established. Pontari et al (2004) analyzed bladder muscle specimens from patients with neurogenic bladder dysfunction to determine whether the muscarinic receptor subtype mediating contraction shifts from M_3 to the M_2 receptor subtype, as found in the denervated, hypertrophied rat bladder. They concluded that although normal detrusor contractions are mediated by the M_3 receptor subtype, in patients with neurogenic bladder dysfunction, contractions can be mediated by the M_2 receptors.

Muscarinic receptors may also be located on the presynaptic nerve terminals and participate in the regulation of transmitter release. The inhibitory prejunctional muscarinic receptors have been classified as M_2 in the rabbit and rat, and M_4 in the guinea pig, rat, and human bladder. Prejunctional facilitatory muscarinic receptors appear to be of the M_1 subtype in the rat and rabbit urinary bladder (Andersson and Arner, 2004). Prejunctional muscarinic facilitation has also been detected in human bladders. The muscarinic facilitatory mechanism seems to be upregulated in OABs from chronic spinal cord–transected rats. The facilitation in these preparations is primarily mediated by M_3 muscarinic receptors (Somogyi et al, 2003).

Muscarinic receptors have also been demonstrated in the urothelium and in the suburothelium (Bschleipfer et al, 2007; Chess-Williams, 2002; Mansfield et al, 2005), but their functional importance has not been clarified. It has been suggested that they may be involved in the release of an unknown inhibitory factor (Chess-Williams, 2002), or they may be directly involved in afferent signaling, and thus a target for antimuscarinic agents, explaining part of the efficacy of these drugs in DO/OAB (Andersson, 2004; Andersson and Yoshida, 2003; Kim et al, 2005; Yokoyama et al, 2005).

▶ Antimuscarinics

In general, antimuscarinics can be divided into tertiary and quaternary amines (Abrams and Andersson, 2007; Guay, 2003). They differ with regard to lipophilicity, molecular charge, and even molecular size, tertiary compounds generally having higher lipophilicity and molecular charge than quaternary agents. *Atropine, darifenacin, fesoterodine* (and its active metabolite 5-hydroxymethyl-tolterodine), *oxybutynin, propiverine, solifenacin,* and *tolterodine* are tertiary amines. They are generally well absorbed from the gastrointestinal tract and should theoretically be able to pass into the CNS, dependent on their individual physicochemical properties. High lipophilicity, small molecular size, and less charge will increase the possibilities to pass the blood–brain barrier, but for some of the drugs, this counteracted by active transport out of the CNS. Quaternary ammonium compounds, like propantheline and trospium, are not well absorbed, pass into the CNS to a limited extent, and have a low incidence of CNS side effects (Guay, 2003). They still produce well-known peripheral antimuscarinic side effects, such as accommodation paralysis, constipation, tachycardia, and dryness of mouth.

Many antimuscarinics are metabolized by the P450 enzyme system to active and/or inactive metabolites (Guay, 2003). The most commonly involved P450 enzymes are CYP2D6 and CYP3A4. The metabolic conversion creates a risk for drug–drug interactions, resulting in either reduced (enzyme induction) or increased (enzyme inhibition, substrate competition) plasma concentration/effect of the antimuscarinic and/or interacting drug. Antimuscarinics secreted by the renal tubules (eg, trospium) may theoretically be able to interfere with the elimination of other drugs using this mechanism.

Antimuscarinics are still the most widely used treatment for urgency and urgency incontinence (Andersson et al, 2009a, 2009b). However, currently used drugs lack selectivity for the bladder, and effects on other organ systems may result in side effects, which limit their usefulness. For example, all antimuscarinic drugs are contraindicated in untreated narrow angle glaucoma.

Theoretically, drugs with selectivity for the bladder could be obtained, if the subtype(s) mediating bladder contraction, and those producing the main side effects of antimuscarinic drugs, were different. Unfortunately, this does not seem to be the case. One way of avoiding many of the antimuscarinic side effects is to administer the drugs intravesically. However, this is practical only in a limited number of patients.

Clinical efficacy. The clinical relevance of efficacy of antimuscarinic drugs relative to placebo has been questioned (Herbison et al, 2003). However, large meta-analyses of studies performed with the currently most widely used drugs (Chapple et al, 2005, 2008; Novara et al, 2008) clearly show that antimuscarinics are of significant clinical benefit.

None of the antimuscarinic drugs in common clinical use (darifenacin, fesoterodine, oxybutynin, propiverine, solifenacin, tolterodine, or trospium) is ideal as a first-line treatment for *all* OAB/DO patients. Optimal treatment should be individualized, implying that the patient's comorbidities and concomitant medications, and the pharmacological profiles of the different drugs, should be taken into consideration (Chapple et al, 2008).

Tolerability and safety. An extensive literature supports that antimuscarinics for the treatment of OAB symptoms are generally well tolerated. The adverse effect profiles of the different drugs are determined by their organ and muscarinic receptor subtype selectivities and pharmacokinetic parameters. The most commonly reported adverse effects are dry mouth, constipation, headache, and blurred vision.

Among the more serious concerns related to antimuscarinic use is the risk of cardiac adverse effects, particularly increases in heart rate and QT prolongation and induction of polymorphic ventricular tachycardia (torsade de pointes). It should be emphasized that QT prolongation and its consequences are not related to blockade of muscarinic receptors, but rather linked to inhibition of the hERG potassium channel in the heart (Roden, 2004). Thus, QT prolongation is not a class effect of antimuscarinics. In general, the cardiovascular safety for antimuscarinic drugs seems to be good. However, the potential of the different agents to increase heart rate or to prolong the QT time has not been extensively explored. Differences between the drugs cannot be excluded, but risk assessments based on available evidence are not possible.

Another concern is that antimuscarinic drugs commonly used to treat OAB can be associated with CNS side effects including cognitive dysfunction, memory impairment, dizziness, fatigue, and headache. With the exception for oxybutynin, CNS-related side effects are not commonly found when investigated. The potential to cause CNS-related adverse effects may differ between drugs, but in the absence of comparative trials, relative risk assessments are not possible.

For detailed discussion of the clinical efficacy, tolerability, and safety of the individual antimuscarinics, see Andersson et al (2009b).

▶ Adrenergic Receptors

A. Alpha-ARs

Most investigators agree that there is a low expression of α-ARs in the human detrusor (Michel, 2006). Malloy et al (1998) found that two-thirds of the α-AR mRNA expressed was α_{1D}, and one-third was α_{1A} (there was no α_{1B}). It has been suggested that a change of subtype distribution may be produced by outflow obstruction. Nomiya and Yamaguchi (2003) confirmed the low expression of α-AR mRNA in normal human detrusor, and further demonstrated, in

contrast to data from animal experiments (Hampet et al, 2000), that there was no upregulation of any of the adrenergic receptors with obstruction. In addition, in functional experiments, they found a small response to phenylephrine at high drug concentrations with no difference between normal and obstructed bladders. Thus, in the obstructed human bladder, there seems to be no evidence for α-AR upregulation or change in subtype, although this finding was challenged by Bouchelouche et al (2005), who found an increased response to α_1-AR stimulation in obstructed bladders. Whether or not this would mean that the α_{1D}-ARs in the detrusor muscle are responsible for DO or OAB is unclear.

Sugaya et al (2002) investigated the effects of intrathecal tamsulosin (blocking $\alpha_{1A/D}$-ARs) and naftopidil (blocking preferably on α_{1D}-ARs) on isovolumetric bladder contractions in rats. Intrathecal injection of tamsulosin or naftopidil transiently abolished these contractions. The amplitude of contraction was decreased by naftopidil but not by tamsulosin. It was speculated that in addition to the antagonistic action of these agents on the α_{1A}-ARs of prostatic smooth muscle, both agents (especially naftopidil) may also act on the lumbosacral cord (α_{1D}-ARs). This observation is of particular interest considering the findings that in the human spinal cord, α_{1D}-AR mRNA predominated overall (Smith et al, 1999). Ikemoto et al (2003) gave tamsulosin and naftopidil to 96 patients with BPH for 8 weeks in a crossover study. Although naftopidil monotherapy decreased the I-PSS for storage symptoms, tamsulosin monotherapy decreased the I-PSS for voiding symptoms. However, this difference (which was suggested to depend on differences in affinity for α_1-AR subtypes between the drugs) could not be reproduced in a randomized head-to-head comparison between the drugs (Gotoh et al, 2005).

B. Beta-ARs

It has been known for a long time that isoprenaline, a non–subtype selective β-AR agonist, can relax bladder smooth muscle (Andersson, 1993). Even if the importance of β-ARs for human bladder function still remains to be established (Andersson and Arner, 2004), this does not exclude that they can be useful therapeutic targets. All three subtypes of β-ARs (β_1, β_2, and β_3) can be found in the detrusor muscle of most species, including humans (Michel and Vrydag, 2006), and also in the human urothelium (Otsuka et al, 2008). However, the expression of β_3-AR mRNA (Nomiya and Yamaguchi, 2003; Michel and Vrydag, 2006) and functional evidence indicate a predominant role for this receptor in both normal and neurogenic bladders (Michel and Vrydag, 2006). The human detrusor also contains β_2-ARs, and most probably both receptors are involved in the physiological effects (relaxation) of noradrenaline in the bladder (Andersson and Arner, 2004; Michel and Vrydag, 2006). β_3-AR agonists have a pronounced effect on spontaneous contractions of isolated detrusor muscle (Biers et al, 2006), which may be the basis for their therapeutic effects in OAB/DO.

It is generally accepted that β-AR-induced detrusor relaxation is mediated by activation of adenylyl cyclase with the subsequent formation of cAMP (Andersson, 1999). However, there is evidence suggesting that in the bladder, β-AR agonists can mediate relaxation via K+ channels (particularly BK_{Ca} channels), independent of cAMP (Frazier et al, 2008; Hristov et al, 2009; Takemoto et al, 2008; Uchida et al, 2005).

The in vivo effects of $β_3$-AR agonists on bladder function have been studied in several animal models. It has been shown that $β_3$-AR agonists increase bladder capacity with no change in micturition pressure and residual volume. For example, Hicks et al (2007) studied the effects of the selective $β_3$-AR agonist, GW427353, in the anesthetized dog and found that the drug evoked an increase in bladder capacity under conditions of acid-evoked bladder hyperactivity, without affecting voiding.

$β_3$-AR selective agonists are currently being evaluated as potential treatment for OAB/DO in humans (Colli et al, 2007). One of these, mirabegron (YM187), was given to patients with OAB in a controlled clinical trial (Chapple et al, 2008). The primary efficacy analysis showed a statistically significant reduction in mean micturition frequency, compared with placebo, and with respect to secondary variables, mirabegron was significantly superior to placebo concerning mean volume voided per micturition, mean number of incontinence episodes, nocturia episodes, urgency incontinence episodes, and urgency episodes per 24 hours. The drug was well tolerated, and the most commonly reported side effects were headache and gastrointestinal adverse effects. The results of this proof of concept study showed that the principle of $β_3$-AR agonism may be useful for treatment of patients with OAB/DO.

▶ Ion Channels

A. Calcium Channels

There is no doubt that an increase in $[Ca^{2+}]_i$ is a key process required for the activation of contraction in the detrusor myocyte. However, it is still uncertain whether this increase is due to influx from the extracellular space and/or release from intracellular stores. Furthermore, the importance of each mechanism in different species, and also with respect to the particular transmitter studied, has not been firmly established (Kajioka et al, 2002).

Theoretically, inhibition of calcium influx by means of calcium antagonists would be an attractive way of inhibiting DO/OAB. However, there have been few clinical studies of the effects of calcium antagonists in patients with DO. Naglie et al (2002) evaluated the efficacy of nimodipine for geriatric urgency incontinence in a randomized, double-blind, placebo-controlled crossover trial, and concluded that this treatment was unsuccessful.

Thus, available information does not suggest that systemic therapy with calcium antagonists is an effective way to treat DO/OAB (Andersson et al, 2009a, 2009b; Andersson and Wein, 2004).

B. Potassium Channels

Potassium channels represent another mechanism to modulate the excitability of the smooth muscle cells. There are several different types of K+-channels and at least two subtypes have been found in the human detrusor: ATP-sensitive K+-channels (K_{ATP}) and large conductance calcium-activated K+-channels (BK_{Ca}). Studies on isolated human detrusor muscle and on bladder tissue from several animal species have demonstrated that K+-channel openers reduce spontaneous contractions as well as contractions induced by carbachol and electrical stimulate. However, the lack of selectivity of presently available K+-channel blockers for the bladder versus the vasculature has thus far limited the use of these drugs. The first generation of K-channel openers, such as cromakalim and pinacidil, were found to be more potent as inhibitors of vascular smooth muscle than of detrusor muscle (Andersson and Arner, 2004). No effects of cromakalim or pinacidil on the bladder were found in studies on patients with spinal cord lesions or detrusor instability secondary to outflow obstruction. Also with more recently developed K_{ATP}-channel openers, claimed to have selectivity toward the bladder, negative results have been obtained in an RTC on patients with idiopathic DO (Chapple et al, 2006).

Thus, at present there is no clinical evidence to suggest that K+-channel openers represent a treatment alternative for DO/OAB (Andersson et al, 2009a, 2009b; Andersson and Wein, 2004).

▶ Vanilloid Receptors

The TRP channel superfamily has been demonstrated to be involved in nociception and mechanosensory transduction in various organ systems, and studies of the LUT have indicated that several TRP channels, including TRPV1, TRPV2, TRPV4, TRPM8, and TRPA1, are expressed in the bladder, and may act as sensors of stretch and/or chemical irritation. However, the roles of these individual receptors for normal LUT function and in LUTS/DO/OAB have not been established. TRPV1 is the channel best investigated. By means of CAP, a subpopulation of primary afferent neurons innervating the bladder and urethra, the "CAP-sensitive nerves," has been identified. It is believed that CAP exerts its effects by acting on specific "vanilloid" receptors (TPVR1), on these nerves. CAP exerts a biphasic effect: initial excitation is followed by a long-lasting blockade, which renders sensitive primary afferents (C-fibers) resistant to activation by natural stimuli. In sufficiently high concentrations, CAP is believed to cause "desensitization" initially by releasing and emptying the stores of neuropeptides, and then by blocking further release. Resiniferatoxin (RTX) is an analogue of CAP, approximately 1000 times more potent for desensitization than CAP, but only a few hundred times more potent for excitation. Possibly, both CAP and RTX can have effects on Aδ-fibers. It is also possible that CAP at high concentrations (mM) has additional nonspecific effects.

The rationale for intravesical instillations of vanilloids is based on the involvement of C-fibers in the pathophysiology of conditions such as bladder hypersensitivity and neurogenic DO. In the healthy human bladder, C-fibers carry the response to noxious stimuli, but they are not implicated in the normal voiding reflex. After spinal cord injury, major neuroplasticity appears within bladder afferents in several mammalian species, including man (de Groat and Yoshimura, 2006). C-fiber bladder afferents proliferate within the suburothelium and become sensitive to bladder distention. Those changes lead to the emergence of a new C-fiber–mediated voiding reflex, which is strongly involved in spinal neurogenic DO. Improvement of this condition by defunctionalization of C-fiber bladder afferents with intravesical vanilloids has been widely demonstrated in humans and animals.

Despite available information (including data from randomized controlled trials) suggests that both capsaicin and RTX may have useful effects in the treatment of neurogenic DO, and that they may have beneficial effects also in nonneurogenic DO in selected cases refractory to antimuscarinic treatment (Andersson et al, 2009a, 2009b), they are no longer widely used.

▶ Botulinum Toxin-Sensitive Mechanisms

Seven immunologically distinct antigenic subtypes of botulinum toxin (BTX) have been identified: A, B, C1, D, E, F, and G. Types A and B are in clinical use in urology, but most studies have been performed with BTX A type. BTX is believed to act mainly by inhibiting acetylcholine release from cholinergic nerve terminals interacting with the protein complex necessary for docking acetylcholine vesicles, but the mechanism of action may be more complex (Apostolidis et al, 2006; Simpson, 2004; Smith et al, 2003; Yokoyama et al, 2002). Apostolidis et al (2006) proposed that a primary peripheral effect of BTX is "the inhibition of release of acetylcholine, ATP, substance P, and reduction in the axonal expression of the CAP and purinergic receptors. This may be followed by central desensitization through a decrease in central uptake of substance P and neurotrophic factors."

The BTX-produced chemical denervation is a reversible process and axons are regenerated in about 3–6 months. Given in adequate amounts BTX inhibits release not only of acetylcholine but also of several other transmitters. The BTX molecule cannot cross the blood–brain barrier and therefore has no CNS effects.

BTX injected into the external urethral sphincter was initially used to treat spinal cord injured patients with detrusor-external sphincter dyssynergia (Smith et al, 2002; Yokoyama et al, 2002). The use of BTX has increased rapidly, and successful treatment of neurogenic DO by intravesical BTX injections has now been reported by several groups (Cruz and Silva, 2004; Leippold et al, 2003; Sahai et al, 2005). BTX may also be an alternative to surgery in children with intractable OAB (Schurch and Corcos, 2005). However, toxin injections may also be effective in refractory idiopathic DO (Anger et al, 2010; Rapp et al, 2004). Intravesical injection of BTX resulted in improvement in medication refractory OAB symptoms. However, the risk of increased postvoid residual and symptomatic urinary retention was significant. Several questions remain concerning the optimal administration of BTX-A for the patient with OAB.

Adverse effects, for example, generalized muscle weakness, have been reported (De Laet and Wyndaele, 2005), but seem to be rare.

SUMMARY AND FUTURE ASPECTS

To effectively control bladder activity, and to treat urinary incontinence, identification of suitable targets for pharmacological intervention is necessary. Such targets may be found within or outside the CNS. LUTSs, including OAB/DO, are all conditions that can have major effects on quality of life and social functioning. Antimuscarinic drugs are still first-line treatment—they have often good initial response rates, but adverse effects and decreasing efficacy cause long-term compliance problems. A new target is TRP channel superfamily, which has been demonstrated to be involved in nociception and mechanosensory transduction in various organ systems. Studies of the LUT have indicated that several TRP channels, including TRPV1, TRPV2, TRPV4, TRPM8, and TRPA1, are expressed in the bladder and may act as sensors of stretch and/or chemical irritation. However, the roles of these individual receptors for normal LUT function and in LUTS/DO/OAB have not been established. There may be several other new possibilities to treat LUTS/OAB/DO. For example, β_3-AR agonists (eg, mirabegron) are in phase 3 trials after promising initial results, and the principle of β_3-AR agonism seems clinically useful.

There is currently increasing interest in drugs modulating the micturition reflex by a central action. However, central nervous mechanisms have so far not been preferred targets for drugs aimed to treat OAB, since selective actions may be difficult to obtain. Drugs with a central mode of action such as NK-1 receptor antagonists, tramadol, and gabapentin have positive proof of concept documented in RCTs. Even if neither of these drugs can be recommended for general use in the treatment of LUTS/OAB/DO, they illustrate that agents with a target in the CNS can be therapeutically useful. Thus, even if antimuscarinic drugs remain the first-line treatment of the OAB, and their favorable efficacy/tolerability–safety ratio has been confirmed, new drugs are needed.

BIBLIOGRAPHY

Abrams P et al: Standardisation Subcommittee of the International Continence Society. The standardisation of terminology of lower urinary tract function: Report from the Standardisation Subcommittee of the International Continence Society. Neurourol Urodyn 2002;21(2):167–178. [PMID: 12114899]

Abrams P, Andersson KE: Muscarinic receptor antagonists for overactive bladder. BJU Int 2007;100(5):987–1006.

Andersson KE: Pathways for relaxation of detrusor smooth muscle. Adv Exp Med Biol 1999;462:241–252.

Andersson KE: Bladder activation: Afferent mechanisms. Urology 2002;59(5, Suppl 1):43. [PMID: 12007522]

Andersson KE: Antimuscarinics for treatment of overactive bladder. Lancet Neurol 2004;3(1):46–53. [PMID: 14693111]

Andersson KE: Mechanisms of disease: Central nervous system involvement in overactive bladder syndrome. Nat Clin Pract Urol 2004;1(2):103–108. [PMID: 16474523]

Andersson KE: LUTS treatment: Future treatment options. Neurourol Urodyn 2007;26(6, Suppl):934–947.

Andersson KE et al: Pharmacological treatment of overactive bladder: Report from the International Consultation on Incontinence. Curr Opin Urol 2009a;19(4):380–394.

Andersson K-E et al: Pharmacological treatment of urinary incontinence. In Abrams P et al (eds) Incontinence, 4th International Consultation on Incontinence. Plymbridge Distributors Ltd, Plymouth, UK, 2009b, pp 631–699.

Andersson KE, Arner A: Urinary bladder contraction and relaxation: Physiology and pathophysiology. Physiol Rev 2004;84(3):935–986. [PMID: 15269341]

Andersson KE, Gratzke C: Pharmacology of alpha1-adrenoceptor antagonists in the lower urinary tract and central nervous system. Nat Clin Pract Urol 2007;4(7):368–378. [PMID: 17615548]

Andersson KE, Pehrson R: CNS involvement in overactive bladder: Pathophysiology and opportunities for pharmacological intervention. Drugs 2003;63(23):2595–2611. [PMID: 14636079]

Andersson KE, Wein AJ: Pharmacology of the lower urinary tract: Basis for current and future treatments of urinary incontinence. Pharmacol Rev 2004;56(4):581–631. [PMID: 15602011]

Andersson KE, Yoshida M: Antimuscarinics and the overactive detrusor—Which is the main mechanism of action? Eur Urol 2003;43(1):1–5. [PMID: 12507537]

Apostolidis A et al: Proposed mechanism for the efficacy of injected botulinum toxin in the treatment of human detrusor overactivity. Eur Urol 2006;49(4):644–650. [PMID: 16426734]

Birder LA et al: Vanilloid receptor expression suggests a sensory role for urinary bladder epithelial cells. Proc Natl Acad Sci USA 2001;98(23):13396–13401. [PMID: 11606761]

Birder LA et al: Altered urinary bladder function in mice lacking the vanilloid receptor TRPV1. Nat Neurosci 2002;5(9):856–860. [PMID: 12161756]

Birder LA: Urothelial signaling. Auton Neurosci 2010;153(1–2):33–40.

Birder L et al: Neural control of the lower urinary tract: Peripheral and spinal mechanisms. Neurourol Urodyn 2010;29(1):128–139.

Birder LA, de Groat WC: Mechanisms of disease: Involvement of the urothelium in bladder dysfunction. Nat Clin Pract Urol 2007;4(1):46–54. [PMID: 17211425]

Blok BF et al: The pontine micturition center projects to sacral cord GABA immunoreactive neurons in the cat. Neurosci Lett 1997;233(2–3):109–112. [PMID: 9350844]

Bouchelouche K et al: Increased contractile response to phenylephrine in detrusor of patients with bladder outlet obstruction: Effect of the alpha1A and alpha1D-adrenergic receptor antagonist tamsulosin. J Urol 2005;173(2):657–661. [PMID: 15643283]

Brading AF, McCloskey KD: Mechanism of disease: Specialized interstitial cells of the urinary tract-an assessment of current knowledge. Nature Clin Pract Urol 2005;11:546–554. [PMID: 16474598]

Braverman AS et al: Interaction between muscarinic receptor subtype signal transduction pathways mediating bladder contraction. Am J Physiol Regul Integr Comp Physiol 2002;283(3):R663–R668. [PMID: 12185001]

Braverman AS, Ruggieri MR Sr: Hypertrophy changes the muscarinic receptor subtype mediating bladder contraction from M3 toward M2. Am J Physiol Regul Integr Comp Physiol 2003;285(3):R701–R708. [PMID: 12763741]

Bschleipfer T et al: Expression and distribution of cholinergic receptors in the human urothelium. Life Sci 2007;80(24–25):2303–2307. [PMID: 17335853]

Candenas L et al: Tachykinins and tachykinin receptors: Effects in the genitourinary tract. Life Sci 2005;76(8):835–862. [PMID: 15589963]

Carbone A et al: The effect of gabapentin on neurogenic detrusor over-activity, a pilot study. Eur Urol 2003;2(Suppl):141 (abstract 555).

Chapple C et al: The effects of antimuscarinic treatments in overactive bladder: A systematic review and meta-analysis. Eur Urol 2005;48:5–26.

Chapple CR et al: Effects of ZD0947, an ATP-sensitive potassium channel opener, in subjects with overactive bladder: A randomized, double-blind, placebo-controlled study (ZD0947IL/0004). Eur Urol 2006;49(5):879–886. [PMID: 16517051]

Chapple CR et al: The effects of antimuscarinic treatments in overactive bladder: An update of a systematic review and meta-analysis. Eur Urol 2008;54(3):543–562.

Chebib M, Johnston GAR: The 'ABC' of GABA receptors: A brief review. Clin Exp Pharmacol Physiol 1999;26(11):937–940. [PMID: 10561820]

Chen Q et al: Function of the lower urinary tract in mice lacking 1D-adrenoceptor. J Urol 2005;174(1):370–374. [PMID: 15947692]

Chess-Williams R: Muscarinic receptors of the urinary bladder: Detrusor, urothelial and prejunctional. Auton Autacoid Pharmacol 2002;22(3):133–145. [PMID: 12452898]

Cockayne DA et al: Urinary bladder hyporeflexia and reduced pain-related behaviour in P2X3-deficient mice. Nature 2000;407(6807):1011–1015. [PMID: 11069181]

Covenas R et al: Mapping of neurokinin-like immunoreactivity in the human brainstem. BMC Neurosci 2003;4(1):3.

Cruz F, Silva C: Botulinum toxin in the management of lower urinary tract dysfunction: Contemporary update. Curr Opin Urol 2004;14(6):329–334. [PMID: 15626874]

Das AK et al: Effect of doxazosin on rat urinary bladder function after partial outlet obstruction. Neurourol Urodyn 2002;21(2):160–166. [PMID: 11857670]

de Groat WC: Influence of central serotonergic mechanisms on lower urinary tract function. Urology 2002;59(5, Suppl 1):30–36. [PMID: 12007520] de Groat WC: The urothelium in overactive bladder: Passive bystander or active participant? Urology 2004;64(6, Suppl 1):7–11. [PMID: 16465182]

de Groat WC: Integrative control of the lower urinary tract: Preclinical perspective. Br J Pharmacol 2006;147(Suppl 2):S25–S40. [PMID: 16465182]

de Groat WC, Yoshimura N: Pharmacology of the lower urinary tract. Annu Rev Pharmacol Toxicol 2001;41:691–721. [PMID: 11264473]

de Groat WC, Yoshimura N: Mechanisms underlying the recovery of lower urinary tract function following spinal cord injury. Prog Brain Res 2006;152:59–84. Review. [PMID: 16198694]

de Groat WC, Yoshimura N: Afferent nerve regulation of bladder function in health and disease. Handb Exp Pharmacol 2009;(194):91–138.

De Laet K, Wyndaele JJ: Adverse events after botulinum A toxin injection for neurogenic voiding disorders. Spinal Cord 2005;43(7):397–399.[PMID: 15741978]

Fowler CJ et al: The neural control of micturition. Nat Rev Neurosci 2008;9(6):453–466.

Frenkl TL et al: A multicenter, double-blind, randomized, placebo controlled trial of a neurokinin-1 receptor antagonist for overactive bladder. J Urol 2010;184(2):616–622.

Gotoh M et al: Comparison of tamsulosin and naftopidil for efficacy and safety in the treatment of benign prostatic hyperplasia: A randomized controlled trial. BJU Int 2005;96(4):581–586. [PMID: 16104914]

Green SA et al: Efficacy and safety of a neurokinin-1 receptor antagonist in postmenopausal women with overactive bladder with urge urinary incontinence. J Urol 2006;176(6, Pt 1):2535–2540.

Griffiths DJ: Cerebral control of bladder function. Curr Urol Rep 2004;5(5):348–352. [PMID: 15461910]

Griffiths D et al: Brain control of normal and overactive bladder. J Urol 2005;174(5):1862–1867. [PMID: 16217325]

Guay DR: Clinical pharmacokinetics of drugs used to treat urge incontinence. Clin Pharmacokinet 2003;42(14):1243–1285.

Hampel C et al: Modulation of bladder alpha1-adrenergic receptor subtype expression by bladder outlet obstruction. J Urol 2002;167:1513–1521. [PMID: 11832780]

Hegde SS et al: Functional role of M-2 and M-3 muscarinic receptors in the urinary bladder of rats in vitro and in vivo. Br J Pharmacol 1997;120:1409–1418. [PMID: 9113359]

Herbison P et al: Effectiveness of anticholinergic drugs compared with placebo in the treatment of overactive bladder: Systematic review. BMJ 2003;326(7394):841–844.

Holstege G: Micturition and the soul. J Comp Neurol 2005;493(1):15–20. [PMID: 16254993]

Ikemoto I et al: Usefulness of tamsulosin hydrochloride and naftopidil in patients with urinary disturbances caused by benign prostatic hyperplasia: A comparative, randomized, two-drug crossover study. Int J Urol 2003;10(11):587–594. [PMID: 08314633]

Kajioka S et al: Ca(2+) channel properties in smooth muscle cells of the urinary bladder from pig and human. Eur J Pharmacol 2002;443(1–3):19–29. [PMID: 12044787]

Kanai A, Andersson KE: Bladder afferent signaling: Recent findings. J Urol 2010;183(4):1288–1295.

Katofiasc MA et al: Comparison of the effects of serotonin selective norepinephrine selective, and dual serotonin and norepinephrine reuptake inhibitors on lower urinary tract function in cats. Life Sci 2002;71(11):1227–1236.

Kim YT et al: Gabapentin for overactive bladder and nocturia after anticholinergic failure. Int Braz J Urol 2004;30(4):275–278. [PMID: 15679954]

Kim Y et al: Antimuscarinic agents exhibit local inhibitory effects on muscarinic receptors in bladder-afferent pathways. Urology 2005;65(2):238–242. [PMID: 15708029]

Kuipers R et al: Afferent projections to the pontine micturition center in the cat. J Comp Neurol 2006;494(1):36–53. [PMID: 16304684]

Lazzeri M et al: Intravesical vanilloids and neurogenic incontinence: Ten years experience. Urol Int 2004;72(2):145–149. [PMID: 14963356]

Lecci A, Maggi CA: Tachykinins as modulators of the micturition reflex in the central and peripheral nervous system. Regul Pept 2001;101(1–3):1–18.

Leippold T et al: Botulinum toxin as a new therapy option for voiding disorders: current state of the art. Eur Urol 2003;44(2):165–174. [PMID: 12875934]

Maggi CA et al: Cystometric evidence that capsaicin-sensitive nerves modulate the afferent branch of micturition reflex in humans. J Urol 1989;142(1):150–154. [PMID: 2733095]

Malloy BJ et al: Alpha1-adrenergic receptor subtypes in human detrusor. J Urol 1998;160:937–943. [PMID: 9720591]

Maneuf YP et al: Cellular and molecular action of the putative GABA-mimetic, gabapentin. Cell Mol Life Sci 2003;60(4):742–750. [PMID: 12785720]

Mansfield KJ et al: Muscarinic receptor subtypes in human bladder detrusor and mucosa, studied by radioligand binding and quantitative competitive RT-PCR: Changes in ageing. Br J Pharmacol 2005;144(8):1089–1099. [PMID: 15723094]

Massaro AM, Lenz KL: Aprepitant: A novel antiemetic for chemotherapy-induced nausea and vomiting. Ann Pharmacother 2005;39(1):77–85.

McCloskey KD: Interstitial cells in the urinary bladder–localization and function. Neurourol Urodyn 2010;29(1):82–87.

Michel MC, Vrydag W: Alpha(1)-, alpha(2)- and beta-adrenoceptors in the urinary bladder, urethra and prostate. Br J Pharmacol 2006;147(Suppl 2):S88–S119. [PMID: 16465187]

Movig KL et al: Selective serotonin reuptake inhibitor-induced urinary incontinence. Pharmacoepidemiol Drug Saf 2002;11(4):271–279. [PMID: 12138594]

Naglie G et al: A randomized, double-blind, placebo controlled crossover trial of nimodipine in older persons with detrusor instability and urge incontinence. J Urol 2002;167(2 Pt 1):586–590. [PMID: 11792]

Nomiya M, Yamaguchi O: A quantitative analysis of mRNA expression of alpha 1 and beta-adrenoceptor subtypes and their functional roles in human normal and obstructed bladders. J Urol 2003;170(2, Pt 1):649–653. [PMID: 12 853849]

Novara G et al: Systematic review and meta-analysis of randomized controlled trials with antimuscarinic drugs for overactive bladder. Eur Urol 2008;54(4):740–763.

O'Reilly BA et al: P2X receptors and their role in female idiopathic detrusor instability. J Urol 2002;167(1):157–164. [PMID: 11743296]

Ouslander JG: Management of overactive bladder. N Engl J Med 2004;350(8):786–799. [PMID: 14973214]

Pandita RK et al: Actions of tramadol on micturition in awake, freely moving rats. Br J Pharmacol 2003;139(4):741–748. [PMID: 12812997]

Pandita RK, Andersson KE: Intravesical adenosine triphosphate stimulates the micturition reflex in awake, freely moving rats. J Urol 2002;168(3):1230–1234. [PMID: 12187273]

Pehrson R, Andersson KE: Effects of tiagabine, a gamma-aminobutyric acid re-uptake inhibitor, on normal rat bladder function. J Urol 2002;167(5):2241–2246. [PMID: 11956486]

Pehrson R et al: Effects of gamma-aminobutyrate B receptor modulation on normal micturition and oxyhemoglobin induced detrusor overactivity in female rats. J Urol 2002;168(6):2700–2705. [PMID: 12442013]

Pehrson R et al: Effects of tramadol on rat detrusor overactivity induced by experimental cerebral infarction. Eur Urol 2003;44(4):495–499. [PMID: 14499688]

Pehrson R, Andersson KE: Tramadol inhibits rat detrusor overactivity caused by dopamine receptor stimulation. J Urol 2003;170(1):272–275. [PMID: 12796703]

Persson K et al: Spinal and peripheral mechanisms contributing to hyperactive voiding in spontaneously hypertensive rats. Am J Physiol 1998;275:R1366–R1373. [PMID: 9756570]

Pontari MA et al: The M2 muscarinic receptor mediates in vitro bladder contractions from patients with neurogenic bladder dysfunction. Am J Physiol Regul Integr Comp Physiol 2004;286(5):R874–R880. [PMID: 14751843]

Raffa RB, Friderichs E: The basic science aspect of tramadol hydrochloride. Pain Rev 1996;3:249–271.

Ramage AG: The role of central 5-hydroxytryptamine (5-HT, serotonin) receptors in the control of micturition. Br J Pharmacol 2006;147(Suppl 2):S120–S131. [PMID: 16465176]

Rapp D et al: Use of botulinum-A toxin for the treatment of refractory overactive bladder symptoms: An initial experience. Urology 2004;63(6):1071–1075. [PMID: 15183952]

Reitz A, Schurch B: Intravesical therapy options for neurogenic detrusor overactivity. Spinal Cord 2004;42(5):267–272. [PMID: 14758352]

Rekling JC et al: Synaptic control of motoneuronal excitability. Physiol Rev 2000;80(2):767–852. [PMID: 10747207]

Roden DM: Drug-induced prolongation of the QT interval. N Engl J Med 2004;350(10):1013–1022.

Safarinejad MR, Hosseini SY: Safety and efficacy of tramadol in the treatment of idiopathic detrusor overactivity: A double-blind, placebo-controlled, randomized study. Br J Clin Pharmacol 2006;61(4):456–463.

Saffroy M et al: Autoradiographic distribution of tachykinin NK2 binding sites in the rat brain: Comparison with NK1 and NK3 binding sites. Neuroscience 2003;116(3):761–773.

Sahai A et al: Botulinum toxin for the treatment of lower urinary tract symptoms: A review. Neurourol Urodyn 2005;24(1):2–12. [PMID: 15578628]

Schneider T et al: Signal transduction underlying carbachol-induced contraction of human urinary bladder. J Pharmacol Exp Ther 2004;309(3):1148–1153. [PMID: 15879883]

Schurch B, Corcos J: Botulinum toxin injections for paediatric incontinence. Curr Opin Urol 2005;15(4):264–267. [PMID: 15928517]

Shefchyk SJ: Spinal cord neural organization controlling the urinary bladder and striated sphincter. Prog Brain Res 2002;137:71–82. [PMID: 16198695]

Silva C et al: Urodynamic effect of intravesical resiniferatoxin in patients with neurogenic detrusor overactivity of spinal origin: Results of a double-blind randomized placebo-controlled trial. Eur Urol 2005;48(4):650–655. [PMID: 15961217]

Simpson LL: Identification of the major steps in botulinum toxin action. Annu Rev Pharmacol Toxicol 2004;44:167–193. [PMID: 14744243]

Smith MS et al: Alpha1-adrenergic receptors in human spinal cord: Specific localized expression of mRNA encoding alpha1-adrenergic receptor subtypes at four distinct levels. Brain Res Mol Brain Res 1999;63(2):254–261. [PMID: 9878769]

Smith CP et al: Effect of botulinum toxin A on the autonomic nervous system of the rat lower urinary tract. J Urol 2003;169(5):1896–1900. [PMID: 12686869]

Somogyi GT et al: Change in muscarinic modulation of transmitter release in the rat urinary bladder after spinal cord injury. Neurochem Int 2003;43(1):73–77. [PMID12605884]

Steers WD et al: Duloxetine compared with placebo for treating women with symptoms of overactive bladder. BJU Int 2007;100(2):337.

Sugaya K et al: Evidence for involvement of the subcoeruleus nucleus and nucleus raphe magnus in urine storage and penile erection in decerebrate rats. J Urol 1998;159(6):2172–2176. [PMID: 9598564]

Sugaya K et al: Effects of intrathecal injection of tamsulosin and naftopidil, alpha-1A and -1D adrenergic receptor antagonists, on bladder activity in rats. Neurosci Lett 2002;328(1):74–76. [PMID: 12123863]

Sugaya K et al: Central nervous control of micturition and urine storage. J Smooth Muscle Res 2005;41(3):117–132. [PMID: 16006745]

Sui GP et al: Gap junctions and connexin expression in human suburothelial interstitial cells. BJU Int 2002;90(1):118–129. [PMID: 12081783]

Sui GP et al: Electrical characteristics of suburothelial cells isolated from the human bladder. J Urol 2004;171(2, Pt 1):938–943. [PMID: 14713858]

Tai C et al: Suppression of bladder reflex activity in chronic spinal cord injured cats by activation of serotonin 5-HT(1A) receptors. Exp Neurol 2006;199(2):427–437. [PMID: 16488413]

Takahashi R et al: Ca2+ sensitization in contraction of human bladder smooth muscle. J Urol 2004;172(2):748–752. [PMID: 15247775]

Thor KB, Donatucci C: Central nervous system control of the lower urinary tract: New pharmacological approaches to stress urinary incontinence in women. J Urol 2004;172(1):27–33. [PMID: 15201731]

Thor KB, de Groat WC: Neural control of the female urethral and anal rhabdosphincter and pelvic floor muscles. Am J Physiol Regul Integr Comp Physiol 2010;299(2):R416–R438.

Thor K, Katofiasc MA: Effects of duloxetine, a combined serotonin and norepinephrine reuptake inhibitor, on central neural control of lower urinary tract function in the chloralose-anesthetized female cat. J Pharmacol Exp Ther 1995;274(2):1014–1024.

Vlaskovska M et al: P2X3 knock-out mice reveal a major sensory role for urothelially released ATP. J Neurosci 2001;21(15):5670–5677. [PMID: 11466438]

Yamaguchi O: Beta3-adrenoceptors in human detrusor muscle. Urology 2002;59(Suppl 1):25–29. [PMID: 12007519]

Yokoyama T et al: Botulinum toxin treatment of urethral and bladder dysfunction. Acta Med Okayama 2002;56(6):271–277. [PMID: 12685855]

Yokoyama O et al: Effects of tolterodine on an overactive bladder depend on suppression of C-fiber bladder afferent activity in rats. J Urol 2005;174(5):2032–2036. [PMID: 16217388]

Yoshiyama M et al: Role of spinal alpha(1)-adrenergic mechanisms in the control of lower urinary tract in the rat. Brain Res 2000;882(1–2):36–44. [PMID: 11056182]

Zinner NR et al: Pharmacotherapy for stress urinary incontinence: Present and future options. Drugs 2004;64(14):1503–1516. [PMID: 15233589]

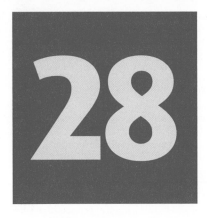

Neuropathic Bladder Disorders

Tom F. Lue, MD, FACS, ScD (Hon), & Emil A. Tanagho, MD

The urinary bladder is a visceral smooth-muscle organ but is under voluntary control from the cerebral cortex. Normal bladder function requires coordinated interaction of afferent and efferent components of both the somatic and autonomic nervous systems. Because many levels of the nervous system are involved in the regulation of voiding function, neurologic diseases often cause changes in bladder function. Examples are multiple sclerosis, spinal cord injury, cerebrovascular disease, Parkinson disease, diabetes mellitus, meningomyelocele, and amyotrophic lateral sclerosis. Injury to the sacral roots or pelvic plexus from spinal surgery, herniation of an intervertebral disk, or pelvic surgery (hysterectomy, abdominoperineal resection) can also cause neuropathic bladder.

Significant bladder dysfunction may occur as a result of poor voiding habits in childhood or of degenerative changes in bladder muscle and nerve endings caused by aging, inflammation, or anxiety disorders. All the above conditions can disrupt efficient reflex coordination between sphincter and bladder, and with time, this leads to symptomatic dysfunction.

NORMAL VESICAL FUNCTION

ANATOMY AND PHYSIOLOGY

▶ The Bladder Unit

The bladder wall is composed of a syncytium of smooth-muscle fibers that run in various directions; however, near the internal meatus, three layers are distinguishable: a middle circular layer and inner and outer longitudinal layers. In females, the outer layer extends down the entire length of the urethra, while in males, it ends at the apex of the prostate. The muscle fibers become circular and spirally oriented around the bladder–urethra junction. The middle circular layer ends at the internal meatus of the bladder and is most developed anteriorly. The inner layer remains longitudinally oriented and reaches the distal end of the urethra in females

and the apex of the prostate in males. The convergence of these muscle fibers forms a thickened bladder neck, which functions as the internal smooth-muscle sphincter.

The normal bladder is able to distend gradually to a capacity of 400–500 mL without appreciable increase in intravesical pressure. When the sensation of fullness is transmitted to the sacral cord, the motor arc of the reflex causes a powerful and sustained detrusor contraction and urination if voluntary control is lacking (as in infants). As myelinization of the central nervous system progresses, the young child is able to suppress the sacral reflex so that he or she can urinate when it is appropriate.

The functional features of the bladder include (1) a normal capacity of 400–500 mL, (2) a sensation of fullness, (3) the ability to accommodate various volumes without a change in intraluminal pressure, (4) the ability to initiate and sustain a contraction until the bladder is empty, and (5) voluntary initiation or inhibition of voiding despite the involuntary nature of the organ.

▶ The Sphincteric Unit

In both males and females, there are two sphincteric elements: (1) an internal involuntary smooth-muscle sphincter at the bladder neck and (2) an external voluntary striated muscle sphincter from the prostate to the membranous urethra in males and at the midurethra in females.

The bladder neck sphincter is a condensation of smooth muscle of the detrusor. This area is rich in sympathetic innervation. Active contraction of the bladder neck region occurs simultaneously with seminal emission, just before ejaculation. In the filling phase, the bladder neck remains closed to provide continence. It opens during both spontaneous contraction and contraction induced by stimulation of the pelvic nerve.

The external sphincter is composed of slow-twitch, small striated muscle fibers in addition to longitudinal and circularly oriented smooth-muscle fibers. This sphincter maintains a constant tonus and is the primary continence mechanism. While the resting tone is maintained by the slow-twitch striated muscle and the smooth muscles, it can be voluntarily increased by contraction of the striated muscles of the pelvic floor (eg, levator ani), which contain both fast- and slow-twitch fibers.

Relaxation of the sphincter is mostly a voluntary act without which voiding is normally inhibited. Nitric oxide released by parasympathetic nerve endings has been proposed to be the neurotransmitter for sphincter relaxation. Failure to initiate sphincteric relaxation is a mechanism of urinary retention often seen in children with dyssynergic voiding. In infancy, the detrusor behaves in an uninhibited fashion. As the central nervous system matures, children learn to suppress or enhance the micturition reflex through voluntary contraction or relaxation of the pelvic musculature.

▶ The Ureterovesical Junction

The function of the ureterovesical junction is to prevent backflow of urine from the bladder to the upper urinary tract. Longitudinal muscle from the ureter contributes to the makeup of the trigone. Stretching of the trigone has an occlusive effect on the ureteral openings. During normal detrusor contraction, the increased pull on the ureters prevents reflux of urine. Conversely, the combination of detrusor hypertrophy and trigonal stretch owing to residual urine can significantly obstruct the flow of urine from the ureters into the bladder.

INNERVATION AND NEUROPHYSIOLOGY

▶ Nerve Supply

The lower urinary tract receives afferent and efferent innervation from both the autonomic and somatic nervous systems. The parasympathetic innervation originates in the second to fourth sacral segments. The cholinergic postganglionic fibers supply both the bladder and smooth-muscle sphincter. The sympathetic nerves originate at T10–L2. The noradrenergic postganglionic fibers innervate the smooth muscles of the bladder base, internal sphincter, and proximal urethra. Somatic motor innervation originates in S2–4 and travels to the striated urethral sphincter via the pudendal nerve. Some motor neurons to the tonic small muscle fibers of the striated sphincter may also project through the pelvic nerve (Crowe et al, 1989).

There are both somatic and visceral afferents from the bladder and urethra. The somatic afferent is carried by the pudendal nerve, while the visceral afferent projects through the sympathetic and parasympathetic nerves to their respective spinal areas.

The normal afferent pathway is mediated largely by Aδ-fibers, which send information about the state of bladder fullness to the pontine micturition center (PMC). C-fibers respond to chemical irritation or cold. After spinal injury, C-fibers become more prominent contributing to

neurogenic detrusor overactivity (NDO). The common sources of afferent information for either pathway are likely to be afferents from the urothelium, lamina propria, and afferents that originate in the bladder wall (Birder et al, 2010; Clemens, 2010; de Groat and Yoshimura, 2010). On the other hand, the thoracolumbar visceral afferents may transmit discomfort and pain.

▶ The Micturition Reflex

Intact reflex pathways via the spinal cord and the pons are required for normal micturition. Afferents from the bladder are essential for the activation of the sacral center, which then causes detrusor contraction, bladder neck opening, and sphincteric relaxation. The periaqueductal gray (PAG) in the rostral brain stem is the integration center for signals from bladder, cerebral cortex, and hypothalamus. The PMC, through its connection with the sacral center, may send either excitatory or inhibitory impulses to regulate the micturition reflex (Tai et al, 2009). Electrical or chemical stimulation of the neurons in the medial PMC generates contraction of the detrusor and relaxation of the external sphincter. Disruption of pontine control, as in upper spinal cord injury, leads to contraction of the detrusor without sphincteric relaxation (detrusor–sphincter dyssynergia).

In pathologic conditions affecting the urethra (eg, urethritis or prostatitis) or the bladder (eg, cystitis or obstructive hypertrophy), overactive detrusor activity may occur because of facilitation of the micturition reflex (Figure 28–1).

▶ The Storage Function

The external sphincter plays an important role in urine storage. The afferent signals from pelvic and pudendal nerves activate both the sacral and lateral PMC; this enhances sphincteric contraction while suppressing the parasympathetic impulse to the detrusor. Voluntary tightening of the sphincter can also inhibit the urge to urinate. In addition, activation of sympathetic nerves increases urethral resistance and facilitates bladder storage (Figure 28–2).

▶ Cerebral (Suprapontine) Control

Although micturition and urine storage are primary functions of the autonomic nervous system, these are under voluntary control from suprapontine cerebral centers, so that other groups of muscles (arm, leg, hand, bulbocavernosus) can be integrated to assist in urination at the appropriate time and place. Cerebral lesions (eg, from tumor, Parkinson's disease, vascular accident) are known to affect the perception of bladder sensation and result in voiding dysfunction.

▶ Neurotransmitters and Receptors

In parasympathetic innervation, acetylcholine and nicotinic receptors mediate pre- to postganglionic transmission, while acetylcholine and M_3 muscarinic receptors mediate the

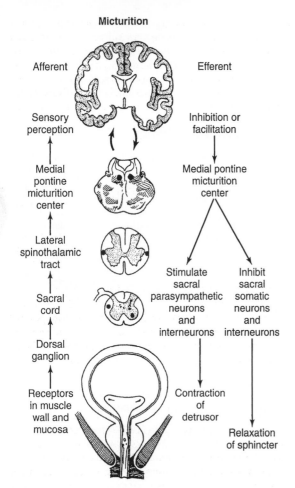

Micturition

Afferent   Efferent

Sensory perception   Inhibition or facilitation

Medial pontine micturition center   Medial pontine micturition center

Lateral spinothalamic tract   Stimulate sacral parasympathetic neurons and interneurons   Inhibit sacral somatic neurons and interneurons

Sacral cord

Dorsal ganglion

Receptors in muscle wall and mucosa   Contraction of detrusor   Relaxation of sphincter

▲ **Figure 28–1.** Afferent and efferent pathways and central nervous system centers involved in micturition.

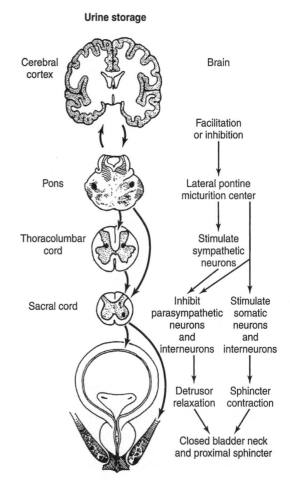

Urine storage

Cerebral cortex   Brain

Facilitation or inhibition

Pons   Lateral pontine micturition center

Thoracolumbar cord   Stimulate sympathetic neurons

Sacral cord   Inhibit parasympathetic neurons and interneurons   Stimulate somatic neurons and interneurons

Detrusor relaxation   Sphincter contraction

Closed bladder neck and proximal sphincter

▲ **Figure 28–2.** Pathways and central nervous system centers involved in urine storage.

postganglionic neuron–smooth muscle transmission. In some species, adenosine triphosphate (ATP) is released with acetylcholine and acts on purinoceptors (P_2) in the smooth-muscle cell. In sympathetic nerves, noradrenaline can act on the beta-3 adrenoreceptors to relax the detrusor or the alpha-1-receptors to contract the bladder neck and the external sphincter (Birder et al, 2010).

In addition, many neuropeptides, which usually colocalize with the classic transmitters, are also found in the genitourinary tract. Neuropeptide Y, enkephalin, and vasoactive intestinal polypeptide (VIP) are found in cholinergic postganglionic neurons, while calcitonin gene-related peptide (CGRP), VIP, substance P, cholecystokinin, and enkephalins are distributed in sacral visceral afferent fibers. These peptides are thought to be involved in modulation of efferent and afferent neurotransmissions.

Please refer to Chapter 27 ("Neurophysiology and Pharmacology of the Lower Urinary Tract") for more detail discussion of the neurophysiology.

URODYNAMIC STUDIES (SEE ALSO CHAPTER 27)

▶ **Micturition**

Urodynamic studies are techniques used to obtain graphic recordings of activity in the urinary bladder, urethral sphincter, and pelvic musculature. The current method involves use of water to transfer pressure to a transducer housed near a polygraph or use of a transducer-tipped catheter to transfer pressure recordings directly to a polygraph. Pressure recordings can be complemented by electromyography of the perineal musculature, ultrasound, or radiography (Figure 28–3).

screening or monitoring procedure. The normal peak flow rate for males is 20–25 mL/s and for females 20–30 mL/s. Lower flow rates suggest outlet obstruction or a weak detrusor; higher flow rates suggest bladder spasticity or excessive use of abdominal muscles to assist voiding. Intermittent flow patterns generally reflect spasticity of the sphincter or straining to overcome resistance in the urethra or the prostate.

▷ Cystometry

Cystometry is the urodynamic evaluation of the reservoir function of the bladder. Cystometry is most informative when combined with studies of the external urethral sphincter and pelvic floor.

Normal bladder capacity is 400–500 mL. Bladder pressure during filling should remain low up to the point of voiding. The first desire to void is generally felt when the volume reaches 150–250 mL, but detrusor-filling pressure should remain unchanged until there is a definite sense of fullness at 350–450 mL, the true capacity of the bladder. Detrusor contractions before this point are considered abnormal. Normal voiding pressures in the bladder should not rise above 30 cm of water pressure. With normal voiding, there should be no residual urine, and voiding should be accomplished without straining.

▷ Urethral Pressure Recordings

Normal voiding requires a synergic action of the bladder (contraction) and urethra (relaxation). High pressures in the bladder during voiding reflect abnormal resistance in the urethral outlet. Increased outlet resistance can result from prostatic enlargement, urethral stricture, bladder neck contracture, or spasm of the external urethral sphincter. Low resistance in the urethral outlet generally reflects compromised function of the sphincter mechanism. Recording of urethral pressures with the bladder at rest as well as during contraction helps determine the presence of functional or anatomic disorders.

▷ Electromyography

With electromyography, the activity of the striated urethral muscles can be monitored without obstructing the urethral lumen. In the normal urethra, activity increases slightly as the bladder fills and falls precipitously just before voiding begins. Denervation results in an overall decrease in activity as well as production of denervation potentials. An overall increase in activity reflects a state of hyperreflexia. The technique provides a sensitive assessment of urethral and pelvic muscle behavior. The disadvantages of the technique are dependence on accurate needle position and a tendency to record artifacts.

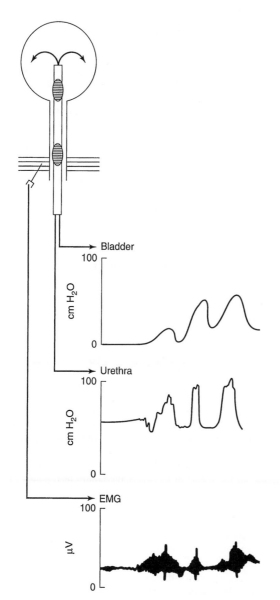

▲ **Figure 28–3.** Simultaneous recording of bladder and urethral pressure as well as electromyographic recording of the external sphincter. Note the dyssynergic response. With bladder contraction, there is increased activity in the external sphincter and pelvic floor, as recorded by the intraurethral pressure and electromyogram tracings.

▷ Uroflowmetry

Uroflowmetry is the study of the flow of urine from the urethra. Uroflowmetry is best performed separately from all other tests and, whenever possible, as a standard office

ABNORMAL VESICAL FUNCTION

CLASSIFICATION OF NEUROPATHIC BLADDER

The traditional classification was according to neurologic deficit. Thus, the terms motor, spastic, upper motor neuron, reflexic, and uninhibited were used to describe dysfunction found with injury above the spinal cord micturition center. The classification system recommended by the standardization committee for the International Continence Society includes description of bladder activity (normal, overactive, areflexic, impaired), bladder compliance (normal, decreased, increased), smooth sphincter activity (synergic, dyssynergic), striated sphincter activity (synergic, dyssynergic, fixed tone), and sensation (normal, absent, impaired) (Abrams et al, 2002).

Descriptions of neuromuscular dysfunction of the lower urinary tract should be individualized because no two neural injuries (no matter how similar) result in the same type of dysfunction.

1. Neuropathic bladder due to lesions above the sacral micturition center—Most lesions above the level of the cord where the micturition center is located will cause bladder overactivity. Sacral reflex arcs remain intact, but loss of inhibition from higher centers results in overactive bladder and sphincter behavior on the segmental level. The degree of spasticity varies between the bladder and sphincter, from lesion to lesion, and from patient to patient with similar lesions.

Common lesions found above the brain stem that affect voiding include dementia, vascular accidents, multiple sclerosis, tumors, and inflammatory disorders such as encephalitis or meningitis. These lesions can produce a wide range of functional changes, including precipitate urge, frequency, residual urine, retention of urine, recurrent urinary tract infections, and gross incontinence. Symptoms range from mild to disabling. Obviously, incontinence is especially troublesome. If the lesion is above the PMC, detrusor–striated sphincter dyssynergia usually does not occur. However, leakage may occur because the need to void cannot be felt or because the sphincter becomes more relaxed and can no longer inhibit spontaneous voiding. Lesions of the internal capsule include vascular accidents and Parkinson's disease. Both spastic and semiflaccid voiding disorders are found with these lesions.

Spinal cord injury can be the result of trauma, herniated intervertebral disk, vascular lesions, multiple sclerosis, tumor, syringomyelia, or myelitis, or it may be iatrogenic. Traumatic spinal cord lesions are of greatest clinical concern. Partial or complete injuries may cause equally severe genitourinary dysfunction. Sphincter spasticity and voiding dyssynergia can lead to detrusor hypertrophy, high voiding pressures, ureteral reflux, or ureteral obstruction. With time, renal function may be compromised. If infection is combined with back pressure on the kidney, loss of renal function can be particularly rapid.

Spinal cord injuries at the high thoracic (above T6) and cervical levels are often associated with (1) detrusor–sphincter (both smooth and striated) dyssynergia and (2) autonomic dysreflexia. Because the lesions occur above the sympathetic outflow from the cord, hypertensive blood pressure fluctuations, bradycardia, and sweating can be triggered by insertion of a catheter, mild overdistention of the bladder with filling, or dyssynergic voiding (see later). When a complete lesion is near the levels of sympathetic outflow, patient may develop bladder overactivity with no sensation, smooth sphincter synergy but striated sphincter dyssynergia.

In summary, the overactive neuropathic bladder is typified by (1) reduced capacity, (2) involuntary detrusor contractions, (3) high intravesical voiding pressures, (4) marked hypertrophy of the bladder wall, (5) spasticity of the pelvic-striated muscle, and (6) autonomic dysreflexia in cervical cord lesions.

2. Neuropathic bladder due to lesions at or below the sacral micturition center

▶ Injury to the Detrusor Motor Nucleus

The most common cause of flaccid neuropathic bladder is injury to the spinal cord at the micturition center, S2–4. Other causes of anterior horn cell damage include infection due to poliovirus or herpes zoster and iatrogenic factors such as radiation or surgery. Herniated disks can injure the micturition center but more commonly affect the cauda equina or sacral nerve roots. Myelodysplasias could also be grouped here, but the mechanism is actually failure in the development or organization of the anterior horn cells. Lesions in this region of the cord are often incomplete, with the result commonly being a mixture of spastic behavior with weakened muscle contractility. Mild trabeculation of the bladder may occur. External sphincter and perineal muscle tone are diminished. Urinary incontinence usually does not occur in these cases because of the compensatory increase in bladder storage. The bladder pressure is low and little outlet resistance is needed to provide continence. Evacuation of the bladder may be accomplished by straining, but with variable success.

▶ Injury to the Afferent Feedback Pathways

Flaccid neuropathic bladder also results from a variety of neuropathies, including diabetes mellitus, tabes dorsalis, pernicious anemia, and posterior spinal cord lesions. Here, the mechanism is not injury of the detrusor motor nucleus but a loss of sensory input to the detrusor nucleus or a change in motor behavior due to loss of neurotransmission in the dorsal horns of the cord. The end result is the same. Loss of perception of bladder filling permits overstretching of the detrusor. Atony of the detrusor results in weak, inefficient contractility. Capacity is increased and residual urine significant.

In summary, the flaccid neuropathic bladder is typified by (1) large capacity, (2) lack of voluntary detrusor contractions, (3) low intravesical pressure, (4) mild trabeculation (hypertrophy) of the bladder wall, and (5) decreased tone of the external sphincter.

▶ Injury Causing Poor Detrusor Distensibility

Another cause of atonic neuropathic bladder is peripheral nerve injury. This category includes injury caused by radical surgical procedures such as low anterior resection of the colon or radical hysterectomy. Impaired innervation of detrusor and both the smooth and striated sphincters create outflow resistance and incomplete voiding. The end result is a bladder that stores poorly owing to failure to accommodate with filling.

Radiation therapy can result in denervation of the detrusor or sphincters. More commonly, it damages the detrusor, resulting in fibrosis and loss of distensibility. Other inflammatory causes of injury to the detrusor include chronic infection, interstitial cystitis, and carcinoma in situ. These lesions produce a fibrotic bladder wall with poor distensibility.

▶ Selective Injury to the External Sphincter

Pelvic fracture often damages the nerves to the external sphincter. Selective denervation of the external sphincter muscle, with incontinence, can follow if the bladder neck is not sufficiently competent. Radical surgery in the perineum may affect sensory but not motor innervation of the external sphincter.

SPINAL SHOCK AND RECOVERY OF VESICAL FUNCTION AFTER SPINAL CORD INJURY

Immediately following severe injury to the spinal cord or conus medullaris, regardless of level, there is a stage of flaccid paralysis, with numbness below the level of the injury. The smooth muscle of the detrusor and rectum is affected. The result is detrusor overfilling to the point of overflow incontinence and rectal impaction.

Spinal shock may last from a few weeks to 6 months (usually 2–3 months). Reflex response in striated muscle is usually present from the time of injury but is suppressed. With time, the reflex excitability of striated muscle progresses until a spastic state is achieved. Smooth muscle is much slower to develop this hyperreflexic activity. Therefore, urinary retention is the rule in the early months following injury.

Urodynamic studies are indicated periodically to monitor the progressive return of reflex behavior. In the early recovery stages, a few weak contractions of the bladder may be found. Later, in injuries above the micturition center, more significant reflex activity will be found. Low-pressure storage can be managed via intermittent catheterization. High-pressure storage should be addressed early to avoid problems with the upper urinary tract.

A seldom used but valuable test is instillation of ice water. A strong detrusor contraction in response to filling with cold saline (3.3°C [38°F]) is one of the first indications of return of detrusor reflex activity. This test is of value in differentiating upper from lower motor neuron lesions early in the recovery phase.

Activity of the bladder after the spinal shock phase depends on the site of injury and extent of the neural lesion. With upper motor neuron (suprasegmental) lesions, there is obvious evidence of spasticity toward the end of the spinal shock phase (eg, spontaneous spasms in the extremities, spontaneous leakage of urine or stool, and, possibly, the return of some sensation). A plan of management can be made at this time. A few patients will retain the ability to empty the bladder reflexively by using trigger techniques, that is, by tapping or scratching the skin above the pubis or external genitalia. More often, detrusor overactivity must be suppressed by anticholinergic medication to prevent incontinence. Evacuation of urine can then be accomplished by intermittent catheterization. Although incomplete lesions are more amenable to this approach than complete lesions, 70% of complete lesions ultimately can be managed using this program. Patients who cannot be managed in this way can be evaluated for sphincterotomy, dorsal rhizotomy, diversion, augmentation, or a bladder pacemaker procedure.

In cases of lower motor neuron lesions, it is difficult to distinguish spinal shock from the end result of the injury. Spontaneous detrusor activity cannot be elicited on urodynamic evaluation. If the bladder is allowed to fill, overflow incontinence will occur. Striated muscle reflexes will be suppressed or absent. The bladder may be partially emptied by the Credé maneuver (ie, by manually pushing on the abdomen above the pubic symphysis) or, preferably, by intermittent catheterization.

▶ Diagnosis of Neurogenic Bladder

The diagnosis of a neuropathic bladder disorder depends on a complete history and physical (including neurologic) examination, as well as use of radiologic studies (voiding cystourethrography, excretory urography, computed tomography scanning, magnetic resonance imaging, when necessary); urologic studies (cystoscopy, ultrasound); urodynamic studies (cystometry, urethral pressure recordings, uroflowmetry); and neurologic studies (electromyography, evoked potentials). Patients should be reevaluated often as recovery progresses.

1. Neurogenic overactive (spastic, hyperreflexic) bladder—Overactive bladder results from extensive neural damage above sacral cord but below the PMC. The bladder functions on the level of spinal segmental reflexes, without efficient regulation from higher brain centers.

▶ Clinical Findings

A. Symptoms

The severity of symptoms depends on the site and extent of the lesion as well as the length of time from injury. Symptoms include involuntary urination, which is often frequent, spontaneous, scant, and triggered by spasms in the lower extremities. A true sensation of fullness is lacking, although vague lower abdominal sensations due to stretch of the overlying peritoneum may be felt. The major nonurologic symptoms are those of spastic paralysis and objective sensory deficits.

B. Signs

A complete neurologic examination is most important. The sensory level of the injury needs to be established, followed by assessment of the anal, bulbocavernosus, knee, ankle, and toe reflexes. These reflexes vary in degree of hyperreflexia on a scale of 1–4. Levator muscle tone and anal tone should be gauged separately, also on a scale of 1–4. Bladder volumes in established lesions are usually <300 mL (not infrequently, <150 mL) and cannot be detected by abdominal percussion. Ultrasound is a useful and rapid means of determining bladder capacity. Voiding often can be triggered by stimulation of the skin of the abdomen, thigh, or genitalia, often with spasm of the lower extremities.

With high thoracic and cervical lesions, distention of the bladder (due to a plugged catheter or during cystometry or cystoscopy) can trigger a series of responses, including hypertension, bradycardia, headache, piloerection, and sweating (autonomic dysreflexia). Inserting a catheter and leaving the catheter on open drainage usually reverses the dysreflexia.

C. Laboratory Findings

Virtually all patients experience one or more urinary tract infections during the recovery phase of spinal shock. This is due to the necessity of catheter drainage, either intermittent or continuous. Urinary stasis, prolonged immobilization, and urinary tract infections can predispose to stone formation. Renal function may be normal or impaired, depending on the efficacy of treatment and the absence of complications (hydronephrosis, pyelonephritis, urinary stones). Red blood cells (erythrocytes) in the urine may reflect a number of abnormalities. Uremia will result if complications are not addressed appropriately and the patient is not checked at regular intervals.

D. X-Ray Findings

Periodic excretory urograms and retrograde cystograms are essential because complications are common. A trabeculated bladder of small capacity is typical of this type of neuropathic dysfunction. The bladder neck may be dilated. The kidneys may show evidence of pyelonephritic scarring, hydronephrosis, or stone disease. The ureters may be dilated from obstruction or reflux. A voiding film may detect a narrowed zone created by the spastic sphincter or identify a strictured segment of the urethra. Magnetic resonance imaging, especially the sagittal view, offers clear delineation of the bladder neck and posterior urethra if pathology if suspected.

E. Instrumental Examination

Cystourethroscopy helps assess the integrity of the urethra and identify stricture sites. The bladder shows variable degrees of trabeculation, occasionally with diverticula. Bladder capacity, stones, competency of the ureteral orifices, changes secondary to chronic infection or indwelling catheters, and the integrity of the bladder neck and external urethral sphincter can be assessed. When indicated, ureteroscopy can also be used to inspect the ureter and the renal pelvis.

F. Urodynamic Studies

Combined recording of bladder and urethral sphincter activity during filling will reveal a low-volume bladder with spastic dyssynergy of the external sphincter (Figure 28–4). High voiding pressures in the bladder are common. Ureteral reflux or obstruction is more likely if voiding pressures exceed 40 cm of water. A high resting pressure is noted in the external sphincter on the urethral pressure profile, and labile spastic behavior is noted during filling and voiding. Various auras replace a true sense of bladder filling, for example, sweating, vague abdominal discomfort, and spasm of the lower extremities. Movement of a catheter in the urethra can trigger detrusor contraction and voiding.

2. Spastic neuromuscular dysfunction—Incomplete lesions of the cerebral cortex, pyramidal tracts, or spinal cord may weaken, but not abolish, cerebral restraint. The patient may have frequency and nocturia or urinary incontinence due to

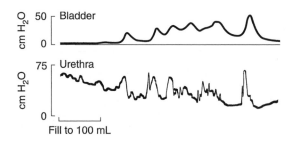

▲ **Figure 28–4.** Spinal cord injury at T12. Simultaneous recording of intravesical and urethral pressure with bladder filling. Note the rise in intravesical pressure associated with unstable activity of the external sphincter, as reflected on the urethral pressure tracing.

precipitous urge or voiding. Common causes include brain tumors, Parkinson's disease, multiple sclerosis, dementias, cerebrovascular accidents, prolapsed disks, or partial spinal injury.

In many cases, the cause is unclear. The hyperreflexic behavior often seems to be associated with a peripheral abnormality (eg, prostatitis, benign prostatic hypertrophy, urethritis) or follows pelvic surgery (eg, anterior colporrhaphy, anteroposterior tumor resection). Symptoms are commonly associated with psychological factors.

► Clinical Findings

A. Symptoms

Frequency, nocturia, and urgency are the principal symptoms. Hesitancy, intermittency, double voiding, and residual urine are also common. Incontinence may vary from pre- or postvoiding dribbling to complete voiding that the patient does not recognize or cannot inhibit once started.

B. Signs

The degree of voiding dysfunction does not parallel neurologic deficits. Slight physical disabilities can be associated with gross disturbances in bladder function, and the reverse is also true. However, it is always important to check lower extremity and perineal reflexes for evidence of hyperreflexia. Sensory or motor deficits may also be detected in the lumbar or sacral segments.

C. X-Ray Findings

In the early stages, radiologically evident change is minimal or absent. Low bladder volume and mild trabeculation of the bladder are usually evident.

D. Instrumental Examination

Cystoscopy and urethroscopy are generally unremarkable. Mild detrusor and sphincter irritability and diminished capacity may be demonstrated.

E. Urodynamic Studies

The behavior patterns of the sphincter and bladder are similar to those of the previous group but on a milder scale. Detrusor overactivity, evident urodynamically, may not be associated with the same symptom pattern on the clinical level. The patient occasionally perceives a sense of urgency and the need to void. However, these sensations may not be present, and the patient may complain of the occasional leakage as the main inconvenience. Morphologic changes in the bladder are slight, with changes in the upper urinary tract occurring rarely and late because of lower pressures in the bladder.

3. Neurogenic areflexic (flaccid, atonic) bladder—Direct injury to the peripheral innervation of the bladder or sacral

cord segments S2–4 results in flaccid paralysis of the urinary bladder. Characteristically, the capacity is large, intravesical pressure low, and involuntary contractions absent. Because smooth muscle is intrinsically active, fine trabeculations in the bladder may be seen. Common causes of this type of bladder behavior are trauma, tumors, tabes dorsalis, and congenital anomalies (eg, spina bifida, meningomyelocele).

► Clinical Findings

A. Symptoms

The patient experiences flaccid paralysis and loss of sensation affecting the muscles and dermatomes below the level of injury. The principal urinary symptom is retention with overflow incontinence. Male patients lose their erections. Surprisingly, despite weakness in the striated sphincter, neither bowel nor urinary incontinence is a major factor. Storage pressures within the bladder remain below the outlet resistance.

B. Signs

Neurologic changes are typically lower motor neuron. Extremity reflexes are hypoactive or absent. Sensation is diminished or absent. It is important to check sensation over the penis (S2) and perianal region (S2–3) for evidence of a mixed or partial injury. Anal tone (S2) should be compared with levator tone (S3–4), again for evidence of a mixed injury.

Similarly, sensation over the outside of the foot (S2), sole of the foot (S2–3), and large toe (S3) should be compared for evidence of mixed injury. Occasionally, extremity findings do not parallel those of the perineum, with the pattern being absent sensation and tone in the feet but partial tone or sensation in the perineum. This is especially true in patients who have spina bifida or meningomyelocele.

C. Laboratory Findings

Repeated urinalysis at regular intervals is no less important in this group than in others. Infection with white blood cells (leukocytes) and bacteria may occur because of the need for bladder catheterization. Advanced renal change is unusual because bladder storage is under low pressure, but chronic renal failure secondary to pyelonephritis, hydronephrosis, or calculus formation is still possible.

D. X-Ray Findings

A plain film of the abdomen may reveal fracture of the lumbar spine or extensive spina bifida. Calcific shadows compatible with urinary stone may be seen. Excretory urograms should be performed initially to check for calculus, hydronephrosis, pyelonephritic scarring, or ureteral obstruction secondary to an overdistended bladder. A cystogram may detect morphologic changes in the detrusor (it is usually large and smooth walled); vesicoureteral reflux may be present. Checks on the integrity of both the lower and upper urinary tracts can subsequently be made using ultrasound.

E. Instrumental Examination

Cystoscopy and urethroscopy performed some months or weeks after the injury will confirm the laxity and areflexia of the sphincter and pelvic floor; the bladder neck is usually funneled and open and the bladder should be large and smooth walled. The integrity of the ureteral orifices should be normal. Fine trabeculation may be evident. Bladder stones and urethral stricture or obstruction may be seen in long-term cases.

F. Urodynamic Studies

The urethral pressure profile reflects low smooth and striated sphincter tone. Bladder filling pressures are low; detrusor contractions are weak or absent; voiding is accomplished by straining or by the Credé maneuver, if at all; and there is a large volume of residual urine. Awareness of filling is markedly diminished and usually results from stretch on the peritoneum or abdominal distention.

G. Denervation Hypersensitivity

This test is classically performed by giving bethanechol chloride (Urecholine) 15 mg subcutaneously. A cystometrogram is performed after 20 minutes, and the results are compared with the findings obtained before the bethanechol was given. If the results are positive, a rise in filling pressure of more than 15 cm of water is noted, with a shift in the filling curve to the left. A finding of no change on filling reflects myogenic damage to the detrusor. The ice water test also checks for detrusor hypersensitivity.

Bethanechol does not facilitate a detrusor contraction; it can only increase tone in the detrusor wall, which in turn might trigger the voiding reflex. The test is not a check on the integrity of the voiding reflex but demonstrates denervation hypersensitivity in flaccid bladders and differentiates this condition from myogenic damage.

The test is not applicable in patients with reduced bladder capacity, decreased compliance (ie, sharp rise in detrusor-filling pressure), or forceful contractions of the detrusor.

DIFFERENTIAL DIAGNOSIS OF NEUROGENIC BLADDER

The diagnosis of neuropathic bladder is usually obvious from the history and physical examination. Neural impairment is evidenced by abnormal sacral reflex activity and decreased perineal sensation. Some disorders with which neuropathic bladder may be confused are cystitis, chronic urethritis, vesical irritation secondary to psychic disturbance, myogenic damage, interstitial cystitis, cystocele, and infravesical obstruction.

▶ Cystitis

Inflammation of the bladder, both nonspecific and tuberculous, causes frequency of urination and urgency, even to the point of incontinence. Infections secondary to residual urine caused by neuropathic behavioral disturbance should be ruled out.

The urodynamics of the inflamed bladder are similar to those of the neurogenic overactive bladder. However, with inflammation, symptoms disappear after definitive antibiotic therapy, and the urodynamic behavior reverts to normal. If symptoms persist or infections return repeatedly, a neuropathic behavioral abnormality should be considered (eg, multiple sclerosis or even idiopathic detrusor–sphincter dyssynergia).

▶ Chronic Urethritis

Symptoms of frequency, nocturia, and burning on urination may be due to chronic inflammation of the urethra not necessarily associated with infection. The urodynamics will show an irritable urethral sphincter zone with labile, spastic tendencies. The cause is unknown.

▶ Vesical Irritation Secondary to Psychic Disturbance

Anxious, tense individuals or those with pathologic psychological fixation on the perineum may present a long history of periodic bouts of urinary frequency or perineal or pelvic pain. The clinical picture and urodynamic findings are similar to those described previously for chronic urethritis. Often, however, if the patient's anxieties can be allayed, the symptoms subside. The underlying problem is one of excessive pelvic muscle tension and inefficient sphincter behavior. Some of the symptoms may improve with manual therapy of pelvic floor myofascial trigger points (Weiss, 2001).

▶ Interstitial Cystitis

Interstitial cystitis is poorly understood chronic inflammation of the bladder (Hanno et al, 2011). The typical patient is a woman older than 40 years, with symptoms of frequency, nocturia, urgency, and suprapubic pain. The symptoms are brought on by bladder distention. Capacity is limited (often <100 mL in the most symptomatic and disabled patients). Urinalysis is normal, and there is no residual urine. Urodynamic studies show a hypertonic, poorly compliant bladder. Distention of the bladder with cystoscopy produces bleeding from petechial hemorrhages and fissuring in the mucosa. The condition represents an end-stage inflammatory process of unknown cause in the detrusor.

▶ Cystocele

Relaxation of the pelvic floor following childbirth may cause some frequency, nocturia, and stress incontinence. Residual urine may be present and predispose to infection. Loss of urine occurs with lifting, standing, or coughing. Pelvic examination usually reveals relaxation of the anterior vaginal wall and descent of the urethra and bladder when the patient strains to void.

▶ Bladder Outlet Obstruction

Urethral strictures, benign or malignant enlargement of the prostate gland, and congenital urethral valves all can produce significant obstruction of the urinary outlet. Hypertrophy (ie, trabeculation) of the detrusor develops, and residual urine can accumulate. Detrusor overactivity is often found at this stage and resembles that of the neurogenic overactive bladder.

If decompensation occurs, the vesical wall becomes attenuated and atonic, and capacity may be markedly increased. Overflow incontinence may develop. The behavior of the bladder is similar to that of the neurogenic areflexic bladder.

If the difficulty is nonneuropathic, the anal sphincter tone is normal and the bulbocavernosus reflex intact. Peripheral sensation, voluntary muscle contraction, and limb reflexes should also be normal. Cystoscopy and urethroscopy reveal the local lesion that causes obstruction. Once the obstruction is relieved, bladder function improves but may never return to normal.

TREATMENT OF NEUROPATHIC BLADDER

The treatment of any form of neuropathic bladder is guided by the need to restore low-pressure activity to the bladder. In doing so, renal function is preserved, continence restored, and infection more readily controlled. Reflex evacuation may develop if detrusor integrity is protected and trigger techniques are practiced.

1. Spinal shock—Following severe injury to the spinal cord, the bladder becomes atonic. During the spinal shock stage, some type of bladder drainage must be instituted immediately and maintained. Chronic overdistention can damage the detrusor smooth muscle and limit functional recovery of the bladder. Intermittent catheterization using strict aseptic technique has proved to be the best form of management. This avoids urinary tract infection as well as the complications of an indwelling catheter (eg, urethral stricture, abscess, erosions, stones).

If a Foley catheter becomes necessary, a few principles need to be followed. The catheter should not be larger than 16F and preferably should be made of silicon, and it should be taped to the abdomen. Taping the catheter to the leg puts unnecessary stress on the penoscrotal junction and bulbous urethra (ie, the curves in the urethra), and this can lead to stricture formation. The catheter should be changed with sterile procedure every 2–3 weeks.

Some urologists advocate the use of suprapubic cystostomy rather than a urethral catheter to avoid the risks associated with permanent indwelling catheters. Certainly, whenever catheter-related complications occur, the physician should not hesitate in resorting to cystostomy drainage.

Irrigation of the bladder with antibiotic solutions, use of systemic antibiotics, or covering the tip of the meatus with antibiotic creams does not significantly lower the long-term risk of bladder infection. However, keeping the meatus lubricated does help avoid meatal stricturing.

As peripheral reflex excitability gradually returns, urodynamic evaluation should be performed. A cystogram is needed to rule out reflux. The urodynamic study should be repeated every 3 months as long as spasticity is improving and then annually to check for complications of the upper urinary tract.

To control infection, a fluid intake of at least 2–3 L/day should be maintained (100–200 mL/h) if at all possible. This reduces stasis and decreases the concentration of calcium in the urine. Renal and ureteral drainage are enhanced by moving the patient frequently, with ambulation in a wheelchair as soon as possible, and even by raising the head of the bed. These measures improve ureteral transport of urine, reduce stasis, and lower the risk of infection.

2. Specific types of neuropathic bladder—Once a neuropathic voiding disorder is established, regardless of cause, the following steps should be taken to attain optimum function.

▶ Neurogenic Overactive Bladder

A. Patient with Reasonable Bladder Capacity

The goal is to rehabilitate the bladder to a functional state, that is, being able to go 2–3 hours between voiding and not be incontinent during this interval. Voiding is initiated using trigger techniques—tapping the abdomen suprapubically; tugging on the pubic hair; squeezing the penis; or scratching the skin of the lower abdomen, genitalia, or thighs. Patients can accomplish this on their own unless they are high quadriplegics with no upper limb function.

Some patients in this category can empty the bladder completely but are incontinent due to inconvenient triggering of the voiding reflex. They may be helped by low-dose anticholinergic medication or by neural stimulation (Gulur and Drake, 2010).

B. Patient with Markedly Diminished Functional Vesical Capacity

If the functional capacity of the bladder is <100 mL, involuntary voiding can occur as often as every 15 minutes. Satisfactory training of the bladder cannot be achieved, and alternative measures must be taken. Of course, one must first determine that reduced functional bladder capacity is not due to a large residual volume of urine. One of the following treatment regimens can then be administered.

1. A permanent indwelling catheter with or without anticholinergic medication.

2. A condom catheter and a leg bag in males if residual urine volumes are small and the patient does not have

bladder pressures above 40 cm of water on urodynamic evaluation. If either of these parameters is found, the upper urinary tract is considered at risk from obstruction or reflux.

3. Performance of a sphincterotomy in males (Perkash, 2007). It is possible to turn the bladder into a urinary conduit by surgically eliminating all outlet resistance from the bladder. This option should be used only when other options have failed, as it is irreversible. Patients having this procedure usually have more serious sequelae of a highly spastic bladder (ie, upper urinary tract dilatation, recurrent urinary tract infections, or marked autonomic dysreflexia).

4. Conversion of the spastic bladder to a flaccid bladder through sacral rhizotomy. Complete surgical section or percutaneous heat fulguration of the S3 and S4 roots is necessary. Chemical rhizotomy is unreliable, as spasticity usually returns after 6–9 months. These procedures may cause loss of reflex erections, and the decision to perform them should be weighed accordingly. These procedures can relieve spasticity, lower intravesical pressures, increase bladder storage, and decrease the risk of damage to the upper urinary tract. The bladder would then be managed as a flaccid bladder (see later).

5. Neurostimulation of the sacral nerve roots to accomplish bladder evacuation (see the following section).

6. Urinary diversion for irreversible, progressive upper urinary tract deterioration. A variety of procedures are available, including the standard ileal conduit, cutaneous ureterostomies, transureteroureterostomy, or nonrefluxing urinary reservoir (eg, Mainz pouch, Koch pouch, or one of several other continent diversions designed to protect the upper urinary tract and kidneys).

7. In females with a spastic bladder, one does not have the option of performing a sphincterotomy. If pharmacologic methods are unsuccessful, surgical conversion to a flaccid, low-pressure system or a urinary diversion should be considered.

C. Muscarinic Receptor Antagonist

Because of the chronic nature of the neuropathic bladder, patients are not always willing to tolerate the side effects of muscarinic receptor antagonist. Several drugs in this category can be alternated to reduce the side effects of either drug. They may also be useful when given with skeletal muscle relaxants. Dosages must be individualized. Commonly used drugs and dosages are as follows: oxybutynin chloride (Ditropan) XL, 10 mg once daily, and tolterodine (Detrol) LA, 4 mg daily or other newer drugs (see Chapter 30). (Andersson, 2010; Andersson et al, 2010). These drugs may not be effective if incontinence is the result of uninhibited sphincter relaxation or compliance changes in the bladder wall.

D. Intravesical Instillation of Medications

Capsaicin and resiniferatoxin are specific C-fiber afferent neurotoxins. After spinal cord injury, C-fiber afferents proliferate in the bladder mucosa and are involved in detrusor hyperreflexia. In patients with NDO from spinal cord injury or multiple sclerosis, both capsaicin and resiniferatoxin showed better effect than placebo. However, the panel of the 4th International Consultation on Incontinence feels that they are of very limited clinical use in detrusor overactivity (Andersson et al, 2009). On the other hand, intravesical oxybutynin has been used successfully in neurogenic bladder (Lazarus, 2009).

E. Botulinum-A Toxin

Several studies have investigated injection of 100–300 units of botulinum-A toxin into 30–40 sites in the bladder in adults who have detrusor hyperreflexia (Alvares et al, 2010; Datta et al, 2010; Smaldone et al, 2010). Most published results conclude that intravesical injection of botulinum toxin resulted in improvement in medication refractory overactive bladder symptoms. However, the risk of increased postvoid residual and symptomatic urinary retention was significant. Several studies also showed the effect of repeated injection and its sustained effect (Png and Toh, 2010). The panel of the 4th International Consultation on Incontinence recommends its use in patients who are resistant to antimuscarinics (Andersson et al, 2009).

F. Neurostimulation (Bladder Pacemaker)

Neuroprosthetics are becoming an established alternative to managing selective neuropathic bladder disorders (Bosch and Groen, 1995; Burks et al, 2010). Patients are evaluated for a bladder pacemaker primarily by urodynamic monitoring of bladder and sphincter responses to trial stimulation of the various sacral nerve roots. Selective blocks are then prepared to the right and left pudendal nerves. If voiding is produced, patients are considered suitable for a neuroprosthesis. Other factors such as detrusor storage capability, sphincter competence, age, kidney function, and overall neurologic and psychological status are also taken into consideration.

Electrodes are implanted on the motor (ventral) nerve roots of those sacral nerves that will produce detrusor contraction on stimulation (always S3, occasionally S4). Steps are then taken to reduce sphincter hyperreflexia by selectively dividing the sensory (dorsal) component of these same sacral nerve roots and selective branches of the pudendal nerves. The electrodes are connected to a subcutaneous receiver that can be controlled from outside the body. Bladder or bowel evacuation or continence can then be controlled selectively by the external transmitter (Brindley, 1995; Tanagh et al, 1989).

The first two goals are to protect upper tract and restore continence. Both can be achieved by combining neurostimulation of the sphincter with selective sacral neurotomies that lead to increased bladder capacity and reduced bladder pressure. This approach preserves sphincter integrity and avoids the need for drugs. Other options include complete bladder denervation or bladder augmentation.

The third goal, restoration of controlled evacuation, eliminates the need for catheters and associated risk of infection. This is the most difficult goal to achieve, and patients need to be carefully evaluated for their suitability.

▶ Neurogenic Areflexic Bladder

If the neurologic lesion completely destroys the micturition center, volitional voiding cannot be accomplished without manual suprapubic pressure, that is, the Credé maneuver. Bladder evacuation can be accomplished by straining, using the abdominal and diaphragmatic muscles to raise intra-abdominal pressures. Partial injuries to the lower spinal cord (T10–11) result in a spastic bladder and a weak or weakly spastic sphincter. Incontinence can then result from spontaneous detrusor contraction.

A. Bladder Training and Care

In partial lower motor neuron injury, voiding should be tried every 2 hours by the clock to avoid embarrassing leakage. This helps protect the bladder from overdistention due to a buildup of residual urine.

B. Intermittent Catheterization

Any patient with adequate bladder capacity can benefit from regular intermittent catheter drainage every 3–6 hours (McGuire and Savastano, 1983). This technique eliminates residual urine, helps prevent infection, avoids incontinence, and protects against damage to the upper urinary tract. It simulates normal voiding and is easily learned and adapted by patients. It is an extremely satisfactory solution to the problems of the flaccid neuropathic bladder. A clean technique is used rather than the inconvenient, expensive, sterile technique. Urinary tract infections are infrequent, but if they occur, an antibiotic can be given. The method is contraindicated if ureteral reflux is present, unless the reflux is mild and the bladder emptied frequently.

C. Surgery

Transurethral resection is indicated for hypertrophy of the bladder neck or an enlarged prostate, either of which may cause obstruction of the bladder outlet and retention of residual urine. It may also be performed in some male patients to weaken the outlet resistance of the bladder to permit voiding by the Credé maneuver or abdominal straining.

Complete urinary incontinence due to sphincter incompetence can be managed by implanting an artificial sphincter (Chung and Cartmill, 2010; Kastler et al, 2010). Bladder pressure should be low, however, for this to be successful. Bladder neck and posterior urethral reconstruction also may be considered as a way to increase outlet resistance (Churchill et al, 2010; Dave and Salle, 2008). Incontinence in this group of patients can be treated with drugs or neurostimulation if it results from mild bladder spasticity.

D. Parasympathomimetic Drugs

The stable derivatives of acetylcholine are at times of value in assisting the evacuation of the bladder. Although they *do not* initiate or effect bladder contraction, they do provide increased bladder tonus. They may be helpful in symptomatic treatment of the milder types of flaccid neuropathic bladder. Drugs may be tried empirically, but usefulness is best gauged during urodynamic evaluation. If filling pressure or resting tonus is increased after bethanechol chloride (Urecholine) is administered, evacuation of the bladder through trigger reflexes or straining should be more effective. The drug then should be clinically helpful.

Bethanechol chloride is the drug of choice. It is given orally, 25–50 mg every 6–8 hours. In special situations (eg, urodynamic study or immediately following operation), it may be given subcutaneously, 5–10 mg every 6–8 hours.

▶ Neurogenic Bladder Associated with Spina Bifida

Spina bifida is incomplete formation of the neural arch at various levels of the spine. The defect is recognized at birth and closed immediately to prevent infection. The scarring that results can entrap and tether nerves in the cauda equina. With failure of the neural arch to close, there is failure of anterior horn cell development and organization. The end result is a mixed type of neuropathic defect. Roughly two-thirds of patients have a spastic bladder with weakness in the feet and toes. About one-third of patients have a flaccid bladder. Often, there is a greater degree of flaccidity in the pelvic floor than in the detrusor. The goals of therapy are to control incontinence and preserve renal function.

A. Conservative Treatment

Clean intermittent catheterization is the best management. Parents can be taught to do this for the child, and eventually the child can take over this function. Frequency should be determined by the storage capacity of the bladder and the fluid intake, usually every 3–6 hours. An anticholinergic drug may be required to mediate bladder spasticity and improve storage function in order to control incontinence.

1. Mild symptoms—If there is occasional dribbling or some residual urine associated with lack of desire to void, the patient should try to void every 2 hours when awake. Manual suprapubic pressure enhances the efficiency of emptying. An external condom catheter or a small pad can be worn to protect against small-volume losses of urine.

2. More severe symptoms—If urinary incontinence is associated with residual urine or if ureteral reflux is found, the following steps should be taken:

a. **Hypotonic bladder**—If reflux has been demonstrated, intermittent self-catheterization four to six times a day may protect the upper urinary tract from deterioration and the consequences of pyelonephritis. Ureteral reimplantation can be considered for bilateral reflux or a transureteroureterostomy for single-sided reflux if all other considerations are favorable. Intermittent catheterization should then be reinstituted.

b. **Hypertonic bladder**—The problem with patients in this category is more serious because the bladder is spastic with reduced capacity and the sphincter is hypotonic. Virtually constant dribbling can result. The cystogram will reveal heavy trabeculation of the bladder, often with reflux and advanced hydroureteronephrosis. Anticholinergic medication should be given, and an indwelling catheter should be inserted for several months. Once upper urinary tract dilatation has been improved and the bladder has been restored to a more spheric shape, intermittent catheterization may be reinstituted. With time and care, many of these children develop a more balanced type of bladder behavior. Continence may be gained without compromising the upper urinary tract.

Most of these patients will not require urinary diversion if they are carefully followed up and if the parents actively participate in their care.

B. Surgical Treatment

If the bladder is of the spastic type with diminished capacity, there are several surgical options short of actual urinary diversion. Sacral nerve block during urodynamic evaluation helps in determining whether sacral nerve root section would be beneficial. This helps in cases of spastic bladder but not in cases of poorly compliant, fibrotic bladder. Sectioning the S3 nerves reduces intravesical pressures, improves storage, and reduces the risk of reflux or obstruction of the ureters.

For patient with a mildly spastic bladder and reasonable storage capacity (>200 mL), urinary incontinence might be controlled via electrostimulation of the pelvic floor. Many of these patients have intact nerves to the sphincter. These can be stimulated to enhance sphincter tone and inhibit voiding. If the bladder has a limited capacity with poor compliance and poor contractility, augmentation cystoplasty (Duel et al, 1998) followed by intermittent self-catheterization is the treatment of choice.

If the refluxing patient has recurrent fever (equivalent to pyelonephritis) despite the presence of an indwelling catheter or if incontinence cannot be controlled because of poor detrusor compliance, urinary diversion must be considered. Nonrefluxing continent reservoirs offer the most favorable long-term outlook for preservation of the upper urinary tract.

In patient with hyperreflexic neurogenic bladder and detrusor external sphincter dyssynergia caused by complete suprasacral spinal cord injury, anastomosis between the L5 and S2/3 ventral roots, or between 11th and 12th intercostal nerves and the S2–S3 roots, has been carried out so that urination can be controlled by somatic afferent (Livshits et al, 2004; Xiao et al, 2003). Varying degree of success has been reported.

3. Control of urinary incontinence—Most men with spastic bladders rely on a condom catheter for protection against leakage and for practical urine collection. The only exception is patients who are predictably dry between catheterizations. The condom catheter attaches to the penis without pressure and has a conduit to a leg bag. The adhesives are nonirritating and long lasting. Problems involved in keeping these catheters in place are limited to noncircumcised patients and those with large suprapubic fat pads that shorten the length of the shaft of the penis. Circumcision or placement of a penile prosthesis will correct for these limitations.

Urethral compression by means of a Cunningham clamp is occasionally preferred by patients. This protects only against low-pressure leakage, however, and if it is applied too tightly, a urethral diverticulum may develop.

Other types of external collection devices are available (McGuire urinal, Texas catheter), but with advancements in adhesive glues for condom catheters and use of penile prostheses, the other methods are being used less frequently.

▶ Neurostimulation

Extensive research continues to be conducted on methods of restoring voluntary control over the storage and evacuation functions of the bladder. Sacral and pudendal nerve anatomy has been determined so that surgical exposure of these nerves and their branches is possible. An electrode can be placed for selective stimulation of the bladder, levator, and urethral or anal sphincters (Schmidt, 1986; Tanagho et al, 1989; Thompson et al, 2010). A number of possibilities exist for neurostimulation or rhizotomy, but only a few are practical. Urodynamic evaluation of bladder function following a nerve block or during neurostimulation can help determine the therapeutic value of these treatments.

Single or multiple electrodes can be placed on selected nerves and coupled to a subcutaneous receiver (Brindley, 1995; Tanagho and Schmidt, 1988). The desired function (continence or evacuation) can be selected. Usually, one or the other is needed in any one patient. Much will change in this approach as technologic advances become adapted to the increased understanding of bladder physiology. Striking successes are also being seen with electroevacuation in highly selected patients.

COMPLICATIONS OF NEUROGENIC BLADDER

The principal complications of the neuropathic bladder are recurrent urinary tract infection, hydronephrosis secondary to ureteral reflux or obstruction, and stone formation

(Pickelsimer et al, 2010). The primary factors contributing to these complications are the presence of residual urine, sustained high intravesical pressures, and immobilization, respectively.

Incontinence in neuropathic disorders may be passive, as in flaccid lesions when outlet resistance is compromised, or may be the result of uninhibited detrusor contractions, as in spastic lesions.

▶ Infection

Infection is virtually inevitable with the neuropathic bladder state. During the stage of spinal shock that follows cord injury, the bladder must be emptied by catheterization. Sterile intermittent catheterization is recommended at this stage, but for practical purposes or for the sake of convenience, a Foley catheter is often left indwelling. Chronic catheter drainage guarantees infection regardless of any preventive measures taken.

The upper urinary tract is usually protected from infection by the integrity of the ureterovesical junction. If this becomes incompetent, infected urine will reflux up to the kidneys. Decompensation of the ureterovesical junction results from the high intravesical pressures generated by the spastic bladder. It is most important that these cases be treated aggressively with an intensive program of self-catheterization and anticholinergic medication. The Credé maneuver should not be used.

A number of infective complications can result from the presence of a chronically indwelling Foley catheter. These include cystitis and periurethritis resulting from mechanical irritation. A periurethral abscess may follow, with formation of a fistula via eventual rupture of the abscess through the perineal skin. Drainage may also take place through the urethra, with the end result being a urethral diverticulum. Infection may travel up into the prostatic ducts (prostatitis) or seminal vesicles (seminal vesiculitis) and along the vas into the epididymis (epididymitis).

A. Treatment of Pyelonephritis

Episodic renal infection should be treated aggressively with appropriate antibiotics to prevent renal loss. The source and cause of infection should be eliminated if possible.

B. Treatment of Epididymitis

This condition is a complication of either dyssynergic voiding or an indwelling catheter. Treatment consists of appropriate antibiotics, bed rest, and scrotal elevation. The indwelling catheter should be removed or replaced with a suprapubic catheter. Preferred long-term management is to place the patient on an intermittent self-catheterization program. Rarely, ligation of the vas is required.

▶ Hydronephrosis

Two mechanisms lead to back pressure on the kidney. Early, the effect of trigonal stretch secondary to residual urine and detrusor hypertonicity becomes compounded by evolving trigonal hypertrophy. The combination causes abnormal pull on the ureterovesical junction, with increased resistance to the passage of urine. A "functional" obstruction results, which leads to progressive ureteral dilatation and back pressure on the kidney. At this stage, this condition can be relieved by continuous catheter drainage or by combined intermittent catheter drainage and use of anticholinergics.

A delayed consequence of trigonal hypertrophy and detrusor spasticity is reflux due to decompensation of the ureterovesical junction. The causative factor appears to be a combination of high intravesical pressure and trabeculation of the bladder wall. The increased stiffness of the ureterovesical junction weakens its valve-like function, slowly eroding its ability to prevent reflux of urine during forceful bladder contractions.

When ureteral reflux is detected by cystography, previous methods of bladder care must be radically adjusted. An indwelling catheter may manage the problem temporarily. However, if the reflux persists after a reasonable period of drainage, antireflux surgery must be considered. In addition, measures to reduce high intravesical pressure are needed (bladder augmentation, sacral rhizotomy, transurethral resection of the bladder outlet, or sphincterotomy). Progressive hydronephrosis may require nephrostomy. Urinary diversion is a last resort, which should be avoidable if the patient is followed up regularly.

▶ Calculus

A number of factors contribute to stone formation in the bladder and kidneys. Bed rest and inactivity cause demineralization of the skeleton, mobilization of calcium, and subsequent hypercalciuria. Recumbency and inadequate fluid intake both contribute to urinary stasis, possibly with increased concentration of urinary calcium. Catheterization of the neurogenic bladder may introduce bacteria. Subsequent infection is usually due to a urea-splitting organism, which causes the urine to become alkaline, with reduced solubility of calcium and phosphate.

A. Bladder Stones

Because these stones are usually soft, they can be crushed and will wash out through a cystoscope sheath. Occasionally, they are large and need to be removed via a suprapubic cystotomy.

B. Ureteral Stones

Virtually, all ureteral stones can now be removed by endoscopy via antegrade or retrograde retrieval methods or by extracorporeal shock wave lithotripsy (ESWL).

C. Renal Stones

In a patient with neurogenic bladder, kidney stones generally are the result of infection; if the infection is untreated, the stones become the source of persistent renal infection and eventual renal loss. Most of the stones in the renal pelvis can be removed by either a percutaneous endoscopic procedure or ESWL. Occasionally, a large staghorn stone may require open surgery.

Renal Amyloidosis

Secondary amyloidosis of the kidney is a common cause of death in patients with neuropathic bladder. It is a result of chronic debilitation in patients with difficult decubitus ulcers and poorly controlled infection. Fortunately, due to better medical care, this is an uncommon finding today.

Sexual Dysfunction

Men who have had traumatic cord or cauda equina lesions experience varying degrees of sexual dysfunction. Those with upper motor lesions fare well, with the majority having reflexogenic erectile capability. Dangerous elevations in blood pressure can occur with erections in patients with high thoracic or cervical lesions. Problems of quality of erection or premature detumescence are found with all levels of injury. Patients with lower motor lesions are, as a rule, impotent, unless the lesion is incomplete. There is a high degree of variability in the sexual capabilities of patients with all levels of spinal injury. Fortunately, sexual function can be restored to most patients by oral phosphodiesterase type 5 inhibitors, transurethral medications, a vacuum erection device, intracavernous injection, or a penile prosthesis.

Often, patients with spinal injury lose the ability to ejaculate even with preservation of functional erections. This is a result of lost coordination between reflexes normally regulated through higher centers. Patients may have the capability to ejaculate after an erection, but they are either unable to trigger this sexual event or are unable to trigger it in proper sequence. Techniques using vibratory stimulation of the penis or transrectal electrical stimulation have been developed to accomplish semen collection in patients with "functional infertility."

Autonomic Dysreflexia

Autonomic dysreflexia is sympathetically mediated reflex behavior triggered by sacral afferent feedback to the spinal cord. The phenomenon is seen in patients with cord lesions above the sympathetic outflow from the cord (Weaver et al, 2006). As a rule, it occurs in rather spastic lesions above T1 but on occasion in lesions of mild spasticity or those as low as T5. Symptoms include dramatic elevations in systolic or diastolic blood pressure (or both), increased pulse pressure, sweating, bradycardia, headache, and piloerection. It can be triggered by pelvic autonomic afferent activity (overdistention of bowel or bladder, erection) or somatic afferent activity (ejaculation, spasm of lower extremities, insertion of a catheter, dilation of the external urethral sphincter). The

headache can be severe and the hypertension can be life threatening. Treatment must be immediate. Immediate catheterization to empty the bladder usually brings about prompt lowering of blood pressure. Oral nifedipine (20 mg) has been shown to alleviate this syndrome when given 30 minutes before cystoscopy (Dykstra et al, 1987) or electroejaculation (Steinberger et al, 1990). The acute hemodynamic effect can be managed with a parenteral ganglionic blocking agent or alpha-adrenergic blockers. Transurethral sphincterotomy (Perkash, 2007) and peripheral rhizotomy have been used by some to prevent recurring autonomic dysreflexia.

PROGNOSIS

The greater threat to the patient with a neuropathic bladder is progressive renal damage (pyelonephritis, calculosis, and hydronephrosis). Advances in the management of the neuropathic bladder, together with better follow-up of patients at regular intervals, have substantially improved the outlook for long-term survival.

BIBLIOGRAPHY

Abrams P et al: Fourth International Consultation on Incontinence Recommendations of the International Scientific Committee: Evaluation and treatment of urinary incontinence, pelvic organ prolapse, and fecal incontinence. Neurourol Urodyn 2010;29(1): 213–240.

Abrams P et al: The standardisation of terminology in lower urinary tract function: Report from the standardisation sub-committee of the International Continence Society. Urology 2003;61(1):37–49.

Alvares RA et al: Botulinum toxin A in the treatment of spinal cord injury patients with refractory neurogenic detrusor overactivity. Int Braz J Urol 2010;36(6):732–737.

Andersson KE: Antimuscarinic mechanisms and the overactive detrusor: An update. Eur Urol 2010;59(3):377–386.

Andersson KE et al: Pharmacological treatment of overactive bladder: Report from the International Consultation on Incontinence. Curr Opin Urol 2009;19(4):380–394.

Birder L et al: Neural control of the lower urinary tract: Peripheral and spinal mechanisms. Neurourol Urodyn 2010;29(1):128–139.

Bosch J, Groen J: Sacral (S3) segmental nerve stimulation as a treatment for urge incontinence in patients with detrusor instability: Results of chronic electrical stimulation using an implantable neural prosthesis. J Urol 1995;154:504.

Brindley GS: The sacral anterior root stimulator as a means of managing the bladder in patients with spinal cord lesions. Baillieres Clin Neurol 1995;4:1.

Burks FN et al: Neuromodulation and the neurogenic bladder. Urol Clin North Am 2010;37(4):559–565.

Chung E, Cartmill RA: 25-year experience in the outcome of artificial urinary sphincter in the treatment of female urinary incontinence. BJU Int 2010;106(11):1664–1667.

Churchill BM et al: Improved continence in patients with neurogenic sphincteric incompetence with combination tubularized posterior urethroplasty and fascial wrap: The lengthening, narrowing and tightening procedure. J Urol 2010;184(4, Suppl):1763–1767.

Clemens JQ. Afferent neurourology: A novel paradigm. Neurourol Urodyn 2010;29(Suppl 1):S29–S31.

Crowe R et al: Adrenergic innervation of the striated muscle of the intrinsic external urethral sphincter from patients with lower motor spinal cord lesion. J Urol 1989;141:47.

Datta SN et al: Immunohistochemical expression of muscarinic receptors in the urothelium and suburothelium of neurogenic and idiopathic overactive human bladders, and changes with botulinum neurotoxin administration. J Urol 2010;184(6):2578–2585.

Dave S, Salle JL: Current status of bladder neck reconstruction. Curr Opin Urol 2008;18(4):419–424.

de Groat WC, Yoshimura N: Changes in afferent activity after spinal cord injury. Neurourol Urodyn 2010;29(1):63–76.

Duel BP et al: Alternative techniques for augmentation cystoplasty. J Urol 1998;159:998.

Dykstra D et al: The effect of nifedipine on cystoscopy induced autonomic hyperreflexia in patients with high spinal cord injuries. J Urol 1987;138:1155.

Gulur DM, Drake MJ: Management of overactive bladder. Nat Rev Urol 2010;7(10):572–582.

Hanno P et al: Bladder pain syndrome. Med Clin North Am 2011; 95(1):55–73.

Kastler EC et al: Treatment of neurogenic male urinary incontinence related to intrinsic sphincter insufficiency with an artificial urinary sphincter: A French retrospective multicentre study. BJU Int 2010;107(3):426–432.

Lazarus J: Intravesical oxybutynin in the pediatric neurogenic bladder. Nat Rev Urol 2009;6(12):671–674.

Livshits A et al: Reinnervation of the neurogenic bladder in the late period of the spinal cord trauma. Spinal Cord 2004;42(4):211–217.

McGuire EJ, Savastano JA: Long-term followup of spinal cord injury patients managed by intermittent catheterization. J Urol 1983; 129(4):775–776.

Perkash I: Transurethral sphincterotomy provides significant relief in autonomic dysreflexia in spinal cord injured male patients: Long-term followup results. J Urol 2007;177(3):1026–1029.

Pickelsimer E et al: Statewide investigation of medically attended adverse health conditions of persons with spinal cord injury. J Spinal Cord Med 2010;33(3):221–231.

Png KS, Toh KL: Sustained clinical efficacy after repeat intradetrusor botulinum toxin type A in the treatment of neurogenic detrusor overactivity. Ann Acad Med Singapore 2010;39(2):152–153.

Schmidt RA: Advances in genitourinary neurostimulation. Neurosurgery 1986;19:1041.

Smaldone MC et al: Botulinum toxin therapy for neurogenic detrusor overactivity. Urol Clin North Am 2010;37(4):567–580.

Steinberger RE et al: Nifedipine pretreatment for autonomic dysreflexia during electroejaculation. Urology 1990;36(3):228–231.

Tai C et al: Brain switch for reflex micturition control detected by FMRI in rats. J Neurophysiol 2009;102(5):2719–2730.

Tanagho EA, Schmidt RA: Electrical stimulation in the clinical management of the neurogenic bladder. J Urol 1988;140:1331.

Tanagho EA et al: Neural stimulation for control of voiding dysfunction: A preliminary report in 22 patients with serious neuropathic voiding disorders. J Urol 1989;142:340.

Thompson JH et al: Sacral neuromodulation: Therapy evolution. Indian J Urol 2010;26(3):379–384.

Weaver LC et al: Autonomic dysreflexia after spinal cord injury: central mechanisms and strategies for prevention. Prog Brain Res 2006;152:245–263.

Weiss JM: Pelvic floor myofascial trigger points: Manual therapy for interstitial cystitis and the urgency-frequency syndrome. J Urol 2001;166:2226.

Xiao CG et al: An artificial somatic-central nervous system-autonomic reflex pathway for controllable micturition after spinal cord injury: Preliminary results in 15 patients. J Urol 2003;170(4 Pt 1): 1237–1241.

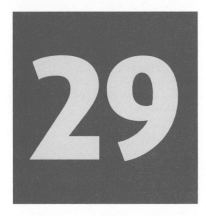

Urodynamic Studies

Sherif R. Absoeif, MD, & Emil A. Tanagho, MD

Urodynamic study is an important part of the evaluation of patients with lower urinary tract obstruction, voiding dysfunctions, urinary incontinence, and neuropathic disorders involving the lower urinary tract. Formerly, the examiner simply observed the act of voiding, noting the strength of the urinary stream, and drawing inferences about the possibility of obstruction of the bladder outlet. In the 1950s, it became possible to observe the lower urinary tract by fluoroscopy during the act of voiding, and in the 1960s, the principles of hydrodynamics were applied to lower urinary tract physiology. In the 1970s, videourodynamic was introduced, where fluoroscopy was incorporated with the pressure measurements to adequately assess both anatomy and function.

The field of urodynamic now has clinical applications in evaluating voiding problems resulting from lower urinary tract disease.

The nomenclature of the tests used in urodynamic studies is not yet settled, and the meanings of urodynamic terms are sometimes overlapping or confusing. In spite of these difficulties, urodynamic tests are extremely valuable. Symptoms elicited by the history or by physical, endoscopic, or even radiographic examination usually delineate the anatomic findings, but the function often must be investigated further by urodynamic tests so that therapy can be devised that is based on an understanding of the altered physiology of the lower urinary tract.

As is true of many high-technology testing procedures (eg, electrocardiography, electroencephalography), urodynamic tests have the greatest clinical validity when their interpretation is left to the treating physician, who should either perform or closely supervise the study or be responsible for correlating all of the findings with personal clinical observations.

FUNCTIONS RELEVANT TO URODYNAMICS AND TESTS APPLICABLE TO EACH

Urodynamic studies in concert with an accurate history and physical examination are the most useful clinical tools available for the evaluation of the lower urinary tract and can provide useful clinical information about the function of the urinary bladder, the sphincteric mechanism, and the voiding pattern itself.

Bladder function. This can be evaluated by simple cystometrogram (CMG) that measures vesical pressure as a function of bladder volume. This can provide important information on cystometric bladder capacity, bladder sensation, bladder compliance, and the presence of involuntary bladder contraction and bladder contractility.

Sphincteric function depends on two elements: the smooth muscle sphincter and the voluntary sphincter. The activity of both elements can be recorded urodynamically by measuring urethral pressure profile or by recording sphincter electromyography.

The act of voiding is a function of the interaction between bladder and sphincter, and the result is the *flow rate*. The flow rate is one major aspect of the total function of the lower urinary tract. It is generally recorded in milliliters per second as well as by total urine volume voided. The simultaneous recording of bladder activity (by intraluminal pressure measurements), sphincteric activity (by electromyography or intraluminal urethral pressure measurements), and flow rate reveals interrelationships among the three elements. Each measurement may give useful information about the normality or abnormality of one specific aspect of lower urinary tract function. A more complete picture is provided by integrating all the three lower tract elements for simultaneous comparison. This comprehensive approach may involve synchronous recordings of variable pressures, flow rate, volume voided, and electrical activity of skeletal musculature around the urinary sphincter (electromyography), along with fluoroscopic imaging of the lower urinary tract. The multiple pressures recorded are quite variable and usually include intravesical pressure, intraurethral pressure at several levels, intra-abdominal pressure, and anal sphincteric pressure as a function of muscular activity of the pelvic floor.

The techniques of urodynamic study must be tailored to the needs of specific patients. Each method has advantages and limitations depending on the requirements of the study. In one patient, results of a single test might be sufficient to establish the diagnosis and suggest appropriate therapy; in another, many more studies might be necessary.

PHYSIOLOGIC AND HYDRODYNAMIC CONSIDERATIONS

URINARY FLOW RATE

Because urinary flow rate is the product of detrusor action against outlet resistance, a variation from the normal flow rate might reflect dysfunction of either. The normal flow rate from a full bladder is about 20–25 mL/s in men and 25–30 mL/s in women. These variations are directly related to the volume voided and the person's age. Obstruction or detrusor dysfunction should be suspected in any adult voiding with a full bladder at a rate of <15 mL/s. A flow rate <10 mL/s is considered definite evidence of obstruction or detrusor dysfunction. Occasionally, one encounters "super-voiders" with flow rates far above the normal range. This may signify low outlet resistance but is of less concern clinically than obstruction. This phenomenon is more commonly seen in women.

▶ Outlet Resistance

Outlet resistance is the primary determinant of flow rate and varies according to mechanical or functional factors.

Functional, outlet resistance is primarily related to sphincteric activity, which is controlled by both the smooth sphincter and the voluntary sphincter. Overactivity of the smooth sphincter is very rare and essentially nonexistent in females. It is rarely seen in men in association with hypertrophy of the bladder neck due to neurogenic dysfunction or distal obstruction. However, such cases must be evaluated before this conclusion is reached.

On the other hand, increased voluntary sphincteric activity is not uncommon. It is often neglected as a primary underlying cause of increased sphincteric resistance. It is manifested either as lack of relaxation or as actual overactivity during voiding. The normal voluntary sphincter provides adequate resistance, along with the smooth sphincter, to prevent escape of urine from the bladder, but it should completely relax during the act of voiding. If the voluntary sphincter does not relax during detrusor contraction, partial functional obstruction occurs. Overactivity of the sphincter, resulting in increased outlet resistance, is usually a neuropathic phenomenon. However, it can also be functional, resulting from irritative phenomena such as infection or other factors—chemical, bacterial, hormonal, or, even more commonly and often not appreciated, psychological and in patients who are infrequent voiders. This is commonly referred to as pelvic floor dysfunction. This is a spectrum of disease that varies from mild difficulty in voiding associated with incomplete emptying and some pelvic/perineal and genital discomfort to extreme cases of urinary retention known as Fowler's syndrome.

▶ Mechanical Outlet Resistance

Mechanical factors resulting in obstruction to urine flow are the easiest to identify by conventional methods. In women, they may take the form of large cystoceles, urethral kinks, or, most commonly, iatrogenic scarring, fibrosis, and compression from previous vaginal or periurethral operative procedures. Mechanical factors in men are well known to all urologists; the classic form is benign prostatic hypertrophy. Urethral stricture from various causes and posterior urethral valves are other common causes of urinary obstruction in men, and there are many others.

Normal voiding with a normal flow rate is the product of both detrusor activity and outlet resistance. Complete sphincteric relaxation usually precedes detrusor contraction by a few seconds, and when relaxation is maximal, detrusor activity starts and is sustained until the bladder is empty. A high intravesical pressure resulting from detrusor contraction is usually an indication of increased outlet resistance and is not necessary to initiate normal voiding.

▶ Variations in Normal Flow Rate

The sequence just described is not essential for normal flow rates. The flow rate may be normal in the absence of any detrusor contraction if sphincteric relaxation is assisted by increased intra-abdominal pressure from straining. Persons with weak outlet resistance and weak sphincteric control can achieve a normal flow rate by complete voluntary sphincteric relaxation without detrusor contraction or straining. A normal flow rate can be achieved in spite of increased sphincteric activity or lack of complete relaxation if detrusor contraction is increased to overcome outlet resistance.

Because a normal flow rate can be achieved in spite of abnormalities of one or more of the mechanisms involved, recording the flow rate alone does not provide insight into the precise mechanisms by which it occurs. Distinction between patterns of flow can be difficult. For practical purposes, if the flow rate is adequate and the recorded pattern and configuration of the flow curve are normal, these variations may not be clinically significant except in rare cases.

▶ Nomenclature

The study of urinary flow rate itself is usually called *uroflowmetry*. The flow rate is generally identified as *maximum flow rate, average flow rate, flow time, maximum flow time* (the time elapsed before maximum flow rate is reached), and *total flow time* (the aggregate of flow time if the flow has been interrupted by periods of no voiding) (Figure 29–1). The *flow rate pattern* is characterized as continuous or intermittent, etc.

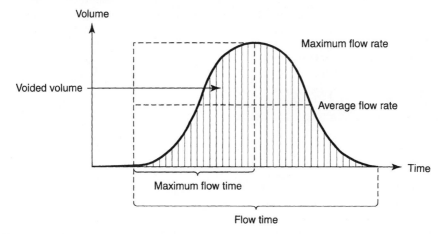

▲ **Figure 29–1.** Uroflowmetry. Basic elements of maximum flow, average flow, total flow time, and total volume voided.

▶ Pattern Measurement of Flow Rate

A normal flow pattern is represented by a bell-shaped curve (Figure 29–1). However, the curve is rarely completely smooth; it may vary within limits and still be normal. Flow rate can be determined by measuring a 5 seconds' collection at the peak of flow and dividing the amount obtained by 5 to arrive at the average rate per second. This rough estimate is useful, especially if the flow rate is normal and the values are above 20 mL/s.

In modern practice, the flow rate is more often recorded electronically: The patient voids into a container on top of a measuring device that is connected to a transducer, the weight being converted to volume and recorded on a chart

in milliliters per second. Figure 29–2 is an example of such a recording from a normal man. The general bell-shaped curve is quite clear, and the tracing shows all of the values discussed previously: total flow time, maximum flow time, maximum flow rate, average flow rate, and total volume voided. Occasional supervoiders can exceed the limits of the chart, but this is usually not of clinical concern (Figure 29–3). A possible variation in the bell appearance is seen in Figure 29–4.

The overall appearance of the flow curve may disclose unsuspected abnormalities. In Figure 29–5, for example, flow time is greatly prolonged. Maximum flow rate may not be low, but the average flow rate is very low—though the maximum flow rate is at one point within the normal range. Such

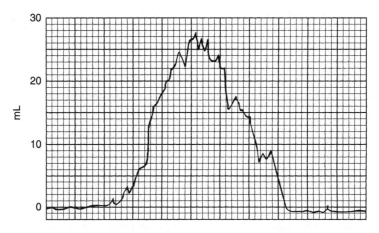

▲ **Figure 29–2.** Classic normal flow rate, with peak of about 30 mL/s and average of about 20 mL/s. On the horizontal scale, one large square equals 5 seconds.

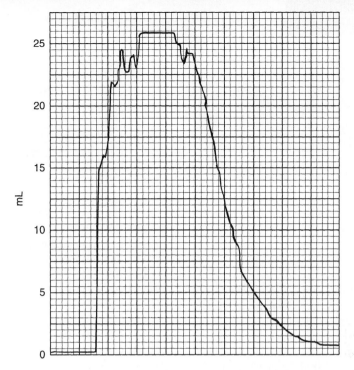

▲ **Figure 29–3.** Flow rate of "supervoider." Maximum flow rate exceeds limits of chart. Tracing shows fast buildup and complete bladder emptying of large volume of urine in a very short period. On the horizontal scale, one large square equals 5 seconds.

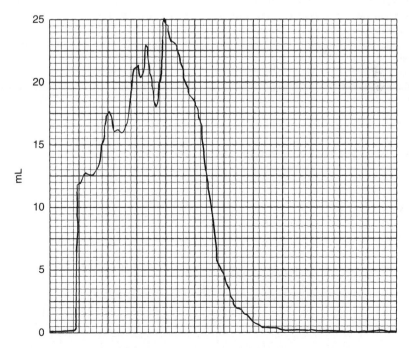

▲ **Figure 29–4.** Normal flow rate with some variation in appearance of curve. Note the rapid pressure rise but progressive increase to maximum, followed by a sharp drop. There is also fluctuation in ascending limb of tracing. On the horizontal scale, one large square equals 5 seconds.

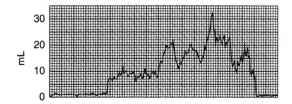

▲ **Figure 29–5.** Rather low flow rate (not exceeding 10 mL/s), yet at one point, the peak reaches 27–32 mL/s. Note again fluctuation in flow. On the horizontal scale, one large square equals 5 seconds.

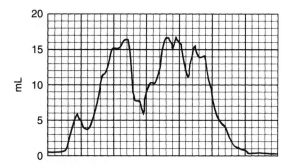

▲ **Figure 29–6.** Very low flow rate of short duration and small volume. Note that maximum flow is not >15 mL/s; however, flow average is <10 mL/s, and flow is almost completely interrupted in the middle. On the horizontal scale, one large square equals 5 seconds.

fluctuation in flow rate is most commonly related to variations in voluntary sphincteric activity. In Figure 29–6, this pattern is extreme: Maximum flow rate never exceeds 15 mL/s, and average flow rate is about 10 mL/s, which is indicative of obstruction. (Again, this fluctuation in pattern probably reflects sphincteric hyperactivity.)

The flow rate pattern reveals a great deal about the forces involved. For example, if the patient is voiding without the aid of detrusor contractions—primarily by straining—this can be easily deduced from the pattern of the flow rate. Figure 29–7 shows an example of intermittent voiding, primarily by straining, with no detrusor activity, and at a rate that sometimes does not reach the usual peaks. With experience, one becomes expert at detecting the mechanisms underlying abnormalities in flow rate. For example, in Figure 29–5, the maximum flow rate is in the normal range, the average flow rate is slightly low, and the curve has a general bell pattern, yet brief partial intermittent obstructions to flow can be readily interpreted as due to overactivity of the voluntary sphincter, a mild form of detrusor/sphincter dyssynergia (see discussion following).

Flow rates in mechanical obstruction are totally different, classically in the range of 5–6 mL/s; flow time is greatly prolonged, and there is sustained low flow with minimal variation (Figure 29–8). Figure 29–9 is a striking example of a curve for a patient with benign prostatic hypertrophy. No simultaneous studies are needed with such a pattern, since the pattern is obviously one of mechanical obstructions.

Reduced flow rate in the absence of mechanical obstruction is due to some impairment of sphincteric or detrusor activity. This is seen in a variety of conditions, for example, normal detrusor contraction with no associated sphincteric relaxation and normal detrusor contraction with sphincteric overactivity, which is more serious. These two entities are commonly referred to as *detrusor/sphincter dyssynergia*. If with detrusor contraction the sphincter does not relax and open up or (worse) if it becomes overactive, urine flow is obstructed (ie, flow rate is reduced and of abnormal pattern). Reduced flow rate may occur even with increased detrusor activity if the latter is not adequate to overcome sphincteric resistance.

So many variations are possible in the shape of the flow curve—no matter how accurately the flow is recorded or how often the study is repeated to confirm abnormal findings—that it is beneficial to relate it to simultaneous recordings,

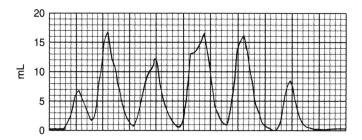

▲ **Figure 29–7.** Classic flow rate due to abdominal straining with no detrusor activity. See effect of spurts of urine with complete interruption between them; patient cannot sustain increased intra-abdominal pressure. On the horizontal scale, one large square equals 5 seconds.

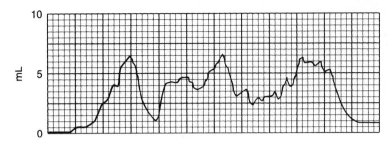

▲ **Figure 29–8.** Flow rate in a case of urinary obstruction showing very low average flow rate (not above 5 or 6 mL/s). Prolonged duration of flow is associated with incomplete emptying. On the horizontal scale, one large square equals 5 seconds.

such as of bladder pressure, pelvic floor electromyography, urethral pressure profile, or simply cinefluoroscopy. Nevertheless, by itself it can be one of the most valuable urodynamic studies undertaken to evaluate a specific type of voiding dysfunction. Flowmetry is not only of diagnostic value but also of valuable in follow-up studies and in deciding on treatment. In some cases, however, flowmetry alone does not provide enough data about the abnormality in the voiding mechanism. More information must then be obtained by evaluation of bladder function.

BLADDER FUNCTION

The basic factors of normal bladder function are bladder capacity, compliance, sensation, contractility, voluntary control, and response to drugs. All of them can be evaluated by cystometry. If all are within the normal range, bladder physiology can be assumed to be normal. Evaluation of every factor has its own implication and, before a definitive conclusion is reached, must be examined in the light of associated manifestations and findings.

Cystometry can be done by either of two basic methods: (1) allowing physiologic filling of the bladder with secreted urine and continuously recording the intravesical pressure throughout a voiding cycle (starting the recording when the patient's bladder is empty and continuing it until the bladder has been filled—at which time the patient is asked to urinate—and voiding begins) or (2) by filling the bladder with

water and recording the intravesical pressure against the volume of water introduced into the bladder.

With the first (physiologic filling) method, the assessment of bladder function is based on voided volume (assuming that the presence of residual urine has been ruled out). The second method permits accurate determination of the volume distending the bladder and of the pressures at each level of filling, yet it has inherent defects: fluid is introduced rather than naturally secreted, and bladder filling occurs more rapidly than it normally does.

▶ Bladder Capacity, Compliance, and Sensation

Bladder capacity: The maximum cystometric bladder capacity is the volume at which the patient feels he/she can no longer delay micturition, uninhibited detrusor contraction occurs leading to micturition or the intravesical pressure rises and the patient leaks. This is different from functional bladder capacity which is the maximum volume that the patient normally void. This is usually more relevant and is assessed from a voiding diary.

▶ Bladder Compliance (Accommodation)

Bladder compliance reflects the ability of the bladder wall to expand to capacity with minimal changes in intravesical pressure. This expansile capability is contributed to by the smooth muscular, collagenous, and elastic components of the

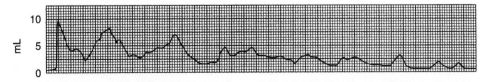

▲ **Figure 29–9.** Classic low flow rate of bladder outlet obstruction (benign prostatic hypertrophy), markedly prolonged flow time, and fluctuation due to attempt at improving flow by increasing intra-abdominal pressure. On the horizontal scale, one large square equals 5 seconds.

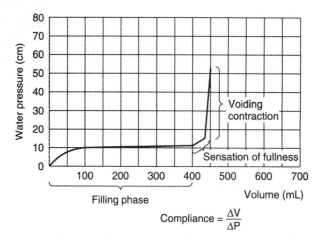

▲ **Figure 29–10.** Cystometrogram of patient with normal bladder capacity. Note the stable intravesical pressure during filling phase; slight rise at end of filling phase, indicating bladder capacity perceived as sense of fullness; and sharp rise at end (voiding contraction).

bladder submucosa and muscularis. The normally innervated bladder without any coexistent pathologic lesions retains this vesicoelastic capability during the storage phase of bladder activity.

The CMG (Figure 29–10) is obtained during the phase of bladder filling; the volume of fluid in the bladder is plotted against the intravesical pressure to show bladder wall compliance to filling. The normal cystometric curve shows a fairly constant low intravesical pressure until the bladder nears capacity, then a moderate rise until capacity is reached, and then a sharp rise as voiding is initiated. Normally, the sensation of fullness is first perceived when the bladder contains 100–200 mL of fluid and strongly felt as the bladder nears capacity; the desire to void occurs when the bladder is full (normal capacity, 400–500 mL). However, the bladder has a power of accommodation; that is, it can maintain an almost constant low intraluminal pressure throughout its filling phase regardless of the volume of fluid present, and this directly influences compliance. As the bladder progressively accommodates larger volumes with no change in intraluminal pressure, the compliance values become higher (compliance = volume/pressure) (Figure 29–10).

▶ Contractility and Voluntary Control

The bladder normally shows no evidence of contractility or activity during the filling phase. However, once it is filled to capacity and the patient perceives the desire to urinate and consciously allows urination to proceed, strong bladder contractions occur and are sustained until the bladder is empty. The patient can of course consciously inhibit detrusor contraction. Both of these aspects of voluntary detrusor control must be assessed during cystometric study in order to rule out uninhibited bladder activity and to determine whether

the patient can inhibit urination with a full bladder and initiate urination when asked to do so. The latter is occasionally difficult to verify clinically because of conscious inhibition by a patient who may be embarrassed by the unnatural circumstances.

▶ Responses to Drugs

Drugs are being used with increasing frequency in the evaluation of detrusor function. They can help to diagnose underlying neuropathy and to determine whether drug treatment might be of value in individual cases. Study of the relationship of bladder capacity to intravesical pressure and bladder contractility gives a rough evaluation of the patient's bladder function. Low intravesical pressure with normal bladder capacity might not be significant, whereas low pressure with a very large capacity might imply sensory loss or a flaccid lower motor neuron lesion, a chronically distended bladder, or a large bladder due to myogenic damage. High pressure (usually associated with reduced capacity) that rises rapidly with bladder filling is most commonly due to inflammation, enuresis, or reduced bladder capacity. However, uninhibited bladder activity during this high-pressure filling phase might indicate neuropathic bladder or an upper motor neuron lesion.

The parasympathetic drug bethanechol chloride (Urecholine) is often used to assess bladder muscle function in patients with low bladder pressure associated with lack of detrusor contraction. No response to bethanechol suggests myogenic damage; a normal response indicates a bladder of large capacity with normal musculature; and an exaggerated response indicates a lower motor neuron lesion. The test has so many variables that it must be done meticulously to give reliable results.

Testing with anticholinergic drugs or muscle depressants may be helpful in the evaluation of uninhibited detrusor contraction or increased bladder tonus and low compliance. The information thus obtained can be useful in choosing drugs for treatment.

▶ Recording of Intravesical Pressure

Intravesical pressure can be measured directly from the vesical cavity, either by a suprapubic approach or via a transurethral catheter. The pressure inside the bladder is actually a function of both intra-abdominal and intravesical pressure. Thus, true detrusor pressure is the pressure recorded from the bladder cavity (intravesical pressure) minus intraabdominal pressure. This point is important because variations in intra-abdominal pressure may alter the recorded intravesical pressure, and if the recorded intravesical pressure is mistakenly considered to reflect only detrusor pressure and not increased intra-abdominal pressure due to straining as well, erroneous conclusions may be reached.

Whenever possible, intra-abdominal pressure should be recorded simultaneously with intravesical pressure, since there is no other way to determine the true detrusor pressure. Intra-abdominal pressure is usually recorded by a small balloon catheter inserted high in the rectum and connected to a separate transducer.

The most valuable part of the cystometric study is the determination of voiding activity or voiding contraction. The characteristics of intravesical pressure can be quite significant. Normally, voiding contractions are not high (20–40 cm of water); this magnitude of intravesical pressure is generally adequate to deliver a normal flow rate of 20–30 mL/s and completely empty the bladder if it is well sustained. A higher voiding pressure is indicative of possible increase in outlet resistance yet denotes an overactive, healthy detrusor musculature. Figure 29–11 shows a normal flow rate associated with normal detrusor contraction at a magnitude of 20 cm of water that is well sustained and of short duration and results in complete bladder emptying.

The quality of bladder pressure can also be informative, even without simultaneous recording of flow rate. In such cases, however, it is preferable to record flow rate under normal circumstances. A well-sustained detrusor contraction, high at initiation and sustained at normal values, is seen in Figure 29–12. In Figure 29–13, the voiding pressure is too high—there is an element of sphincteric dyssynergia triggering variations in voiding pressures and flow rate. Simultaneous recording of bladder and intra-abdominal pressures would provide more information. As suggested previously, recording the intravesical pressure alone does not give as much information as may be required, and increased intra-abdominal pressure might be mistaken for detrusor action. This situation is illustrated in Figure 29–14. The bladder pressure appears to indicate good detrusor function; nevertheless, simultaneous recording of intra-abdominal pressure

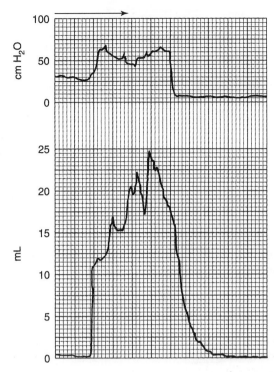

▲ **Figure 29–11.** Simultaneous recording of voiding contraction and resulting flow rate. Note the normal range of intravesical pressure during voiding phase as well as adequate normal flow rate (shown in Figure 29–4). On the horizontal scale, one large square equals 5 seconds.

makes it clear that all of the apparent changes in vesical intraluminal pressure in fact represent variations in intra-abdominal pressure.

Figure 29–15 shows the two pressures recorded on the same chart, on the same channel, by having the writing pen share the time between two transducers—one recording intra-abdominal pressure; the other, intravesical pressure.

A. Pathologic Changes in Bladder Capacity

The bladder capacity is normally 400–500 mL, but it can be reduced or increased in a variety of disorders and lesions (Table 29–1). Some common causes of reduced bladder capacity are enuresis, urinary tract infection, contracted bladder, upper motor neuron lesion, and defunctionalized bladder. Reduced capacity also may occur in association with incontinence and in postsurgical bladder. Increased bladder capacity is not uncommon in women who have trained themselves to retain large volumes of urine. Bladder capacity is increased also in sensory neuropathic disorders, lower motor neuron lesions, and chronic obstruction from myogenic damage. It is important to relate bladder capacity to the

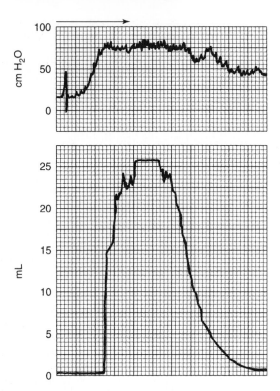

▲ **Figure 29–12.** Recording of bladder pressure simultaneously with flow rate. Note the slightly higher intravesical pressure with high flow rate, which, at its maximum, is that of a supervoider (see Figure 29–3). On the horizontal scale, one large square equals 5 seconds.

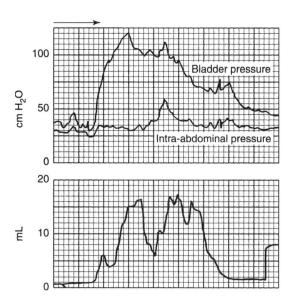

▲ **Figure 29–13.** Simultaneous recording of flow rate and intra-abdominal pressure; intravesical pressure overlap in top recording. Note the very high voiding pressure. However, flow rate is relatively low, with some interruption most likely due to sphincteric overactivity. On the horizontal scale, one large square equals 5 seconds.

intravesical pressure (Table 29–2). Slight variations in bladder capacity with no change in bladder pressure might be of less significance than the reverse. What is usually of greatest significance is the bladder with reduced capacity associated with normal pressure or, more important, with increased pressure, or the bladder with large capacity associated with decreased pressure.

B. Pathologic Changes in Accommodation (Compliance)

Compliance is a measurement of the elasticity of the bladder wall and usually reflects change in intravesical pressure in response to filling. In a bladder with normal compliance—in which case the micturition center of the spinal cord is controlled by the central nervous system—intravesical pressure does not vary with progressive bladder filling until capacity is reached; in other words, when compliance is reduced secondary to fibrosis of the bladder wall, there will be a progressive increase in intravesical pressure and loss of accommodation. This usually occurs at smaller volumes and

with reduced capacity. Poor compliance can be seen in cases of long-standing urinary obstruction or iatrogenically after extensive pelvic surgery.

The patient being studied by cystometry can always note the presence or absence of a sensation of fullness. One

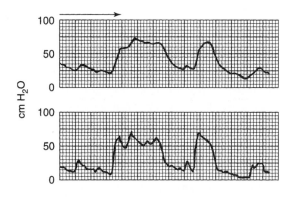

▲ **Figure 29–14.** Simultaneous recording of intra-abdominal and intravesical pressures. If one considers only intravesical pressure (**upper recording**), one might assume adequate detrusor contraction. Comparison with intra-abdominal pressure (**lower recording**) shows that they are almost identical and that there is no detrusor contraction at all.

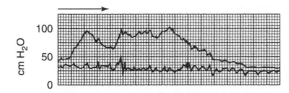

▲ **Figure 29–15.** Simultaneous recording of two measurements—intravesical pressure (**top**) and intra-abdominal pressure (**bottom**)—on a single channel. The difference between the two can be clearly seen as pure detrusor contraction.

normally does not sense volumes in the bladder but only changes in pressure.

Compliance plays a crucial role in the long-term function of the upper urinary tract. The direct effect of intravesical pressure on ureteral urine transport and the long-term effects from the elevated pressure are significant.

C. Pathologic Changes in Sensation

A slight rise in intravesical pressure on cystometry signifies that the bladder is full to normal capacity and that the patient is perceiving it. This sign is usually absent in pure sensory neuropathy and in mixed sensory and motor loss. (Other sensations can be tested for in different ways; see Chapter 26.)

D. Pathologic Changes in Contractility

The bladder is normally capable of sustaining contraction until it is empty. Absence of residual urine after voiding usually denotes well-sustained contractions. Neuropathic dysfunction is usually associated with residual urine of variable amount depending on the type of dysfunction. Significant outlet resistance—mechanical or functional—is also a cause of residual urine.

Table 29–1. Causes of reduced or increased bladder capacity.

Causes of reduced bladder capacity
Enuresis or incontinence
Bladder infections
Bladder contracture due to fibrosis (from tuberculosis, interstitial cystitis, etc)
Upper motor neuron lesions
Defunctionalized bladder
Postsurgical bladder
Neuropathic disorders
Lower motor neuron lesions
Megacystis (congenital)
Chronic urinary tract obstruction

Note: Normal capacity in adults is 400–500 mL.

Table 29–2. Relationship between intravesical pressure and capacity in various diseases.

Low intravesical pressure
Normal capacity
Large capacity
Sensory deficits (diabetes mellitus, tabes dorsalis)
Flaccid lower motor neuron lesions
Large bladder (due to repeated stretching)
High intravesical pressure
Rapidly rising
Reduced capacity
Inflammation
Enuresis
Uninhibited contraction
Uninhibited neurogenic bladder
Upper motor neuron lesions

Cystometric study may disclose complete absence of detrusor contractility due to motor or sensory deficits or conscious inhibition of detrusor activity (Table 29–3). Detrusor hyperactivity is shown as uninhibited activity, usually due to interruption of the neural connection between spinal cord centers and the higher inhibitory midbrain and cortical centers.

An integrated picture of bladder capacity, intravesical pressure, and contractility is useful for general assessment of the basic physiologic mechanisms of the bladder. Low intravesical pressure in a patient with normal bladder capacity may have no clinical significance, whereas low pressure with a very large capacity may signify sensory loss or a flaccid lower motor neuron lesion, a chronically distended bladder, or a large bladder due to myogenic damage. High pressure (usually associated with reduced capacity) that rises rapidly with bladder filling is most commonly associated with inflammation, enuresis, or reduced bladder capacity. However, uninhibited activity during the interval of rising pressure that occurs with bladder filling may indicate a neurogenic bladder or an upper motor neuron lesion.

Table 29–3. Variations in detrusor contractility in various diseases.

Normal contractions
Normal volume
Well-sustained contractions
Absent or weak contractions
Sensory neuropathic disorders
Conscious inhibition of contractions
Lower motor neuron lesions
Uninhibited contractions
Upper motor neuron lesions
Cerebrovascular lesions

SPHINCTERIC FUNCTION

Urinary sphincteric function can be evaluated either by recording the electromyographic activity of the voluntary component of the sphincteric mechanism or by recording the activity of both smooth and voluntary components by measuring the intraurethral pressure of the sphincteric unit. The latter method is called *pressure profile measurement (profilometry)*. With the use of videourodynamic, abdominal/Valsalva leak point pressure (ALPP) is another way to evaluate the sphincteric function: This test measures the ability of the urethra to resist abdominal pressure as an expulsive force. This will be discussed more in Section "Videourodynamic."

▶ Profilometry

The urethral pressure profile is determined by recording the pressure in the urethra at every level of the sphincteric unit from the internal meatus to the end of the sphincteric segment. Water profilometry, which requires a flow rate of about 2 mL/min, gives fairly accurate results. It may be used for screening patients with incontinence or functional obstruction, but it is not very sensitive and only provides information about total urethral pressure. The membrane catheter and microtransducer techniques of profilometry described in the following sections provide much more accurate and detailed information.

A. Membrane Catheter Technique

Membrane catheters used for recording pressure profiles usually have several channels, so several measurements can be obtained simultaneously. One such catheter used at UCSF has four lumens and an outside diameter of 7F. Two of the four lumens are open at the end, one for bladder filling and the other for recording bladder pressure; the other two lumens, which are situated 7 cm and 8 cm from the catheter tip, are covered by a thin membrane with a small chamber underneath (Figure 29–16). The space under the membrane and the lumen connected to it are filled with fluid, free of any gas, and connected to a pressure transducer. The pressure under this membrane should be zero at the level of the transducer so that it can register any pressure applied to the membrane whatever its level at any time. The catheter also has radiopaque markers at 1-cm intervals starting at the tip, with a heavier marker every 5 cm; it also has a special marker showing the site of each membrane. The markers permit fluoroscopic visualization of the catheter and the membrane levels during the entire study.

B. Microtransducer Technique

The results of microtransducer profilometry are as accurate as those obtained with the membrane catheter. Two microtransducers can be mounted on the same catheter, one at the tip for recording of bladder pressure and the other about 5–7 cm from the tip to record the urethral pressure profile as

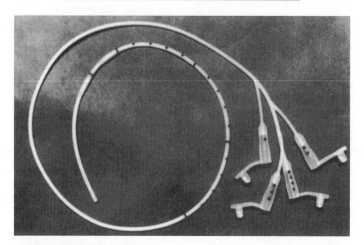

▲ **Figure 29–16.** Membrane catheter showing radiopaque markers. Note the two membrane chambers for urethral pressure measurements and four separate channels—two channels for urethral pressure recording, one for bladder pressure recording, and one for bladder filling—each of which is connected to a separate ending. (Reproduced, with permission, from Tanagho EA, Jonas U: Membrane catheter: Effective for recording pressure in lower urinary tract. Urology 1977;10:173.)

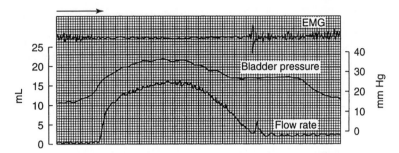

▲ **Figure 29–17.** Simultaneous recording of bladder pressure, flow rate, and electromyography of anal sphincter. With rise in bladder pressure for voiding, start of flow rate has a smooth, continuous, bell-shaped curve. Note also the complete absence of electromyographic activity of the anal sphincter throughout the voiding act. On the horizontal scale, one large square equals 5 seconds.

the catheter is gradually withdrawn from the bladder cavity to below the sphincteric segment.

▶ Electromyographic Study of Sphincteric Function

Electromyography alone gives useful information about sphincteric function, but it is most valuable when done in conjunction with cystometry. There are several techniques for electromyographic studies of the urinary sphincter: either surface electrodes or needle electrodes are used. Surface electrode recordings can be obtained either from the lumen of the urethra in the region of the voluntary sphincter or, preferably, from the anal sphincter by using an anal plug electrode. Recording via needle electrodes can be obtained from the anal sphincter, from the bulk of the musculature of the pelvic floor, or from the external sphincter itself, though in the latter case, the placement is difficult and the accuracy of the results is questionable.

Direct needle electromyography of the urethral sphincter provides the most accurate information. Because the technique is difficult, however, simpler approaches are generally used. The anal sphincter is readily accessible for electromyographic testing, and testing of any area of the pelvic floor musculature generally reflects the overall electrical activity of the pelvic floor, including the external sphincter. Electromyography is not simple, and the assistance of an experienced electromyographer is probably essential. Electromyographic study makes use of the electrical activity that is constantly present within the pelvic floor and external urinary sphincter at rest and that increases progressively with bladder filling. If the bladder contracts for voiding, electrical activity ceases completely, permitting free flow of urine, and is resumed at the termination of detrusor contraction to secure closure of the bladder outlet (Figure 29–17). Electromyography is important in showing this effect and, along with bladder pressure measurement, can pinpoint the exact time of detrusor contraction. Persistence of electromyographic activity during the phase of detrusor contraction for voiding—or, even worse, its overactivity during that phase—interferes with the voiding mechanism and leads to in coordination between detrusor and sphincter (*detrusor/sphincter dyssynergia*). During the interval of detrusor contraction, increased electromyographic activity interferes with the free flow of urine, as can be shown by simultaneous recording of flow rate.

Electromyographic recording shows only the activity of the voluntary component of the urinary sphincteric mechanism and the overall activity of the pelvic floor. More information is gained when the electromyogram is recorded simultaneously with detrusor pressure or flow rate. However, this method gives no information about the smooth component of the urinary sphincter.

▶ Pressure Measurement for Evaluation of Sphincteric Function

Perfusion profilometry, usually performed with the patient supine and with an empty bladder, provides a simple pressure profile that allows determination of the maximum pressure within the urethra. This is adequate for screening patients with incontinence or functional obstruction. However, in order to determine the maximum closure pressure (see section following), the bladder pressure must be recorded simultaneously with the urethral pressure profile. Such simultaneous recording is not possible with perfusion profilometry.

The membrane catheter and microtransducer techniques of profilometry, because they use multichannel recording, routinely provide much more detailed information; at least four distinct sets of measurements can be obtained from the simplest pressure profile made using the membrane catheter or microtransducer (Figure 29–18): (1) the maximum pressure exerted around the sphincteric segment, (2) the net closure pressure of the urethra, (3) the distribution of this closure pressure along the entire length of the sphincter, and (4) the exact functional length of the sphincteric unit and its relation to the anatomic length.

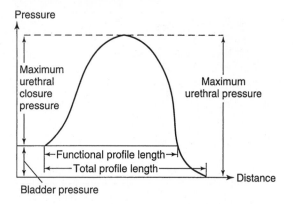

▲ **Figure 29–18.** Urethral pressure profile and its components. Note the functional length, anatomic length, and the shape of the profile, with maximum closure pressure in the middle segment of the urethra rather than at the level of the internal meatus. (Reproduced, with permission, from Bradley W: Cystometry and sphincter electromyography. Mayo Clin Proc 1976;329:335.)

A. Total Pressure

The urethral pressure profile recording shows the pressure directly recorded within the urethral lumen along the entire length of the urethra from internal to external meatus. From this measurement, the maximum pressure exerted around the sphincteric segment can be determined.

B. Closure Pressure

The urethral closure pressure is the difference between intravesical pressure (bladder pressure) and urethral pressure, that is, the net closure pressure. The *maximum closure pressure* is the most important measurement in evaluating the activity of the sphincteric unit and its responses to various factors.

C. Distribution of Closure Pressure

As the catheter is withdrawn down the urethra, the closure pressure at various levels along the entire length of the sphincteric segment is recorded.

D. Functional Length of Sphincteric Unit

The functional length of the sphincteric unit is the portion with positive closure pressure, that is, where urethral pressure is greater than bladder pressure. The distinction between anatomic length and functional length is important. Regardless of the anatomic length, the effectiveness of the urethral sphincter may be limited to a shorter segment. In women, the pressure is normally rather low at the level of the internal meatus but builds up gradually until it reaches its maximum in the midurethra, where the voluntary sphincter is concentrated; it

slowly drops until it is at its lowest at the external meatus. On the basis of these measurements, it is clear that the anatomic and functional lengths of the normal urethra in women are about the same and that the maximum closure pressure is at about the center of the urethra—not at the level of the internal meatus. In men, the pressure profile is slightly different: the functional length is longer, and the maximum closure pressure builds up in the prostatic segment, reaches a peak in the membranous urethra, and drops as it reaches the level of the bulbous urethra (Figure 29–19). The entire functional length in men is about 6–7 cm; in women, it is about 4 cm.

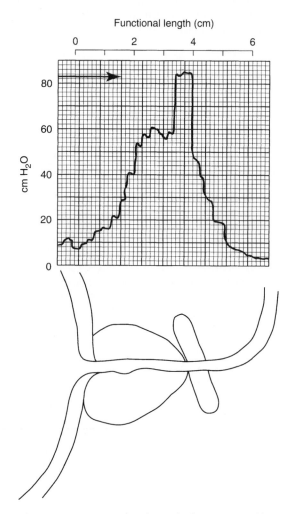

▲ **Figure 29–19.** Normal male urethral pressure profile showing progressive rise throughout prostatic segment and peak being reached in membranous urethra. (Reproduced, with permission, from Tanagho EA: Membrane and microtransducer catheters: Their effectiveness for profilometry of the lower urinary tract. Urol Clin North Am 1979;6:110.)

Dynamic Changes in Pressure Profile

The usefulness of the pressure profile is enhanced if the examiner notes the sphincteric responses to various physiologic stimuli: (1) postural changes (supine, sitting, and standing), (2) changes in intra-abdominal pressure (sharp increase with coughing; sustained increase with bearing down), (3) voluntary contractions of the pelvic floor musculature to assess activity of the voluntary sphincter, and (4) bladder filling. The latter test consists of making baseline recordings with both an empty bladder and a full bladder and comparing these recordings with recordings made under conditions of stress (coughing, bearing down) and during voluntary contraction with an empty bladder and a full bladder.

A simple pressure profile is informative but does not provide data that will delineate and identify specific sites of sphincteric dysfunction. The advantage of using a membrane catheter or microtransducer is that the pressure profile can be expanded by slowing down the rate of withdrawal of the catheter and speeding up the motion of the recording paper. Since the catheter can be held at different levels for any length of time, other tests can be made and their effects monitored. Response to stress (particularly when standing), response to bladder distention, response to changes in position, the effects of drugs, and the effects of nerve stimulation can all be evaluated if needed. Bladder filling normally leads to increase in tonus of the sphincteric element, with some rise in closure pressure, especially when bladder filling approaches maximum capacity. Stress from coughing or straining also normally results in sustained or increased closure pressure (Figure 29–20). When the patient stands up, closure pressure is usually substantially increased (Figure 29–21). Testing for activity of the voluntary sphincter by the hold maneuver (asking the patient to actively contract the perineal muscles) produces a significant rise in urethral pressure (Figure 29–22). When the effects of all of these responses are recorded concomitantly with intravesical pressure, the data can be interrelated and the exact closure pressure at any given time can be ascertained.

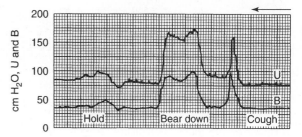

▲ **Figure 29–20.** Simultaneous recording of intraurethral (U) and intravesical (B) pressures and their responses to coughing and bearing down. Rise in intravesical pressure as a result of increase in intra-abdominal pressure is associated with simultaneous rise in intraurethral pressure, maintaining a constant closure pressure.

The response to stress with the patient standing usually should also be recorded. Especially in cases of stress incontinence, weakness of the sphincteric mechanism may not be apparent with the patient sitting or supine but becomes clear when the patient stands up.

The effectiveness of drugs in increasing or reducing the urethral pressure profile can also be tested. For example, phenoxybenzamine (Regitine) can be administered and the urethral pressure profile recorded; a drop in pressure indicates that alpha-blockers may be an effective means of decreasing urethral resistance, with obvious implications for the management of urinary obstruction. Anticholinergic drugs can be tested for possible use as detrusor depressants. Detrusor activity can be investigated by administering bethanechol chloride (Urecholine) and simultaneously recording bladder and urethral pressures.

Characteristics of Normal Pressure Profile (Figure 29–23)

The basic features of the ideal pressure profile are not easily defined. In women, the normal urethral pressure profile has a

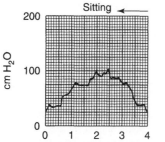 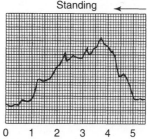

▲ **Figure 29–21.** Urethral pressure profile of normal woman in sitting and standing positions. Note the marked improvement in closure pressure (in both functional length and magnitude) when patient stands up. (Reproduced, with permission, from Tanagho EA: Urodynamics of female urinary incontinence with emphasis on stress incontinence. J Urol 1979;122:200.)

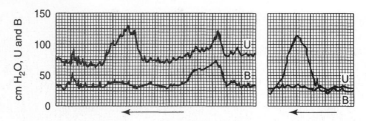

▲ **Figure 29–22.** ***Right:*** Urethral pressure profile in normal range. U, urethra; B, bladder. ***Left:*** Main point of effect of hold maneuver is significant increase in closure pressure of urethra (U) without change in bladder pressure (B)—act of voluntary sphincter.

peak of 100–120 cm of water and the closure pressure is in the range of 90–100 cm of water. Closure pressure is lowest at the level of the internal meatus, gradually builds up in the proximal 0.5 cm, and reaches its maximum about 1 cm below the internal meatus. It is sustained for another 2 cm and then starts to drop in the distal urethra. The functional length of a normal adult female urethra is about 4 cm. The response to stress with coughing and bearing down is sustained or augmented closure pressure. Standing up also increases this pressure, with maximum rise in the midsegment.

▶ Pressure Profile in Pathologic Conditions

A. Urinary Stress Incontinence

The classic pressure changes noted in this type of incontinence are as follows:

1. Low urethral closure pressure.
2. Short urethral functional length at the expense of the proximal segment.

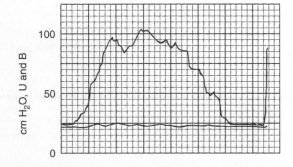

▲ **Figure 29–23.** Recording of normal female urethral pressure profile, showing basic features and actual values, including anatomic as well as functional length. U, urethra; B, bladder. (Reproduced, with permission, from Tanagho EA: Membrane and microtransducer catheters: Their effectiveness for profilometry of the lower urinary tract. Urol Clin North Am 1979;6:110.)

3. Weak responses to stress.
4. Loss of urethral closure pressure with bladder filling.
5. Fall in closure pressure on assuming the upright position.
6. Weak responses to stress in the upright position.

B. Urinary Urge Incontinence

The most pertinent pressure changes in urinary urge incontinence are normal or high closure pressures with normal responses to stress, normal responses to bladder filling, and normal responses when the patient stands up. Urge incontinence can result from any of the following mechanisms (Figure 29–24):

1. Detrusor overactivity, with active detrusor contractions overcoming urethral resistance and leading to urine leakage.
2. The exact reverse, that is, a constant detrusor pressure with no evidence of detrusor overactivity but with urethral instability in that urethral pressure becomes less than bladder pressure, so that urine leakage occurs without any detrusor contraction.
3. A combination of the two preceding mechanisms (the most common form), that is, some drop in closure pressure and some rise in bladder pressure. In such cases, the drop in urethral pressure is often the initiating factor.

C. Combination of Stress and Urge Incontinence

In this common clinical condition, profilometry is used to determine the magnitude of each component, that is, whether the incontinence is primarily urge, primarily stress, or both equally. As a guide to treatment, profilometric studies sometimes show that stress incontinence precipitates urge incontinence. The stress elements initiate urine leakage in the proximal urethra, exciting detrusor response and sphincteric relaxation and ending with complete urine leakage. Once the stress components are corrected, the urge element disappears. This combination cannot be detected clinically.

D. Postprostatectomy Incontinence

After prostatectomy, there is usually no positive pressure in the entire prostatic fossa, minimal closure pressure at the

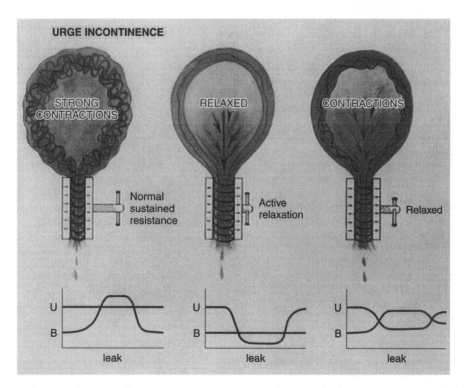

▲ **Figure 29–24.** Three mechanisms of urinary urge incontinence. **Left:** Normal sphincter activity exceeded by hyperactive detrusor. **Center:** Normal detrusor, without any overactivity, yet unstable urethra with marked drop in urethral pressure leading to leakage. **Right:** Most common combination—some rise in intravesical pressure due to detrusor hyperirritability associated with drop in urethral pressure due to sphincteric relaxation. U, urethra; B, bladder.

apex of the prostate, and normal or greater than normal pressure within the voluntary sphincteric segment of the membranous urethra. It is the functional length of the sphincteric segment above the genitourinary diaphragm that determines the degree of incontinence; the magnitude of closure pressure in the voluntary sphincteric segment has no bearing on the patient's symptoms. High pressure is almost always recorded within the voluntary sphincter despite the common belief that what someone termed "iatrogenically induced incontinence" is due to damage to the voluntary sphincter—which is definitely not the case.

E. Detrusor/Sphincter Dyssynergia

In this situation, findings of cystometric studies are normal at the filling phase, with possible closure pressure above average. However, the pathologic entity becomes clear when the patient attempts to void: Detrusor contraction is associated with a simultaneous increase in urethral closure pressure instead of a drop in pressure. This is a direct effect of overactivity of the voluntary component, leading to obstructive voiding or low flow rate and frequent interruption of

voiding. This phenomenon is commonly seen in patients with supraspinal lesions. It can be encountered in several other conditions as well.

▶ Value of Simultaneous Recordings

Measurement of each of the physiologic variables described previously gives useful clinical information. A rise in intravesical pressure has greater significance when related to intra-abdominal pressure. The urine flow rate is more significant if recorded in conjunction with the total volume voided as well as with evidence of detrusor contraction. The urethral pressure profile is more significant when related to bladder pressure and to variations in intra-abdominal pressure and voluntary muscular activity. And for greatest clinical usefulness, all data must be recorded simultaneously so that the investigator can analyze the activity involved in each sequence.

At a minimum, a proper urodynamic study should include recordings of intravesical pressure and intra-abdominal pressure (true detrusor pressure is intravesical pressure minus intra-abdominal pressure), urethral pressure or electromyography, flow rate, and, if possible, voided volume. For a complete study, the following are necessary: intra-abdominal pressure, intravesical pressure, urethral sphincteric pressure at various (usually 2) levels, flow rate, voided volume, anal sphincteric pressure (as a function of pelvic floor activity), and electromyography of the anal or urethral striated sphincter. These physiologic data are recorded with the patient quiet as well as during activity (ie, voluntary increase in intra-abdominal pressure, changes in the state of bladder filling, voluntary contraction of perineal muscles, or—more comprehensively—an entire voiding act starting from an empty bladder; continuing through complete filling of the bladder, and initiation of voiding; and ending when the bladder is empty).

The data derived from urodynamic studies are descriptive of urinary tract function. Simultaneous visualization of the lower urinary tract as multiple recordings are made gives more precise information about the pathologic changes underlying the symptoms. By means of cinefluoroscopy, the examiner can observe the configuration of the bladder, bladder base, and bladder outlet during bladder filling (usually with radiopaque medium). The information obtained can then be correlated with the level of catheters, with pressure recordings, and with changes in pelvic floor support during voiding. Combined cinefluoroscopy and pressure measurements thus represent the ultimate in urodynamic studies.

VIDEOURODYNAMIC

This involves the use of fluoroscopy with concurrent measurement of bladder and urethral pressure. Although simple urodynamic can make the diagnosis in many cases, the use of videourodynamic is essential when simultaneous evaluation of structure and function is necessary to make the diagnosis. The simultaneous pressure measurement with fluoroscopic visualization reduces the possibility of misinterpretation of findings because artifactual errors are minimized. In addition, the study is available on videotape, so it can be reviewed to restudy particular portions of the examination. McGuire et al have demonstrated that combination of radiographic imaging and urodynamic studies is extremely valuable in many situations, including male and female incontinence, neurologic conditions, assessment of bladder compliance, and bladder outlet obstruction. In neurologic or obstructive conditions, evaluation of bladder compliance is of great importance because poor compliance is associated with a direct risk to ureteral and renal function. During simple urodynamic, undetected leakage per urethra or vesicoureteral reflux can occur, both of which may allow detrusor compliance to appear better than it really is as they act as a vent to lower bladder pressure. Evaluating compliance with fluoroscopy obviates these problems (Figure 29–25).

▶ Videourodynamic Equipment

Videourodynamic studies can be performed with almost any fluoroscopic unit as long as the table can be tilted to place the patient in the upright position. Fluoroscopy time is generally under 1 minute with minimal radiographic exposure. The urodynamic machine is equipped with a video capability that allows capturing and playing images slowly and correlating pressure and events as straining and coughing with fluoroscopic images.

▶ Indications for Videourodynamic

A videourodynamic evaluation is indicated when the diagnosis cannot be achieved using standard urodynamic testing. Conditions in which videourodynamic is particularly helpful include the evaluation of incontinence in females and various neurologic and obstructive conditions.

In females with urinary incontinence, in addition to evaluation of bladder and sphincteric function, videourodynamic provides valuable information about anatomical

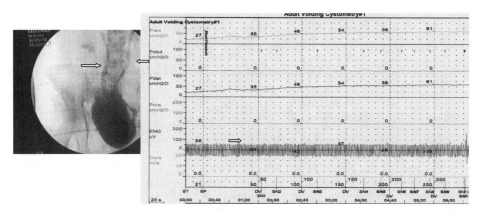

▲ **Figure 29–25.** Videourodynamic showing bilateral ureteral reflux and urinary incontinence in a small contracted bladder. The bladder compliance is poor; however, it is masked by both the reflux and urinary leakage.

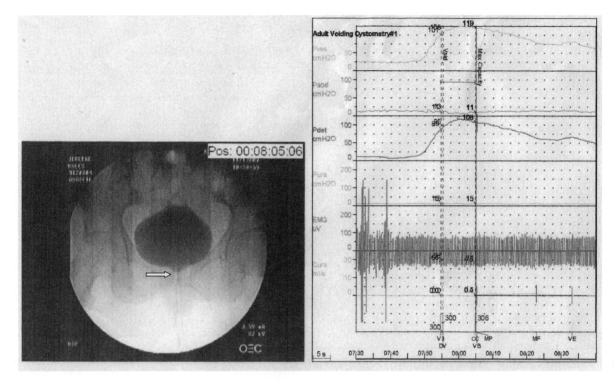

▲ **Figure 29–26.** Videourodynamic after pubovaginal sling in a patient with urinary retention showing high voiding pressure and dilation of proximal urethra above the sling during voiding.

findings, such as degree of urethral hypermobility, and any associated significant prolapse that may mask coexisting stress incontinence.

Diagnosis of urethral obstruction in females can be very difficult with standard urodynamic methods. The diagnosis can be derived much easier with the use of videourodynamic because in addition to high detrusor pressure during voiding, the level of obstruction can be documented (Figure 29–26).

In neurologic and obstructive conditions, evaluation of bladder compliance is considered to be the most important part of the bladder evaluation, as poor compliance is associated with direct risk to ureteral and kidney functions. Poor compliance with its detrimental effect on the renal function can be masked by the presence of vesicoureteral reflux or leakage per urethra. Both can be easily seen on fluoroscopy (Figure 29–25).

LEAK POINT PRESSURE

A great amount of credit should be given to Dr. McGuire and his colleagues who popularized the use of leak point pressure measurement. They developed and defined leak point pressure measurement based on videourodynamic studies done over many years in a broad cross section of

patients with various types of incontinence and neurogenic conditions.

There are two leak point pressure tests that measure different aspects of lower urinary tract function. Bladder or detrusor leak point pressure (DLPP) and abdominal or Valsalva leak point pressure.

▶ Detrusor Leak Point Pressure

This is a measurement of the detrusor pressure required to induce leakage across the urethra. It measures bladder compliance, and the higher the DLPP, the worse the compliance. It is not very useful to determine if obstruction exists or not, nor it is useful to characterize bladder contractility. Both are measured by pressure flow studies.

In late 1970s, McGuire and his group from Michigan noted that myelodysplastic children with detrusor leak pressure of 40 cm H_2O or more at the instant of leakage invariably developed upper tract disease if not treated. These findings were later confirmed by another retrospective study by the same group that showed that all children with abnormal upper tracts demonstrated very poor bladder compliance. Because poor compliance was not likely to impair ureteral function unless outlet resistance was high, it seemed likely that elevated outlet resistance led to the development of poor compliance in the first place. Furthermore, it has been shown by Wang et al that control of detrusor pressure below 40 cm H_2O prevented the development of upper urinary tract disease in myelodysplastic children.

In children with high DLPP and poor compliance, urethral dilation resulted in an immediate fall in leak point pressure and surprisingly a gradual but significant improvement in bladder compliance.

▶ Abdominal/Valsalva Leak Point Pressure

This test measures the ability of the urethra to resist abdominal pressure as an expulsive force. This is usually equal to detrusor pressure plus the abdominal pressure generated by the Valsalva maneuver. McGuire et al have shown that low ALPP is associated with poor intrinsic sphincteric function (intrinsic sphincteric deficiency); however, this has no or poor relationship to simultaneously measured maximum urethral closure pressure. They believed that measuring the urethral intraluminal pressure, particularly in the high-pressure zone, cannot tell how good or bad the urethra is.

The abdominal pressure required to induce leakage appears to be inversely proportional to urethral weakness. A normal urethra does not leak at any achievable pressure, whereas a very bad urethra leaks at a very low pressure. Between these two points, lie most of incontinent patients.

Although this test is widely used to assess patients with urinary incontinence, it has inherent flaws that need to be addressed including volume in the bladder, pelvic organ prolapse, and ability of the individual to generate the required pressure to complete the testing.

Volume in the bladder is very important, as an empty bladder will not leak and a very full bladder can induce a pronounced detrusor component that can make a good urethra look very bad. Measuring the ALPP should be done at moderate volume, between 200 and 250 mL.

Pelvic organ prolapse can dissipate the effect of the abdominal pressure on the urethra and mask the stress incontinence. It is very important to determine whether genital prolapse exists and if present, the prolapse should be reduced in order to properly interpret the leak point pressure.

▶ How to Measure the Abdominal Leak Point Pressure

The bladder is filled slowly to approximately 200 mL while the patient is in the upright position. The patient is asked to do a progressive Valsalva maneuver until he or she leaks. If no leakage can be demonstrated with the Valsalva maneuver, then repetitive coughing may be tried. If still no leakage is seen, the same is repeated at a higher volume. In the absence of significant pelvic organ prolapse, low leak point pressure of 65 cm H_2O or less indicates intrinsic sphincteric deficiency. A high leak point pressure of 100 or more usually associated with urethral hypermobility.

BIBLIOGRAPHY

Urethra and Bladder

Aboseif SR et al: Continence mechanism of the ileal neobladder in women. A urodynamic study. World J Urol 1998;16(6):400–404.

Abrams P: Managing lower urinary tract symptoms in older men. Br Med J 1995;310:1113.

Abrams P: Objective evaluation of bladder outlet obstruction. Br J Urol 1995;76(Suppl 1):11.

Abrams P: Lower urinary tract symptoms in women: Who to investigate and how. Br J Urol 1997;80(Suppl 1):43.

Abrams P et al; Standardisation Sub-Committee of the International Continence Society: The standardisation of terminology in lower urinary tract function: Report from the standardisation sub-committee of the International Continence Society. Urology 2003;61(1):37–49.

Artibani W: Diagnosis and significance of idiopathic overactive bladder. Urology 1997;50(6A, Suppl):25.

Awad SA et al: Urethral pressure profile in female stress incontinence. J Urol 1978;120:475.

Bazeed MA et al: Histochemical study of urethral striated musculature in the dog. J Urol 1982;128:406.

Beck RP et al: Intraurethral-intravesical cough-pressure spike differences in 267 patients surgically cured of genuine stress incontinence of urine. Obstet Gynecol 1988;72:302.

Berger Y et al: Urodynamic findings in Parkinson's disease. J Urol 1987;138:836.

Borirakchanyavat S et al: Continence mechanism of the isolated female urethra. An anatomical study of the intrapelvic somatic nerves. J Urol 1997;158(3, Pt 1):822–826.

Bruschini H et al: Effect of urethral stretch on urethral pressure profile. Invest Urol 1977;15:107.

Bruskewitz R, Raz S: Urethral pressure profile using microtip catheter in females. Urology 1979;14:303.

Bump RC et al: Dynamic urethral pressure profilometry pressure transmission ratio determinations after continence surgery: Understanding the mechanism of success, failure, and complications. Obstet Gynecol 1988;72:870.

Cameron AP et al: Combination drug therapy improves compliance of the neurogenic bladder. J Urol 2009;182(3):1062–1067.

Cardenas DD et al: Residual urine volumes in patients with spinal cord injury: Measurement with a portable ultrasound instrument. Arch Phys Med Rehabil 1988;69:514.

Cho SY et al: The clinical significance of poor bladder compliance. Neurourol Urodyn 2009;28(8):1010–1014.

Coolsaet B: Bladder compliance and detrusor activity during the collection phase. Neurourol Urodyn 1985;4:263.

DeGroat WC: A neurologic basis for the overactive bladder. Urology 1997;50(6A, Suppl):36.

Desai P: Bladder pressure studies combined with micturating cysto-urethrography. Radiography 1985;52:2.

Desmond AD, Ramayya GR: The adaptation of urethral pressure profiles to detect sphincter incompetence and sphincter obstruction using a microcomputer. J Urol 1987;137:457.

Dwyer PL, Rosamilia A: Evaluation and diagnosis of the overactive bladder. Clin Obstet Gynecol 2002;45:193.

Glen ES et al: Urethral closure pressure profile measurements in female urinary incontinence. Acta Urol Belg 1984;52:174.

Gosling JA et al: A comparative study of the human external sphincter and periurethral levator ani muscles. Br J Urol 1981;53:35.

Graber P et al: Effect of abdominal pressure rise on the urethral profile: An experimental study on dogs. Invest Urol 1974;12:57.

Griffiths D: Clinical aspects of detrusor instability and the value of urodynamics: A review of the evidence. Eur Urol 1998;34(Suppl 1):13.

Harvey MA, Versi E: Predictive value of clinical evaluation of stress urinary incontinence: A summary of the published literature. Int Urogynecol J Pelvic Floor Dysfunct 2001;12:31.

Henriksson L et al: The urethral pressure profiles in continent and stress-incontinent women. Scand J Urol Nephrol 1979;13:5.

Henriksson L et al: Combined urethrocystometry and cinefluorography in continent and incontinent women. Radiology 1979;130:607.

Jepsen JV, Bruskewitz RC: Comprehensive patient evaluation for benign prostatic hyperplasia. Urology 1998;51(4A, Suppl):13.

Jonas U, Klotter HJ: Study of three urethral pressure recording devices: Theoretical considerations. Urol Res 1978;6:119.

Kelly MJ et al: Transurethral incision of the prostate: A preoperative and postoperative analysis of symptoms and urodynamic findings. J Urol 1989;142:1507.

Kim YH et al: Bladder leak point pressure: The measure for sphincterotomy success in spinal cord injured patients with external detrusor-sphincter dyssynergia. J Urol 1998;159:493.

Koefoot RB Jr, Webster GD: Urodynamic evaluation in women with frequency, urgency symptoms. Urology 1983;21:648.

Koelbl H, Bernaschek G: A new method for sonographic urethrocystography and simultaneous pressure-flow measurements. Obstet Gynecol 1989;74:417.

Langer R et al: Detrusor instability following colposuspension for urinary stress incontinence. Br J Obstet Gynaecol 1988;95:607.

Lim CS, Abrams P: The Abrams-Griffiths nomogram. World J Urol 1995;13:34.

Lose G: Urethral pressure measurement. Acta Obstet Gynecol Scand Suppl 1997;166:39.

McGuire EJ: The role of urodynamic investigation in the assessment of benign prostatic hypertrophy. J Urol 1992;148:1133.

McGuire EJ et al: Leak-point pressures. Urol Clin North Am 1996;23:253.

Narayan P et al: Neuroanatomy of the external urethral sphincter implications for urinary continence preservation during radical prostate surgery. J Urol 1995;153(2):337–341.

Nevéus T et al: The standardization of terminology of lower urinary tract function in children and adolescents: report from the Standardisation Committee of the International Children's Continence Society. J Urol 2006;176(1):314–324.

Nørgaard JP et al: Standardization and definitions in lower urinary tract dysfunction in children. International Children's Continence Society. Br J Urol 1998;81(Suppl 3):1.

Ouslander J et al: Simple versus multichannel cystometry in the evaluation of bladder function in an incontinent geriatric population. J Urol 1988;140:1482.

Saxton HM: Urodynamics: The appropriate modality for the investigation of frequency, urgency, incontinence, and voiding difficulties. Radiology 1990;175:307.

Schafer W: Analysis of bladder-outlet function with the linearized passive urethral resistance relation, linPURR, and a disease-specific approach for grading obstruction: From complex to simple. World J Urol 1995;13:47.

Schafer W: Principles and clinical application of advanced urodynamic analysis of voiding function. Urol Clin North Am 1990;17:553.

Schmidt RA et al: Recording urethral pressure profile. Urology 1977;10:390.

Schmidt RA et al: Urethral pressure profilometry with membrane catheter compared with perfusion catheter systems. Urol Int 1978;33:345.

Schmidt RA, Tanagho EA: Urethral syndrome or urinary tract infection? Urology 1981;18:424.

Snyder JA, Lipsitz DU: Evaluation of female urinary incontinence. Urol Clin North Am 1991;18:197.

Sullivan MP et al: Micturitional urethral pressure profilometry. Urol Clin North Am 1996;23:263.

Tanagho EA et al: Urethral resistance: Its components and implications. 2. Striated muscle component. Invest Urol 1969;7:136.

Tanagho EA: Interpretation of the physiology of micturition. In: Hinman F Jr (ed) Hydrodynamics. Thomas, 1971.

Tanagho EA: Vesicourethral dynamics. In: Lutzeyer W, Melchior H (eds) Urodynamics. Springer-Verlag, 1974.

Tanagho EA: Membrane and microtransducer catheters: Their effectiveness for profilometry of the lower urinary tract. Urol Clin North Am 1979;6:110.

Tanagho EA: Neurophysiology of urinary incontinence. In: Cantor EB (ed) Female Urinary Stress Incontinence. Thomas, 1979.

Tanagho EA: Urodynamics of female urinary incontinence with emphasis on stress incontinence. J Urol 1979;122:200.

Tanagho EA, Jones U: Membrane catheter: Effective for recording pressure in lower urinary tract. Urology 1977;10:173.

Tanagho EA, Miller ER: Functional considerations of urethral sphincteric dynamics. J Urol 1973;109:273.

Turner WH, Brading AF: Smooth muscle of the bladder in the normal and the diseased state: Pathophysiology, diagnosis and treatment. Pharmacol Ther 1997;75:77.

van Geelen JM et al: The clinical and urodynamic effects of anterior vaginal repair and Burch colposuspension. Am J Obstet Gynecol 1988;159:137.

Versi E: Discriminant analysis of urethral pressure profilometry data for the diagnosis of genuine stress incontinence. Br J Obstet Gynaecol 1990;97:251.

Woodside JR, McGuire EJ: A simple inexpensive urodynamic catheter. J Urol 1979;122:788.

Yalla SV et al: Striated sphincter participation in distal passive urinary continence mechanisms: Studies in male subjects deprived of proximal sphincter mechanism. J Urol 1979;122:655.

Urinary Flow Rate

Bates CP et al: Synchronous cine-pressure-flow cystourethrography with special reference to stress and urge incontinence. Br J Urol 1970;42:714.

Gleason DM, Bottaccini MR: Urodynamic norms in female voiding. 2. Flow modulation zone and voiding dysfunction. J Urol 1982;127:495.

Griffiths D: Basics of pressure-flow studies. World J Urol 1995;13:30.

Griffiths DJ: Pressure-flow studies of micturition. Urol Clin North Am 1996;23:279.

Jensen KM-E et al: Relationship between uroflowmetry and prostatism. Proc Int Continence Soc 1985;15:134.

Jørgensen JB, Jensen KM: Uroflowmetry. Urol Clin North Am 1996; 23:237.

Kavia RB et al: Urinary retention in women. BJU Int 2006;97(2): 281–287.

Kavia R et al: A functional magnetic resonance imaging study of the effect of sacral neuromodulation on brain responses in women with Fowler's syndrome. BJU Int 2010;105(3):366–372.

Meyhoff HH et al: The effects of transurethral resection on the urodynamics of prostatism. J Urol 1989;142:785.

Nording J: A clinical view of pressure-flow studies. World J Urol 1995;13:70.

Siroky MB et al: The flow rate nomogram. 2. Clinical correlation. J Urol 1980;23:208.

Siroky MB: Interpretation of urinary flow rates. Urol Clin North Am 1990;17:537.

Stubbs AJ, Resnic MI: Office uroflowmetry using maximum flow rate purge meter. J Urol 1979;122:62.

Tanagho EA, McCurry E: Pressure and flow rate as related to lumen caliber and entrance configuration. J Urol 1971;105:583.

van Mastrigt R, Kranse M: Analysis of pressure-flow data in terms of computer-derived urethral resistance parameters. World J Urol 1995;13:40.

Electromyography

Colstrup H et al: Urethral sphincter EMG activity registered with surface electrodes in the vagina. Neurourol Urodyn 1985;4:15.

King DG, Teague CT: Choice of electrode in electromyography of external urethral and anal sphincter. J Urol 1980;124:75.

Koyanagi T et al: Experience with electromyography of the external urethral sphincter in spinal cord injury patients. J Urol 1982;127:272.

Nielsen KK et al: A comparative study of various electrodes in electromyography of the striated urethral and anal sphincter in children. Br J Urol 1985;57:557.

Siroky MB: Electromyography of the perineal floor. Urol Clin North Am 1996;23:299.

Steward JE et al: Quantitative evaluation of electrodes for external urethral sphincter electromyography during bladder-to-urethral guarding reflex. World J Urol 2010;28(3):365–371.

Urodynamic Testing

Barrent DM, Wein AJ: Flow evaluation and simultaneous external sphincter electromyography in clinical urodynamics. J Urol 1981; 125:538.

Blaivas JG: Multichannel urodynamic studies. Urology 1984;23:421.

Blaivas JG et al: The role of urodynamic testing in the evaluation of subtle neurologic lesions. Neurourol Urodyn 1985;4:211.

Blaivas JG: Multichannel urodynamic studies in men with benign prostatic hyperplasia: Indications and interpretation. Urol Clin North Am 1990;17:543.

Blaivas JG, Fischer DM: Combined radiographic and urodynamic monitoring: Advances in technique. J Urol 1981;125:693.

Cassidenti AP, Ostergard DR: Multichannel urodynamics: Ambulatory versus standard urodynamics. Curr Opin Obstet Gynecol 1999;11:485.

Daneshgari F: Valsalva leak point pressure: Steps toward standardization. Curr Urol Rep 2001;2:388.

Everaert K et al: Urodynamic assessment of voiding dysfunction and dysfunctional voiding in girls and women. Int Urogynecol J Pelvic Floor Dysfunct 2000;11:254.

Gasthuisberg KU, Vereecken RL: A critical view on the value of urodynamics in non-neurogenic incontinence in women. Int Urogynecol J Pelvic Floor Dysfunct 2000;11:188.

Gerber GS: The role of urodynamic study in the evaluation and management of men with lower urinary tract symptoms secondary to benign prostatic hyperplasia. Urology 1996;48:668.

Kulseng-Hanssen S: Reliability and validity of stationary cystometry, stationary cysto-urethrometry and ambulatory cysto-urethrovaginometry. Acta Obstet Gynecol Scand Suppl 1997;166:33.

Lane TM, Shah PJ: Leak-point pressures. BJU Int 2000;86:942.

Lewis P, Abrams P: Urodynamic protocol and central review of data for clinical trials in lower urinary tract dysfunction. BJU Int 2000;85(Suppl 1):20.

Massey A, Abrams P: Urodynamics of the female lower urinary tract. Urol Clin North Am 1985;12:231.

McGuire EJ, Woodside JR: Diagnostic advantages of fluoroscopic monitoring during urodynamic evaluation. J Urol 1981;125:830.

McLellan A, Cardozo L: Urodynamic techniques. Int Urogynecol J Pelvic Floor Dysfunct 2001;12:266.

O'Donnell PD: Pitfalls of urodynamic testing. Urol Clin North Am 1991;18:257.

Sand PK et al: Uninhibited urethral relaxation: An unusual cause of incontinence. Proc Int Continence Soc 1985;15:117.

Schafer W: Urethral resistance? Urodynamic concepts of physiological and pathological bladder outlet function during voiding. Neurourol Urodyn 1985;4:161.

Schafer W et al: Good urodynamic practices: Uroflowmetry, filling cystometry, and pressure-flow studies. Neurourol Urodyn 2002;21(3):261–274.

Siroky MB: Urodynamic assessment of detrusor denervation and areflexia. World J Urol 1984;2:181.

Sutherst JR, Brown MC: Comparison of single and multichannel cystometry in diagnosing bladder instability. Br Med J 1984;288:1720.

Tanagho EA: Membrane and microtransducer catheters: Their effectiveness for profilometry of the lower urinary tract. Urol Clin North Am 1979;6:110.

Thüroff JW: Mechanism of urinary continence: Animal model to study urethral responses to stress conditions. J Urol 1982;127:1202.

Turner-Warwick R, Brown AD: A urodynamic evaluation of urinary incontinence in the female and its treatment. Urol Clin North Am 1979;6:203.

Turner-Warwick R, Milroy E: A reappraisal of the value of routine urological procedures in the assessment of urodynamic function. Urol Clin North Am 1979;6:63.

van Waalwijk van Doorn ES et al: Ambulatory urodynamics: Extramural testing of the lower and upper urinary tract by Holter monitoring of cystometrogram, uroflowmetry, and renal pelvic pressures. Urol Clin North Am 1996;23:345.

Wein AJ et al: Effects of bethanechol chloride on urodynamic parameters in normal women and in women with significant residual urine volumes. J Urol 1980;124:397.

Videourodynamic

McGuire EJ et al: Upper urinary tract deterioration in patients with myelodysplasia and detrusor hypertonia: A follow up study. J Urol 1983;129:183.

McGuire EJ et al: Clinical assessment of urethral sphincter. J Urol 1993;150:1452–1454.

McGuire EJ, Woodside JR: Diagnostic advantages of fluoroscopic monitoring during urodynamic evaluation. J Urol 1981;125: 830.

Sinha D et al: Value of leak point pressure study in women with incontinence. J Urol 2006;176(1):186–188; discussion 188.

Türker P et al: The presence of transurethral cystometry catheter and type of stress test affect the measurement of abdominal leak point pressure (ALPP) in women with stress urinary incontinence (SUI). Neurourol Urodyn 2010;29(4):536–539.

Wang SC et al: A bladder pressure management system for myelodysplasia-clinical outcome. J Urol 1988;140:1499–1502.

White T et al: Correlation of maximum urethral closure pressure with Valsalva leak point pressure using air-charged urodynamic catheters. Int Urogynecol J Pelvic Floor Dysfunct 2009;20(9): 1109–1112.

Urinary Incontinence

Tom F. Lue, MD, FACS, ScD (Hon), & Emil A. Tanagho, MD

It is estimated that 45.2%, 10.7%, 8.2%, and 21.5% of the 2008 worldwide population (4.3 billion) was affected by at least one lower urinary tract symptoms (LUTS), overactive bladder (OAB), urinary incontinence, and LUTS/bladder outlet obstruction (BOO), respectively (Irwin et al, 2011). Urinary incontinence is a major health issue and the total direct and indirect cost in the United States alone was estimated at $19.5 billion in 2000, of which 75% is for the management of women with this condition. Incontinence also results in psychological and medical morbidity, significantly impacting health-related quality of life in a manner similar to other chronic medical conditions including osteoporosis, chronic obstructive pulmonary disease, and stroke. Overall prevalence of female incontinence is reported at 38%, increasing with age from 20–30% during young adult life to almost 50% in the elderly (Anger et al, 2006; Hawkins et al, 2010). Recent advances in the understanding of pathophysiology, as well as development of novel pharmacotherapy and surgical techniques for stress, mixed, and urge incontinence (UI), have redefined contemporary care of this patient group.

To facilitate comparisons of results and enable effective communication by investigators, the International Continence Society (ICS) has proposed standard terminology to be used to describe symptoms, signs, conditions, urodynamic findings, as well as treatment (Abrams et al, 2003). The ICS defines the symptom of urinary incontinence as "the complaint of any involuntary loss of urine." It is also recommended, when describing incontinence, to specify relevant factors such as type, severity, precipitating factors, social impact, effect on hygiene and quality of life, measures used to contain the leakage, and whether or not the individual experiencing incontinence desires help.

PATHOPHYSIOLOGY

Incontinence can be transient or chronic. Transient incontinence may occur after childbirth or during an acute lower urinary tract infection and usually resolved spontaneously.

Chronic incontinence can result from a multitude of causes and is often persistent and progressive. From a functional and anatomic perspective, it is intuitive to consider the lower urinary tract as a two-part system: the urinary bladder as a reservoir and the bladder outlet as a sphincteric mechanism. Incontinence occurs when either part or both malfunction. Several common types of incontinence are discussed herein: stress urinary incontinence (SUI), urgency urinary incontinence, mixed urinary incontinence (MUI), neuropathic incontinence, and overflow incontinence (OI).

GENERAL APPROACH

A step-wise management algorithm has been recommended for the management of male and female incontinence by the scientific committee of the 4th International Consultation on Incontinence (Abrams et al, 2010). In principle, the committee recommends an initial management and a specialized management algorithm for all types of incontinence. In initial assessment, one should identify the complicated incontinence group for specialized management. This includes recurrent or total incontinence, incontinence associated with pain, hematuria, recurrent infection, prostate irradiation, and radical pelvic surgery, suspected of fistula and significant postvoid residual. The following groups are suitable for initial management: stress incontinence, urgency incontinence, and incontinence with mixed symptoms. The initial clinical assessment should include general, urinary, pelvic floor, symptom scores, quality of life, desire for treatment, physical examination, urinalysis, and postvoid residual urine. The initial management consists of lifestyle intervention, bladder and pelvic floor muscle training, and incontinence products and medications. Specialized management is recommended for patients who failed the above-mentioned managements or those with specialized conditions. The assessment includes imaging of urinary tracts, urodynamics, and cystourethroscopy, and more invasive treatments including surgery, neuromodulation, and prosthetics are recommended for these patients.

STRESS URINARY INCONTINENCE

The ICS defines it as involuntary urine leakage on effort or exertion, or on sneezing or coughing. In men, stress incontinence is mostly due to surgery (eg, after radical prostatectomy) or trauma to the bladder neck/urethral sphincter. The causes of stress incontinence in women are more complicated and somewhat controversial and therefore the following discussion is mostly related to female stress incontinence. The vast majority of stress incontinence occurs in women after middle age (with repeated vaginal deliveries and obstructed labor). It is usually a result of weakness/disruption of the pelvic floor muscle and ligaments leading to poor support of the vesicourethral sphincteric unit. An increase in urethral closure pressure is normally seen during bladder filling; when assuming an upright position; or in stressful events such as coughing, sneezing, or bearing down. During exertion, both passive pressure transmission from increased abdominal pressure and reflexic contraction of the sphincteric mechanism augment urethral resistance to prevent urine leakage.

▶ Anatomy

Stress incontinence is thought to be caused by two major anatomical deficits: hypermobility of the sphincteric unit and intrinsic sphincter deficiency. In hypermobility, the assumption is that the intrinsic structure of the sphincter itself is intact. It loses closing efficiency because of excessive mobility and loss of support. Thus, the anatomic feature of stress incontinence is hypermobility or a lowering of the position of the vesicourethral segment (or a combination of the two factors) (Figure 30–1). On the other hand, some women who have undergone multiple retropubic or urethral operations have a deficient intrinsic sphincteric mechanism characterized by an open bladder neck and proximal urethra at rest with minimal or no urethral descent during stress. Nevertheless, many women maintain normal continence with hypermobility, and a recent dynamic magnetic resonance imaging (MRI) study finds no correlation between perineal descent and patients' symptoms of urinary incontinence (Broekhuis et al, 2010). Therefore, contemporary opinion suggests that all women with stress incontinence have some degree of intrinsic sphincter deficiency.

The relationships between the urethra, the bladder base, and various bony points have been the object of much study. For many years, the posterior vesicourethral angle has been considered a key factor indicating the presence of anatomic stress incontinence. Some authors, however, have emphasized the axis of inclination, that is, the angle between the urethral line and the vertical plane. Other investigators stress bony landmarks in the pelvis in their descriptions of the relationship of the bladder base and the

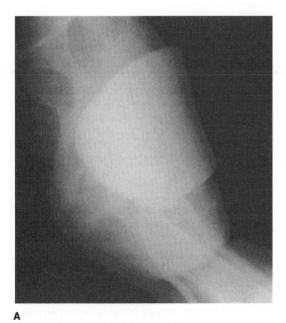 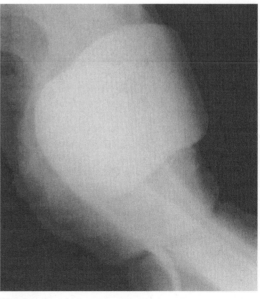

A   **B**

▲ **Figure 30–1.** Lateral cystograms in a 53-year-old woman with stress incontinence. **A:** Preoperative, relaxed. Note slightly low-lying vesicourethral junction. The posterior vesicourethral angle is near normal. **B:** With straining, excessive downward and posterior mobility of the vesicourethral segment is shown. Posterior angle almost disappears.

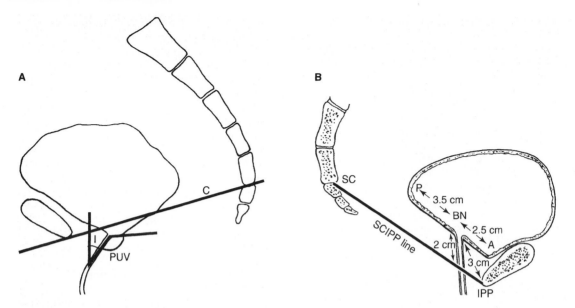

▲ **Figure 30–2.** Diagrammatic representation of (**A**) the angles considered when assessing adequacy of bladder support (posterior vesicourethral angle; angle of inclination) and (**B**) the "SCIPP line" (sacrococcygeal inferior pubic point) and its relationship to the bladder base and the vesicourethral segment as a reference to adequate pelvic support.

vesicourethral junction to the sacrococcygeal inferior pubic point (Figure 30–2).

These descriptions illustrate that abnormal anatomic position and excessive mobility are essential elements in the diagnosis of stress incontinence due to hypermobility. To evaluate this aspect of incontinence, a simplified cystographic study (a lateral cystogram with a urethral catheter in place) is recommended. With the patient lying on the flat x-ray table, a lateral film is obtained, first at rest to determine the position of the vesicourethral segment in relation to the pubic bone and then with straining to ascertain its degree of mobility (Figures 30–3 and 30–4). Normally, the vesicourethral junction is opposite the lower third of the pubic bone and moves 0.5–1.5 cm with straining. This demonstration of abnormal position or excessive mobility of the vesicourethral segment is helpful in identifying the cause of existing urinary incontinence.

The urethral pressure profile is a measure of the activity of the external sphincter. A static profile demonstrates the resting tonus of both components of the sphincteric mechanism (see Figure 30–5); a dynamic profile gives the responses of these sphincteric elements to various activities, such as an increase in bladder volume, assumption of the upright position (Figure 30–6), the prolonged stress of bearing down, or the sudden stress of coughing and sneezing (Figure 30–7). Normally, the urethral closure pressure—the net difference between the intraurethral and intravesical pressures—is maintained or augmented during stress.

Detailed research of the role of smooth and striated components of the bladder and urethra were performed in animal experiments in the 1980's. Electrical stimulation of the pelvic nerve induces contraction of the smooth muscle of the bladder and urethra (Figure 30–8) while stimulation of the sacral nerve contracts smooth muscle of the bladder and urethra as well as striated muscle of the external sphincter (Figure 30–9). The contribution of smooth and striated muscle to urethral opening/closure pressure is further demonstrated in Figures 30–10 to 30–12.

The high rate of success from midurethral sling surgery led some to believe that the midurethral support is the key element in preventing stress incontinence and raise doubts about the relevance of the cystographic study. Petros and Ulmstem (1990) proposed that support of the anterior vaginal wall is provided by three separate but synergistic mechanisms: the anterior pubococcygeus muscle; the bladder neck; and the pelvic floor musculature, which acts like a hammock to help close the bladder neck during stress. Laxity of the anterior vaginal wall causes dissipation of all of three forces, resulting in stress incontinence. Delancey (1994) proposes that the stability of the supporting layer rather than the position of the urethra determines stress continence. During rises in intra-abdominal pressure, the urethra is compressed against the supporting structures, which act like a backboard and prevent loss of urine. The fact that both bladder neck and midurethral slings have been shown to be successful in treating stress incontinence

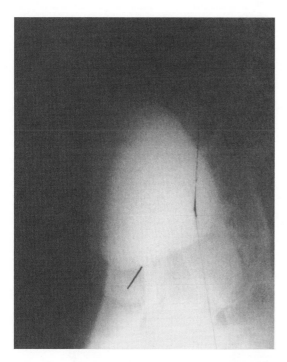
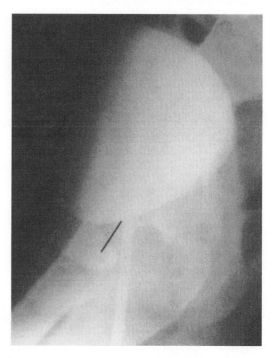

▲ **Figure 30–3.** Lateral cystograms in two continent women in the relaxed state. A perpendicular line from the anterior vesicourethral angle over the long axis of the pubic bone crosses the bone near the junction of the middle and lower thirds.

supports the above-mentioned theories (Novara et al, 2010; Ulmsten et al, 1998).

A recent report of a clinical study concludes that low urethral closure pressure is the best predictor of SUI in women (DeLancey et al, 2008). An MRI study also revealed that the striated urogenital sphincter in women with stress incontinence was 12.5% smaller than that in asymptomatic continent women (Morgen et al, 2009). A study on dulox-etine, a serotonin and norepinephrine reuptake inhibitor, showed that it elevates both baseline urethral pressure (adrenergic innervation on the smooth muscle) and active pressure rise with sneezing (Onuf' nucleus activated striated muscle contraction (Miyazato et al, 2008). These observa-tions reaffirm the original observation by Tanagho that smooth muscle, striated muscle, and mucosa and submuco-sal vessels each contribute about one-third of the urethral closure pressure and all are important in sphincter function.

▶ Diagnosis

A detailed history is important, including the degree of leak-age; its relation to activity, position, and state of bladder full-ness; the timing of its onset; and the course of its progression. Knowledge of past surgical and obstetric history, medications taken, dietary habits, and systemic diseases (eg, diabetes) can be helpful in the diagnosis. A micturition diary that records the

time of micturition, voided volume, and type of incontinence is recommended by the ICS as a useful supplement (Abrams et al, 2010). A pad test over 1 hour or 24 hours has also been recommended. In addition, history should also include the degree of bother and effect on quality of life. Many question-naires and diaries are available for clinical and research use.

Physical examination is essential especially if urine leakage is witnessed by the examiner. In women, the pelvic examina-tion demonstrates laxity of pelvic support, presence of any degree of prolapse, cystocele, rectocele, and mobility of the anterior vaginal wall. A neurologic examination should be done if neuropathy is suspected. Cystographic study for dem-onstration of the anatomic abnormality is helpful, as is urody-namic study to confirm the classic features of urinary incontinence and determine its cause. The goals of cysto-graphic and urodynamic study are, first, to demonstrate the anatomic abnormality and its extent and, second, to assess the activity of the sphincteric mechanism and hence the potential for improvement by correcting the anatomic abnormality. The degree of hypermobility in women can also be assessed by a simple Q-tip test (Swift et al, 2010). This is done by inserting a well-lubricated sterile cotton-tipped applicator gently through the urethra into the bladder and then pulling it back to the level of the bladder neck. The angle from the horizontal at rest and after straining is recorded. Hypermobility is defined as a resting or straining angle >30° from the horizontal.

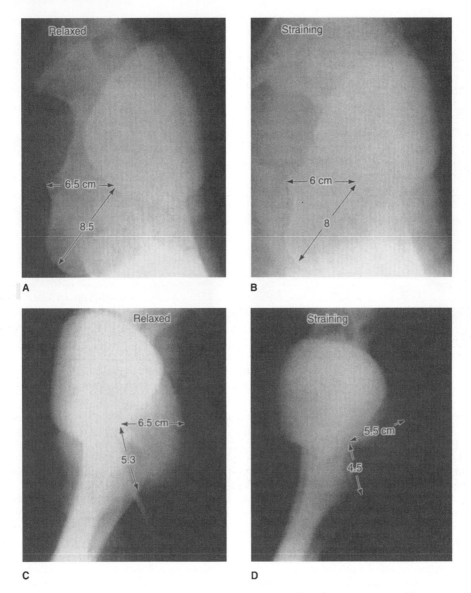

▲ **Figure 30–4.** Lateral cystograms in two young continent women. **A:** Relaxed state, 28-year-old woman. **B:** With straining, the vesicourethral segment is displaced 0.5 cm downward and posteriorly. **C:** Relaxed state, 34-year-old woman. **D:** With straining, the vesicourethral segment is displaced 0.8 cm downward and 1 cm posteriorly.

▶ Urodynamic Characteristics of Stress Incontinence

A. Urethral Pressure Profile

The ICS defines urodynamic stress incontinence as the involuntary leakage of urine during increased abdominal pressure, in the absence of a detrusor contraction (Abrams et al, 2003).

As would be expected, most patients with stress incontinence have a low urethral pressure profile with reduced closure pressure. This factor varies with the severity of the sphincteric impairment. Not infrequently, this weakness of the pressure profile is not demonstrable when the bladder is relatively empty. It becomes more significant when the bladder has been distended (Figure 30–13). Also, the pressure profile may appear normal when the patient is in the resting (sitting) position;

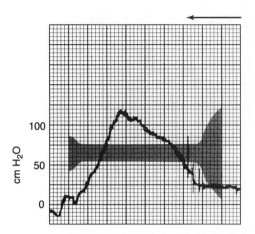

▲ **Figure 30–5.** Normal urethral pressure. Closure pressure at the level of the internal meatus is very low; the pressure rises progressively to reach its maximum at approximately the middle third of the urethra—the site of maximal condensation of striated muscle.

when he or she assumes the upright position in the dynamic pressure profile, the weakness becomes apparent (Figure 30–14).

B. Functional Urethral Length

The anatomic length of the urethra is usually maintained, yet the functional length is shorter due to loss in the proximal urethral segment (Figure 30–15). Although it might not appear funneled on the cystogram, this segment has very low closure efficiency and its pressure is almost equal to intravesical pressure. The functional shortening might be minimal or it might involve more than one-half of the length of the urethra. It is important to note that the functional length, like the pressure profile, might appear normal when the bladder is not filled or the patient is in the sitting position.

C. Response to Stress

With the sustained stress of bearing down or the sudden stress of coughing or sneezing, the net urethral closure pressure is reduced, depending on the degree of sphincteric weakness. In severe urinary stress incontinence, any strain or increase in intravesical pressure leads to urinary leakage (Figure 30–16).

D. Voluntary Increase in Urethral Closure Pressure

Patients with mild stress incontinence might be capable of activating their external sphincter maximally and generating a high urethral closure pressure. However, with progression of the anatomic problem and hypermobility, this voluntary increase progressively diminishes.

E. Response to Bladder Distention and Change in Position

It must be emphasized that, although the features described might be normal in the resting position with minimal bladder filling, all of them can become aggravated with a full bladder or the upright position (Figures 30–14 and 30–17).

F. Abdominal Leak Point Pressure

Abdominal leak point pressure (ALPP) is defined as the intravesical pressure at which urine leakage occurs because of increased abdominal pressure in the absence of a detrusor contraction (Abrams et al, 2003). This test assesses the intrinsic urethral function, and thus the lower the ALPP, the weaker the sphincter.

▶ Treatment

In mild and moderate cases, the ICS recommends lifestyle interventions, such as weight loss, caffeine reduction, pelvic floor muscle training, or duloxetine, a serotonin and norepinephrine reuptake inhibitor that has been approved in many

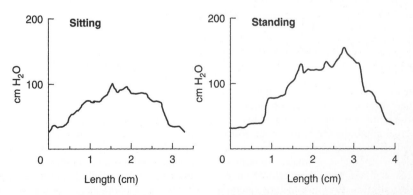

▲ **Figure 30–6.** Urethral pressure profile for a patient in sitting and upright positions. An approximately 50% increase in urethral closure pressure occurs when the patient assumes the upright position. Urethral functional length is well sustained.

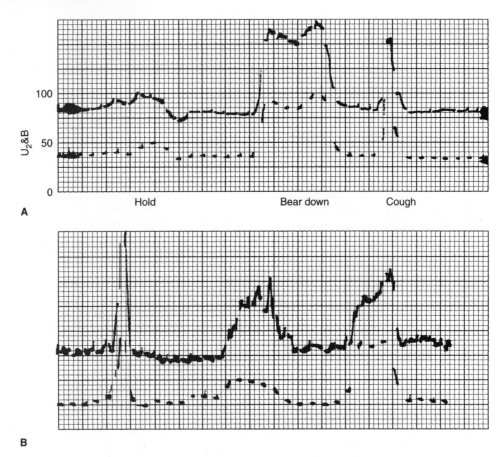

A

B

▲ **Figure 30–7.** **A:** Intravesical and urethral pressure responses to the stresses of coughing, bearing down, and the hold maneuver. Note the sharp increase in intra-abdominal pressure reflected in intravesical pressure with coughing and the simultaneous greater increase in urethral pressure. The response is similar with bearing down. Closure pressure is maintained and even augmented during these periods of stress. The hold maneuver (recording membrane is in the proximal urethra) produces a minimal response in closure pressure of the proximal urethra. **B:** Recording comparable with that in **A**, but the membrane is in the midurethra. Note again the sustained closure pressure as a result of coughing and bearing down and the marked pressure increase in the midurethral segment with the hold maneuver.

countries but not in the United States. Electrical stimulation, vaginal devices, and urethral inserts may also help some women.

If the initial management fails, the principal surgical treatment of female urinary stress incontinence is to provide proper support of the vesicourethral segment or the midurethra.

There are numerous approaches to restoring the normal position and providing adequate support—some vaginal, others suprapubic. The suprapubic approach was popularized by the classic Marshall-Marchetti-Krantz (MMK) retropubic suspension described in 1949, in which periurethral tissue is attached to the back of the pubic symphysis. A modification was introduced by Burch in 1961, in which the anterior vaginal wall is fixed to Cooper's ligament. Many urologic surgeons today have found that the latter technique, with modifications, provides the most lasting results (Drouin et al, 1999; Kulseng-Hanssen and Berild, 2002) (Figures 30–18 and 30–19).

The other approach is to suspend the bladder neck or support the midurethra with an abdominal or transobturator sling. Numerous sling materials are being used: for example, cadaveric fascia lata and various synthetic materials. Tension-free vaginal tape (TVT) has been gaining popularity. Early results for TVT with follow-up to 11 years demonstrate comparable or improved versus traditional surgical approaches (suburethral slings, urethropexy, colposuspension, or

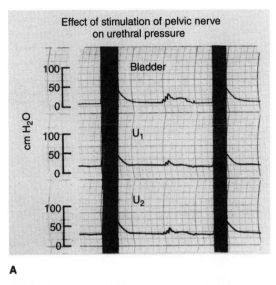

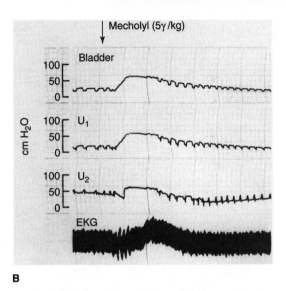

Figure 30-8. **A:** Response to pelvic nerve stimulation. Note the simultaneous, equal pressure rise in the bladder, proximal urethra (U_1), and midurethra (U_2). **B:** Vesical and sphincteric responses to an injection of the parasympathetic drug methacholine chloride. Note again the simultaneous rise in pressure at the bladder, proximal urethra (U_1), and midurethra (U_2).

injectable bulking agents) and reported success rates of up to 77% (Fong and Netti, 2010; Novara et al, 2010). Potential complications include bladder injury, infection, urinary retention, hemorrhage or hematoma, erosion (vaginal or urethral), and dyspareunia.

In patients with significant intrinsic sphincteric damage, local injection of bulking material, such as hyaluronic acid/

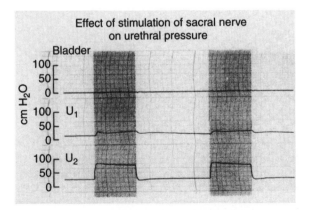

Figure 30-9. Response of the striated component to sacral nerve stimulation. Note that bladder pressure does not change and proximal urethral pressure (U_1) rises only slightly, compared with the sharp and sustained increase in midurethral pressure (U_2).

dextranomer gel, polydimethylsiloxane (Macroplastique), pyrolytic carbon-coated beads suspended in a water-based carrier gel (*Durasphere®*), and collagen, is used to increase the bladder outlet resistance for patients in whom vesicourethral mobility is not excessive and whose primary problem is intrinsic sphincteric weakness (Ghoniem et al, 2010; Lightner et al, 2009). Recently, myoblast, fibroblast, and adult stem cells have been injected into periurethral tissue with very promising results (Carr et al, 1988; Mitterberger et al, 2007, 2008; Yamamoto et al, 2010). Besides the bulking effect, the injected stem cells seem to be able to stimulate local tissue proliferation (smooth muscle, collagen and elastic fibers) and thus improve the competence of the sphincter (Lin et al, 2010).

URGE INCONTINENCE

UI is defined as involuntary loss of urine, accompanied or immediately preceded by urgency. The basic feature of UI is detrusor overactivity or low bladder compliance and the loss of urine while attempting to inhibit micturition. Sphincteric instability is less common. The focus of this section is restricted to UI; OAB, which has replaced the term unstable bladder, and is clinically defined by symptoms of urgency, frequency, and nocturia with or without UI, is addressed only in the context of UI.

Neurogenic, myogenic, or urothelial bladder dysfunction can lead to UI or the constellation of symptoms that define OAB. OAB, with or without UI, is common in both men and women and can result from neuropathic injuries (brain or spinal cord deficit), obstruction, inflammation (interstitial

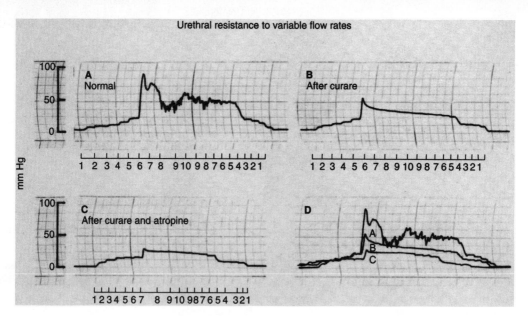

▲ **Figure 30–10. A:** The resistance required to force the urethra open, overcoming both voluntary and involuntary sphincteric elements. With progressively increasing pressure, the urethra opens at the **critical opening pressure** (in this recording, about 85 mm Hg). Once the urethra is forced open, the resistance to flow drops precipitously and becomes sustained at the level of **sustained urethral resistance** (in this recording, roughly 50 mm Hg). **B:** A similar recording obtained after administration of curare, which completely blocks voluntary sphincteric responses. Note the appreciable drop in both critical opening pressure and sustained resistance. **C:** Recording after administration of both curare and atropine (a combination that eliminates the activity of smooth and voluntary sphincteric elements). The critical opening pressure drops markedly and is now equal to the sustained resistance; both are very low. **D:** An overlap of the three recordings shows the contribution of each muscular element: the voluntary component contributes roughly 50% of the total resistance, while the smooth component contributes the other 50%. The minimal residual resistance is a function of the collagen elastic element of the urethral wall; this collagen element has no sphincteric significance.

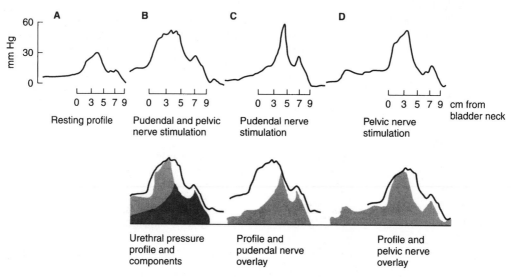

▲ **Figure 30–11.** Urethral pressure profile. **A:** At rest. **B:** Stimulation of both the pudendal and the pelvic nerves incites the maximal response from both smooth and voluntary sphincteric elements. **C:** Pudendal stimulation alone demonstrates the contribution of the voluntary component. **D:** Pelvic nerve stimulation shows the response of the smooth-muscle component alone. **Bottom tracings:** Total maximal pressure profile obtained by stimulation of pelvic and pudendal nerves depicted by overlapping the profile of simultaneous stimulation of both nerves. The contribution and anatomic distribution of each element are clearly seen. Their summation results in the overall total responses recorded in **B** above.

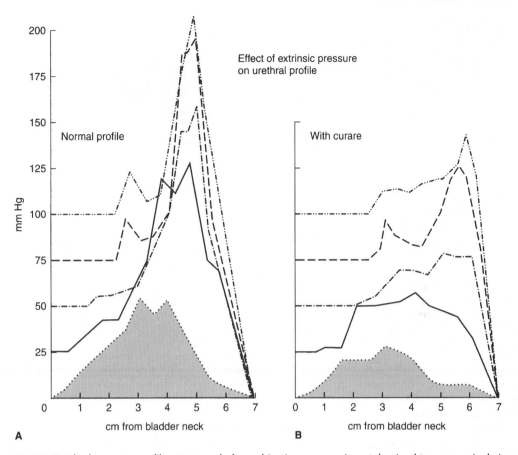

▲ **Figure 30–12.** Urethral pressure profile at rest and after subjecting an experimental animal to progressively increasing extrinsic pressure applied around the abdomen—not involving any muscular activity. **A:** Extrinsic pressure was increased by 25-mm Hg increments. Note the sharp increase in urethral closure pressure with each increment, marked after 25 and 50 mm Hg, less so after 75 and 100 mm Hg. The increase in urethral closure pressure is far higher than the increase in extrinsic pressure, which denotes not simple transmitted pressure but active muscular function. **B:** Curare administration demonstrates that much of the rise in closure pressure recorded in **A** results from the activity of the voluntary sphincter, which is lost after blockade by curare.

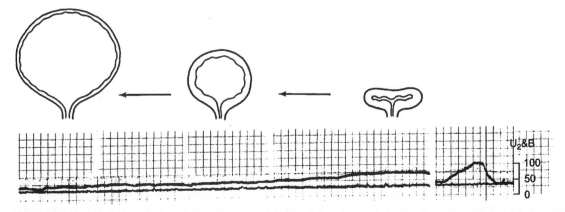

▲ **Figure 30–13.** Urethral pressure profile with minimally filled bladder. Bladder pressure remains constant, but urethral pressure drops progressively. Closure pressure becomes minimal at the end of bladder filling.

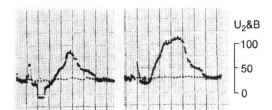

▲ Figure 30–14. Urethral pressure profile in moderately severe stress incontinence: closure pressure with patient in the sitting position with half-distended bladder, then after the upright position is assumed. Note that closure pressure is close to 75 cm H_2O with the patient in the sitting position but decreases to approximately 35 cm H_2O with the upright position. Note also the marked shortening of functional urethral length once the upright position is assumed.

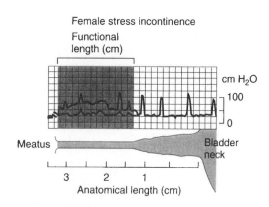

▲ Figure 30–15. Urethral pressure profile in a female patient with moderate urinary stress incontinence. Note the relatively low closure pressure, the short functional urethral length, and the loss of closure pressure of the proximal 1.5 cm of urethra.

cystitis), diabetes, benign prostatic hyperplasia (BPH), and so on, or be iatrogenic. Bladder overactivity may originate from the urothelium, detrusor muscle, or altered neural activation.

▶ Diagnosis

Assessment of patients with symptoms of UI, or OAB, should include detailed history, including an assessment of the impact of the disorder on daily life; physical examination; urinalysis; and identification of modifiable causes such as impaired mobility. A sudden urge with uncontrolled loss of urine not associated with physical activity and leak of urine prior to reaching the bathroom are common patient complaints. Because cough-induced urinary leakage may be symptomatic of urgency and stress urinary incontinence, this simple stress incontinence test should be performed in the

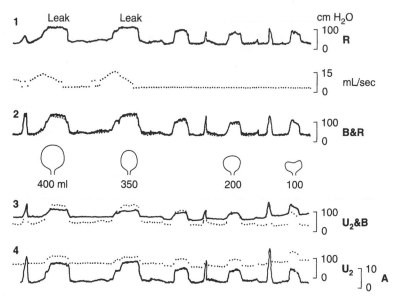

▲ Figure 30–16. Urethral pressure profile in moderate stress incontinence. Note that, with the bladder relatively empty, closure pressure is close to the normal range. At the start of bladder filling, resting pressure is again normal; as filling progresses, bladder pressure remains stable and urethral closure pressure decreases progressively to a minimum with full bladder distention.

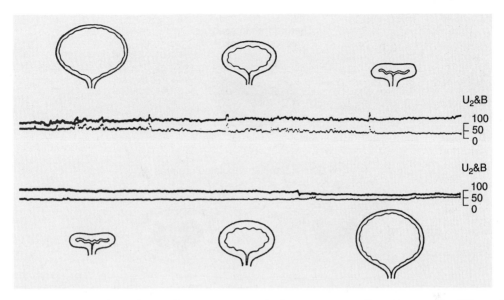

▲ **Figure 30–17.** Effect of bladder filling and emptying on urethral pressure. ***Top:*** Effect of progressive filling, which leads to a gradual drop in urethral pressure. At the end of filling, urethral closure pressure is only a fraction of the relatively normal initial closure pressure. ***Bottom:*** At the start, the bladder is full. With gradual emptying, note the progressive buildup in urethral resistance and closure pressure.

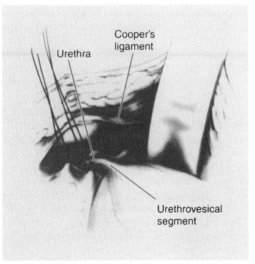

A

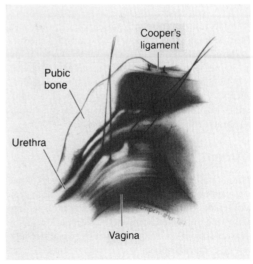

B

▲ **Figure 30–18.** ***A:*** Diagrammatic depiction of the retropubic space after mobilization of the anterior vaginal wall and placement of sutures, two on either side and far from the midline laterally. Distal sutures are opposite the midurethra, while proximal sutures are at the end of the vesicourethral junction. Sutures are attached to Cooper's ligament. ***B:*** Side view of suture placement with one side tied. The anterior vaginal wall acts as a broad sling, supporting and lifting the vesicourethral segment. The urethra is free in the retropubic space.

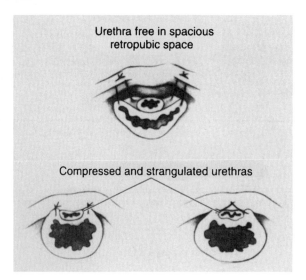

Urethra free in spacious
retropubic space

Compressed and strangulated urethras

▲ **Figure 30–19.** ***Top:*** Cross section shows the urethra free in the retropubic space with the anterior vaginal wall lifting and supporting it. ***Bottom:*** The urethra is compressed against the pubic bone when vaginal sutures are applied close to the urethra and fixed to the symphysis pubis. The vaginal suspension has various forms; in some, the tissue is gathered behind the bladder neck (eg, the Kelly procedure), while others rely on sutures in the paravaginal tissues that are passed bluntly to the suprapubic area by a needle to be tied over the rectus sheath. This technique was originally described by Pereyra in 1959 and subsequently was modified—in 1973 by Stamey, who added endoscopic confirmation of suture placement and the degree of compression, and in 1981 by Raz. Most of these techniques have a high initial success rate; however, there is some concern about the long-term results. Hence, the retropubic approach remains the recommended procedure.

office setting to rule out mixed incontinence (Dmochowski, 2006). Most women with uncomplicated urinary incontinence can be given a preliminary diagnosis at this point and treatment is initiated. Should initial management fail (usually after 8–12 weeks trial), or if complex conditions are present (eg, pelvic organ prolapse, significant postvoid residual), urodynamics or other specialized investigations are recommended (Abrams et al, 2010).

▶ Treatment

The treatment of UI often progresses from lifestyle change, behavioral techniques (bladder training) to anticholinergic pharmacotherapy. Options for nonresponders to drug therapy may include implanted sacral nerve stimulation (SNS). More invasive surgical procedures, including bladder augmentation or urinary diversion for persistent severe UI, are rarely indicated.

Lifestyle modification includes fluid management, as large volumes can exacerbate urinary incontinence, and bladder training to correct voiding patterns, improve the ability to suppress urge, and increase bladder capacity. Maneuvers included pelvic muscle training, scheduled voiding, and relaxation

techniques. The International Consultation on Continence recommends an initial voiding interval of 1 hour during waking hours, with weekly increases of 15–30 minutes until a 2–3-hour interval is achieved (Norton and Brubaker, 2006).

Anticholinergic agents, such as oxybutynin (Ditropan), tolterodine (Detrol), fesoterodine (Toviaz), propiverine, and trospium (Sanctura), suppress involuntary bladder contractions and thus reduce the symptoms of OAB and are considered first-line therapy for UI (Andersson et al, 2009). Controlled clinical trials have demonstrated improvements in micturition frequency and episodes of incontinence, although side effects of dry mouth and constipation can lead to discontinuation of treatment. Extended release formulations of oxybutynin (Ditropan XL) and tolterodine (Detrol LA) can be dosed once daily, increasing patient compliance. More selective M3 receptor antagonists, solifenacin (Vesicare) darifenacin (Enablex), have also demonstrated good efficacy, safety, and patient tolerance (Dmochowski, 2006). A new oxybutynin 10% gel (Gelnique) has also been available with similar effect but has less incidence of dry mouth and constipation.

Intravesical botulinum toxin A has shown significant benefits for UI, OAB, prostatic enlargement, and neurogenic detrusor overactivity, and it may offer an important alternative to long-term oral pharmacotherapy or more invasive treatments. Quality of life, urgency, frequency, and bladder capacity improvements have been impressive to date (Chancellor, 2010; Kuo and Liu, 2009). Resiniferatoxin and capsaicin are two other agents currently under investigation but are not recommended by the International Consultation on Incontinence (Andersson et al, 2009). Others have proposed beta-3 adrenoceptor agonist as a potential agent for OAB (Igawa et al, 2010).

The results of randomized control trials provide evidence of SNS in decreasing episodes of incontinence, pad use, voiding frequency, and improvement of bladder capacity and voided volume (Tanagho and Schmidt, 1988; Thompson et al, 2010). Although surgical revision was required for one-third of cases, no major irreversible complications were reported and benefits of SNS were reported to persist at follow-up of 3–5 years.

MIXED URINARY INCONTINENCE

MUI *refers to the* complaint of an involuntary leakage of urine associated with urgency and also with exertion, effort, sneezing, or coughing. This disorder comprises an element of detrusor dysfunction (motor or sensory) and is associated with urethral sphincter underactivity. About one-third of incontinent patients have both UI linked to idiopathic overactivity and genuine SUI. Some experts believe that MUI is now the predominant symptom grouping, with rates >50% reported in large population studies (Dmochowski, 2006). The relative incidence increases with advancing age and occurs most commonly in women older than 60 years.

▶ Diagnosis

The definition of MUI by the ICS emphasizes the presence of SUI and components of OAB (frequency and urgency) with or without UI, in the absence of known instigating factors. Urodynamically, detrusor overactivity is often noted. However, it should be emphasized that the underlying source of MUI may be a reflex response initiated by urine released into the proximal urethra during stress events. In this way, some individuals with SUI may mimic MUI due to a significant urge component associated with spontaneous urine loss. The diagnostic steps for MUI are the same as for SUI and are described in Section "Stress Urinary Incontinence." In those individuals with equal bother (UI and SUI), or difficulty defining their symptoms, urodynamics may help define dysfunction and therapy.

▶ Treatment

The presenting symptoms serve as a guide to initial therapeutic approach. The most bothersome aspect, SUI versus UI, is usually addressed first. If both types of incontinence are equally bothersome, treatment of the urge component is preferred in most cases.

Initial approaches include behavioral therapy, biofeedback, and treatment with anticholinergics, with approximately 70% of patients experiencing symptomatic improvement with this class of medications; the notable exception is the patient with severe stress incontinence. In men, antimuscarinics for treatment of storage LUTS and prostate enlargement have also been shown to be effective with <3% chance of developing urinary retention (Kaplan et al, 2011). Once the initial treatment response is determined, further therapies can be initiated for persistent or secondary symptoms as outlined in Sections "Stress Urinary Incontinence" and "Urge Incontinence," respectively.

Surgical outcomes for MUI have been reviewed for various sling techniques. Correction of a low-pressure outlet may benefit at least some patients with detrusor overactivity, although results for pure SUI remain superior. MUI symptom resolution has been demonstrated for upward of 70% of patients in some series, including a 4-year cure rate of 85% reported for the TVT approach (Dmochowski and Staskin, 2005; Lleberia, 2011). Current data support the use of either midurethral or pubovaginal slings for MUI.

OVERFLOW INCONTINENCE

OI is defined as the involuntary loss of urine associated with bladder overdistension. Two primary processes are involved: urinary retention caused by BOO or inadequate bladder contractions. Outflow obstruction may be secondary to BPH, bladder neck contracture or urethral stricture, or, less commonly, prostate cancer in men and due to cystocele, pelvic organ prolapse, or previous incontinence surgery in women. Impaired bladder emptying caused by decreased detrusor contractility may be the result of medications, spinal or peripheral nerve injuries, or due to long-standing overdistension. Diabetic cystopathy can result in OI, as both sensory and contractile functions may be compromised. OI may also occur following transurethral prostatectomy (TURP), as urine flow is impeded by stricture, contracture, or residual adenoma.

▶ Diagnosis

A similar approach is followed as outlined previously for the other incontinence subtypes. Reversible causes can usually be identified by patient history. Specific to OI, overflow bladder is detected by measuring postvoid residual urine volume with ultrasonography (preferred) or urethral catheterization immediately after the patient urinates. Normally, <50 mL of urine remains in the bladder immediately following voiding and residual volumes of >200 mL indicate overflow bladder. Urodynamic testing and cystourethroscopy are used to determine the underlying cause or differentiate OI from other incontinence states.

▶ Treatment

Initial treatment of OI focuses on addressing reversible causes identified during patient evaluation such as cystocele, pelvic organ prolapse, impaired mobility, and so on.

Should such precipitating elements not be found, outlet obstruction may be treated conservatively, with adjustment of fluid intake and timed voiding. However, male patients will often require further intervention, including pharmacotherapy with alpha-adrenergic antagonists or 5α-reductase (finasteride)/dual 5α-reductase (dutasteride) inhibitors. If stricture or prostatic obstruction is present, surgical intervention (transurethral resection of prostate, incision of the bladder neck, visual internal urethrotomy) may offer definitive treatment.

For OI secondary to nonobstructive underactive detrusor, the first step is to decompress the bladder with an indwelling catheter or clean intermittent catheterization (CIC) for 7–14 days, while addressing potential reversible causes such as medications, infection, or constipation. An alpha-blocker may be initiated during this time period. Should voiding trials fail repeatedly in the patient with an acontractile detrusor, CIC is the treatment of choice versus a permanent indwelling catheter (if feasible).

NEUROPATHIC INCONTINENCE

Many diseases or conditions involving the brain, spinal cord, and peripheral nerve can affect the function and structure of the bladder and sphincter as well as the synergic action of the two structures. Although complete lesions at different levels of the nervous system may produce typical urodynamic findings, the symptoms of patients suffering from the same lesion may vary due to nerve plasticity, secondary changes from infection, fibrosis, etc. Many diseases can also involve both peripheral and central nervous system to varying degrees. Incontinence can also be due to patient's inability to respond to sensory cue from bladder or having no perception of bladder fullness at all.

A. Failure of Bladder Storage Function

Loss of reservoir function in a contracted bladder can be caused by poor compliance in the detrusor muscle. Intravesical pressure rises with minimal bladder filling, exceeding the outlet resistance and causing urinary leakage. Failure of reservoir function may be found in patients who have meningomyelocele or exhibit other upper motor neuron lesions. Although these patients may have partial lesions with significant striated sphincteric activity offering some degree of resistance, early loss of bladder compliance increases intravesical pressure with minimal bladder filling and overcomes remaining outlet resistance (Figure 30–20). These patients,

once recognized, must be managed aggressively because they often have a significant risk to the upper urinary tract, which can lead to possible vesicoureteral reflux, early renal deterioration, or lower ureteral obstruction.

B. Failure of Sphincter Function

Complete lesions of the sacral segment or the cauda equina result in a total loss of smooth and striated sphincteric activity. The external sphincter offers minimal resistance. Most patients experiencing such failure can retain some volume, because the bladder musculature becomes atonic and intravesical pressure remains low, but any increase in intravesical pressure can cause leakage and the bladder never reaches full capacity. Consequently, the integrity of the upper urinary tract is not endangered, as in cases of reservoir failure.

▶ Diagnosis

Diagnostic evaluation of neuropathic urinary incontinence determines whether the condition arises from detrusor or sphincteric dysfunction, or from a combination of the two. In many patients with multiple sclerosis, spinal stenosis, herniated disk, or partial traumatic damage to the spinal cord, the contribution of neural deficit to urinary incontinence can be difficult to determine.

A complete urologic and neurologic history, physical examination, and urodynamics (cystometry, urethral pressure recordings, uroflowmetry) should be performed. Ultrasound evaluation, which can accurately measure renal size and identify scarring, calculi, and hydronephrosis (obstruction or vesicoureteral reflux), is an appropriate baseline study for all patients with neuropathic lesions. Other radiologic studies (voiding cystourethrography, excretory urography, computed tomography scanning, MRI) and neurologic studies (electromyography, evoked potentials) are performed as indicated. Cystourethroscopy is not recommended as part of the routine screening evaluation; if clinically indicated, it is used to assess the integrity of the urethra and identify stricture sites, diverticula, calculi, or other anatomic abnormalities.

The following are valuable in determining the underlying cause of incontinence:

1. Bladder responses to progressive filling.
2. Sphincteric pressure profile and its response to progressive filling and the initiation of voiding.
3. The presence of detrusor overactivity.
4. Electromyographic studies of the striated urinary sphincter.
5. In selected patients, response to neurostimulation of the sacral roots and pudendal nerve and measurement of latencies.

Differentiation among incontinence caused by neurogenic detrusor overactivity and poor bladder compliance is a straightforward process. Significant findings include sphincteric weakness, precipitous sphincteric relaxation, and

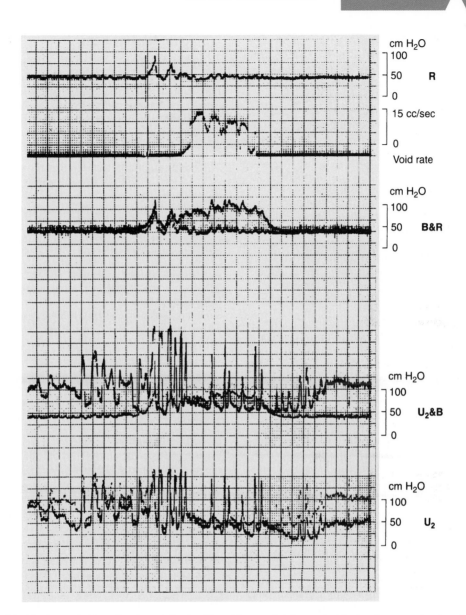

▲ **Figure 30–20.** Urodynamic recording in a patient with evidence of detrusor/sphincter dyssynergia, showing spontaneous activity in the bladder associated with a burst of activity in the external sphincter interrupting voiding. This represents a classic demonstration of upper motor neuron dysfunction leading to urinary incontinence as a result of detrusor hyperactivity or hyperreflexia. R, rectal pressure; B, bladder pressure; U2, distal urethral pressure.

decrease in pressure, as well as a lack of electromyographic activity of the pelvic floor musculature and external sphincter.

The proper diagnosis can be achieved by establishing the integrity of the sacral root reflex arc by neurostimulation of the sacral roots, with simultaneous recording of intravesical and intraurethral pressures at the levels of the internal and the external sphincter. The extent of one cause relative to another (eg, sphincteric weakness versus detrusor overactivity) should

be taken into consideration, and management should be directed toward the predominating cause of incontinence.

▶ **Treatment**

The management of neurogenic urinary incontinence can be challenging. The rehabilitation of the neuropathic condition and the alleviation of potentially damaging sequelae must be the guiding principles of management (see also Chapter 28—Neuropathic Bladder Disorders). Choices must be made according to the severity and potential progression of the lesion and the integrity of the system, with great care taken to prevent deterioration of the upper tracts. In patients with spinal cord injury and meningomyelocele, early treatment provides the best chance of preserving the integrity of the entire urinary system.

A. Failure of Storage Function

Anticholinergic agents are commonly used to treat detrusor overactivity. These medications inhibit the binding of acetylcholine to muscarinic receptors in the detrusor muscle, increasing bladder capacity and inhibiting involuntary contractions. Treatment with oxybutynin chloride (Ditropan) 5 mg three times daily, tolterodine tartrate (Detrol) 2 mg twice daily, and single-dose extended release daily formulations (Ditropan XL 10 mg and Detrol ER 4 mg) has proven to be highly effective and well tolerated. Fesoterodine fumarate (Toviaz), propiverine hydrochloride (Detrunorm), trospium chloride (Sanctura), and the more selective M3 receptor antagonists (darifenacin hydrochloride [Enablex] and solifenacin succinate [Vesicare]) are newer anticholinergic options (Andersson et al, 2009). Dosages can be increased above these levels in some patients, dependent on tolerance of adverse effects and treatment response. Common side effects include dry mouth, palpitations, constipation, nausea, or drowsiness, although newer extended-release formulations provide a reduced incidence versus immediate-release anticholinergics.

Propantheline bromide (Pro-Banthine) and imipramine hydrochloride (Tofranil) are considered second-line treatments for some patients, while the efficacy of flavoxate hydrochloride (Urispas) is unclear (Corcos et al, 2006).

Injection of botulinum-A toxin into the detrusor muscle for both children and adults who have failure of reservoir function is a promising new treatment that has demonstrated a significant increase in bladder capacity and compliance as well as symptomatic improvement for several weeks after cystoscopic injection (Chancellor, 2010). This neurotoxin binds to the presynaptic nerve endings of cholinergic neurons and leads to a temporary chemodenervation and the reduction of neural activity, as well as changes the muscarinic receptors in the bladder (Datta et al, 2010).

B. Failure of Sphincter Mechanism

CIC is the first line of conservative management in this group. Although such patients have very low outlet resistance, atonic bladder function may result in some retention. Most of the time, CIC every 4–6 hours avoids leakage. When CIC is not possible and the increase in intravesical pressure becomes excessive, the patient can wear pads or diapers. Pharmacotherapy has proven unsuccessful to date.

C. Surgical Management

1. Sphincterotomy—For spastic hyperreflexive male patients, this procedure can eliminate outlet resistance so that, with an external appliance or condom catheter, the bladder will remain empty (Perkash, 2007). Although many consider this procedure the easiest way to preserve the upper urinary tract, it is clearly not rehabilitative and might interfere with other treatments.

2. Bladder augmentation—In patients with poor compliance owing to bladder wall hypertrophy or fibrosis, augmentation improves reservoir function. If the sphincteric mechanism is adequate, detubularized bowel segments can be used to expand a small contracted bladder. Usually, patients will be required to perform CIC to empty the bladder postoperatively.

3. Artificial urinary sphincter (AUS)—For patients with severe sphincteric damage and a low-pressure, large-capacity bladder, the AUS is a useful option. In males, it is applied around the bulbous urethra. When the device is deflated, the patient can void either by detrusor contraction (if some capability is preserved) or by straining and the Valsalva maneuver. A complete sphincterotomy can be performed first.

4. Continent urinary diversion—This method should be considered only with progressively deteriorating upper urinary tract function, and even then, a simple conduit is often preferable.

5. Neurostimulation—In selected patients with detrusor overactivity, stimulation of the sacral roots can be used to suppress the overactive detrusor. If such patients with spinal cord injury, meningomyelocele, multiple sclerosis, and other neuropathies show significant improvement after temporary testing, a permanent electrode can be placed over the most responsive root, usually S_3.

6. Dorsal rhizotomy—Complete dorsal rhizotomy of S_2–S_4 extra- or intradurally effectively eliminates detrusor hyperreflexia and increases bladder capacity. Increases have been seen from a capacity of 150 or 200 mL to 600–800 mL. In patients with suprasegmental lesions and spastic upper motor neuron lesions, sacral root electrode (bladder pacemaker) implantation promotes detrusor contraction and bladder evacuation.

BIBLIOGRAPHY

Abrams P et al; Standardisation Sub-Committee of the International Continence Society: The standardisation of terminology in lower urinary tract function: Report from the standardisation subcommittee of the International Continence Society. Urology 2003;61(1):37–49.

Abrams P et al: Fourth International Consultation on Incontinence Recommendations of the International Scientific Committee: Evaluation and treatment of urinary incontinence, pelvic organ prolapse, and fecal incontinence. Neurourol Urodyn 2010;29(1):213–240.

Andersson KE et al: Pharmacological treatment of overactive bladder: Report from the International Consultation on Incontinence. Curr Opin Urol 2009;19(4):380–394.

Anger JT et al: The prevalence of urinary incontinence among community dwelling adult women: Results from the National Health and Nutrition Examination Survey. J Urol 2006;175:601.

Broekhuis SR et al: Perineal descent and patients' symptoms of anorectal dysfunction, pelvic organ prolapse, and urinary incontinence. Int Urogynecol J Pelvic Floor Dysfunct 2010;21(6):721–729.

Carr LK et al: 1-year follow-up of autologous muscle-derived stem cell injection pilot study to treat stress urinary incontinence. Int Urogynecol J Pelvic Floor Dysfunct 2008;19(6):881–883.

Chancellor MB: Ten years single surgeon experience with botulinum toxin in the urinary tract; clinical observations and research discovery. Int Urol Nephrol 2010;42(2):383–391.

Corcos J et al: Canadian Urological Association guidelines on urinary incontinence. Can J Urol 2006;13:3127.

Datta SN et al: Immunohistochemical expression of muscarinic receptors in the urothelium and suburothelium of neurogenic and idiopathic overactive human bladders, and changes with botulinum neurotoxin administration. J Urol 2010;184(6):2578–2585.

DeLancey JO: Structural support of the urethra as it relates to stress urinary incontinence: The hammock hypothesis. Am J Obstet Gynecol 1994;170(6):1713–1720.

Dmochowski R, Staskin D: Mixed incontinence: Definitions, outcomes, and interventions. Curr Opin Urol 2005;15:374.

Drouin J et al: Burch colposuspension: Long-term results and review of published reports. Urology 1999;54:808.

Fong ED, Nitti VW: Review article: Mid-urethral synthetic slings for female stress urinary incontinence. BJU Int 2010;106(5):596–608.

Ghoniem G et al: Durability of urethral bulking agent injection for female stress urinary incontinence: 2-year multicenter study results. J Urol 2010;183(4):1444–1449.

Hawkins K et al: The prevalence of urinary incontinence and its burden on the quality of life among older adults with Medicare supplement insurance. Qual Life Res 2010;20(5):723–732.

Igawa Y et al: Beta3-adrenoceptor agonists: Possible role in the treatment of overactive bladder. Korean J Urol 2010;51(12):811–818.

Irwin DE et al: Worldwide prevalence estimates of lower urinary tract symptoms, overactive bladder, urinary incontinence and bladder outlet obstruction. BJU Int 2011;108(7):1138–1139.

Kaplan SA et al: Antimuscarinics for treatment of storage lower urinary tract symptoms in men: A systematic review. Int J Clin Pract 2011;65(4):487–507.

Kulseng-Hanssen S, Berild GH: Subjective and objective incontinence 5 to 10 years after Burch colposuspension. Neurourol Urodyn 2002;21:100.

Kuo HC, Liu HT: Therapeutic effects of add-on botulinum toxin A on patients with large benign prostatic hyperplasia and unsatisfactory response to combined medical therapy. Scand J Urol Nephrol 2009;43(3):206–211.

Lightner D et al: Randomized controlled multisite trial of injected bulking agents for women with intrinsic sphincter deficiency: Mid-urethral injection of Zuidex via the Implacer versus proximal urethral injection of Contigen cystoscopically. Urology 2009;74(4):771–775.

Lin G et al: Treatment of stress urinary incontinence with adipose tissue-derived stem cells. Cytotherapy 2010;12(1):88–95.

Lleberia J et al: Surgical treatment of mixed urinary incontinence: Effect of anterior colpoplasty. Int Urogynecol J Pelvic Floor Dysfunct 2011;22(8):1025–1030.

Mitterberger M et al: Autologous myoblasts and fibroblasts for female stress incontinence: A 1-year follow-up in 123 patients. BJU Int 2007;100(5):1081–1085.

Mitterberger M et al: Myoblast and fibroblast therapy for postprostatectomy urinary incontinence: 1-year followup of 63 patients. J Urol 2008;179(1):226–231.

Miyazato M, et al: Effect of duloxetine, a norepinephrine and serotonin reuptake inhibitor, on sneeze-induced urethral continence reflex in rats. Am J Physiol Renal Physiol 2008;295(1):F264–F271.

Morgan DM et al: Urethral sphincter morphology and function with and without stress incontinence. J Urol 2009;182(1):203–209.

Norton R, Brubaker L: Urinary incontinence in women. Lancet 2006;367:57.

Novara G et al: Updated systematic review and meta-analysis of the comparative data on colposuspensions, pubovaginal slings, and midurethral tapes in the surgical treatment of female stress urinary incontinence. Eur Urol 2010;58(2):218–238.

Perkash I: Transurethral sphincterotomy provides significant relief in autonomic dysreflexia in spinal cord injured male patients: Long-term followup results. J Urol 2007;177(3):1026–1029.

Petros PE, Ulmsten UI: An integral theory of female urinary incontinence. Experimental and clinical considerations. Acta Obstet Gynecol Scand Suppl 1990;153:7–31.

Swift S et al: Test-retest reliability of the cotton swab (Q-tip) test in the evaluation of the incontinent female. Int Urogynecol J Pelvic Floor Dysfunct 2010;21(8):963–967.

Tanagho EA, Schmidt RA: Electrical stimulation in the clinical management of the neurogenic bladder. J Urol 1988;140(6):1331–1339.

Thompson JH et al: Sacral neuromodulation: Therapy evolution. Indian J Urol 2010;26(3):379–384.

Ulmsten U et al: A multicenter study of tension-free vaginal tape (TVT) for surgical treatment of stress urinary incontinence. Int Urogynecol J Pelvic Floor Dysfunct 1998;9(4):210–213.

Yamamoto T et al: Periurethral injection of autologous adipose-derived stem cells for the treatment of stress urinary incontinence in patients undergoing radical prostatectomy: Report of two initial cases. Int J Urol 2010;17(1):75–82.

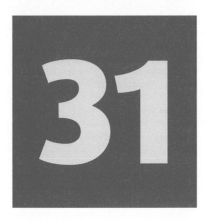

31

Disorders of the Adrenal Glands

Christopher J. Kane, MD, FACS

Disorders of the adrenal glands result in classic endocrine syndromes such as Cushing's syndrome, hyperaldosteronism, and catechol excess from pheochromocytoma (Figure 31–1). The diagnosis of these disorders requires careful endocrine evaluation and imaging with computed tomography (CT) or magnetic resonance imaging (MRI).

In addition, many adrenal lesions are discovered on cross-sectional imaging performed for other reasons. These "incidentalomas" require metabolic evaluation and assessment to determine their need for treatment.

DISEASES OF THE ADRENAL CORTEX

CUSHING'S SYNDROME

Cushing's syndrome is the clinical disorder caused by overproduction of cortisol. Most cases (80%) are due to bilateral adrenocortical hyperplasia stimulated by overproduction of pituitary adrenocorticotropic hormone (ACTH, corticotropin), known as Cushing's disease. About 10% of cases are due to the ectopic production of ACTH from nonpituitary tumors. Ectopic ACTH production occurs most frequently in small-cell lung carcinoma; other tumors producing ACTH include carcinoids (lung, thymic, gastrointestinal tract), islet cell tumors of the pancreas, medullary thyroid carcinoma, pheochromocytoma, and small-cell carcinoma of the prostate. Adrenal adenoma is the cause in 5% of cases and carcinoma in 5%. In children, adrenocortical carcinoma is the most common cause of Cushing's syndrome.

▶ Pathophysiology

Overproduction of cortisol by adrenocortical tissue leads to a catabolic state. This causes liberation from muscle tissue of amino acids, which are transformed into glucose and glycogen in the liver by gluconeogenesis. The resulting weakened protein structures (muscle and elastic tissue) cause a protuberant abdomen and poor wound healing, generalized muscle weakness, and marked osteoporosis, which is made worse by excessive loss of calcium in the urine.

In addition, glucose is transformed largely into fat and appears in characteristic sites such as the abdomen, supraclavicular fat pads, and cheeks. There is a tendency to diabetes, with an elevated fasting plasma glucose level in 20% of cases and abnormal glucose tolerance in 80% of patients.

The cortisol excess also suppresses the immune mechanisms, making patients susceptible to infection. Inhibition of fibroblast function by excess cortisol further interferes with wound healing.

Hypertension is present in 90% of cases. Although the aldosterone level is not usually elevated, cortisol itself exerts a hypertensive effect when present in excessive amounts, as does 11-deoxycorticosterone. The hypertension may be accompanied by manifestation of mineralocorticoid excess (hypokalemia and alkalosis), especially in patients with ectopic ACTH syndrome or adrenocortical carcinoma.

▶ Pathology

The cells in adrenal hyperplasia resemble those of the zona fasciculata of the normal adrenal cortex. Frank adenocarcinoma reveals pleomorphism and invasion of the capsule, the vascular system, or both (Figure 31–2). Local invasion may occur, and metastases are common to the liver, lungs, bone, or brain. Histologic differentiation between adenoma and adenocarcinoma is frequently difficult.

In the presence of adenoma or malignant tumor, atrophy of the cortices of both adrenals occurs because the main secretory product of the tumor is cortisol, which inhibits the pituitary secretion of ACTH. Thus, although the tumor continues to grow, the contralateral adrenal cortex undergoes atrophy.

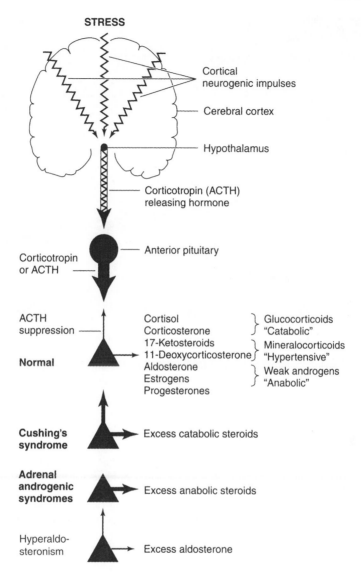

▲ **Figure 31–1.** The hypothalamic–pituitary–adrenocortical relationships in various adrenocortical syndromes.

▶ Clinical Findings

A. Symptoms and Signs (Figures 31–3 and 31–4)

The presence of at least three of the following strongly suggests Cushing's syndrome:

1. Obesity (with sparing of the extremities), moon face, and fat pads of the supraclavicular and dorsocervical areas (buffalo hump).

2. Striae (red and depressed) over the abdomen and thighs.

3. Hypertension (almost always present).

4. Proximal myopathy with marked weakness, especially in the quadriceps femoris, making unaided rising from a chair difficult.

5. Emotional lability, irritability, difficulty in sleeping, and sometimes psychotic personality.

6. Osteoporosis (common), with back pain from compression fractures of the lumbar vertebrae as well as rib fractures.

7. In 80% of cases, postprandial hyperglycemia is present, and in 20%, there is an elevated fasting plasma glucose level.

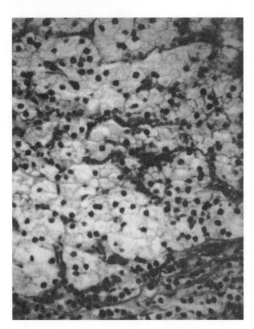 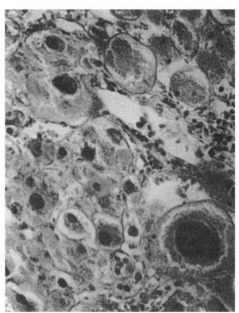

▲ **Figure 31–2.** ***Left:*** Histologic appearance of a typical benign adenoma of the adrenal cortex made up of a large number of identical cells from the zona fasciculata removed from a 39-year-old woman with Cushing's syndrome. ***Right:*** Section of an adenocarcinoma removed from a 36-year-old woman with metastatic adenocarcinoma showing significant pleomorphism of the cells. Invasion of a large vein is not shown in this micrograph. Note that benign adenomas will occasionally have this appearance but without invasion of the bloodstream. (Reproduced, with permission, from Forsham PH: The adrenal cortex. In: Williams RH [ed.] Textbook of Endocrinology. 4th ed. Saunders, 1968.)

8. To a variable extent, there are features of adrenal androgen excess in women with Cushing's syndrome; these are absent in the case of adenoma, most severe with carcinoma, and present to an intermediate degree with Cushing's disease. They consist of recession of the hairline, hirsutism, small breasts, and generalized muscular overdevelopment, with deepening of the voice.

It is not possible to differentiate the cause from the clinical presentation alone.

B. Laboratory Findings

The leukocyte count may be elevated to the range of 12,000–20,000/μL, usually with fewer than 20% lymphocytes. Polycythemia is present in over half the cases, with the hemoglobin ranging from 14 to 16 g/dL. Anemia, however, may occur in patients with malignant tumors ectopically secreting ACTH.

Blood chemical analyses may show an increase in serum Na^+ and CO_2 levels and a decrease in serum K^+ levels. Hyperglycemia may occur.

1. Specific tests for Cushing's syndrome—The following tests are performed to determine whether the patient has Cushing's syndrome.

a. **24-Hour urinary cortisol level**—Urine cortisol is measured in a 24-hour urine collection (normal range, 10–50 μg/24 h). A urine cortisol value more than twofold elevated is typical of Cushing's syndrome. False-positive elevations can occur in acute illness, depression, and alcoholism. However, obesity does not raise the level of urinary-free cortisol above normal.

b. **Suppression of ACTH and plasma cortisol by dexamethasone**—Dexamethasone in low doses is used to assess the feedback suppression of ACTH and cortisol production by glucocorticoids. If dexamethasone is given at 11 pm, ACTH is suppressed in normal persons but not in those with Cushing's syndrome. Dexamethasone is useful because it has 30 times the potency of cortisol as an ACTH suppressant and it is not measured in current plasma or urine cortisol methods.

The procedure is to give 1 mg of dexamethasone by mouth at 11 pm and to draw blood at 8:00 to 9:00 am for measurement of plasma cortisol. If the level is <5 μg/dL (normal is 5–20 mg/dL), Cushing's syndrome can be ruled out. If the value is >10 μg/dL, Cushing's syndrome is present. A level in the range of 5–10 μg/dL is equivocal, and the test should be repeated or the urine cortisol may be measured.

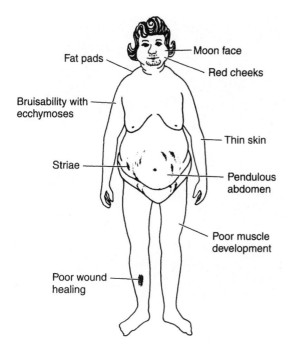

▲ **Figure 31–3.** Drawing of a typical case of Cushing's syndrome showing the principal clinical features. (Reproduced, with permission, from Forsham PH: The adrenal cortex. In: Williams RH [ed.] Textbook of Endocrinology, 4th ed. Saunders, 1968.)

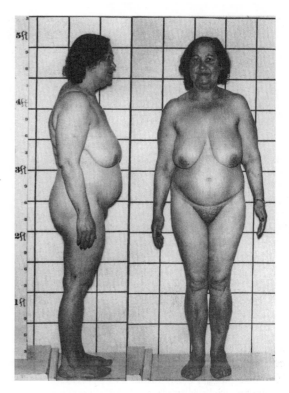

▲ **Figure 31–4.** A patient with Cushing's disease. Note the red moon face, receding hairline, buffalo hump over the seventh vertebra, protuberant abdomen, and inappropriately thin arms and legs.

Women taking birth-control pills have high plasma cortisol levels because, as in pregnancy, the estrogen stimulates production of cortisol-binding globulin. The pills must be withheld for at least 3 weeks before the dexamethasone suppression test. Other conditions causing false-positive responses are acute illness, depression, and alcoholism. Also, about 15% of obese patients do not suppress cortisol with this test.

2. Specific tests for differentiation of causes of Cushing's syndrome—The various causes of Cushing's syndrome can be determined with great accuracy (95% of cases).

a. **Plasma ACTH level**—If the diagnosis of Cushing's syndrome has been established, this test will differentiate ACTH-dependent causes (Cushing's disease and the ectopic ACTH syndrome) from adrenal tumors, which are ACTH independent. The normal range is 10–50 pg/mL. Patients with Cushing's disease have ACTH levels that range from 10 to 200 pg/mL; in the ectopic ACTH syndrome, levels are usually >200 pg/mL; and patients with adrenal tumors have suppressed ACTH levels (<5 pg/mL).

b. **Plasma androgen levels**—In patients with adrenal adenomas, androgen levels are normal or low, and in

adrenocortical carcinoma, these levels are often markedly elevated.

C. X-Ray Findings and Special Examinations

1. Localization of source of ACTH excess—When tests suggest Cushing's disease or the ectopic ACTH syndrome and an elevated plasma level of ACTH is present, the source of ACTH must be identified. Because the great majority of these patients have Cushing's disease and because most of the patients with ectopic ACTH secretion have an obvious malignancy, the first step is to perform *pituitary MRI*. These are positive in 50–60% of patients with Cushing's disease; in the remainder, the diagnosis should be established by the sampling of ACTH levels in the venous drainage of the anterior pituitary, that is, the cavernous sinuses and inferior petrosal sinuses. If the MRI and venous sampling do not reveal a pituitary source of ACTH, CT scans of the chest and abdomen are used to localize an ectopic tumor.

2. Localization of adrenal lesions—Patients with Cushing's syndrome with suspected adrenal tumors and

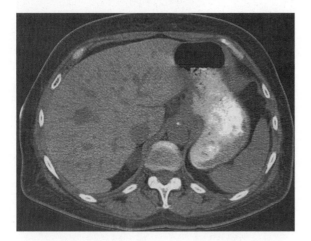

▲ **Figure 31–5.** Noncontrast CT image of a right benign adrenal adenoma. Hounsfield units under 10. (Image courtesy of Fergus Coakley, MD, UCSF Radiology Department.)

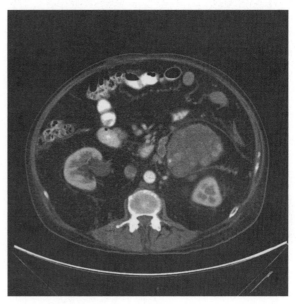

▲ **Figure 31–6.** Contrast CT image of a left adrenocortical carcinoma. Note the irregular border and small satellite masses medially. (Image courtesy of Fergus Coakley, MD, UCSF Radiology Department.)

suppressed ACTH levels should undergo a CT scan of the abdomen with 3-mm sections through the adrenals. Adrenal tumors causing Cushing's syndrome are usually >3 cm in diameter (Figure 31–5) and are therefore easily visualized. Adenomas are usually 3–6 cm in diameter; carcinomas are usually >5 cm in diameter (Figure 31–6) and are frequently locally invasive or metastatic to the liver and lungs at the time of diagnosis. In patients with adrenal tumors, the contralateral adrenal is suppressed and therefore appears atrophic or normal on CT scan. The finding of bilateral adrenal enlargement is typical of Cushing's disease or the ectopic ACTH syndrome. Ultrasound or MRI may also be used for adrenal localization, although these techniques do not appear to offer significant advantage over CT.

▶ **Treatment**

A. Cushing's Disease

A pituitary microadenoma, which is the most common cause of bilateral adrenocortical hyperplasia, must be located and removed surgically. *Transsphenoidal resection* performed by an experienced neurosurgeon is the method of choice. Success is reported in >80% of cases, and in most instances, the endocrine functions of the pituitary gland are preserved.

B. Ectopic ACTH Syndrome

The treatment of these patients is difficult because most have an advanced malignancy and severe hypercortisolism. Removal of the primary tumor is clearly the therapy of choice; however, curative resection is limited to the few patients with benign tumors such as bronchial carcinoids. Patients with residual or metastatic tumors should be managed first

with adrenal inhibitors, and if that is not successful, bilateral adrenalectomy should be considered.

C. Total Bilateral Adrenalectomy

Total bilateral adrenalectomy is indicated in patients with Cushing's disease in whom the pituitary tumor is not resectable and in whom medical therapy fails to control the cortisol excess. A laparoscopic approach to adrenalectomy is preferred, since it significantly decreases morbidity and length of hospital stay compared with open adrenalectomy. Bilateral adrenalectomy is also indicated in patients with ectopic ACTH syndrome who have life-threatening hypercortisolism that cannot be controlled by inhibitors of adrenal secretion.

1. Preoperative preparation—Because removal of the source of excessive cortisol will inevitably lead to temporary or permanent adrenal insufficiency, it is of the utmost importance to administer cortisol preoperatively and to continue substitution therapy after surgery to control Addison's disease. In the postoperative period, the dose is tapered downward until oral medication provides sufficient control.

2. Postoperative status—The patient feels moderately well following removal of the source of excess ACTH or adrenalectomy or while receiving a high dose of hydrocortisone in excess of the usual daily output of approximately 20 mg. It is important to reduce the steroid substitution gradually over a period of several days. On the day of operation, 200 mg of cortisol is given; the dosage is then reduced gradually on successive days (150, 100, 80, 60, and 40 mg) until a maintenance dosage of 20–30 mg cortisol combined with 0.1 mg fludrocortisone is reached.

D. Adrenal Adenoma and Adenocarcinoma

Virtually all adrenal adenomas and smaller adrenal carcinomas are now removed laparoscopically, again allowing decreased hospital stay and more rapid recovery from surgery. Most patients now have a 1-day hospitalization after laparoscopic adrenalectomy if their metabolic management allows. There is some emerging evidence that select small adrenal tumors can be percutaneously ablated with radiofrequency ablation (RFA). The long-term efficacy of this approach is not known. Adrenal carcinomas that are large, locally invasive or involve the inferior vena cava are best approached by an open operation.

1. Preoperative preparation—Preoperative preparation is the same as that for bilateral hyperplasia, since, in this case, the remaining adrenal gland will be atrophic and thus the patient will be hypoadrenal.

2. Postoperative treatment and follow-up—Cortisol is administered perioperatively in the doses described earlier and then tapered to a replacement dose of 20–30 mg/day. Hydrocortisone is given orally in a dosage of 10 mg three times daily initially and reduced within 2–3 weeks to 10 mg daily given at 7 or 8 am. Substitution therapy may be necessary for 6 months to 2 years depending on the rate of recovery of the residual gland. Mineralocorticoid therapy is rarely necessary, since the atrophic adrenal usually produces sufficient aldosterone. Patients with adrenocortical carcinoma are usually not cured by surgery and require additional therapy.

E. Medical Therapy

There is no effective method of inhibiting ACTH secretion; however, adrenal hypersecretion can be controlled in many patients by inhibitors of adrenal cortisol secretion. Medical therapy is indicated in patients who either cannot undergo surgery (eg, because of debility, recent myocardial infarction) or in those who have had unsuccessful resection of their pituitary, ectopic, or adrenal tumor.

Ketoconazole is the current drug of choice; it blocks cortisol secretion by inhibiting P450c11 and P450scc. The total dose required is 800–1600 mg/day given in two divided doses. Side effects are adrenal insufficiency, abnormal liver function tests, and hepatotoxicity in a few patients.

Metyrapone may be used alone or may be added if ketoconazole alone is unsuccessful in normalizing cortisol levels. The usual dosage is 1–4 g daily given in four divided doses.

Aminoglutethimide and trilostane also inhibit adrenal secretion, but they are uncommonly used at present.

Mitotane (o,p′-DDD, Lysodren) is both an inhibitor of adrenal secretion and a cytotoxic agent that damages adrenocortical cells. It is used almost exclusively in patients with residual adrenocortical carcinoma, in whom it helps to reduce cortisol hypersecretion. The usual dosage is 6–12 g daily in three to four divided doses. About 70% of patients achieve a reduction in steroid secretion and 35% achieve a reduction in tumor size; however, there is no convincing evidence that the drug prolongs survival. Side effects occur in 80% of patients and include nausea, vomiting, diarrhea, depression, and somnolence.

▶ Prognosis

Treatment of hypercortisolism usually leads to disappearance of symptoms and many signs within days to weeks, but osteoporosis usually persists in adults, whereas hypertension and diabetes often improve. Cushing's disease treated by pituitary adenomectomy has an excellent early prognosis, and long-term follow-up shows a recurrence rate of about 10%. Patients with the ectopic ACTH syndrome and malignant tumors in general have a poor prognosis. Patients with benign lesions may be cured by resection of the tumor. Removal of an adrenal adenoma offers an excellent prognosis, and these patients are cured by unilateral adrenalectomy.

The outlook for patients with adrenocortical carcinoma is poor. The antineoplastic drug mitotane reduces the symptoms and signs of Cushing's syndrome but does little to prolong survival. Radiotherapy and chemotherapy are not successful in these patients.

ADRENAL ANDROGENIC SYNDROMES

Adrenal androgenic syndromes are more common in females. Congenital bilateral adrenal hyperplasia and tumors, both benign and malignant, may be observed. In contrast to Cushing's syndrome, which is protein catabolic, the androgenic syndromes are anabolic. In untreated cases, there is a marked recession of the hairline, increased beard growth, and excessive growth of pubic and sexual hair, in general, in both sexes. In males, there is enlargement of the penis, usually with atrophic testes; in females, enlargement of the clitoris occurs, with atrophy of the breasts and amenorrhea. Muscle mass increases and fat content decreases, leading to a powerful but trim figure. The voice becomes deeper, particularly in females; this condition is irreversible, because it is due to enlargement of the larynx. In both sexes, there may be increased physical sexual aggressiveness and libido.

1. Congenital bilateral adrenal androgenic hyperplasia

▶ Pathophysiology

A congenital defect in certain adrenal enzymes results in the production of abnormal steroids, causing *a disorder of sexual differentiation (DSD)* in females and *macrogenitosomia* in males. The enzyme defect is associated with excess androgen production in utero. In females, the Müllerian duct structures (eg, ovaries, uterus, and vagina) develop normally, but the excess androgen exerts a masculinizing effect on the urogenital sinus and genital tubercle, so that the vagina is connected to the urethra, which, in turn, opens at the base of the enlarged clitoris. The labia are often hypertrophied. Externally, the appearance is that of severe hypospadias with cryptorchidism.

The adrenal cortex secretes mostly anabolic and androgenic steroids, leading to various degrees of cortisol deficiency depending on the nature of the enzyme block. This increases the secretion of ACTH, which causes hyperplasia of both adrenal cortices. The cortices continue to secrete large amounts of inappropriate anabolic, androgenic, or hypertensive steroids. Absence or reduction of the usual tissue concentration of various enzymes accounts for blocks in the adrenocortical synthetic pathways. 21-Hydroxylase deficiency, which is the most common cause of congenital adrenal hyperplasia, does not allow for the transformation of 17α-hydroxyprogesterone to cortisol. This common deficiency occurs in two forms: the salt-losing variety, with low-to-absent aldosterone, and the more frequent non–salt-losing type. Infants present with adrenal insufficiency and DSD; older children develop pseudoprecocious puberty and accelerated growth and skeletal maturation. Other enzymatic defects cause specific defects in sexual differentiation, adrenal insufficiency, hypertension, or salt wasting.

▶ Clinical Findings

A. Symptoms and Signs

In newborn girls, the appearance of the external genitalia resembles severe hypospadias with cryptorchidism. Infant boys may appear normal at birth. The earlier in intrauterine life the fetus has been exposed to excess androgen, the more marked the anomalies.

In untreated cases, hirsutism, excess muscle mass, and, eventually, amenorrhea are the rule. Breast development is poor. In males, growth of the phallus is excessive. The testes are often atrophic because of inhibition of gonadotropin secretion by the elevated androgens. On rare occasions, hyperplastic adrenocortical rests in the testes make them large and firm. In most instances, there is azoospermia after puberty.

In both males and females with androgenic hyperplasia, the growth rate is initially increased so that they are taller than their classmates. At about age 9–10 years, premature fusion of the epiphyses caused by excess androgen causes termination of growth so that these patients are short as adults.

B. Laboratory Findings

Urinary 17-ketosteroid levels are higher than normal for sex and age, and plasma androstenedione, DHEA, DHEA-S, and testosterone are elevated. Plasma ACTH is also elevated, and in patients with the most common defect (ie, 21-hydroxylase deficiency), plasma 17α-hydroxyprogesterone is markedly elevated. Chromosome studies are normal.

C. X-Ray Findings

X-rays show acceleration of bone age.

D. CT Scans

Scans usually show the hypertrophied adrenals.

▶ Treatment

It is imperative to make the diagnosis early. Treatment of the underlying cause is medical, with the goal of suppressing excessive ACTH secretion, thus minimizing excess androgenicity. This is accomplished by adrenal replacement with cortisol or prednisone in doses sufficient to suppress adrenal androgen production and therefore prevent virilization and rapid skeletal growth. In patients with mineralocorticoid deficiency, fludrocortisone (0.05–0.3 mg, depending on severity and age) together with good salt intake is necessary to stabilize blood pressure and body weight.

After puberty, the vagina can be surgically separated from the urethra and opened in the normal position on the perineum. Judicious administration of estrogens or birth-control pills feminizes patients.

▶ Prognosis

If the condition is recognized early and ACTH suppression is begun even before surgical repair of the genital anomaly, the outlook for normal linear growth and development is excellent. Delay in treatment inevitably results in stunted growth. In some female patients, menses begins after treatment, and conception and childbirth can occur when the anatomic abnormalities are minimal or have been surgically repaired.

2. Adrenocortical tumors—Adrenocortical tumors producing androgens are most frequently carcinomas; however, a few benign adenomas have been reported. Most of the carcinomas also hypersecrete other hormones (ie, cortisol or 11-deoxycorticosterone), and thus, the clinical presentation is variable. Female patients present with androgen excess, which may be severe enough to cause virilization; many of these patients also have Cushing's syndrome and mineralocorticoid excess (hypertension and hypokalemia). In adult males, excess androgens may cause no clinical manifestations, and diagnosis in these patients may be delayed until there is abdominal pain or an abdominal mass. These patients may also present with Cushing's syndrome and mineralocorticoid excess.

THE HYPERTENSIVE, HYPOKALEMIC SYNDROME (PRIMARY ALDOSTERONISM)

Excessive production of aldosterone, due mostly to aldosteronoma or spontaneous bilateral hyperplasia of the zona glomerulosa of the adrenal cortex, leads to the combination of hypertension, hypokalemia, nocturia, and polyuria. A syndrome resembling nephrogenic diabetes insipidus may occur as a result of reversible damage to the renal collecting tubules. The alkalosis may produce tetany.

▶ Pathophysiology

Excessive aldosterone, acting on most cell membranes in the body, produces typical changes in the distal renal tubule and the small bowel that lead to urinary potassium loss together with increased renal sodium reabsorption and hydrogen ion secretion. This results in potassium depletion, metabolic alkalosis, increased plasma sodium concentration, and hypervolemia. With low serum levels of potassium, the concentrating ability of the kidney is lowered and the tubules no longer respond to the administration of vasopressin by increased reabsorption of water. Finally, impairment of insulin release secondary to potassium depletion increases carbohydrate intolerance in about 50% of cases.

Plasma renin and, secondarily, plasma angiotensin are depressed by excess aldosterone as a result of blood volume expansion. Early in the course of excess aldosterone production, there may be hypertension with a normal serum potassium level. Later, the potassium level will be low as well, and this suggests the diagnosis.

▶ Clinical Findings

A. Symptoms and Signs

Hypertension is usually the presenting manifestation, and the accompanying hypokalemia suggests mineralocorticoid excess. Headaches are common, nocturia is invariably present, and rare episodes of paralysis occur with very low serum potassium levels. Numbness and tingling of the extremities are related to alkalosis that may lead to tetany.

B. Laboratory Findings

Before the tests (outlined later in the chapter) are done, one must ascertain that the patient is not taking oral contraceptives or other estrogen preparations, since these may increase renin and angiotensin levels and therefore aldosterone levels, thus raising the blood pressure artificially. Withdrawal of these medications for 1 week is mandatory. Diuretics must also be discontinued, since they lower blood volume and induce secondary aldosteronism and hypokalemia. Also, if the patient is following a salt-restricted diet, aldosterone is normally elevated.

In true aldosterone excess, serum sodium is slightly elevated and CO_2 increased, whereas serum potassium is very low, for example, ≤3 mEq/L. Urine and serum potassium

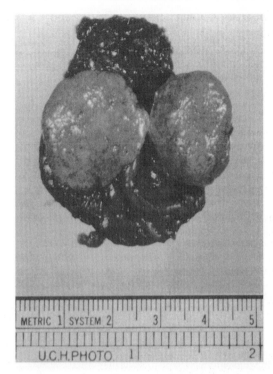

▲ **Figure 31–7.** A typical canary yellow aldosteronoma associated with the syndrome of hypertension, hypokalemia, and alkalosis. Note the relatively small size of this tumor compared with other types of adrenocortical tumors.

determinations while the patient is receiving good sodium replacement provide a screening test. Potassium wasting is established if the urinary potassium level is <30 mEq/L/24 h, but the serum potassium level is low (≤3 mEq/L).

Definitive diagnosis rests on demonstration of an elevated urine or plasma aldosterone level. The initial step is to obtain simultaneous plasma aldosterone and plasma renin levels. If the aldosterone is elevated and the renin is suppressed with a ratio of <20:1, the diagnosis is established. Further confirmation can be obtained by demonstrating an elevated aldosterone level in a 24-hour urine sample.

C. Localization

A thin-section CT scan is the initial procedure and will localize an adenoma in approximately 90% of patients (Figure 31–7). If no adenoma is visualized, adrenal vein sampling of aldosterone and cortisol will correctly differentiate adenoma from hyperplasia in virtually all cases.

▶ Differential Diagnosis

Secondary hyperaldosteronism may accompany renovascular hypertension. This too is associated with hypokalemic alkalosis; however, the renin level is elevated rather than suppressed.

Essential hypertension does not cause changes in the electrolyte pattern. Definitive tests for hyperaldosteronism show negative results.

▶ Treatment

A. Aldosteronoma

If the site of the tumor has been established, only the affected adrenal need be removed. Again, the procedure of choice is laparoscopic unilateral adrenalectomy, which is highly successful at resolving the metabolic defect.

B. Bilateral Nodular Hyperplasia

Most authorities do not recommend resection of both adrenals, since the fall in blood pressure is only temporary and electrolyte imbalance may continue. Medical treatment is recommended.

C. Medical Treatment

If surgery must be postponed, if the hypertension is mild in an older person, or if bilateral hyperplasia is the cause, one may treat medically with spironolactone (Aldactone), 25–50 mg orally four times daily. Amiloride, a potassium-sparing diuretic, may be given in doses of up to 20–40 mg/day. Other antihypertensive agents may also be necessary.

▶ Prognosis

Following removal of an adrenal adenoma, the hypokalemia resolves. Seventy percent of patients become normotensive and 50% of patients show some lowering of hypertension. Bilateral nodular hyperplasia is not amenable to surgical treatment, and the results of medical treatment are variable.

DISEASES OF THE ADRENAL MEDULLA

PHEOCHROMOCYTOMA

Pheochromocytoma, derived from the neural crest, is one of the surgically curable hypertensive syndromes. There is no gender predilection. Pheochromocytoma accounts for fewer than 1% of cases of hypertension, but it is readily diagnosed and treated. It usually occurs spontaneously, but 10% of cases occur in patients with other disorders such as neurofibromatosis or familial syndromes such as multiple endocrine neoplasia type II or von Hippel–Lindau disease. The tumor is bilateral or extra-adrenal in 10% of cases in adults and in an even greater percentage in children and is then most often familial.

▶ Clinical Findings

A. Symptoms and Signs

Hypertension may be either sustained and indistinguishable from ordinary blood pressure elevation, or paroxysmal, coming on for variable lengths of time and then subsiding to normal levels. Such attacks are usually precipitated by trigger mechanisms of various sorts, for example, emotional upsets or straining at stool.

Headache is a frequent complaint and is commensurate in severity with the degree of hypertension. Increased sweating is common. Tachycardia with palpitations may occur. Postural hypotension is a frequent finding, as a result of diminished plasma volume. Profound weakness may occur after an attack of hypertension. Weight loss is common.

Decreased gastrointestinal motility, anxiety, and psychic instability are also common and due to excess circulating catechols.

B. Biochemical Diagnosis

Free-fractionated plasma metanephrines and the 24-hour urinary-fractionated metanephrine tests are the mainstay for pheochromocytoma testing. The 2005 International Symposium on pheochromocytoma concluded that one of these two tests should be used for the initial diagnosis and screening for pheochromocytoma. The choice of biochemical test and whether to measure plasma or urine values remain controversial, but certain principles are clear: (1) Screening the hypertensive population is not recommended because of the low incidence of pheochromocytoma (about 0.1%). (2) Patients with pheochromocytoma who have sustained hypertension usually have clearly elevated catecholamines or metabolites in both urine and plasma. More than 80% of these patients have urine values two times greater than normal and total plasma catecholamine (Epi + Norepi) >2000 ng/L. Levels of this magnitude are unusual in patients without pheochromocytoma except in acute major illness. (3) Patients with only episodic hypertension may have normal random plasma catecholamine levels and normal 24-hour urine values. Evaluation of these patients must be directed to obtaining plasma catecholamine during an episode or having the patient collect timed urine values (eg, 2–4 hours) from the onset of an episode. (4) Suppression or stimulation tests are not recommended except in the rare instances when the diagnosis cannot be established by routine procedures.

1. Urinary measurements—Urine measurements are the traditional diagnostic procedure. Normal values are shown in Table 31–1, and recent series in patients with pheochromocytoma are summarized in Table 31–2. These data suggest that measurements of metanephrines (MNs) or catecholamine are more useful than measurement of vanillylmandelic acid, since >80% of patients have values that were elevated more than two times. Spot urinary MNs and normetanephrines (NMNs) measured by radioimmunoassay are very simple and highly accurate. At a cutpoint of 500 ng/mL creatinine for either MN or NMN, Ito et al (1998) reported 100% sensitivity and specificity. Patients with only episodic symptoms or episodic hypertension should be studied with shorter urine collections if 24-hour studies are normal.

Table 31–1. 24-Hour urine measurements in patients with pheochromocytoma.

Urine
    Norepinephrine: 10–100 μg/24 h
    Epinephrine: Up to 20 μg/24 h
    Normetanephrine and metanephrine: <1.5 mg/24 h
    Vanillylmandelic acid (VMA): 2–9 mg/24 h

Plasma
    Norepinephrine: 100–200 pg/mL
    Epinephrine: 30–50 pg/mL

Source: Reprinted with permission from Stein PP, Black HR: A simplified diagnostic approach to pheochromocytoma. Medicine 1991;70:46.

2. Plasma catecholamines—These values, when measured by specific methods, are elevated in most patients with pheochromocytoma; however, the frequency of false-positive values limits diagnostic utility. Thus, in patients with pheochromocytoma and sustained hypertension, 85% have plasma catecholamine values >2000 ng/L. When patients with only paroxysmal hypertension are included, however, only 75% have values >2000 ng/L. Values between 600 and 2000 ng/mL are commonly obtained in stressed or anxious patients without pheochromocytoma. This is especially true if samples are obtained by venipuncture without prior placement of an intravenous line with the patient supine for 30 minutes. Plasma catecholamine measurements do have a role, though, because markedly elevated levels during an episode may be diagnostic; conversely, the finding of normal values during episodes of severe hypertension essentially excludes the diagnosis.

▶ **Tumor Localization**

Pheochromocytomas are intra-abdominal in 98% of cases, and 90% are intra-adrenal (10% are bilateral, especially in familial syndromes). Extra-adrenal pheochromocytomas are

Table 31–2. Catecholamines in urine and plasma.

	Normal no. (%)	1–2X Elevated no. (%)	>2X Elevated no. (%)
VMA (*n* = 384)	41 (11)	86 (22)	257 (67)
MN (*n* = 271)	12 (5)	33 (12)	226 (83)
UFC (*n* = 319)	14 (4)	30 (10)	275 (86)

VMA, vanillylmandelic acid; MN, metanephrine; UFC, urinary-free cortisol.
Note: The values listed represent the means of the normal ranges, which vary for each laboratory.
Source: Reprinted with permission from Stein PP, Black HR: A simplified diagnostic approach to pheochromocytoma. Medicine 1991;70:46.

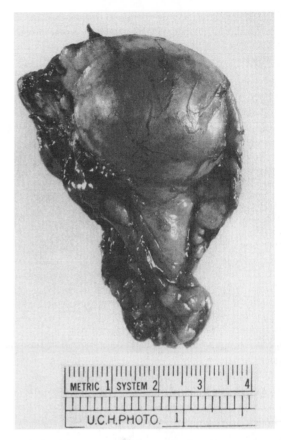

▲ **Figure 31–8.** A typical large pheochromocytoma. Removal was followed by complete remission of hypertension.

usually within the abdomen and are located along the sympathetic chain, the periaortic areas, and at the bifurcation of the aorta. The tumors may also arise from the bladder. Extra-abdominal pheochromocytomas occur in posterior mediastinum, rarely in the heart or pericardium and rarely in the neck. Tumors <2 cm in diameter are rare, and most are >3 cm (Figure 31–8). Thus, the vast majority of pheochromocytomas are larger than the lower limits of resolution of current imaging techniques.

A. CT Scans

CT scan is currently the initial imaging procedure of choice; with current technology, it demonstrates virtually all intra-abdominal tumors and most of those that are extra-adrenal. Small tumors in the abdomen, pelvis, and chest may be obscured by surrounding structures. CT scan is not useful in determining whether an adrenal mass is in fact a pheochromocytoma (ie, if the adrenal mass is found coincidentally or the catechol determinations are equivocal, the adrenal mass could be a nonfunctioning adenoma). In this case, MRI or metaiodobenzylguanidine (MIBG) techniques may be useful.

B. MRI

The accuracy of detecting pheochromocytoma with MRI is as good as that obtained with CT, but the cost is greater at most institutions. MRI has the advantage of greater diagnostic specificity in that T2-weighted images or those obtained with gadolinium enhancement show greater signal intensity of the pheochromocytoma (compared with liver) than that obtained with adrenal adenomas. Limited data suggest that MRI may be superior to CT in localizing extra-adrenal tumors.

C. MIBG Scanning

Radionuclide scanning with MIBG has assumed a prominent role in the localization of pheochromocytomas. The compound is taken up by pheochromocytomas, ganglioneuromas, neuroblastomas, and other neural crest tumors, as well as some carcinoids. MIBG scans are positive in about 85–90% of patients with pheochromocytomas. MIBG scans have great utility in the localization of (1) small lesions, (2) extra-adrenal lesions, (3) bilateral lesions, and (4) metastatic deposits in patients with malignant tumors.

▶ Diagnostic Strategy

Patients in whom there is a high index of clinical suspicion and those who have a greater than twofold elevation of urine catechols should undergo an adrenal CT. If the CT reveals a unilateral tumor and the contralateral adrenal is normal, the diagnosis is established. Patients with familial syndromes and those in whom cancer is suspected should undergo MIBG scanning to determine the extent of disease. If the adrenal CT is negative, MIBG scanning or MRI of the chest and abdomen is indicated to localize the tumor.

If the clinical suspicion is low and urine catechols are normal, imaging procedures are not indicated. However, it is not infrequent that patients at low risk on the basis of clinical manifestations have persisting mild elevations of catecholamines. In this situation, a single negative adrenal imaging procedure should suffice to terminate the evaluation, and the patient may be followed clinically and reevaluated if appropriate.

▶ Therapy

A. Preoperative Management

Once the diagnosis of pheochromocytoma is established, the patient should be prepared for surgery to reduce the incidence of intraoperative complications and postoperative hypotension. The greatest experience is with the long-acting alpha-adrenergic blocker phenoxybenzamine, and its use has

minimized surgical mortality and morbidity. The initial dosage is 10 mg twice daily, and patients may require hospitalization for bed rest and intravenous fluids to overcome the initially increased orthostatic hypotension that occurs in most patients. The dose may then be titrated upward every 2–3 days over several weeks until the blood pressure is <160/90 mm Hg and symptoms are abolished. Doses in the range of 100–200 mg/day are routinely used; however, no data are available that establish the superiority of these dosage levels. Higher doses of phenoxybenzamine are not associated with a higher risk of postoperative hypotension. Beta-blockers are generally unnecessary unless tachycardia and arrhythmias are present.

Metyrosine (alpha-methylparatyrosine), an inhibitor of catecholamine synthesis, is also useful for preoperative management, although current experience is limited. Initial dosage is 250 mg every 6 hours, and total daily dosages of 2–4 g are required. Preoperative treatment for 1–2 weeks appears to be sufficient to prevent operative complications. Metyrosine can be used in conjunction with alpha-blockers.

Successful preoperative management with prazosin, calcium channel blockers, and labetalol has been reported.

B. Surgery

Surgery is the mainstay of therapy for pheochromocytoma; it requires adequate preoperative control of symptoms and hypertension with alpha-blockers or metyrosine. Intraoperatively, hypertension is controlled with nitroprusside, and antiarrhythmics are used as needed. Adequate volume replacement is essential and in conjunction with preoperative medical therapy prevents postoperative hypotension.

If CT and MIBG show only a solitary adrenal lesion in patients with sporadic disease, a unilateral laparoscopic approach is preferred. For small tumors or patients at risk for bilateral disease, partial adrenalectomy can usually be performed and is associated with similar outcomes as total adrenalectomy. Bilateral or malignant disease may require a transabdominal approach, and even if total resection is not feasible, debulking of tumor mass facilitates subsequent medical management of catecholamine excess.

▶ Malignant Pheochromocytoma

The incidence of cancer in pheochromocytoma has been traditionally estimated to be approximately 10%, although recent series describe a higher incidence. Thus, all patients should undergo serial follow-up to detect early recurrences. Patients with known metastatic disease should undergo surgical debulking of accessible disease. Catecholamine excess can be controlled in most patients with alpha-blockade, metyrosine, or both. Despite encouraging reports of chemotherapy or ^{131}I-MIBG therapy, it appears that only a minority of patients have sustained remissions.

Prognosis

In general, the prognosis is good. With better understanding of the disease, surgical deaths are now rare. Blood pressure falls to normal levels in most patients with benign tumors. Patients with cancer have persisting hypertension and require the multiple therapies described earlier.

INCIDENTALOMA

The most common presentation of adrenal masses is incidental detection on cross-sectional imaging performed for other reasons. The differential diagnosis is quite broad (see Table 31–3) and includes benign adenoma, functional adrenal tumors as previously discussed, metastasis and benign adrenal lesions such as myelolipoma, and neurofibroma. A systematic approach is required to differentiate functional adrenal masses that deserve removal and those lesions with a significant risk of carcinoma from the more common benign nonfunctional adenoma.

Metabolic Evaluation

A careful history and physical examination with focus on obesity pattern, virilization, glucose intolerance, and hypertension is warranted. The NIH consensus statement recommends metabolic testing for all adrenal incidentalomas. Laboratory examination with serum electrolytes including glucose and potassium should be done. If hypokalemia exists, then further tests for aldosteronoma are indicated. There are three first line tests to screen patients with incidentalomas for Cushing syndrome: an overnight low dose dexamethasone suppression test, a late-night salivary cortisol test and traditional 24-hour urinary-free cortisol test. The Endocrine society recommends either of the first two tests as the urinary-free cortisol test may not be sufficiently sensitive to detect subclinical Cushing syndrome. Patient should also have free-fractionated plasma metenephrines or the 24-hour urinary fractionated metanephrine test to rule out pheochromocytoma. Additional metabolic

Table 31–3. Differential diagnosis of adrenal incidentaloma.

Adenoma
Metastasis
Lymphoma
Pheochromocytoma
Neuroblastoma
Adrenocortical carcinoma
Hematoma
Myelolipoma
Adrenal hyperplasia
Adrenal cyst
Granulomatous disease
Hemangioma
Ganglioneuroma

tests are performed when there are suspicious signs or symptoms or when screening tests are abnormal.

If the test identified the adrenal mass was an ultrasound or CT, an MRI may be helpful to differentiate the various causes of adrenal masses. Because adrenal adenomas have abundant intracytoplasmic lipid, they can often be confirmed on CT and MRI.

Imaging

Lesions that are primarily cystic on CT or MRI are typically benign and can be followed with serial imaging. Benign adrenal cysts are characterized by thin nonenhancing walls; fluid attenuation on CT and thin calcifications may be present peripherally in about 50%.

Characteristics suspicious for malignancy include solid masses that are large, hemorrhagic, or necrotic. MRI is usually heterogeneous on T1- and T2-weighted images due to internal bleeding.

Masses with gross fat on CT (Hounsfield unit [HU] <30) are myelolipomas (Figure 31–9), benign nonfunctional adrenal lesions with lipid and myeloid components. Myelolipomas are usually asymptomatic or present with pain if they bleed.

Noncontrast CT sensitivity for benign adenomas ranges from 50% to 80% depending on the HU attenuation value threshold chosen (Figure 31–5). If a threshold of <10 HU is chosen, the specificity is 84–100%. Chemical-shift imaging is an MR technique to identify intracellular lipid. In-phase

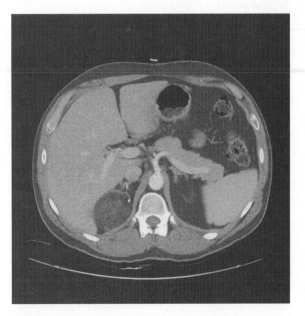

▲ **Figure 31–9.** A large right adrenal myelolipoma. Note the similar CT density to perinephric and subcutaneous fat. (Image courtesy of Fergus Coakley, MD, UCSF Radiology Department.)

A

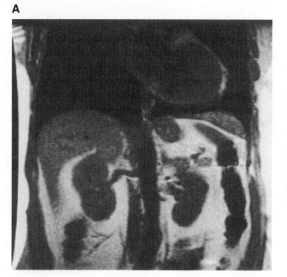

B

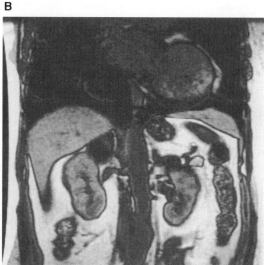

▲ **Figure 31–10.** In-phase (**A**) and out-of-phase (**B**) coronal MRI of a patient with bilateral benign nonfunctional adrenal adenomas. (Image courtesy of Fergus Coakley, MD, UCSF Radiology Department.)

and out-of-phase T1-weighted images can distinguish water and fat protons from water photons only. Sensitivities of 81–87% with specificities of 92–100% have been reported for chemical-shift MRI (Figure 31–10).

Diagnostic Algorithm

Percutaneous CT-guided biopsy may be appropriate for adrenal masses with imaging characteristics suspicious for metastasis or in patients with known malignancy. All functional adrenal masses and those >5 cm should be removed. Laparoscopic adrenalectomy is the preferred technique and is used in most cases except very large masses suspicious for malignancy or with evidence of local extension. Nonfunctional adrenal masses <5 cm should be assessed for radiographic features concerning for malignancy and removed if they are irregular or hemorrhagic or have demonstrated growth. An individualized approach for nonsuspicious nonfunctional masses <5 cm can be taken. It may be appropriate to remove lesions in the 3–5 cm range in well-informed younger patients in order to avoid the burden of radiographic follow-up. Those <3 cm can generally be followed. There is growing evidence that some incidentalomas that have initial negative screening tests may be causing "subclinical" Cushing's disease. Therefore, if a patient with an incidentaloma has symptoms or signs of Cushing's disease, additional or repeat screening tests may be appropriate.

NEUROBLASTOMA

Neuroblastomas are of neural crest origin and may therefore develop from any portion of the sympathetic chain. Most arise in the retroperitoneum, and 45% involve the adrenal

gland. The latter offer the poorest prognosis. In childhood, neuroblastoma is the third most common neoplastic disease after leukemia and brain tumors. Most are encountered in the first 2½ years of life, but a few are seen as late as the sixth decade, when they seem to be less aggressive. Abnormalities of muscle and heart and hemihypertrophy have been observed in association with neuroblastoma.

Metastases spread through both the bloodstream and lymphatics. Common sites in children include the skull and long bones, regional lymph nodes, liver, and lungs. Local invasion is common. In infants, who enjoy the best prognosis, metastases are usually limited to the liver and subcutaneous fat.

The following staging of neuroblastoma is generally accepted:

Stage I: Tumors confined to the structure of origin.

Stage II: Tumors extending in continuity beyond the organ but not crossing the midline. Ipsilateral lymph nodes may be involved.

Stage III: Tumors extending in continuity beyond the midline. Regional lymph nodes may be involved.

Stage IV: Remote disease involving skeletal organs, soft tissues, and distant lymph node groups.

Stage IV-S: Stage I or II patients with remote spread of tumor confined to one or more of the following sites: liver, skin, or bone marrow.

Clinical Findings

A. Symptoms

An abdominal mass is usually noted by parents, the physician, or the patient. About 70% of patients have metastases when first seen. Symptoms relating to metastases include fever, malaise, bone pain, failure to thrive, and constipation or diarrhea.

B. Signs

A flank mass is usually palpable and may even be visible; it often extends across the midline. The tumor is usually nodular and fixed, since it tends to be locally invasive. Evidence of metastases may be noted: ocular proptosis from metastases to the skull, enlarged nodular liver, or a mass in bone. Hypertension is often found.

C. Laboratory Findings

Anemia is common. Urinalysis and renal function are normal. Because 70% of neuroblastomas elaborate increased levels of norepinephrine and epinephrine, urinary vanillylmandelic acid and homovanillic acid levels should be measured. Serial estimations of these substances during definitive treatment can be used as tumor markers. A return to normal levels is encouraging, while rising levels imply residual or progressive tumor. Bone marrow aspiration may reveal tumor cells.

D. X-Ray Findings

Plain radiographs may show a mass and displacement of the kidneys or other organs. CT scans are used to define tumor size, vascular invasion (eg, of the vena cava), local tumor spread, and distant metastases. Further evaluation includes CT scan of the chest to determine whether lung metastases are present and a bone scan to define skeletal metastases. Many of these tumors take up ^{131}I–MIB; thus, this test can be used for staging.

Differential Diagnosis

Wilms tumor is also a disease of childhood. Imaging shows the caliceal distortion characteristic of an intrinsic renal tumor; no such distortion is shown in neuroblastoma, which merely displaces the kidney. Hydronephrosis, polycystic renal disease, and neonatal adrenal hemorrhage may be confused with neuroblastoma. CT scan is very useful in differentiating the various lesions.

▶ Treatment

Surgical excision of a tumor is standard care of stage I and stage II patients. Although neuroblastoma is radiosensitive, radiation therapy is typically used as part of multimodality therapy of high-risk disease. In stage IV and high-risk stage III disease, chemotherapy is typically given followed by surgery and radiation therapy for residual disease. Useful drugs include cisplatin, cyclophosphamide, doxorubicin, and etoposide. There is evidence that after chemotherapy and surgery/radiation for residual disease, bone marrow transplant followed by 13-*cis*-retinoic acid prolongs disease-specific survival in high-risk patients and is now standard care.

▶ Prognosis

Patients with stage I and II diseases have an 80% survival rate. Including all patients, however, long-term survival occurs in only 15% of patients. Infants have the best prognosis; their 2-year survival rate approaches 60%, and if the tumor is confined to the primary site with or without adjacent regional spread, the cure rate is about 80%. Factors that define high-risk neuroblastoma include age >1 year, metastasis, amplification of the MYCN oncogene, and particular histologic findings.

In a few infants, spontaneous maturation of neuroblastoma to ganglioneuroma has been observed.

BIBLIOGRAPHY

General

Brunt LM et al: Outcomes analysis in patients undergoing laparoscopic adrenalectomy for hormonally active adrenal tumors. Surgery 2001;130:629.

Hsu TH, Gill IS: Bilateral laparoscopic adrenalectomy: Retroperitoneal and transperitoneal approaches. Urology 2002;59:184.

Kaye DR et al: Partial adrenalectomy: Underused first line therapy for small adrenal tumors. J Urol 2010;184(1):18–25.

Lin DD et al: Diagnosis and management of surgical adrenal diseases. Urology 2005;66:476.

Lockhart ME et al: Imaging of adrenal masses. Eur J Radiol 2002;41:95.

MacGillivray DC et al: Laparoscopic resection of large adrenal tumors. Ann Surg Oncol 2002;9:480.

Smith CD et al: Laparoscopic adrenalectomy: New gold standard. World J Surg 1999;23:389.

Winfield HN et al: Laparoscopic adrenalectomy: The preferred choice? A comparison to open adrenalectomy. J Urol 1998;160:325.

Cushing's Syndrome and Adrenocortical Tumors

Atkinson AB: The treatment of Cushing's syndrome. Clin Endocrinol (Oxf) 1991;34:507.

Boushey RP, Dackiw AP: Adrenal cortical carcinoma. Curr Treat Options Oncol 2001;2:355.

Decker RA et al: Eastern Cooperative Oncology Group Study 1879: Mitotane and Adriamycin in patients with advanced adrenocortical carcinoma. Surgery 1991;110:1006.

Doherty GM et al: Time to recovery of the hypothalamic-pituitary-adrenal axis after curative resection of adrenal tumors in patients with Cushing's syndrome. Surgery 1990;108:1085.

Findling JW, Raff H: Diagnosis and differential diagnosis of Cushing's syndrome. Endocrinol Metab Clin North Am 2001;30:729.

Grus JR, Nelson DH: ACTH-producing pituitary tumors. Endocrinol Metab Clin North Am 1991;20:319.

Luton JP et al: Clinical features of adrenocortical carcinoma, prognostic factors, and the effect of mitotane therapy. N Engl J Med 1990;322:1195.

Mendiratta-Lala M et al: Efficacy of radiofrequency ablation in the treatment of small functional adrenal neoplasms. Radiology 2010; 258(1):308–316.

Ng L, Libertino JM: Adrenocortical carcinoma diagnosis, evaluation and treatment. J Urol 2003;169:5.

Nieman LK et al: The diagnosis of Cushing's syndrome: An Endocrine Society Clinical Practice Guideline. J Clin Endocrinol Metab 2008;93(5):1526–1540.

Raff H, Findling, JW: A physiologic approach to diagnosis of the Cushing syndrome. Ann Intern Med 2003;138:980.

Styne DM et al: Treatment of Cushing's disease in childhood and adolescence by transsphenoidal microadenomectomy. N Engl J Med 1984;B310:889.

Trainer PJ, Grossman A: The diagnosis and differential diagnosis of Cushing's syndrome. Clin Endocrinol (Oxf) 1991;34:317.

Tyrrell JB et al: An overnight high-dose dexamethasone suppression test: Rapid differential diagnosis of Cushing's syndrome. Ann Intern Med 1986;104:180.

Adrenal Androgenic Syndromes

Azziz R. The evaluation and management of hirsutism. Obstet Gynecol 2003;101(5, Pt 1):995–1007.

Masiakos PT et al: Masculinizing and feminizing syndromes caused by functioning tumors. Semin Pediatr Surg 1997;6:147.

Mendonca BB et al: Clinical, hormonal and pathological findings in a comparative study of adrenocortical neoplasms in childhood and adulthood. J Urol 1995;154:2004.

Miller WL: Genetics, diagnosis, and management of 21-hydroxylase deficiency. J Clin Endocrinol Metab 1994;78:241.

Siegel SF et al: ACTH stimulation tests and plasma dehydroepiandrosterone sulfate levels in women with hirsutism. N Engl J Med 1990;323:849.

Primary Aldosteronism

Ganguly A: Primary aldosteronism. N Engl J Med 1998;339:1828.

Gomez-Sanchez CE: Primary aldosteronism and its variants. Cardiovasc Res 1998;37:8.

Gordon RD: Primary aldosteronism. J Endocrinol Invest 1995;18:495.

Shen WT et al: Laparoscopic vs open adrenalectomy for the treatment of primary hyperaldosteronism. Arch Surg 1999;134:628.

Siren J et al: Laparoscopic adrenalectomy for primary aldosteronism. Surg Laparosc Endosc 1999;9:9.

Vallotton MB: Primary aldosteronism. Part I. Diagnosis of primary hyperaldosteronism. Clin Endocinol (Oxf) 1996;45:47.

Vallotton MB: Primary aldosteronism. Part II. Differential diagnosis of primary hyperaldosteronism and pseudoaldosteronism. Clin Endocrinol (Oxf) 1996;45:53.

Young WF Jr et al: Primary aldosteronism: Adrenal venous sampling. Surgery 1996;120:913.

Pheochromocytoma

Eigelberger MS, Duh QY: Pheochromocytoma. Curr Treat Options Oncol 2001;2:321.

Grossman A et al: Biochemical diagnosis and localization of pheochromocytoma: Can we reach a consensus? Ann NY Acad Sci 2006;1073:332–347.

Ito Y et al: Efficacy of single voided urine metanephrine and normetanephrine assay for diagnosing pheochromocytoma. World J Surg 1998;22:684.

Joris JL et al: Hemodynamic changes and catecholamine release during laparoscopic adrenalectomy for pheochromocytoma. Anesth Analg 1999;88:16.

Kebebew E, Duk QY: Benign and malignant pheochromocytoma: Diagnosis, treatment and follow-up. Surg Oncol Clin N Am 1998; 7:765.

Kercher KW et al: Laparoscopic curative resection of pheochromocytomas. Ann Surg 2005;241:919.

Lenders JW et al: Biochemical diagnosis of pheochromocytoma: Which test is best? JAMA 2002;287:1427.

Loh KC et al: The treatment of malignant pheochromocytoma with iodine-131 metaiodobenzylguanidine (131I-MIBG): A comprehensive review of 116 reported patients. J Endocrinol Invest 1997;20:648.

Peaston RT et al: Overnight excretion of urinary catecholamines and metabolites in the detection of pheochromocytoma. J Clin Endocrinol Metab 1996;81:1379.

Incidentaloma

Grumbach MM et al: Management of the clinically inapparent adrenal mass. Ann Intern Med 2003;138(5):424–429.

Kievit J, Haak HR: Diagnosis and treatment of adrenal incidentaloma: A cost-effectiveness analysis. Endocrinol Metab Clin North Am 2000;29:69.

Korobkin M et al: Characterization of adrenal masses with chemical shift and gadolinium-enhanced MR imaging. Radiol 1995; 197:411.

Nieman LK: Approach to the patient with an adrenal incidentaloma. J Clin Endocrinol Metab 2010;95(9):4106–4113.

Terzolo M et al: Adrenal incidentaloma: A new cause of the metabolic syndrome? J Clin Endocrinol Metab 2002;87:998.

Neuroblastoma

Maris JM et al: Neuroblastoma. Lancet 2007;369:2106–2120.

Matthay KK: Neuroblastoma: Biology and therapy. Oncology (Huntingt) 1997;11:1857.

Matthay KK et al: Treatment of high-risk neuroblastoma with intensive chemotherapy, radiotherapy, autologous bone marrow transplantation, and 13-*cis*-retinoic acid. N Engl J Med 1999;341: 1165.

Matthay KK et al: Long-term results for children with high-risk neuroblastoma treated on a randomized trial of myeloablative therapy followed by 13-cis-retinoic acid: A children's oncology group study. J Clin Oncol 2009;27:1007–1013.

Disorders of the Kidneys

32

Jack W. McAninch, MD, FACS, FRCS(E)(Hon)

CONGENITAL ANOMALIES OF THE KIDNEYS

Congenital anomalies occur more frequently in the kidney than in any other organ. Some cause no difficulty, but many (eg, hypoplasia, polycystic kidneys) cause impairment of renal function. It has been noted that children with a gross deformity of an external ear associated with ipsilateral maldevelopment of the facial bones are apt to have a congenital abnormality of the kidney (eg, ectopy, hypoplasia) on the same side as the visible deformity. Lateral displacement of the nipples has been observed in association with bilateral renal hypoplasia.

A significant incidence of renal agenesis, ectopy, malrotation, and duplication has been observed in association with congenital scoliosis and kyphosis. Unilateral agenesis, hypoplasia, and dysplasia are often seen in association with supralevator imperforate anus. For a better understanding of these congenital abnormalities, see the discussion of the embryology and development of the kidney in Chapter 2.

AGENESIS

Bilateral renal agenesis is extremely rare; no more than 400 cases have been reported. The children do not survive. The condition does not appear to have any predisposing factors. Prenatal suspicion of the anomaly exists when oligohydramnios is present on fetal ultrasound examination. Pulmonary hypoplasia and facial deformities (Potter facies) are usually present. Abdominal ultrasound examination usually establishes the diagnosis.

One kidney may be absent (estimated incidence: 1 in 450–1000 births). In some cases, this may be because the ureteral bud (from the Wolffian duct) failed to develop or, if it did develop, did not reach the metanephros (adult kidney). Without a drainage system, the metanephric mass undergoes atrophy. The ureter is absent on the side of the unformed kidney in 50% of cases, although a blind ureteral duct may be found (see Chapter 2).

Renal agenesis causes no symptoms; it is usually found by accident on abdominal or renal imaging. It is not an easy diagnosis to establish even though on inspection of the bladder,

the ureteral ridge is absent and no orifice is visualized, for the kidney could be present but be drained by a ureter whose opening is ectopic (into the urethra, seminal vesicle, or vagina). If definitive diagnosis seems essential, isotope studies, ultrasonography, and computed tomography (CT) should establish the diagnosis.

There appears to be an increased incidence of infection, hydronephrosis, and stones in the contralateral organ. Other congenital anomalies associated with this defect include cardiac, vertebral column, and anal anomalies, as well as anomalies of the long bones, hands, and genitalia.

HYPOPLASIA

Hypoplasia implies a small kidney. The total renal mass may be divided in an unequal manner, in which case one kidney is small and the other correspondingly larger than normal. Some of these congenitally small kidneys prove, on pathologic examination, to be dysplastic. Unilateral or bilateral hypoplasia has been observed in infants with fetal alcohol syndrome, and renal anomalies have been reported in infants with in utero cocaine exposure.

Differentiation from acquired atrophy is difficult. Atrophic pyelonephritis usually reveals typical distortion of the calyces. Vesicoureteral reflux in infants may cause a dwarfed kidney even in the absence of infection. Stenosis of the renal artery leads to shrinkage of the kidney.

Such kidneys have small renal arteries and branches and are associated with hypertension, which is relieved by nephrectomy. Selective renal venography is helpful in differentiating between a congenitally absent kidney and one that is small and nonvisualized.

SUPERNUMERARY KIDNEYS

The presence of a third kidney is very rare; the presence of four separate kidneys in one individual has been reported only once. The anomaly must not be confused with duplication (or triplication) of the renal pelvis in one kidney, which is not uncommon.

DYSPLASIA AND MULTICYSTIC KIDNEY

Renal dysplasia has protean manifestations. Multicystic kidney of the newborn is usually unilateral, nonhereditary, and characterized by an irregularly lobulated mass of cysts; the ureter is usually absent or atretic. It may develop because of faulty union of the nephron and the collecting system. At most, only a few embryonic glomeruli and tubules are observed. The only finding is the discovery of an irregular mass in the flank. Nothing is shown on urography, but in an occasional case, some radiopaque fluid may be noted. If the cystic kidney is large, its mate is usually normal. However, when the cystic organ is small, the contralateral kidney is apt to be abnormal. The cystic nature of the lesion may be revealed by sonography, and the diagnosis can be established in utero. If the physician feels that the proper diagnosis has been made, no treatment is necessary. If there is doubt about the diagnosis, nephrectomy is considered the procedure of choice. Neoplastic changes in multicystic renal dysplasia have been noted, but this is accepted as a benign condition.

Multicystic kidney is often associated with contralateral renal and ureteral abnormalities. Contralateral ureteropelvic junction obstruction is one of the common problems noted. Diagnostic evaluation of both kidneys is required to establish the overall status of anomalous development.

Dysplasia of the renal parenchyma is also seen in association with ureteral obstruction or reflux that was probably present early in pregnancy. It is relatively common as a segmental renal lesion involving the upper pole of a duplicated kidney whose ureter is obstructed by a congenital ureterocele. It may also be found in urinary tracts severely obstructed by posterior urethral valves; in this instance, the lesion may be bilateral.

Microscopically, the renal parenchyma is "disorganized." Tubular and glomerular cysts may be noted; these elements are fetal in type. Islands of metaplastic cartilage are often seen. The common denominator seems to be fetal obstruction.

ADULT POLYCYSTIC KIDNEY DISEASE

Adult polycystic kidney disease is an autosomal dominant hereditary condition and almost always bilateral (95% of cases). The disease encountered in infants is different from that seen in adults, although the literature reports a small number of infants with the adult type. The former is an autosomal recessive disease in which life expectancy is short, whereas that diagnosed in adulthood is autosomal dominant; symptoms ordinarily do not appear until after age 40. Cysts of the liver, spleen, and pancreas may be noted in association with both forms. The kidneys are larger than normal and are studded with cysts of various sizes.

▶ Etiology and Pathogenesis

The evidence suggests that the cysts occur because of defects in the development of the collecting and uriniferous tubules and in the mechanism of their joining. Blind secretory tubules that are connected to functioning glomeruli become cystic. As the cysts enlarge, they compress adjacent parenchyma, destroy it by ischemia, and occlude normal tubules. The result is progressive functional impairment.

▶ Pathology

Grossly, the kidneys are usually much enlarged. Their surfaces are studded with cysts of various sizes (Figure 32–1). On section, the cysts are found to be scattered throughout the parenchyma. Calcification is rare. The fluid in the cyst is usually amber colored but may be hemorrhagic.

Microscopically, the lining of the cysts consists of a single layer of cells. The renal parenchyma may show peritubular fibrosis and evidence of secondary infection. There appears to be a reduction in the number of glomeruli, some of which may be hyalinized. Renal arteriolar thickening is a prominent finding in adults.

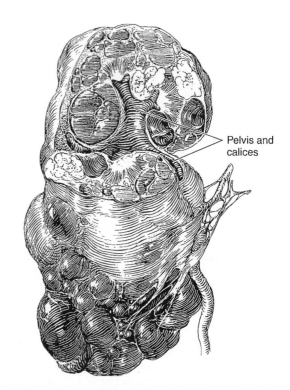

Pelvis and calices

▲ **Figure 32–1.** Polycystic kidney. Multiple cysts deep in the parenchyma and on the surface. Note distortion of the calyces by the cysts.

Clinical Findings

A. Symptoms

Pain over one or both kidneys may occur because of the drag on the vascular pedicles by the heavy kidneys, from obstruction or infection, or from hemorrhage into a cyst. Gross or microscopic total hematuria is not uncommon and may be severe; the cause for this is not clear. Colic may occur if blood clots or stones are passed. The patient may notice an abdominal mass.

Infection (chills, fever, renal pain) commonly complicates polycystic disease. Symptoms of vesical irritability may be the first complaint. When renal insufficiency ensues, headache, nausea and vomiting, weakness, and loss of weight occur.

B. Signs

One or both kidneys are usually palpable. They may feel nodular. If infected, they may be tender. Hypertension is found in 60–70% of these patients. Evidence of cardiac enlargement is then noted.

Fever may be present if pyelonephritis exists or if cysts have become infected. In the stage of uremia, anemia and loss of weight may be evident. Ophthalmoscopic examination may show changes typical of moderate or severe hypertension.

C. Laboratory Findings

Anemia may be noted, caused either by chronic loss of blood or, more commonly, by the hematopoietic depression accompanying uremia. Proteinuria and microscopic (if not gross) hematuria are the rule. Pyuria and bacteriuria are common.

Progressive loss of concentrating power occurs. Renal clearance tests show varying degrees of renal impairment. About one-third of patients with polycystic kidney disease are uremic when first seen.

D. X-Ray Findings

Both renal shadows are usually enlarged on a plain film of the abdomen, even as much as five times normal size. Kidneys >16 cm in length are suspect.

The renal masses are usually enlarged and the calyceal pattern is quite bizarre (spider deformity). The calyces are broadened and flattened, enlarged, and often curved, as they tend to hug the periphery of adjacent cysts. Often, the changes are only slight or may even be absent on one side, leading to the erroneous diagnosis of tumor of the other kidney. If cysts are infected, perinephritis may obscure the renal and even the psoas shadows.

E. CT Scanning

CT is an excellent noninvasive technique used to establish the diagnosis of polycystic disease. The multiple thin-walled cysts filled with fluid and the large renal size make this imaging method extremely accurate (95%) for diagnosis.

F. Isotope Studies

Photoscans reveal multiple "cold" avascular spots in large renal shadows.

G. Ultrasonography

Sonography appears to be superior to both excretory urography and isotope scanning in diagnosis of polycystic disorders.

H. Instrumental Examination

Cystoscopy may show evidence of cystitis, in which case the urine will contain abnormal elements. Bleeding from a ureteral orifice may be noted. Ureteral catheterization and retrograde urograms are rarely indicated.

Differential Diagnosis

Bilateral hydronephrosis (on the basis of congenital or acquired ureteral obstruction) may present bilateral flank masses and signs of impairment of renal function, but ultrasonography shows changes quite different from those of the polycystic kidney.

Bilateral renal tumor is rare but may mimic polycystic kidney disease perfectly on urography. Tumors are usually localized to one portion of the kidney, whereas cysts are quite diffusely distributed. The total renal function should be normal with unilateral tumor but is usually depressed in patients with polycystic kidney disease. CT scan may be needed at times to differentiate between the two conditions.

In **von Hippel-Lindau disease** (angiomatous cerebellar cyst, angiomatosis of the retina, and tumors or cysts of the pancreas), multiple bilateral cysts or adenocarcinomas of both kidneys may develop. The presence of other stigmas should make the diagnosis. CT, angiography, sonography, or scintiphotography should be definitive.

Tuberous sclerosis (convulsive seizures, mental retardation, and adenoma sebaceum) is typified by hamartomatous tumors often involving the skin, brain, retinas, bones, liver, heart, and kidneys (see Chapter 21). The renal lesions are usually multiple and bilateral and microscopically are angiomyolipomas. The presence of other stigmas and use of CT or sonography should make the differentiation.

A **simple cyst** (see section following) is usually unilateral and single; total renal function should be normal. Urograms usually show a single lesion (Figure 32–2), whereas polycystic kidney disease is bilateral and has multiple filling defects.

Complications

For reasons that are not clear, pyelonephritis is a common complication of polycystic kidney disease. It may be asymptomatic; pus cells in the urine may be few or absent. Stained smears or quantitative cultures make the diagnosis. A gallium-67 citrate scan will definitely reveal the sites of infection, including abscess.

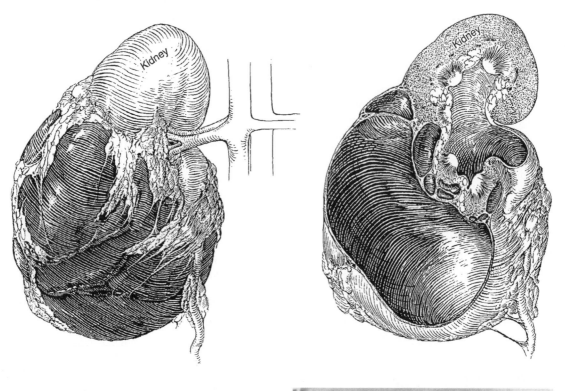

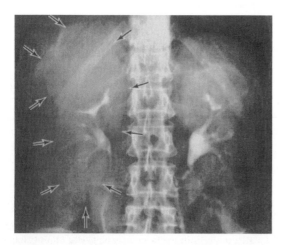

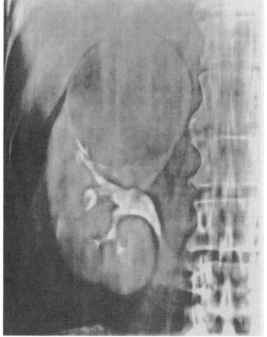

▲ **Figure 32–2.** Simple cyst. ***Upper left:*** Large cyst displacing lower pole laterally. ***Upper right:*** Section of kidney showing one large and a few small cysts. ***Lower left:*** Excretory urogram showing soft-tissue mass in upper pole of right kidney. Elongation and distortion of upper calyces by cyst. ***Lower right:*** Infusion nephrotomogram showing large cyst in upper renal pole distorting upper calyces and dislocating upper portion of kidney laterally.

Infection of cysts is associated with pain and tenderness over the kidney and a febrile response. The differential diagnosis between infection of cysts and pyelonephritis may be difficult, but here again a gallium scan will prove helpful. In rare instances, gross hematuria may be so brisk and persistent as to endanger life.

▶ Treatment

Except for unusual complications, the treatment is conservative and supportive.

A. General Measures

The patient should be put on a low-protein diet (0.5–0.75 g/kg/day of protein) and fluids forced to 3000 mL or more per day. Physical activity may be permitted within reason, but strenuous exercise is contraindicated. When the patient is in the state of absolute renal insufficiency, one should treat as for uremia from any cause. Hypertension should be controlled. Hemodialysis may be indicated.

B. Surgery

There is no evidence that excision or decompression of cysts improves renal function. If a large cyst is found to be compressing the upper ureter, causing obstruction and further embarrassing renal function, it should be resected or aspirated. When the degree of renal insufficiency becomes life threatening, chronic dialysis or renal transplantation should be considered.

C. Treatment of Complications

Pyelonephritis must be rigorously treated to prevent further renal damage. Infection of cysts requires surgical drainage. If bleeding from one kidney is so severe that exsanguination is possible, nephrectomy or embolization of the renal or, preferably, the segmental artery must be considered as a life-saving measure. Concomitant diseases (eg, tumor, obstructing stone) may require definitive surgical treatment.

▶ Prognosis

When the disease affects children, it has a very poor prognosis. The large group presenting clinical signs and symptoms after age 35–40 has a somewhat more favorable prognosis. Although there is wide variation, these patients usually do not live longer than 5 or 10 years after the diagnosis is made, unless dialysis is made available or renal transplantation is done.

SIMPLE (SOLITARY) CYST

Simple cyst (Figures 32–2 and 32–3) of the kidney is usually unilateral and single but may be multiple and multilocular and, more rarely, bilateral. It differs from polycystic kidneys both clinically and pathologically.

▶ Etiology and Pathogenesis

Whether simple cyst is congenital or acquired is not clear. Its origin may be similar to that of polycystic kidneys, that is, the difference may be merely one of degree. On the other hand, simple cysts have been produced in animals by causing tubular obstruction and local ischemia; this suggests that the lesion can be acquired.

As a simple cyst grows, it compresses and thereby may destroy renal parenchyma, but rarely does it destroy so much renal tissue that renal function is impaired. A solitary cyst

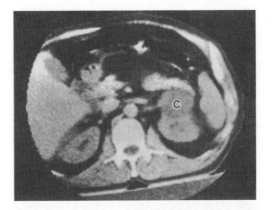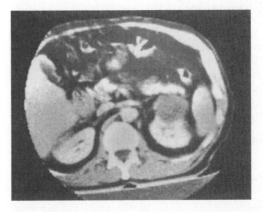

▲ **Figure 32–3.** Left renal cyst. ***Left:*** Computed tomography (CT) scan shows a homogeneous low-density mass (C) arising from anterior border of left kidney just posterior to tail of the pancreas. The CT attenuation value was similar to that of water, indicating a simple renal cyst. ***Right:*** After intravenous injection of contrast material, the mass did not increase in attenuation value, adding further confirmatory evidence of its benign cystic nature.

may be placed in such a position as to compress the ureter, causing progressive hydronephrosis. Infection may complicate the picture.

Acquired cystic disease of the kidney can arise as an effect of chronic dialysis. The spontaneous regression of cysts has occasionally been noted.

▶ Pathology

Simple cysts usually involve the lower pole of the kidney. Those that produce symptoms average about 10 cm in diameter, but a few are large enough to fill the entire flank. They usually contain a clear amber fluid. Their walls are quite thin, and the cysts are "blue-domed" in appearance. Calcification of the sac is occasionally seen. About 5% contain hemorrhagic fluid, and possibly one-half of these have papillary cancers on their walls.

Simple cysts are usually superficial but may be deeply situated. When a cyst is situated deep in the kidney, the cyst wall is adjacent to the epithelial lining of the pelvis or calyces, from which it may be separated only with great difficulty. Cysts do not communicate with the renal pelvis (Figure 32–2). Microscopic examination of the cyst wall shows heavy fibrosis and hyalinization; areas of calcification may be seen. The adjacent renal tissue is compressed and fibrosed. A number of cases of simple cysts have been reported in children. However, large cysts are rare in children; the presence of cancer must therefore be ruled out.

Multilocular renal cysts may be confused with tumor on urography. Sonography usually makes the diagnosis. Occasionally, CT and magnetic resonance imaging (MRI) may be necessary.

The Bosniak classification of simple renal cysts is an aid to determining the chance of malignancy based on imaging criteria. Type I cysts are simple and smooth walled, with clear fluid; Type II cysts are also benign, but may have minimal septations and a small fine rim of calcification; Type III cysts are more complex, with more calcification, increasing septations, and a thick cyst wall; Type IV cysts have a thickened irregular wall, often with calcifications, and a mass may be noted inside the cyst, suggesting carcinoma. Numerous variations of the findings are used as a guide in the diagnosis of renal cancer.

▶ Clinical Findings

A. Symptoms

Pain in the flank or back, usually intermittent and dull, is not uncommon. If bleeding suddenly distends the cyst wall, pain may come on abruptly and be severe. Gastrointestinal symptoms are occasionally noted and may suggest peptic ulcer or gallbladder disease. The patient may discover a mass in the abdomen, although cysts of this size are unusual. If the cyst becomes infected, the patient usually complains of pain in the flank, malaise, and fever.

B. Signs

Physical examination is usually normal, although occasionally a mass in the region of the kidney may be palpated or percussed. Tenderness in the flank may be noted if the cyst becomes infected.

C. Laboratory Findings

Urinalysis is usually normal. Microscopic hematuria is rare. Renal function tests are normal unless the cysts are multiple and bilateral (rare). Even in the face of extensive destruction of one kidney, compensatory hypertrophy of the other kidney will maintain normal total function.

D. CT Scanning

CT scan appears to be the most accurate means of differentiating renal cyst and tumor (Figure 32–3). Cysts have an attenuation approximating that of water, whereas the density of tumors is similar to that of normal parenchyma. Parenchyma is made more dense with the intravenous injection of radiopaque fluid, but a cyst remains unaffected. The wall of a cyst is sharply demarcated from the renal parenchyma; a tumor is not. The wall of a cyst is thin, and that of a tumor is not. CT scan may well supplant cyst puncture in the differentiation of cyst and tumor in many cases.

E. Renal Ultrasonography

Renal ultrasonography is a noninvasive diagnostic technique that in a high percentage of cases differentiates between a cyst and a solid mass. If findings on ultrasonography are also compatible with a cyst, a needle can be introduced into the cyst under ultrasonographic control and the cyst can be aspirated.

F. Isotope Scanning

A rectilinear scan clearly delineates the mass but does not differentiate cyst from tumor. The technetium scan, made with the camera, reveals that the mass is indeed avascular.

G. Percutaneous Cyst Aspiration with Cystography

If the studies listed leave some doubt about the differentiation between cyst and tumor, aspiration may be done (see Section "Treatment," given later).

▶ Differential Diagnosis

Carcinoma of the kidney also occupies space but tends to lie more deeply in the organ and therefore causes more distortion of the calyces. Hematuria is common with tumor, rare with cyst. If a solid tumor overlies the psoas muscle, the edge of the muscle is obliterated on the plain film; it can be seen through a cyst, however. Evidence of metastases (ie, loss of weight and strength, palpable supraclavicular nodes, chest film showing metastatic nodules), erythrocytosis, hypercalcemia, and increased sedimentation rate suggest cancer. It must be remembered, however, that the walls of a simple cyst may undergo cancerous degeneration. Sonography, CT scan, or MRI should be almost definitive in differential diagnosis. It is wise to assume that all space-occupying lesions of the kidneys are cancers until proved otherwise.

Polycystic kidney disease is almost always bilateral. Diffuse calyceal and pelvic distortion is the rule. Simple cyst is usually solitary and unilateral. Polycystic kidney disease is usually accompanied by impaired renal function and hypertension; simple cyst is not.

Renal cortical abscess is rare. A history of skin infection a few weeks before the onset of fever and local pain may be obtained. CT scan of the kidney will usually show signs of the abscess. The kidney may be fixed; this can be demonstrated by comparing the position of the kidney when the patient is supine and upright. Angiography demonstrates an avascular lesion. A gallium-67 scan demonstrates the inflammatory nature of the lesion, but an infected simple cyst might have a similar appearance.

Hydronephrosis may present the same symptoms and signs as simple cyst, but the urograms are quite different. Cyst causes calyceal distortion; with hydronephrosis, dilatation of the calyces and pelvis due to an obstruction is present. Acute or subacute hydronephrosis usually produces more local pain because of increased intrapelvic pressure and is more apt to be complicated by infection.

Extrarenal tumor (eg, adrenal, mixed retroperitoneal sarcoma) may displace a kidney, but rarely does it invade it and distort its calyces. If an echinococcal cyst of the kidney does not communicate with the renal pelvis, it may be difficult to differentiate from solitary cyst, for no scoleces or hooklets will be present in the urine. The wall of a hydatid cyst often reveals calcification on x-ray examination (see Figure 14–5). A skin sensitivity test (Casoni) for hydatid disease may prove helpful.

▶ Complications (Rare)

Spontaneous infection in a simple cyst is rare, but when it occurs, it is difficult to differentiate from carbuncle. Hemorrhage into the cyst sometimes occurs. If sudden, it causes severe pain. The bleeding may come from a complicating carcinoma arising on the wall of the cyst.

Hydronephrosis may develop if a cyst of the lower pole impinges on the ureter. This in itself may cause pain from back pressure of urine in the renal pelvis. This obstruction may lead to renal infection.

▶ Treatment

A. Specific Measures

1. If renal sonography, CT, or MRI does not lead to a definitive diagnosis, renal angiography or needle aspiration of the cyst may be necessary. Should aspiration be necessary, it can be done under sonographic guidance. The recovery of clear fluid is characteristic of a benign cyst, which should be confirmed by cytologic evaluation. In some centers, contrast radiopaque fluid is injected into the cyst after aspiration for a more thorough evaluation of the cyst wall. A smooth cyst wall, free of irregularities, supports the presence of a benign cyst. If the aspirate contains blood, surgical exploration should be considered, because the chances are great that the growth is cancerous.

2. If the diagnosis can be clearly established, one should consider leaving the cyst alone, since it is rare for a cyst to harm the kidney. Sonography is useful in follow-up of patients with cysts.

B. Treatment of Complications

If the cyst becomes infected, intensive antimicrobial therapy should be instituted; antimicrobial drugs have been found to attain very low concentrations in the cyst fluid. Therefore, percutaneous drainage is often required. Surgical excision of the extrarenal portion of the cyst wall and drainage are curative when percutaneous drainage fails.

If hydronephrosis is present, excision of the obstructing cyst will relieve the ureteral obstruction. Pyelonephritis in the involved kidney should suggest urinary stasis secondary to impaired ureteral drainage. Removal of the cyst and consequent relief of urinary back pressure make antimicrobial therapy more effective.

▶ Prognosis

Simple cysts can be diagnosed with great accuracy using sonography and CT scan. Yearly sonography is recommended as a method of following the cyst for changes in size, configuration, and internal consistency. CT scan may be done if changes suggest carcinoma, and aspiration may then be performed if necessary to establish a diagnosis. Most cysts cause little difficulty.

RENAL FUSION

About 1 in 1000 individuals has some type of renal fusion, the most common being the horseshoe kidney. The fused renal mass almost always contains two excretory systems and therefore two ureters. The renal tissue may be divided equally between the two flanks, or the entire mass may be on one side. Even in the latter case, the two ureters open at their proper places in the bladder.

▶ Etiology and Pathogenesis

It appears that this fusion of the two metanephroi occurs early in embryologic life, when the kidneys lie low in the pelvis. For this reason, they seldom ascend to the high position that normal kidneys assume. They may even remain in the true pelvis. Under these circumstances, such a kidney may derive its blood supply from many vessels in the area (eg, aorta, iliacs). In patients with both ectopia and fusion, 78% have extraurologic anomalies and 65% exhibit other genitourinary defects.

▶ Pathology (Figure 32–4)

Because the renal masses fuse early, normal rotation cannot occur; therefore, each pelvis lies on the anterior surface of its organ. Thus, the ureter must ride over the isthmus of a horseshoe kidney or traverse the anterior surface of the fused kidney. Some degree of ureteral compression may arise from this or from obstruction by one or more aberrant blood vessels. The incidence of hydronephrosis and, therefore, infection is high. Vesicoureteral reflux has frequently been noted in association with fusion.

In horseshoe kidney, the isthmus usually joins the lower poles of each kidney; each renal mass lies lower than normal. The axes of these masses are vertical, whereas the axes of normal kidneys are oblique to the spine, because they lie along the edges of the psoas muscles. On rare occasions, the two nephric masses are fused into one mass containing two pelves and two ureters. The mass may lie in the midline in order to open into the bladder at the proper point (crossed renal ectopy with fusion).

▶ Clinical Findings

A. Symptoms

Most patients with fused kidneys have no symptoms. Some, however, develop ureteral obstruction. Gastrointestinal symptoms (renodigestive reflex) mimicking peptic ulcer, cholelithiasis, or appendicitis may be noted. Infection is apt to occur if ureteral obstruction and hydronephrosis or calculus develops.

B. Signs

Physical examination results are usually negative unless the abnormally placed renal mass can be felt. With horseshoe kidney, it may be possible to palpate a mass over the lower lumbar spine (the isthmus). In the case of crossed ectopy, a mass may be felt in the flank or lower abdomen.

C. Laboratory Findings

Urinalysis is normal unless there is infection. Renal function is normal unless disease coexists in each of the fused renal masses.

D. X-Ray Findings

In the case of horseshoe kidney, the axes of the two kidneys, if visible on a plain film, are parallel to the spine. At times, the isthmus can be identified. The plain film may also reveal a large soft-tissue mass in one flank, yet not show a renal shadow on the other side. Excretory urograms establish the diagnosis if the renal parenchyma has been maintained. The increased density of the renal tissue may make the position or configuration of the kidney more distinct. Urograms also visualize the pelvis and ureters.

1. With horseshoe kidney, the renal pelves lie on the anterior surfaces of their kidney masses, whereas the normal kidney has its pelvis lying mesial to it. The most valuable clue to the diagnosis of horseshoe kidney is the presence of calyces in the region of the lower pole that point medially and lie medial to the ureter (Figure 32–4).

2. Crossed renal ectopy with fusion shows two pelves and two ureters. One ureter must cross the midline in order to empty into the bladder at the proper point (Figure 32–4).

3. A cake or lump kidney may lie in the pelvis (fused pelvis kidney), but again its ureters and pelves will be shown (Figure 32–4). It may compress the dome of the bladder.

CT scan clearly outlines the renal mass but is seldom necessary for diagnosis. With pelvic fused kidney or one lying in the flank, the plain film taken with ureteral catheters in place gives the first hint of the diagnosis. Retrograde urograms show the position of the pelves and demonstrate changes compatible with infection or obstruction. Renal scanning delineates the renal mass and its contour, as does sonography.

▶ Differential Diagnosis

Separate kidneys that fail to undergo normal rotation may be confused with horseshoe kidney. They lie along the edges of the psoas muscles, whereas the poles of a horseshoe kidney lie parallel to the spine and the lower poles are placed on the psoas muscles. The calyces in the region of the isthmus of a horseshoe kidney point medially and lie close to the spine.

The diagnosis of fused or lump kidney may be missed on excretory urograms if one of the ureters is markedly obstructed, so that a portion of the kidney, pelvis, and ureter fails to visualize. Infusion urograms or retrograde urograms demonstrate both excretory tracts in the renal mass.

▶ Complications

Fused kidneys are prone to ureteral obstruction because of a high incidence of aberrant renal vessels and the necessity for one or both ureters to arch around or over the renal tissue. Hydronephrosis, stone, and infection, therefore, are common. A large fused kidney occupying the concavity of the sacrum may cause dystocia.

▶ Treatment

No treatment is necessary unless obstruction or infection is present. Drainage of a horseshoe kidney may be improved by dividing its isthmus. If one pole of a horseshoe is badly damaged, it may require surgical resection.

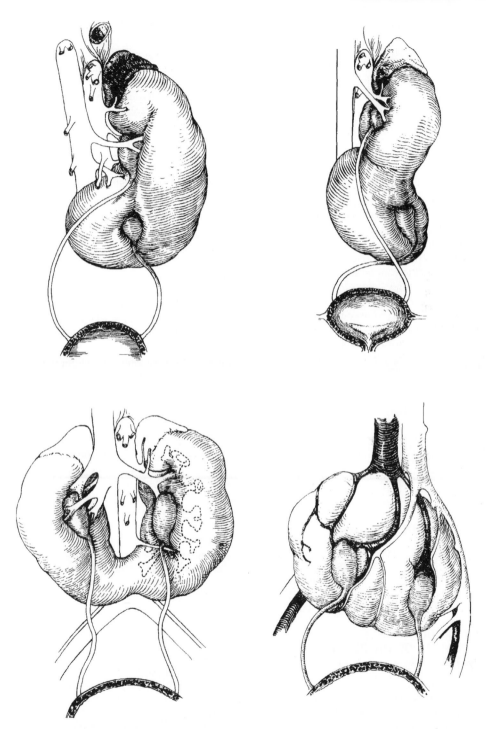

▲ **Figure 32–4.** Renal fusion. **Upper left:** Crossed renal ectopy with fusion. The renal mass lies in the left flank. The right ureter must cross over the midline. **Upper right:** Example of "sigmoid" kidney. **Lower left:** Horseshoe kidney. Pelves are anterior. Note the aberrant artery obstructing the left ureter and the low position of renal mass. **Lower right:** Pelvic kidney. Pelves are placed anteriorly. Note the aberrant blood supply.

▶ **Prognosis**

In most cases, the outlook is excellent. If ureteral obstruction and infection occur, renal drainage must be improved by surgical means so that antimicrobial therapy will be effective.

ECTOPIC KIDNEY

Congenital ectopic kidney usually causes no symptoms unless complications such as ureteral obstruction or infection develop.

▶ **Simple Ectopy**

Simple congenital ectopy usually refers to a low kidney on the proper side that failed to ascend normally. It may lie over the pelvic brim or in the pelvis. Rarely, it may be found in the chest. It takes its blood supply from adjacent vessels, and its ureter is short. It is prone to ureteral obstruction and infection, which may lead to pain or fever. At times, such a kidney may be palpable, leading to an erroneous presumptive diagnosis (eg, cancer of the bowel, appendiceal abscess).

Excretory urograms reveal the true position of the kidney. Hydronephrosis, if present, is evident. There is no redundancy of the ureter, as is the case with nephroptosis or acquired ectopy (eg, displacement by large suprarenal tumor). Obstruction and infection may complicate simple ectopy and should be treated by appropriate means.

CROSSED ECTOPY WITHOUT FUSION

In crossed ectopy without fusion, the kidney lies on the opposite side of the body but is not attached to its normally placed mate. Unless two distinct renal shadows can be seen, it may be difficult to differentiate this condition from crossed ectopy with fusion (Figure 32–4). Sonography, angiography, or CT should make the distinction.

ABNORMAL ROTATION

Normally, when the kidney ascends to the lumbar region, the pelvis lies on its anterior surface. Later, the pelvis comes to lie mesially. Such rotation may fail to occur, although this seldom leads to renal disease. Urography demonstrates the abnormal position.

MEDULLARY SPONGE KIDNEY (CYSTIC DILATATION OF THE RENAL COLLECTING TUBULES)

Medullary sponge kidney is a congenital autosomal recessive defect characterized by widening of the distal collecting tubules. It is usually bilateral, affecting all of the papillae, but it may be unilateral. At times, only one papilla is involved. Cystic dilatation of the tubules is also often present. Infection and calculi are occasionally seen as a result of urinary stasis in the tubules. It is believed that medullary sponge kidney is related to polycystic kidney disease. Its occasional

association with hemihypertrophy of the body has been noted.

The only symptoms are those arising from infection and stone formation. The diagnosis is made on the basis of excretory urograms or contrast-enhanced CT scan (Figure 32–5). The pelvis and calyces are normal, but dilated (streaked) tubules are seen just lateral to them; many of the dilated tubules contain round masses of radiopaque material (the cystic dilatation). If stones are present, a plain film will reveal small, round calculi in the pyramidal regions just beyond the calyces.

The differential diagnosis includes tuberculosis, healed papillary necrosis, and nephrocalcinosis. Tuberculosis is usually unilateral, and urography shows ulceration of calyces; tubercle bacilli are found on bacteriologic study. Papillary necrosis may be complicated by calcification in the healed stage but may be distinguished by its typical calyceal deformity, the presence of infection, and, usually, impaired renal function. The tubular and parenchymal calcification seen in nephrocalcinosis is more diffuse than that seen with sponge kidney (see Figure 16–3); the symptoms and signs of primary hyperparathyroidism or renal tubular acidosis may be found.

There is no treatment for medullary sponge kidney. Therapy is directed toward the complications (eg, pyelonephritis and renal calculi). Only a small percentage of people with sponge kidney develop complications. The overall prognosis is good. A few patients may pass small stones occasionally.

ABNORMALITIES OF RENAL VESSELS

A single renal artery is noted in 75–85% of individuals and a single renal vein in an even higher percentage. Aberrant veins and, especially, arteries occur. An aberrant artery passing to the lower pole of the kidney or crossing an infundibulum can cause obstruction and hydronephrosis. These causes of obstruction can be diagnosed on angiography or spiral CT.

ACQUIRED LESIONS OF THE KIDNEYS

ANEURYSM OF THE RENAL ARTERY

Aneurysm of the renal artery usually results from degenerative arterial disease that weakens the wall of the artery so that intravascular pressure may balloon it out. It is most commonly caused by arteriosclerosis or polyarteritis nodosa, but it may develop secondary to trauma or syphilis. Well over 300 cases have been reported. Congenital aneurysm has been recorded. Most cases represent an incidental finding on angiography.

Aneurysmal dilatation has no deleterious effect on the kidney unless the mass compresses the renal artery, in which case some renal ischemia and, therefore, atrophy are to be expected. A true aneurysm may rupture, producing a false aneurysm. This is especially likely to occur during pregnancy.

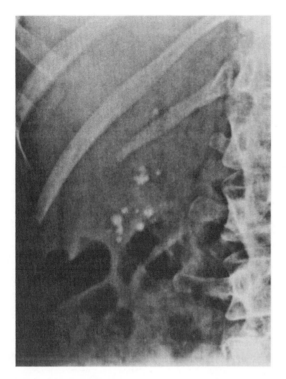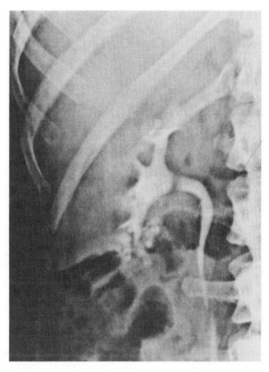

▲ **Figure 32–5.** Medullary sponge kidneys. ***Left:*** Plain film of right kidney showing multiple small stones in its mid portion. ***Right:*** Excretory urogram showing relationship of calculi to calyces. Typically, the calyces are large; the stones are located in the dilated collecting tubules.

The extravasated blood in the retroperitoneal space finally becomes encapsulated by a fibrous covering as organization occurs. An aneurysm may involve a small artery within the renal parenchyma. It may rupture into the renal pelvis or a calyx.

Most aneurysms cause no symptoms unless they rupture, in which case, there may be severe flank pain and even shock. If an aneurysm ruptures into the renal pelvis, marked hematuria occurs. The common cause of death is severe hemorrhage from rupture of the aneurysm. Hypertension is not usually present. A bruit should be sought over the costovertebral angle or over the renal artery anteriorly. If spontaneous or traumatic rupture has occurred, a mass may be palpated in the flank.

A plain film of the abdomen may show an intrarenal or extrarenal ringlike calcification (Figure 32–6). Urograms may be normal or reveal renal atrophy. Some impairment of renal function may be noted if compression or partial obstruction of the renal artery has developed. Aortography delineates the aneurysm. Sonography and CT scanning may prove helpful.

The differential diagnosis of rupture of an aneurysm and injury to the kidney is difficult unless a history or evidence of trauma is obtained. A hydronephrotic kidney may present a mass, but renal imaging clarifies the issue.

Because a significant number of noncalcified and large calcified aneurysms rupture spontaneously, the presence of such a lesion is an indication for operation, particularly during pregnancy. The repair of extrarenal aneurysms may be considered, but complications (eg, thrombosis) are not uncommon. If an intrarenal aneurysm is situated in one pole, heminephrectomy may be feasible. If it is in the center of the organ, however, nephrectomy is required. Therapeutic occlusion of an aneurysm by intra-arterial injection of autologous muscle tissue has been reported. Those few patients with hypertension may become normotensive following definitive surgery.

RENAL INFARCTS

Renal infarcts are caused by arterial occlusion. The major causes are subacute infective endocarditis, atrial or ventricular thrombi, arteriosclerosis, polyarteritis nodosa, and trauma. A thrombotic process in the abdominal aorta may gradually extend upward to occlude the renal artery. Renal infarcts may be unilateral or bilateral.

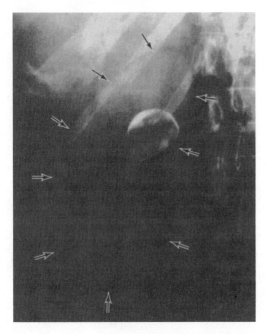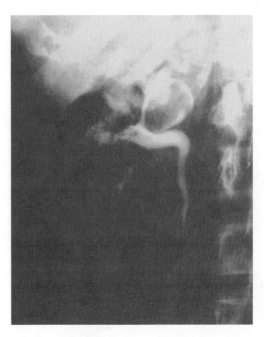

▲ **Figure 32–6.** Intrarenal aneurysm of renal artery. ***Left:*** Plain film showing calcified structure over right renal shadow. ***Right:*** Excretory urogram relating calcific mass to pelvis and upper calyx. (Courtesy of CD King.)

If smaller arteries or arterioles become obstructed, the tissue receiving blood from such a vessel will first become swollen and then undergo necrosis and fibrosis. Multiple infarcts are the rule. If the main renal artery becomes occluded, the entire kidney will react in kind. The kidney may become functionless and atrophic, therefore, as it undergoes necrosis and fibrosis.

Partial renal infarction is a silent disease, but it can result in flank pain and microscopic or gross hematuria. Sudden and complete infarction may cause renal or chest pain and at times gross or microscopic hematuria. Proteinuria and leukocytosis are found. "Epitheluria," representing sloughing of renal tubular cells, has been noted. Tenderness over the flank may be elicited. The kidney is not significantly enlarged by arterial occlusion.

CT scan may fail to have contrast enhancement in a portion of the kidney with partial infarction; with complete infarction, none of the radiopaque fluid is excreted. If complete renal infarction is suspected, a radioisotope renogram should be performed. A completely infarcted kidney shows little or no radioactivity. A similar picture is seen on CT scans performed after injection of radiopaque contrast medium. Even though complete loss of measurable function has occurred, renal circulation may be restored spontaneously in rare instances. Renal angiography or CT makes the definitive diagnosis. A dynamic technetium scan will reveal no perfusion of the affected renal vasculature.

During the acute phase, infarction may mimic ureteral stone. With stone, the excretory urogram may also show lack of renal function, but even so, there is usually enough medium in the tubules for a "nephrogram" to be obtained (see Figure 16–3). This will not occur with complete infarction. Evidence of a cardiac or vascular lesion is helpful in arriving at a proper diagnosis.

The complications are related to those arising from the primary cardiovascular disease, including emboli to other organs. In a few cases, hypertension may develop a few days or weeks after the infarction. It may later subside.

Although emergency surgical intervention has been done, it has become clear that anticoagulation therapy is the treatment of choice. It has been shown that an infusion of streptokinase may dissolve the embolus. Renal function returns in most cases.

THROMBOSIS OF THE RENAL VEIN

Thrombosis of the renal vein is rare in adults. It is frequently unilateral and usually associated with membranous glomerulonephritis and nephrotic syndrome. Invasion of the renal vein by tumor or retroperitoneal disease can be the cause. Thrombosis of the renal vein may occur as a complication of severe dehydration and hemoconcentration in children with severe diarrhea from ileocolitis. The thrombosis may extend from the vena cava into the peripheral venules or may originate in the peripheral veins and propagate to the main renal vein. The severe passive congestion that develops causes the kidney to swell and become engorged. Degeneration of the nephrons ensues. There is usually flank pain, and hematuria may be noted. A large, tender mass is often felt in the flank. Thrombocytopenia may be noted. The urine contains albumin and red cells. In the acute stage, urograms show poor or absent secretion of the radiopaque material in a large kidney. Stretching and thinning of the calyceal infundibula may be noted. Clots in the pelvis may cause filling defects. Later, the kidney may undergo atrophy.

Ultrasonography shows the thrombus in the vena cava in 50% of cases. The involved organ is enlarged. CT scan is also a valuable diagnostic tool; visualization of the thrombus can be noted in a high percentage of cases. Recently, MRI has proved to be a very sensitive diagnostic tool. Renal angiography reveals stretching and bowing of small arterioles. In the nephrographic phase, the pyramids may become quite dense. Late films may show venous collaterals. Venacavography or, preferably, selective renal venography demonstrates the thrombus in the renal vein (Figure 32–7) and, at times, in the vena cava.

The symptoms and signs resemble obstruction from a ureteral calculus. The presence of a stone in the ureter should be obvious; some degree of dilatation of the ureter and pelvis also should be expected. Clot obstruction in the ureter must be differentiated from an obstructing calculus.

While thrombectomy and even nephrectomy have been recommended in the past, it has become increasingly clear that medical treatment is usually efficacious. The use of heparin anticoagulation in the acute phase and warfarin chronically offers satisfactory resolution of the problems in most patients. In infants and children, it is essential to correct fluid and electrolyte problems and administer anticoagulants. Fibrinolytic therapy has also been successful. Renal function is usually fully recovered.

ARTERIOVENOUS FISTULA

Arteriovenous fistula may be congenital (25%) or acquired. A number of these fistulas have been reported following needle biopsy of the kidney or trauma to the kidney. A few have occurred following nephrectomy secondary to suture or ligature occlusion of the pedicle. These require surgical repair. A few have been recognized in association with adenocarcinoma of the kidney.

A thrill can often be palpated and a murmur heard both anteriorly and posteriorly. In cases with a wide communication, the systolic blood pressure is elevated and a widened pulse pressure is noted. Renal angiography or isotopic scan establishes the diagnosis. CT scan, sonography, and, recently, duplex ultrasound with color flow are particularly helpful. Arteriovenous fistula involving the renal artery and vein requires surgical repair or nephrectomy. Most, however, can be occluded by embolization, balloon, or steel coil. Those that develop secondary to renal biopsy tend to heal spontaneously.

ARTERIOVENOUS ANEURYSM

About 100 instances of this lesion have been reported (Figure 32–8). Most follow trauma. Hypertension is to be expected and is associated with high-output cardiac failure.

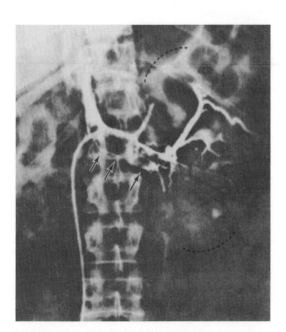

▲ **Figure 32–7.** Thrombosis of renal vein. Selective left renal venogram showing almost complete occlusion of vein. Veins to lower pole failed to fill. Note the large size of kidney.

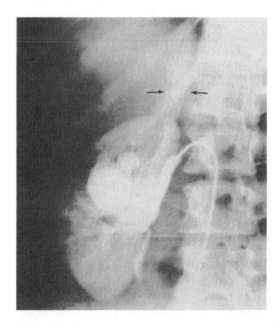

▲ **Figure 32–8.** Arteriovenous aneurysm. Selective renal angiogram. Note the aneurysm in center of kidney, with prompt filling of the vena cava (shown by **arrows**).

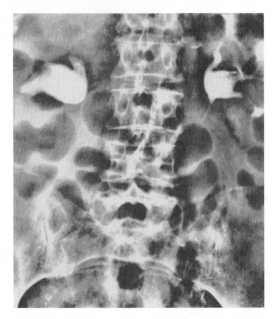
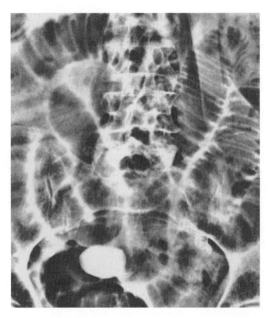

▲ **Figure 32–9.** Nephroduodenal fistula and small-bowel obstruction from renal staghorn calculus. *Left:* Excretory urogram showing nonfunction of right kidney; staghorn stone. *Right:* Patient presented with symptoms and signs of bowel obstruction 4 years later. Plain film showing dilated loops of small bowel down to a point just proximal to ileocecal valve. Obstruction due to stone extruded into duodenum. (Courtesy of CD King.)

A bruit is usually present. Nephrectomy is usually indicated.

RENOALIMENTARY FISTULA

Over 100 instances of renoalimentary fistula have been reported. They usually involve the stomach, duodenum, or adjacent colon, although fistula formation with the esophagus, small bowel, appendix, and rectum has been reported.

The underlying cause is usually a pyonephrotic kidney or renal cell carcinoma that becomes adherent to a portion of the alimentary tract and then ruptures spontaneously, thus creating a fistula (Figure 32–9). A few cases following trauma have been reported. The patient is apt to have symptoms and signs of acute pyelonephritis. Urography may show radioopaque material escaping into the gastrointestinal tract. Gastrointestinal series may also reveal the connection with the kidney. The treatment is nephrectomy with closure of the opening into the gut.

RENOBRONCHIAL FISTULA

Renobronchial fistulas are rare. They are caused by rupture of an infected, calculous kidney through the diaphragm.

BIBLIOGRAPHY

Congenital Anomalies of the Kidneys

General

Calisti A et al: The risk of associated urological abnormalities in children with pre and postnatal occasional diagnosis of solitary, small or ectopic kidney: Is a complete urological screening always necessary? World J Urol 2008;26(3):281–284.

Donohue RE, Fauver HE: Unilateral absence of the vas deferens: A useful clinical sign. JAMA 1989;261:1180.

Hálek J et al: Diagnostic accuracy of postnatal ultrasound screening for urinary tract abnormalities. Pediatr Nephrol 2010;25(2):281–287.

Sheih CP et al: Renal abnormalities in schoolchildren. Pediatrics 1989;84:1086.

Yoshida J et al: Mass screening for early detection of congenital kidney and urinary tract abnormalities in infancy. Pediatr Int 2003;45:142.

Agenesis

Kaneyama K et al: Associated urologic anomalies in children with solitary kidney. J Pediatr Surg 2004;39:85.

Ouden van den D et al: Diagnosis and management of seminal vesicle cysts associated with ipsilateral renal agenesis: A pooled analysis of 52 cases. Eur Urol 1998;33:433.

Spira EM et al: Sonographic long-term study: Paediatric growth charts for single kidneys. Arch Dis Child 2009;94(9):693–698.

Hypoplasia

Saborio P, Scheinman J: Genetic renal disease. Curr Opin Pediatr 1998;10:174.

Dysplasia and Multicystic Kidney

Alconcher L, Tombesi M: Multicystic dysplastic kidney detected by prenatal ultrasonography: Conservative management. Pediatr Nephrol 2005;20:1024.

Mattioli G et al: Nephrectomy for multicystic dysplastic kidney and renal hypodysplasia in children: Where do we stand? Pediatr Surg Int 2010;26(5):523–528.

McMann LP et al: Magnetic resonance urography in the evaluation of prenatally diagnosed hydronephrosis and renal dysgenesis. J Urol 2006;176(4, Pt 2):1786–1792.

Shaheen IS et al: Multicystic dysplastic kidney and pelviureteric junction obstruction. Pediatr Surg Int 2005;21:282.

Singh S et al: Clinico-pathological profile of 22 cases of cystic renal dysplasia. Indian J Pathol Microbiol 2007;50(1):6–10.

Welch TR, Wacksman J: The changing approach to multicystic dysplastic kidney in children. J Pediatr 2005;146:723.

Adult Polycystic Kidney Disease

Avni FE, Hall M: Renal cystic diseases in children: New concepts. Pediatr Radiol 2010;40(6):939–946.

Dambreville S et al; Consortium for Radiologic Imaging Studies of Polycystic Kidney Disease (CRISP): Renal arterial blood flow measurement by breath-held MRI: Accuracy in phantom scans and reproducibility in healthy subjects. Magn Reson Med 2010;63(4):940–950.

Deacu M et al: Urothelial carcinoma of the renal pelvis associated with cystic disease of the kidney. Rom J Morphol Embryol 2011;52(1, Suppl):497–501.

Dunn MD et al: Laparoscopic cyst marsupialization in patients with autosomal dominant polycystic kidney disease. J Urol 2001;165:1888.

Ekser B, Rigotti P: Images in clinical medicine. Autosomal dominant polycystic kidney disease. N Engl J Med 2010;363(1):71.

Lentine KL et al: Renal function and healthcare costs in patients with polycystic kidney disease. Clin J Am Soc Nephrol 2010;5(8):1471–1479.

Meijer E et al: Early renal abnormalities in autosomal dominant polycystic kidney disease. Clin J Am Soc Nephrol 2010;5(6):1091–1098.

Punia RP et al: Unilateral and segmental cystic disease of the kidney. Int J Urol 2005;12:308.

Serra AL et al: Sirolimus and kidney growth in autosomal dominant polycystic kidney disease. N Engl J Med 2010;363(9):820–829.

Taskinen S et al: Segmental cystic kidney tumours in children. Scand J Urol Nephrol 2009;43(6):476–481.

Simple (Solitary) Cyst

Israel GM et al: Evaluation of cystic renal masses: Comparison of CT and MR imaging by using the Bosniak classification system. Radiology 2004;231:365.

Israel GM, Bosniak MA: An update of the Bosniak renal cyst classification system. Urology 2005;66:484.

Patel NS et al: The characterization of small hypoattenuating renal masses on contrast-enhanced CT. Clin Imaging 2009;33(4):295–300.

Ryu DS, Oh TH: Laparoscopic decortication of large renal cysts: A comparison between the transperitoneal and retroperitoneal approaches. J Laparoendosc Adv Surg Tech A 2009;19(5):629–632.

Terada N et al: The 10-year natural history of simple renal cysts. Urology 2008;71(1):7–11; discussion 11–12.

Warren KS, McFarlane J: The Bosniak classification of renal cystic masses. BJU Int 2005;95:939.

White WM et al: Single-port urological surgery: Single-center experience with the first 100 cases. Urology 2009;74(4):801–804.

Acquired Lesions of the Kidneys
General

Nanda S et al: Inferior vena cava anomalies—A common cause of DVT and PE commonly not diagnosed. Am J Med Sci 2008;335(5):409–410.

Rawashdeh YF et al: The intrarenal resistive index as a pathophysiological marker of obstructive uropathy. J Urol 2001;165:1397.

Zhang JQ et al: Etiology of spontaneous perirenal hemorrhage: A meta-analysis. J Urol 2002;167:1593.

Infection-Related Renal Disorders

Best CD et al: Clinical and radiological findings in patients with gas-forming renal abscess treated conservatively. J Urol 1999;162:1273.

Cheng CH et al: Renal abscess in children: A 10-year clinical and radiologic experience in a tertiary medical center. Pediatr Infect Dis J 2008;27(11):1025–1027.

Cheng CH et al: Clinical courses of children with acute lobar nephronia correlated with computed tomographic patterns. Pediatr Infect Dis J 2009;28(4):300–303.

Demertzis J, Menias CO: State of the art: Imaging of renal infections. Emerg Radiol 2007;14(1):13–22.

Guzzo TJ et al: Xanthogranulomatous pyelonephritis: Presentation and management in the era of laparoscopy. BJU Int 2009;104(9):1265–1268.

Hussein N et al: Xanthogranulomatous pyelonephritis in pediatric patients: Effect of surgical approach. Urology 2009;73(6):1247–1250.

Lee BE et al: Recent clinical overview of renal and perirenal abscesses in 56 consecutive cases. Korean J Intern Med 2008;23(3):140–148.

Li L, Parwani AV: Xanthogranulomatous pyelonephritis. Arch Pathol Lab Med 2011;135(5):671–674.

Loffroy R et al: Xanthogranulomatous pyelonephritis in adults: Clinical and radiological findings in diffuse and focal forms. Clin Radiol 2007;62(9):884–890.

Meng MV et al: Current treatment and outcomes of perinephric abscesses. J Urol 2002;168:1337.

Rogers C et al: Robotic nephrectomy for the treatment of benign and malignant disease. BJU Int 2008;102(11):1660–1665.

Vourganti S et al: Ultrasonographic evaluation of renal infections. Radiol Clin North Am 2006;44(6):763–775.

Aneurysm of the Renal Artery

Cura M et al: Renal aneurysms and pseudoaneurysms. Clin Imaging 2011;35(1):29–41.

Helck A et al: Diagnosis, therapy monitoring and follow up of renal artery pseudoaneurysm with contrast-enhanced ultrasound in three cases. Clin Hemorheol Microcirc 2010;46(2–3):127–137.

Ikeda O et al: Endovascular management of visceral artery pseudoaneurysms: Transcatheter coil embolization using the isolation technique. Cardiovasc Intervent Radiol 2010;33(6):1128–1134.

Keddis MT et al: Ischaemic nephropathy secondary to atherosclerotic renal artery stenosis: Clinical and histopathological correlates. Nephrol Dial Transplant 2010;25(11):3615–3622.

Robinson WP III et al: Favorable outcomes with in situ techniques for surgical repair of complex renal artery aneurysms. J Vasc Surg 2011;53(3):684–691.

Thrombosis of the Renal Vein

Akin O et al: Bland and tumor thrombi in abdominal malignancies: Magnetic resonance imaging assessment in a large oncologic patient population. Abdom Imaging 2011;36(1):62–68.

Al-Said J, Kamel O: Changes in renal cortical and medullary perfusion in a patient with renal vein thrombosis. Saudi J Kidney Dis Transpl 2010;21(1):123–127.

Cai S et al: Evaluation of acute renal artery thrombosis or embolism with color Doppler sonography. Clin Imaging 2008;32(5):367–371.

Ciancio G et al: Long-term survival in patients undergoing radical nephrectomy and inferior vena cava thrombectomy: single-center experience. Eur Urol 2010;57(4):667–672.

Decoster T et al: Renal colic as the first symptom of acute renal vein thrombosis, resulting in the diagnosis of nephrotic syndrome. Eur J Emerg Med 2009;16(4):170–171.

Demirel N et al: Neonatal thrombo-embolism: Risk factors, clinical features and outcome. Ann Trop Paediatr 2009;29(4):271–279.

Douma RA et al: Incidental venous thromboembolism in cancer patients: Prevalence and consequence. Thromb Res 2010;125(6): e306–e309.

Mehta S, Vijayakumar M: Spontaneous renal vein thrombosis with anti-thrombin III deficiency. Indian J Pediatr 2009;76(9):964–965.

Mahmoodi BK et al; Prevention of Renal and Vascular End-stage Disease (PREVEND) Study Group: Microalbuminuria and risk of venous thromboembolism. JAMA 2009;301(17):1790–1797.

Wahlgren CM et al: Endovascular treatment in postthrombotic syndrome. Vasc Endovascular Surg 2010;44(5):356–360.

Diagnosis of Medical Renal Diseases

33

Brian K. Lee, MD, & Flavio G. Vincenti, MD

MEDICAL RENAL DISEASE—OVERVIEW

Medical renal diseases are those that involve principally the parenchyma of the kidneys. Hematuria, proteinuria, pyuria, oliguria, polyuria, pain, renal insufficiency with azotemia, acidosis, anemia, electrolyte abnormalities, and hypertension may occur in a wide variety of disorders affecting any portion of the parenchyma of the kidney, the blood vessels, or the excretory tract.

A complete medical history and physical examination, a thorough examination of the urine, and blood and urine chemistry examinations as indicated are essential initial steps in the workup of any patient.

▶ History and Examination

A. Family History

The family history may reveal disease of genetic origin, for example, tubular metabolic anomalies, polycystic kidneys, unusual types of nephritis, or vascular or coagulation defects that may be essential clues to the diagnosis. First-degree relatives of patients with diabetic renal disease have an enhanced risk of end-stage renal disease, inherited independently of diabetes mellitus.

B. Past History

The past personal history should cover infections, injuries, and exposure to toxic agents, anticoagulants, or drugs that may produce toxic or sensitivity reactions. A history of diabetes, hypertensive disease, or autoimmune disease may be obtained. The inquiry may also elicit symptoms of uremia, debilitation, and the vascular complications of chronic renal disease, but often, the patient is asymptomatic and the diagnosis of renal disease is made incidentally on abnormal laboratory findings.

▶ Physical Examination

Pallor, edema, hypertension, retinopathy (either hypertensive or diabetic changes), or stigmas of congenital and hereditary disease may be detected.

▶ Laboratory Findings

A. Urinalysis

Examination of the urine is the essential part of any investigation of renal disease.

1. Proteinuria—Proteinuria of any significant degree (2–4+) is suggestive of medical renal disease (parenchymal involvement). Formed elements present in the urine additionally establish the diagnosis. Significant proteinuria occurs in immune-mediated glomerular diseases or disorders with glomerular involvement such as diabetes mellitus, myeloma, or amyloidosis. Interstitial nephritis, polycystic kidneys, and other tubular disorders are not usually associated with significant proteinuria. To better quantify the degree of proteinuria, one could either collect a 24-hour urine sample or use a spot urine protein to creatinine ratio (measured in milligrams of protein/mg creatinine) as a surrogate (see Figure 33–1).

2. Erythrocyte casts—Red blood cell casts point to glomerulonephritis. If red blood cell (erythrocyte) casts are not present, microscopic hematuria may or may not be of glomerular origin. Phase contrast microscope study may reveal dysmorphic changes in the erythrocytes present in the urine in patients with glomerular disorders.

3. Fatty casts and oval fat bodies—Tubular cells showing fatty changes occur in degenerative diseases of the kidney (nephrosis, glomerulonephritis, autoimmune disease, amyloidosis, and damage due to toxins such as lead or mercury).

4. Granular casts—These types of casts result from degeneration of cellular casts. They are nondiagnostic of a specific

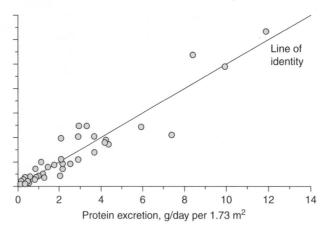

▲ **Figure 33–1.** This graph illustrates the relation between total 24-hour urinary protein excretion and the total protein-to-creatinine ratio (mg/mg) determined on a random urine specimen. Although there appears to be a close correlation, there can be wide variability in 24-hour protein excretion at a given total protein-to-creatinine ratio. At a ratio of 2, for example, 24-hour protein excretion varied from 2 to almost 8 g/d. (Data from Ginsberg JM et al: N Engl J Med 1983;309:1543.)

renal disorder but do reflect an inflammatory condition in the kidneys.

B. Other Findings

Abnormal urinary chemical constituents may be the only indication of a metabolic disorder involving the kidneys. These disorders include diabetes mellitus, renal glycosuria, aminoacidurias (including cystinuria), oxaluria, gout, hyperparathyroidism, hemoglobinuria, and myoglobinuria.

▶ Examination of the Kidneys and Urinary Tract

Roentgenographic, sonographic, and radioisotopic studies provide information about the size, structure, blood supply, and function of the kidneys.

▶ Renal Biopsy

Renal biopsy is a valuable diagnostic procedure. The technique has become well established, providing sufficient tissue for light and electron microscopy and for immunofluorescence examination. Relative contraindications for percutaneous kidney biopsy may include the patients with a congenitally solitary kidney, severe malfunction of one kidney even though function is adequate in the other, bleeding diathesis, and an unco-operative patient. Poorly controlled blood pressure (systolically >160 or diastolically >100 mm Hg) should be controlled prior to performing an invasive procedure such as renal biopsy.

Clinical indications for renal biopsy, in addition to the necessity for establishing a diagnosis, include the need to determine prognosis, to follow progression of a lesion and response to treatment, to confirm the presence of a generalized disease (autoimmune disorder, amyloidosis, sarcoidosis), and to diagnose renal dysfunction in a transplanted kidney. Ultrasound or computed tomography (CT) guidance provides a more effective biopsy result. More recently, laparoscopic approach has been used by some urologists.

With the increasing demand for renal biopsies in patients with a bleeding diathesis, especially in those with concomitant liver dysfunction, a transjugular approach has been advocated. However, the success of this procedure is highly dependent on the experience of the center and operators, and diagnostic yield on samples obtained range from 73% to 97%.

GLOMERULONEPHRITIS

The clinical manifestations of glomerular renal disease are apt to consist only of varying degrees of hematuria, excretion of characteristic formed elements in the urine, proteinuria, and renal insufficiency and its complications. Excluding diabetes, purported immunologic renal diseases are the most common cause of proteinuria and the nephrotic syndrome.

Alterations in glomerular architecture as observed in tissue examined by light microscopy alone can be minimal, nonspecific, and difficult to interpret. For these reasons, specific diagnoses of renal disease require targeted immune fluorescent techniques for demonstrating a variety of antigens, antibodies, and complement fractions. Electron microscopy has complemented these immunologic methods. Tissue analysis can be assisted by blood tests of immunoglobulins (Ig), complement, and other mediators of inflammation.

There are two important humoral mechanisms leading to deposition of antibodies within the glomerulus. These are based on the location of the antigen, whether fixed within the kidney or present in soluble form in circulation. The fixed antigens are either a natural structural element of the glomerulus or foreign materials that have been trapped within the glomerulus for a variety of immunologic or physiochemical reasons. The best examples of the fixed natural antigens are those associated with the glomerular basement membrane (GBM). These antigens are evenly distributed in the GBM and cause characteristic linear IgG deposition, as determined in immunofluorescence studies. This process represents 5% of cases of immune-mediated glomerular disease and is referred to as anti-GBM disease. When this is coupled with pulmonary symptoms (antibodies directed against the alveolar membrane), it is known as Goodpasture's syndrome. However, most patients with glomerular immune deposits have discontinuous immune aggregates caused by antibody binding to native renal cell antigens or to antigens trapped within the glomerulus. In addition, immune complexes formed in the circulation can deposit and accumulate in the GBM and the mesangium.

A group of immune-mediated nephritides characterized by necrotizing and crescentic architecture and rapid progression are referred to as pauci-immune glomerular nephritides because, while antibodies may contribute to the pathogenesis of the disease, they are rarely demonstrated within the glomeruli. These are known as antineutrophil cytoplasmic antibody (ANCA) diseases. Circulating antibodies against myeloperoxidase (MPO, P-ANCA) and proteinase 3 (PR3, C-ANCA) have been noted in microscopic angiitis and Wegener's granulomatosis, respectively.

Cellular immune processes are likely to be stimulated and contribute in different ways in various other forms of glomerulonephritides.

The current classification of glomerulonephritis is based on the mechanism, the presence, and the localization of immune aggregates in the glomeruli.

▶ Immunologic Mechanisms Likely

A. Subepithelial Immune Deposits

1. Glomerulonephritis associated with postinfectious glomerulonephritis such as poststreptococcal glomerulonephritis.

2. Membranous nephropathy idiopathic or secondary to other causes such as systemic lupus erythematosus, cancer, gold, penicillamine.

B. Subendothelial Immune Deposits

Glomerulonephritis associated with systemic lupus erythematosus, type I idiopathic membranoproliferative glomerulonephritis (MPGN), glomerulonephritis associated with hepatitis C infection, bacterial endocarditis, and shunt nephritis.

C. Mesangial Immune Deposits

IgA nephropathy, Schönlein–Henoch purpura.

D. Anti-GBM Disease

Diffuse linear deposition of Ig.

▶ Immunologic Mechanisms Not Clearly Established

1. Minimal change nephropathy.

2. Focal, segmental glomerulosclerosis.

3. Hemolytic–uremic syndrome and thrombotic thrombocytopenic purpura.

4. ANCA-associated disease: Wegener's granulomatosis and small-vessel vasculitis.

5. Type II MPGN (dense deposit disease).

▶ Poststreptococcal Glomerulonephritis

A. Essentials of Diagnosis

- History of streptococcal infection.
- Mild generalized edema, mild hypertension, retinal hemorrhages.
- Gross hematuria; protein, erythrocyte casts, granular and hyaline casts, white blood cells (leukocytes), and renal epithelial cells in urine.
- Elevated antistreptolysin O titer, hypocomplementemia.

B. General Considerations

Poststreptococcal glomerulonephritis is a disease affecting both kidneys. In most cases, recovery from the acute stage is complete, but progressive involvement may destroy renal tissue, leading to renal insufficiency. Acute glomerulonephritis is most common in children aged 3–10 years. By far the most common cause is an antecedent infection of the pharynx and tonsils or of the skin with group A beta-hemolytic streptococci, certain strains of which are nephritogenic. Nephritis occurs in 10–15% of children and young adults who have clinically evident infection with a nephritogenic strain. In children younger than 6 years, pyoderma (impetigo) is the most common antecedent; in older children and young adults, pharyngitis is a common antecedent. Occasionally, nephritis may follow infection due to other agents, hence the more general term postinfectious glomerulonephritis.

The pathogenesis of the glomerular lesion has been further elucidated by the use of new immunologic techniques (immunofluorescence) and electron microscopy. A likely sequel to infection is injury to the mesangial cells in the intercapillary space. The glomerulus may then become more easily damaged by antigen-antibody complexes developing from the immune response to the infection. Complement is deposited in association with IgG or alone in a granular pattern on the epithelial side of the basement membrane.

Gross examination of the involved kidney shows only punctate hemorrhages throughout the cortex. Microscopically, the primary alteration is in the glomeruli, which show proliferation and swelling of the mesangial and endothelial cells of the capillary tuft. The proliferation of capsular epithelium occurs, and around the tuft, there are collections of leukocytes, erythrocytes, and exudate. Edema of the interstitial tissue and cloudy swelling of the tubular epithelium are common. When severe, typical histologic findings in glomerulitis are enlarging crescents that become hyalinized and converted into scar tissue and obstruct the circulation through the glomerulus. Degenerative changes occur in the tubules, with fatty degeneration, necrosis, and ultimately scarring of the nephron.

C. Clinical Findings

1. Symptoms and signs—Often the disease is mild, and there may be no reason to suspect renal involvement unless the urine is examined. In severe cases, about 2 weeks after the acute streptococcal infection, the patient has headache, malaise, mild fever, puffiness around the eyes and face, flank pain, and oliguria. Hematuria is usually noted as "bloody" or, if the urine is acid, as "brown" or "coca-cola colored." There may be moderate tachycardia, dyspnea, and moderate to marked elevation of blood pressure. Tenderness in the costovertebral angle is common.

2. Laboratory findings—The diagnosis is confirmed by examination of the urine, which may be grossly bloody or coffee colored (acid hematin) or may show only microscopic hematuria. In addition, the urine contains protein (1–3+) and casts. Hyaline and granular casts are commonly found in large numbers, but the classic sign of glomerulitis, occasionally noted, is the erythrocyte cast. The erythrocyte cast is usually of small caliber, is intensely orange or red, and may show the mosaic pattern of the packed erythrocytes held together by the clot of fibrin and plasma protein.

With the impairment of renal function (decrease in glomerular filtration rate and blood flow) and with oliguria, plasma or serum urea nitrogen and creatinine become elevated, the levels varying with the severity of the renal lesion. A mild normochromic anemia may result from fluid retention and dilution.

Infection of the throat with nephritogenic streptococci is frequently followed by increasing antistreptolysin O titers in the serum, whereas high titers are usually not demonstrable following skin infections. The streptozyme test is available consisting of five antistreptococcal antibodies, and has a diagnostic yield of 95% among those with pharyngitis and 80% of those with a skin infection as precipitating events.

Serum complement levels are usually low.

Confirmation of diagnosis is made by examination of the urine, although the history and clinical findings in typical cases leave little doubt. The finding of erythrocytes in a cast is proof that erythrocytes were present in the renal tubules and did not arise from elsewhere in the genitourinary tract.

3. Microbiologic cultures—Due to the lag in symptoms weeks after the antecedent infection, only 25% of patients will have positive throat or skin cultures.

4. Renal biopsy—This is often not necessary; however, if the pattern of presentation deviates significantly from expected, a tissue diagnosis may help differentiate between differential diagnoses. For example, recurrent hematuria may indicate IgA nephropathy, whereas a persistently depressed complement (C3) level 6 weeks and beyond suggests a diagnosis of membrano-proliferative glomerulonephritis.

5. Treatment—There is no specific treatment. Eradication of infection, prevention of overhydration and hypertension, and prompt treatment of complications such as hypertensive encephalopathy and heart failure require careful management. Some have used intravenous (IV) methylprednisolone in patients with significant crescents at biopsy, but this is not a universal practice.

6. Prognosis—Most patients with the acute disease recover completely; 5–20% show progressive renal damage. This damage may be evident only years after the immune injury. If oliguria, heart failure, or hypertensive encephalopathy is severe, death may occur during the acute attack. Even with severe acute disease, however, recovery is the rule, particularly in children.

▶ Immunoglobulin A Nephropathy

Primary hematuria (idiopathic benign and recurrent hematuria, Berger's disease) is now known to be an immune complex glomerulopathy in which deposition of IgA occurs in a granular pattern in the mesangium of the glomerulus. The associated light microscopic findings are variable and range from normal to extensive crescentic glomerulonephritis.

Recurrent macroscopic and microscopic hematuria and mild proteinuria are usually the only manifestations of renal disease. Most patients with IgA nephropathy are between the ages of 16 and 35 years at the time of diagnosis. The disease occurs much more frequently in males than in females and is the most common cause of glomerulonephritis among Asians and in the developed world. While most patients continue to have episodes of gross hematuria or microscopic hematuria, renal function is likely to remain stable. However, approximately 30% of patients will have progressive renal dysfunction and develop end-stage renal disease. Clinical features that indicate a poor prognosis include male sex, older age at onset of disease, the presence of nephrotic-range proteinuria, hypertension, or renal dysfunction at presentation.

There is no satisfactory therapy for IgA nephropathy. Use of angiotensin-converting enzyme (ACE) inhibitors and angiotensin receptor blockade in an effort to lower proteinuria and delay progression of chronic kidney disease should be first-line therapy. The role of immunosuppressive drugs such as steroids and cytotoxic agents is not clear, and there have been few rigorously performed controlled trials. A more intriguing approach is the use of omega-3 fatty acids (fish oils) to delay progression of the renal disease. A large, prospective, randomized, placebo-controlled trial in patients with IgA nephropathy using 12 g of omega-3 fatty acids has shown that fish oils probably can reduce the deterioration of renal function and the number of patients in whom end-stage renal disease develops.

After renal transplantation, recurrent IgA disease has been described. The risk varies from 21% to 58%. Of those who develop graft dysfunction attributable to recurrence, eventual graft loss occurred in 46–71% of patients. It is disputable whether allografts from living related donors confer a greater risk of recurrence than deceased or living unrelated donors.

Rapidly Progressive Glomerulonephritis

This condition has several pulmonary-renal diseases. The patient usually gives a history of recent hemoptysis and often of malaise, anorexia, and headache. A severe acute glomerulonephritis may be accompanied by diffuse hemorrhagic inflammation of the lungs. The urine shows gross or microscopic hematuria, and laboratory findings of severely suppressed renal function are usually evident. Biopsy shows glomerular crescents, glomerular adhesions, and inflammatory infiltration interstitially. Electron microscope examination shows an increase in basement membrane material and deposition of fibrin beneath the capillary endothelium. In cases of anti-GBM disease, circulating antibody against GBM can be identified. IgG, C3, and, often, other components of the classic complement pathway can be demonstrated as linear deposits on the basement membranes of the glomeruli and the lung. This was formerly called *Goodpasture's disease.*

Large doses of corticosteroids in combination with immunosuppressive therapy may be useful. Plasmapheresis to remove circulating antibody has been reported to be effective in some patients. Transplantation should be delayed until circulating antiglomular basement antibodies have disappeared.

In contrast, some patients have crescenteric glomerulonephritis but do not show any immune deposits or antibody deposition by immunofluorescence studies. They have pauci-immune idiopathic rapidly progressive glomerulonephritis (RPGN). Many of these patients are serologically ANCA

positive. High-dose prednisone pulse therapy and cytotoxic agents may result in prolonged remission.

NEPHROTIC SYNDROME E

▶ Essentials of Diagnosis and General Considerations

- Edema.
- Proteinuria >3.5 g/d.
- Hypoalbuminemia <3 g/dL.
- Hyperlipidemia: cholesterol >300 mg/dL.
- Lipiduria: free fat, oval fat bodies, fatty casts.

Because treatment and prognosis vary with the cause of nephrotic syndrome, renal biopsy is important. Light microscopy, electron microscopy, and immunofluorescence identification of immune mechanisms diagnose most causes of nephrosis.

Glomerular diseases associated with nephrosis include the following.

▶ Minimal Glomerular Lesions

Minimal-change nephropathy (nil disease) accounts for about 20% of cases of nephrosis in adults and 90% in children. No abnormality is visible by examination of biopsy material with the light microscope. With the electron microscope, alterations of the GBM, with effacement of foot processes of the epithelial cells, are evident. There is no evidence of immune disease by immunofluorescence studies. The response to treatment with corticosteroids is good; however, in adults, a longer course of prednisone is normally required compared with the pediatric population. For patients who have frequent relapses with steroids or are steroid resistant, a course of cyclophosphamide or chlorambucil may induce a prolonged remission. Patients who do not respond to these agents may show a favorable response with cyclosporine or tacrolimus. Renal function usually remains stable. Partial response is uncommon, which should prompt a search for misdiagnosed FSGS due to sampling error on biopsy.

▶ Focal Glomerulosclerosis

Focal glomerulosclerosis is the second most common cause of nephrotic syndrome in children and an increasing cause of the nephrotic syndrome in adults. Some regard this to be in the same spectrum of disease as minimal change nephropathy. The diagnosis is based on light microscope findings of segmental hyalinosis and sclerosis associated with effacement of the foot processes on electron microscopy. Focal glomerulosclerosis is frequently idiopathic but can be associated with human immunodeficiency virus infection and heroin use. There is much debate about a circulating permeability factor as the causative agent, but its true identity has remained elusive. A secondary form of focal glomerulosclerosis without the diffuse changes in foot processes may occur in patients with a solitary kidney, hyperfiltration syndromes, and reflux nephropathy. There are reports of familial variants (due to nephrin and podocin mutations). The response of the idiopathic form of focal glomerulosclerosis to therapy is suboptimal. Prolonged corticosteroid therapy produces remission in approximately 40% of patients. Over a 10-year period, approximately 50% of patients will develop chronic kidney disease. Idiopathic focal glomerulosclerosis has a recurrence rate of 25% after transplantation. With a history of recurrence in a prior failed transplant, the risk of recurrence in a second transplant increases substantially.

▶ Membranous Nephropathy

Examination of biopsy material with the light microscope shows thickening of the glomerular cells but no cellular proliferation. With the electron microscope, irregular lumpy deposits appear between the basement membrane and the epithelial cells, and new basement membrane material protrudes from the GBM as spikes or domes. Immunofluorescence studies show diffuse granular deposits of Ig (especially IgG) and complement (C3 component). As the membrane thickens, glomeruli become sclerosed and hyalinized.

The pathogenesis of most cases of membranous nephropathy in humans is unclear. Several mechanisms have been suggested. They include trapping of circulating immune complexes or binding of an antibody to scattered glomerular antigens (either present already or "planted" after a nonrenal-source antigen lodges in the glomerulus).

There is considerable controversy regarding the effectiveness of therapy with steroids or immunosuppressive agents. Therapy should be most often used in patients high risk of progressive renal failure with the following criteria: proteinuria >5 g/d, hypertension, and elevated serum creatinine. Initial protocols consisted of using prednisone/methylprednisolone and chlorambucil, but head-to-head trials showed equal outcomes with cyclophosphamide, which is preferred given the multitude of side effects with chlorambucil.

▶ Membranoproliferative Glomerulonephritis—Types I and II

In type I MPGN, light microscopy shows thickening of glomerular capillaries, accompanied by mesangial proliferation and obliteration of glomeruli. Some cases show the characteristic double-contour glomerular capillary membranes. With the electron microscope, subendothelial deposits and growth of mesangium into capillary walls are demonstrable. Immunofluorescence studies show the presence of C3 component of complement and, rarely, Ig. The most common cause of MPGN type I is chronic hepatitis C virus infection. This condition is usually associated with high levels of IgG/IgM. Cryoimmunoglobulins may be present with normal or slightly reduced levels of complement. There is no known effective treatment. Treatment of hepatitis C using pegylated

interferon-α and ribavirin (in those with eGFR >50 mL/min) may slow down progression or prompt regression of renal lesions.

Type II MPGN is characterized by dense deposits visible by electron microscopy and lack of findings by immunofluorescence studies. Treatment is unsatisfactory, and there is a high rate of recurrence after kidney transplantation (80–100%).

▶ Miscellaneous Diseases

Many medical illnesses that are metabolic, autoimmune, or infectious, as well as neoplastic diseases and reactions to drugs and other toxic substances can produce glomerular disease. These include diabetic glomerulopathy, systemic lupus erythematosus, ANCA-positive renal disease (including Wegener's granulomatosis), amyloid disease, multiple myeloma, lymphomas, carcinomas, syphilis, reaction to toxins, reaction to drugs (eg, trimethadione), and exposure to heavy metals.

A rare glomerular illness has been recently described with nephrotic syndrome: fibrillary and immunotactoid glomerular nephritis. The lesions of fibrillary glomerulonephritis are characterized by randomly oriented fibril deposits 10–30 nm in diameter located within the mesangium and capillary wall. Immunotactoid glomerulopathy is characterized by deposits of microtubular structures of 18–19 nm and has been associated with lymphoproliferative disorders. In contrast to amyloid, the deposits in both diseases are Congo red negative. Treatment is generally unsatisfactory.

▶ Clinical Findings in Nephrosis

A. Symptoms and Signs

Edema may appear insidiously and increase slowly or can appear suddenly and accumulate rapidly. Symptoms other than those related to the mechanical effects of edema are not remarkable.

On physical examination, massive peripheral edema is apparent. Signs of hydrothorax and ascites are common. Pallor is often accentuated by the edema, and striae commonly appear.

B. Laboratory Findings

The urine contains large amounts of protein, 4–10 g/24 h or more. There is a good correlation between the urine protein to creatinine ratio (from a "spot" morning urine) and the 24-hour urine collections. For example, a ratio in excess of 3:1 in the spot urine usually correlates to a 24-hour proteinuria of 3 g. The sediment contains casts, including the characteristic fatty and waxy varieties; renal tubular cells, some of which contain fatty droplets (oval fat bodies); and variable numbers of erythrocytes. A mild normochromic anemia is common, but anemia may be more severe if renal damage is great. Nitrogen retention varies with the severity of impairment of renal function. The plasma is often lipemic, and the blood cholesterol is usually greatly elevated. Plasma protein is greatly reduced. The albumin fraction may fall to <2 g/dL. Serum complement is usually low in active disease. The serum electrolyte concentrations are often normal, although the serum sodium may be slightly low; total serum calcium may be low, in keeping with the degree of hypoalbuminemia and decrease in the protein-bound calcium moiety. During edema-forming periods, urinary sodium excretion is very low and urinary aldosterone excretion is elevated. If renal insufficiency (see preceding discussion) is present, the blood and urine findings are usually altered accordingly.

Renal biopsy is often essential to establish the diagnosis between the various conditions and to indicate prognosis.

C. Differential Diagnosis

The nephrotic syndrome (nephrosis) may be associated with a variety of primary renal diseases or may be secondary to a systemic process: collagen-vascular diseases (eg, disseminated lupus erythematosus, polyarteritis), diabetic nephropathy, amyloid disease, thrombosis of the renal vein, myxedema, multiple myeloma, malaria, syphilis, reaction to toxins or heavy metals, reactions to drugs, and constrictive pericarditis.

D. Treatment

An adequate diet with restricted sodium intake (0.5–1 g/d) and prompt treatment of intercurrent infection are the basis of therapy. Diuretics may be given but are often only partially effective. Salt-free albumin and other oncotic agents are of little help, and their effects are transient. The corticosteroids have been shown to be of value in treating nephrotic syndrome when the underlying disease is of minimal change—focal segmental glomerulosclerosis, systemic lupus erythematosus, or proliferative and crescentic glomerulonephritis. Steroids are often less effective in the treatment of membranous disease and membranoproliferative lesions of the glomerulus.

Alkylating agents, azathioprine, mycophenolate mofetil, cyclosporine, and tacrolimus, have been used in the treatment of nephrotic syndrome. Encouraging early results have been reported in children and adults with proliferative or membranous lesions and with systemic lupus erythematosus. It is not known what percentage of patients can be expected to benefit from these drugs.

Both corticosteroids and cytotoxic agents are commonly associated with serious side effects. At present, this form of therapy should be employed only in patients in whom the disease has proved refractory to well-established treatment regimens.

Reduction in proteinuria and improvement in nephrotic edema have been reported using low-protein diets and ACE inhibitors or angiotensin receptor blockers (ARBs). Most recently, studies have shown some improvements with lipid-lowering drugs.

E. Prognosis

The course and prognosis depend on the basic disease responsible for nephrotic syndrome. In most children with nephrosis (usually secondary to minimal change nephropathy), the disease appears to run a rather benign course when properly treated and to leave insignificant sequelae. Of the remaining children, most go inexorably into renal insufficiency. Adults with nephrosis fare less well. Hypertension, heavy proteinuria, and renal dysfunction are poor prognosticators.

RENAL INVOLVEMENT IN COLLAGEN DISEASES

Although it may not be accurate to classify all of these disorders as collagen diseases, systemic lupus erythematosus, polyarteritis nodosa, microscopic angiitis, scleroderma, Wegener's granulomatosis, Henoch–Schönlein purpura, and thrombotic thrombocytopenic purpura have been implicated in cases of glomerulonephritis. The urine sediment is often diagnostic, containing erythrocytes and erythrocyte casts; renal tubular cells, including some filled with fat droplets; and waxy and granular broad casts. The presence of these formed elements is indicative of active glomerular and tubular disease. The symptoms and signs of the primary disease, involving extrarenal findings (eg, pulmonary or ear, nose, or throat changes with Wegener's granulomatosis; dermatologic abnormalities or carditis with systemic lupus erythematosus; dysphagia with scleroderma), as well as the presence of ANCA and other serologic tests, help to differentiate the form of collagen disease present. Complete renal recovery from the disease is not likely to occur, although steroid and immunosuppressive drugs (alone or in combination) may be effective for long-term amelioration.

DISEASES OF THE RENAL TUBULES AND INTERSTITIUM

▶ Interstitial Nephritis

Acute interstitial diseases are usually due to sensitivity to drugs, including antibiotics (penicillin, sulfonamides), nonsteroidal anti-inflammatory drugs, and phenytoin. The pathologic hallmark of acute interstitial nephritis is the infiltration of inflammatory cells in the interstitium. A typical presentation is a rapid deterioration in renal function associated with a recent introduction of a new drug. The finding of eosinophiluria is very suggestive of allergic interstitial nephritis. Recovery may be complete, especially if the offending drug is withdrawn. A short course with corticosteroids may hasten the recovery.

Chronic interstitial nephritis is characterized by focal or diffuse interstitial fibrosis accompanied by infiltration, with inflammatory cells ultimately associated with extensive tubular atrophy. It represents a nonspecific reaction to a variety of causes: analgesic abuse, lead and cadmium toxicity, nephrocalcinosis, urate nephropathy, radiation nephritis, sarcoidosis, Balkan nephritis, and some instances of obstructive uropathy.

▶ Analgesic Nephropathy

Analgesic nephropathy typically occurs in patients with chronic and recurrent headaches or with chronic arthritis who habitually consume large amounts of the drugs. Phenacetin was implicated initially, but with elimination of phenacetin from the mixtures, the incidence of analgesic nephropathy has not decreased. Chronic use of nonsteroidal anti-inflammatories is a frequent cause of this condition. The ensuing damage to the kidneys usually is detected late, after renal insufficiency has developed. Careful history taking or the detection of analgesic metabolites in the urine can lead to this diagnosis. The history of excessive use of analgesics may be concealed by the patient. The effects of the drug appear to be cumulative (ie, life-time total dose of intake).

The kidney lesion is pathologically nonspecific, consisting of peritubular and perivascular inflammation with degenerative changes of the tubular cells (chronic interstitial nephritis). There are often no glomerular changes. Renal papillary necrosis extending into the medulla may involve many papillae.

Hematuria can be a common presenting complaint, but it is usually microscopic. Renal colic occurs when necrotic renal papillae slough away. Polyuria may be prominent. Signs of acidosis (hyperpnea), dehydration, and pallor are common. Infection is a frequent complication. The urine usually is remarkable only for the presence of blood and small amounts of protein. Elevated blood urea nitrogen and creatinine and the electrolyte changes characteristic of metabolic acidosis and renal failure are typically present. Urinary concentrating impairments are usually present. Urograms show cavities and ring shadows typical of areas of destruction of papillae.

▶ Uric Acid Nephropathy

Crystals of urate produce an interstitial inflammatory reaction. Urate may precipitate out in acid urine in the calyces to form uric acid stones. Patients with myeloproliferative disease under treatment are subject to occlusion of the upper urinary tract by uric acid crystals. Alkalinization of the urine and a liberal fluid intake help prevent crystal formation. Allopurinol is a useful drug to prevent hyperuricemia and hyperuricosuria. Recombinant urate oxidase (rasburicase) has been used in those with severe tumor lysis syndrome to lower the uric acid load.

Recently, it has been suggested that many instances considered to be chronic "gouty nephropathy" are instead related to chronic lead renal injury and not due to primary uric acid depositions.

▶ Obstructive Uropathy

Interstitial nephritis due to obstruction may not be associated with infection. Tubular conservation of salt and water is impaired. Partial to full renal recovery follows relief of the obstruction but is inversely related to the duration of obstruction.

▶ Kidney Diseases in Multiple Myeloma

Features of myelomatosis that contribute to renal disease include proteinuria (including filterable Bence-Jones protein and κ and λ chains) with precipitation in the tubules leading to accumulation of abnormal proteins in the tubular lumen. A Fanconi-like syndrome may develop.

Plugging of tubules, tubular atrophy, and, occasionally, the accumulation of amyloid may also be present. Renal failure may occur acutely or develop slowly. Hemodialysis may rescue the patient during efforts to control the myeloma with chemical agents.

Another related primary renal disorder is termed light chain deposition disease. Patients have nephritic range proteinuria and usually progressive renal failure. In contrast to multiple myeloma, there is no malignant hematopoietic process. Either κ or λ light chains are measurable via urine and serum immunofixation studies. Light chain deposits are seen in the glomeruli. There is no effective treatment.

HEREDITARY RENAL DISEASES

The importance of inheritance and the familial incidence of disease warrant the inclusion of a classification of hereditary renal diseases. Although relatively uncommon in the population at large, hereditary renal disease must be recognized to permit early diagnosis for detection and genetic counseling.

▶ Chronic Hereditary Nephritis

Evidence of the disease usually appears in childhood, with episodes of hematuria. Renal insufficiency commonly develops in males but only rarely in females. Survival beyond age 40 is rare.

In many families, deafness and abnormalities of the eyes accompany the renal disease (so-called Alport's disease). Another form of the disease is accompanied by polyneuropathy. Infection of the urinary tract is a common complication.

There is splitting and thickening of the GBM or podocyte proliferation and thickening of Bowman's capsule. Recently, kindreds have been described that have "thin-membrane disease." This condition is characterized by microscopic hematuria and, often, later progression to chronic renal failure. This, like Alport's disease, may represent inherited abnormalities or deficiencies in type IV collagen in the GBM. This affects both genders.

Laboratory findings with these conditions are commensurate with existing renal function. Treatment is symptomatic.

► Cystic Diseases of the Kidney

Congenital structural anomalies of the kidney must be considered in any patient with hypertension, pyelonephritis, or renal insufficiency. Many of these patients are at increased risk of urinary tract infection.

A. Polycystic Kidneys

Polycystic kidney disease is familial and often involves not only the kidney but the liver and pancreas as well. It is clear that at least two genetic loci can lead to autosomal dominant polycystic kidney disease.

The formation of cysts on the cortex of the kidney is thought to result from failure of union of the collecting tubules and convoluted tubules of some nephrons. Intrarenal cysts may be of a proximal or a distal luminal type, differing on analysis by their cyst electrolyte content. This is important if one or more of these cysts become infected, and an antibiotic (with varying cyst-type penetrance) is chosen. New cysts do not form, but those present enlarge and, by exerting pressure, cause destruction of adjacent renal tissue. The incidence of cerebral vessel aneurysms and mitral valve prolapse is higher than normal.

Cases of polycystic disease are discovered during the investigation of hypertension, by diagnostic study in patients presenting with pyelonephritis or hematuria, or by investigation of families of patients with known polycystic disease. At times, flank pain due to hemorrhage into a cyst occurs. Otherwise the symptoms and signs are those commonly seen in hypertension or renal insufficiency. On physical examination, the enlarged, irregular kidneys are often easily palpable.

The urine may contain leukocytes and erythrocytes. With bleeding into the cysts, there may also be bleeding into the urinary tract. The blood chemistry findings reflect the degree of renal insufficiency. Examination by sonography, CT scan, or x-ray shows the enlarged kidneys, and urography demonstrates the classic elongated calyces and renal pelves stretched over the surface of the cysts. Researchers have established ultrasonographic criteria for the diagnosis of autosomal dominant polycystic kidney disease (when genetic testing is not available or unknown genotype). See Table 33–1.

No specific therapy is available, and surgical interference is only indicated to decompress very large cysts in patients with severe pain. Initial excitement with mTOR inhibitors in limiting cyst growth did not translate into improved renal function in recent studies, dampening enthusiasm for its clinical applicability.

Patients with polycystic kidney disease live in reasonable comfort with slowly advancing uremia. Both hemodialysis and renal transplantation extend the life of these patients. Nephrectomy is indicated only in patients with recurrent

Table 33–1. Ultrasonographic criteria for the diagnosis of autosomal dominant polycystic kidney disease.

Age	Diagnostic criteria	Sensitivity	Specificity
15–29	Three unilateral/bilateral cysts	82	100
30–39	Three unilateral/bilateral cysts	96	100
40–59	Two cysts in each kidney	90	100
>60	Four cysts in each kidney	100	100

Source: Adapted from Pei Y et al: Unified criteria for ultrasonographic diagnosis of ADPKD. J Am Soc Nephrol 2009;20(1):205–12.

infections, severe recurrent bleeding, or markedly enlarged kidneys causing compressive symptoms.

B. Cystic Disease of the Renal Medulla

1. Medullary cystic disease—Medullary cystic disease is a familial disease that may become symptomatic during adolescence. Anemia is usually the initial manifestation, but azotemia, acidosis, and hyperphosphatemia soon become evident. Urine findings are not remarkable, although there is often an inability to concentrate and renal salt wasting often occurs. Many small cysts are scattered through the renal medulla. Renal transplantation is indicated by the usual criteria.

2. Medullary sponge kidney—Medullary sponge kidney is asymptomatic and is discovered by the characteristic appearance of tubular ectasia in the urogram. Enlargement of the papillae and calyces and small cavities within the pyramids is demonstrated by the contrast media in the excretory urogram. Many small calculi often occupy the cysts, and infection may be troublesome. Life expectancy is not affected and only therapy for ureteral stone or for infection is required.

ANOMALIES OF THE PROXIMAL TUBULE

► Defects of Amino Acid Reabsorption

A. Congenital Cystinuria

Increased excretion of cystine results in the formation of cystine calculi in the urinary tract. Ornithine, arginine, and lysine are also excreted in abnormally large quantities. There is also a defect in absorption of these amino acids in the jejunum. Nonopaque stones should be examined chemically to provide a specific diagnosis.

Treatment goals include a large fluid intake and keeping the urine pH above 7 by giving sodium bicarbonate and sodium citrate plus acetazolamide at bedtime to ensure an alkaline night urine. In refractory cases, a low methionine (cystine precursor) diet may be necessary. Penicillamine has proved useful in some cases.

B. Aminoaciduria

Many amino acids may be poorly absorbed, resulting in unusual losses. Failure to thrive and the presence of other tubular deficits suggest the diagnosis. There is no treatment.

C. Hepatolenticular Degeneration (Wilson's Disease)

In this congenital familial disease, aminoaciduria and renal tubular acidosis (RTA) are associated with cirrhosis of the liver and neurologic manifestations. Hepatomegaly, evidence of impaired liver function, spasticity, athetosis, emotional disturbances, and Kayser–Fleischer rings around the cornea constitute a unique syndrome. There is a decrease in synthesis of ceruloplasmin, with a deficit of plasma ceruloplasmin and an increase in free copper that may be etiologically specific.

Penicillamine is given to chelate and remove excess copper. Edathamil (EDTA) may also be used to remove copper.

D. Multiple Defects of Tubular Function (de Toni-Fanconi-Debré Syndrome)

Aminoaciduria, phosphaturia, glycosuria, and a variable degree of RTA characterize this syndrome. Osteomalacia is a prominent clinical feature; other clinical and laboratory manifestations are associated with specific tubular defects described previously.

Treatment consists of replacing cation deficits (especially potassium), correcting acidosis with bicarbonate or citrate, replacing phosphate loss with isoionic neutral phosphate (mono- and disodium salts) solution, and ensuring a liberal calcium intake. Vitamin D is useful, but the dose must be controlled by monitoring levels of serum calcium and phosphate.

E. Defects of Phosphorus and Calcium Reabsorption

Several sporadic, genetically transmitted, and acquired disorders are grouped under this category and are characterized by persisting hypophosphatemia because of excessive phosphaturia and an associated metabolic bone disorder, rickets in childhood, and osteomalacia in adulthood. Response to vitamin D therapy (1,25,-dihydroxycholecalciferol, the active analog of vitamin D) is variable.

F. Defects of Glucose Absorption (Renal Glycosuria)

Renal glycosuria results from an abnormally poor ability to reabsorb glucose and is present when blood glucose levels are normal. Ketosis is not present. The glucose tolerance response is normal. There is no treatment for renal glycosuria, just reassurance.

G. Defects of Bicarbonate Reabsorption

Proximal RTA, type II, is due to reduced bicarbonate reclamation in the proximal tubule, with resultant loss of bicarbonate in the urine and decreased bicarbonate concentration in extracellular fluid. There are increased K^+ losses into the urine and retrieval of Cl^- instead of HCO_3. The acidosis is therefore associated with hypokalemia and hyperchloremia. Transport of glucose, amino acids, phosphate, and urate may be deficient as well (Fanconi syndrome).

ANOMALIES OF THE DISTAL TUBULE

▶ Defects of Hydrogen Ion Secretion and Bicarbonate Reabsorption (Classic Renal Tubular Acidosis, Type I)

Failure to secrete hydrogen ion and to form ammonium ion results in loss of "fixed base," sodium, potassium, and calcium. There is also a high rate of excretion of phosphate. Vomiting, poor growth, and symptoms and signs of chronic metabolic acidosis are accompanied by weakness due to potassium deficit and bone discomfort due to osteomalacia. Nephrocalcinosis, with calcification in the medullary portions of the kidney, occurs in about one-half of cases. The urine is alkaline and contains larger than normal quantities of sodium, potassium, calcium, and phosphate. An abnormality in urinary anion gap ($U.Na^+ + U.K^+ - U.Cl^-$) is noted (low), which is associated with the reduced NH_4^+ production. This abnormality differentiates this condition from type II RTA and from the metabolic acidosis seen with diarrhea. The blood chemistry findings are those of metabolic acidosis with low serum potassium.

Treatment consists of replacing deficits and increasing the intake of sodium, potassium, calcium, and phosphorus. Sodium and potassium should be given as bicarbonate or citrate. Additional vitamin D may be required.

▶ Excess Potassium Secretion (Potassium "Wastage" Syndrome)

Excessive renal secretion or loss of potassium may occur in four situations: (1) moderate renal insufficiency with diminished H^+ secretion; (2) RTA (proximal and distal RTA); (3) hyperaldosteronism and hyperadrenocorticism; and (4) tubular secretion of potassium, the cause of which is unknown. Hypokalemia indicates that the deficit is severe. Muscle weakness and polyuria and dilute urine are signs attributable to hypokalemia. Treatment consists of correcting the primary disease and giving supplementary potassium.

▶ Reduced Potassium Secretion

Reduced potassium secretion is noted in conditions in which extrarenal aldosterone is reduced or when intrarenal production of renin (and secondary hypoaldosteronism) occurs. The latter condition is termed RTA, type IV, and is associated with impaired H^+ and K^+ secretion in the distal tubule. Drug-induced interstitial nephritis, gout, and diabetes mellitus are clinical circumstances that may produce type IV RTA and resulting hyperkalemia and mild metabolic acidosis. Treatment is to promote kaliuresis (with loop diuretics) to prescribe potassium-binding gastrointestinal resins (Kayexalate), or to provide the patient with a mineralocorticoid, fludrocortisone acetate.

▶ Defects of Water Absorption (Renal Diabetes Insipidus)

Nephrogenic diabetes insipidus occurs more frequently in males than in females. Unresponsiveness to antidiuretic hormone is the key to differentiate from central (pituitary) diabetes insipidus.

In addition to congenital refractoriness to antidiuretic hormone, obstructive uropathy, lithium, methoxyflurane, and demeclocycline also may render the tubule refractory to vasopressin.

Symptoms are related to inability to reabsorb water, with resultant polyuria and polydipsia. The urine volume approaches 12 L/d, and osmolality and specific gravity are low.

Treatment consists primarily of an adequate water intake. Chlorothiazide may ameliorate the polyuria; the mechanism of action is unknown, but the drug may act by increasing isosmotic reabsorption in the proximal segment of the tubule.

UNSPECIFIED RENAL TUBULAR ABNORMALITIES

In idiopathic hypercalciuria, decreased reabsorption of calcium predisposes to the formation of renal calculi. Serum calcium and phosphorus are normal. Urine calcium excretion is high; urine phosphorus excretion is low. Microscopic hematuria may be present. For treatment of urinary stones containing calcium, see Chapter 17 ("Urinary Stone Disease")

BIBLIOGRAPHY

Adler S: Diabetic nephropathy: Linking histology, cell biology, and genetics. Kidney Int 2004;66:2095.

Alric L et al: Influence of antiviral therapy in hepatitis C virus-associated cryoglobulinemic MPGN. Am J Kidney Dis 2004;43:617.

Appel GB et al: Membranoproliferative glomerulonephritis Type II (dense deposit disease): An update. J Am Soc Nephrol 2005;16:1392.

Barratt J, Feehally J: IgA nephropathy. J Am Soc Nephrol 2005;16:2088.

Braden GL et al: Tubulointerstitial diseases. Am J Kidney Dis 2005; 46:560.

Buhaescu I et al: Systemic vasculitis: Still a challenging disease. Am J Kidney Dis 2005;46:173.

Chesney R: The changing face of childhood nephrotic syndrome. Kidney Int 2004;66:1294.

Couser WG (guest editor): Frontiers in nephrology: Membranous nephropathy. J Am Soc Nephrol 2005;16:1184.

Flanc RS et al: Treatment of diffuse proliferative lupus nephritis: A meta-analysis of randomized controlled trials. Am J Kidney Dis 2004;43:197.

Ginzler EM et al: Mycophenolate mofetil or intravenous cyclophosphamide for lupus nephritis. N Engl J Med 2005;353:2219.

Grantham JJ: Advancement in the understanding of polycystic kidney disease: A system approach. Kidney Int 2003;64:1154.

Heering P et al: Cyclosporine A and chlorambucil in the treatment of idiopathic focal segmental glomerulosclerosis. Am J Kidney Dis 2004;43:10.

Hruska KA: Treatment of chronic tubulointerstitial disease: A new concept. Kidney Int 2002;61:1911.

Imaging the kidney—Radiologic imaging 2006. (Excerpts) Nephron Clin Pract 2006;103:c19.

Izzedine H et al: Oculorenal manifestations in systemic autoimmune diseases. Am J Kidney Dis 2004;43:209.

Javaid B, Quigg RJ: Treatment of glomerulonephritis: Will we ever have options other than steroids and cytotoxics? Kidney Int 2005;67:1692.

Nair R, Walker PD: Is IgA nephropathy the commonest primary glomerulopathy among young adults in the USA? Kidney Int 2006; 69:1455.

Noris M, Remuzzi G: Hemolytic uremic syndrome. J Am Soc Nephrol 2005;16:1035.

Perna A et al: Immunosuppressive treatment for idiopathic membranous nephropathy: A systematic review. Am J Kidney Dis 2004;44: 385.

Pettitt DJ et al: Familial predisposition to renal disease in two generations of Pima Indians with type 2 (non-insulin-dependent) diabetes mellitus. Diabetologia 1990;33(7):438–443.

Ponticelli C et al: A randomized study comparing methylprednisolone plus chlorambucil versus methylprednisolone plus cyclophosphamide in idiopathic membranous nephropathy. J Am Soc Nephrol 1998;9(3):444–450.

Rosner MH, Bolton WK: Renal function testing. Am J Kidney Dis 2006;47:174.

Rossert J: Drug-induced acute interstitial nephritis. Kidney Int 2001; 60:804.

Tenenhouse HS, Murer H: Disorders of renal tubular phosphate transport. J Am Soc Nephrol 2003;14:240.

Troyanov S et al: Renal pathology in idiopathic membranous nephropathy: A new perspective. Kidney Int 2006;69:1641.

Wilmer WA et al: Management of glomerular proteinuria: A commentary. J Am Soc Nephrol 2003;14:3217.

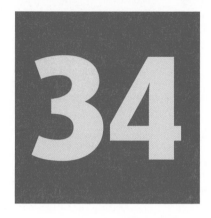

Acute Kidney Injury & Oliguria

Brian K. Lee, MD, & Flavio G. Vincenti, MD

Oliguria literally means "reduced" urine volume—less than that necessary to remove endogenous solute loads that are the end products of metabolism. If the patient concentrates urine in a normal fashion while consuming a regular Western diet, oliguria (for that person) is present at urine volumes <400 mL/day, or approximately 6 mL/kg body weight. If the kidney concentration is impaired and the patient can achieve a specific gravity of only 1.010, oliguria is present at urine volumes <1000–1500 mL/day.

In an attempt to standardize the diagnosis of acute renal failure, the new terminology acute kidney injury (AKI) was coined. New staging systems have been devised to compare severity of the damage sustained across different study groups and for prognostication.

AKI is a condition in which the glomerular filtration rate is abruptly reduced, causing a sudden retention of endogenous and exogenous metabolites (urea, potassium, phosphate, sulfate, creatinine, administered drugs) that are normally cleared by the kidneys. The urine volume is usually low (<400 mL/day). If renal concentrating mechanisms are impaired, the daily urine volume may be normal or even high (*high-output or nonoliguric renal failure*). In extreme cases, anuria occurs (urine output completely shuts down) in acute kidney injury.

The causes of AKI are listed in Table 34–1. Prerenal causes are usually reversible if treated promptly, but a delay in therapy may allow it to progress to a fixed intrinsic renal failure (eg, acute tubular necrosis). The other causes of AKI are classified on the basis of their involvement with vascular lesions, intrarenal disorders, or postrenal disorders.

PRERENAL KIDNEY INJURY

The term *prerenal* denotes inadequate renal perfusion or lowered effective arterial circulation. The most common cause of this form of AKI is dehydration due to renal or extrarenal fluid losses from diarrhea, vomiting, excessive use of diuretics, and so on. Less common causes are septic shock, "third spacing" with extravascular fluid pooling (eg, pancreatitis),

and excessive use of antihypertensive drugs. Heart failure with reduced cardiac output also can reduce effective renal blood flow. Careful clinical assessment may identify the primary condition responsible for the prerenal state, but many times several conditions can coexist. In the hospital setting, these circulatory abnormalities often are prolonged, leading to a more sustained injury (acute tubular necrosis).

Acute reductions in glomerular filtration rate may also be noted in patients with cirrhosis (hepatorenal syndrome) or in patients taking cyclosporine, tacrolimus, nonsteroidal anti-inflammatory drugs, or angiotensin-converting enzyme inhibitors. It is felt that these conditions represent significant intrarenal hemodynamic functional derangements. In these clinical circumstances, the urinary findings may mimic prerenal renal failure, but the patient's clinical assessment does not demonstrate the extrarenal findings seen in common prerenal conditions, as noted in the following section. Improvements in glomerular filtration rate are usually noted after drug discontinuance or, in cases of hepatorenal syndrome, with management of the liver disease or following liver transplantation.

▶ Clinical Findings

A. Symptoms and Signs

Except for rare cases with associated cardiac or "pump" failure, patients usually complain of thirst or of dizziness in the upright posture (orthostatic dizziness). There may be a history of overt fluid loss. Weight losses reflect the degree of dehydration. Physical examination frequently reveals decreased skin turgor, collapsed neck veins, dry mucous membranes, and, most importantly, excessive orthostatic or postural changes in blood pressure (defined as a systolic drop >20 or a diastolic drop >10 mm Hg) and pulse.

B. Laboratory Findings

1. Urine—The urine volume is usually low. Accurate assessment may require bladder catheterization followed by hourly

Table 34–1. Causes of acute kidney injury.

I. Prerenal
 1. Dehydration
 2. Vascular collapse due to sepsis, antihypertensive drug therapy, "third spacing"
 3. Reduced cardiac output

II. Functional-hemodynamic
 1. Angiotensin-converting enzyme inhibitor drugs
 2. Nonsteroidal anti-inflammatory drugs
 3. Cyclosporine; tacrolimus (calcineurin inhibitors)
 4. Hepatorenal syndrome

III. Vascular
 1. Atheroembolism
 2. Dissecting arterial aneurysms
 3. Malignant hypertension

IV. Parenchymal (intrarenal)
 1. Specific
  a. Glomerulonephritis
  b. Interstitial nephritis
  c. Toxin, dye induced
  d. Hemolytic uremic syndrome
 2. Nonspecific
  a. Acute tubular necrosis
  b. Acute cortical necrosis

V. Postrenal
 1. Calculus in patients with solitary kidney
 2. Bilateral ureteral obstruction
 3. Outlet obstruction
 4. Leak, posttraumatic

output measurements (which will also rule out lower urinary tract obstruction; see discussion following). High urine specific gravity (>1.025) and urine osmolality (>600 mOsm/kg) are also noted in this form of acute apparent renal failure. Routine urinalysis usually shows a bland sediment. However, as it progresses to acute tubular necrosis, sloughed off tubular cells and muddy brown casts may become apparent.

2. Urine and blood chemistries—The blood urea nitrogen–creatinine ratio, normally 10:1, is usually increased with prerenal renal failure. Other findings are set forth in Table 34–2. Because mannitol, radiocontrast dyes, and diuretics affect the delivery and tubular handling of urea, sodium, and creatinine, urine and blood chemistry tests performed after these agents have been given can be misleading.

3. Central venous pressure—A low central venous pressure indicates hypovolemia. If severe cardiac failure is the principal cause of prerenal renal failure (it is rarely the sole cause), reduced cardiac output and high central venous pressure are apparent.

4. Fluid challenge—An increase in urine output in response to a carefully administered fluid challenge is both diagnostic

and therapeutic in cases of prerenal renal failure. Rapid intravenous administration of 300–500 mL of physiologic saline is the usual initial treatment. Urine output is measured over the subsequent 1–3 hours. A urine volume increase of >50 mL/h is considered a favorable response that warrants continued intravenous infusion. If the urine volume does not increase, the physician should carefully review the results of blood and urine chemistry tests, reassess the patient's fluid status, and repeat the physical examination to determine whether an additional fluid challenge (with or without furosemide) might be worthwhile.

▶ **Treatment**

In states of dehydration, fluid losses must be rapidly corrected to treat oliguria. Inadequate fluid management may cause further renal hemodynamic deterioration and eventual renal tubular ischemia (with fixed acute tubular necrosis; see discussion following). If oliguria and hypotension persists in a well-hydrated patient, vasopressor drugs are indicated in an effort to correct the hypotension associated with sepsis or cardiogenic shock. Pressor agents that restore systemic blood pressure while maintaining renal blood flow and renal function are most useful. However, the previously touted benefits of renally dosed dopamine (1–5 µg/kg/min) have not been proven. A more promising agent might be fenoldopam, a direct dopamine A-1 receptor agonist. However, this will have to be tested more rigorously in a randomized trial before it could be widely recommended. Discontinuance of antihypertensive medications or diuretics can, by itself, cure the apparent acute kidney injury resulting from prerenal conditions.

VASCULAR RENAL FAILURE

Common causes of acute kidney injury due to vascular disease include atheroembolic disease, dissecting arterial aneurysms, and malignant hypertension. Atheroembolic disease is rare before age 60 and precipitating events include vascular procedures, angiographic studies, and administration of heparin anticoagulation. Dissecting arterial aneurysms and malignant hypertension are usually clinically evident.

Rapid assessment of the arterial blood supply to the kidney requires arteriography or other noncontrasted blood flow studies (eg, magnetic resonance imaging or Doppler ultrasound). The cause of malignant hypertension may be identified on physical examination (eg, scleroderma). Primary management of the vascular process is necessary to affect the course of these forms of acute kidney injury.

INTRARENAL CAUSES

Diseases in this category can be divided into specific and nonspecific parenchymal processes.

1. Specific intrarenal disease states—The most common causes of intrarenal acute kidney injury are acute or rapidly progressive glomerulonephritis, acute interstitial nephritis, toxic nephropathies, and hemolytic uremic syndrome.

▶ Clinical Findings

A. Symptoms and Signs

Usually the history shows some salient data such as sore throat or upper respiratory infection, diarrheal illness, use of antibiotics, or intravenous use of drugs (often illicit types). Bilateral back pain, at times severe, is occasionally noted. Gross hematuria may be present. It is unusual for pyelonephritis to present as acute kidney injury unless there is associated sepsis, obstruction, or involvement of a solitary kidney. Systemic diseases in which acute kidney injury occurs include Henoch-Schönlein purpura, systemic lupus erythematosus, and scleroderma. Human immunodeficiency virus (HIV) infection may present with acute kidney injury from HIV-associated nephropathy.

B. Laboratory Findings

I. Urine—Urinalysis discloses variably active sediments: many red or white cells and multiple types of cellular and granular casts. Phase contrast microscopy usually reveals dysmorphic red cells in the urine. In allergic interstitial nephritis, eosinophils may be noted. The urine sodium concentration may range from 10 to 40 mEq/L.

II. Blood test—Components of serum complement are often diminished (due to activation and consumption). In a few conditions, circulating immune complexes can be identified. Serologic tests may disclose systemic diseases such as lupus erythematosus (eg, anti-neutrophil antibody, anti-double-stranded DNA antibodies, anti-Smith antibodies). Thrombocytopenia and altered red cell morphologic structure are noted in peripheral blood smears in the hemolytic uremic syndrome. Rapidly progressive glomerulonephritis can be evaluated with tests for ANCA (antineutrophil cytoplasmic antibodies) and anti-GBM titers (anti-glomerular basement membrane antibodies).

III. Renal biopsy—Light microscopic examination shows characteristic changes of glomerulonephritis (ie, crescents within Bowman's capsule, see Figure 34–1), acute interstitial nephritis, or glomerular capillary thrombi (in hemolytic uremic syndrome). Immunofluorescence microscopy showing immune deposits helps toward the diagnosis of rapidly progressive glomerulonephritis. The immune deposits can further be divided into subendothelial (lupus nephritis), subepithelial (postinfectious glomerulonephritis), or mesangial (IgA nephropathy).

C. X-Ray Findings

Dye studies should be avoided because of the risk of contrast-induced renal injury. For this reason, sonography is preferable to rule out obstruction.

Rapidly progressive glomerulonephritis

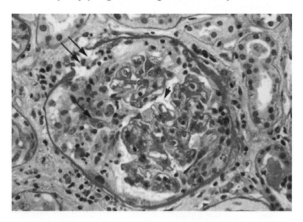

▲ **Figure 34–1.** High power light micrograph showing an active hypercellular crescent containing fibrin, which has a bright red appearance (*long arrow*). Note that the severe inflammatory injury has led to fragmentation of the glomerular tuft (*short arrow*) and to creation of a rent in the capsule (*double arrow*). (Courtesy of Helmut Rennke, MD.)

▶ Treatment

Therapy is directed toward removing the underlying injurious constituent, for example, eradication of infection, removal of antigen, elimination of toxic materials and drugs, suppression of autoimmune mechanisms, removal of autoimmune antibodies, or a reduction in effector-inflammatory responses. Immunotherapy may involve drugs (corticosteroids) or the temporary use of plasmapheresis. Initiation of supportive dialysis may be required (see discussion following).

2. Nonspecific intrarenal states—Nonspecific intrarenal causes of acute kidney injury include acute tubular necrosis and acute cortical necrosis. The latter is associated with intrarenal intravascular coagulation and has a poorer prognosis than the former. These forms of acute kidney injury usually occur in hospital settings. Various morbid conditions leading to septic syndrome–like physiologic disturbances are often present.

Degenerative changes of the distal tubules (lower nephron nephrosis) are believed to be due to ischemia. With dialysis, most of these patients recover—usually completely—provided intrarenal intravascular coagulation and cortical necrosis does not occur.

Elderly patients, who are more prone to have this form of oliguric acute kidney injury, develop following hypotensive episodes. It appears that exposure to some drugs such as nonsteroidal anti-inflammatory agents may increase the risk of acute tubular necrosis. Although the classic picture of lower nephron nephrosis may not develop, a similar nonspecific acute kidney injury is noted in some cases of mercury (especially mercuric chloride) poisoning and following exposure to radiocontrast agents, especially in patients with preexisting renal impairment, diabetes mellitus, or myeloma.

▶ Clinical Findings

A. Symptoms and Signs

Usually the clinical picture is that of the associated clinical state. Dehydration and shock may be present concurrently, but the urine output and acute kidney injury fail to improve following administration of intravenous fluids, in contrast to patients who have prerenal renal failure (see preceding discussion). On the other hand, there may be signs of excessive fluid retention in patients with acute kidney injury following radiocontrast exposure. Symptoms of uremia per se (eg, altered mentation or gastrointestinal symptoms) are unusual in acute kidney injury (in contrast to chronic kidney disease).

B. Laboratory Findings (Table 34–2)

I. Urine—The specific gravity is usually low or fixed in the 1.005–1.015 range. Urine osmolality is also low (<450 mOsm/kg and U/P osmolal ratio <1.5:1). Urinalysis often discloses tubular cells and granular casts; the urine may be muddy brown. If the urine is heme positive, but no red cells are seen on microscopy, one must be concerned about the presence of pigment nephropathy (myoglobinuria or hemoglobinuria). Tests for differentiating myoglobin pigment are available.

II. Central venous pressure—This is usually normal to slightly elevated.

III. Fluid challenges—There is no increase in urine volume following intravenous administration of mannitol or physiologic

Table 34–2. Intrinsic versus prerenal azotemia.

	Intrinsic	Prerenal
Urine osmolality (mOsm/L)	<350	>500
Urine/Plasma urea	<3	>8
Urine/Plasma creatinine	<20	>40
Urine Na (mEq/L)	>40	<20
$FE_{Na} = \dfrac{U/P_{Na}}{U/P_{cr}} \times 100$	>1	<1
$FE_{urea} = \dfrac{U/P_{urea}}{U/P_{cr}}$	>50	<35
$FE_{uric\ acid} = \dfrac{U/P_{uric\ acid}}{U/P_{cr}}$	>15	<7

Miller TR et al: Urinary diagnostic indices in acute renal failure: A prospective study. Ann Intern Med 1978;89:47; and Safirstein RL: Pathophysiology of acute renal failure. In: Greenburg A, Cheung AK, Coffman TM et al. Primer on Kidney Diseases. 4th ed., National Kidney Foundation, Elsevier Saunders, 2005, pp. 280–292.

saline. Occasionally, following the use of furosemide or "renal doses" of dopamine (1–5 μg/kg/min), a low urine output is converted to a high fixed urine output. Although, traditionally, it was thought that by converting patients with oliguric AKI into nonoliguric states by the above means translates into better prognosis, this does not appear to be evidence based. In fact, recent studies seem to suggest worse outcomes in those administered loop diuretics in the midst of AKI.

▶ Treatment

If there is no response to the initial fluid or mannitol challenge, the volume of administered fluid must be sharply curtailed to noted losses. An assessment of serum creatinine and blood urea nitrogen and of the concentrations of electrolytes is necessary to predict the possible use of dialysis. With appropriate regulation of the volume of fluid administered, maintenance of nutritional intake to provide a caloric content of 30–35 kcal/kg is used to correct or reduce the severity of the catabolic state accompanying acute tubular necrosis.

Serum potassium must be closely monitored to ensure early recognition of hyperkalemia. This condition can be treated with (1) intravenous sodium bicarbonate administration; (2) Kayexalate, 25–50 g (with sorbitol) orally (enema preparations are less favored due to the risk of bowel ischemia); (3) intravenous glucose and insulin; and (4) intravenous calcium preparations to prevent cardiac irritability (usually given with electrocardiographic changes, eg, peaked T waves, widening of QRS complexes).

Strategies to prevent the development of contrast-induced nephropathy include administration of normal saline and sodium bicarbonate infusions, N-acetylcysteine and preemptive hemodialysis and hemodiafiltration. None has been definitively shown in randomized trials to confer protective effects, except for maybe volume expansion. The use of low-osmolar contrast dye has been adopted as standard, although no added benefits can be shown with iso-osmolar (iodixanol) contrast material.

Peritoneal dialysis or hemodialysis should be used as necessary to avoid or correct uremia, hyperkalemia, or fluid overload. Hemodialysis in patients with AKI can be either intermittent or continuous (with arteriovenous or venovenous hemofiltration techniques). Vascular access is obtained with percutaneous catheters. The continuous dialysis techniques allow for easier management in many hemodynamically unstable patients in intensive care units.

There remains no consensus over what the best modality of renal replacement therapy is amongst patients with AKI. Continuous venovenous hemofiltration/hemodialysis/hemodiafiltration did not confer a more favorable survival or renal recovery benefit compared with intermittent forms of dialysis. Earlier reports of more intensive dialysis prescriptions (6 days per week vs every other day dialysis) showing superior survival are not substantiated by more recent evidence. What has emerged, however, is the need for meticulous attention to the delivered dialysis dose with each session and to minimize interruptions in dialytic therapy because of poor vascular access.

▶ Prognosis

Most cases are reversible within 7–14 days. Residual renal damage may be noted, particularly in elderly patients.

POSTRENAL AKI

The conditions listed in Table 34–1 involve primarily the need for urologic diagnostic and therapeutic interventions. Following lower abdominal surgery, urethral or ureteral obstruction should be considered as a cause of AKI. The causes of bilateral ureteral obstruction are (1) peritoneal or retroperitoneal neoplastic involvement, with masses or nodes; (2) retroperitoneal fibrosis; (3) renal calculi; and (4) postsurgical or traumatic interruption. With a solitary kidney, ureteral stones can produce total urinary tract obstruction and acute kidney injury. Urethral or bladder neck obstruction is a frequent cause of renal failure, especially in elderly men (prostatic enlargement). Posttraumatic urethral tears are discussed in Chapter 17.

▶ Clinical Findings

A. Symptoms and Signs

Pain and tenderness over the costovertebral angle often are present. If there has been an operative ureteral injury with associated urine extravasation, urine may leak through a wound. Edema from overhydration may be noted. Ileus is often present along with associated abdominal distention and vomiting.

B. Laboratory Findings

Urinalysis is usually not helpful. A large volume of urine obtained by catheterization may be both diagnostic and therapeutic for lower tract obstruction.

C. X-Ray Findings

Radionuclide renal scans may show a urine leak or, in cases of obstruction, retention of the isotope in the renal pelvis. Ultrasound examination often reveals a dilated upper collecting system with deformities characteristic of hydronephrosis.

D. Instrumental Examination

Cystoscopy and retrograde ureteral catheterization demonstrate ureteral obstruction.

▶ Treatment

For further discussion of ureteral injuries, see Chapter 17.

BIBLIOGRAPHY

Bellomo R et al; Acute Dialysis Quality Initiative Workup: Acute renal failure-definition, outcome measures, animal models, fluid therapy and information technology needs: The Second International Consensus Conference of the Acute Dialysis Quality Initiative (ADQI) Group. Crit Care 2004;8:R204–R212.

Forni LG, Hilton PJ: Continuous hemofiltration in the treatment of acute renal failure. N Engl J Med 1997;336:1303.

Fredrich JO et al: Meta-analysis: Low-dose dopamine increases urine output but does not prevent renal dysfunction or death. Ann Intern Med 2005;142(7):510–524.

Gines P, Arroyo V: Hepatorenal syndrome. J Am Soc Nephrol 1999; 10:1833.

Gonzales DA et al: A meta-analysis of N-acetylcysteine in contrast-induced nephrotoxicity: Unsupervised clustering to resolve heterogeneity. BMC Med 2007;5:32.

Intensive care nephrology. J Am Soc Nephrol 2001;12(Suppl 17):S1.

Lassnigg A et al: Lack of renoprotective effects of dopamine and furosemide during cardiac surgery. J Am Soc Nephrol 2000; 11(1): 97–104.

Marik PE et al: Low-dose dopamine does not prevent acute renal failure in patients with septic shock and oliguria. Am J Med 1999; 107:387.

Merten GJ et al: Prevention of contrast-induced nephropathy with sodium bicarbonate: A randomized controlled trial. JAMA 2004; 291:2328–2334.

Murphy SW et al: Contrast nephropathy. J Am Soc Nephrol 2000; 11:177.

Nolan CR, Anderson RJ: Hospital-acquired acute renal failure. J Am Soc Nephrol 1998;9:710.

Palevsky PM et al: Intensity of renal support in critically ill patients with acute kidney injury. N Engl J Med 2008;359:7–20.

Pannu N et al: Renal replacement therapy in patients with acute renal failure: A systematic review. JAMA 2008;299:793–805.

Schiffl H et al: Daily hemodialysis and the outcome of acute renal failure. N Engl J Med 2002;346:305.

Schor N: Acute renal failure and the sepsis syndrome. Kidney Int 2002;61:764.

Star RA: Treatment of acute renal failure. Kidney Int 1998;54:1817.

Tepel M et al: Prevention of radiographic-contrast-agent-induced reductions in renal function by acetylcysteine. N Engl J Med 2000; 343:180.

Chronic Kidney Disease & Renal Replacement Therapy

Brian K. Lee, MD, & Flavio G. Vincenti, MD

OVERVIEW

In chronic kidney disease (CKD), reduced clearance of certain solutes principally excreted by the kidney results in their retention in the body fluids. The solutes are end products of endogenous metabolism as well as exogenous substances (eg, drugs). The most commonly measured indicators of renal failure are blood urea nitrogen and serum creatinine. The renal clearance of creatinine (as calculated from a 24-hour urine collection) is often used as a surrogate measure of glomerular filtration rate (GFR).

Renal failure may be classified as acute or chronic depending on the rapidity of onset and the subsequent course of azotemia. An analysis of the acute or chronic development of renal failure is important in understanding physiologic adaptations, disease mechanisms, and ultimate therapy. In individual cases, it is often difficult to establish the duration of renal failure. Historical clues such as preceding hypertension or radiologic findings such as small, shrunken kidneys tend to indicate a more chronic process. Acute renal failure may progress to irreversible chronic renal failure. For a discussion of acute renal failure, see Chapter 33.

A new classification has been made by the National Kidney Foundation–Kidney Disease Outcomes Quality Initiative (K/DOQI). This delineates CKD by varying degrees of reduced GFR, either in the presence or absence of structural or functional renal abnormalities (available on the NFK Web site: http://www.kidney.org/professionals/KDOQI/guidelines_ckd/p4_class_g1.htm). This has been useful in studies of the progression of CKD, especially in varying drug regimens to reduce the rate of worsening of GFRs.

There are now numerous online calculators that can estimate a person's GFR (eGFR) based on the creatinine value, one example of which is available through the National Kidney Foundation (http://www.kidney.org/professionals/kdoqi/gfr_calculator.cfm). Although not perfect, these calculations help us to alert patients with subtle renal function impairment in the face of creatinine values within the normal reference ranges.

The incidence of end-stage renal disease (ESRD) reached 360 cases per million population in 2006, after a period of relative stability between 2001 and 2005. Almost all of this increase can be explained by the uptake in incidence of diabetic nephropathy over the same period (Figure 35–1). Particularly affected are older patients (75+ years old) and African Americans (3.6 times higher than Caucasians, Figure 35–2). The severity and the rapidity of development of uremia are hard to predict. The use of dialysis and transplantation is expanding rapidly worldwide. As of 2007, more than 340,000 prevalent ESRD patients in the United States are currently treated with hemodialysis, with around 26,000 patients treated with peritoneal dialysis. There are approximately 158,000 patients with a functioning kidney transplant.

▶ Historical Background

There are various causes of progressive renal dysfunction leading to end-stage or terminal renal failure. In the 1800s, Bright described several dying patients who presented with edema, hematuria, and proteinuria. Chemical analyses of sera drew attention to retained nitrogenous compounds and an association was made between this and the clinical findings of uremia. Although the pathologic state of uremia was well described, long-term survival was not achieved until chronic renal dialysis and renal transplantation became available after 1960–1970. Significant improvements in patient survival have been made in the past 50 years.

▶ Etiology

A variety of disorders are associated with CKD. Either a primary renal process (eg, glomerulonephritis, pyelonephritis, congenital hypoplasia) or a secondary one (owing to a systemic process such as diabetes mellitus or lupus

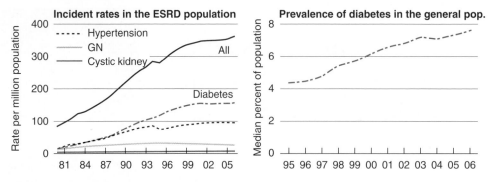

▲ **Figure 35–1.** Incident ESRD patients; rates adjusted for age, gender, and race. Data on the prevalence of diabetes in the general population obtained from the CDC's Behavioral Risk Factor Surveillance System, at www.cdc.gov/brfss.

erythematosus) may be responsible. Once there is kidney injury, it is now felt that the initially adaptive hyperfiltration to undamaged nephron units produces further stress and injury to remnant kidney tissue, ultimately leading to worsening renal function and urinary abnormalities (ie, proteinuria). The patient will show progression from one stage of CKD severity to the next. Superimposed physiologic alterations secondary to dehydration, infection, obstructive uropathy, or hypertension may put a borderline patient into uncompensated chronic uremia.

▶ Clinical Findings

A. Symptoms and Signs

With milder CKD, there may be no clinical symptoms. Symptoms such as pruritus, generalized malaise, lassitude, forgetfulness, loss of libido, nausea, and easy fatigability are frequent and nonfocal complaints in moderate to severe CKD. Growth failure is a primary complaint in preadolescent patients. Symptoms of a multisystem disorder (eg, systemic lupus erythematosus) may be present coincidentally.

Most patients with CKD have elevated blood pressure secondary to volume overload or from hyperreninemia. However, the blood pressure may be normal or low if patients have marked renal salt-losing tendencies (eg, medullary cystic disease). The pulse and respiratory rates are rapid as manifestations of anemia and metabolic acidosis. Clinical findings of uremic fetor, pericarditis, neurologic findings of asterixis, altered mentation, and peripheral neuropathy are present only with severe, stage V CKD. Palpable kidneys suggest polycystic disease. Ophthalmoscopic examination may show hypertensive or diabetic retinopathy. Alterations involving the cornea/lens have been associated with metabolic disease (eg, Fabry disease, cystinosis, and Alport hereditary nephritis).

B. History

In 20% of cases, there is a family history of CKD. A report of antecedent nephritis episodes or a history of previous proteinuria may be elicited. It is important to review drug usage and possible toxic exposures (eg, lead).

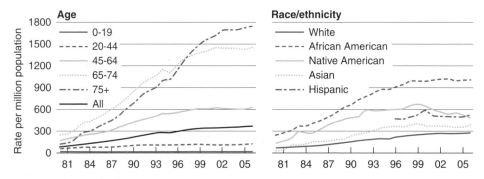

▲ **Figure 35–2.** Incident ESRD patients; rates by age adjusted for gender and race; rates by race and ethnicity adjusted for age and gender.

C. Laboratory Findings

1. Urine composition—The urine volume varies depending on the type of renal disease. Quantitatively normal amounts of water and salt losses in urine can be associated with polycystic and interstitial forms of disease. Usually, however, urine volumes are quite low when the GFR falls below 5% of normal. The urinary concentrating (fixed, low value specific gravity) and acidification (high urinary pH) mechanisms may be impaired. Daily salt losses become less regulated, and, if they are low, a state of positive sodium balance results in edema. Proteinuria can be variable. Urinalysis examinations may reveal mononuclear white blood cells (leukocyturia) and occasionally broad waxy casts, but usually the urinalysis is nonspecific and inactive.

2. Blood testing—Often seen is a picture of normocytic, normochromic anemia, the so-called anemia of chronic disease. With worsening renal function, iron deficiency may ensue. Despite normal platelet counts, patients suffer from dysfunction (thrombasthenia), characterized by abnormal bleeding times.

Several abnormalities in serum electrolytes and mineral metabolism become manifest when the GFR drops below 30 mL/min (in the case of secondary hyperparathyroidism, impairment may begin with GFR < 60 mL/min). Progressive reduction of body buffer stores and an inability to excrete titratable acids result in progressive metabolic acidosis characterized by reduced serum bicarbonate and compensatory respiratory hyperventilation. The metabolic acidosis of uremia is associated with a normal anion gap, hyperchloremia, and normokalemia. However, as renal dysfunction progresses, some patients may develop an anion gap acidosis (due to the buildup of organic anions). Hyperkalemia is not usually seen unless the GFR is below 5 mL/min. In patients with interstitial renal diseases, gouty nephropathy, or diabetic nephropathy, hyperchloremic metabolic acidosis with hyperkalemia (renal tubular acidosis, type IV) may develop. In these cases, the acidosis and hyperkalemia are out of proportion to the degree of renal failure and are related to a decrease in renin and aldosterone secretion. In moderate to severe CKD, multiple factors lead to an increase in serum phosphate and a decrease in serum calcium. The hyperphosphatemia develops as a consequence of reduced phosphate clearance by the kidney. In addition, vitamin D activity is diminished because of reduced conversion of 25-OH vitamin D to the active form, 1,25-OH vitamin D in the kidney by the enzyme 1α- hydroxylase. These alterations lead to secondary hyperparathyroidism with skeletal changes of both osteomalacia and osteitis fibrosa cystica. Uric acid levels are frequently elevated but rarely lead to calculi or gout during chronic uremia.

D. X-Ray Findings

Patients with reduced renal function should not be routinely subjected to radiographic studies involving iodinated contrast (nephrotoxic). Renal sonograms are helpful in determining renal size (usually small) and cortical thickness (usually thin) and in localizing tissue for percutaneous renal biopsy. Bone x-rays may show retarded growth, osteomalacia (renal rickets), or osteitis fibrosa (brown tumors). Soft-tissue or vascular calcification may be noted on plain films. Patients with polycystic kidney disease will have variably large kidneys with evident cysts (on sonograms or abdominal CT scans).

E. Renal Biopsy

Renal biopsies may not reveal much except nonspecific interstitial fibrosis and glomerulosclerosis. There may be pronounced vascular changes consisting of thickening of the media, fragmentation of elastic fibers, and intimal proliferation, which may be secondary to uremic hypertension or due to primary arteriolar nephrosclerosis. Percutaneous biopsies of end-stage shrunken kidneys may be complicated by bleeding (due to the uremic platelet dysfunction; see Section "Blood testing"). The bleeding tendency can be ameliorated once patient starts on dialysis, or through the use of desmopressin (mediates release of endothelial stores of Factor VIII:von Willebrand Factor multimers).

▶ Treatment

Recent studies indicate some benefit of drugs to reduce progression of CKD. The use of angiotensin-converting enzyme inhibitors and angiotensin receptor blockers in slowing down renal decline has been well documented, especially in the diabetic population with significant proteinuria. With the addition of aldosterone antagonists to optimize blood pressure control, patients need to be followed closely for potential hyperkalemia. Lipid lowering agents should be employed to lower the already accelerated risk of atherosclerotic disease in the ESRD population and can potentially retard the progression of renal dysfunction.

Overall, management should be conservative until it becomes impossible for patients to continue their customary lifestyles. Restriction of dietary protein (0.8–1.0 g/kg/d), potassium, and phosphorus is recommended. As well, maintenance of close sodium balance in the diet is necessary so that patients become neither sodium expanded nor depleted. This is best done by the accurate and frequent monitoring of the patient's weight. Use of oral bicarbonate (0.5–1 mEq/kg/d) can be helpful when moderate acidemia occurs (aim for serum HCO_3 level ≥ 23 mEq/L). Anemia can be treated with recombinant erythropoietin given subcutaneously (aiming for hemoglobin levels between 11.0 and 12.0 g/dL per the K/DOQI guidelines). Prevention of possible uremic osteodystrophy and secondary hyperparathyroidism requires close attention to calcium and phosphorus balance. Phosphate-retaining antacids and calcium or vitamin D supplements may be needed to maintain the balance. Cinacalcet can directly reduce parathyroid hormone secretion. If severe secondary hyperparathyroidism occurs, subtotal parathyroidectomy may be needed.

A. Chronic Peritoneal Dialysis

Chronic peritoneal dialysis is used electively or when circumstances (ie, no available vascular access) prohibit chronic hemodialysis. Ten percent of dialysis is done with this treatment. Improved soft catheters can be used for repetitive peritoneal lavages. In comparison to hemodialysis, small molecules (such as creatinine and urea) are cleared less effectively than larger molecules, but excellent treatment can be accomplished. Intermittent thrice-weekly treatment (IPPD), continuous cycler-assisted peritoneal dialysis (CCPD), or chronic ambulatory peritoneal dialysis (CAPD) is possible. With the latter, the patient performs 3–5 daily exchanges using 1–2 L of dialysate at each exchange. The dialysate contains a high glucose concentration and the peritoneal surface serves as the semipermeable membrane. Bacterial contamination and peritonitis are becoming less common with improvements in connection technology. Over time, many patients will transition to hemodialysis due to either peritoneal membrane failure (eg, peritoneal sclerosis, adhesions) or inadequate dialysis as native renal clearance of solutes deteriorates.

B. Chronic Hemodialysis

Chronic hemodialysis using semipermeable dialysis membranes is now widely performed. Access to the vascular system is provided by an arteriovenous fistula, vascular grafts (with autologous saphenous vein or synthetic material), or by a percutaneous permcatheter (placed either surgically or with interventional radiology). Most dialyzer membranes nowadays are made with biocompatible materials (less blood–membrane reactions). Body solutes and excessive body fluids can be easily cleared by using dialysate fluids of known chemical composition. Newer, high-efficiency membranes (high/flux) are serving to reduce dialysis treatment time.

Treatment is intermittent—usually 3–5 hours three times weekly. Computer modeling, using measurements of urea kinetics, has provided more precise hemodialysis prescriptions. Treatments may be given in a kidney center, a satellite unit, or the home. Home dialysis is optimal because it provides greater scheduling flexibility and is generally more comfortable and convenient for the patient, but only 20% of dialysis patients meet the requirements for this type of therapy. There is rising interest in this modality of treatment given better patient survival and quality of life.

More widespread use of dialytic techniques has permitted greater patient mobility. Treatment on vacations and business trips can be provided by prior arrangement. There are even dedicated cruise ships that provide dialysis.

Common problems with either type of chronic dialysis include infection, bone symptoms, technical accidents, persistent anemia, and psychological disorders. The excessive morbidity and mortality associated with atherosclerosis often occurs with long-term treatment. It is now recognized that occasionally uremic patients, despite dialysis, can develop wasting syndrome, cardiomyopathy, polyneuropathy, and secondary dialysis-amyloidosis so that kidney transplant must be urgently done. Routine bilateral nephrectomy should be avoided because it increases the transfusion requirements of dialysis patients. Nephrectomy in dialysis patients should be performed in cases of refractory hypertension, reflux with infection, and cystic disease with recurrent bleeding and pain. The dialysis patient can occasionally have acquired renal-cystic disease. Such patients need close monitoring for the development of in situ renal cell carcinoma.

Yearly costs range from an average of $50,000 for patients who receive dialysis at home to as much as $50,000–$75,000 for patients treated at dialysis centers (with those dialyzing through an AV graft or catheter incurring more cost), but much of this is absorbed under HR-1 (Medicare) legislation. If the patient has no other systemic problems (eg, diabetes), the mortality rate is 8–10%/year once maintenance dialysis therapy is instituted. Despite these medical, psychological, social, and financial difficulties, most patients lead productive lives while receiving dialysis treatment.

C. Renal Transplantation

After immunosuppression techniques and genetic matching were developed, renal allotransplantation became an acceptable alternative to maintenance hemodialysis. Improved short-term transplant results are now noted owing to the development of newer immunosuppressant drugs. Currently employed posttransplant drugs include prednisone, mycophenolate mofetil (and its enteric-coated formulation), cyclosporine, tacrolimus, and sirolimus. There are a number of novel medications under investigation that inhibit different pathways in the allorecognition mechanism, including a variety of injectable bioagents. The great advantage of transplantation is reestablishment of nearly normal and constant body physiology and chemistry. Diet can be less restrictive. The disadvantages include bone marrow suppression, susceptibility to infection, oncogenesis risks, and the psychological uncertainty of the allograft's future. Most of the disadvantages of transplantation are related to the medicines given to counteract the rejection. Later problems with transplantation include recurrent disease in the transplanted kidney and an increased incidence of cancer. Genitourinary infection appears to be of minor importance if structural urologic complications (eg, leaks) do not occur. However, the shortage of organ supply continues to plague the transplant community. As of 2007, there

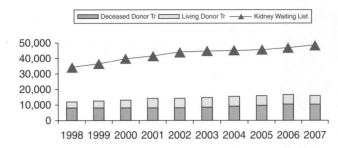

▲ **Figure 35–3. Number of transplants and size of active waiting list.** There was a very large gap between the number of patients waiting for a transplant and the number receiving a transplant. This gap widened over the decade, meaning that the waiting times from listing to transplant continued to increase. The number of living donor transplants grew until 2004, while the number of deceased donor transplants continued to rise gradually. Source: *2008 OPTN/SRTR Annual Report,* Tables 1.7, 5.1a.

were more than 70,000 patients on the kidney transplant waiting list, with annual death rates of 65 patients/1000 patient-years at risk (Figure 35–3).

Nephrology centers, with close cooperation between medical and surgical staff, attempt to use these treatment alternatives of dialysis and transplantation in an integrated fashion.

For a more detailed review, see Chapter 35.

BIBLIOGRAPHY

Astor BC et al: Type of vascular access and survival among incident hemodialysis patients. J Am Soc Nephrol 2005;16:1449.

Atkins RC et al: Proteinuria reduction and progression to renal failure in patients with type 2 diabetes mellitus and overt nephropathy. Am J Kidney Dis 2005;45:281.

Clinical Practice Guidelines and Clinical Practice Recommendations 2006: K/DOQI Advisory Panel (Excerpts). Am J Kidney Dis 2006;48(Suppl 1):1.

Coresh J et al: Chronic kidney disease awareness, prevalence and trends among U.S. adults. J Am Soc Nephrol 2005;16:180.

Daugas E et al: HAART-related nephropathies in HIV-infected patients. Kidney Int 2005;67:393.

El Nahas M: The global challenge of chronic kidney disease. Kidney Int 2005;68:2918.

Go AS et al: Chronic kidney disease and the risks of death, cardiovascular events, and hospitalization. N Engl J Med 2004;351:1296.

Hsu CY et al: Elevated blood pressure and risk of end-stage renal disease in subjects without baseline kidney disease. Arch Int Med 2005;165:923.

K/DOQI Clinical Practice Guidelines for Chronic Kidney Disease: Evaluation, classification, and stratification (excerpts). Am J Kidney Dis 2002;39(Suppl 1):1.

Levey AS et al: A new equation to estimate glomerular filtration rate. Ann Intern Med 2009;150:604–612.

Muntner P et al: Association of Serum Intact Parathyroid Hormone with Lower Estimated Glomerular Filtration Rate. Clin J Am Soc Nephrol 2009;4:186–194.

2008 OPTN/SRTR Annual Report 1998–2007. HHS/HRSA/HSB/DOT; UNOS; Arbor Research Collaborative for Health.

Remuzzi G et al: Chronic renal disease: Renoprotection benefits of renin-angiotensin system inhibition. Ann Intern Med 2002;136:304.

Stewart JH et al: Cancers of the kidney and urinary tract in patients on dialysis for end-stage renal disease. J Am Soc Nephrol 2003;14:197.

U.S. Renal Data Systems: 2008–2009 Annual Data Report. Available at: http://www.usrds.org/adr.htm. Accessed July 6, 2010.

Woods JD et al: Comparison of mortality with home hemodialysis and center hemodialysis: A national study. Kidney Int 1996;49(5):1464–1470.

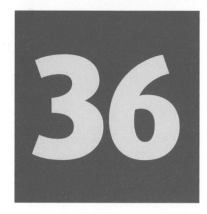

Renal Transplantation

Stuart M. Flechner, MD, FACS

The first successful kidney transplant from a live donor to his identical twin brother was done in 1954. Since then, kidney transplantation has progressed from an experimental procedure to the preferred method of renal replacement therapy around the world. There are three primary reasons for the worldwide acceptance of renal transplantation: (1) transplant recipients enjoy a prolongation of survival compared with dialysis (Wolfe et al, 1999), (2) recipients report an improved quality of life (Joseph et al, 2003), and (3) it is less costly than that of dialysis (USRDS, 2010). At the end of 2010 in the United States, there were about 382,000 patients receiving dialysis therapy, with an incident rate of about 342 per million population, and over 165,000 living with a kidney transplant (USRDS, 2010). In 2010, there were 16,889 kidney transplants performed in the United States, 10,622 from deceased donors and 6277 from live donors (UNOS Web page). However, more than 88,847 patients were actively waiting for a kidney, and the gap between the number waiting and available organs widens every year (Wolfe et al, 2010). Currently, 1- and 5-year kidney graft survival ranges between 89–95% and 66–80%, depending on donor source (Figure 36–1). The major reasons leading to improved outcomes are more potent, yet selective immunosuppression, better surgical techniques, more sensitive tissue typing and crossmatching, and better prophylaxis and treatment of morbid infections. There is also an emerging consensus that preemptive transplantation, immediately prior to the need to dialysis, is advantageous, reducing much morbidity and even mortality (Kasiske et al, 2002).

SELECTION AND PREPARATION OF RECIPIENTS

The most frequent diagnoses of renal failure for patients on the transplant waiting list are diabetes, 28% (the fastest growing); all types of glomerulonephritis/focal sclerosis, 25%; hypertension nephrosclerosis, 23%; cystic kidney diseases, 9%; interstitial/pyelonephritis, 5%; urologic diseases, 4%; and unknown causes, 7% (USRDS, 2010). Children <age 18

with renal failure often have congenital urologic conditions such as obstruction, valves, dysplasia, cystic disease reflux, prune-belly syndrome, inborn errors of metabolism (stones), or neurogenic bladders (NAPRTCS, 2009). Patients older than 65–70 years, the fastest growing recipient group, are commonly transplanted today, as physiological age is considered more important than chronological age (Flechner, 2002). Most patients with end-stage renal disease (ESRD) can be suitable transplant candidates with a few absolute contraindications. These include active infections or cancer, severe vasculopathy from atherosclerosis, and metabolic diseases likely to recur (oxalosis, cystinosis). However, all decisions must be individualized, and patients with a life expectancy of less than 3–5 years probably should be maintained on dialysis. Other factors such as psychosocial status, environment, and ability to follow a complex medical regimen are also important considerations. Prior to transplant, it is important to identify correctable conditions that may increase morbidity and diminish outcomes after the transplant (Flechner, 2002).

▶ Genitourinary Tract Evaluation

It is important that the native urinary tract will function properly after transplant, and an accurate urologic history is essential. Potential recipients without a history of urologic symptoms or prior interventions do not need an extensive evaluation. Upper tract ultrasound and urine cultures usually suffice; some recommend voided cytology. An age appropriate screening prostate specific antigen (PSA) in males. Patients with a history of urologic symptoms (especially hematuria, infections, stones, and incontinence), prior interventions, or a neurogenic bladder should have a full urologic evaluation including upper tract/pelvic imaging, a voiding cystogram, cystoscopy and retrograde studies, cytology, and if indicated a urodynamic study. If patients are dialyzed, upper tract computed tomography (CT) scans with intravenous contrast can be done, while noncontrast images are

Kidney-only Graft Survival-
according to donor source

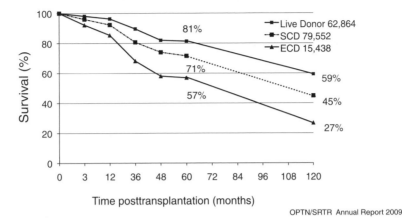

Live Donor 62,864
SCD 79,552
ECD 15,438

OPTN/SRTR Annual Report 2009

▲ **Figure 36–1.** Ten-year UNOS/OPTN.

appropriate prior to dialysis. Gadolinium enhanced magnetic resonance imaging studies remain contraindicated in patients with glomerular filtration rates (GFRs) <60 cc/min, due to the risk of nephrogenic systemic fibrosis (Thomsen, 2009).

A. Upper Tract Abnormalities

Removal of the native kidneys is usually not necessary, done in 10% or fewer patients. Residual urine output and potassium excretion, even if small, as well as production of erythropoietin and vitamin D3 via the retained kidneys are considered beneficial. Medical indications for nephrectomies are rare and include heavy proteinuria (>10 g/day), intractable hypertension (4–5 drugs), and persistent hematuria. Kidneys with chronic hydronephrosis, high-grade reflux, stones, abscesses, filling defects, enhancing masses, complex or very large cysts, etc., that may lead to persistent infections or harbor potential cancers should be removed prior to transplant. In addition, very large polycystic kidneys may need removal for relief of symptoms or size considerations. Potential recipients with acquired renal cystic disease, found in 1/3 to 1/2 of all dialyzed patients, need intervention for contrast enhancing lesions. In most instances, nephrectomy or nephroureterectomy can be done laparoscopically with diminished morbidity (Ghasemian et al, 2005; Ismail et al, 2005). Lesions not removed prior to transplant will need surveillance after the transplant.

B. Lower Tract Abnormalities

It is important to remember that dialyzed patients often have a diminished urine volume, resulting in a small capacity bladder with low compliance. Such bladders will resume normal

function, even 25 years later, once urine volume is restored (Serrano et al, 1996). However, small capacity bladders that are fibrotic and scarred from prior surgery, radiation, old TB, and congenital anomalies (posterior urethral valves, meningomyelocele, etc.) will not recover. In these rare cases, often children, the preferred option is a bladder augmentation with bowel (ileum, stomach, colon, or dilated ureter) or a continent neobladder to produce a compliant reservoir with adequate volume (Mendizabal et al, 2004; Nahas et al, 2002; Rigamonti et al, 2005). Bladder augmentation is not without risk, as mucous production, residual urine, and infection often require subsequent intermittent catheterization. If the bladder is absent or destroyed, an ileal conduit can be created for transplantation (Hatch et al, 1993). It is advisable that major surgery is completed and healed prior to transplantation. Experience has taught that operations on a dry urinary tract, that is, bladder neck incisions, urethral stricture repair, and prostatectomy will lead to restricturing and further scarring. Therefore, they should only be done when urine volume is more than a liter per day; or if not, delayed for about 3 months after the transplant. This includes older males who experience progressive prostatic growth absent urine output while on dialysis. These recipients may experience symptoms of prostatism or even urinary retention after the transplant, which will require treatment. During this interval when immunosuppression is reduced and stable engraftment is evolving, recipients are preferably managed by intermittent clean catheterization (Flechner et al, 1983). An indwelling Foley catheter or a suprapubic tube may be necessary if self-cath is not possible. As an alternative, a Spanner stent can be used (Shore et al, 2007).

▶ Infection

A. Bacterial

Active infections are a contraindication to transplantation, which need to be appropriately treated and resolved. This may include surgical drainage of abscesses or removal of a chronic nidus such as infected bone, teeth, maxillary sinus, etc. The urinary tract should be sterile for transplantation. Recurrent urinary tract infections require a full urologic evaluation including upper tract imaging, a voiding cystogram, cystoscopy, and retrograde studies. Recipients with a prior history of tuberculous disease or exposure should receive a year of isoniazid prophylaxis. ESRD patients may be anergic to skin testing.

B. Viral

Herpes family DNA viruses such as cytomegalovirus (CMV), Epstein–Barr virus (EBV), varicella zoster virus (VZV), and herpes simplex virus (HSV) can be transmitted with the donor organ or reactivated from a latent state in the recipient. Therefore, recipients are usually given prophylaxis with a nucleoside inhibitor such as oral valganciclovir for 3–6 months, especially when they are seronegative and the donor is seropositive. Those patients with serologic evidence of prior hepatitis B or C exposure have diminished outcomes, especially if their liver has evidence of cirrhosis. However, those recipients with inactive liver disease who have antibodies to either virus may receive organs from donors that are also positive for either hepatitis B core or hepatitis C antibody (Akalin et al, 2005; Aroldi et al, 2005). A relationship between hepatitis C infection and posttransplant diabetes is also emerging (Bloom and Lake, 2006). Renal failure patients with active and untreated human immunodeficiency virus (HIV) should not be further immunosuppressed by transplant. However, those stable HIV-positive individuals treated with current antiretroviral drug therapy can do well at 1 and 3 years after kidney transplant (Stock et al, 2010).

▶ Malignant Disease

Active or recurrent malignant disease is an absolute contraindication to renal transplantation. The bulk of evidence suggests that immunosuppressive therapy facilitates the growth of residual cancers. The safe waiting period for transplantation after surgical removal of solid tumors varies and depends on the grade and stage of tumor on presentation and the associated risk of recurrence. Penn (1997) reported that of 1137 neoplasms treated prior to transplantation, the overall recurrence rate was 21%. Fifty-four percent recurred for those waiting only 2 years before transplantation, 33% in those waiting 2–5 years before transplantation, and 13% among those waiting more than 5 years. The highest recurrence rates occurred with breast carcinomas (23%), symptomatic renal carcinomas (27%), sarcomas (29%), bladder carcinomas (29%), nonmelanoma skin cancers (53%), and multiple myeloma (67%).

Therefore, with some exceptions, a minimum waiting period of 2 years for cancers with a favorable prognosis is desirable. A waiting period of 5 years is desirable for lymphomas, most carcinomas of the breast, colon, or for large (>5 cm) symptomatic renal carcinomas. No waiting period is necessary for incidentally discovered small renal carcinomas, in situ carcinomas, and possibly tiny focal neoplasms. More recently, it has been suggested that rather than using fixed waiting times, it is more logical to use cancer recurrence nomograms to establish risk. For example, such nomograms have been well established for localized prostate cancer (Kattan, 2008).

▶ Systemic and Metabolic Disease

Patients with certain metabolic diseases affecting the kidney such as Fabry's disease, hemolytic uremic syndrome, vasculitis, systemic lupus erythematosus, amyloidosis, etc., as well as various forms of glomerulonephritis and focal sclerosis may experience recurrence, and patients should be counseled regarding this possibility (Couser, 2005). Those with severe metabolic stone disease that resulted in kidney loss may experience recurrent stones and a poor outcome. A combined hepatic and kidney transplant is now commonly recommended for primary hyperoxaluria (Jamieson, 2005) and less so for cystinosis (Rogers et al, 2001).

▶ Cardiovascular Status

Cardiovascular disease represents the leading cause of death after kidney transplantation, and is ubiquitous among renal failure patients, especially diabetics and those older than 50 years. Potential recipients should be thoroughly screened and have symptomatic lesions corrected prior to transplant, since those with ESRD are at high risk for ischemic events (Pilmore, 2006). Since many dialysis patients are sedentary, already have abnormal EKG patterns and diabetics may not experience angina with exertion, provocative stress tests are necessary. However, patients should reach their target heart rate for these tests to have an accurate predictive value, but may be limited in long-standing diabetics (Welsh et al, 2011). If any uncertainty exists, the gold standard remains coronary angiography. In an analysis of dialysis patients undergoing coronary revascularization, Herzog et al (2002) found that although the in-hospital mortality was greatest for those undergoing coronary artery bypass graft (CABG) (8.6%) compared with patients having stents (4.1%) or percutaneous transluminal coronary angioplasty (PTCA) (6.4%), the 2-year patient all-cause survival was significantly superior for those after CABG (56.4%) than after stenting (48.4%) or PTCA (48.2%). Patients with a history of strokes or transient ischemic attacks should be screened with a carotid ultrasound and receive neurology clearance. Those with adult polycystic kidney disease need a brain magnetic resonance angiogram to screen for aneurysms. Peripheral vascular disease is common in renal failure, especially diabetics, and pulse volume recordings (PVRs) of the lower extremities can be helpful. A pelvic CT scan without contrast can determine the degree of calcification of the target pelvic vessels and aid in kidney placement. Active claudication, femoral bruits, or diminished pulses demands a complete vascular surgical assessment.

Gastrointestinal Disease

Patients with ESRD often have a history of gastrointestinal problems such as peptic ulcer disease, gastroesophageal reflux, cholecystitis, pancreatitis, inflammatory bowel disease, diverticulosis, chronic diarrhea or constipation, or hemorrhoids. If present, these should be evaluated and resolved prior to transplant. Upper or lower gastrointestinal endoscopy, and/or contrast imaging of the bowel, may be required. Routine cholecystectomy for asymptomatic cholelithiases is no longer advised (Jackson et al, 2005).

Modifiable Risk Factors

A. Obesity

In North America, obesity is affecting a greater number of patients with renal failure each year. Numerous reports have identified obesity (body mass index [BMI] >30 kg/m^2) and morbid obesity (BMI >35 kg/m^2) as an independent risk factor for increased cardiovascular mortality, decreased graft survival, delayed graft function (DGF), wound complications, posttransplant diabetes, proteinuria, and prolonged hospitalization (Armstrong et al, 2005; Gore et al, 2006; Modlin et al, 1997). Weight reduction to lower the morbidly obese range is desirable and may require bariatric surgery in extreme circumstances (Modanlou et al, 2009).

B. Smoking

Tobacco smoking is particularly deleterious for transplant recipients, and patients need to stop prior to transplantation. Smoking accelerates the progression of atherosclerotic cardiovascular disease and is nephrotoxic to the kidney resulting in proteinuria (Orth, 2004; Tozawa et al, 2002).

Blood Transfusion

The use of intentional third-party blood transfusions to modulate the immune system is no longer done. In fact, transfusions are generally avoided to prevent the possibility of disease transmission (hepatitis, HIV, etc.) and recipient sensitization to human leukocyte antigen (HLA) phenotypes that may diminish the chance of a negative cross match with a potential donor. Anemia of renal failure is effectively treated with recombinant erythropoietin for most patients (Cody et al, 2005).

Transplant Allograft Nephrectomy

After a failed transplant, immunosuppression is weaned off and the patient returns to dialysis. If graft loss occurs after a year, it is usually not necessary to remove the failed graft, as a new kidney can be placed on the contralateral side. In a few cases, when graft failure is early or is due resistant rejection, the kidney tissue may undergo necrosis and the graft needs to be removed. Indications for allograft nephrectomy include fevers, graft tenderness, gross hematuria, malaise, infection, and uncontrolled hypertension. The subcapsular allograft nephrectomy is the safest approach to prevent iliac vessel injury. This technique can be augmented with presurgical angioinfarction of the allograft to reduce surgical blood loss and the need for transfusion (Westesson et al, 2011).

SELECTION OF DONORS

Living Donors

A. Directed Living Kidney Donors

Living kidney donation provides better patient and allograft survival when compared with deceased-donor transplantation, especially when the live-donor transplant is performed before the onset of dialysis (Figures 36–1 and 36–2) (Meier-Kriesche et al, 2002). Living donation rates vary worldwide, but in many Western countries, Asia, and the Middle East, it has become the predominant form of kidney transplantation. In the United States, the annual number of live kidney donors has surpassed the number of deceased donors since 2001, although the absolute number of transplants from deceased donors still outnumbers those from living donors (Klein et al, 2010). Living donors are most often directed; they have an established relationship with the intended recipient. Based on tissue typing disparities (HLA mismatches), an immunologic hierarchy can be established for the best "match" (Table 36–1). The advantages for identical twins and HLA-identical siblings are quite significant, while all other live-donor combinations are similar and provide significant advantages to the deceased donor. More than 30% of live

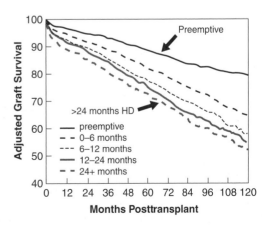

▲ **Figure 36–2.** Preemptive.

Table 36–1. Immunologic hierarchy of kidney donors.

Monozygotic twins
HLA-identical siblings
Haploidentical: siblings, parents, children, other relatives
Zero haplotype relatives
Living unrelated: spouses, friends
Deceased donors

donors are genetically unrelated to their recipient, and represent the fastest growing category of donors. These living unrelated donors (LURDs) (Figure 36–3) come from a spouse, a friend, or even someone anonymous to their recipient (nondirected). The ethical underpinning of this evolving practice is the excellent survival achieved by LURD transplantation, which is similar to the survival of a kidney from a parent or child, from a haploidentical sibling, or from a completely mismatched related donor (Cecka, 2004). These observations have influenced decisions regarding the suitability of live donors who are spouses, friends of the recipients, or anonymous. Today, there is little concern about the degree of HLA match if the ABO blood type and T-cell cross match are compatible. The gender of the living donor in the United States is more frequently female, constituting 60% of the live-donor population (Axelrod et al, 2010). This pattern is similar to what has been observed worldwide, with more male recipients undergoing live-donor transplantation. However, among similarly matched groups, kidneys that provide a greater "nephron dose" (anatomically ideal, young, large, male donors) are often preferred.

B. Nondirected Living Kidney Donors

The extreme shortage of kidneys to meet the demand of waiting recipients coupled with the success of LURD kidney transplantation has opened up creative ways to expand the pool of live donors. In particular, there are individuals who wish to be anonymous donors, that is, "nondirected or altruistic donor." However, in the United States, living-donor exchanges must adhere to section 301 of the National Organ Transplant Act of 1984 (NOTA), which states, "It shall be unlawful for any person to knowingly acquire, receive, or otherwise transfer any human organ for valuable consideration for use in human transplantation." Valuable consideration according to this Act has traditionally been considered to be monetary transfer or a transfer of valuable property between the donor and the recipient. The donation of an organ is properly considered to be a legal gift. With these constraints, any person who is competent, willing to donate, free of coercion, and found to be medically and psychosocially suitable may be a live kidney donor (Adams et al, 2002). Three protocols of nondirected living donation have been developed to accommodate such donors: (1) a live-donor paired exchange, (2) a live-donor/deceased-donor exchange, and (3) altruistic donation.

C. Live-Donor Paired Exchange

This approach involves exchanging donors who are ABO or cross match incompatible with their intended recipients so that each donates a kidney to a compatible recipient (Delmonico, 2004). The exchange derives the benefit of live donation but avoids the risk of incompatibility; several computer algorithms have been modeled to execute the exchange (Montgomery et al, 2005). The best example is two families, one with an A donor to a B recipient and the second with B donor to an A recipient. Swapping donors solves the dilemma. Live-donor exchange procedures have been performed worldwide and are best performed with large sharing pools (Segev et al, 2005). The popularity of paired kidney donor exchanges has been bolstered by the demonstrated safety of shipping live donor kidneys between centers.

D. Live-Donor/Deceased-Donor Exchange

Another system of exchange of donors was devised by centers in UNOS region 1, by permitting the live donor to be used by another compatible individual on the waiting list in "exchange" for the next blood type compatible deceased donor in the region, for the live donor's recipient. With this method, two patients will be transplanted instead of only one, although some fine-tuning of donor organ quality and age is necessary (Delmonico, 2004).

E. Altruistic Living Donors

Altruistic kidney donation (to a complete stranger) is developmental in several centers and must be approached with utmost sensitivity, especially today when organ exchanges are advertised on the Internet. Participating centers usually offer the kidney to the highest wait listed patient at their center after a match run. However, the use of such altruistic donors may aid the formation of live donor "chains" (Rees et al, 2009). The motives of the nondirected donor should be established with care to avoid a prospective donor's intention of remedying a

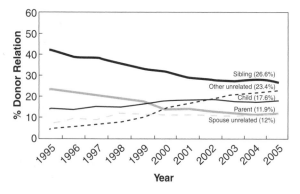

▲ **Figure 36–3.** Living donor (LD) groups.

psychological disorder via donation. Many who inquire about altruistic donation have only a limited understanding of these issues, and upon learning these basic realities, about 60% withdraw from the process (Jacobs et al, 2004).

F. Living-Donor Safety

From its inception, the removal of a kidney from a healthy individual to benefit another has been problematic. The practice is based upon the belief that the removal of one kidney is safe and does not diminish survival or significantly harm long-term kidney function. This notion derives from follow-up of patients up to 45 years after nephrectomy for trauma (Narkun-Burgess et al, 1993). Ibrahim et al (2009) reported the follow-up of 3698 kidney donors between 1963 and 2007 and found that survival and the risk of ESRD appeared to be similar to those in the general population. They found that ESRD developed in 11 donors, a rate of 180 cases per million per year versus 268 cases per million in the general population. At a mean (±SD) of 12.2 ± 9.2 years after donation, 85.5% of a subgroup of 255 donors had a measured GFR >60 mL/min/1.73 m^2, 32.1% had hypertension, and 12.7% had albuminuria. Older age and higher BMI, but not a longer time since donation, were associated with both a GFR <60 mL/min and hypertension. In addition, a recent analysis of 4650 donors between 1987 and 2007 in which 76.3% were white, 13.1% black, 8.2% Hispanic, and 2.4% other found that both black and Hispanic donors had an increased risk of hypertension, diabetes mellitus requiring drug therapy, and chronic kidney disease (Lentine et al, 2010). ESRD developed more frequently in blacks, but it was <1% for the donor population studied. These recent studies are in line with prior reports that unilateral nephrectomy caused an average decrease of 30% in the GFR that tended to improve with each 10 years of follow-up (average increase 1.4 mL/min per decade); a small, progressive increase in proteinuria (average 76 mg/decade); and variable effects on hypertension (Kasiske et al, 1995). Thus, the published evidence indicates that there is little long-term medical risk to a healthy donor after unilateral nephrectomy. Nevertheless, Ellison et al (2002) identified 56 live kidney donors who were subsequently listed for a kidney transplant. The rate of ESRD in donors was calculated to be 0.04%, comparable with the rate (0.03%) in the general population. The renal diagnosis in these patients was hypertension, focal sclerosis, chronic glomerulonephritis, familial nephropathy, diabetes, and other. Recently, some have advocated the use of donors with isolated medical abnormalities such as hypertension, obesity, dyslipidemia, or stones, which may not result in the safety profiles previously reported. As of 2011, prior living donors get preference for deceased donor kidneys should they develop ESRD (UNOS Web site).

▶ Deceased Donors

The imbalance between the supply of brain dead deceased donors and the growing demand for kidneys has created many innovative uses of organs that were excluded in the past. These generally include kidneys from donors older than 60 years; the presence of systemic disease such as atherosclerosis, hypertension, or early diabetes; donors with cardiac arrest or significant hypotension; and some with prior exposure to virus and/or infections that have resolved (Ismail and Flechner, 2006). While kidneys that are severely traumatized or come from donors with active cancer, sepsis, or HIV–AIDS are excluded, a number of donor organs with extended criteria that convey about a 10% worse overall graft survival have been incorporated into the donor pool. To maximize kidney usage, the following categories have been developed.

A. Standard Criteria Donors

Most individuals that meet the criteria for brain death from age 5 to 60 years with normal kidney function and no history of systemic or infectious disease.

B. Expanded Criteria Donors

Kidneys from brain dead donors with 1.7 times relative risk of graft failure. These criteria were developed from a consensus conference that analyzed registry survival data (Rosengard et al, 2002). These include any donor older than 60 years or older than 50 years with a history of hypertension, cerebrovascular accident (CVA) death, or creatinine >1.5 mg/dL (Table 36–2). Informed consent of the recipient is requested to receive an expanded criteria donor (ECD) kidney.

Table 36–2. Expanded criteria kidney donors.

Donor	Condition	Donor <10	Age 10–39	Category 40–49	(Years) 50–59	(Years) ≥60
CVA + HTN	Cr >1.5				X	X
CVA + HTN					X	X
CVA + Cr >1.5					X	X
HTN + Cr >1.5					X	X
CVA						X
HTN						X
Cr >1.5						X
None of above						X

CVA, cerebrovascular accident; HTN, hypertension; Cr >1.5, creatinine >1.5 mg/dL.

Note: The decision matrix using relative risk for graft failure >1.7 for donors older than 10 years. Used for organ allocation in the United States.

Source: http://optn.transplant.hrsa.gov.

C. Donation After Cardiac Death

When a potential donor does not meet brain death criteria but has an irretrievable head injury, viable organs for transplant can be procured after a controlled cardiac arrest. Such kidneys experience a greater incidence of DGF, but long-term function is comparable with standard donor kidneys (Rudich et al, 2002).

D. Dual Transplants

At the extremes of life, one kidney may not be sufficient to deliver an adequate GFR (nephron dose) to an adult recipient. In these instances, using both kidneys from a single donor can overcome these limitations.

1. Pediatric en bloc—Kidneys from donors younger than 5 years (often <6 cm in length) have a historically higher failure rate from technical problems and develop hyperfiltration injury (proteinuria) when transplanted into adults (Bresnahan et al, 2001). Both kidneys can be transplanted en bloc, attached to the donor aorta and vena cava, in a more reliable fashion (Hobart et al, 1998). Such kidneys will grow to adult size in 6–12 months.

2. Adult dual transplants—When kidneys have extremely unfavorable risk factors for graft success due to insufficient nephron mass, both may provide for successful outcome (Bunnapradist et al, 2003). Such adult dual transplants can be placed in either iliac fossa or preferably on the same side through one incision (Flechner, 2008). The criteria established for dual kidney allocation appear in Table 36–3. This approach utilizes kidneys that in the past were often discarded.

E. Extracorporeal Renal Preservation

1. Simple hypothermic storage and flush solutions—Once removed, kidneys are flushed to remove blood and stored in a hyperosmolar, hyperkalemic, and hyponatremic solution at (4–10°C) to minimize ischemic injury (cellular

Table 36–3. Criteria for adult dual cadaveric kidney transplants.

(A) Donor age >60 years
(B) Estimated donor creatinine clearance <65 mL/min based upon serum creatinine upon admission
(C) Rising serum creatinine (>2.5 mg/dL) at the time of retrieval
(D) History of medical disease in donor (defined as either long-standing hypertension or diabetes mellitus)
(E) Adverse donor kidney histology (defined as moderate-to-severe glomerulosclerosis (>15% and <50%).

Note: Kidneys from adult donors must be offered singly unless the donor meets at least two of the following conditions and the OPO would not otherwise use the kidneys singly.
Source: http://optn.transplant.hrsa.gov.

swelling). This is usually sufficient for up to 24 hours of preservation although longer cold ischemic times (up to 40 hours) have been reported, but result in higher rates of DGF. A commercial storage solution from the University of Wisconsin (UW) is frequently used, which contains inert substrates such as lactobionate, raffinose, hydroxyethyl starch, and adenosine as an energy substrate. Recently, a less viscous alternative histidine-tryptophan-ketoglutarate (HTK) solution has been shown to yield similar results with cold ischemia times <24 and >24 hours (Agarwal et al, 2006).

2. Pulsatile perfusion—Hypothermic pulsatile perfusion is an alternative method of preservation, which takes advantage of a continuous pulsatile flow through the graft. Some feel that such hydrodistention is therapeutic in dilating the ischemic renal microcirculation and permits the delivery of vasodilator drugs (ie, verapamil, beta-blockers). It also permits measurement of flow, pulse pressure, and resistance through the graft, which is an accurate method to determine viability of the kidney (Schold et al, 2005). Pulsatile perfusion is more costly and requires investment in a preservation unit (Waters Co, Rochester, MN) and a technologist, but has been gaining popularity due to the increasing number of ECD and donation after cardiac death (DCD) donors that are considered for transplant (Matsuoka et al, 2009; Shah et al, 2008).

▶ The Major Histocompatibility Complex

A. Tissue Typing

The major histocompatibility complex (MHC) describes a region of genes located on chromosome 6 in man, which encode proteins that are responsible for the rejection of tissue between different species or members of the same species (Flechner et al, 2011). The cell surface MHC markers are called human leukocyte antigens (HLAs), because they were first identified on white blood cells. There are two major types of HLA antigens termed class I and class II. Virtually all nucleated cells express HLA class I antigens, while class II antigens are primarily found on B cells, monocytes, macrophages, and antigen-presenting cells. Each individual inherits two serologically defined class I (named A and B) and one class II (named Dr) antigen from each parent, so six HLA antigens constitute an individual's tissue type. One set of HLA A, B, and Dr antigens inherited on one chromosome from a parent is called a haplotype so that HLA-identical siblings have inherited both haplotypes. The HLA molecules are polymorphic (over 170 defined), so it is very unusual if two unrelated individuals have the same tissue type of six HLA antigens. HLA antigens not shared between two individual will generate an immune response. Therefore, the term HLA matching describes the number of shared antigens. One can generate a hierarchical rating of genetic HLA similarities, which roughly correlate to the risk for rejection and eventual kidney transplant outcomes ranging from identical twins to deceased donor (DD) (Table 36–1). In clinical practice, the impact of HLA on graft survival is small in the initial years but may play an important role after 5–10 years. No doubt other factors affect survival: especially donor organ quality (age, function, size, etc) as well as recipient age and comorbidities. However, at present, six Ag-matched (or zero HLA mismatched) deceased donor kidneys are shared nationally due to the beneficial effect on immunological outcomes. In addition, HLA antigen matches also play a role in the algorithm for distribution of deceased donor kidneys with more points assigned for better matches.

B. Crossmatching

Preformed circulating anti-HLA antibodies against the specific phenotype of the donor will lead to acute (if not hyperacute) rejection. Such antibodies (usually IgG) are detected by crossmatching the sera of the recipient with lymphocytes of the donor and adding complement. Such complement-dependent cytotoxicity (CDC) will kill the donor cells and is indicative of deleterious clinical outcome. A similar, yet more sensitive, test has been developed using flow cytometry to identify the presence of anti-HLA antibodies bound to the surface of donor lymphocytes. A crossmatch against both donor T and B lymphocytes is performed within 24 hours of surgery, and transplants are not done if these antibodies are strongly present. In addition, the ABO system will trigger CDC against the mismatched blood group antigens (glycoproteins) present on many tissues. Therefore, transplants are usually done only between ABO compatible individuals. In the last few years, more transplants have been done with weak ABO incompatibilities (low anti-A or anti-B titers) with good outcomes (Montgomery et al, 2009).

C. Serum Screening

At monthly intervals waiting, patients have their serum screened for the presence of anti-HLA antibodies against a panel of HLA phenotypes (lymphocytes) that represent the general population. The result is reported as a percentage of the total referred to as percent reactive antibody (PRA). Those with high titers (>50%) of anti-HLA antibody against the broad population are said to be sensitized and will find it very hard to find a cross-match negative donor. Sensitized patients waiting for an organ depend on better HLA matches to find a cross-match negative donor (McCune et al, 2002). Sensitization to HLA can occur from prior blood transfusions, viral infections, pregnancy, or previous transplants.

D. Posttransplant Antibodies

The development of de novo donor-specific or nondonor-specific anti-HLA antibodies after the transplant has a deleterious effect on outcomes. Both a greater frequency of acute and chronic rejection as well as lower graft survival have been reported among those patient with these antibodies detected by flow cytometry (El Fettouh et al, 2001; Hourmant et al,

2005). The presence of these antibodies may identify those recipients that need more rather than less immunosuppression. The recent introduction of solid phase technology in which specific HLA antigens bound to synthetic beads can be used as a target to screen sera for the presence of HLA antibodies has expanded our ability to monitor recipients before and after transplant (Lefaucheur et al, 2010).

▶ Donor Nephrectomy for Transplantation

Removal of a kidney for transplant depends upon minimizing both surgical injury and warm ischemia, which will hasten the recovery of function in the recipient. It is best to ensure a brisk diuresis in the donor before the kidney is removed, which can be enhanced by the use of volume expansion with saline and albumin, osmotic diuretics (mannitol), and loop diuretics (furosemide) in order to maximize immediate graft function in the recipient. Minimal dissection of the renal hilum is preferred (Flechner et al, 2008).

A. Living Donors

1. Evaluation—All donors should be evaluated both medically and surgically to ensure donor safety. An outline of the usual donor evaluation is shown in Table 36–4. First, a thorough history and physical examination is needed to rule out hypertension, diabetes, obesity, infections, cancers, and specific renal/urologic disorders. Second, laboratory testing of blood and urine, chest x-ray, electrocardiogram, and appropriate cardiac stress testing is done. Several methods to measure GFR and urine protein excretion can be used. Finally, radiographic assessment of the renal anatomy is done, which is usually accomplished by a CT angiogram (Kapoor et al, 2004). A catheter angiogram is reserved for complex vascular anatomy. If anatomic differences are detected between the two kidneys, the donor should always be left with the better kidney. If the two kidneys are equal, the left is preferred for transplant due to its longer and often thicker renal vein. However, in cases when one kidney has three or more renal arteries, the kidney with the single artery is selected. In younger fertile female donors, concern about physiologic hydronephrosis of the right kidney is taken into consideration.

2. Surgical technique—Today, the most commonly used approach is intraperitoneal laparoscopic donor nephrectomy, primarily due to patient choice (Moinzadeh and Gill, 2006). This technique has all but supplanted open donor nephrectomy via an extraperitoneal flank incision due to reports of reduced pain and shorter recovery time. The hand-assisted laparoscopic approach, where the extraction incision is used during the dissection is the most common technique used in the US (Fisher et al, 2006). Nevertheless, in cases with a short right vein or three or more arteries, we prefer an open nephrectomy using 12th rib-sparing flank incision (Turner-Warwick, 1965). When multiple renal arteries are

Table 36–4. Standard evaluation of the potential live donor.

History: Focus on relation to renal disease
  Hypertension, diabetes, family history, use of NSAIDs, other chronic drugs, environmental exposure (heavy metals), chronic UTI, stones, prior surgery, prior cardiovascular or pulmonary events (TB), begin to explore desire to donate

Physical exam: Focus on relation to renal disease
  Blood pressure, weight/height (BMI), lymph nodes, joints, breast, prostate
  Cardiovascular disease assessment

Laboratory testing:
  Urinalysis and culture, electrolytes, BUN creatinine, calcium, phosphorus, magnesium, liver panel, fasting blood glucose, and lipid profile
  CBC with platelets, coagulation screen
  24-hour urine, creatinine clearance, and protein excretion (albumin/creatinine ratio) or GFR measurement (iothalamate clearance)
  Remote stone history: 24-hour urine calcium, uric acid, oxalate, citrate
  Viral serology: Hepatitis C; hepatitis B; HIV; Epstein-Barr virus; cytomegalovirus; herpes simplex; and RPR (rapid plasmin reagent)
  Electrocardiogram, chest x-ray
  Females PAP, mammogram—age appropriate
  Males PSA (age >40-50, family history)
  Colonoscopy (age appropriate)

Imaging of the kidneys: Local availability
  Computed tomography angiogram
  Magnetic resonance angiogram
  Catheter arteriogram

NSAIDs, nonsteroidal anti-inflammatory drugs; UTI, urinary tract infection; BMI, body mass index; BUN, blood urea nitrogen.

encountered, they should be conjoined ex vivo while the kidney is on ice, in order to minimize the number of anastomoses in the recipient and reduce ischemia times (Flechner and Novick, 2002). Smaller upper pole arteries (<2 mm) often can be sacrificed, while lower pole vessels should be retained because of a risk to the ureteral blood supply.

B. Deceased Donors

Today, most donors are multiple-organ donors, and they require removal of the liver, heart, lungs, and pancreas, in addition to the kidneys. The retrieval needs to be coordinated, and it is often performed by several teams representing each organ for transplant. Usually, the thoracic organs are removed first while the abdominal organs are cooled and perfused with UW or HTK perfusion solution. The kidneys are removed en bloc with the aorta and vena cava and a large amount of retroperitoneal tissue. They are separated on the backbench by dividing the great vessels with the renal vessels attached. Donor characteristics and projected cold ischemia

time may influence the use of cold storage or pulsatile perfusion preservation.

▶ Standard Renal Transplant Surgery

There are several different methods for surgical revascularization of the kidney; the following is one reliable method (Flechner, 2008). While either iliac fossa is acceptable for the transplant, the right side is often preferred due to the longer and more horizontal segments of external iliac artery and vein compared with the left side. A lower quadrant curvilinear (Gibson) incision is made, and the iliac vessels are exposed through a retroperitoneal approach, a self-retaining retractor is used. The renal-to-iliac vein anastomosis is usually performed first, in an end-to-side fashion with 5–0 nonabsorbable monofilament suture, using a running quadrant technique. The renal artery can be anastomosed end to end to the internal iliac using 6–0 nonabsorbable monofilament suture. However, in older recipients and diabetic patients, this vessel often has significant arterial plaque causing poor runoff. In addition, concern about compromising arterial flow to the penis via the pudendal artery with subsequent erectile dysfunction limits this approach in older males. Because of these factors, an end-to-side anastomosis of the renal artery to the external iliac artery is more frequently done with 6–0 nonabsorbable monofilament suture using a running quadrant technique. An extravesical ureteroneocystostomy (variation of Lich technique) is the preferred method to reimplant the ureter. When healthy appearing ureter is short or the bladder is defunctionalized and small, a native to transplant ureteroureterostomy can be done. An internal double J ureteral stent is usually placed, and a closed suction drain is left in the deep pelvis.

▶ Imaging of the Transplant Kidney

Immediately after the transplant, it is advisable to obtain a baseline duplex Doppler ultrasound to confirm patency of the renal vessels, blood flow to the parenchyma, and to identify large fluid collections, hematomas, or hydronephrosis. This is especially important when the graft is oliguric. Similar information can be obtained using an isotopic (mercaptoacetyltriglycerine, 99mTc-MAG-3) renal scan, which is especially helpful to identify urinary extravasation. Kidneys with DGF demonstrate a typical pattern of isotopic uptake with little clearance or excretion. If fluid collections or intraperitoneal problems are suspected, finer definition can be obtained with a computed axial tomography (CAT) scan. The use of 3-D CAT scans or MR angiography can delineate actual vascular lesions (stenoses, aneurysms, a-v fistula). Catheter angiography is reserved for interventions that require access to the renal vessels such as angioplasty. Imaging with intravenous iodinated contrast should be limited when the creatinine is >1.8 mg/dL, but cystograms and antegrade nephrostograms can be helpful to identify urinary fistulas or obstructions.

▶ Immediate Posttransplant Care

A. Hemodynamic Management

Initial postsurgical care in the first hours and days focuses on the urine output and eventual recovery of GFR. It is important to avoid hypotension, dehydration, or use of alpha-adrenergic drugs, which will exacerbate surgical and preservation injury. It is helpful to monitor central venous pressures to maintain adequate preload (10–15 cm water). Urine output >1 cc/kg/h is desirable, and hourly intravenous replacement at cc/cc of urine is usually sufficient. Some live donor kidneys may generate outputs up to a liter per hour, which will drop the blood pressure and should be managed with only 1/2–2/3 volume replaced. Alternatively, fluid overload and pulmonary edema may cause renal hypoperfusion and should be avoided. Treatment with fluid restriction, diuretics, and even dialysis may be needed. Even when hemodynamically stable, many deceased donor recipients (and a few living donor recipients) will experience delayed recovery of graft function, which is a consequence of extended cold preservation times or warm ischemia in the donor or prolonged anastomosis time in the recipient.

B. Delayed Recovery of Graft Function

DGF is more formally defined as the need for dialysis during the first week after transplant and occurs in about a third of deceased donor recipients. The term slow graft function (SGF) is said to occur if the recipient creatinine is not <3 mg/dL by day 5, and occurs in another third of deceased donor recipients (Humar et al, 2002). Patients with DGF may produce liters of urine a day (nonoliguric DGF), but have a rising creatinine and need dialysis. Others produce <300 cc a day of urine and are described as oliguric DGF, which is usually an indication of a more prolonged recovery time. These clinical events are associated with specific histological findings referred to as acute tubular necrosis (ATN), the hallmark of which is tubular epithelial swelling, necrosis, and regeneration with mitotic figures. If kidneys are in oliguric DGF for over a week and imaging studies demonstrate good blood flow, a biopsy should be done to rule out rejection and confirm ATN. Transplant DGF due to ATN resolves in most cases but may take up to several weeks, while about 1–2% of grafts never function (primary nonfunction) and may progress to cortical necrosis. Since the definition of DGF encompasses not just ATN but all causes of early graft dysfunction, it does have a negative impact on both short- and long-term graft survival compared with kidneys that function immediately (Shoskes et al, 1997). During DGF, it is helpful to delay the introduction of calcineurin inhibitor (CNI) drugs for 7–10 days until some recovery of function is evident. This usually requires the use of an induction antibody as an umbrella of protection until the graft heals.

C. Sudden Drop in Urine Output

During the first few days, a sudden loss of urine output after an initial diuresis demands prompt attention to ensure patency of the Foley catheter, and if easily obtainable, a repeat ultrasound to confirm vascular flow and exclude hydronephrosis. If there is any question of abnormal blood flow or a delay in obtaining an imaging study, the kidney should be promptly reexplored, since vascular compromise of a few hours will result in allograft necrosis. Loss of urine output from the bladder catheter with increased drain output may suggest a urine fistula. The drainage fluid can be sent for creatinine, and if 5–10 times the serum level suggests urine. If the above problems are excluded with imaging studies, renal biopsy is needed to rule out acute rejection or thrombotic microangiopathy and to ensure graft viability.

▶ Transplant Rejection

The disparate HLA phenotypes on donor tissue trigger an immune response that leads to renal dysfunction and histological changes in the transplanted kidney called rejection. These responses are both humoral and cellular, and depend upon the presentation of processed donor HLA antigens via either donor (direct) or host (indirect) antigen-presenting cells to the recipient's immunocompetent T cells (Flechner et al, 2011). The clinical signs and symptoms of acute renal allograft rejection may include fever, chills, lethargy, hypertension, pain and swelling of the graft, diminished urine output, edema, an elevated serum creatinine and blood urea nitrogen (BUN), and proteinuria. Immunosuppression is designed to prevent these events. Rejection can also be divided in three distinct clinical entities based on the timing and mechanism responsible for triggering these events.

Hyperacute rejection occurs immediately after revascularization of a kidney when preformed cytotoxic anti-HLA antibody is present. It will lead to graft thrombosis, and the kidney must be removed. While there is no treatment, it can be prevented almost completely by using the sensitive crossmatching techniques available today.

Acute rejection episodes can occur at anytime after the transplant, but most occur in the first 3 months. Such episodes can be mild or severe and cause the symptoms previously described to a variable degree. With the currently available immunosuppression, about 20% or less of transplant recipients experience acute rejection, and most episodes are reversible with treatment. Less than 5% of recipients lose their graft due to unresponsive acute rejection. These episodes are predominantly cellular and cause graft infiltration of cytotoxic cells, but humoral mechanisms contribute to the process. Treated acute rejections that result in a return to baseline renal function appear to have little impact on long-term graft survival (Meier-Kriesche et al, 2004).

Chronic rejection defines a process of gradual, progressive, decline in renal function over time. It is associated with

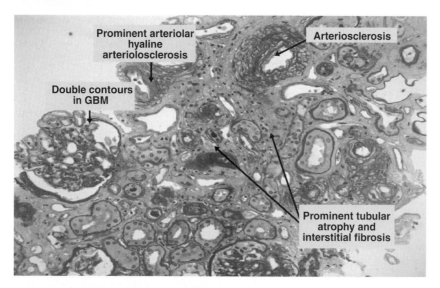

Prominent arteriolar
hyaline
arteriolosclerosis

Arteriosclerosis

Double contours
in GBM

Prominent tubular
atrophy and
interstitial fibrosis

▲ **Figure 36–4.** Chronic allograft nephropathy.

hypertension and proteinuria, and is accompanied by histological features of tubular atrophy, interstitial fibrosis, and an occlusive arteriolopathy (Figure 36–4). It can be detected as early as 6 months after transplant, and is thought to have a strong humoral response against the graft. Some, but not all, recipients have had prior acute rejections or have donor-specific antibody (DSA) detected. There is a role for alloimmunity (antigen-dependent factors), since it does not occur in identical twins, is rare in HLA-identical sibling transplants, and is most common among deceased donor recipients (Kreiger et al, 2003). However, many of these histologic changes are found with older donor age, ischemic injury, viral infections, and other systemic comorbidities, referred to as antigen-independent factors. Therefore, the process remains less well characterized, is no doubt multifactorial, and is often given the name chronic allograft nephropathy (CAN). Treatment is not often effective and consists of tight control of blood pressure, the use of angiotensin converting enzyme (ACE) inhibitor or angiotensin receptor blocker (ARB) drugs for proteinuria, and sparing or elimination of CNI drugs.

▶ Immunosuppression

The holy grail of transplantation is to develop methods that permit a recipient to keep a transplanted organ in a state of "tolerance" or donor-specific unresponsiveness. Until that day arrives, clinical practice is dependent on our ability to interrupt the host immune response using agents that are not precise. It is a constant struggle to deliver enough immunosuppression to prevent rejection, but not too much to render the patient susceptible to infection and cancer. In addition, immunosuppressive drugs have unique mechanisms of action and their own specific toxicities (Halloran, 2004). Immunosuppressive agents can be used in one of three ways: (1) induction or high-dose therapy to prevent a primary immune response immediately after transplantation, (2) low-dose or maintenance therapy once engraftment has stabilized, or (3) additional high-dose therapy to treat acute rejection should it arise.

A. Chemical Immunosuppression with Small Molecules

1. Corticosteroids—Since the initial observations almost 50 years ago that corticosteroids could prevent and treat renal allograft rejection (Hume et al, 1963), they have become the cornerstone of immunosuppressive therapy. Corticosteroids have numerous effects on the immune system that include sequestration of lymphocytes in lymph nodes and the bone marrow resulting in lymphopenia. Glucocorticoids become bound to intercellular receptors, and conformational changes in the steroid–receptor complex interfere with cytokine production. Their primary immunosuppressive effect is inhibition of monocyte production and release of interleukin (IL-1), with subsequent inhibition of T-cell IL-2 and interferon-gamma, thus interfering with lymphocyte activation and production of effector cells. However, systemic toxicities of steroids are myriad, including cushingoid features, hypertension, hyperlipidemia, hyperglycemia, weight gain, osteoporosis, poor wound healing, growth retardation, psychiatric disturbances, etc, and have resulted in intense efforts to reduce steroid dosage. Alternate-day steroid dosing appears beneficial for growth in children, but complete steroid withdrawal or avoidance has become more appealing. The potential benefits include lower blood pressure, improved lipid profiles, and diminished physical side effects attributed to steroids. Today, standard maintenance therapy is achieved with as little as 5 mg prednisone daily. There have been several reviews of trials attempting to withdraw steroids 3 months or later from stable transplant patients. Initial graft stability is often followed by acute rejection requiring the reintroduction of steroids (Pascual et al, 2004). If attempted, withdrawal should be entertained in well-matched recipients, 1 year or more after transplant, with no prior episodes of rejection. Avoidance of steroids after 1 week may be favorable if accompanied by depleting antibody induction (Khwaja et al, 2004), although randomized trials confirm few if any lasting benefits (Woodle et al, 2008).

2. Antiproliferative drugs

A. Azathioprine—Introduced first in the 1960s, 6-mercaptopurine and its imidazole derivative azathioprine represent antimetabolites that blocks purine biosynthesis and cell division. The developers of azathioprine, Gertrude Elion and George Hitchings, received the 1988 Nobel Prize. Azathioprine is most effective if given immediately after antigen presentation to prevent rejection and is ineffective in treating established rejection. Adverse effects of azathioprine include bone marrow suppression (primarily leukopenia), alopecia, hepatoxicity, and increased risk of infection and neoplasia. When compared directly with another antiproliferative agent, mycophenolate mofetil (MMF), azathioprine is not as potent in rejection prophylaxis. Therefore, its use has been diminishing rapidly over the past few years but serves as a secondary agent replacing MMF for intractable toxicity.

B. Mycophenolate mofetil—MMF is a morpholinoethyl ester of the fungal antibiotic mycophenolic acid, which is a noncompetitive inhibitor of the enzyme inosine monophosphate dehydrogenase. MMF inhibits purine biosynthesis preventing the proliferation of activated T and B cells, thereby blocking both cellular and humoral immune responses. It is thought to be more specific for those lymphocytes that rely primarily on *de novo* purine synthetic pathways, and has replaced azathioprine as an antimetabolite. MMF is usually well tolerated at dosages up to 2 g (divided dosing), with gastrointestinal disorders (nausea, vomiting, cramps, and diarrhea) and bone marrow suppression (leukopenia, anemia) being its major toxicities. Therapeutic drug monitoring of blood levels has demonstrated wide interpatient variability, but it may provide some benefit by preventing rejections due to poor exposure. An additional enteric coated product, mycophenolate sodium, is also available.

C. Cyclophosphamide—Cyclophosphamide has historically been used in place of azathioprine, although it is much less commonly used today. It is an alkylating agent that is biotransformed by the hepatic microsomal oxidase system to active alkylating metabolites. It inhibits DNA replication and, like azathioprine, affects rapidly dividing cells and is most effective immediately after antigen presentation.

Cyclophosphamide has a narrower therapeutic-to-toxic ratio than azathioprine, and adverse effects include myelosuppression with leukopenia, fertility disorders, and hemorrhagic cystitis.

D. Leflunomide—Leflunomide is an oral agent that inhibits the enzyme dihydro-orotate dehydrogenase, essential for de novo pyrimidine synthesis. The drug exhibits both antiproliferative and anti-inflammatory activity, and was initially approved for the treatment of rheumatoid and psoriatic arthritis. Its use in organ transplantation as an adjunctive agent is limited. The most common side effects include diarrhea, nausea, dyspepsia, rash, abnormal liver function test results, or marrow suppression. Interestingly, the major metabolite has antiviral activity against CMV and polyoma virus, which can infect transplant recipients (Josephson et al, 2006). It can be substituted for MMF or azathioprine in patients infected with the BK virus.

3. Antilymphocyte drugs

A. Calcineurin inhibitor drugs—Cyclosporine, a lipophilic small molecule, has been the cornerstone of transplant immunosuppression since the early 1980s and is the prototype CNI drug. It binds to a specific intracellular immunophilin (cyclophilin) causing conformational changes and subsequent engaging of the enzyme calcineurin phosphatase, thereby preventing the downstream gene transcription of IL-2 and other cytokines required for T-cell activation and proliferation. The adverse effects of cyclosporine, which are related to the concentration of the drug, include nephrotoxicity, hypertension, hyperlipidemia, gingival hyperplasia, hirsutism, and the hemolytic uremic syndrome. CNI drugs are metabolized by the hepatic cytochrome P-450 (3A4) system, and other drugs that inhibit or stimulate this enzyme system (ie, diltiazem and ketoconazole, or phenytoin and isoniazid) can significantly affect blood levels, thus favoring therapeutic drug monitoring. Recent developments include monitoring of the peak cyclosporine levels 2 hours after administration to better reflect exposure to the drug. A microemulsion that exhibits more reproducible absorption and metabolism has replaced the initial oral formulation.

Tacrolimus is another CNI drug that engages a different immunophilin, FK-binding protein 12 (FKBP12), to create a complex that inhibits calcineurin with greater molar potency than does cyclosporine. Although quite similar to cyclosporine in efficacy, both can cause nephrotoxicity and the hemolytic uremic syndrome. Tacrolimus is more likely to induce new onset diabetes after transplant, hyperkalemia, hypomagnesemia, and tremors. It seems less likely to cause hyperlipidemia, hypertension, and cosmetic problems. In some regimens, tacrolimus is reported to reduce subclinical rejection, and its use has increased steadily. In the United States, Tacrolimus is now the predominant CNI drug, given to 90% of new recipients. However, the most distressing feature of continuous CNI use is acute and chronic nephrotoxicity. Acute CNI nephrotoxicity is mediated by pronounced vascular and, to a lesser degree, tubular alterations, manifested by oligoanuria and azotemia, with associated hyperkalemia, hyperuricemia, hypertension, hypomagnesia, and renal tubular acidosis. A dose-dependent reduction in renal blood flow and glomerular filtration is well documented. Chronic CNI nephrotoxicity is more insidious, associated with progressive deterioration of graft histology (scarring) in more than 50% by 5 years and virtually all treated patients by 10 years (Nankivell et al, 2003). CNI-treated recipients have a profile of upregulated genes associated with profibrotic/fibrotic activity and tissue remodeling (Flechner et al, 2004). Dosage reduction will often mitigate against some of these effects, and numerous regimens have been tested to try to minimize or eliminate CNI drugs, although it must be done carefully to avoid increased risk of rejection (Ekberg et al, 2007; Russ et al, 2005). In a carefully controlled comparison of monitored exposure to cyclosporine versus tacrolimus, Rowshani et al (2006) reported a similar degree of scarring at 1 year after transplant. Calcium channel blockers are often used to ameliorate CNI nephrotoxicity due to their ability to reduce the dosage requirements, treat the associated hypertension, and reverse the calcium-dependent afferent arteriolar vasoconstriction.

B. TARGET OF RAPAMYCIN INHIBITORS—Sirolimus and everolimus form a class of immunosuppressive agents that have similar molecular structure to the CNIs and bind to the same immunophilin protein (FKBP-12) as tacrolimus. However, their mode of action appears to be distinct, as the sirolimus-FKBP-12 complex does not inhibit calcineurin. Instead, the sirolimus-FKBP-12 complex engages a distinct serine/threonine p70 kinase called mTOR (molecular target of rapamycin). The inhibition of mTOR blocks downstream signal transduction pathways that prevent cell-cycle progression from G-, to S-phase in activated T cells. The principal nonimmune toxic effects of sirolimus and everolimus include hyperlipidemia, bone marrow suppression, and impaired wound healing and lymphoceles. Other reported side effects include aggravation of proteinuria, mouth ulcers, reduced testosterone and pneumonitis. Sirolimus and everolimus may also reduce CMV infection. Sirolimus and everolimus were initially registered for use with cyclosporine, but the combination increased nephrotoxicity, the hemolytic–uremic syndrome, and hypertension. Sirolimus has been combined with tacrolimus, but this combination also produced renal dysfunction and hypertension, which indicates that sirolimus potentiates CNI nephrotoxicity. Nephrotoxicity can be reduced by using very low doses of CNI (Tedesco-Silva et al, 2007), or by withdrawing the CNI (Russ et al, 2005). The mTOR inhibitors also possess antifibrotic, antineoplastic, and arterial protective effects. The combination of de novo sirolimus with MMF in a CNI-free regimen can result in improved renal function with less CAN. However, some have had a hard time using this combination due to tolerability issues (Flechner, 2009). The mTOR inhibitors have been demonstrated to slow down the growth of established experimental tumors and have potential applications in oncology (Guba et al, 2002). In fact, the mTOR inhibitors (temsirolimus and everolimus) are approved for treatment of kidney cancer (Figlin, 2008). The possibility that sirolimus and everolimus can protect arteries is suggested by two observations: mTOR inhibitors can reduce restenosis when eluted from coronary artery stents (Morice et al, 2002) and TOR inhibitors plus CNI inhibitors reduce the incidence of graft coronary artery disease after heart transplant (Eisen et al, 2003).

B. Antilymphocyte Antibodies

1. Polyclonal antibodies—Polyclonal antibodies are produced by injecting (immunizing) animals such as horses, goats, sheep, or rabbits with cells from human lymphoid tissue. Immune sera from several animals are pooled and the gamma globulin fractions extracted and purified. A rabbit-derived antithymocyte antibody (Thymoglobulin, Sanofi) is the most frequently used preparation. Once injected, the antibodies bind to lymphocytes resulting in a rapid lymphopenia or *depletion* due to complement-mediated cell lysis, as well as masking of surface antigens or induction of suppressor populations that block cell function. Polyclonal antibodies are used primarily as induction therapy and to treat vascular or antibody-mediated rejection (AMR). Because of their strong immunosuppressive effects, polyclonal antibodies are limited to short courses of 3–10 days, but their depletion may last 6–12 months. Although designed to deplete T cells, they may also affect B cells, NK cells, other mononuclear cells, platelets, etc. Adverse effects include fever, chills, and arthralgias related to the injection of foreign proteins and the release of cytokines. These effects can be minimized by pretreatment with corticosteroids and antihistamines. More serious adverse effects include increased susceptibility to infections (especially viral) and neoplasia.

2. Monoclonal antibodies that deplete lymphocytes—The introduction of murine hybridoma technology opened the door to the development of highly specific antibodies directed against functional cell surface targets. These antibodies, like polyclonal antibodies, exert their effects through a variety of immune mechanisms. In addition to complement-mediated lysis, blockade and inactivation of cell surface molecules, and opsonization with phagocytosis, these antibodies can induce cytotoxicity and modulation of cell surface molecules on target tissues.

A. MUROMONAB-CD3—Muromonab-CD3, a mouse monoclonal antibody against CD3, was the first commercially available selective monoclonal antibody used in transplantation for both induction and to treat rejection. Muromonab-CD3 binds to the T-cell receptor associated CD3 complex, which first triggers a massive cytokine-release syndrome before depleting and functionally modulating T cells. Although potent in rejection prophylaxis and its reversal, the toxicity exhibited during use has led to the development of safer products, and the drug is no longer in production.

B. Alemtuzumab—Alemtuzumab is a humanized monoclonal antibody (IgG1) that specifically interacts with the 21–28-kd lymphocyte cell surface glycoprotein CD52, which is predominantly expressed on peripheral blood lymphocytes, monocytes, and macrophages. Once engaged with CD52, it produces a profound depletion of lymphocyte populations (T, B, and NK) that can persist for over a year. Although multiple doses are FDA approved for treating B-cell chronic lymphocytic leukemia, one or two 30 mg doses have been introduced as an induction agent in organ transplantation. Side effects of alemtuzumab include first-dose reactions, bone marrow suppression, and autoimmunity. Worries concerning prolonged immunodeficiency (infections and cancer) with alemtuzumab persist, although it is commonly used with lower doses of other maintenance agents. Early predictions that the agent would induce prope or "almost" tolerance were not confirmed, as some reports suggested a higher than expected incidence of rejection episodes, including AMR.

C. Rituximab—Rituximab is chimeric anti-CD20 monoclonal antibody that eliminates most B cells, and it was initially FDA approved for treating refractory non-Hodgkin's B-cell lymphomas. It was introduced in transplantation to treat a similar tumor, posttransplantation lymphoproliferative disease (PTLD). Rituximab is currently being evaluated to treat donor-specific alloantibody responses such as AMR or in transplanting sensitized recipients. It is used in combination with maintenance immunosuppressive drugs, plasmapheresis, and intravenous immune globulin (IVIG). While plasma cells are usually CD20 negative, some precursors are CD20 positive and their elimination may reduce some antibody responses. Such therapy may provide the first of future tools to control humoral rejection.

3. Monoclonal antibodies that are nondepleting

A. Daclizumab and basiliximab—Another selective site for monoclonal antibody targeting of the immune response is the IL-2 receptor (CD25), present on the surface of activated T cells and responsible for further signal transduction and T-cell proliferation. Both a chimeric (basiliximab) and a humanized (daclizumab) anti-CD25 have been genetically engineered to produce a hybrid IgG that retains the specific anti-CD25 binding characteristics with a less xenogenic (murine) backbone. These agents cause minimal cytokine release upon first exposure and exhibit a prolonged elimination half-life resulting in weeks to months of CD25 suppression. Because expression of CD25 (IL-2 receptor α chain) requires T-cell activation, anti-CD25 antibody causes little depletion of T cells. Anti-CD25 antibodies are useful as safe induction agents in low-to-moderate risk recipients, but have little effect in treating an established rejection episode. Their use appear to offer a favorable risk–benefit compared with

depleting agents, providing for improved graft survival with a lower risk of posttransplant cancers. In 2010, daclizumab (Zenapax) was removed from commercial production.

B. Belatacept—Basic immunology generated the concept that blocking costimulation (signal 2) could prevent the activation of antigen primed T cells, thus providing a new avenue for control of allograft rejection. A first generation of monoclonal antibodies designed to block costimulation proved the concept in animals, but lacked sufficient efficacy in initial clinical trials. Belatacept is a second-generation cytotoxic T-lymphocyte–associated antigen 4 (CTLA-4) immune globulin, engineered as a fusion protein combining CTLA-4 with the Fc portion of an IgG molecule. This biological agent engages CD80 and CD86 on the surface of antigen-presenting cells, thereby blocking costimulation through T-cell CD28. The 2-year results of a phase 3 trial in renal transplant recipients given MMF, steroids, and anti-CD25 antibody demonstrated that belatacept versus cyclosporine resulted in increased acute rejection (23% vs 7%) but better, 10–15 cc/min GFR, renal function (Larsen et al, 2010). However, a higher incidence of PTLD was observed, especially for recipients who were naïve to the EBV at transplant (Vincenti et al, 2010). Belatacept was FDA approved in 2011, and is given at intervals of 2–4 weeks as an intravenous preparation and may be further evaluated in CNI-sparing regimens.

C. Baseline Immunosuppression

Current regimens vary according to center preference and are often subject to center experience and willingness to participate in clinical trials. Two areas of current investigative interest include CNI sparing or avoidance (to minimize CNI nephrotoxicity) and steroid sparing or avoidance trials (to minimize steroid side effects). A very typical regimen applicable to HLA mismatched deceased or live donor recipients would include an induction agent, either a nondepleting (basiliximab) or a depleting (Thymoglobulin/alemtuzumab) antibody. Maintenance therapy would include an antilymphocytic agent (tacrolimus, cyclosporine, or sirolimus), an antiproliferative agent (MMF or azathioprine), and steroids. The most common initial regimen today is tacrolimus–MMF–steroids. Delayed introduction of CNI drugs for 7–10 days is often selected for recipients with DGF to permit early healing of the ischemic injury, assuming an induction antibody has been administered. Steroid elimination after a week and CNI conversion to an mTOR inhibitor at 2–4 months is done in many centers.

D. Treatment of Rejection

1. Cellular rejection—Acute rejection leads to graft injury and eventual CAN if untreated. Therefore, it requires prompt and accurate diagnosis, which is best provided from a percutaneous renal transplant biopsy. One of the remarkable achievements of the last 10 years has been the universal acceptance of the Banff schema to diagnose and characterize renal allograft rejection (Racusen et al, 1999). The scoring system is semiquantitative, based on light microscopy, and describes features for acute rejection and chronic/sclerosing nephropathy as well as features attributed to both cellular and antibody-mediated mechanisms. For patients with Banff I or II acute rejections, high-dose intravenous steroid pulses of 5–7 mg/kg/d for 3 days will reverse about 85%. Some clinicians also prefer to add a 10–14-day recycle of oral prednisone at 2 mg/kg tapered to baseline. If rejections are unresponsive to steroids or histology confirms a component of Banff II or III vascular changes, a depleting antibody such as Thymoglobulin is given at 7–8 mg/kg over a week. It is not generally prudent to treat more than two to three acute rejections in any one recipient.

2. Antibody-mediated rejection—If distinct evidence of AMR is present, which includes biopsy evidence of deposition of the complement split product C4d in the peritubular capillaries coupled with the presence of circulating donor specific antibody (DSA), additional treatments are needed to recover renal function (Colvin, 2007). These include plasmapheresis to remove existing anti-HLA antibody and blocking IVIG (2 g/kg). The anti-CD20 monoclonal antibody rituximab has also been used, although it does not target the plasma cell. Some optimism has been generated by the use of proteasome inhibitor bortezomib, which directly targets plasma cells, the source of DSA. This drug, approved for the treatment of B-cell chronic leukemias, can reduce titers of the DSA and may reverse AMR episodes when clinically combined with plasmapheresis and IVIG over a 2-week course (Flechner et al, 2010).

▶ Results of Kidney Transplantation

There have been dramatic improvements in short-term kidney transplant outcomes since the inception of clinical practice five decades ago. For recipients of living donor kidneys, 1-year patient and graft survival has increased to about 98.7% and 96.5%, and for recipients of standard criteria deceased donors 96.3% and 91.4% (Figure 36–1). The major reasons for this improvement are a reduction of acute rejection episodes (better immunosuppression and crossmatching techniques) with fewer complications from its treatment, and better prophylaxis and treatment of the common posttransplant infections. However, long-term graft loss beyond 5–10 years has not changed much, with stagnant survival half-lives of 7–8 years for deceased donor and 10–11 years for living donor kidneys. Factors that are statistically associated with graft failure are listed in Table 36–5. Ultimately, these factors lead to a multifaceted process of graft scarring (Figure 36–4) resulting in decline of function termed CAN, which is the major reason for late graft loss. The etiologies of CAN include processes that are immune related as well as those associated with nonspecific renal injury (Colvin, 2003). The second leading cause of late graft loss is death with a functioning graft, primarily due to the consequences of

Table 36–5. Major factors that affect long-term graft outcome.

HLA match between donor and recipient
Age of donor and recipient
Rejection-both acute and chronic
Prior failed transplants
Sensitization (preformed anti-HLA antibodies)
Recipient race (Asians > whites > blacks)
Comorbidities (DM, obesity, hyperlipidemia)
Immunosuppressive drugs utilized

HLA, human leukocyte antigen.

atherosclerotic cardiovascular disease, less so infections and cancers. Some risk factors for CAN and cardiovascular disease overlap (hypertension, hyperlipidemia, smoking, diabetes, etc). Graft loss secondary to patient noncompliance with medications has been estimated at 5–10%.

▶ Complications of Kidney Transplantation

A. Surgical

The majority of significant surgical problems posttransplant are either vascular or urologic. They include renal artery thrombosis, disruption, stenosis, or mycotic aneurysm; renal vein thrombosis or disruption; urinary fistula or ureteral stenosis; pelvic lymphocele or hematoma; scrotal hydrocele or abscess; and wound abscess, dehiscence, or hernia (Flechner, 2011). Prevention is the best way to avoid these problems using meticulous surgical and antiseptic techniques, including the routine use of preoperative broad-spectrum antibiotics.

1. Vascular problems—In the early posttransplant period, vascular problems may prevent a new kidney from ever functioning, and questions raised from imaging studies often require surgical reexploration. Anastomotic bleeding requires immediate repair; twisting or compression of the vessels may require reanastomosis, while complete thrombosis necessitates nephrectomy. Early large hematomas should be surgically drained and hemostasis confirmed. Significant transplant renal artery stenosis can occur from poor surgical technique, damage of the vessel intima at procurement, atherosclerosis or fibrous disease, or immune injury, but it is fairly uncommon (1–5% of transplants). Poorly controlled hypertension, renal dysfunction (especially after ACE inhibitors or beta-blockers), and a new pelvic bruit are clinical clues. Percutaneous transluminal angioplasty is the treatment of choice and restores kidney perfusion in 60–90% of cases. The risk of restenosis can be minimized with an internal stent (Bruno et al, 2004). Pseudoaneurysms of the renal or iliac artery and A-V fistula after biopsy are often amenable to embolization or endovascular stenting. Large (>5 cm) or mycotic aneurysms, inability to dilate a vascular stenosis, or unusual lesions may require open operative repair to prevent rupture.

2. Urologic problems—Urologic complications are reported in 2–10% of kidney transplants (Streeter et al, 2002), and usually do not result in graft loss if promptly treated (van Roijen et al, 2001). Recent meta-analysis has confirmed that the routine placement of an indwelling ureteral stent will aid healing and reduce early ureteral fistula or obstruction (Wilson et al, 2005). It is advisable to leave a Foley catheter for 10–14 days for thin walled, poorly vascularized, or small-defunctionalized bladders. Ureteral fistulas and stenoses are usually a consequence of ischemia to the distal ureter from surgical dissection, overzealous electrocautery, or immune injury. CMV and BK virus infection of the urinary tract have been associated with ureteral stenosis (Fusaro et al, 2003; Mylonakis et al, 2001). For large fistulas, rapid surgical repair and drainage is advised, either by ureteral reimplantation to the bladder or native ureteroureterostomy or ureteropyelostomy. Small fistulas are occasionally amenable to long-term stenting with or without a proximal diverting nephrostomy, or bladder catheter. Ureteral stenoses are often amenable to balloon dilation and stenting but, if recurrent, require open repair. Urinary retention is more common in recent years as older males with prostatism are transplanted. It is advisable to wait a few months if prostatectomy is needed to ensure healing of the graft. Hydroceles, usually ipsilateral to the transplant and a consequence of spermatic cord transection, may cause discomfort or enlarge. They are best repaired by hydrocelectomy, although successful aspiration and sclerotherapy has been reported.

3. Wound problems—Wound complications are reported in 5–20% of transplants, and are best prevented since they can cause significant morbidity and take many months to resolve. Since immunosuppression delays wound healing, especially sirolimus and MMF, the use of nonabsorbable sutures in the fascia and more conservative surgical technique in the obese are warranted (Flechner et al, 2003; Humar et al, 2001). A closed suction pelvic drain is also helpful immediately posttransplant. Early fascial defects or late incisional hernias require operative repair; synthetic mesh or Alloderm may be required (Buinewicz, 2004). Suprafascial dehiscence or infection can resolve slowly by secondary intention, which may be hastened by the use of vacuum-assisted closure (Argenta et al, 2006). Lymphocele formation in the retroperitoneum can develop from disruption of small lymphatic channels in the pelvis or around the kidney. The reported incidence of symptomatic lymphoceles ranges from 6% to 18% and is influenced by obesity, immunosuppression (mTOR inhibitors, steroids), and treatment of rejection (Goel et al, 2004). Most are asymptomatic and resolve spontaneously over several months. Clinical presentation may include abdominal swelling, ipsilateral leg edema, renal dysfunction, or lower urinary voiding symptoms depending upon which pelvic structures are being compressed. Simple aspiration tends to recur; definitive treatments include prolonged tube drainage, sclerotherapy (povidone iodine, fibrin

glue, tetracycline, etc), or marsupialization and drainage into the peritoneal cavity via laparoscopy or open surgery (Flechner, 2011).

B. Medical Complications

1. Bacterial infections—Renal failure and immunosuppression make recipients more susceptible to infections after the transplant that includes bacterial, viral, fungal, and opportunistic pathogens. It is not surprising that such infections occur more often during the first 6 months when doses of immunosuppression are greatest. It is therefore common practice to give recipients prophylaxis against those infective agents that occur with the greatest frequency. Bacterial urinary tract infections are the most common and are controlled by the use of daily prophylaxis with oral trimethoprim/sulfa for the first year. This antibiotic is particularly useful since it also provides excellent prophylaxis of *Pneumocystis carinii* pneumonia, an opportunistic infection that is usually restricted to transplant patients, or others immunocompromised by HIV–AIDS, cancer chemotherapy, etc. Breakthrough infections and transplant pyelonephritis need further workup to identity, obstruction, reflux, foreign body, stones, or voiding dysfunction.

2. Viral infections—One of the most significant advances in transplant practice during the last decades has been the control of viral infections, in particular the Herpes viruses (CMV, EBV, VZV, and HSV), which caused major morbidity and even mortality in past years. These DNA viruses are characterized by transmission from donor to host, resulting in primary infections, as well as reactivation of latent virus in the host (Rubin, 2001). Therefore, recipients that have had no prior exposure (serologically negative at transplant) are at the greatest risk for infections. CMV is the most frequently encountered pathogen (10–40% of recipients), and donor and recipient serology (anti-CMV IgG) define risk of infection (D+R– > D+R+ > D–R+ > D–R–) and treatment strategies (Flechner et al, 1998). The virus can cause an asymptomatic infection (viral DNA copies in the blood); CMV syndrome with fever and leukopenia; and tissue invasive disease with the liver, lung, gastrointestinal tract–colon, and retina often infected. The introduction of the potent nucleoside inhibitors—acyclovir, ganciclovir, and valganciclovir—has largely controlled these infections. Those who receive organs from CMV-positive donors or have had prior exposure are routinely given 3 months of prophylaxis with oral valganciclovir. Six months is recommended for the high-risk D+R– group (Humar et al, 2010). Some prefer the use of preemptive therapy, awaiting detection by screening for virus (Khoury et al, 2006). The use of intravenous ganciclovir is often coadministered with anti–T-cell antibodies for patients at risk.

3. Fungal infections—Candida urinary infections or esophagitis occur with some frequency, especially in diabetic patients. The use of oral fluconazole or Mycelex troche provides prophylaxis during the first few months. Systemic fungal infections are uncommon, but sporadic cases of aspergillosis, cryptococcosis, histoplasmosis, mucormycosis, etc, are reported. Invasive fungal infections usually require treatment with Amphotericin B, or its liposomal formulation.

4. Posttransplant diabetes—New onset diabetes after renal transplantation is a growing problem (10–20% of adults) that mimics the features of diabetes type 2. It is a result of both impaired insulin production as well as peripheral insulin resistance, and includes patients that have hyperglycemia responsive to oral agents as well as those that require exogenous insulin. It can be diagnosed up to several years after transplant and is attributed to the use of CNI drugs (tacrolimus > cyclosporine) as well as glucocorticoids. Family history, older age, weight gain, hyperlipidemia, sedentary lifestyle, and viral infections are contributing factors (Duclos et al, 2006).

5. Posttransplant cancer—Immunosuppression impairs immune surveillance, and not surprisingly, it is associated with an increased incidence of de novo cancers. In particular, those oncogenic viruses that are cleared by T cells become the primary agents that induce posttransplant cancers. These include EBV, HHV-8, HPV, and hepatitis B and C. Kasiske et al (2004) examined malignancy rates among first-time recipients of deceased or living donor kidney transplantations in 1995–2001 ($n = 35,765$) using Medicare billing claims. They found that compared with the general population, a 20-fold increase for non-Hodgkin's lymphomas (including PTLD), nonmelanoma skin cancers, and Kaposi's sarcoma; 15-fold for kidney cancers; 5-fold for melanoma, leukemia, hepatobiliary tumors, cervical tumors, and vulvovaginal tumors; 3-fold for testicular and bladder cancers; and 2-fold for most common tumors, for example, colon, lung, prostate, stomach, esophagus, pancreas, ovary, and breast. PTLDs comprise a spectrum of diseases characterized by lymphoid proliferation ranging from benign lymphoid hyperplasia to high-grade invasive lymphoma. Most PTLDs are B-cell lymphomas arising as a result of immunosuppression and many of these are associated with EBV infections. PTLD is reported to occur in up to 3% of adults and up to 10% of children after kidney or liver transplantation (Oplez et al, 2003). Registry data has emerged that identify the use of a depleting anti–T-cell antibody for induction therapy as a significant risk factor for PTLD (Opelz et al, 2006). Since the rates for most malignancies remain higher after kidney transplantation compared with the general population, cancer should continue to be a major focus of prevention.

BIBLIOGRAPHY

Adams P et al: The nondirected live-kidney donor: Ethical considerations and practice guidelines: A National Conference Report. Transplantation 2002;74:582–589.

Agarwal A et al: Comparison of HTK solution and University of Wisconsin solution in prolonged cold preservation of kidney allografts. Transplantation 2006;81:480–482.

Akalin E et al: Safety of using hepatitis B virus core antibody or surface antigen-positive donors in kidney or pancreas transplantation. Clin Transpl 2005;19:364–366.

Araki M et al: Posttransplant diabetes mellitus in kidney transplant recipients receiving calcineurin or mTOR inhibitor drugs. Transplantation 2006;81:335–341.

Argenta LC et al: Vacuum-assisted closure: State of clinic art. Plast Reconstr Surg 2006;117:127S–142S.

Armstrong K et al: Obesity is associated with worsening cardiovascular risk factor profiles and proteinuria progression in renal transplant recipients. Am J Transplant 2005;5:2710–2718.

Aroldi A et al: Natural history of hepatitis B and C in renal allograft recipients. Transplantation 2005;79:1132–1136.

Axelrod D et al: Kidney and pancreas transplantation in the United States, 1999–2008: The changing face of living donation. Am J Transplant 2010;10(Pt 2):987–1002.

Bloom R, Lake J: Emerging issues in hepatitis C virus-positive liver and kidney transplant recipients. Am J Transplant 2006;6(10):2232–2237.

Bresnahan BA et al: Risk factors for renal allograft survival from pediatric cadaver donors: An analysis of united network for organ sharing data. Transplantation 2001;72:256–261.

Bruno S et al: Transplant renal artery stenosis. J Am Soc Nephrol 2004;15:134–141.

Buinewicz B, Rosen B: Acellular cadaveric dermis (AlloDerm): A new alternative for abdominal hernia repair. Ann Plast Surg 2004;52:188–194.

Bunnapradist S et al: Dual kidneys from marginal adult donors as a source for cadaveric renal transplantation in the United States. J Am Soc Nephrol 2003;14:1031–1036.

Cecka JM: The OPTN/UNOS renal transplant registry. Clin Transpl 2004;1–12.

Cody J et al: Recombinant human erythropoietin for chronic renal failure anemia in pre-dialysis patients. Cochrane Database Syst Rev 2005;3:CD003266.

Colvin RB: Chronic allograft nephropathy. N Engl J Med 2003;349:2288–2293.

Colvin RB: Antibody-mediated renal allograft rejection: Diagnosis and pathogenesis. J Am Soc Nephrol 2007;18:1046–1056.

Couser W: Recurrent glomerulonephritis in the renal allograft: An update of selected areas. Exp Clin Transpl 2005;3:283–288.

Davis C: Evaluation of living kidney donor: Current perspectives. Am J Kidney Dis 2004;53:508–530.

Davis C, Delmonico F: Living-donor kidney transplantation: A review of the current practices for the live donor. J Am Soc Nephrol 2005;16:2098–2110.

Delmonico FL: Exchanging kidneys—Advances in living donor transplantation. N Engl J Med 2004;350:1812–1814.

Duclos A et al: Post transplant diabetes mellitus: Risk reducing strategies in the elderly. Drugs Aging 2006;23(9):1–13.

Eisen HJ et al: Everolimus for the prevention of allograft rejection and vasculopathy in cardiac-transplant recipients. N Engl J Med 2003;349:847–858.

Ekberg H et al: Cyclosporine sparing with mycophenolate mofetil, daclizumab and corticosteroids in renal allograft recipients: The CAESAR Study. Am J Transplant 2007;7:560–570.

El Fettouh HA et al: Early and late impact of a positive flow cytometry crossmatch on graft outcome in primary renal transplantation. Transplant Proc 2001;33:2968–2970.

Ellison MD et al: Living kidney donors in need of kidney transplants: A report from the OPTN. Transplantation 2002;74:1349–1351.

Fehrman-Ekholm I et al: Kidney donors live longer. Transplantation 1997;64:976–978.

Figlin RA: Mechanisms of disease: Survival benefit of temsirolimus validates a role for mTOR in the management of advanced RCC. Nat Clin Pract Oncol 2008;5:601–609.

Fisher P et al: 200 consecutive hand assisted laparoscopic donor nephrectomies: Evolution of operative technique and outcomes. J Urol 2006;175:1439–1443.

Flechner SM et al: Intermittent clean catheterization: An alternative to diversion in continent renal transplant recipients with lower urinary tract dysfunction. J Urol 1983;130:878–880.

Flechner SM et al: A prospective randomized, controlled trial of oral acyclovir vs. oral ganciclovir for CMV prophylaxis in high risk kidney transplant recipients. Transplantation 1998;66:1682–1688.

Flechner SM: Transplantation in the Elderly. Will You Still List Me When I'm 64? J Am Geriatr Soc 2002;50:195–197.

Flechner SM, Novick AC: Renal transplantation. In: Gillenwater JY et al (eds) Adult and Pediatric Urology, 4th edn. Lippincott Williams & Wilkins, Philadelphia, PA, 2002, pp. 907–972, Chapter 22.

Flechner SM et al: The impact of sirolimus, mycophenolate mofetil, cyclosporine, azathioprine, and steroids on wound healing in 513 kidney transplant recipients. Transplantation 2003;76:1729–1734.

Flechner SM et al: De novo kidney transplantation without use of calcineurin inhibitors preserves renal structure and function at two years. Am J Transplantation 2004;4:1776–1785.

Flechner SM, Duclos A: Renal transplantation. In: Montague DK et al (eds) Reconstructive Urologic Surgery: Adult and Pediatric. Taylor and Francis Books Ltd, Oxford, 2008, pp. 133–142, Chapter 15.

Flechner SM: Sirolimus in kidney transplantation Indications and practical guidelines: De novo sirolimus based therapy without calcineurin inhibitors. Transplantation 2009;87:S1–S6.

Flechner SM et al: The role of proteasome inhibition with bortezomib in the treatment of antibody mediated rejection after kidney-only or kidney-combined organ transplantation. Transplantation 2010;90(12):1486–1492.

Flechner SM et al: Basic principles of immunology in urology. In Campbell's Urology, 10th edn, Vol. 1, Chapter 17. Elsevier Health Sciences, Philadelphia, PA, 2011 (in press).

Flechner SM: Surgical complications after kidney transplantation. In: Srinivas T, Shoskes D (eds) Kidney and Pancreas Transplantation—A Practical Guide. Humana Press, Springer-Science, New York, 2011, pp. 281–299, Chapter 15.

Fusaro F et al: CMV and BKV ureteritis: Which prognosis for the renal graft? J Nephrol 2003;16:591–594.

Ghasemian S et al: Bilateral laparoscopic radical nephrectomy for renal tumors in patients with acquired cystic kidney disease. J Laparoendosc Adv Surg Tech A 2005;15:606–610.

Goel M et al: The influence of various maintenance immunosuppressive drugs on lymphocele formation and treatment after kidney transplantation. J Urol 2004;171:1788–1792.

Gore J et al: Obesity and outcome following renal transplantation. Am J Transplant 2006;6:357–363.

Guba M et al: Rapamycin inhibits primary and metastatic tumor growth by antiangiogenesis: Involvement of vascular endothelial growth factor. Nat Med 2002;8:128.

Halloran PF: Immunosuppressive drugs for kidney transplantation. N Engl J Med 2004;351:2715–2729.

Hatch DA et al: Fate of renal allograft transplanted in patients with urinary diversion. Transplantation 1993;56:838–843.

Herzog CA et al: Comparative survival of dialysis patients in the United States after coronary angioplasty, coronary artery stenting, and coronary artery bypass surgery and impact of diabetes. Circulation 2002;106:2207–2221.

Hobart MG: Transplantation of pediatric en bloc cadaver kidneys into adult recipients. Transplantation 1998;66:1689–1694.

Hourmant M et al: Frequency and clinical implications of development of donor-specific and non-donor-specific HLA antibodies after kidney transplantation. J Am Soc Nephrol 2005;16:2804–2812.

Humar A et al: Are wound complications after a kidney transplant more common with modern immunosuppression? Transplantation 2001;72:1920.

Humar A et al: Risk factors for slow graft function after kidney transplants: A multivariate analysis. Clin Transpl 2002;16:425–429.

Humar A et al: Extended valganciclovir prophylaxis in D+/R- kidney transplant recipients is associated with long-term reduction in cytomegalovirus disease: Two-year results of the IMPACT study. Transplantation 2010;90:1427–1431.

Hume DM et al: Renal homotransplantation in man in modified recipients. Ann Surg 1963;158:608–613.

Ibrahim H et al: Long-term consequences of kidney donation. N Engl J Med 2009;360:459–469.

Ismail HR et al: Simultaneous vs. sequential laparoscopic bilateral native nephrectomy and renal transplantation. Transplantation 2005;80:1124–1127.

Ismail HR, Flechner SM: Expanded criteria donors: An emerging source of kidneys to alleviate the organ shortage. Curr Opin Organ Transplant 2006;11:395–400.

Jacobs CL et al: Twenty two nondirected kidney donors: An update on a single center's experience. Am J Transplant 2004;4:1110–1116.

Jackson T et al: Management of asymptomatic cholelithiasis for patients awaiting renal transplantation. Surg Endosc 2005;19:510–513.

Jamieson NV: A 20-year experience of combined liver/kidney transplantation for primary hyperoxaluria (PH1): The European PH1 transplant registry experience 1984–2004. Am J Nephrol 2005;25:282–289.

Joseph JT et al: Quality of life after kidney and pancreas transplantation. Am J Kidney Dis 2003;42(3):431–445.

Josephson MA et al: Treatment of renal allograft polyoma BK virus infection with leflunomide. Transplantation 2006;81:704–710.

Kapoor A et al: Multi-spiral computed tomographic angiography of renal arteries of live potential renal donors: A review of 118 cases. Transplantation 2004;77:1535–1539.

Kasiske BL et al: Long-term effects of reduced renal mass in humans. Kidney Int 1995;48:814–819.

Kasiske BL et al: Preemptive kidney transplantation: The advantage and the advantaged. J Am Soc Nephrol 2002;13:1358–1364.

Kasiske BL et al: Cancer after kidney transplantation in the United States. Am J Transplant 2004;4:905–913.

Kattan M: A nomogram for predicting 10-year life expectancy in men with prostate cancer after definitive therapy. Nat Clin Pract Urol 2008;5(3):138–139.

Kaufman DB et al: Alemtuzumab induction and prednisone-free maintenance immunotherapy in kidney transplantation: Comparison with basiliximab induction–long-term results. Am J Transplant 2005;5:2539–2548.

Khauli RB et al: Treatment of lymphocele and lymphatic fistula following renal transplantation by laparoscopic peritoneal window. J Urol 1992;147:1353–1355.

Khoury JA et al: Prophylactic versus preemptive oral valganciclovir for the management of cytomegalovirus infection in adult renal transplant recipients. Am J Transplant 2006;6:2134–2143.

Khwaja K et al: Outcome at 3 years with a prednisone-free maintenance regimen: A single-center experience with 349 kidney transplant recipients. Am J Transplant 2004;4:980–987.

Klein A et al: Organ donation and utilization in the United States, 1999–2008. Am J Transplant 2010;10:973–986.

Kreiger N et al: Chronic allograft nephropathy uniformly affects recipients of cadaveric, nonidentical living related, and living-unrelated grafts. Transplantation 2003;75:1677–1682.

Larsen C et al: Belatacept-based regimens versus a cyclosporine A-based regimen in kidney transplant recipients: 2-year results from the BENEFIT and BENEFIT-EXT studies. Transplantation 2010;90:1528–1535.

Lefaucheur C et al: Preexisting donor-specific HLA antibodies predict outcome in kidney transplantation. J Am Soc Nephrol 2010; 21:1398–1406.

Lentine K et al: Racial variation in medical outcomes among living kidney donors. N Engl J Med 2010;363:724–732.

Matsuoka L et al: Pulsatile perfusion of kidney allografts. Curr Opin Organ Transplant 2009;14:365–369.

McCune TR et al: Sensitized patients require sharing of highly matched kidneys. Transplantation 2002;73:1891–1896.

Meier-Kriesche H et al: Lack of improvement in renal allograft survival despite a marked decrease in acute rejection rates over the most recent era. Am J Transplant 2004;4:378–383.

Meier-Kriesche HU, Kaplan B: Waiting time on dialysis as the strongest modifiable risk factor for renal transplant outcomes: A paired donor kidney analysis. Transplantation 2002;74:1377–1381.

Mendizabal S et al: Renal transplantation in children with severe bladder dysfunction. J Urol 2004;173:226–229.

Modanlou K et al: Bariatric surgery among kidney transplant candidates and recipients: Analysis of the United States renal data system and literature review. Transplantation 2009;87:1167–1173.

Modlin CS et al: Should obese patients lose weight prior to receiving a kidney transplant? Transplantation 1997;64:599–604.

Moinzadeh A, Gill I: Living laparoscopic donor nephrectomy. In: Novick AC, Jones SA (eds) Operative Urology at the Cleveland Clinic. Humana Press, Totowa, NJ, 2006, pp. 117–120, Chapter 10.

Montgomery RA et al: Clinical results from transplanting incompatible live kidney donor/recipient pairs using kidney paired donation. JAMA 2005;294:1655–1663.

Montgomery RA et al: ABO incompatible renal transplantation: A paradigm ready for broad implementation. Transplantation 2009; 87:1246–1255.

Morice M-C et al: A randomized comparison of a sirolimus eluting stent with a standard stent for coronary revascularization. N Engl J Med 2002;346:1773–1780.

Mylonakis E et al: BK virus in solid organ transplant recipients: An emerging syndrome. Transplantation 2001;72:1587–1592.

Nahas W et al: Augmentation cystoplasty in renal transplantation: A good and safe option–experience with 25 cases. Urology 2002; 60:770–774.

Nankivell B et al: The natural history of chronic allograft nephropathy. N Engl J Med 2003;349:2326–2333.

Narkun-Burgess DM et al: Forty-five year follow-up after uninephrectomy. Kidney Int 1993;43:1110–1115.

North American Pediatric Renal Transplant Cooperative Study (NAPRTCS) 2009 Annual Report. Available at http://www.naprtcs .org.

Opelz G et al: Disassociation between risk of graft loss and risk of non-Hodgkin lymphoma with induction agents in renal transplant recipients. Transplantation 2006;81:1227–1233.

Opelz G, Dohler B: Lymphomas after solid organ transplantation: A Collaborative Transplant Study Report. Am J Transplant 2003;4: 222–230.

Orth SR: Effects of smoking on systemic and intrarenal hemodynamics: Influence on renal function. J Am Soc Nephrol 2004;15 (Suppl 1):S58–S63.

Pascual J et al: Steroid withdrawal in renal transplant patients on triple therapy with a calcineurin inhibitor and mycophenolate mofetil: A meta-analysis of randomized, controlled trials. Transplantation 2004;78:1548–1556.

Penn I. Evaluation of transplant candidates with pre-existing malignancies. Ann Transplant 1997;2:14–17.

Pilmore H, Pilmore H. Cardiac assessment for renal transplantation. Am J Transplant 2006;6:659–665.

Port FK et al: Recent trends and results for organ donation and transplantation in the United States, 2005. Am J Transplant 2006;6(5, Pt 2):1095–1100.

Racusen LC et al: The Banff working classification of renal allograft pathology. Kidney Int 1999;55:713–723.

Rees MA et al: A nonsimultaneous, extended, altruistic-donor chain. N Engl J Med 2009;360:1096–1101.

Rigamonti W et al: Kidney transplantation into bladder augmentation or urinary diversion: Long-term results. Transplantation 2005;80:1435–1440.

Rogers J et al: Results of simultaneous and sequential pediatric liver and kidney transplantation. Transplantation 2001;72:1666–1670.

Rosengard BR et al: Report of the crystal city meeting to maximize the use of organs recovered from the cadaver donor. Am J Transplant 2002;2:1–10.

Rowshani AT et al: No difference in degree of interstitial sirius Red-stained area in serial biopsies from AUC over time curves-guided CsA vs. tac treated renal transplant recipients at one year. J Am Soc Nephrol 2006;17:305–312.

Rubin RH: Cytomegalovirus in solid organ transplantation. Transpl Infect Dis 2001;3(Suppl 2):1–5.

Rudich SM et al: Renal transplantations performed using non-heart-beating organ donors: Going back to the future? Transplantation 2002;74:1715–1720.

Russ G et al: Superior outcomes in renal transplantation after early cyclosporine withdrawal and sirolimus maintenance therapy, regardless of baseline renal function. Transplantation 2005;80: 1204–1211.

Schold JD et al: Are we frozen in time? Analysis of the utilization and efficacy of pulsatile perfusion in renal transplantation. Am J Transplant 2005;5:1681–1688.

Segev DL et al: Kidney paired donation and optimizing the use of live donor organs. JAMA 2005;293:1883–1890.

Serrano D et al: Transplantation into the long-term defunctionalized bladder. J Urol 1996;156:885–888.

Shah A et al: Comparison of pulsatile perfusion and cold storage for paired kidney allografts. Transplantation 2008;86:1006–1009.

Shore ND et al: A temporary intraurethral prostatic stent relieves prostatic obstruction following transurethral microwave thermotherapy. J Urol 2007;177(3):1040–1046.

Shoskes DA, Cecka JM: Effect of delayed graft function on short- and long-term kidney graft survival. Clin Transpl 1997;11:297–303.

Stock PG et al: Outcomes of kidney transplantation in HIV-infected recipients. N Engl J Med 2010;363:2004–2014.

Streeter E et al: The urological complications of renal transplantation: A series of 1535 patients. BJU Int 2002;90:627–634.

Tedesco-Silva H et al: 12-month safety and efficacy of everolimus with reduced exposure cyclosporine in de novo renal transplant recipients. Transpl Int 2007;20:27–36.

Thomsen HS: Nephrogenic systemic fibrosis: History and epidemiology. Radiol Clin North Am 2009;47(5):827–831.

Tozawa M et al: Influence of smoking and obesity on the development of proteinuria. Kidney Int 2002;62:956–962.

Turner-Warwick RT: The supracostal approach to the renal area. Br J Urol 1965;37:671–672.

UNOS Web page: Available at http://optn.transplant.hrsa.gov.

United States Renal Data System: 2010 Annual Data Report. Available at http://www.usrds.org/2010/ADR_booklet_2010_lowres.pdf.

van Roijen JH et al: Long-term graft survival after urological complications of 695 kidney transplantations. J Urol 2001;165:1884–1887.

Vincent F et al: Five-year safety and efficacy of belatacept in renal transplantation. J Am Soc Nephrol 2010;21:1587–1596.

Welsh R et al: Cardiovascular assessment of diabetic end-stage renal disease patients before renal transplantation. Transplantation 2011; 91:213–218.

Westesson K et al: The role of embolization prior to transplant nephrectomy to reduce transfusion requirements and sensitization. Am J Transplant 2011;11(S2):1284.

Wilson CH et al: Routine intraoperative stenting for renal transplant recipients. Transplantation 2005;80:877–882.

Wolfe RA et al: Comparison of mortality in all patients on dialysis, patients on dialysis awaiting transplantation, and recipients of a first cadaver transplant. N Engl J Med 1999;341:1725–1730.

Wolfe RA et al: Trends in organ donation and transplantation in the United States, 1999–2008. Am J Transplant 2010;10(4, Pt 2):961–972.

Woodle ES et al: A prospective, randomized, double-blind, placebo-controlled multicenter trial comparing early (7 day) corticosteroid cessation versus long-term, low-dose corticosteroid therapy. Ann Surg 2008;248:564–577.

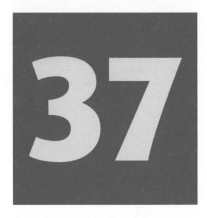

37

Disorders of the Ureter & Ureteropelvic Junction

Barry A. Kogan, MD

The ureter is a complex functional conduit carrying urine from the kidneys to the bladder. Any pathologic process that interferes with this activity can cause renal abnormalities, the most common sequels being hydronephrosis (see Chapter XXX) and infection. Disorders of the ureter can be classified as congenital or acquired.

CONGENITAL ANOMALIES OF THE URETER

Congenital ureteral malformations are common and range from complete absence to duplication of the ureter. They may cause severe obstruction requiring urgent attention, or they may be asymptomatic and of no clinical significance. The nomenclature can be confusing and has been standardized to prevent ambiguity (Glassberg et al, 1984).

URETERAL ATRESIA

The ureter may be absent entirely, or it may end blindly after extending only part of the way to the flank. These anomalies are caused during embryologic development, by failure of the ureteral bud to form from the mesonephric duct or by an arrest in its development before it comes in contact with the metanephric blastema. The genetic determinants of ureteral bud development and the causes of bud abnormalities are being elucidated and it is known that GDNF signaling via the RET receptor is generally required (Michos et al, 2010). In any event, the end result of an atretic ureteral bud is an absent or multicystic dysplastic kidney. The multicystic kidney is usually unilateral and asymptomatic and of no clinical significance. In rare cases, it can be associated with hypertension, infection, or tumor. Contralateral vesicoureteral reflux is common, and many clinicians recommend a voiding cystourethrogram as part of the initial workup. There has been a concern about the risk of malignancy in these cases; however, the preponderance of evidence now suggests that no treatment is necessary and indeed no

follow-up is needed from a urological standpoint (Onal and Kogan, 2006).

DUPLICATION OF THE URETER

Complete or incomplete duplication of the ureter is one of the most common congenital malformations of the urinary tract. Nation (1944) found some form of duplication of the ureter in 0.9% of a series of autopsies. The condition occurs more frequently in females than in males and is often bilateral.

Incomplete (Y) type of duplication is caused by branching of the ureteral bud before it reaches the metanephric blastema. In most cases, this anomaly is associated with no clinical abnormality. However, disorders of peristalsis may occur near the point of union (Figure 37–1).

In complete duplication of the ureter, the presence of two ureteral buds leads to the formation of two totally separate ureters and two separate renal pelves. Because the ureter to the upper segment arises from a cephalad position on the mesonephric duct, it remains attached to the mesonephric duct longer and consequently migrates farther, ending medial and inferior to the ureter draining the lower segment (Weigert-Meyer law). Thus, the ureter draining the upper segment may migrate too far caudally and become ectopic and obstructed, whereas the ureter draining the lower segment may end laterally and have a short intravesical tunnel that leads to vesicoureteral reflux (Figure 37–2) (Tanagho, 1976). More recent studies have suggested that apoptosis of the common nephric duct cells is essential for separation of the ureter from the Wolffian duct; failure of this likely is the root cause of an ectopic ureter (Mendelsohn, 2009). Moreover, it is the urogenital sinus that induces this apoptosis and separation, and it appears that the upper ureteral bud may, in some cases, be too far from the urogenital sinus to receive the signal, thereby failing to separate from the Wolffian duct.

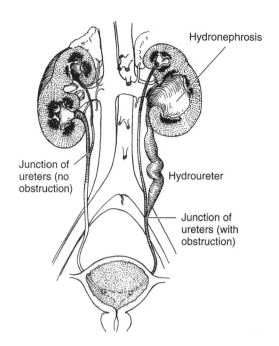

▲ Figure 37–1. Duplication of the ureter. Incomplete (Y) type with hydronephrosis of lower pole of left kidney. Ureteroureteral (yo-yo) reflux can also occur and account for the radiographic appearance.

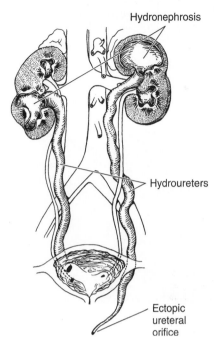

▲ Figure 37–2. Duplication of the ureter. Complete duplication with reflux to lower pole of right kidney and chronic pyelonephritic scarring. Upper-pole ureter of left kidney is ectopic, and its associated renal parenchyma is often dysplastic.

Although many patients with duplication of the ureter are asymptomatic, a common presentation is persistent or recurrent infections. In females, the ureter to the upper pole may be ectopic, with an opening distal to the external sphincter or even outside the urinary tract. Such patients have classic symptoms: incontinence characterized by constant dribbling and at the same time, a normal pattern of voiding. In males, because the mesonephric duct becomes the vas and seminal vesicles, the ectopic ureter is always proximal to the external sphincter, and associated incontinence does not occur. In recent years, prenatal ultrasonography has led to the diagnosis in many asymptomatic neonates.

At the present time, ultrasound is the study of choice in these children. Generally, a hydronephrotic upper pole and a dilated distal ureter are seen, and in addition, one can readily evaluate parenchymal thickness and the presence of a ureterocele or other bladder anomalies. A voiding cystourethrogram is important to determine the presence of vesicoureteral reflux and confirm the presence of a ureterocele. Renal scanning (especially with ^{99m}Tc-dimercaptosuccinic acid) is helpful for estimating the degree of renal function in each renal segment (Figure 37–3).

The treatment of reflux is controversial (Chapter XXXX), but the treatment should not be influenced by the presence of ureteral duplication. Lower grades of reflux are generally treated medically and higher grades of reflux are more likely to be treated surgically. Because of anatomic variations, many surgical options are available. If upper-pole obstruction or ectopy is present, surgery is almost always required. Numerous operative approaches have been recommended (Belman et al, 1974). If renal function in one segment is very poor, heminephrectomy is the most appropriate procedure. In an effort to preserve renal parenchyma, treatments by pyeloureterostomy, ureteroureterostomy, and ureteral reimplantation are all appropriate (Amar, 1970, 1978). This can be done laparoscopically or open (Lowe et al, 2008; Prieto et al, 2009).

URETEROCELE

A ureterocele is a sacculation of the terminal portion of the ureter (Figure 37–4). It may be either intravesical or ectopic; in the latter case, some portion is located at the bladder neck or in the urethra. Intravesical ureteroceles are associated most often with single ureters, whereas ectopic ureteroceles nearly always involve the upper pole of duplicated ureters. Ectopic ureteroceles are four times more common than those

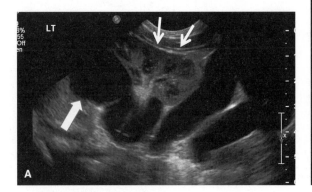

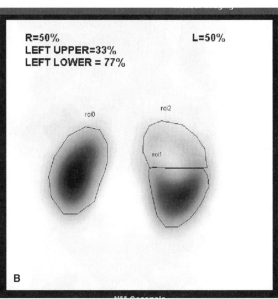

▲ **Figure 37–3.** Duplicated left kidney. *A:* Ultrasound showing marked hydronephrosis of the left upper pole (*large arrow*) in continuity with a large tortuous ureter. The lower pole of the kidney is well preserved (*small arrows*). *B:* 99mTc-DMSA scan showing the relative function of the different renal segments.

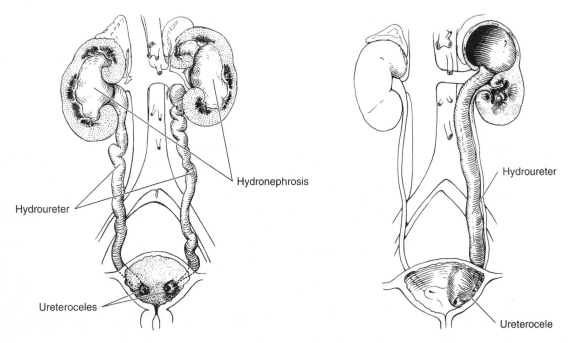

▲ **Figure 37–4.** Ureterocele. *Left:* Orthotopic ureterocele associated with a single ureter. *Right:* Ureterocele associated with ureteral duplication and poor function of upper pole of kidney.

that are intravesical (Snyder and Johnston, 1978). Ureterocele occurs seven times more often in girls than in boys, and about 10% of cases are bilateral. Mild forms of ureterocele are found occasionally in adults examined for unrelated reasons.

Ureterocele has been attributed to delayed or incomplete canalization of the ureteral bud leading to an early prenatal obstruction and expansion of the ureteral bud prior to its absorption into the urogenital sinus (Tanagho, 1976). The cystic dilation forms between the superficial and deep muscle layers of the trigone. Large ureteroceles may displace the other orifices, interfere with the muscular backing of the bladder, or even obstruct the bladder outlet. There is nearly always significant hydroureteronephrosis, and a dysplastic segment of the upper pole of the kidney may be found in association with a ureterocele.

Clinical findings vary considerably. In the past, patients presented with infection, bladder outlet obstruction, or incontinence (and rarely a ureterocele may prolapse through the female urethra). However, most of the current cases are diagnosed by antenatal maternal ultrasound. After birth, sonography and voiding cystourethrography should be performed. The former confirms the diagnosis and defines the renal anatomy and the latter demonstrates whether there is reflux into the lower pole or contralateral ureter (Figures 37–5 and 37–6). Renal scanning is helpful for estimating renal function and the combination of findings is critical in planning therapy.

Treatment must be individualized. Transurethral incision has been recognized as the definitive procedure in many instances, particularly in patients with intravesical ureteroceles and may be the initial therapy in neonates. When an open operation is needed, the procedure must be chosen on the basis of the anatomic location of the ureteral meatus, the position of the ureterocele, and the degree of hydroureteronephrosis and impairment of renal function. In general, choices range from heminephrectomy and ureterectomy to excision of the ureterocele, vesical reconstruction, and ureteral reimplantation. When the ureterocele is ectopic, definitive treatment often entails excision of the ureterocele and reconstruction (Wang, 2008). Often, more than one procedure is necessary.

ECTOPIC URETERAL ORIFICE

Although an ectopic ureteral orifice most commonly occurs in association with duplication of the ureter (see preceding sections), single ectopic ureters do occur. They are caused by a delay or failure of separation of the ureteral bud from the mesonephric duct during embryologic development. Again, the genetic determinants of these ureteral bud abnormalities are currently being determined, but at least GDNF signaling via the RET receptor is needed and apoptosis of the common nephric duct is critical (Michos et al, 2010). In anatomic terms, the primary anomaly may be an abnormally located ureteral bud; that also explains the high incidence of dysplastic kidneys associated with single ectopic ureters.

The clinical picture varies according to the sex of the patient and the position of the ureteral opening. Boys are seen because of urinary tract infection or epididymitis. In these cases, the ureter may drain directly into the vas deferens or seminal vesicle. In girls, the ureteral orifice may be in the urethra, vagina, or perineum. Although infection may be present, incontinence is the rule. Continual dribbling despite normal voiding is pathognomonic, but urgency and urge incontinence may confound the diagnosis.

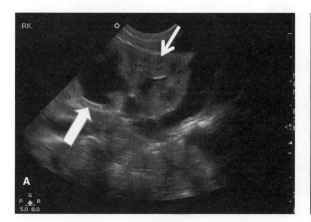 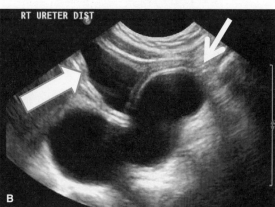

▲ **Figure 37–5.** Ureterocele in a girl with a duplication. **A:** Ultrasound showing marked hydronephrosis of the right upper pole (*large arrow*). The lower pole of the kidney is well preserved (*small arrow*). **B:** In contrast to an ectopic ureter, the dilated distal right ureter ends in a large ureterocele (*small arrow*) within the bladder (*large arrow*).

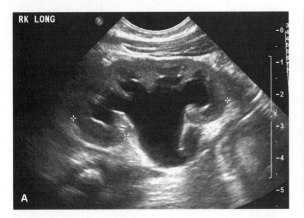

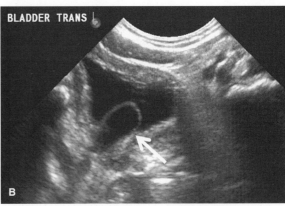

▲ **Figure 37–6.** Ureterocele in a boy with a single system. **A:** Ultrasound showing moderate right hydronephrosis with a dilated proximal ureter. **B:** The right distal ureter ends in a small orthotopic ureterocele within the bladder (*arrow*).

Sonography and voiding cystourethrography help delineate the problem. If the ureter is ectopic to the urethra, the ectopic ureter may be seen on the voiding film from the voiding cystourethrography (Figure 37–7). However, because an ectopic kidney may be both tiny and in an abnormal location, it may be difficult to find by ultrasound, and magnetic resonance imaging, cystoscopy, or laparoscopy may be necessary to confirm the diagnosis (Lipson et al, 2008). During cystoscopy, a hemitrigone may be seen and the ectopic orifice may be visualized directly or demonstrated by retrograde catheterization. Renal scanning is also helpful in estimating relative renal function. As in ureteroceles and duplication of the ureter, the clinical picture and the degree of renal function dictate the therapeutic approach.

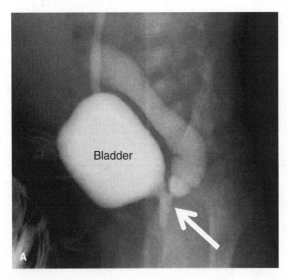

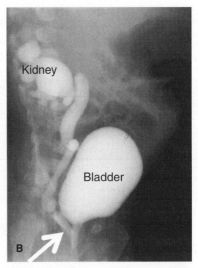

▲ **Figure 37–7.** Ectopic ureter. **A:** Voiding cystourethrogram in a boy showing voiding into the posterior urethra with reflux into a very dilated ureter, seen entering the prostatic urethra (*arrow*). **B:** A voiding cystourethrogram in a girl showing voiding with reflux into a very dilated ureter and continuing all the way up to a dilated lower pole of the right kidney. Note that the ureter is ectopic, entering the proximal urethra (*arrow*).

ABNORMALITIES OF URETERAL POSITION

Retrocaval ureter (also called circumcaval ureter and postcaval ureter) is a rare condition in which an embryologically normal ureter becomes entrapped behind the vena cava because of abnormal persistence of the right subcardinal (as opposed to the supracardinal) vein. This forces the right ureter to encircle the vena cava from behind. The ureter descends normally to approximately the level of L3, where it curves back upward in the shape of a reverse J to pass behind and around the vena cava (Figure 37–8). Obstruction generally results.

The diagnosis of retrocaval ureter is still made by excretory urography in some cases. However, since sonography is now usually the first test performed, the radiologist must be suspicious of the anomaly based on a dilated proximal (but not distal) ureter. Currently, magnetic resonance imaging may be the best single study to delineate the anatomy clearly and noninvasively. Surgical repair for retrocaval ureter, when indicated, consists of dividing the ureter (preferably across the dilated portion), bringing the distal ureter from behind the vena cava, and reanastomosing it to the proximal end. The procedure has been performed laparoscopically to reduce morbidity (Bagheri, 2009).

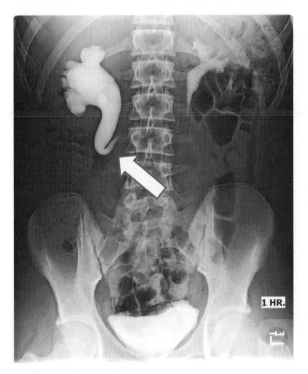

▲ **Figure 37–8.** Retrocaval ureter. An intravenous urogram showing the classic appearance of a J-hooking of the ureter behind the inferior vena cava (*arrow*).

OBSTRUCTION OF THE URETEROPELVIC JUNCTION

In children, primary obstruction of the ureter usually occurs at the ureteropelvic junction or the ureterovesical junction (Figure 37–9). Obstruction of the ureteropelvic junction is probably the most common congenital abnormality of the ureter. In children, it is seen more often in boys than in girls (5:2 ratio), but it has recently been discovered that in adults, it is more common in women than in men (Capello, 2005). In unilateral cases, it is more often on the left than on the right side (5:2 ratio). Bilateral obstruction occurs in 10–15% of cases and is especially common in infants (Johnston et al, 1977). The abnormality may occur in several members of the same family, but it shows no clear genetic pattern.

The exact cause of obstruction of the ureteropelvic junction often is not clear. Ureteral polyps and valves are seen but are rare. There is almost always an angulation and kink at the junction of the dilated renal pelvis and ureter. This by itself can cause obstruction, but it is unclear whether this is primary or merely secondary to another obstructive lesion. True stenosis is found rarely; however, a thin-walled, hypoplastic proximal ureter is observed frequently. Characteristic histologic and ultrastructural changes are observed in this area and could account for abnormal peristalsis through the ureteropelvic junction and consequent interference with pelvic emptying (Hanna et al, 1976). Current basic research suggests that decreased BMP4 signaling leads to disruption of smooth muscle investment of the ureter and may be involved (Wang, 2009). In addition, there seems to be an overexpression of extracellular matrix and depleted numbers of nerves (Kaya et al, 2010). Two other findings sometimes seen at operation are a high origin of the ureter from the renal pelvis and an abnormal relationship of the proximal ureter to a lower-pole renal artery. It is debatable whether these findings are the cause or the result of pelvic dilatation, but Stephens (1982) has suggested that abnormal rotation of the renal pelvis allows the ureter to become entrapped in the blood vessels of the lower pole of the kidney, ultimately leading to obstruction. Using careful studies at the time of operation, it is possible to define whether the principal lesion is intrinsic or extrinsic (Johnston, 1969; Koff et al, 1986).

Clinical findings vary depending on the patient's age at diagnosis. Many cases are now diagnosed in utero. These tend to be primarily intrinsic lesions and many resolve spontaneously. Later, pain and vomiting are the most common symptoms; however, hematuria and urinary infection also may be seen. A few patients have complications such as calculi, trauma to the enlarged kidney (Figure 37–10), or (rarely) hypertension. Most of the latter are extrinsic lesions but it is unclear whether they originated from intrinsic problems earlier in development.

The diagnosis is made most often by sonography. In equivocal cases, diuretic renography or (rarely) antegrade urography with pressure-flow studies is helpful (Thrall et al, 1981;

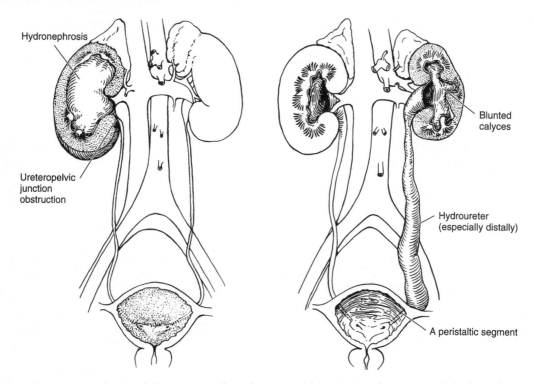

▲ **Figure 37–9.** Congenital ureteral obstruction. *Left:* Right ureteropelvic junction obstruction with hydronephrosis. *Right:* Left ureterovesical junction obstruction (obstructed megaureter) with hydroureteronephrosis.

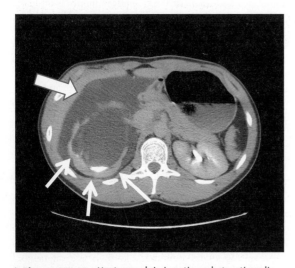

▲ **Figure 37–10.** Ureteropelvic junction obstruction discovered after trauma. CT scan in an 18-year-old boy performed after abdominal trauma shows a markedly hydronephrotic right kidney (*small arrows*) and a urinoma due to urinary extravasation from a rupture of the renal pelvis (*large arrow*).

Whitaker, 1973) (Figure 37–11). Many surgeons consider a voiding cystourethrogram a routine part of the preoperative workup, since radiographic findings in vesicoureteral reflux may be similar to those in ureteropelvic junction obstruction. This fact is especially relevant when the ureter is well seen or dilated (or both) below the ureteropelvic junction.

Symptomatic obstruction of the ureteropelvic junction should be treated surgically. Because most cases are now detected by hydronephrosis on prenatal ultrasonography and the infants are asymptomatic, it becomes important to assess the significance of the hydronephrosis. On the one hand, early surgery may prevent future urinary tract infections, stones, or other complications; on the other hand, many of the patients could live their whole lives without experiencing a consequence of the hydronephrosis. This remains an area of considerable controversy. Early surgery is recommended for patients who have kidneys with diminished function, massive hydronephrosis, infection, or stones. Nonoperative surveillance with good follow-up is thought to be safe, although about 25% of patients will ultimately require an operative repair for pain, urinary infection, or reduced renal function on repeat nuclear scan. Clinicians and scientists are searching for biomarkers of obstruction, and urinary proteome analysis seems promising (Drube et al, 2010). This subject remains

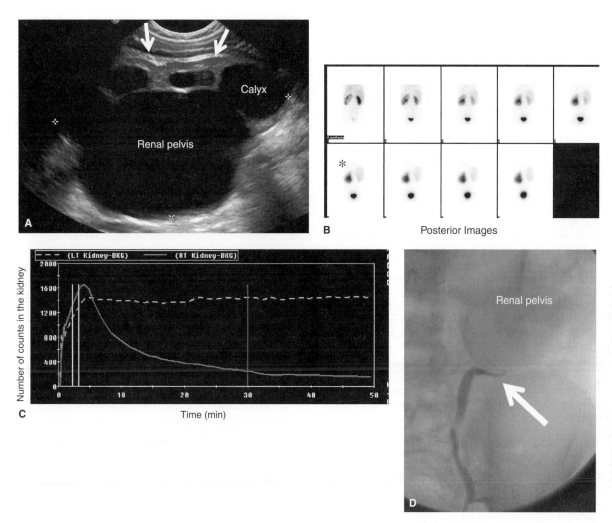

▲ **Figure 37–11.** Ureteropelvic junction obstruction after prenatal hydronephrosis. **A:** An ultrasound shows marked hydronephrosis with a large renal pelvis and dilated calyces. There is some preservation of renal parenchyma (*arrows*). **B:** Images taken every 5 minutes from the 99mTc-MAG-3 diuretic renogram showing good function on the left kidney, but hydronephrosis and slow drainage from the kidney. The *asterisk* indicates when furosemide is given. Of note, there is no increase in drainage from the left kidney after furosemide. **C:** The computer calculated time/activity curves from the renogram pictures. Both kidneys have good function (high counts in the first couple of minutes). The right kidney (*solid line*) excretes the radioisotope rapidly. There is poor drainage of the left kidney (*dotted line*). **D:** A retrograde pyelogram demonstrates a normal ureter with obstruction at the ureteropelvic junction (*arrow*) and a large renal pelvis above the obstruction.

particularly controversial, but there are some data suggesting that early childhood treatment reduces the risk of ureteropelvic junction obstruction in adults (Capello, 2005).

Because of anatomic variations, no single procedure is sufficient for all situations (Smart, 1979). Regardless of the technique used, all successful repairs have in common the creation of a dependent and funnel-shaped ureteropelvic junction of adequate caliber. Although preservation of the intact ureteropelvic junction is feasible in some circumstances, when the obstruction appears to be caused by a dyskinetic segment of proximal ureter, the most popular operation is a dismembered pyeloureteroplasty (Anderson, 1963). Dismembered pyeloureteroplasty is also favored when the proximal ureter is hooked over a lower-pole blood vessel. When there is a dilated extrarenal renal pelvis, dismembered pyeloureteroplasty can be combined with a Foley Y-V plasty to create a more funnel-shaped ureteropelvic junction (Foley, 1937). Pelvic flap procedures (Culp and DeWeerd, 1951; Scardino and Prince, 1953) are suited ideally to cases in which the ureteropelvic junction has remained in a dependent position despite significant pelvic dilatation. They also have the advantage of interfering less with the ureteral blood supply; this is particularly relevant when distal ureteral surgery (eg, ureteral reimplantation) is contemplated in the future. In most centers, the dismembered pyeloureteroplasty is the mainstay of repairs.

Both the Y-V plasty and the flap techniques are useful in managing ureteropelvic junction obstructions in horseshoe or pelvic kidneys, in which the anatomy may prevent creation of a dependent ureteropelvic junction if a dismembered technique is attempted. The use of stenting catheters and proximal diversion at the time of pyeloplasty has been the subject of debate, and the issue has not been resolved. Excellent results have been reported both with and without stents and diversions (Smith et al, 2002).

The prognosis is generally good. In several large series, the reported reoperation rate has been only 2–4%, but the postoperative radiographic appearance of the area may be disappointing. There can be marked improvement when a large extrarenal pelvis has prevented massive calyceal distortion; however, in most cases, considerable deformity persists despite adequate drainage of the kidney. Furthermore, it is usually many years before the radiographic appearance improves.

The progressive move to minimally invasive surgery has resulted in a number of trends in the repair of ureteropelvic junction obstruction. Endopyelotomy can be performed percutaneously or via ureteroscopy and treats the problem by incising directly through the obstruction, stenting the area and allowing healing via secondary intention. The technique is similar to that reported by Davis (1943) but is done entirely endoscopically. Unfortunately, the success rate is only 80–85% at best, and currently, it is primarily used for cases that have failed an initial repair. Another selected indication is when there are stones in the kidney with a ureteropelvic junction obstruction. Both conditions can be dealt within one endoscopic procedure. However, these procedures have largely been supplanted by laparoscopic repair. In particular, the remarkable growth of robotic urological surgery has allowed for many more surgeons to become proficient with robotic-assisted pyeloplasty and this has become a viable option. It remains unclear whether the long-term results are as good as open procedures, but there is a clear trend towards performing an increasing number of repairs this way. Although the morbidity of open surgery is decreasing, success rates with laparoscopic and robotic approaches are comparable and parents seem to prefer the robotic approach (Braga et al, 2009; Chacko et al, 2006; Freilich et al, 2010).

OBSTRUCTED MEGAURETER

Obstruction at the ureterovesical junction is four times more common in boys than in girls. It may be bilateral and is usually asymmetric. The left ureter is slightly more often involved than the right.

The embryogenesis of the lesion is uncertain. It is clear that in most cases, there is no stricture at the ureterovesical junction. At operation, a retrograde catheter or probe can usually be passed through the area of obstruction. Close observation either at operation or by fluoroscopy reveals a failure of the distal ureter to transmit the normal peristaltic wave, resulting in a functional obstruction. Moreover, on fluoroscopy, retrograde peristalsis is seen. This transmits abnormal pressures up to the kidney, resulting in calyceal dilation out of proportion with the renal pelvic dilation. Histologic findings include an excess of circular muscle fibers and collagen in the distal ureter that may account for the problem (Tanagho et al, 1970). Ultrastructural studies show that this obstruction is similar in appearance to obstruction of the ureteropelvic junction.

Currently, most of the cases are discovered on prenatal sonography. Sonography usually shows the pathognomonic configuration of a dilated distal ureter, a less dilated proximal ureter, a relatively normal-appearing renal pelvis, and calyces blunted out of proportion to the renal pelvis (Figure 37–12).

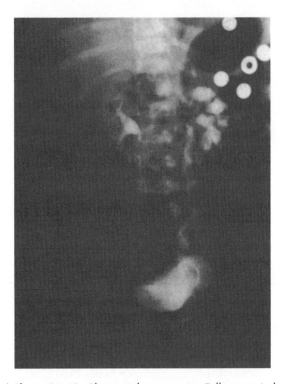

▲ **Figure 37–12.** Obstructed megaureter. Follow-up study in a 9-month-old boy with unilateral hydronephrosis detected by ultrasonography in utero. Excretory urogram shows the classic configuration of a dilated distal ureter, a less dilated proximal ureter, and blunted calyces.

It was assumed previously that surgery was indicated in most cases. Ureteral reimplantation with excision of the distal ureter is curative. Because of the excessive dilation of the ureter, ureteral tapering or folding may be necessary (Ehrlich, 1985; Hanna, 1982; Hendren, 1969). Because the ureteral muscle is generally healthy, these cases have an excellent prognosis. However, in recent years, it has become obvious that at least 50% of cases will undergo spontaneous resolution. A period of observation is nearly always appropriate when the diagnosis is made in an asymptomatic patient (Baskin et al, 1994; Chertin et al, 2008). Because of the high risk of infection, 1–2 years of prophylactic antibiotics are recommended in neonates.

UPPER URINARY TRACT DILATATION WITHOUT OBSTRUCTION

It should not be assumed that every dilated upper urinary tract is obstructed. A voiding cystourethrogram is an essential part of the evaluation, not only to rule out reflux but also to ensure that no abnormality of the lower urinary tract is responsible for the upper urinary tract dilatation. Other cases in which diagnosis may be difficult include residual dilatation in a previously obstructed system, dilatation associated with bacterial infection (presumably related to a direct effect of endotoxin on the ureteral musculature), neonatal hydronephrosis, and prolonged polyuria in patients with diabetes insipidus.

In such cases, the usual investigations may not provide sufficient information. A radionuclide diuretic renogram is especially helpful in distinguishing nonobstructive from obstructive dilation and in determining whether renal functional injury has occurred (Figure 37–13) (Thrall et al, 1981). However, the procedure must be performed carefully, as technical problems may confuse the results (Gungor et al, 2002; Nguyen et al, 1997). Use of percutaneous renal puncture is occasionally beneficial; in the dilated system, it carries minimal risk, making antegrade urography and pressure-flow studies feasible in selected cases. Measurement of the renal pelvic pressure during infusion of saline into the renal pelvis at high rates (10 mL/min) (*the Whitaker test*) may help differentiate nonobstructive from obstructive dilation (Wolk and Whitaker, 1982). Unfortunately, there is no true "gold standard," and these studies do not always agree; clinical judgment is the final arbiter.

ACQUIRED DISEASES OF THE URETER

Nearly all acquired diseases of the ureter are obstructive in nature. Although they are seen frequently, their actual incidence is unknown. Their clinical manifestations, effects on the kidney, complications, and treatment are similar to those described previously. The lesions can be broadly categorized as either intrinsic or extrinsic.

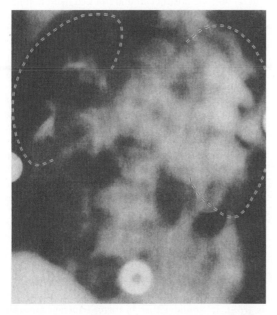 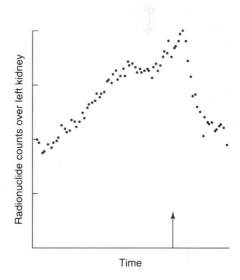

▲ **Figure 37–13.** Upper urinary tract dilatation. *Left:* Three months after resection of posterior urethral valves, hydronephrosis in the right kidney has completely resolved. The left collecting system remains dilated. (*Dashed lines* outline kidneys.) *Right:* Radionuclide diuretic renography was performed to determine if there was secondary ureteropelvic or ureterovesical obstruction. Renogram demonstrates clear-cut "washout" of radionuclide following injection of furosemide (*arrow*). There is no significant obstruction.

▶ Intrinsic Ureteral Obstruction

The most common causes of intrinsic ureteral obstruction are as follows:

1. Ureteral stones (see Chapter 17)

2. Transitional cell tumors of the ureter (see Chapter 21)

3. Chronic inflammatory changes of the ureteral wall (usually due to tuberculosis or schistosomiasis) leading to contracture or insufficient peristalsis (see Chapter 15 and Figures 15–2 and 15–4)

▶ Extrinsic Ureteral Obstruction

The most frequent causes of extrinsic ureteral obstruction are as follows:

1. Severe constipation, sometimes with bladder obstruction, seen primarily in children but in adult women as well.

2. Secondary obstruction due to kinks or fibrosis around redundant ureters. The primary process is either distal obstruction or massive reflux.

3. Benign gynecologic disorders such as endometriosis or right ovarian vein syndrome.

4. Local neoplastic infiltration associated with carcinoma of the cervix, bladder, or prostate.

5. Pelvic lymphadenopathy associated with metastatic tumors.

6. Iatrogenic ureteral injuries, primarily after extensive pelvic surgery (Figure 37–14) and also after extensive radiotherapy.

7. Retroperitoneal fibrosis.

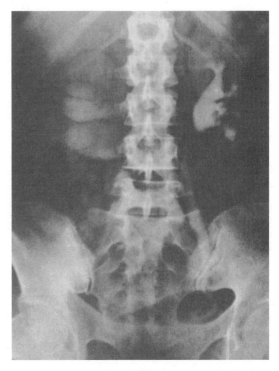

▲ **Figure 37–14.** Ureteral obstruction. Excretory urogram obtained 2 weeks after a radical hysterectomy shows bilateral ureteral obstruction and marked hydronephrosis on right.

RETROPERITONEAL FIBROSIS (RETROPERITONEAL FASCIITIS, CHRONIC RETROPERITONEAL FIBROPLASIA, ORMOND DISEASE)

One or both ureters may be compressed by a chronic inflammatory process that involves the retroperitoneal tissues over the lower lumbar vertebrae. There are numerous causes of retroperitoneal fibrosis. Malignant diseases (most commonly Hodgkin's disease, carcinoma of the breast, and carcinoma of the colon) should always be suspected and ruled out. Some medications have been implicated, most notably methysergide (Sansert), an ergot derivative used to treat migraine headaches. Rarely, membranous glomerulonephritis (Shirota et al, 2002), inflammatory bowel disease (Siminovitch and Fazio, 1980), or an aortic aneurysm (Brock and Soloway, 1980) is responsible. The remainder of cases are idiopathic, a condition sometimes referred to as Ormond disease. It is most recently thought to be autoimmune, and in men especially, IgG4 is likely involved (Zen, 2009).

The symptoms are nonspecific and include low back pain, malaise, anorexia, weight loss, and, in severe cases, uremia (Swartz, 2009). Infection is uncommon. Although the diagnosis is usually made by Computed tomography (CT) scan, an intravenous urogram (or delayed plain x-ray from the CT scan) is pathognomonic (Figure 37–15). There is medial deviation of the ureters with proximal dilation. A long segment of ureter is usually involved, and, in some cases, in the CT urogram reconstructions, there is a pipestem appearance caused by aperistalsis related to the fibrosis. Ultrasonography is useful for monitoring the response to therapy. CT scanning or magnetic resonance imaging is essential for evaluating the retroperitoneum itself, in addition to imaging the ureters (Hricak et al, 1983). Recently, positron emission tomography scanning has been advocated to diagnose metastatic cancer and to follow the severity of the inflammatory lesions (Piccoli, 2010).

Spontaneous regression has been reported (Kume and Kitamura, 2001); however, treatment is usually surgical. A course of corticosteroids may be successful, but recurrence is high if not continued (Swartz, 2009). When the response to corticosteroids is poor or the obstruction is severe, the ureter must be dissected surgically from the fibrous plaque. After it is freed, it should either be placed intraperitoneally or wrapped in omentum in an attempt to prevent recurrence; this procedure can also be performed laparoscopically (Stein, 2010). Numerous biopsies of the fibrous tissue should be obtained at the time of operation to determine whether there is a malignant tumor.

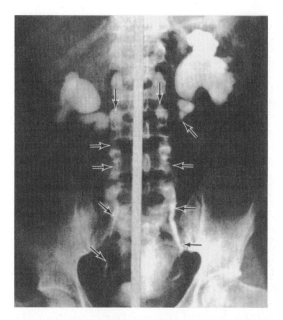

▲ **Figure 37–15.** Retroperitoneal fibrosis. Right and left kidneys of same patient as shown by excretory urography. Note medial marked obstruction. (Courtesy of JA Hutch.)

URETERAL OBSTRUCTION SECONDARY TO MALIGNANT DISEASE

Ureteral obstruction associated with widespread malignant disease was at one time a terminal event. Because therapy for malignant diseases has improved, however, urinary diversion is indicated more frequently in such cases. Diversion usually is necessary for relatively short periods of time; either the tumor is progressive or if therapy is effective, the obstruction resolves. Thus, the goal of treatment is to leave the urinary tract intact and effect as little morbidity as possible. This can be accomplished with indwelling stents passed either retrograde during cystoscopy or antegrade using percutaneous techniques. Plastic stents can easily become obstructed and metal stents may be considered for long-term use (Sountoulides, 2010).

BIBLIOGRAPHY

Congenital Anomalies of the Ureter

Glassberg KI et al: Suggested terminology for duplex systems, ectopic ureters and ureteroceles. J Urol 1984;132:1153.

Ureteral Atresia

Michos O et al: Kidney development in the absence of Gdnf and Spry1 requires Fgf10. PLoS Genet 2010;6(1):e1000809.

Onal B, Kogan BA: Natural history of patients with multicystic dysplastic kidney: What follow-up is needed? J Urol 2006;176: 1607–1611.

Duplication of the Ureter

Amar AD: Ureteropyelostomy for relief of single ureteral obstruction due to retroperitoneal fibrosis in a patient with ureteral duplication. J Urol 1970;103(3):296–297.

Amar AD: Ipsilateral ureteroureterostomy for single ureteral disease in patients with ureteral duplication: A review of 8 years of experience with 16 patients. J Urol 1978;119(4):472–475.

Belman AB et al: Surgical management of duplication of the collecting system. J Urol 1974;112(3):316–321.

Lowe GJ et al: Laparoscopic reconstructive options for obstruction in children with duplex renal anomalies. BJU Int 2008;101(2): 227–230.

Mendelsohn C: Using mouse models to understand normal and abnormal urogenital tract development. Organogenesis 2009; 5(1):306–314.

Nation EF: Duplication of the kidney and ureter: A statistical study of 230 new cases. J Urol 1944;51:456.

Prieto J et al: Ureteroureterostomy via inguinal incision for ectopic ureters and ureteroceles without ipsilateral lower pole reflux. J Urol 2009;181(4):1844–1848; discussion 1848–1850.

Tanagho EA: Embryologic basis for lower ureteral anomalies: A hypothesis. Urology 1976;7(5):451–464.

Ureterocele

Snyder HM, Johnston JH: Orthotopic ureteroceles in children. J Urol 1978;119(4):543–546.

Tanagho EA: Embryologic basis for lower ureteral anomalies: A hypothesis. Urology 1976;7(5):451–464.

Wang MH et al: Ectopic ureteroceles in duplex systems: Long-ectopic ureteral orifice. J Pediatr Urol 2008;4:183–187.

Ectopic Ureteral Orifice

Lipson JA et al: Subtle renal duplication as an unrecognized cause of childhood incontinence: Diagnosis by magnetic resonance urography. J Pediatr Urol 2008;4(5):398–400.

Michos O et al: Kidney development in the absence of Gdnf and Spry1 requires Fgf10. PLoS Genet 2010;6(1):e1000809.

Abnormalities of Ureteral Position

Bagheri F et al: Laparoscopic repair of circumcaval ureter: One-year follow-up of three patients and literature review. Urology 2009; 74(1):148–153.

Obstruction of the Ureteropelvic Junction

Anderson JC: Hydronephrosis. Heinemann, Portsmouth, New Hampshire, 1963.

Braga LH et al: Systematic review and meta-analysis of robotic-assisted versus conventional laparoscopic pyeloplasty for patients with ureteropelvic junction obstruction: Effect on operative time, length of hospital stay, postoperative complications, and success rate. Eur Urol 2009;56:848–858.

Capello SA et al: Prenatal ultrasound has led to earlier detection and repair of ureteropelvic junction obstruction. J Urol 2005;174(4, Pt 1):1425–1428.

Chacko JK et al: The minimally invasive open pyeloplasty. J Pediatr Urol 2006;2(4):368–372.

Culp OS, De WJ: A pelvic flap operation for certain types of ureteropelvic obstruction: Preliminary report. Mayo Clin Proc 1951; 26(25):483–488.

Davis DM: Intubated ureterotomy: A new operation for ureteral and ureteropelvic strictures. Surg Gynecol Obstet 1943;76:513.

Drube J et al: Urinary proteome analysis identifies infants but not older children requiring pyeloplasty. Pediatr Nephrol 2010; 25:1673–1678.

Foley FEB: A new plastic operation for stricture at the ureteropelvic junction. J Urol 1937;38:643.

Freilich DA et al: Parental satisfaction after open versus robot assisted laparoscopic pyeloplasty: Results from modified Glasgow Children's Benefit Inventory Survey. J Urol 2010;183(2):704–708.

Hanna MK et al: Ureteral structure and ultrastructure. Part II. Congenital ureteropelvic junction obstruction and primary obstructive megaureter. J Urol 1976;116(6):725–730.

Johnston JH: The pathogenesis of hydronephrosis in children. Br J Urol 1969;41(6):724–734.

Johnston JH et al: Pelvic hydronephrosis in children: A review of 219 personal cases. J Urol 1977;117(1):97–101.

Kaya C et al: Extracellular matrix degradation and reduced neural density in children with intrinsic ureteropelvic junction obstruction. Urology 2010;76:185–189.

Koff SA et al: Pathophysiology of ureteropelvic junction obstruction: Experimental and clinical observations. J Urol 1986;136(1, Pt 2): 336–338.

Scardino PL, Prince CL: Vertical flap ureteropelvioplasty. South Med J 1953;46(4):325–331.

Smart WR: Surgical correction of hydronephrosis. In: Harrison JH (ed.) Campbell's Urology, Vol. 3. Saunders, Philadelphia, 1979.

Smith KE et al: Stented versus nonstented pediatric pyeloplasty: A modern series and review of the literature. J Urol 2002;168(3): 1127–1130.

Stephens FD: Ureterovascular hydronephrosis and the "aberrant" renal vessels. J Urol 1982;128(5):984–987.

Thrall JH et al: Diuretic radionuclide renography and scintigraphy in the differential diagnosis of hydroureteronephrosis. Semin Nucl Med 1981;11(2):89–104.

Wang GJ et al: Antagonism of BMP4 signaling disrupts smooth muscle investment of the ureter and ureteropelvic junction. J Urol 2009;181(1):401–407.

Whitaker RH: Methods of assessing obstruction in dilated ureters. Br J Urol 1973;45(1):15–22.

Obstructed Megaureter

Baskin LS et al: Primary dilated megaureter: Long-term followup. J Urol 1994;152:618.

Chertin B et al: Long-term follow up of antenatally diagnosed megaureters. J Pediatr Urol 2008;4:188.

Ehrlich RM: The ureteral folding technique for megaureter surgery. J Urol 1985;134:668.

Hanna MK: Recent advances and further experience with surgical techniques for one-stage total remodeling of massively dilated ureters. Urology 1982;19:495.

Hendren WH: Operative repair of megaureter in children. J Urol 1969; 101:491.

Tanagho EA et al: Pathophysiology of functional ureteral obstruction. J Urol 1970;104:73.

Upper Urinary Tract Dilatation without Obstruction

Gungor F et al: Effect of the size of regions of interest on the estimation of differential renal function in children with congenital hydronephrosis. Nucl Med Commun 2002;23:147.

Nguyen HT et al: Changing the technique of background subtraction alters calculated renal function on pediatric mercaptoacetyltriglycine renography. J Urol 1997;158:1252.

Thrall JH et al: Diuretic radionuclide renography and scintigraphy in the differential diagnosis of hydroureteronephrosis. Semin Nucl Med 1981;11:89.

Wolk FN, Whitaker RH: Late follow-up of dynamic evaluation of upper urinary tract obstruction. J Urol 1982;128:346.

Acquired Diseases of the Ureter

Retroperitoneal Fibrosis (Retroperitoneal Fasciitis, Chronic Retroperitoneal Fibroplasia, Ormond Disease)

Brock J, Soloway MS: Retroperitoneal fibrosis and aortic aneurysm. Urology 1980;15(1):14–16.

Hricak H et al: Nuclear magnetic resonance imaging in retroperitoneal fibrosis. AJR Am J Roentgenol 1983;141(1):35–38.

Kume H, Kitamura T: Spontaneous regression of bilateral hydronephrosis due to retroperitoneal fibrosis. Scand J Urol Nephrol 2001;35(3):255–256.

Piccoli GB et al: Positron emission tomography as a tool for the 'tailored' management of retroperitoneal fibrosis: A nephro-urological experience. Nephrol Dial Transplant 2010;25:2603–2610.

Shirota S et al: Retroperitoneal fibrosis associated with membranous nephropathy effectively treated with steroids. Intern Med 2002;41(1):20–25.

Siminovitch JM, Fazio VW: Ureteral obstruction secondary to Crohn's disease: A need for ureterolysis? Am J Surg 1980;139(1): 95–98.

Stein RJ et al: Laparoscopic ureterolysis with omental wrap for idiopathic retroperitoneal fibrosis. BJU Int 2010;106(5):703–707.

Swartz RD: Idiopathic retroperitoneal fibrosis: A review of the pathogenesis and approaches to treatment. Am J Kidney Dis 2009;54(3):546–553.

Zen Y et al: Retroperitoneal fibrosis: a clinicopathologic study with respect to immunoglobulin G4. Am J Surg Pathol 2009;33(12): 1833–1839.

Ureteral Obstruction Secondary to Malignant Disease

Sountoulides P et al: Current status of metal stents for managing malignant ureteric obstruction. BJU Int 2010;105:1066–1072.

Disorders of the Bladder, Prostate, & Seminal Vesicles

38

Katsuto Shinohara, MD

CONGENITAL ANOMALIES OF THE BLADDER

▶ Exstrophy

Exstrophy of the bladder is a rare congenital anomaly with complete ventral defect of the urogenital sinus and the overlying skeletal system (Gambhir et al, 2008). Incidence of this anomaly is reported to be 3.3 per 100,000 births. Male to female ratio is about 1.5:1 (Anon, 1987).

A. Signs and Symptoms

The lower central abdomen is occupied by the inner surface of the posterior wall of the bladder, whose mucosal edges are fused with the skin. Urine spurts onto the abdominal wall from the ureteral orifices.

The rami of the pubic bones are widely separated. The pelvic ring thus lacks rigidity, the femurs are rotated externally, and the child "waddles like a duck."

The rectus muscles are widely separated from each other caudally. A hernia, made up of the exstrophic bladder and surrounding skin, is present.

Epispadias is almost always associated. Undescended testicles may be seen, and the anus and vagina located anteriorly. Urinary tract infection and hydronephrosis are common.

B. Diagnosis

Prenatal diagnosis is difficult (Austin et al, 1998; Emanuel et al, 1995). Obvious anomaly of exposed bladder mucosa makes diagnosis easy at birth. X-ray studies will reveal separation of pubic bones.

C. Treatment

Historical treatment includes staged repair of this anomaly (Stec et al, 2011). The first stage is to close the abdominal wall, the bladder, and the posterior urethra. Orthopedic procedure of sacral osteotomy in order to close the abdominal

wall may be necessary (Meldrum et al, 2003; Suson et al, 2011; Vining et al, 2011). Mollard (1980) recommends the following steps for satisfactory repair of bladder exstrophy (Mollard, 1980): (1) bladder closure with sacral osteotomy in order to close the pelvic ring at the pubic symphysis (Cervellione, 2011), plus lengthening of the penis; (2) antiureteral reflux procedure and bladder neck reconstruction; and (3) repair of the epispadiac penis. Treatment needs to be initiated prior to the fibrosis of the bladder mucosa in order to repair this anomaly completely (Oesterling and Jeffs, 1987). When the bladder is small, fibrotic, and inelastic, functional closure becomes inadvisable, and urinary diversion with cystectomy is the treatment of choice. Modern approach is to perform primary repair of this anomaly completely (Mitchell, 2005; Mourtzinos and Borer, 2004). Recent studies show better outcomes with primary repair (Grady et al, 1999; Kiddoo et al, 2004; Lowentritt et al, 2005).

D. Prognosis

Common complications after surgical repair include incontinence (Gargollo et al, 2011; Light and Scott, 1983; Perlmutter et al, 1991; Toguri et al, 1978), infertility, vesicoureteral reflux, and urinary tract infection (Ebert et al, 2008; Gargollo and Borer, 2007). Complete primary closure appears to be the best choice for improved continence. Adenocarcinoma of the bladder and rectum are noted in higher frequency (Husmann and Rathbun, 2008).

▶ Persistent Urachus

Embryologically, the allantois connects the urogenital sinus with the umbilicus. Normally, the allantois is obliterated and is represented by a fibrous cord (urachus) extending from the dome of the bladder to the navel (Bauer and Retik, 1978). Urachal formation is directly related to bladder descent. Lack of descent is more commonly associated with patent urachus than with bladder outlet obstruction (Scheye et al, 1994).

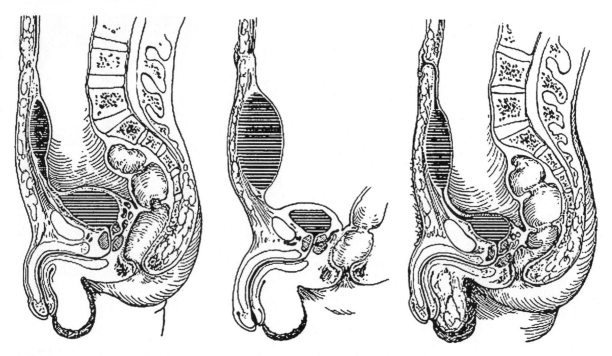

▲ **Figure 38-1.** Diagrams showing various types of patent urachus. ***Left:*** Complete atresia toward umbilicus but patent toward bladder. ***Center:*** Atresia on both ends leading cystic dilation in the middle. ***Right:*** Completely patent urachus with cystic dilation.

A. Sign and Symptoms

If the urachal obliteration is complete except at the superior end, a draining umbilical sinus may be noted. If it becomes infected, the drainage will be purulent. If the inferior end remains open, it will communicate with the bladder, but this does not usually produce symptoms. Rarely, the entire tract remains patent, in which case urine drains constantly from the umbilicus. This is apt to become obvious within a few days of birth. If only the ends of the urachus seal off, a cyst of that body may form and may become quite large, presenting a low midline mass (Figure 38–1) (al-Hindawi and Aman, 1992). If the cyst becomes infected, signs of general and local sepsis will develop (Mesrobian et al, 1997).

Adenocarcinoma may occur in an urachal cyst, particularly at its vesical extremity (Figure 38–2), and tends to invade the tissues beneath the anterior abdominal wall.

B. Diagnosis

Physical examination reveals opening sinus or lower abdominal mass. Computed tomography (CT) scan, magnetic resonance imaging (MRI), or ultrasound may show cystic structure adjacent to the bladder dome (Chouhan et al, 2011; Cilento et al, 1998; Holten et al, 1996). Cystoscope may show extrinsic compression from the mass. Stones may develop in a cyst of the urachus and can be identified on a plain x-ray film.

C. Treatment

Treatment consists of excision of the urachus, which lies on the peritoneal surface (Chan et al, 2009; Destri et al, 2011; Stone et al, 1995; Yohannes et al, 2003). If adenocarcinoma is present, radical resection is required. Unless other serious congenital anomalies are present, the prognosis is good (Upadhyay and Kukkady, 2003). The complication of adenocarcinoma offers a poor prognosis (Gopalan et al, 2009).

▶ Other Bladder Anomalies

A. Diverticulum

Congenital diverticulum is found in approximately 1.7% of children (Blane et al, 1994). This is caused by the congenital weakness of Waldeyer fascial sheath. Most of the cases are asymptomatic; however, it can cause urinary tract infection, and in rare cases, it can cause ureteral or bladder outlet obstruction (Bhat et al, 2011; Bogdanos et al, 2005; Pieretti and Pieretti-Vanmarcke, 1999).

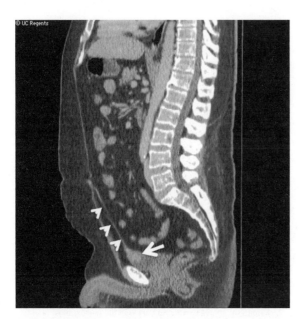

▲ **Figure 38–2.** MRI midline sagittal view of a case with adenocarcinoma of the urachus. A cord like urachus is seen connecting the bladder dome and umbilicus (*arrow heads*). A soft tissue mass is seen in the dome of the bladder (*arrow*). (Image Courtesy of Dr. Fergus Coakley.)

B. Bladder Ears

One side of the bladder may become involved in an inguinal hernia (Figure 38–3). Such a mass may recede on urination. The condition can be found during contrast x-ray studies of urinary tract (Bjurlin et al, 2011; Catalano, 1997). However, it is more commonly found as a previously unsuspected complication during surgical correction of a hernia (McCormack et al, 2005; Patle et al, 2011).

C. Megacystis

Megacystis is a condition with enlarged bladder due to overdistention during the development, commonly associated with massive reflux with hydronephrosis (Burbige et al, 1984). This condition can be associated with other conditions, such as posterior valve (Confer et al, 2011), Ehlers–Danlos syndrome (Sato et al, 1993), and meningomyelocele (Blane et al, 1994).

ACQUIRED DISEASES OF THE BLADDER

▶ Interstitial Cystitis or Bladder Pain Syndrome

Interstitial cystitis is unknown etiology syndrome characterized by urinary frequency, urgency, and bladder pain (Nickel, 2004). In the past, it was reported to be frequently affecting

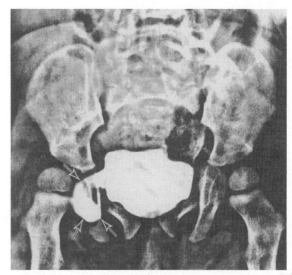

▲ **Figure 38–3.** Cystogram demonstrating sliding hernia of the bladder in the inguinal canal (*arrows*).

middle-aged women; however, recent studies revealed that it affect men and women in all ages (Kusek and Nyberg, 2001). Recent study showed that as high as 12% of women may be affected with early symptoms of interstitial cystitis/bladder pain syndrome (IC/BPS) (Rosenberg and Hazzard, 2005).

A. Sign and Symptoms

Common symptoms with IC/BPS are bladder pain worsened with bladder filling, certain food intake, and burning on urination. Urinary frequency, nocturia, and urgency are also common.

B. Etiology

The etiology of IC/BPS is unknown and various causes are proposed. These include increased mast cell in the bladder wall, deficiency of glycosaminoglycan layer over bladder mucosa leading to bladder wall inflammation by urine stimulation, unknown virus infection, toxic substance in the urine, autoimmune disorder, etc (Buffington, 2004; Burkman, 2004; Clemens et al, 2008; Elbadawi, 1997; Wesselmann, 2001).

C. Diagnosis

Laboratory test: The urine is almost always free of infection. Microscopic hematuria may be noted. Results of renal function tests are normal except in the occasional patient in whom vesical fibrosis has led to vesicoureteral reflux or obstruction. No urine cytology or markers are found to be specific to IC/BPS (Hurst et al, 1993). No serologic tests are shown to be diagnostic for this condition.

Imaging: No radiographic findings are found to be specific to IC/BPS. Excretory urograms are usually normal unless reflux has occurred, in which case hydronephrosis is found. The accompanying cystogram reveals a bladder of small capacity; reflux into a dilated upper tract may be noted on cystography.

Urodynamic study: Urodynamic study is not required for diagnosis of IC/BPS; however, it can be used to rule out other condition, such as neurogenic bladder or bladder outlet obstruction.

Cystoscopy: Diagnostic cystoscopy is commonly performed under anesthesia in order to adequately distend the bladder. Typical cystoscopic findings associated with IC/BPS are reduced capacity, scarring and cracking of the mucosa with distention (Hunner's ulcer), and appearance of glomerulation (diffuse petechial hemorrhages in the mucosa) after distension. However, classic Hunner's ulcer is rare. Glomerulation can be seen with other conditions, and the finding is not specific to IC/BPS (Ottem and Teichman, 2005; Simon et al, 1997).

Histology: Bladder biopsy has been shown to have increase mast cell in the bladder wall (Sant and Theoharides, 1994). However, this finding does not include or exclude the diagnosis (Johansson and Fall, 1990).

KCl test: Patients with deficiency of the urothelial defense layer (Nickel et al, 1993) may experience severe pain with instillation of potassium chloride solution in the bladder. However, this test is controversial and not widely used.

Validated questionnaires: The Wisconsin Interstitial Cystitis Scale and The Interstitial Cystitis symptom and Problem Index (O'Leary et al, 1997) are validated questionnaires and useful in diagnosis and evaluation of treatment effectiveness (Lubeck et al, 2001; Sirinian et al, 2005).

National Institute of Diabetes and Digestive and Kidney Disease criteria: Since IC/BPS is unknown etiology clinical symptom complex, National Institute of Diabetes and Digestive and Kidney Disease criteria was created to rule in/out this diagnosis (Gillenwater and Wein, 1988; Nordling, 2004; Oberpenning et al, 2002) (Table 38–1).

D. Differential Diagnosis

Tuberculosis of the bladder may cause true ulceration but is most apt to involve the region of the ureteral orifice that drains the tuberculous kidney. Vesical ulcers due to schistosomiasis cause symptoms similar to those of interstitial cystitis. The diagnosis is suggested if the patient lives in an area in which schistosomiasis is endemic. Nonspecific vesical infection seldom causes ulceration. Pus and bacteria are found in the urine. Antimicrobial treatment is effective.

E. Treatment

Oral medication: Pentosan polysulfate provides protective coating in the bladder and suppose to reduce IC/

Table 38–1. National Institute of Diabetes and Digestive and Kidney Diseases Criteria for interstitial cystitis.

To be diagnosed with interstitial cystitis, patients must have either
Glomerulations on cystoscopic examination or a classic Hunner's ulcer

And either
Pain associated with the bladder or urinary urgency

An examination for glomerulations should be undertaken after distention of the bladder under anesthesia to 80–100 cm of water pressure for 1–2 minutes

The bladder may be distended up to two times before evaluation.

The glomerulations must
Be diffuse—present in at least 3 quadrants of the bladder
Be present at a rate of at least 10 glomerulations per quadrant
Not be along the path of the cystoscope (to eliminate artifact from contact instrumentation)

The presence of any one of the following criteria excludes the diagnosis of interstitial cystitis:
1. Bladder capacity of >350 cc on awake cystometry using either a gas or liquid filling medium
2. Absence of an intense urge to void with the bladder filled to 100 cc of gas or 150 cc of water during cystometry, using a fill rate of 30–100 cc/min
3. The demonstration of phasic involuntary bladder contractions on cystometry using the fill rate described above
4. Duration of symptoms <9 months
5. Absence of nocturia
6. Symptoms relieved by antimicrobials, urinary antiseptics, anticholinergics, or antispasmodics
7. A frequency of urination, while awake, of less than eight times per day
8. A diagnosis of bacterial cystitis or prostatitis within a 3-month period
9. Bladder or ureteral calculi
10. Active genital herpes
11. Uterine, cervical, vaginal, or urethral cancer
12. Urethral diverticulum
13. Cyclophosphamide or any type of chemical cystitis
14. Tuberculous cystitis
15. Radiation cystitis
16. Benign or malignant bladder tumors
17. Vaginitis
18. Younger than 18 years

BPS-related pain (Parsons and Mulholland, 1987). However, a randomized study has shown no significant benefit of the medicine over placebo (Nordling, 2004; Sairanen et al, 2005; Sant et al, 2003). Cyclosporine A has been shown to be more effective than pentosan polysulfate; however, its toxicity limits the usage (Sairanen et al, 2005). Anticholinergics are frequently used to control frequency and urgency. Amitriptyline has shown to improve IC/BPS symptoms including pain and frequency.

Instillation therapy: Hydrodistention under anesthesia can improve symptoms. Intravesical instillations of dimethyl sulfoxide (DMSO), heparin, bacille Calmett-Guerrin (Mayer et al, 2005), and sodium hyaluronate (Riedl et al, 2008) are also used with some benefits (Chancellor and Yoshimura, 2004).

Other therapy: Other nonspecific medications, such as analgesics, anti-inflammatory agents, gabapentin, and serotonin reuptake inhibitors, can be used. Transcutaneous electrical nerve stimulation (Comiter, 2003) and biofeedback therapy may have some benefit for controlling the symptoms (Peters et al, 2007). Diet modification to avoid certain foods or drinks may have a role in the treatment (Chaiken et al, 1993).

Surgical therapy: Surgical therapy is rarely indicated. Even after cystectomy, some patients continue to experience pain (Baskin and Tanagho, 1992). For those who have small bladder capacity, augmentation procedure can be indicated. Recent trials of botulinum toxin A injection in the bladder wall have shown to improve symptoms and bladder capacity.

F. Prognosis

Most patients respond to one of the conservative measures mentioned previously. IC/BPS is a chronic condition and requires patient understanding and support.

▶ Foreign Body Inserted into the Bladder

Numerous objects have been found in the urethra and bladder of both men and women. Some of them find their way into the urethra in the course of inquisitive self-exploration (Cardozo, 1997; Mastromichalis et al, 2011). Other objects can migrate in the bladder through erosion. Commonly reported objects are intrauterine contraceptive devices (Bjornerem and Tollan, 1997; Chuang et al, 2010; Hick et al, 2004). Other foreign bodies placed during surgery include hernia repair mesh (Bjurlin and Berger, 2011), drain, vaginal sling material, and bone fragments after trauma (Stone et al, 1995).

The presence of a foreign body causes cystitis. Hematuria is not uncommon. Embarrassment may cause the victim to delay medical consultation. A plain x-ray of the bladder area discloses metal objects. Nonopaque objects sometimes become coated with calcium. Cystoscopy visualizes them all.

Cystoscopic or suprapubic removal of the foreign body is indicated. If not removed, the foreign body will lead to infection of the bladder. If the infecting organisms are urea splitting, the alkaline urine (which causes increased insolubility of calcium salts) contributes to rapid formation of stone on the foreign object.

▶ Vesical Manifestations of Allergy

So many mucous membranes are affected by allergens that the possibility of allergic manifestations involving the bladder must be considered. Hypersensitivity is occasionally suggested in cases of recurrent symptoms of acute "cystitis" in the absence of urinary infection or other demonstrable

abnormality. During the attack, general erythema of the vesical mucosa may be seen and some edema of the ureteral orifices noted. Sometimes, lesions mimic malignancy (Salman et al, 2006; Thompson et al, 2005). Biopsy of the bladder wall reveals diffuse eosinophilic cell infiltrations (eosinophilic cystitis) (Popescu et al, 2009; Rubin and Pincus, 1974).

A careful history may reveal that these attacks follow the ingestion of a food not ordinarily eaten (eg, fresh lobster). Sensitivity to spermicidal creams is occasionally observed. If vesical allergy is suspected, it may be aborted by the subcutaneous injection of 0.5–1 mL of 1:1000 epinephrine. Control may also be afforded by the use of one of the antihistamines. Steroid therapy is effective for severe cases (Watanabe et al, 2009). Skin testing has shown positive in some cases.

▶ Diverticula

Most vesical diverticula are acquired and are secondary to either obstruction distal to the vesical neck or the upper motor neuron type of neurogenic bladder. Increased intravesical pressure causes vesical mucosa to insinuate itself between hypertrophied muscle bundles, so that a mucosal extravesical sac develops (Figure 38–4). Often this sac lies just superior to the ureter and causes vesicoureteral reflux. The diverticulum is devoid of muscle and therefore has no expulsive power; residual urine is the rule, and infection is perpetuated. If the diverticulum has a narrow opening that

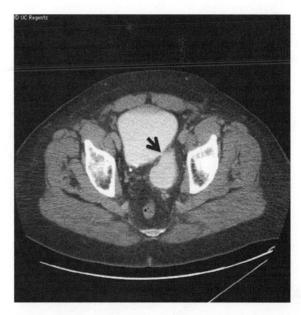

▲ **Figure 38–4.** CT scan of the pelvis with contrast depicts a large bladder diverticulum filled with contrast and its orifice (*arrow*). (Image Courtesy of Dr. Fergus Coakley.)

interferes with its emptying, transurethral resection of its neck will improve drainage. Carcinoma occasionally develops on its wall (Prakash et al, 2010). Micic (1983) discovered 13 diverticula harboring malignant tumors: nine transitional cell tumors, two squamous cell tumors, and two adenocarcinomas. Gerridzen and Futter (1982) saw 48 cases of vesical diverticula. Transitional cell tumors were found in five of these patients, but almost all the rest had abnormal histopathology: chronic inflammation and metaplasia. These authors stress the need for visualizing the interior of diverticula during endoscopy. Lack of wall thickness in diverticula makes potential early invasion of tumor and can results in poor prognosis (Yu et al, 1993). Diverticulectomy can be successfully performed laparoscopically (Khonsari et al, 2004; Kural et al, 2009; Macejko et al, 2008). Endoscopic management of bladder outlet obstruction must be performed, if a diverticulectomy is performed.

▶ Vesical Fistulas

Vesical fistulas are common. The bladder may communicate with the skin, intestinal tract, or female reproductive organs (Figure 38–5). The primary disease is usually not urologic. The causes are as follows: (1) primary intestinal disease—diverticulitis, 50–60%; cancer of the colon, 20–25%; and Crohn's disease, 10% (Badlani et al, 1980; Simoneaux and Patrick, 1997); (2) primary gynecologic disease—pressure necrosis during difficult labor; advanced cancer of the cervix (Chapple and Turner-Warwick, 2005; Gilmour et al, 1999); (3) treatment for gynecologic disease following hysterectomy, low cesarean section, or radiotherapy for tumor (Ayhan et al, 1995); and (4) trauma. Ablative therapy of prostate cancer such as, cryosurgery or high intensity focused ultrasound therapy, is a frequent cause of rectourethral fistula, but development of rectovesical fistula is rare.

Malignant tumors of the small or large bowel, uterus, or cervix may invade and perforate the bladder. Inflammations of adjacent organs may also erode through the vesical wall. Severe injuries involving the bladder may lead to perivesical abscess formation, and these abscesses may rupture through the skin of the perineum or abdomen. The bladder may be inadvertently injured during gynecologic or intestinal surgery; cystotomy for stone or prostatectomy may lead to a persistent cutaneous fistula.

A. Sign and Symptoms

Symptoms arising from a vesicointestinal fistula include vesical irritability, the passage of debris (fecauria) and gas through the urethra (pneumaturia), and usually a change in bowel habits (eg, constipation, abdominal distention, diarrhea) caused by the primary intestinal disease (Kirsh et al, 1991). Signs of bowel obstruction may be elicited; abdominal tenderness may be found if the cause is inflammatory.

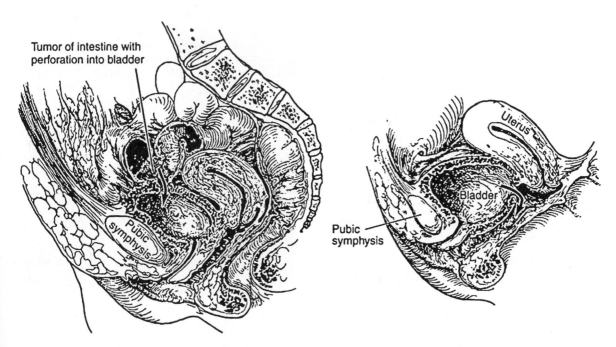

▲ **Figure 38–5.** Diagrams showing vesicoenteric fistula due to tumor in the sigmoid colon (**left**) and vesicovaginal fistula (**right**).

B. Laboratory Findings

Urinalysis shows increased WBC and RBC with bacteria. Urine culture commonly grow mixed bacterial flora.

C. Diagnosis

Imaging studies: CT scan and MRI are sensitive test for enterovesical fistula. It may show thickening of the bladder wall, mass adjacent to the bladder, and air in the bladder (Figure 38–6) (Moon et al, 2001). However, air in the bladder can be seen in an infection caused by gas forming bacteria or instrumentation and is not solely diagnostic (Joseph et al, 1996). Barium enema is not sensitive to describe fistula. However, it may show diverticulosis or malignancy. Cystography may show contrast in the bowel, although the sensitivity of cystography for enterovesical fistula is low. Radionuclide voiding cystography is reported to be sensitive test for enterovesical fistula diagnosis (Tamam et al, 2009).

Cystoscopy: Cystoscopic examination shows a severe localized inflammatory reaction from which bowel contents may exude. Catheterization of the fistulous tract may be feasible; the instillation of radiopaque fluid often establishes the diagnosis.

Other test: Charcoal (Huettner et al, 1992) or poppy seed test (Kwon et al, 2008) is to detect orally ingested charcoal or poppy seeds in patient urine. Bourne test detects barium particle in urine after barium enema (Amendola et al, 1984). Those tests may show the evidence of fistula; however, anatomical characterization cannot be achieved.

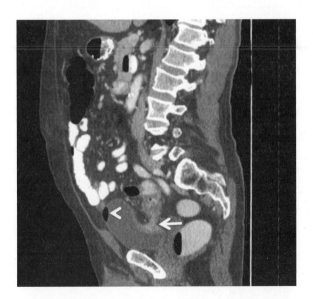

▲ **Figure 38–6.** CT scan of a case with vesicoenteric fistula due to diverticulitis demonstrates tissue thickening of the bladder wall with adhered sigmoid colon (*arrow*). Free air is seen in the bladder (*arrow head*). (Image Courtesy of Dr. Fergus Coakley.)

D. Differential Diagnosis

It is necessary to differentiate ureterovaginal from vesicovaginal fistula. Phenazopyridine (Pyridium) is given by mouth to color the urine orange. One hour later, three cotton pledgets are inserted into the vagina, and methylene blue solution is instilled into the bladder. The patient should then walk around, after which the pledgets are examined. If the proximal cotton ball is wet or stained orange, the fistula is ureterovaginal. If the deep cotton pledget contains blue fluid, the diagnosis is vesicovaginal fistula. If only the distal pledget is blue, the patient probably has urinary incontinence (Raghavaiah, 1974).

E. Treatment

Conservative management: Fistula caused by Crohn's disease is commonly managed with medical therapy with steroid, sulfasalazine, and antibiotics. Patients with poor surgical candidate with fistula from diverticulosis can be managed with antibiotics therapy.

Surgical therapy: Enterovesical fistula is commonly treated with affected portion of bowel resection with or without bladder repair (Melchior et al, 2009). If inflammation by diverticulosis is severe, staged approach with fecal diversion can be performed (Moss and Ryan, 1990). If malignancy is the cause of the fistula, partial or total cystectomy with affected bowel is necessary.

For vesicovaginal fistula, tiny openings may become sealed following the introduction of an electrode into the fistula to ablate mature tract epithelium. An indwelling catheter should be left in place for 2 weeks or more. Larger fistulas secondary to obstetric or surgical injuries respond readily to surgical repair, which may be done either through the vagina or transvesically (Huang et al, 2002; McKay, 2004). Persky et al (1979) advised repairing such fistulas immediately rather than waiting for 3–6 months as counseled by most surgeons (Blaivas et al, 1995). Fistulas that develop following radiation therapy for cancer of the cervix are much more difficult to close because of the avascularity of the tissues. Surgical closure of fistulas that arise from direct invasion of the bladder by cervical carcinoma is impossible; diversion of the urinary stream above the level of the bladder (example ureterosigmoidostomy) is therefore necessary.

F. Prognosis

The surgical repair of fistulas caused by benign disease or operative trauma is highly successful. Postirradiation necrosis offers a more guarded prognosis. Fistulas secondary to invading cancers present difficult problems.

▶ Pelvic Lipomatosis

The cause of pelvic lipomatosis is not known. The disorder seems to affect principally black men in the 20–40-year age group with hypertension (Heyns, 1991). There are no pathognomonic symptoms. There may be some dysuria or mild urinary obstructive symptoms. Examination may demonstrate microscopic hematuria, a distended or enlarged pear-shaped bladder. Excretory urograms and cystography may show dilatation of both upper tracts and an upward displacement and lateral compression of the bladder (Miglani et al, 2010; Mordkin et al, 1997). In the perivesical area, x-ray reveals areas of radiolucency compatible with fatty tissue. A barium x-ray may show extrinsic pressure on the rectosigmoid. CT scan in association with the preceding findings establishes the diagnosis by clearly demonstrating the fatty nature of the perivesical tissue. Ultrasonography may be equally helpful. Cystitis glandularis is frequently associated with pelvic lipomatosis (Heyns et al, 1991; Masumori and Tsukamoto, 1999). Adenocarcinoma of the bladder can develop in the bladder in this condition (Sozen et al, 2004).

Noninfectious Hemorrhagic Cystitis

Some patients, following radiotherapy for carcinoma of the cervix, bladder, or prostate, are prone to intermittent, often serious vesical hemorrhage. The same is true of those given cyclophosphamide or ifosfamide. Cyclophosphamide is metabolized in liver to acrolein. This is excreted in urine to cause bladder damage (Cox, 1979). About 5–10% of patients with a history of pelvic irradiation (Levenback et al, 1994) and up to 70% of patients exposed to high dose of cyclophosphamide or iphosphamide are at risk of hemorrhagic cystitis (Efros et al, 1990).[16] Penicillins (Bracis et al, 1977), and danazol (Andriole et al, 1986) are reported to be associated with hemorrhagic cystitis (deVries and Freiha, 1990).

A. Signs and Symptoms

Gross hematuria with clots without evidence of typical urinary infection symptoms.

B. Differential Diagnosis

Malignancy, urinary tract infection, calculi, and benign prostate hyperplasia can cause gross hematuria.

C. Diagnosis

Cystoscopy shows abnormal neovascularity that is easy to bleed with distention. Diffuse mucosal bleeding is common (Figure 38–7).

D. Prevention

For prevention of cyclophosphamide or iphosphamide induced hemorrhage, hydration and continuous bladder drainage during chemotherapy are recommended (Ballen et al, 1999). 2-Mercaptoethanesulfonate binds to acrolein to

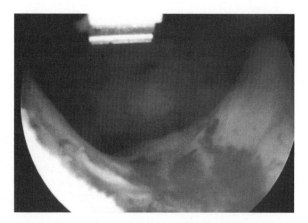

▲ **Figure 38–7.** Cystoscopy of a patient with gross hematuria after radiation therapy of prostate cancer reveals diffuse bleeding at the bladder neck due to radiation induced cystitis.

reduce toxic effect, and it can be administered during the chemotherapy (Goren et al, 1997).

E. Treatment

Bladder irrigation with three-way catheter is essential. Oral epsilon aminocaproic acid can be tried. Conservative therapy includes bladder irrigation with alum or silver nitrate. For severe hemorrhage with clots retention, cystoscopic clots evacuation, electro fulguration (Kaplan and Wolf, 2009), and formalin instillation in the bladder can be done under anesthesia (Donahue and Frank, 1989).[19] A cystogram to confirm no association of vesicoureteral reflux prior to instillation is important since formalin can damage renal function if it is induced in the kidneys.[17]

Giulani et al have reported success by selective transcatheter embolization of the internal iliac arteries (Giuliani et al, 1979). Ostroff and Chenault (1982) believe that the best and least harmful method of treatment is continuous irrigation with 1% alum solution (the ammonium or potassium salt) through a three-way Foley catheter (Giuliani et al, 1979). Alum can induce encephalopathy in renal failure patients, and careful monitoring of serum aluminum level in such patients is recommended (Andriole et al, 1986).[15]

Hyperbaric oxygen therapy has been used for both radiation-induced and chemotherapy-induced hemorrhagic cystitis with encouraging results (Chong et al, 2005).[18,20] Conjugated estrogen therapy has also demonstrated some effect (Liu et al, 1990).[14]

Bilateral nephrostomy to reduce urinary contact to the bladder lumen is moderately effective. For severe refractory hematuria, cystectomy with urinary diversion or neobladder creation is considered as a last resort.

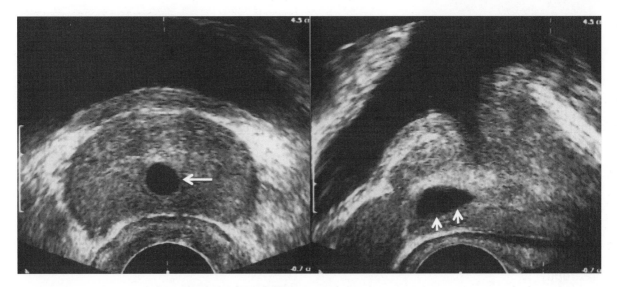

▲ **Figure 38–8.** Transrectal ultrasonography demonstrating typical utricular cyst. Transverse image at the base shows a round cyst (*arrow*) in the midline posterior to the urethra (***left***). On sagittal view, the cyst is typical teardrop shape (*arrow heads*) with the narrow end extends toward the urethra (***right***).

ANOMALIES OF THE PROSTATE AND SEMINAL VESICLES

▶ Prostatic Cyst and Calculi

Cysts in the prostate gland are very common. Enlargements of the prostatic utricle are often found at the time of transrectal ultrasonography. Those cysts are usually small, lying in the midline posterior to the prostatic urethra and typically in teardrop shape in sagittal view (Figure 38–8). These cysts represent embryologic remnants of the distal end of the Müllerian ducts. Those midline cysts commonly have communication with the urethra; however, some variants are known to exist (Furuya et al, 2008).[6] Most of these cysts are asymptomatic and found incidentally. Occasionally, cysts may contain hemorrhage and cause hematospermia (Coppens et al, 2002). Rarely, they become large enough to be easily palpable rectally or even abdominally. Through local pressure, they may cause symptoms of obstruction of the bladder neck (Desautel et al, 1999). Utricular cyst may cause obstruction of the ejaculatory ducts.[9] This condition can be discovered during the male infertility workup. Ejaculatory ducts may open in the midline cyst (Furuya et al, 2008). Other common cysts in the prostate are degenerative cysts. Those cysts are commonly seen in the transition zone of the enlarged gland; however, multiple cysts can also be seen in the peripheral zone. Those cysts cause no symptoms.

Prostatic calculi are very common condition. Almost all men in middle age will have more or less prostatic calculi. Prostatic calculi commonly develop in the prostatic duct near prostatic urethra. Prostatic calculi are commonly found during transrectal ultrasonography of the prostate (Figure 38–9). In general, prostatic calculi cause no symptoms. However, patients with massive prostatic calculi may have voiding dysfunction to cause urine reflux into the prostatic ducts.[7]

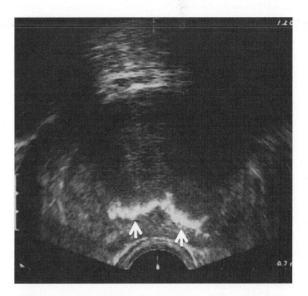

▲ **Figure 38–9.** Typical prostatic calculi on transrectal ultrasonography are seen as curved bright lines (*arrows*) with acoustic shadows.

▶ Anomalies of the Seminal Vesicle

Unilateral or bilateral agenesis of the seminal vesicle is often discovered during an infertility workup. Agenesis of the seminal vesicle is generally asymptomatic except for low ejaculatory volume. On examination, vas deferens on the affected side may be absent. Agenesis or ectopic location of the affected side kidney can be also found.

Ectopic ureteral opening in the ejaculatory duct causes extremely dilated ampulla of vas deferens and seminal vesicle. These patients often have a history of recurrent epididymitis on the affected side. The kidney on the affected side is frequently ectopic and dysplastic or agenesis (Carbone et al, 2007; Cherullo et al, 2002).

BIBLIOGRAPHY

Exstrophy

Anon: Epidemiology of bladder exstrophy and epispadias: A communication from the International Clearinghouse for Birth Defects Monitoring Systems. Teratology 1987;36(2):221–227.

Austin PF et al: The prenatal diagnosis of cloacal exstrophy. J Urol 1998;160(3, Pt 2):1179–1181.

Cervellione RM: The use of pelvic osteotomy in cloacal exstrophy. Semin Pediatr Surg 2011;20(2):119–122.

Ebert AK et al: Genital and reproductive function in males after functional reconstruction of the exstrophy-epispadias complex—long-term results. Urology 2008;72(3):566–569; discussion 569–570.

Emanuel PG et al: Prenatal detection of anterior abdominal wall defects with US. Radiographics 1995;15(3):517–530.

Gambhir L et al: Epidemiological survey of 214 families with bladder exstrophy-epispadias complex. J Urol 2008;179(4):1539–1543.

Gargollo P et al: Bladder neck reconstruction is often necessary after complete primary repair of exstrophy. J Urol 2011;185(6, Suppl):2563–2571.

Gargollo PC, Borer JG: Contemporary outcomes in bladder exstrophy. Curr Opin Urol 2007;17(4):272–280.

Grady RW et al: Complete primary closure of bladder exstrophy. Epispadias and bladder exstrophy repair. Urol Clin North Am 1999;26(1):95–109, viii.

Husmann DA, Rathbun SR: Long-term follow up of enteric bladder augmentations: The risk for malignancy. J Pediatr Urol 2008;4(5):381–385; discussion 386.

Kiddoo DA et al: Initial management of complex urological disorders: Bladder exstrophy. Urol Clin North Am 2004;31(3):417–426, vii–viii.

Light JK, Scott FB: Treatment of the epispadias-exstrophy complex with the AS792 artificial urinary sphincter. J Urol 1983;129(4):738–740.

Lowentritt BH et al: Variants of the exstrophy complex: A single institution experience. J Urol 2005;173(5):1732–1737.

Meldrum KK et al: Pelvic and extremity immobilization after bladder exstrophy closure: Complications and impact on success. Urology 2003;62(6):1109–1113.

Mitchell ME: Bladder exstrophy repair: Complete primary repair of exstrophy. Urology 2005;65(1):5–8.

Mollard P: Bladder reconstruction in exstrophy. J Urol 1980;124(4):525–529.

Mourtzinos A, Borer JG: Current management of bladder exstrophy. Curr Urol Rep 2004;5(2):137–141.

Oesterling JE, Jeffs RD: The importance of a successful initial bladder closure in the surgical management of classical bladder exstrophy: Analysis of 144 patients treated at the Johns Hopkins Hospital between 1975 and 1985. J Urol 1987;137(2):258–262.

Perlmutter AD et al: Vesical neck reconstruction in patients with epispadias-exstrophy complex. J Urol 1991;146(2, Pt 2):613–615.

Stec AA et al: The modern staged repair of classic bladder exstrophy: A detailed postoperative management strategy for primary bladder closure. J Pediatr Urol 2011.

Suson KD et al: Bony abnormalities in classic bladder exstrophy: The urologist's perspective. J Pediatr Urol 2011.

Toguri AG et al: Continence in cases of bladder exstrophy. J Urol 1978;119(4):538–540.

Vining NC et al: Classic bladder exstrophy: Orthopaedic surgical considerations. J Am Acad Orthop Surg 2011;19(9):518–526.

Persistent Urachus

al-Hindawi MK, Aman S: Benign non-infected urachal cyst in an adult: Review of the literature and a case report. Br J Radiol 1992;65(772):313–316.

Bauer SB, Retik AB: Urachal anomalies and related umbilical disorders. Urol Clin North Am 1978;5(1):195–211.

Chan ES et al: Novel approach of laparoscopic transperitoneal en bloc resection of urachal tumor and umbilectomy with a comparison of various techniques. J Laparoendosc Adv Surg Tech A 2009;19(3):423–426.

Chouhan M et al: Utility of diffusion-weighted imaging in the presurgical diagnosis of an infected urachal cyst. Pediatr Radiol 2011;41(1):125–128.

Cilento BG Jr et al: Urachal anomalies: Defining the best diagnostic modality. Urology 1998;52(1):120–122.

Destri GL et al: The urachal pathology with umbilical manifestation: overview of laparoscopic technique. J Laparoendosc Adv Surg Tech A 2011;21(9):809–814.

Gopalan A et al: Urachal carcinoma: A clinicopathologic analysis of 24 cases with outcome correlation. Am J Surg Pathol 2009;33(5):659–668.

Holten I et al: The ultrasonic diagnosis of urachal anomalies. Australas Radiol 1996;40(1):2–5.

Mesrobian HG et al: Ten years of experience with isolated urachal anomalies in children. J Urol 1997;158(3, Pt 2):1316–1318.

Scheye T et al: Anatomic basis of pathology of the urachus. Surg Radiol Anat 1994;16(2):135–141.

Stone NN et al: Laparoscopic excision of a urachal cyst. Urology 1995;45(1):161–164.

Upadhyay V, Kukkady A: Urachal remnants: An enigma. Eur J Pediatr Surg 2003;13(6):372–376.

Yohannes P et al: Laparoscopic radical excision of urachal sinus. J Endourol 2003;17(7):475–479; discussion 479.

Other Bladder Anomalies

Bhat A et al: Congenital bladder diverticulum presenting as bladder outlet obstruction in infants and children. J Pediatr Urol 2011.

Bjurlin MA et al: Clinical and radiographic findings of a sliding inguinoscrotal hernia containing the urinary bladder. Hernia 2011; 14(6):635–638.

Blane CE et al: Bladder diverticula in children. Radiology 1994;190(3):695–697.

Bogdanos J et al: The large bladder diverticulum in children. J Pediatr Urol 2005;1(4):267–272.

Burbige KA et al: The megacystis-megaureter syndrome. J Urol 1984;131(6):1133–1136.

Catalano O: US evaluation of inguinoscrotal bladder hernias: Report of three cases. Clin Imaging 1997;21(2):126–128.

Confer SD et al: Megacystis with an anterior urethral valve: Case report and review of literature. J Pediatr Urol 2011;6(5): 459–462.

McCormack K et al: Laparoscopic surgery for inguinal hernia repair: Systematic review of effectiveness and economic evaluation. Health Technol Assess 2005;9(14):1–203, iii–iv.

Patle NM et al: Sliding inguinal hernias: Scope of laparoscopic repair. J Laparoendosc Adv Surg Tech A 2011;21(3):227–231.

Pieretti RV, Pieretti-Vanmarcke RV: Congenital bladder diverticula in children. J Pediatr Surg 1999;34(3):468–473.

Sato T et al: Megacystis and megacolon in an infant with Ehlers-Danlos syndrome. Acta Paediatr Jpn 1993;35(4):358–360.

Interstitial Cystitis or Bladder Pain Syndrome

Baskin LS, Tanagho EA: Pelvic pain without pelvic organs. J Urol 1992;147(3):683–686.

Buffington CA: Comorbidity of interstitial cystitis with other unexplained clinical conditions. J Urol 2004;172(4, Pt 1):1242–1248.

Burkman RT: Chronic pelvic pain of bladder origin: Epidemiology, pathogenesis and quality of life. J Reprod Med 2004;49(3, Suppl): 225–229.

Chaiken DC et al: Behavioral therapy for the treatment of refractory interstitial cystitis. J Urol 1993;149(6):1445–1448.

Chancellor MB, Yoshimura N: Treatment of interstitial cystitis. Urology 2004;63(3, Suppl 1):85–92.

Clemens JQ et al: Case-control study of medical comorbidities in women with interstitial cystitis. J Urol 2008;179(6):2222–2225.

Comiter CV: Sacral neuromodulation for the symptomatic treatment of refractory interstitial cystitis: A prospective study. J Urol 2003;169(4):1369–1373.

Elbadawi A: Interstitial cystitis: A critique of current concepts with a new proposal for pathologic diagnosis and pathogenesis. Urology 1997;49(5A, Suppl):14–40.

Gillenwater JY, Wein AJ: Summary of the National Institute of Arthritis, Diabetes, Digestive and Kidney Diseases Workshop on Interstitial Cystitis, National Institutes of Health, Bethesda, Maryland, August 28–29, 1987. J Urol 1988;140(1):203–206.

Hurst RE et al: Urinary glycosaminoglycan excretion as a laboratory marker in the diagnosis of interstitial cystitis. J Urol 1993;149(1): 31–35.

Johansson SL, Fall M: Clinical features and spectrum of light microscopic changes in interstitial cystitis. J Urol 1990;143(6):1118–1124.

Kusek JW, Nyberg LM: The epidemiology of interstitial cystitis: Is it time to expand our definition? Urology 2001;57(6, Suppl 1): 95–99.

Lubeck DP et al: Psychometric validation of the O'leary-Sant interstitial cystitis symptom index in a clinical trial of pentosan polysulfate sodium. Urology 2001;57(6, Suppl 1):62–66.

Mayer R et al: A randomized controlled trial of intravesical bacillus calmette-guerin for treatment refractory interstitial cystitis. J Urol 2005;173(4):1186–1191.

Nickel JC: Interstitial cystitis: A chronic pelvic pain syndrome. Med Clin North Am 2004;88(2):467–481, xii.

Nickel JC et al: The bladder mucus (glycosaminoglycan) layer in interstitial cystitis. J Urol 1993;149(4):716–718.

Nordling J: Interstitial cystitis: How should we diagnose it and treat it in 2004? Curr Opin Urol 2004;14(6):323–327.

O'Leary MP et al: The interstitial cystitis symptom index and problem index. Urology 1997;49(5A, Suppl):58–63.

Oberpenning F et al: Interstitial cystitis: An update. Curr Opin Urol 2002;12(4):321–332.

Ottem DP, Teichman JM: What is the value of cystoscopy with hydrodistension for interstitial cystitis? Urology 2005;66(3):494–499.

Parsons CL, Mulholland SG: Successful therapy of interstitial cystitis with pentosanpolysulfate. J Urol 1987;138(3):513–516.

Peters KM et al: Prevalence of pelvic floor dysfunction in patients with interstitial cystitis. Urology 2007;70(1):16–18.

Riedl CR et al: Hyaluronan treatment of interstitial cystitis/painful bladder syndrome. Int Urogynecol J Pelvic Floor Dysfunct 2008;19(5):717–721.

Rosenberg MT, Hazzard M: Prevalence of interstitial cystitis symptoms in women: A population based study in the primary care office. J Urol 2005;174(6):2231–2234.

Sairanen J et al: Cyclosporine A and pentosan polysulfate sodium for the treatment of interstitial cystitis: A randomized comparative study. J Urol 2005;174(6):2235–2238.

Sant GR et al: A pilot clinical trial of oral pentosan polysulfate and oral hydroxyzine in patients with interstitial cystitis. J Urol 2003;170(3):810–815.

Sant GR, Theoharides TC: The role of the mast cell in interstitial cystitis. Urol Clin North Am 1994;21(1):41–53.

Simon LJ et al: The Interstitial Cystitis Data Base Study: Concepts and preliminary baseline descriptive statistics. Urology 1997; 49(5A, Suppl):64–75.

Sirinian E et al: Correlation between 2 interstitial cystitis symptom instruments. J Urol 2005;173(3):835–840.

Wesselmann U: Neurogenic inflammation and chronic pelvic pain. World J Urol 2001;19(3):180–185.

Foreign Body Inserted into the Bladder

Bjornerem A, Tollan A: Intrauterine device—primary and secondary perforation of the urinary bladder. Acta Obstet Gynecol Scand 1997;76(4):383–385.

Bjurlin MA, Berger AD: Herniorrhaphy mesh as nidus for bladder calculi. Urology 2011;78(2):329–330.

Cardozo L: Recurrent intra-vesical foreign bodies. Br J Urol 1997; 80(4):687.

Chuang YT et al: Laparoscopic removal of a migrated intrauterine contraceptive device with bladder penetration. Taiwan J Obstet Gynecol 2010;49(4):518–520.

Hick EJ et al: Bladder calculus resulting from the migration of an intrauterine contraceptive device. J Urol 2004;172(5, Pt 1):1903.

Mastromichalis M et al: Urethral foreign body insertion for secondary gain in the incarcerated population. Can J Urol 2011;18(5):5916–5917.

Stone NN et al: Laparoscopic excision of a urachal cyst. Urology 1995;45(1):161–164.

Vesical Manifestations of Allergy

Popescu OE et al: The spectrum of eosinophilic cystitis in males: Case series and literature review. Arch Pathol Lab Med 2009;133(2):289–294.

Rubin L, Pincus MB: Eosinophilic cystitis: The relationship of allergy in the urinary tract to eosinophilic cystitis and the pathophysiology of eosinophilia. J Urol 1974;112(4):457–460.

Salman M et al: Eosinophilic cystitis simulating invasive bladder cancer: A real diagnostic challenge. Int Urol Nephrol 2006;38(3–4):545–548.

Thompson RH et al: Clinical manifestations and functional outcomes in children with eosinophilic cystitis. J Urol 2005;174(6):2347–2349.

Watanabe M et al: A case of eosinophilic cystitis that was treated with oral suplatast tosilate (IPD-1151T). Hinyokika Kiyo 2009;55(11):715–719.

Diverticula

Gerridzen RG, Futter NG: Ten-year review of vesical diverticula. Urology 1982;20(1):33–35.

Khonsari S et al: Intraoperative catheter management during laparoscopic excision of a giant bladder diverticulum. J Laparoendosc Adv Surg Tech A 2004;14(1):47–50.

Kural AR et al: Robot-assisted laparoscopic bladder diverticulectomy combined with photoselective vaporization of prostate: a case report and review of literature. J Endourol 2009;23(8):1281–1285.

Macejko AM et al: Cystoscope- and robot-assisted bladder diverticulectomy. J Endourol 2008;22(10):2389–2391; discussion 2391–2382.

Prakash et al: Urinary bladder diverticulum and its association with malignancy: An anatomical study on cadavers. Rom J Morphol Embryol 2010;51(3):543–545.

Yu CC et al: Intradiverticular tumors of the bladder: surgical implications—An eleven-year review. Eur Urol 1993;24(2):190–196.

Vesical Fistulas

Amendola MA et al: Detection of occult colovesical fistula by the Bourne test. AJR Am J Roentgenol 1984;142(4):715–718.

Ayhan A et al: Results of treatment in 182 consecutive patients with genital fistulas. Int J Gynaecol Obstet 1995;48(1):43–47.

Badlani G et al: Enterovesical fistulas in Crohn disease. Urology 1980;16(6):599–600.

Blaivas JG et al: Early versus late repair of vesicovaginal fistulas: Vaginal and abdominal approaches. J Urol 1995;153(4):1110–1112; discussion 1112–1113.

Chapple C, Turner-Warwick R: Vesico-vaginal fistula. BJU Int 2005;95(1):193–214.

Gilmour DT et al: Lower urinary tract injury during gynecologic surgery and its detection by intraoperative cystoscopy. Obstet Gynecol 1999;94(5, Pt 2):883–889.

Huang WC et al: Surgical repair of vesicovaginal fistulas. Urol Clin North Am 2002;29(3):709–723.

Huettner PC et al: Colouterine fistula complicating diverticulitis: Charcoal challenge test aids in diagnosis. Obstet Gynecol 1992;80(3, Pt 2):550–552.

Joseph RC et al: Genitourinary tract gas: Imaging evaluation. Radiographics 1996;16(2):295–308.

Kirsh GM et al: Diagnosis and management of vesicoenteric fistulas. Surg Gynecol Obstet 1991;173(2):91–97.

Kwon EO et al: The poppy seed test for colovesical fistula: big bang, little bucks! J Urol 2008;179(4):1425–1427.

McKay HA: Vesicovaginal fistula repair: Transurethral suture cystorrhaphy as a minimally invasive alternative. J Endourol 2004;18(5):487–490.

Melchior S et al: Diagnosis and surgical management of colovesical fistulas due to sigmoid diverticulitis. J Urol 2009;182(3):978–982.

Moon SG et al: Pelvic fistulas complicating pelvic surgery or diseases: spectrum of imaging findings. Korean J Radiol 2001;2(2):97–104.

Moss RL, Ryan JA Jr: Management of enterovesical fistulas. Am J Surg 1990;159(5):514–517.

Persky L et al: Nondelay in vesicovaginal fistula repair. Urology 1979;13(3):273–275.

Raghavaiah NV: Double-dye test to diagnose various types of vaginal fistulas. J Urol 1974;112(6):811–812.

Simoneaux SF, Patrick LE: Genitourinary complications of Crohn's disease in pediatric patients. AJR Am J Roentgenol 1997;169(1):197–199.

Tamam M et al: Direct radionuclide cystography imaging in colovesical fistula due to inguinal hernia operation complication. Ann Nucl Med 2009;23(7):693–696.

Pelvic Lipomatosis

Heyns CF: Pelvic lipomatosis: A review of its diagnosis and management. J Urol 1991;146(2):267–273.

Heyns CF et al: Pelvic lipomatosis associated with cystitis glandularis and adenocarcinoma of the bladder. J Urol 1991;145(2):364–366.

Masumori N, Tsukamoto T: Pelvic lipomatosis associated with proliferative cystitis: Case report and review of the Japanese literature. Int J Urol 1999;6(1):44–49.

Miglani U et al: Rare etiology of obstructive uropathy: Pelvic lipomatosis. Urol Int 2010;84(2):239–241.

Mordkin RM et al: The radiographic diagnosis of pelvic lipomatosis. Tech Urol 1997;3(4):228–230.

Sozen S et al: The importance of re-evaluation in patients with cystitis glandularis associated with pelvic lipomatosis: A case report. Urol Oncol 2004;22(5):428–430.

Noninfectious Hemorrhagic Cystitis

Andriole GL et al: Danazol-induced cystitis: An undescribed source of hematuria in patients with hereditary angioneurotic edema. J Urol 1986;135(1):44–46.

Ballen KK et al: Safety and cost of hyperhydration for the prevention of hemorrhagic cystitis in bone marrow transplant recipients. Oncology 1999;57(4):287–292.

Bracis R et al: Methicillin hemorrhagic cystitis. Antimicrob Agents Chemother 1977;12(3):438–439.

Chong KT et al: Early hyperbaric oxygen therapy improves outcome for radiation-induced hemorrhagic cystitis. Urology 2005;65(4):649–653.

Cox PJ: Cyclophosphamide cystitis—Identification of acrolein as the causative agent. Biochem Pharmacol 1979;28(13):2045–2049.

deVries CR, Freiha FS: Hemorrhagic cystitis: A review. J Urol 1990; 143(1):1–9.

Donahue LA, Frank IN: Intravesical formalin for hemorrhagic cystitis: Analysis of therapy. J Urol 1989;141(4):809–812.

Efros M et al: Cyclophosphamide-induced hemorrhagic pyelitis and ureteritis associated with cystitis in marrow transplantation. J Urol 1990;144(5):1231–1232.

Giuliani L et al: Gelatin foam and isobutyl-2-cyanoacrylate in the treatment of life-threatening bladder haemorrhage by selective transcatheter embolisation of the internal iliac arteries. Br J Urol 1979;51(2):125–128.

Goren MP et al: Combined intravenous and oral mesna in outpatients treated with ifosfamide. Cancer Chemother Pharmacol 1997;40(5):371–375.

Kaplan JR, Wolf JS Jr: Efficacy and survival associated with cystoscopy and clot evacuation for radiation or cyclophosphamide induced hemorrhagic cystitis. J Urol 2009;181(2):641–646.

Levenback C et al: Hemorrhagic cystitis following radiotherapy for stage Ib cancer of the cervix. Gynecol Oncol 1994;55(2):206–210.

Liu YK et al: Treatment of radiation or cyclophosphamide induced hemorrhagic cystitis using conjugated estrogen. J Urol 1990;144(1):41–43.

Anomalies of the Prostate and the Seminal Vesicles

Carbone A et al: Renal aplastic dysplasia and ipsilateral ectopic ureter obstructing the seminal via: A possible cause of male infertility. Eur Urol 2007;52(1):268–272.

Cherullo EE et al: Laparoscopic management of congenital seminal vesicle cysts associated with ipsilateral renal agenesis. J Urol 2002; 167(3):1263–1267.

Coppens L et al: Adult mullerian duct or utricle cyst: Clinical significance and therapeutic management of 65 cases. J Urol 2002;167(4):1740–1744.

Desautel MG et al: Mullerian duct remnants: surgical management and fertility issues. J Urol 1999;162(3, Pt 2):1008–1013; discussion 1014.

Furuya R et al: New classification of midline cysts of the prostate in adults via a transrectal ultrasonography-guided opacification and dye-injection study. BJU Int 2008;102(4):475–478.

39

Male Sexual Dysfunction

Tom F. Lue, MD, FACS, ScD (Hon)

It is estimated that more than half of men aged 40–70 years in the United States are unable to attain or maintain a penile erection sufficient for satisfactory sexual performance. Advances in pharmacologic therapy for erectile dysfunction (ED), coupled with a better understanding of male sexual dysfunction, have resulted in greater numbers of patients seeking care for sexual concerns. Oral phosphodiesterase type-5 inhibitors (PDE-5Is) have emerged as the preferred first-line treatment of ED worldwide due to their efficacy, ease of use, and patient safety. Erectile function can now be evaluated by the response to these agents at home or intracavernous injection (ICI) of vasoactive agents in the office, and improved diagnostic tests can differentiate among types of impotence. Patient satisfaction with penile prostheses is high, as the latest generation of devices is more sophisticated and durable than ever. Current treatments continue to evolve and new therapies such as stem cells and gene therapies may represent the next generation of more physiologic and disease-specific solutions to various types of ED (Bahk et al, 2010; Lin et al, 2009; Melman et al, 2007).

PHYSIOLOGY OF PENILE ERECTION

▶ Innervation of the Penis

The autonomic spinal erection center is located in the intermediolateral nuclei of the spinal cord at levels S2–S4 and T12–L2. Nerve fibers from the thoracolumbar (sympathetic) and sacral (parasympathetic) spinal segments join to form inferior hypogastric and pelvic plexuses, which send branches to the pelvic organs. The fibers innervating the penis (cavernous nerves) travel along the posterolateral aspect of the seminal vesicles and prostate and then accompany the membranous urethra through the genitourinary diaphragm (Figure 39–1). Some of these fibers enter the corpora cavernosa and corpus spongiosum with the cavernous and bulbourethral arteries. Others travel distally with the dorsal nerve

and enter the corpus cavernosum and corpus spongiosum in various locations to supply the mid- and distal portions of the penis. The terminal branches of the cavernous nerves innervate the helicine arteries and trabecular smooth muscle, and are responsible for vascular events during tumescence and detumescence.

The center for somatic motor nerves is located at the ventral horn of the S2–S4 segments (Onuf's nucleus). The motor fibers join the pudendal nerve to innervate the bulbocavernosus and ischiocavernosus muscles. The somatic sensory nerves originate at receptors in the penis to transmit pain, temperature, touch, and vibratory sensations. The brain has a modulatory effect on the spinal pathways of erection, specifically the medial preoptic area and paraventricular nucleus of the hypothalamus, periaqueductal gray of the midbrain, and the nucleus paragigantocellularis of the medulla. Positron emission tomography and functional magnetic resonance imaging have allowed for greater understanding of brain activation during sexual arousal and orgasm by measuring regional cerebral blood flow or activity. These powerful tools, used in the study of higher brain function and central activation of sexual arousal, may better define pathophysiology associated with varied conditions including psychogenic ED, premature ejaculation, and orgasmic dysfunction (Georgiadis and Holstege, 2005).

Three types of erections are noted in humans: genital stimulated (contact or reflexogenic), central stimulated (noncontact or psychogenic), and central originated (nocturnal). Genital-stimulated erection is induced by tactile stimulation of the genital area. This kind of erection can be preserved in upper spinal cord lesions, although erections are usually short in duration and poorly controlled by the individual. Central-stimulated erection is more complex, resulting from memory, fantasy, visual, or auditory stimuli. Centrally originated erections can occur spontaneously without stimulation or during sleep; most sleep erections occur during rapid eye movement (REM) sleep. During REM sleep,

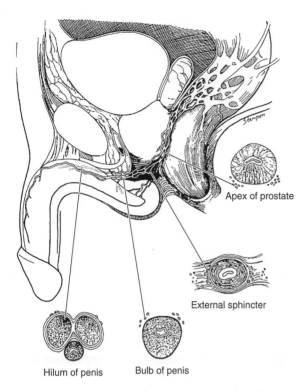

▲ **Figure 39–1.** Location of cavernous nerves in relation to urethra.

Apex of prostate

External sphincter

Hilum of penis   Bulb of penis

the cholinergic neurons in the lateral pontine tegmentum are activated while the adrenergic neurons in the locus coeruleus and the serotonergic neurons in the midbrain raphe are silent. This differential activation may be responsible for the nocturnal erections during REM sleep. Of note, the number and duration of erections for men with hypogonadism or receiving antiandrogen therapy is markedly reduced (Granata et al, 1997).

▶ Anatomy and Hemodynamics of Penile Erection

The tunica of the corpora cavernosa is a bilayered structure with multiple sublayers. The inner circular bundles support and contain the cavernous tissue. From this inner layer, intra-cavernosal pillars that act as struts radiate to augment the septum; both structures provide structural support to the corpus cavernosum. The outer-layer bundles are oriented longitudinally and extend from the glans penis to the proximal crura. These fibers insert into the inferior pubic ramus but are absent between the 5- and 7-o'clock positions. In contrast, the corpus spongiosum lacks an outer layer or intracorporeal struts, ensuring a lower pressure structure during erection. The tunica is composed of elastic fibers forming a

network on which the collagen fibers rest. Emissary veins run between the inner and outer layers for a short distance, often piercing the outer bundles obliquely. Branches of the dorsal artery take a more direct perpendicular route and are surrounded by a periarterial fibrous sheath (Hsu et al, 2004).

The paired internal pudendal artery is the major carrier of the blood supply to the penis, dividing into three branches: the bulbourethral artery, dorsal artery, and the cavernous artery (deep artery). The cavernous artery supplies the corpora cavernosa; the dorsal artery, the skin, subcutaneous tissue, and the glans penis; and the bulbourethral artery, the corpus spongiosum. In some cases, accessory pudendal arteries from external iliac or obturator arteries may supply a major portion of the penis, with collaterals among the three branches often observed. The venous drainage of the glans is mainly through the deep dorsal vein. The corpus spongiosum is drained via the circumflex, urethral, and bulbar veins, but the drainage of the corpora cavernosa is more complex: the mid- and distal shaft are drained by the deep dorsal and periarterial veins to the preprostatic plexus while the proximal portion is drained by the cavernous and crural veins to the preprostatic plexus and internal pudendal vein. The drainage of all three corpora originates in the subtunical venules, which unite to form emissary veins. The glans penis possesses numerous large and small veins that communicate freely with the dorsal veins. The penile skin and subcutaneous tissue are drained by superficial dorsal veins, which then empty into the saphenous veins.

Activation of the autonomic nerves produces a full erection secondary to filling and trapping of blood in the cavernous bodies. After full erection is achieved, contraction of the ischiocavernosus muscle (from activation of the somatic nerves) compresses the proximal corpora and raises the intracorporal pressure well above the systolic blood pressure, resulting in rigid erection (Table 39–1). This rigid phase occurs naturally during masturbation or sexual intercourse but can also occur from slight bending of the penis, without muscular action. The erection process can be divided into phases as shown in Table 39–1 and Figure 39–2. The hemodynamics of the penile glans is somewhat different. Arterial flow increases in a manner similar to that in the shaft. Because it lacks the tunica albuginea, however, the glans functions as an arteriovenous fistula during the full erection phase. Nevertheless, during rigid erection, most of the venous channels are temporarily compressed, and further engorgement of the glans can be observed (Lue, 2000).

▶ Mechanism of Penile Erection

The penile erectile tissue, specifically cavernous, arteriolar, and arterial wall smooth musculature, is key to the erectile process. In the flaccid state, these smooth muscles are tonically contracted due to intrinsic smooth-muscle tone and possibly tonic adrenergic discharge, allowing only a small amount of arterial flow for nutritional purposes. The blood

Table 39-1. Phases of the erection process.[a]

Flaccid phase (1)
  Minimal arterial and venous flow; blood gas values equal those of venous blood.

Latent (filling) phase (2)
  Increased flow in the internal pudendal artery during both systolic and diastolic phases. Decreased pressure in the internal pudendal artery; unchanged intracavernous pressure. Some elongation of the penis.

Tumescent phase (3)
  Rising intracavernous pressure until full erection is achieved. Penis shows more expansion and elongation with pulsation. The arterial flow decreases as the pressure rises. When intracavernous pressure rises above diastolic pressure, flow occurs only in the systolic phases.

Full erection phase (4)
  Intracavernous pressure can rise to as much as 90-100% of the systolic pressure. Arterial flow is less than that in the initial filling phase but is still higher than in the flaccid phase. Although the venous channels are mostly compressed except the proximal ones, the total venous flow is slightly higher than venous flow in the flaccid phase. Blood gas values approach those of arterial blood.

Rigid erection phase (5)
  As a result of contraction of the ischiocavernous muscle, the intracavernous pressure rises well above the systolic pressure, resulting in rigid erection. During this phase, no blood enters the corpus cavernosum. The duration of this phase is short and does not cause ischemia or tissue damage.

Detumescent phase (6)
  After ejaculation or cessation of erotic stimuli, sympathetic tonic discharge resumes, resulting in contraction of the smooth muscles around the sinusoids and arterioles. This diminishes the arterial flow to flaccid level, reopens the venous channels, and expels blood from the sinusoidal spaces. The penis returns to its flaccid length and girth.

[a]Numbers 1–6 correspond to phases shown in Figure 39-2.

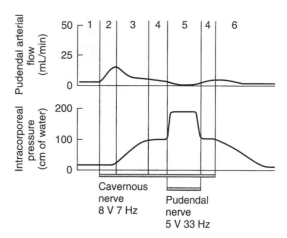

▲ **Figure 39-2.** Phases of penile erection (induced in monkeys via neurostimulation). Numbers correspond to phases outlined in Table 39-1. (Lower tracing = intracavernous pressure; upper tracing = flow within the internal pudendal artery.)

partial pressure of oxygen (PO_2) is about 35 mm Hg. When smooth muscles relax due to the release of neurotransmitters, resistance to incoming flow drops to a minimum. Arterial and arteriolar vasodilatation occurs, and sinusoids expand to receive a large increase of flow. Trapping of blood causes the penis to lengthen and widen rapidly until the capacity of the tunica albuginea is reached. Expansion of the sinusoidal walls against one another and the tunica albuginea results in compression of the subtunical venous plexus. As well, uneven stretching of the layers of the tunica albuginea compresses the emissary veins and effectively reduces the venous flow to a minimum (Lue, 2000; Figures 39–3A and B). Intracavernous pressure (ICP) and PO_2 increase to about 100 and 90 mm Hg, respectively, raising the penis from a dependent position to the erect state; further pressure increases (to several hundred millimeters of mercury) due to

contraction of the ischiocavernosus muscles result in the rigid-erection phase (Dean and Lue, 2005; Gratzke et al, 2010).

▶ Hormones and Sexual Function

Androgens are essential for male sexual maturity. Testosterone (T) regulates gonadotropin secretion and muscle development; dihydrotestosterone mediates male sexual maturation, including hair growth, acne, male pattern baldness, and spermatogenesis. In adults, androgen deficiency results in decreased libido (sexual interest) and impaired seminal emission. Aging is associated with a progressive decline of testosterone, dehydroepiandrosterone, thyroxine, melatonin, and growth hormone and increased levels of sex hormone-binding globulin, pituitary gonadotropins, and prolactin (Morales, 2005). In a longitudinal study of middle-aged men for 7–10 years, total T levels declined at 0.8%/year of age, whereas both free and albumin-bound T declined at about 2%/year. Sex hormone-binding globulin increased at 1.6%/year (Feldman et al, 2002). Testosterone levels do not correspond to severity of ED; however, lower levels are observed in men with reduced libido. Although frequency, magnitude, and latency of nocturnal penile erections are reduced with decreased T, erectile response to visual sexual stimulation is preserved in men with hypogonadism, suggesting that androgen is not essential for erection. Due to the inhibitory action of prolactin on central dopaminergic activity and resultant decreases in gonadotropin-releasing hormone secretion, hyperprolactinemia of any cause results in both reproductive and sexual dysfunction (Corona et al, 2004).

Tunica albuginea:
outer longitudinal layer
inner circular layer

Emissary vein

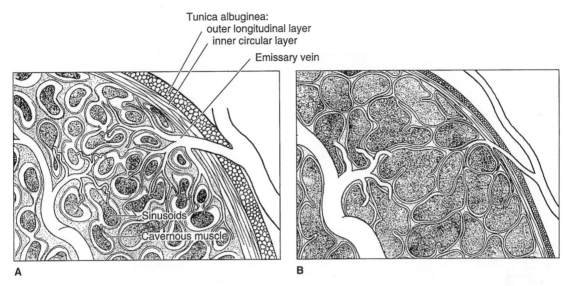

Sinusoids
Cavernous muscle

A

B

▲ **Figure 39–3.** The mechanism of penile erection. In the flaccid state **(A)**, the arteries, arterioles, and sinusoids are contracted. The intersinusoidal and subtunical venular plexuses are wide open, with free flow to the emissary veins. In the erect state **(B)**, the muscles of the sinusoidal wall and the arterioles relax, allowing maximal flow to the compliant sinusoidal spaces. Most of the venules are compressed between the expanding sinusoids. Even the larger intermediary venules are sandwiched and flattened by distended sinusoids and the noncompliant tunica albuginea. This effectively reduces the venous capacity to a minimum.

Neurotransmitters and Pharmacology of Erection

Neural control of penile erection involves adrenergic, cholinergic, and nonadrenergic–noncholinergic (NANC) neuroeffector systems. Adrenergic nerves mediate intracavernous smooth-muscle contraction, maintaining the penis in a nonerect state. Currently, it is suggested that sympathetic contraction is mediated by activation of postsynaptic alpha-1a- and alpha-1d-adrenergic receptors and modulated by presynaptic alpha-2-adrenergic receptors (Giuliano et al, 2004). Cholinergic nerves may contribute to smooth-muscle relaxation and penile erection through inhibition of adrenergic nerves via inhibitory interneurons and the release of nitric oxide (NO) from the endothelium by acetylcholine (Saenz de Tejada et al, 2004).

The principal neurotransmitter for penile erection is NO from parasympathetic, NANC nerve terminals. Once blood rushes into the sinusoids, shear stress can also release NO from endothelium to augment smooth-muscle relaxation and erection. In addition, oxygen tension and substances secreted by endothelial cells lining the sinusoidal spaces, prostaglandins, endothelins, and angiotensin may also be involved in penile erection and detumescence (Musicki and Burnett, 2006). The agents capable of inducing erection and causing detumescence are summarized in Table 39–2.

Although mechanisms of action vary, erection-inducing substances cause smooth muscle to relax and detumescing agents cause them to contract.

Molecular Mechanism of Smooth-Muscle Contraction and Relaxation

Smooth-muscle contraction is regulated by Ca^{2+}. As cytosolic free Ca^{2+} increases from resting levels of 120–270 to 500–700 nM, calmodulin-4 Ca^{2+} complex binds to myosin light-chain kinase. The activated kinase then phosphorylates the light chain and initiates a contraction cycle (Gratzke et al, 2010). Once cytosolic Ca^{2+} returns to basal levels, calcium-sensitizing pathways take over. Activation of excitatory receptors coupled to G proteins causes contraction by increasing calcium sensitivity without changes in cytosolic Ca^{2+} levels. This pathway involves RhoA, a small monomeric G protein that activates Rho-kinase. Activated Rho-kinase phosphorylates, and thereby inhibits, the regulatory subunit of smooth-muscle myosin phosphatase, preventing dephosphorylation of myofilaments and maintaining contractile tone (Jin and Burnett, 2006). The emerging consensus is that phasic contraction of penile smooth muscle is regulated by increased cytosolic Ca^{2+} and tonic contraction is governed by calcium-sensitizing pathways.

Table 39–2. Agents that have been reported to induce or inhibit penile erection.

Inducers	Inhibitors
Papaverine	Phenylephrine
Phentolamine	Epinephrine
Phenoxybenzamine	Norepinephrine
Thymoxamine	Metaraminol
Alprostadil (prostaglandin E1)	Ephedrine
Vasoactive intestinal polypeptide (VIP)	Prostaglandin I 2
Calcitonin gene-related peptide (CGRP)	Prostaglandin F 2α
Nitric oxide donor	Thromboxane A 2 (TXA2)
Guanylate cyclase activator	Endothelin
Dopamine receptor agonist	Angiotensin II
Phosphodiesterase inhibitors	
Rho-kinase inhibitors	
Melanocortin receptors agonist	

▶ Signal Transduction in Penile Erection

During sexual stimulation, NO released from nerve endings and endothelium diffuses into the trabecular and arterial smooth-muscle cells to activate guanylyl cyclase, catalyzing the formation of second messenger cyclic guanosine monophosphate (cGMP). cGMP in turn activates protein kinase G, phosphorylating potassium and calcium channels; the end result is hyperpolarization, reduced intracytosolic calcium, and dissociation of the myosin head from actin as smooth muscle relaxes. Cyclic adenosine monophosphate (cAMP) is another second messenger involved in smooth-muscle relaxation and is activated by cAMP-signaling molecules including adenosine, calcitonin gene-related peptides, and prostaglandins (Lin et al, 2005).

Both of these second messengers activate cAMP- and cGMP-dependent protein kinases, resulting in a drop of cytosolic free calcium and smooth-muscle relaxation via the (1) opening of the potassium channels and hyperpolarization, (2) sequestration of intracellular calcium by the endoplasmic reticulum, and (3) blockage of calcium influx through inhibition of voltage-dependent calcium channels (Dean and Lue, 2005). On the other hand, norepinephrine, phenylephrine, and endothelin appear to activate phospholipase C, leading to the formation of inositol triphosphate and diacylglycerol. The net result is increased cytoplasmic calcium and subsequent smooth-muscle contraction. Detumescence occurs following degradation of cGMP and cAMP to GMP and AMP, respectively, by specific phosphodiesterases. Eleven classes of phosphodiesterases have been identified. The penis is rich in PDE-5 (GMP specific), and therefore, the selective PDE-5Is (sildenafil, vardenafil, and tadalafil) are able to improve penile erections in patients with ED.

▶ Intercellular Communication

Gap junctions are aqueous intercellular channels that have been demonstrated to interconnect the cytoplasm of adjacent cells in many tissues. In the penis, smooth-muscle cells are sparsely innervated by the terminal branches of the cavernous nerves. Therefore, gap junctions play a vital role in the intercellular communication within the corpus cavernosum, enabling the penis to function as a unit (Melman et al, 2007).

MALE SEXUAL DYSFUNCTION

Male sexual dysfunction, denoting the inability to achieve a satisfactory sexual relationship, may involve inadequacy of erection or problems with emission, ejaculation, or orgasm.

Premature (rapid) ejaculation refers to persistent or recurrent occurrence of ejaculation with minimal sexual stimulation before, on, or shortly after penetration and before the person wishes it.

Retarded ejaculation is undue delay in reaching a climax during sexual activity.

Retrograde ejaculation denotes backflow of semen into the bladder during ejaculation owing to an incompetent bladder neck mechanism.

Anorgasmia is the inability to achieve an orgasm during conscious sexual activity, although nocturnal emission may occur.

EPIDEMIOLOGY

In the Massachusetts Male Aging Study, a community-based survey of men between 40 and 70 years of age, 52% of respondents reported some degree of ED: 17% mild, 25% moderate, and 10% complete. Although the prevalence of mild ED remained constant (17%) between the age of 40 and 70, there was a doubling in the number of men reporting moderate ED (from 17% to 34%) and a tripling in the number of men reporting complete ED (from 5% to 15%) (Feldman et al, 1994). More than 70% of men older than 65 years report that they are sexually active; however, 40% are dissatisfied with their sexual function (Braun et al, 2000). Among the major predictors of ED are hypertension, hyperlipidemia, diabetes mellitus, and heart disease. Risk of ED appears to increase with smoking, and may occur in a dose-dependent manner (Polsky et al, 2005). There is a higher prevalence of ED in men who have undergone radiation or surgery for prostate cancer or other pelvic malignancies. The psychological correlates of ED include decreased self-esteem, depression, anxiety, anger, and relationship dissatisfaction (Althof et al, 2006). Other male sexual dysfunctions have also been found to be highly prevalent: premature ejaculation and decreased libido (lack of sexual interest) are common patients' concerns.

Table 39–3. New classification of ED recommended by the International Society for Sexual Medicine.

I. Psychogenic
    1. Generalized type
       A. Generalized unresponsiveness
          a. Primary lack of sexual arousability
          b. Aging-related decline in sexual arousability
       B. Generalized inhibition
          a. Chronic disorder of sexual intimacy
    2. Situational type
       A. Partner related
          a. Lack of arousability in specific relationship
          b. Lack of arousability due to sexual object preference
          c. High central inhibition due to partner conflict or threat
       B. Performance related
          a. Associated with other sexual dysfunction/s (eg, rapid ejaculation)
          b. Situational performance anxiety (eg, fear of failure)
       C. Psychological distress or adjustment related
          a. Associated with negative mood state (eg, depression) or major life stress (eg, death of partner)

II. Organic
    1. Neurogenic
    2. Hormonal
    3. Arterial
    4. Cavernosal (venogenic)
    5. Drug induced

III. Mixed organic/psychogenic (most common type)

CLASSIFICATION AND PATHOGENESIS

The classification system of ED most commonly used encompasses organic, psychogenic, and mixed etiologies of ED and is endorsed by the International Society of Impotence Research (Table 39–3). In the 1950s, 90% of cases of ED were believed to be psychogenic. Most authors now believe that mixed organic and psychogenic ED is the most common.

Psychological Disorders

Many psychologic conditions (performance anxiety, strained relationship, lack of sexual arousal, depression, and schizophrenia) can either cause or aggravate ED. Sexual behavior and penile erection are controlled by the hypothalamus, cerebral cortex, and limbic systems. Given the number and complexity of known and as yet unidentified factors involved, it is not surprising that the pathogenesis of psychogenic ED is still speculative. Possible mechanisms proposed include an imbalance of central neurotransmitters, overinhibition of spinal erection center by the brain, inadequate NO release, and sympathetic overactivity (Bodie et al, 2003).

Neurogenic Disorders

It has been estimated that up to 20% of all ED is neurogenic in origin, resulting from peripheral (cavernous and pudendal nerve) or central pathologies. In men with spinal cord injury, the degree of erectile function depends on the nature, location, and the extent of the lesion. Brain lesions associated with ED include dementias, Parkinson's disease, stroke, tumors, trauma, and Shy-Drager syndrome (Papatsoris et al, 2006). Peripheral neuropathy due to diabetes mellitus, chronic alcohol abuse, or vitamin deficiency may affect the nerve endings and result in a deficiency of neurotransmitters. Direct injury to the cavernous or pudendal nerves from trauma, radical pelvic surgeries for malignancy, or pelvic irradiation can also cause ED. It is important to note that even with nerve-sparing approaches to prostatic and rectal surgery, erectile recovery can take up to 24 months or longer.

Hormonal Disorders

Historically, hypogonadism as a cause of ED was thought to be rare, but recent data support a significant increase of hypogonadism with age. Hypogonadism due to hypothalamic or pituitary tumors, estrogen or antiandrogen therapy, or orchiectomy can suppress sexual interest and nocturnal erections. As mentioned earlier, erections are usually preserved to some extent. Hyperprolactinemia, Cushing's syndrome, and Addison's disease can cause decreased libido and ED. Hyperthyroidism is commonly associated with decreased libido, likely due to elevated estrogen levels, while hypothyroidism can contribute to ED through diminished testosterone secretion and elevated prolactin levels (Veronelli et al, 2006).

Arterial Disorders

Although arteriogenic ED may be congenital or posttraumatic, more often it is part of a generalized systemic arterial disease. Traumatic arterial occlusive or atherosclerotic disease of the hypogastric (iliac)–pudendal–cavernous arterial tree can decrease flow to the sinusoidal spaces and perfusion pressure, thus decreasing the rigidity or prolonging time to maximal erection. Some patients with severe arterial disease may retain erectile function as long as arterial flow exceeds venous flow; conversely, some patients with minimal arterial disease may develop partial or complete ED because of large venous outflow, cavernous smooth-muscle dysfunction, or inadequate neurotransmitter release (Dean and Lue, 2005).

High prevalence of ED has been reported in men with coronary, cerebral, and peripheral vascular diseases (Chai et al, 2009; Kloner et al, 2003). Among men with coronary arterial disease, the prevalence of ED increases as the severity of coronary arterial lesions increase. In patients with chronic coronary disease who also had ED, onset of sexual dysfunction occurred before coronary artery disease (CAD) onset in 93%, with a mean time interval of 24 [12–36] months (Montorsi et al, 2006). When ED occurs in a younger man, it is associated with a marked increase in the risk of future cardiac events, whereas in older men, ED appears to be of little prognostic importance (Inman et al, 2009).

Common risk factors associated with arterial insufficiency include hypertension, hyperlipidemia, diabetes mellitus, and metabolic syndrome. Long-distance cycling is also a likely risk factor for vasculogenic and neurogenic ED (Huang et al, 2005). Several modifiable life style factors such as physical inability, smoking, and alcohol consumption may also contribute to ED (Kupelian et al, 2009).

Arterial disease is classified as extra- or intrapenile arterial insufficiency. Extrapenile disease may be amenable to surgical repair in selected patients, and comprises diseases of the internal pudendal artery, internal and common iliac arteries, aorta, the pelvic steal syndrome, and pelvic trauma. Intrapenile arterial disease secondary to aging, arteriosclerosis, or diabetes mellitus does not respond well to currently available surgical techniques.

▶ Cavernosal Disorders

Cavernous veno-occlusive dysfunction (CVOD) may result from a variety of pathophysiologic processes. Degenerative changes (Peyronie's disease, aging, and diabetes) and traumatic injury to the tunica albuginea (penile fracture) can impair the compression of the subtunical and emissary veins. Fibroelastic alteration of the trabeculae, cavernous smooth muscle, and endothelium may result in venous leakage (Deveci et al, 2006). Men with diabetes mellitus and atherosclerosis are at increased risk of smooth-muscle atrophy, fibrous replacement, and endothelial disruption. In men with no symptoms of coronary disease, the presence of CVOD was reported to have the greatest chance of predicting abnormal exercise stress echocardiography (Mulhall et al, 2009).

CVOD can be divided into five types according to cause: In type 1, large veins exit the corpus cavernosum (etiology is likely congenital); in type 2, venous channels are enlarged as a result of distortion of the tunica albuginea (secondary to Peyronie's disease or weakening associated with aging); in type 3, the cavernous smooth muscle is unable to relax because of fibrosis, degeneration; in type 4, there is inadequate neurotransmitter release (neurologic or psychologic impotence, or endothelial dysfunction) (Watts et al, 2007); and in type 5, there is abnormal communication between the corpus cavernosum and the spongiosum or glans (congenital, traumatic, or secondary to shunt procedures for priapism) (Dean and Lue, 2005).

▶ Medication-Induced Erectile Dysfunction

Many drugs have been reported to cause ED, although the mechanism of action is often unknown and there are few controlled studies on the sexual side effects of a particular agent. As ED is common among older men, it will coexist with other conditions that are themselves risk factors for ED, such as cardiovascular disease, diabetes, or depression. Sexual symptoms related to medications can also involve a combination of complaints concerning desire, arousal, and orgasm rather than being limited to impaired erection.

In general, drugs that interfere with central neuroendocrine or local neurovascular control of penile smooth muscle have the potential to cause ED. Central neurotransmitter pathways, including serotonergic, noradrenergic, and dopaminergic pathways involved in sexual function, may be disturbed by antipsychotics, antidepressants, and centrally acting antihypertensive drugs (Balon, 2005). Selective serotonin reuptake inhibitors are the most common class of drugs currently used to treat depression; it is estimated that up to 50% of patients using these agents experience a change in sexual function. Nonspecific beta-adrenergic blocking drugs may cause ED by potentiating alpha-1 adrenergic activity in the penis. Conversely, alpha-1 blockers and angiotensin-II-receptor blockers both tend to improve sexual function during treatment and may therefore be useful when commencing antihypertensive therapy in men with preexisting ED. Thiazide diuretics have been reported to cause ED; spironolactone can also cause a decrease in libido and gynecomastia. Alpha-adrenergic blocking drugs, such as doxazosin, terazosin, and tamsulosin, may cause retrograde ejaculation owing to relaxation of the bladder neck (Guiliano, 2006). Other drugs thought to cause ED include opiates, antiretroviral agents, and histamine H_2-receptor antagonists (cimetidine).

Antiandrogens modify sexual behavior by varying degrees, ranging from complete loss to normal function, chiefly by modulating sexual desire via central nervous system androgen receptors. Finasteride, a 5-alpha-reductase inhibitor commonly used to treat benign prostatic hypertrophy, is the antiandrogen with the least effect on circulating testosterone and sexual function. Sexual symptoms are reported in approximately 5% of men treated with a 5-mg dose (Miner et al, 2006). Estrogens and drugs with antiandrogenic action such as ketoconazole, luteinizing hormone-releasing hormone (LHRH) agonists, nonsteroidal (bicalutamide), and steroidal (cyproterone acetate) acetate can diminish sexual function. The near-complete androgen deprivation achieved by medical castration with LHRH agonists results in a profound loss of sexual desire, which is usually accompanied by ED.

Cigarette smoking may induce vasoconstriction and penile venous leakage because of its contractile effect on the cavernous smooth muscle and is seen to approximately double the rate of ED in coronary artery disease, hypertension, and atherosclerosis (Korenman, 2004). Alcohol in small amounts improves erection and increases libido because of its vasodilatory effect and the suppression of anxiety; however, large amounts can cause central sedation, decreased libido, and transient ED. Chronic alcoholism may cause hypogonadism and polyneuropathy, which may affect penile nerve function.

Aging and Systemic Disease

Sexual function progressively declines in "healthy" aging men. Longitudinal studies demonstrate a nonlinear decline for most aspects of sexual function as age increases, with a more pronounced decline in older groups (Araujo et al, 2004). The latent period between sexual stimulation and erection increases, erections are less turgid, ejaculation is less forceful, ejaculatory volume decreases, and the refractory period between erections lengthens. There is also a decrease in penile sensitivity to tactile stimulation, a decrease in serum testosterone concentration, and an increase in cavernous muscle tone. While psychologic and organic factors are important contributors to ED across age groups, organic issues tend to play a more profound role as men age.

ED in men with diabetes mellitus occurs approximately threefold that of the general population, and can be the presenting symptom for diabetes mellitus and/or predict later neurologic sequelae (Fonseca and Java, 2005). Diabetes may affect small vessels, cavernous nerve terminals, smooth muscle, and endothelial cells; neurovascular sequelae of long-term diabetes results in decreased responsiveness to oral PDE-5 inhibitor therapy. Obesity, a component of metabolic syndrome, has been linked to endothelial dysfunction, androgen deficiency, and ED (Traish et al, 2009). Alteration of protein levels in the corpus cavernousum has also been proposed as a cause of ED (Chiou et al, 2010).

Men with severe pulmonary disease may have ED because of fear of aggravating dyspnea during sexual intercourse (Koseoglu et al, 2005) Patients with angina, myocardial infarction (MI), or heart failure may have ED from anxiety, depression, or concomitant penile arterial insufficiency, which is quite common in these patients. Chronic renal failure has frequently been associated with diminished erectile function, impaired libido, and infertility (Shamsa et al, 2005). In men with chronic renal failure and ED, many were found to have cavernous artery occlusive disease and veno-occlusive dysfunction. The mechanism is likely multifactorial: low serum testosterone concentration, diabetes mellitus, vascular insufficiency, multiple medications, autonomic and somatic neuropathy, and psychological stress. Other systemic disorders such as cirrhosis, chronic debilitation, and cachexia can cause ED due to loss of libido or neurovascular dysfunction.

DIAGNOSIS AND TREATMENT

The management of ED is built on a patient-centered and evidence-based principle. A detailed medical, sexual, and psychosocial history and a thorough physical examination are the most important steps in the differential diagnosis of sexual dysfunction. Interviewing the partner, if available, is helpful in eliciting a reliable history, planning treatment, and obtaining a successful outcome.

Medical, Sexual, and Psychosocial History

The goals of the medical history are to evaluate the potential role of underlying medical conditions, differentiate between organic and psychogenic causes, and to assess the role of medication(s), both causative and therapeutic. The patient's past surgical history may similarly yield insights. A sexual history confirms the diagnosis, and should ascertain the severity, onset, and duration of the problem, as well as the presence of concomitant medical or psychosocial factors. It is necessary to determine whether the presenting complaint (eg, ED, premature ejaculation) is the primary sexual problem or if some other aspects of the sexual response cycle (desire, ejaculation, orgasm) are involved. Psychosocial assessment of past and present partner relationships is essential given the interpersonal context of sexual problems. Sexual dysfunction may affect the patient's self-esteem and coping ability, as well as social relationships and occupational performance.

Physical and Laboratory Examination

A focused physical examination is performed on each patient, assessing the genitourinary, endocrine, neurologic, and vascular systems, and includes a complete genital examination including digital rectal and measurement of blood pressure and heart rate. Examination may yield a diagnosis of Peyronie's disease, prostatic enlargement, malignancy, or evidence of hypogonadism (decreased testes size, altered secondary sex characteristics).

Recommended tests include fasting glucose, lipid profile, and morning testosterone (calculated free testosterone is more reliable to establish hypogonadism). Diabetic patients should have hemoglobin A_{1C} measured and additional hormonal testing (prolactin, follicle-stimulating hormone [FSH], and luteinizing hormone [LH]) is required when low testosterone levels are noted or for clinical suspicion of abnormality. Optional tests, including prostate-specific antigen (PSA), thyroid-stimulating hormone (TSH), complete blood cell count, and creatinine, must be tailored to the patient's complaints and risk factors.

Self-Reported Questionnaires and Laboratory Investigations

The most commonly used validated questionnaires are the 15-item International Index of Erectile Function (IIEF) or an abridged 5-item version (IIEF-5) more suited for office use. Sexual domain functions measured by the IIEF include erectile function, orgasmic function, sexual desire, intercourse satisfaction, and overall satisfaction. These tools are useful to determine baseline erectile function and to assess the impact of a specific treatment modality. ED severity is classified in five categories based on the IIEF-5: severe (5–7), moderate (8–11), mild to moderate (12–16), mild (17–21), no ED (22–25) (Rosen, 2004).

The physician should review the findings, inquire about the goals and preferences of the man (and his partner), and discuss further diagnostic and therapeutic options such that his (or their) participation in the decision-making process is well informed. For a minority of patients, referral for further testing and/or assessment may be appropriate. Indications for referral include patient request, treatment failure, complex gonadal or other endocrine disorders, neurologic deficits suggestive of brain or spinal cord disease, deep-seated psychologic or psychiatric problems, and active cardiovascular disease. Patients deemed to be at intermediate or higher cardiac risk (cardiac status uncertain, moderate-to-severe symptoms, or unable to perform exercise of modest intensity) should be assessed by a cardiologist/internist and sexual activity deferred until cardiac condition is stabilized or resumption of sexual activity is deemed safe by the consultant. Low-risk patients, those able to perform exercise of modest intensity (six or more metabolic equivalents) without symptoms, do not generally require cardiologic assessment (Jackson et al, 2006).

▶ Follow-up Strategy

Regardless of the treatment regimen chosen, follow-up is essential to ensure optimal outcomes. Modification of life style, diet change, regular exercise, and smoking cessation should be reassessed and encouraged at each clinic visit. Monitoring adverse events, assessing satisfaction or failure with a given treatment, identifying a partner's sexual dysfunction, and assessing overall health and psychosocial function are key considerations. In patients who do not respond to first-line therapy (oral PDE-5 inhibitor therapy), consideration should also be given to whether an alteration in dose or treatment might be of value, as most second- and third-line options have demonstrated reasonable response and satisfaction rates in controlled studies (Lue et al, 2004).

ADVANCED TESTING FOR ERECTILE DYSFUNCTION

For patients with more complex problems, including penile deformity, history of pelvic or perineal trauma, ED of unknown etiology, cases requiring vascular or neurosurgical intervention, complicated endocrinopathy, complicated psychiatric disorder, complex relationship problems, and medicolegal concerns or at the patient's request, a variety of vascular and neurologic diagnostic tests are available to identify the cause of ED or plan treatment (Table 39–4).

▶ Tests for Penile Vascular Function

The goal of vascular evaluation is to identify and evaluate arterial and veno-occlusive dysfunction. The most commonly utilized tests include combined intracavernous injection and stimulation (CIS), duplex ultrasound, dynamic infusion cavernosometry and cavernosography (DICC), and selective penile angiography. A test for endothelium

Table 39–4. Tests Suggested for Various Treatment Options.[a]

1. **Oral medication, transurethral therapy, or vacuum constriction device**
   No further testing
2. **Intracavernous injection therapy**
   CIS test
3. **Penile prosthesis**
   CIS test or NPT test or duplex scanning
4. **Venous surgery**
   CIS test
   Duplex scanning or cavernous arterial occlusion pressure test
   Cavernosometry and cavernosography
5. **Arterial surgery (or combined arterial and venous surgery)**
   CIS test
   Duplex scanning or cavernous arterial occlusion pressure
   Cavernosometry and cavernosography
   Pharmacologic arteriography

CIS, combined injection and stimulation; NPT, nocturnal penile tumescence.

[a]Regardless of desired treatment, all patients must undergo history, physical examination, and basic laboratory testing.

dependent flow-mediated dilation of the brachial artery has been proposed but will not be discussed here because it is not specific for penile function (Yavuzgil et al, 2005).

A. Combined Intracavernous Injection and Stimulation Test

This is a commonly performed diagnostic procedure for ED. It consists of an ICI, visual or manual sexual stimulation, and a rating of the subsequent erection. Before injection, the patient should be informed about the purpose, alternatives, risks, and benefits of the test. Neurogenic and hormonal influences are bypassed, as the vascular status of the penis is assessed by direct injection of medication into the corpus cavernosum. The most commonly used vasodilator is 10 µg of alprostadil or 0.3 mL of a mixture of papaverine and phentolamine. A rigid erection lasting >10 minutes is indicative of normal venous function. However, the same conclusion cannot be made for arterial function, as some men with mild arterial insufficiency can also have the same response. Although some researchers have modified this test by using an oral PDE-5 inhibitor and audiovisual sexual stimulation, the normal criteria have not been established.

B. Color Duplex Ultrasonography

Color duplex ultrasound, the most popular vascular assessment of ED, is utilized when accurate vascular diagnostic testing is indicated. It consists of an intracavernous pharmacotest and measurement of blood flow by color duplex

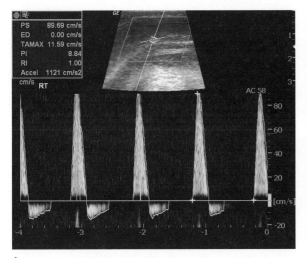
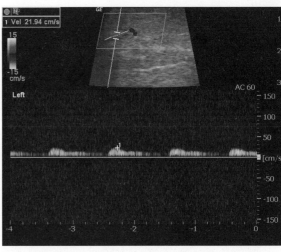

▲ **Figure 39–4.** Color duplex ultrasonography analysis of the arterial response to intracavernous vasodilator injection. In a man with normal vascular response **(A)**, the peak flow velocity of the cavernous artery is 89.69 cm/s with negative diastolic wave indicating that his intracavernous pressure is higher than his diastolic blood pressure. In another man with arterial disease **(B)**, the peak flow velocity is 21.94 cm/s with positive diastolic wave.

ultrasound (Aversa and Sarteschi, 2007; Figure 39–4). High-resolution (7–12 MHz) real-time ultrasonography and color pulsed Doppler enable the ultrasonographer to visualize the dorsal and cavernous arteries selectively, perform dynamic blood flow analysis, and is the best tool available for the diagnosis of high-flow priapism and localization of a ruptured artery. Normal arterial response is a peak flow velocity measured at the base of penis of >30 cm/s, a sharp upstroke of the waveform and absence of diastolic flow after sexual stimulation. Ultrasound can also be used to detect penile abnormalities such as Peyronie's plaque, calcifications, thickened vessel walls, and intracavernous fibrosis. When the Doppler waveform exhibits high systolic flow (>30 cm/s peak systolic velocity [PSV]) and persistent end-diastolic flow velocity (EDV) >5 cm/s accompanied by quick detumescence after self-stimulation, the patient is considered to have venogenic impotence. The parameters useful in diagnosing venous leakage include a diastolic venous flow velocity of >5 cm/s and/or a resistive index (RI) of <0.75. RI = PSV–EDV/PSV.

The Pulsed Doppler Study is performed using the Midus portable unit, which is specifically designed for use in the urologist's office. Penile blood flow is evaluated in a fashion similar to duplex ultrasound by recording the waveform of the cavernous arteries without providing a real-time ultrasound image (UroMetrics, Anoka, MN).

C. Cavernosometry and Cavernosography

Pharmacologic cavernosometry involves ICI of a potent vasodilator combination (papaverine + phentolamine + alprostadil) followed by saline infusion and simultaneous monitoring of ICP to assess the penile outflow system. In men with normal venous function, the maintenance flow should be <10 mL/min at an ICP of 100 mm Hg and the rate ICP drops after infusion ceases should be <50 mm Hg in 30 seconds. Veno-occlusive dysfunction is indicated by either the inability to increase ICP to the level of the mean systolic blood pressure with saline infusion or a rapid drop of ICP after cessation of infusion.

Cavernosography is used to visualize the site of venous leakage. Following the induction of an artificial erection by ICI of vasodilators (activation of the veno-occlusive mechanism), diluted radiocontrast solution is infused into the corpora cavernosa (Mulhall et al, 2004). Minimal or no contrast is seen outside the corpora cavernosa with normal veno-occlusive function. In patients with venous leakage of congenital or traumatic origin, the leakage is seen most often in the crura or at the site of injury, respectively (Figure 39–5). Leakage sites to the glans, corpus spongiosum, superficial dorsal veins, and cavernous and crural veins can be detected. In the majority of patients, more than one site is visualized. The typical finding in men with intrinsic disease of the corpus cavernosum or the tunica albuginea is a diffuse leakage through all penile venous channels.

D. Cavernous Arterial Occlusion Pressure

Cavernous arterial occlusion pressure, a variation of penile blood pressure measurement, involves infusing saline solution into the corpora after ICI of vasodilators to raise the ICP above the systolic blood pressure. A pencil Doppler

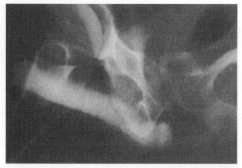

A

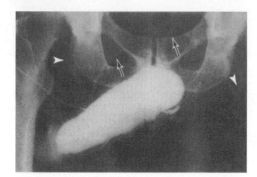

B

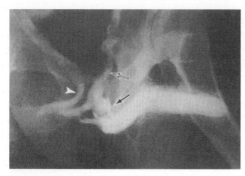

C

▲ **Figure 39–5.** Cavernosography after intracavernous injection of papaverine. In a normal man **(A)**, the cavernosogram shows opacification of the erect corpora cavernosa and nonvisualization of penile veins. In **(B)**, the patient has a large leak through both superficial dorsal veins (*arrows*) to the saphenous veins (*arrowheads*). Film **(C)** shows abnormal venous drainage via the cavernous veins (*solid arrow*) into the preprostatic plexus (*open arrow*) and the internal pudendal veins (*arrowhead*). (Reproduced, with permission, from Lue TF, Tanagho EA: Physiology of erection and pharmacological management of impotence. J Urol 1987;137:829. By Williams & Wilkins, 1987.)

transducer is then applied to the side of the penile base, saline infusion is stopped, and the ICP is allowed to fall. The pressure at which the cavernous arterial flow becomes detectable is defined as the cavernous artery systolic occlusion pressure (CASOP). A gradient between the cavernous and brachial artery pressures of <35 mm Hg and equal pressure between the right and left cavernous arteries are defined as normal.

E. Arteriography

Arteriography is reserved for the evaluation of the complex patient for whom revascularization surgery is contemplated; indications include the young patient with ED secondary to a traumatic arterial disruption or a patient with a history of perineal compression injury. The study is performed by ICI of a vasodilating agent (papaverine, papaverine + phentolamine, or alprostadil) followed by selective cannulation of the internal pudendal artery and injection of a diluted contrast solution of low osmolarity. The anatomy and radiographic appearance of the cavernous arteries is then evaluated (Figure 39–6), as

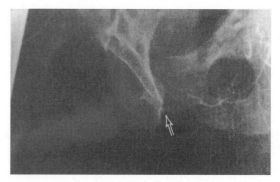

A

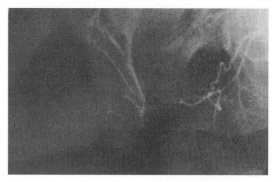

B

▲ **Figure 39–6.** Internal iliac arteriogram in the flaccid penis **(A)** shows poor visualization of penile arteries, simulating occlusion (*arrow*). After intracavernous injection of 60 mg of papaverine **(B)**, all the branches of the penile artery are well visualized.

are the iliac vessels, dorsal penile arteries, and the size and length of the inferior epigastric arteries.

▶ Neurologic Tests

The effect of a neurologic deficit on penile erection is a complicated phenomenon and with few exceptions, neurologic testing rarely changes management. Testing is recommended for specific research protocols or medicolegal investigations, including cases of trauma or surgical complications, or can be used in selected cases to (1) uncover reversible neurologic disease such as dorsal nerve neuropathy secondary to long-distance bicycling, (2) assess the extent of neurologic deficit from a known neurologic disease such as diabetes mellitus or pelvic injury, and (3) determine whether a referral to a neurologist is necessary (eg, workup for possible spinal cord tumor). Based on best-available evidence, neurologic tests lack adequate sensitivity and reliability for routine clinical diagnosis.

Somatic nerves are evaluated by testing nerve conduction velocities and evoked potentials, and these tests have well-known reproducibility and validity. Autonomic function tests are less reliable because they simultaneously measure a chain of events or reactions involving receptors, small fibers, and target organs. The complex interactions among central and peripheral sympathetic and parasympathetic nerve systems make autonomic testing difficult. Currently available tests are not well standardized and lack validity, reproducibility, and comparability.

A. Biothesiometry

This test is designed to measure the sensory perception threshold to various amplitudes of vibratory stimulation produced by a hand-held electromagnetic device (biothesiometer) placed on the pulp of the index fingers, big toes, both sides of the penile shaft, and the glans penis.

B. Bulbocavernosus Reflex Latency

This test is performed by placing two stimulating ring electrodes around the penis, one near the corona and the other 3 cm proximal. Concentric needle electrodes are placed in the right and left bulbocavernous muscles to record the response to square-wave impulses delivered via a direct current stimulator. The latency period for each stimulus response is measured from the onset of the stimulus to the beginning of the response. An abnormal bulbocavernosus reflex (BCR) latency time, defined as a value >3 standard deviations above the mean (30–40 ms), carries a high probability of neuropathology.

C. Penile Thermal Sensory Testing

Thermal threshold measurements quantify conductance of small sensory nerve fibers, which can indirectly reflect autonomic disturbances in the context of diffuse neuropathies, such as diabetic polyneuropathy.

▶ Nocturnal Penile Tumescence Test

Nocturnal erections, 80% of which occur during REM sleep, occur in healthy males of all ages and are relatively free of psychologically mediated effects. The average man has three to five episodes of nocturnal penile tumescence (NPT) each night, with episodes ranging from 30 to 60 minutes. Total NPT time declines with increasing age. Classically, NPT has been measured by several methods including the stamp test, snap or strain gauges, and sleep lab nocturnal penile tumescence rigidity (NPTR). Contemporary NPT testing is performed with simpler outpatient devices such as Rigiscan NPTR (Rigiscan; Timm Medical Technologies, Inc., Eden Prairie, MN). These newer devices electronically record the number, duration, rigidity, and circumference of penile erections: although sleep lab NPTR concurrently records nasal air flow; oxygen saturation; and electroencephalographic, -myographic, and -oculographic data to document REM sleep, hypoxia, and/or abnormal limb movement, it has been replaced by outpatient Rigiscan due to prohibitive expense.

NPT was originally designed to differentiate psychogenic from organic ED, as a full erection indicates a functionally intact neurovascular axis. In the United States, it is now mostly used in medicolegal or complicated cases, as well as for research purposes.

▶ Psychological Evaluation

Psychogenic ED is defined as the persistent inability to achieve or maintain an erection satisfactory for sexual performance, which is due predominantly or exclusively to psychological or interpersonal factors. Clinical subtypes of psychogenic ED include generalized versus situational and lifelong (primary) versus acquired (secondary, including substance abuse or major psychiatric illness). The psychological and interpersonal dimensions of sexual function and dysfunction are complex; therefore, a skillful diagnostic interview is the mainstay of a good psychological evaluation. A suggestive history of psychogenic ED includes sudden onset, selective dysfunction (eg, rigid erection with one partner and poor erection with others, or normal erection during masturbation or fantasy but not during intercourse), and a normal pattern of nocturnal erections coupled with an abnormal pattern during waking hours. This is often associated with anxiety, guilt, fear, emotional stress, religious, or parental inhibition. If the medical and sexual histories suggest a combination of organic and psychological risk factors, these patients should be diagnosed as having mixed organic/psychogenic ED; successful treatment must address both components.

Although psychological consultation is not indicated for most patients, it is very useful in evaluating and treating men with deep-seated psychological problems. Three groups of psychometric instruments are commonly used: (1) personality questionnaires, (2) the depression inventory, and (3) questionnaires for sexual dysfunction and relationship factors. The Minnesota Multiphasic Personality Inventory (MMPI)-2 is a valuable tool for evaluating the patient's personality and its relevance to sexual dysfunction. The self-reported Beck Depression Inventory is a validated test for which a score exceeding 18 is considered indicative of significant clinical depression. Overall quality of relationships can be assessed using the Short Marital Adjustment Test (married couples) and the Dyadic Adjustment Inventory (unmarried individuals) (Mallis et al, 2005).

NONSURGICAL TREATMENT OF ERECTILE DYSFUNCTION

Advances in pharmacologic therapy for ED have resulted in greater numbers of patients seeking primary and specialty care for sexual concerns. Oral PDE-5Is have emerged as the preferred first-line treatment of ED worldwide due to their efficacy, ease of use, and patient safety. Prior to their release, efficacious oral therapies for ED were unavailable and patient options were limited to nonspecific modalities including lifestyle modification, medication changes, vacuum devices, intraurethral agents, intracavernosal injection therapy, or penile prosthesis insertion. Over the last decade, nonsurgical approaches have replaced prosthetic surgery as the preferred choice of management. In most cases, nonspecific therapies appear to be more effective for ED; however, the patient should also be aware of specific therapies so that an informed treatment decision can be made.

▶ Lifestyle Changes

The beneficial effect of lifestyle change (total body weight loss of 10% or more by reducing caloric intake and increasing physical activity) was demonstrated in a randomized, single-blinded trial of 110 obese men (body mass index ≥30) aged 35–55 years, without diabetes, hypertension, or hyperlipidemia, but with ED (a score of 21 or less on the IIEF). The mean IIEF score improved in the intervention group (from 13.9 ± 4.0 to 17 ± 5; $p < .001$), but remained stable in the control group who were given general information about healthy food choices and exercise (Esposito et al, 2004). The beneficial effect was reproduced in a larger study of 209 non-obese men randomly assigned to interventional versus control group (Esposito et al, 2009).

It is well known that ED is intimately related to the atherosclerotic coronary and peripheral vascular diseases, as well as the metabolic syndrome, characterized by central obesity, abnormal lipids, insulin dysregulation, and borderline hypertension. Regular exercise, a healthy diet, smoking cessation, and limiting use of alcohol can reduce the risk of ED or improve underlying dysfunction. A Mediterranean-style diet (fruits, vegetables, nuts, whole grain, olive oil, and decreased saturated lipids) has recently been shown to improve endothelial function scores and inflammatory markers (C-reactive protein) when compared with men on a control diet (Esposito et al, 2010). Obesity and smoking have been prospectively

identified as risk factors for ED, while physical activity is inversely associated with the development of ED.

Perineal compression on penile arteries from long-distance cycling may also represent a modifiable risk factor for ED. Changing the bicycle seat or riding practices will often improve erectile function if penile vascular compromise is identified; specific strategies include replacing a protruding nose with a noseless seat, changing posture to a more upright/reclining position, using a gel saddle, and tilting the seat downward (Huang et al, 2005).

▶ Changing Medications

When a patient complains of sexual dysfunction after taking a particular medication, it is important to determine whether the problem is related to loss of sexual drive, impaired erection, or rapid/delayed ejaculation. In many situations, changing the medication to a different class of agents is a feasible first step. Antihypertensive agents therapeutically lower blood pressure; this primary effect has long been thought the mechanism of their adverse actions on erection. Switching patients to agents including alpha-adrenoceptor antagonists, calcium channel blockers, and angiotensin-converting enzyme (ACE) inhibitors may reverse ED in some patients. Patients complaining of sexual dysfunction while taking antidepressants may benefit from substitution (bupropion, nefazodone, buspirone, mirtazapine), drug holidays, selective serotonin reuptake inhibitor (SSRI) dosage reduction, and/or PDE-5 inhibitors.

▶ Psychosexual Therapy

Therapies such as PDE-5Is or ICIs may provide more rapid relief for patients with ED compared with a prolonged course of psychosexual therapy. However, in patients with evidence of psychological problems, referral to a psychologist or sex therapist is highly recommended because the elimination of a specific underlying cause may result in a cure. Recent approaches to sex therapy have included cognitive-behavioral interventions focused on challenging or correcting maladaptive cognitions, behavioral techniques (desensitization and assertiveness exercises), exploration of past developmental experiences on present behavior, and couples' therapy. Moreover, in some patients with mixed psychogenic and organic ED, psychosexual therapy may help relieve the anxiety and remove unrealistic expectations associated with medical or surgical therapy.

▶ Hormonal Therapy

Referral to an endocrinologist is recommended for patients with thyroid, adrenal, pituitary, or hypothalamic dysfunction. Aging men with ED may show a variety of symptoms when hypogonadism coexists: low libido, depression, decreased intellectual abilities, lean body mass, bone mineral density, or skin turgor, changes in body hair distribution, changes in sleep patterns, and increased visceral fat. In the patient with documented hypogonadism and ED, it is reasonable to initiate androgen therapy; for hypogonadal patients unresponsive to PDE-5 inhibitor therapy alone, the addition of testosterone may enhance the treatment effect and improve erectile function (Morales, 2005). This discussion is limited to treatment of hypogonadism and hyperprolactinemia as they relate to ED.

Parenteral depo-preparations of testosterone (T), such as testosterone cypionate and enanthate, are the least expensive form of androgen supplementation and are effective in restoring serum levels to normal. A normal circadian rhythm is not replicated by these agents. Rather, they are administered through deep intramuscular injection (200–250 mg every 2 weeks) and result in supraphysiologic levels of T for 72 hours with steady exponential decline to subphysiologic levels in 10–12 days; the initial supraphysiologic "rush" may be disconcerting to some patients, but others enjoy an improved sense of well-being, aggression, and libido.

Transdermal delivery more closely simulates normal circadian levels of testosterone if patients apply a patch in the morning, as the higher initial absorption mimics normal diurnal variations. Several U.S. Food and Drug Administration (FDA)-approved preparations are available in the United States. Testoderm TTS, which has largely replaced the Testoderm scrotal patch, is convenient to use, as it is applied daily to the arm, back, or upper buttocks as a 5-mg patch. Another product, Androderm, comes as a patch that delivers 2.5 or 5 mg T per day. The most common adverse reactions to both are itching, chronic skin irritation, and allergic contact dermatitis. Patients should alternate application sites and avoid sun-exposed areas. Local application of cortisone cream may relieve irritated skin. AndroGel is a 1% gel pack (containing 50 mg, 75 mg, or 100 mg of T), which is also applied daily in the morning to clean, dry skin over the shoulders, upper arms, or abdomen. Hands should be washed thoroughly after application, as skin contact can transmit testosterone. Testim topical gel also contains 1% T, providing continuous transdermal delivery for 24 hours after a single application to intact, clean, dry skin of the shoulders and upper arms. One 5-g tube of Testim contains 50 mg of testosterone.

When taken orally, methyl testosterone preparations are largely rendered metabolically inactive during "first pass" circulation through the liver. The large dosages (exceeding 200 mg/d) required to achieve therapeutic levels can be hepatotoxic, leading to hepatitis, cholestatic jaundice, hepatomas, hemorrhagic liver cysts, and hepatocarcinoma. Although unavailable in the United States, the only orally active and safe form of T is Andriol (testosterone undecanoate [TU] in oleic acid), which, owing to its lipophilic side chain, is partly taken up by the lymph and partially escapes hepatic inactivation. The maximal plasma concentration is generally observed within 2–3 hours, but after 6–8 hours, levels have returned to pretreatment values. A dosage of 40 mg three times a day generally provides adequate androgen replacement, yielding T levels within the (low) normal range, whereas dihydrotestosterone (DHT) levels are moderately increased (2–4 nmol/L). Absorption varies with food consumption and the dose required should be based

upon plasma levels and clinical effects. Other FDA-approved delivery systems include Testopel subcutaneous pellets (dosage of 2–6 pellets [150–450 mg T]), which lasts for 4–6 months, and Striant, a tablet-like mucoadhesive buccal system used to deliver 30 mg of T twice daily.

In patients with hyperprolactinemia with or without hypogonadism, androgen therapy does not improve sexual function. Treatment should first be aimed at eliminating the offending drugs, such as estrogens, sedatives, neuroleptics, or morphine. Bromocriptine, a dopamine agonist that lowers prolactin levels and restores T to normal, is used to reduce the size of prolactin-secreting adenomas. Surgical ablation may occasionally be required if the bromocriptine response is unsatisfactory or if visual field changes secondary to optic nerve compression occur.

▶ Potential Adverse Effects of Testosterone Replacement

Testosterone replacement is clearly the treatment of choice for young hypogonadal men without contraindications. However, the potential risks of androgen therapy may outweigh the benefits for some patients. Supraphysiologic levels of T suppress LH and FSH production and can lead to infertility, breast tenderness, and gynecomastia. Erythrocytosis is the most common laboratory alteration noted with long-term therapy; increases in red cell mass, thromboxane A2, and platelet aggregation may increase cardiovascular risk. Androgens may also induce or worsen sleep apnea. Long-term therapy requires a commitment from the patient and the specialist for continued follow-up, as outlined in the following.

Regarding *prostate safety*, a number of studies in the literature suggest that androgen replacement does not induce prostate cancer in men with normal prostates, and placebo-controlled studies show little difference in prostate volume, PSA, and obstructive symptoms. No increased risk of prostate cancer has been noted in (1) clinical trials of T supplementation, (2) longitudinal population-based studies, or (3) in a high-risk population of hypogonadal men receiving T treatment (Morgentaler, 2006). Although the fear of exacerbating an occult cancer of the prostate remains a concern, many older hypogonadal patients whose libido and erectile function can be restored by T therapy likely should not be denied this treatment option. When a patient desires T replacement, a digital rectal examination and a serum PSA level should be obtained. When in doubt, ultrasound-guided biopsy is performed before T therapy is given. The presence of prostate or breast cancer is an absolute contraindication to androgen supplementation. Patients are followed every 6 months with a rectal examination and serum PSA indefinitely while on therapy. Laboratory surveillance should also include hemoglobin/hematocrit levels, liver function tests, and cholesterol and lipid profile. The efficacy of supplementation is determined by clinical response rather than blood levels of testosterone.

▶ Oral Pharmacologic Therapy

A. Phosphodiesterase Inhibitors

Sildenafil (Viagra), vardenafil (Levitra), and tadalafil (Cialis), the three selective PDE-5Is currently approved for clinical use in the United States, have become the preferred first-line therapy for most men with ED due to their efficacy, safety, and ease of use. All are highly effective in enhancing erectile function across a wide range of outcome measures, causes of ED, patient subgroups, and regional populations. The three PDE-5Is appear to have equivalent efficacy in the treatment of ED, are generally well tolerated, and have similar contraindications and warnings (Carson and Lue, 2005).

1. Mechanism of action—Sexual stimulation results in the release of NO from nerve endings and vascular endothelial cells in the penis, which then diffuses into vascular and cavernous smooth-muscle cells of the corpus cavernosum. Stimulation of guanylyl cyclase by NO elevates levels of cGMP, lowering cytoplasmic calcium and resulting in smooth-muscle relaxation and subsequent penile erection. PDE-5Is amplify the NO-cyclic cGMP pathway through competitive inhibition of cGMP degradation by type 5 phosphodiesterase. Without sexual stimulation and resultant NO release, however, these inhibitors are ineffective.

2. Clinical efficacy—The clinical efficacy and safety of sildenafil, vardenafil, and tadalafil has been evaluated in many placebo-controlled, double-blinded trials and open label studies (Brock et al, 2002; Carson and Lue, 2005; Goldstein et al, 1998; Porst et al, 2003). Treatment effect was principally assessed by items 3 and 4 of the IIEF-15 questionnaire (ability to attain and maintain erection, respectively). For sildenafil, improvements in erectile function were reported by 56–84% of subjects taking 25–100 mg of sildenafil versus 25% in the placebo group. Little ED benefit and considerably more side effects were noted above 100 mg. For specific etiologies, sildenafil was effective in 70% of hypertensive patients, 57% of diabetic patients, 43% of radical prostatectomy patients, and 80% of spinal cord injury patients. The efficacy of vardenafil was similarly evaluated with 10-mg and 20-mg dose. Mean IIEF scores increased from 12.8 at baseline to 21 at week 12 of treatment (compared with 13.6 to 15.0 for placebo). Similarly, integrated phase III studies of tadalafil involving 1112 patients demonstrated IIEF erectile domain scores of 24 in men receiving a 20-mg dose versus 15 for placebo. More than 70% of intercourse attempts were successfully completed from >30 minutes to 36 hours after dosing. For difficult to treat groups, including diabetics, severe ED, and postradical prostatectomy, the three PDE-5Is represent effective therapies for many men.

3. Time of onset—The onset of activity, in reports with similar methods, is 14 minutes with sildenafil, 10 minutes with vardenafil, and 16 minutes with tadalafil. However, success rates after 20 minutes are much less than after 1 hour; therefore, if patients do not experience a rapid beneficial effect, they should be advised to delay sexual intercourse for one (sildenafil or vardenafil) or 2 hours (tadalafil)—when serum concentrations have peaked. High-fat meal intake has been shown to delay absorption of vardenafil and sildenafil; this effect is not seen with tadalafil (Carson and Lue, 2005).

4. Period of efficacy—Tadalafil therapy has a broader window of clinical responsiveness than either sildenafil or vardenafil because of its longer half-life (17.5 vs 4–5 hours for sildenafil or vardenafil). Tadalafil enhances erectile function in men with ED for up to 36 hours and may mean less planning and pressure to have sexual intercourse according to a schedule.

5. Adverse events—Eleven distinct families (PDE-1–PDE-11) are known to have or are implicated in a broad range of cellular functions. PDE-5 is present in high concentrations in the smooth muscle of the penile corpora cavernosa. Sildenafil and vardenafil cross-react slightly with PDE-6, that is, the IC50s for PDE-5 are only four- to tenfold lower than those for PDE-6. This may explain why some patients using sildenafil complain of visual disturbances. Tadalafil minimally cross-reacts with PDE-11. Most side effects associated with PDE-5Is result from inhibition of PDE-5 in other tissue or organs. In randomized controlled trials, flushing (10%) and visual side effects were more common in patients receiving sildenafil or vardenafil, and back pain/myalgia (1–4%) was more common for tadalafil users. These events were mostly mild, *abated with time* (within 2–4 weeks), and prompted treatment discontinuation in only a small number of patients (Brock et al, 2002; Goldstein et al, 1998; Porst et al, 2003). Except for visual disturbances, the other reported side effects of PDE-5Is (headaches 15%, flushing, rhinitis 5–10% for vardenafil and sildenafil, slight lowering of blood pressure, dyspepsia, etc.) are likely caused by PDE-5 inhibition in vascular or gastrointestinal smooth muscle.

ED is common among men who have atherosclerotic coronary artery disease. With regard to overall cardiac safety, controlled and postmarketing studies of the three FDA-approved PDE-5Is demonstrated no increase in MI or death rates in double-blinded, placebo-controlled, or open-label studies when compared with expected study population rates. Patients who develop angina during sexual activity with a PDE-5I should discontinue sexual activity, relax for 5–10 minutes and if pain persists, seek emergency care and inform emergency medical personnel that a PDE-5I was taken. Patients who have an acute MI after a PDE-5I may be given standard therapies (except for organic nitrates). Nitroglycerin should not be given with 24 hours of sildenafil or vardenafil use, or 48 hours for tadalafil. Patients who develop hypotension after organic nitrates and PDE-5Is should be placed in the Trendelenburg position and given IV fluids, with alpha-agonists (such as phenylephrine) added as needed. In patients with refractory hypotension, intra-aortic balloon counterpulsation should be administered, as suggested by the American College of Cardiology/American Heart Association (ACC/AHA) guidelines. At present, there is no pharmacologic antidote to the PDE-5 inhibitor/nitrate interaction (Kostis et al, 2005).

Because of its effect on QTc interval, vardenafil is not recommended for patients who take type-1A antiarrhythmics (such as quinidine or procainamide), type-3 antiarrhythmics (such as sotalol or amiodarone), or with congenital prolonged QT syndrome.

Finally, there have been reports of the development of nonarteritic anterior ischemic optic neuropathy (NAION) in men using PDE-5Is. Epidemiologically, NAION is the second most common acquired optic neuropathy in men aged 50 years and older. Risk factors for NAION, cardiovascular disease, and ED are shared and include age, dyslipidemia, diabetes, hypertension, and cigarette smoking. Given the large number of men safely using these agents and a limited number of events, it is not possible to determine whether NAION is directly linked to the use of PDE-5Is. Nevertheless, physicians should continue to advise patients to stop use of a PDE-5 inhibitor and seek immediate medical attention in the event of a sudden loss of vision as a safety measure (Laties, 2009).

6. Warnings and drug interaction—PDE-5Is are contraindicated for patients using nitrates, as a precipitous and potentially life-threatening hypotensive episode may occur with concurrent use. PDE-5Is are either not recommended or are to be used with caution in men with unstable angina, cardiac failure, recent MI, uncontrolled or life-threatening arrhythmia, or poorly controlled blood pressure (resting BP <90/50 mm Hg or >170/100–110 mm Hg). Caution is also advised when an alpha-blocker and a PDE-5 inhibitor are given together, as interaction can lead to excessive vasodilation and hypotension.

7. Starting doses—The recommended starting doses are 50 mg for sildenafil and 10 mg for vardenafil and tadalafil. The dose may be increased to 100 mg (sildenafil) or 20 mg (vardenafil and tadalafil) or decreased to 25 mg or 5 mg, respectively, based on individual efficacy and tolerability. Several reports have shown that daily dose of 5 mg of tadalafil was able to reduce side effects while matching the effectiveness of 20 mg of tadalafil taken as needed (Seftel et al, 2009). Patients should also be counseled to trial a PDE-5I several times before declaring it "ineffective"; for instance, the cumulative probability of success with sildenafil increases with the first nine to ten attempts, after which it stabilizes (McCullough et al, 2002).

B. Centrally Acting Oral Agents

Apomorphine is a proerectile D1/D2 dopamine receptor agonist, but it may also stimulate 5-HT(2C) receptor to enhance penile erection (Kimura et al, 2008). Uprima, a sublingual form designed for buccal absorption, has been approved for ED in Europe (but not in the United States) and reported to induce erection in 67% of men with psychogenic ED. Apomorphine has a rapid onset of action, with a window of sexual opportunity of approximately 2 hours from ingestion. Maximal plasma concentrations are reached in 50 minutes. In a double-blind placebo-controlled study of 2- and 4-mg dosages, erections firm enough for intercourse were reported by 45% and 55% of patients, respectively, with placebo responses of 35% and 36%. Adverse events included nausea 16.9%, dizziness 8.3%, sweating 5%, somnolence 5.8%, yawning 7.9%, and emesis 3.7%. There were no documented food/drug interactions in clinical trials (with the exception of ethanol) and, specifically, no documented pharmacologic interactions for subjects using nitrate drugs.

Yohimbine is a centrally acting alpha-2-adrenergic antagonist that is not recommended for use in the treatment of ED by the 2005 American Urological Association (AUA) guidelines. Side effects include gastrointestinal intolerance, palpitations, headache, agitation, anxiety, and increased blood pressure (precautions are advised in men with cardiovascular disease). Trazodone is also not recommended; efficacy in pooled analyses was statistically equivalent to placebo. Side effects include drowsiness, nausea, emesis, blood pressure changes (both hypotension and hypertension are reported), urinary retention, and priapism (especially at therapeutic antidepressant levels) (Montague et al, 2005).

▶ Transurethral Therapy

Alprostadil, a synthetic formulation of prostaglandin E-1, is the only FDA-approved pharmacologic agent approved for the management of ED via intracavernous and transurethral routes. After absorption from the urethra to the corpus spongiosum and then corpus cavernosum, alprostadil stimulates adenyl cyclase to increase intracellular levels of cAMP and lower levels of intracellular calcium, thereby relaxing arterial and trabecular smooth muscle. MUSE (medicated urethral system for erection) consists of a small semisolid pellet (3 × 1 mm) administered into the distal urethra (2–3 cm) by a proprietary applicator (MUSE; VIVUS Inc., Menlo Park, CA). Clinical studies showed that 66% of men responded to in-office trials; however, postmarketing studies have produced less successful results of about 50% (Mulhall et al, 2001). Penile rigidity can be enhanced by placing an elastic ring at the base of the penis (ACTIS, VIVUS Inc.) to mechanically assist veno-occlusion. Penile and/or scrotal pain or discomfort is a ubiquitous side effect of alprostadil-based therapies and is clearly dosage related and was reported in 33% of men in MUSE trials. Hypotension and syncope have been noted in 1–5.8% of patients, thus mandating initial trial dose administration in the office setting. Some female partners also report vaginal discomfort (about 10%) after ejaculation by a man using MUSE.

Table 39–5. Intracavernous vasodilator injection therapy.[a]

Drug	Test dose	Therapeutic dose
Papaverine	15-30 mg	15-60 mg
Alprostadil	5-10 µg	5-60 µg
Papaverine (30 mg) + phentolamine (1 mg)	0.1-0.3 mL	0.1-1 mL
Papaverine (30 mg) + phentolamine (1 mg) + alprostadil (10 µg)	0.1-0.3 mL	0.1-1 mL

[a]Lower doses for management of neurogenic and psychogenic impotence.

▶ Intracavernous Injection

ICI of vasoactive drugs is considered the most effective nonsurgical therapy for ED. It remains the first-line therapy for select patients and a valuable treatment option for PDE-5I nonresponders or those that cannot tolerate side effects of oral agents. ICI treatment offers several potential advantages to the patient, including a rapid onset of action, essentially no systemic side effects and drug interactions, and dependable efficacy for all forms of ED. Men who have failed first-line oral pharmacotherapy constitute the largest group of ICI-treated patients, with a significant erectile response rate of >80% demonstrated among PDE-5I nonresponders indicating that progression to second-line injection therapy is appropriate. A list of drugs that have been used clinically is presented in Table 39–5, and the most commonly used agents and combinations are discussed later.

A. Papaverine

Papaverine, an alkaloid isolated from the opium poppy, induces relaxation of cavernous smooth muscle and penile vessels via nonspecific inhibition of phosphodiesterase. It is metabolized by the liver, with a plasma half-life of 1–2 hours. Monotherapy doses range from 15 to 60 mg. Advantages include low cost and stability at room temperature, while adverse effects include priapism (up to 6%), corporal fibrosis (6–30%; thought to be associated with poor technique, minimal injection site compression time, >1 cc injection volume, pH 3–4), and occasional elevation of liver enzymes (Bella and Brock, 2004).

B. Alprostadil (Prostaglandin E1)

Alprostadil causes smooth-muscle relaxation, vasodilation, and inhibition of platelet aggregation through elevation of intracellular cAMP. It is metabolized by the enzyme prostaglandin 15-hydroxydehydrogenase, which has been shown to be active in human corpus cavernosum. After ICI, 96% of alprostadil is locally metabolized within 60 minutes and no change in peripheral blood levels is observed. Alprostadil have been approved by the FDA for intracavernous therapy as Caverject (Pfizer, NYC) and Edex (Schwarz Pharma, Milwaukee, WI). Cumulative data yield a success rate of 70–75% across ED etiologies, utilizing a median dose of 12–15 mg. Common adverse effects include pain at the injection site or during erection (11–15%), small hematoma or bruising, penile fibrosis (1–3%), and burning sensation at the time of injection. Rates of priapism are low (1–3%) and systemic side effects are rare (Bella and Brock, 2004).

C. Drug Combinations

The most commonly used drug combinations for ICI in the United States are bimix (papaverine/phentolamine) and trimix (papaverine/phentolamine/alprostadil) in various concentrations (Montorsi et al, 2010). A combination of vasoactive intestinal polypeptide and phentolamine has also been used in other countries. Multiple series have demonstrated patient satisfaction rates of >75% and low rates of priapism or fibrosis. Side effects are reduced, as smaller amounts of each agent are required, and the targeting of multiple pathways increases therapeutic efficacy.

D. Adverse Effects

Priapism and fibrosis are the two serious side effects associated with ICI therapy. Priapism occurred in 1.3% of 8090 patients in 48 studies with alprostadil, which is about five times lower than with papaverine or bimix (Linet and Ogrinc, 1996). Fibrosis can occur as a nodule, diffuse scarring, plaque or curvature. Scar tissue can be prevented by >5 minutes compression of the injection site to reduce bleeding and trauma. Priapism is best prevented by careful dosage titration.

E. Dosage and Administration

Patients must have the first injection performed by medical personnel and receive appropriate training and education before home injection. An initial dose of 2.5 µg for alprostadil is recommended. If the response is inadequate, increases in 2.5-µg increments can be given until a full erection is achieved or a maximum of 60 µg is reached. For drug combinations, treatment is initiated with a small dose (eg, 0.1 mL) and titrated according to erectile response. The goal is to achieve a full erection of <1-hour duration to avoid priapism.

F. Treatment of Prolonged Erection or Priapism

The best treatment is prevention; prolonged erections, a potentially devastating adverse effect of ICI, are often secondary to rapid dose escalation by the patient, missed initial injection with second attempt, or use among neurogenic and/or young patients. It is imperative that the clinician prescribing intracavernous therapies emphasizes to the patient that priapism represents a urologic emergency, and any erection lasting >4 hours necessitates urgent medical evaluation. The best regimen for averting priapism is ICI of diluted phenylephrine 250–500 µg every 3–5 minutes until detumescence. In patients with cardiovascular disease, monitoring of blood pressure and pulse is recommended (Montague et al, 2003). If the priapism lasts for more than 2–3 days, T-shunt with intracavernous tunneling may be required (Brant et al, 2009).

G. Contraindications

ICI is contraindicated in patients with sickle cell anemia, schizophrenia, or a severe psychiatric disorder. Because monoamine oxidase (MAO) in involved in catecholamine (including phenylephrine) metabolism, if a man on an MAO inhibitor developed prolonged erection/priapism after ICI, a simple T-shunt might be a better treatment than ICI of phenylephrine. For patients using an anticoagulant or aspirin, compressing the injection site for 7–10 minutes after injection is recommended. In patients with poor manual dexterity, the sexual partner can be instructed to perform the injection.

▶ Vacuum Constriction Device

The vacuum constriction device consists of a plastic cylinder connected directly or by tubing to a vacuum-generating source (manual or battery-operated pump). Only devices containing a vacuum limiter should be used, as injury to the penis may occur with extremely high negative pressures (Montague et al, 2005). After the penis is engorged, a constricting ring is applied to the base to maintain the erection. The ring may be uncomfortable or painful; to avoid injury, it should not be left in place for <30 minutes. The erection produced differs from a physiologic or ICI-induced erection as the portion of the penis proximal to the ring is not rigid, which may result in a pivoting effect. The penile skin may be cold and dusky, and ejaculation may be trapped by the constricting ring. Complications include penile pain and numbness, difficult ejaculation, ecchymosis, and petechiae. Patients taking aspirin or Coumadin should exercise caution when using these devices.

In some patients, the device can produce an erection that is of sufficient rigidity for coitus or engorge the glans for men with glanular insufficiency. In patients with severe vascular insufficiency, the device may not produce adequate erection. Although it is a safe and less costly means of treating ED when used properly, low patient acceptability limits the application or use of this therapy.

PENILE VASCULAR SURGERY

Isolated stenosis or occlusion of extrapenile arteries may be amenable to surgical repair. Arterial reconstructive surgery is a treatment option for healthy men, usually aged 55 or younger, with acquired ED secondary to focal arterial occlusion and the absence of severe veno-occlusive disorder or generalized vascular disease secondary to hyperlipidemia,

diabetes mellitus, chronic hypertension (Montague et al, 2005). The most commonly used technique for penile revascularization is a bypass from the inferior epigastric artery to the dorsal artery or deep dorsal vein of the penis.

Penile venous surgery is also indicated only in young men with congenital or traumatic venous leakage. In congenital venous leakage, the venous insufficiency is typically through abnormal crural veins or superficial dorsal vein and is amendable to surgical cure. Traumatic venous leak is usually due to localized damage to the tunica albuginea or formation of a "fistula" between the corpus cavernosum and corpus spongiosum. Repair of the tunica or closure of the fistula can result in significant improvement of erectile function. In older men with chronic systemic diseases, venous leakage is usually caused by atrophy of the cavernous smooth muscle and degeneration of tunica albuginea; ligation of penile vein will only produce transient improvement and is not recommended.

PENILE PROSTHESIS

Patients considered for prosthesis implantation should be made aware of types of prosthesis available, efficacy, and potential complications including infection, mechanical failures, cylinder or tubing leaks, perforation, persistent pain, penile shortening, and autoinflation. Penile prostheses are divided into three general types: malleable (semirigid), mechanical, and inflatable devices. The malleable devices are made of silicone rubber, and several models contain a central intertwined metallic core. The mechanical device is also made of silicone rubber but contains polytetrafluoroethylene-coated interlocking polysulfone rings in a rod column, which provides rigidity when the rings are lined up in a straight line and flaccidity when the penis is bent. Inflatable (hydraulic) devices are further divided into two-piece and three-piece devices. Two-piece inflatable prostheses consist of a pair of cylinders attached to a scrotal pump reservoir. The most commonly used device, the three-piece inflatable penile prostheses, consists of paired penile cylinders, a scrotal pump, and a retropubic fluid reservoir (Table 39–6).

In general, the malleable devices last longer than the inflatable ones. Modern three-piece prostheses are extremely durable and reliable. However, patients should be informed

Table 39–6. Types of penile protheses.

Semirigid
American Medical System (AMS) Spectra
Coloplast genesis
Two-piece inflatable
AMS Ambicor, Coloplast Excel
Three-piece inflatable
Coloplast Titan and Titan OTR
AMS 700 MS series: CX, CXR, LGX

that a 5–15% failure rate is expected within the first 5 years for inflatable implants, and the majority of devices will fail in 10–15 years and need replacement. Patient satisfaction with the three-piece device is high, exceeding 85–90% in appropriately selected patients. Recent innovations in penile prosthetics include antibiotic- and hydrophilic-coated devices (infection rate <1%), lockout valves to prevent autoinflation, and a more patient-friendly pump (Knoll et al, 2009; Wolter and Hellstrom, 2004).

MALE SEXUAL DYSFUNCTION INVOLVING EMISSION, EJACULATION, AND ORGASM

▶ Physiology of Emission, Ejaculation, and Orgasm

Different mechanisms are involved in erection, emission, ejaculation, and orgasm, and these events can be dissociated from one another (eg, a frequent complaint of men with ED is ejaculating through a "limp penis"). Except for nocturnal emissions, or "wet dreams," emission and ejaculation require stimulation of the external genitalia. Impulses traveling from the pudendal nerves reach the upper lumbar spinal sympathetic nuclei. Efferent signals traveling in the hypogastric nerve activate secretions and transport sperm from the distal epididymis, vasa deferentia, seminal vesicles, and prostate to the prostatic urethra. Coordinated closing of the internal urethral sphincter and relaxation of the external sphincter direct the semen into the bulbous urethra (emission). Subsequent rhythmic contractions of the bulbocavernosus muscles force the semen through a pressurized conduit—the constricted urethral lumen compressed by the engorged corpus spongiosum—to produce the 2–5-mL ejaculate. The external ejaculation process involves the somatomotor efferent of the pudendal nerve to contract the bulbocavernosus muscle. Since this action is involuntary, however, integrated autonomic and somatic action is required.

The mechanism of orgasm is the least understood of the sexual processes. It probably involves cerebral interpretation and response to sexual stimulation. Along with emission and ejaculation, several nongenital responses also occur. These include involuntary rhythmic contractions of the anal sphincter, hyperventilation, tachycardia, and elevation of blood pressure.

▶ Disorders Affecting Ejaculation, Emission, and Orgasm

Premature or rapid ejaculation, a persistent or recurrent occurrence of ejaculation with minimal sexual stimulation before, on, or shortly after penetration and before the person wishes it, is reported by up to 20–30% of men (Althof, 2006). Some propose that the definition of premature ejaculation should include rapidity of ejaculation, lack of control, and negative consequences (McMahon et al, 2008). In addition to

psychotherapy or behavioral therapy, current guidelines suggest an SSRI, such as paroxetine (10–40 mg daily or 20 mg 3–4 hours before intercourse), may be used as pharmacotherapy for premature ejaculation, although this indication is not FDA approved (Montague et al, 2004). Penile sensitivity may be reduced with use of a condom or topical anesthetizing cream (lidocaine–prilocaine). Although time to ejaculation is prolonged, a significant percentage of men experience decreased pleasure (penile numbness) or loss of erection. A short acting SSRI, dapoxetine hydrochloride, has been developed for on-demand use in premature ejaculation but has not been approved by FDA. Its pharmacokinetic profile is characterized by rapid absorption, a short initial half-life of 1.3–1.4 hours and rapid elimination with minimal accumulation even after multiple dosing. Several large phase III studies have demonstrated that dapoxetine can increase intravaginal ejaculatory latency time and improve several patient-reported outcomes relevant to control of ejaculation and satisfaction with intercourse. The most common adverse events were nausea, dizziness, diarrhea, and headache. There were no signals for treatment-emergent anxiety or SSRI discontinuation syndrome after abrupt withdrawal (Owen, 2009).

Successful emission and ejaculation without orgasm occur in some patients with spinal cord injury. A history of disease or surgery is helpful in differentiating emission failure from retrograde ejaculation. If microscopic examination confirms the presence of sperm in bladder urine after a dry ejaculation, retrograde ejaculation can be diagnosed. If no sperm is found, emission failure is the cause. Bilateral sympathectomy at the L2 level may result in ejaculatory dysfunction in about 40% of patients while high bilateral retroperitoneal lymphadenectomy causes an even higher percentage of emission failures. Retrograde ejaculation is usually the result of dysfunction of the internal sphincter or the bladder neck, as seen after prostatectomy, with alpha-blocker therapy, and in autonomic neuropathy due to diabetes.

Elimination of alpha-adrenergic blockers may cure some patients with emission failure or retrograde ejaculation. Alpha-sympathomimetics, such as ephedrine or a combination of chlorpheniramine maleate and phenylpropanolamine hydrochloride (Ornade), have been used successfully in patients with retrograde ejaculation (McMahon et al, 2008). Electroejaculation via a rectal probe has been applied in patients suffering from spinal cord injury with some success. Psychosexual counseling is appropriate for patients who have normal wet dreams but cannot achieve orgasm and ejaculation.

BIBLIOGRAPHY

Althof SE: Prevalence, characteristics and implications of premature ejaculation/rapid ejaculation. J Urol 2006;175(3, Pt 1):842.

Althof SE et al: Sildenafil citrate improves self-esteem, confidence, and relationships in men with erectile dysfunction: Results from an international, multi-center, double-blind, placebo-controlled trial. J Sex Med 2006;3:521.

Araujo AB et al: Changes in sexual function in middle-aged and older men: Longitudinal data from the Massachusetts Male Aging Study. J Am Geriatr Soc 2004;52:1502.

Aversa A, Sarteschi LM: The role of penile color-duplex ultrasound for the evaluation of erectile dysfunction. J Sex Med 2007;4(5): 1437–1447.

Bahk JY et al: Treatment of diabetic impotence with umbilical cord blood stem cell intracavernosal transplant: preliminary report of 7 cases. Exp Clin Transplant 2010;8(2):150–160.

Balon R: Sexual function and dysfunction during treatment with psychotropic medications. J Clin Psychiatry 2005;66:1488.

Bella AJ, Brock GB: Intracavernous pharmacotherapy for erectile dysfunction. Endocrine 2004;23:149.

Bodie JA et al: Psychogenic erectile dysfunction. Int J Psychiatry Med 2003;33:273.

Brant WO et al: T-shaped shunt and intracavernous tunneling for prolonged ischemic priapism. J Urol 2009;181(4):1699–1705.

Braun M et al: Epidemiology of erectile dysfunction: Results of the 'Cologne Male Survey'. Int J Impot Res 2000;12:305.

Brock GB et al: Efficacy and safety of tadalafil for the treatment of erectile dysfunction: Results of integrated analysis. J Urol 2002;168:1332.

Carson CC, Lue TF: Phosphodiesterase type 5 inhibitors for erectile dysfunction. BJU Int 2005;96:257.

Chai SJ et al: Small-vessel lower extremity arterial disease and erectile dysfunction: The Rancho Bernardo study. Atherosclerosis 2009; 203:620–625.

Chiou WF et al: Abnormal protein expression in the corpus cavernosum impairs erectile function in type 2 diabetes. BJU Int 2010; 105(5):674–680.

Corona G et al: Aging and pathogenesis of erectile dysfunction. Int J Impot Res 2004;16(5):385.

Dean RC, Lue TF: Physiology of penile erection and pathophysiology of erectile dysfunction. Urol Clin North Am 2005;32:379.

Esposito K et al: Effect of lifestyle changes on erectile dysfunction in obese men: A randomized controlled trial. JAMA 2004;291:2978.

Esposito K et al: Effects of intensive lifestyle changes on erectile dysfunction in men. J Sex Med 2009;6(1):243–250.

Esposito K et al: Dietary factors, Mediterranean diet and erectile dysfunction. J Sex Med 2010;7(7):2339–2345.

Feldman HA et al: Impotence and its medical and psychosocial correlates: Results of the Massachusetts Male Aging Study. J Urol 1994;151:54.

Feldman HA et al: Age trends in the level of serum testosterone and other hormones in middle-aged men: longitudinal results from the Massachusetts male aging study. J Clin Endocrinol Metab 2002;87:589.

Fonseca A, Java V: Endothelial and erectile dysfunction, diabetes mellitus, and the metabolic syndrome: Common pathways and treatments? Am J Cardiol 2005;96(12B):13M.

Georgiadis JR, Holstege G: Human brain activation during sexual stimulation of the penis. J Comp Neurol 2005;493:33.

Giuliano F: Impact of medical treatments for benign prostatic hyperplasia on sexual function. BJU Int 2006;97(Suppl 2):34.

Goldstein I et al: Oral sildenafil in the treatment of erectile dysfunction. Sildenafil study group. N Engl J Med 1998;338:1387.

Granata AR et al: Relationship between sleep-related erections and testosterone levels in men. J Androl 1997;18(5):522–527.

Gratzke C et al: Anatomy, physiology, and pathophysiology of erectile dysfunction. J Sex Med 2010;7(1, Pt 2):445–475.

Heaton JP: Characterising the benefit of apomorphine SL (Uprima) as an optimized treatment for representative populations with erectile dysfunction. Int J Impot Res 2001;13(Suppl 3):S35.

Hsu GL et al: Anatomy of the human penis: The relationship of the architecture between skeletal and smooth muscles. J Androl 2004;25:426.

Huang V et al: Bicycle riding and erectile dysfunction: An increase in interest (and concern). J Sex Med 2005;2:596.

Inman BA et al: A population-based, longitudinal study of erectile dysfunction and future coronary artery disease. Mayo Clin Proc 2009;84(2):108–113.

Jackson G et al: The second Princeton consensus on sexual dysfunction and cardiac risk: New guidelines for sexual medicine. J Sex Med 2006;3:28.

Jin L, Burnett AL: RhoA/Rho-kinase in erectile tissue: Mechanisms of disease and therapeutic insights. Clin Sci (Lond) 2006;110: 153.

Kimura Y et al: 5-HT(2C) receptor activation is a common mechanism on proerectile effects of apomorphine, oxytocin and Melanotan-II in rats. Eur J Pharmacol 2008;589(1–3):157–162.

Kloner RA et al: Erectile dysfunction in the cardiac patients: How common and should we treat? J Urol 2003;170:S46–S50.

Knoll LD et al: Physician and patient satisfaction with the new AMS 700 momentary squeeze inflatable penile prosthesis. J Sex Med 2009;6(6):1773–1778.

Korenman SG: Epidemiology of erectile dysfunction. Endocrine 2004;23(2–3):87.

Koseoglu N et al: Erectile dysfunction prevalence and sexual function status in patients with chronic obstructive pulmonary disease. J Urol 2005;174:249.

Kostis JB et al: Sexual dysfunction and cardiac risk (the Second Princeton Consensus Conference). Am J Cardio 2005;96:85M.

Kupelian V et al: Relative contributions of modifiable risk factors to erectile dysfunction: Results from the Boston Area Community Health (BACH) Survey. Prev Med 2009;50(1–2):19–25.

Laties AM: Vision disorders and phosphodiesterase type 5 inhibitors: A review of the evidence to date. Drug Saf 2009;32(1):1–18.

Lin CS et al: Cyclic nucleotide signaling in cavernous smooth muscle. J Sex Med 2005;2:478.

Lin G et al: Potential of adipose-derived stem cells for treatment of erectile dysfunction. J Sex Med 2009;6(Suppl 3):320–327.

Linet OI, Ogrinc FG: Efficacy and safety of intracavernosal alprostadil in men with erectile dysfunction: The Alprostadil Study Group. N Engl J Med 1996;334:873.

Lue TF: Erectile dysfunction. N Engl J Med 2000;342:1802.

Lue TF et al: Summary of the recommendations on sexual dysfunctions in men. J Sex Med 2004;1:6–23.

Mallis D et al: Psychiatric morbidity is frequently undetected in patients with erectile dysfunction. J Urol 2005;174:1913.

McCullough AR et al: Achieving treatment optimization with sildenafil citrate (Viagra) in patients with erectile dysfunction. Urology 2002;60(2, Suppl 2):28.

McMahon CG et al: An evidence-based definition of lifelong premature ejaculation: Report of the International Society for Sexual Medicine (ISSM) ad hoc committee for the definition of premature ejaculation. J Sex Med 2008;5(7):1590–1606.

Melman A et al: Plasmid-based gene transfer for treatment of erectile dysfunction and overactive bladder: Results of a phase I trial. Isr Med Assoc J 2007;9(3):143–146.

Miner M et al: Treatment of lower urinary tract symptoms in benign prostatic hyperplasia and its impact on sexual function. Clin Ther 2006;28:13.

Montague DK et al: American Urological Association guideline on the management of priapism. J Urol 2003;(4, Pt 1):1318.

Montague DK et al: AUA Erectile Dysfunction Guideline Update Panel. AUA guideline on the pharmacologic management of premature ejaculation. J Urol 2004;172:290.

Montague DK et al: Erectile Dysfunction Guideline Update Panel. Chapter 1: The management of erectile dysfunction: An AUA update. J Urol 2005;174:230.

Montorsi P et al: Association between erectile dysfunction and coronary artery disease. Role of coronary clinical presentation and extent of coronary vessels involvement: the COBRA trial. Eur Heart J 2006;27:2632–2638.

Montorsi F et al: Summary of the recommendations on sexual dysfunctions in men. J Sex Med 2010;7(11):3572–3588.

Morgentaler A: Testosterone replacement therapy and prostate risks: Where's the beef? Can J Urol 2006;13(Suppl 1):40.

Mulhall JP et al: Analysis of the consistency of intraurethral prostaglandin E(1) (MUSE) during at-home use. Urology 2001;58: 262.

Mulhall JP et al: Congruence between veno-occlusive parameters during dynamic infusion cavernosometry: Assessing the need for cavernosography. Int J Impot Res 2004;16:146.

Mulhall J et al: Vasculogenic erectile dysfunction is a predictor of abnormal stress echocardiography. J Sex Med 2009;6(3):820–825.

Musicki B, Burnett AL: eNOS function and dysfunction in the penis. Exp Biol Med 2006;231:154.

Owen RT: Dapoxetine: A novel treatment for premature ejaculation. Drugs Today (Barc) 2009;45(9):669–678.

Papatsoris AG et al: Erectile dysfunction in Parkinson's disease. Urology 2006;67:447.

Polsky JY et al: Smoking and other lifestyle factors in relation to erectile dysfunction. BJU Int 2005;96:1355.

Porst H et al: Efficacy and tolerability of vardenafil for treatment of erectile dysfunction in patient subgroups. Urology 2003;62:519.

Saenz de Tejada et al: Physiology of erection and pathophysiology of erectile dysfunction. In: Lue TF et al (eds) Sexual Medicine: Sexual Dysfunctions in Men and Women. Health Publications, Paris, 2004, pp. 287.

Seftel AD et al: Improvements in confidence, sexual relationship and satisfaction measures: Results of a randomized trial of tadalafil 5 mg taken once daily. Int J Impot Res 2009;21(4):240–248.

Shamsa A et al: Erectile function in end-stage renal disease before and after renal transplantation. Transplant Proc 2005;37:3087.

Traish AM et al: Mechanisms of obesity and related pathologies: Androgen deficiency and endothelial dysfunction may be the link between obesity and erectile dysfunction. FEBS J 2009;276(20): 5755–5767.

Veronelli A et al: Prevalence of erectile dysfunction in thyroid disorders: Comparison with control subjects and with obese and diabetic patients. Int J Impot Res 2006;18:111.

Watts GF et al: The erectile-endothelial dysfunction nexus: New opportunities for cardiovascular risk prevention. Nat Clin Pract Cardiovasc Med 2007;4(5):263–273.

Wolter CE, Hellstrom WJ: The hydrophilic-coated inflatable penile prosthesis: 1-year experience. J Sex Med 2004;1(2):221–224.

Yavuzgil O et al: Endothelial function in patients with vasculogenic erectile dysfunction. Int J Cardiol 2005;103(1):19–26.

Female Urology & Female Sexual Dysfunction

40

Donna Y. Deng, MD, MS, & Alan W. Shindel, MD

INTRODUCTION

Female urology encompasses urinary incontinence as well as pelvic reconstructive medicine for prolapse. It is common for urinary incontinence and pelvic organ prolapse to coexist in the same woman or to develop subsequently. This chapter will concentrate on pelvic organ prolapse as urinary incontinence has been discussed in detail in Chapter 29.

Pelvic organ prolapse is the protrusion of the pelvic organs (uterus, bladder, and bowel) into or past the vaginal introitus. Estimates of prevalence vary widely depending on definition used, whether the patient is symptomatic, the epidemiologic methods used, and the population studied. The U.S. National Center for Health Statistics estimates over 250,000 operations performed for genital prolapse apart from hysterectomy. With aging of the population, these quality of life issues and their treatment assume additional importance.

ANATOMY

▶ Bony Pelvis

The maintenance of continence and prevention of pelvic organ prolapse rely on the support mechanisms of the pelvic floor. The bony pelvis is the rigid foundation to which all of the pelvic structures are ultimately anchored. These bones are the ilium, ischium, pubic rami, sacrum, and coccyx. It is important to understand and discuss the bony pelvis from the perspective of a standing woman. In the upright position, the bony arches of the pelvic inlet are oriented in an almost vertical plane (Figure 40–1). This directs the pressure of the intra-abdominal and pelvic contents toward the bones of the pelvis instead of the muscles and fascial attachments of the pelvic floor. This dispersion of forces minimizes the pressure on the pelvic musculature and transmits them to the bones that are better suited to the long-term cumulative stress of daily life.

▶ Musculofascial Support

The muscles of the pelvic floor, particularly the levator ani muscles, have a critical role in supporting the pelvic organs and play an integral role in urinary, defecatory, and sexual function. The levator muscle complex consists of the pubococcygeus, the puborectalis, and the iliococcygeus (Figure 40–2). The pubococcygeus originates on the posterior inferior pubic rami and inserts on the midline organs and the anococcygeal raphe. The puborectalis also originates on the pubic bone, but its fibers pass posteriorly and form a sling around the vagina, rectum, and perineal body, resulting in the anorectal angle and promoting closure of the urogenital hiatus. The iliococcygeus originates from the arcus tendineus levator ani (ATLA) and inserts in the midline onto the anococcygeal raphe.

The ATLA is a linear fascial covering of the obturator internus muscle, and extends from the ischial spine to the posterior area of the superior ramus (Figure 40–2). The levator ani muscle group forms a broad hammock upon which the bladder, proximal vagina, and intrapelvic rectum lie, providing the musculofascial support for a large portion of the anterior pelvis. The space between the levator ani musculature through which the urethra, vagina, and rectum pass is called the urogenital hiatus. The fusion of levator ani where they meet in the midline creates the so-called levator plate.

The pelvic diaphragm has investing connective tissue, which is often referred to as "fascia"; it is, however, less organized and less distinct than traditional fascia (eg, rectus abdominis fascia). This visceropelvic fascia consists of collagen, smooth muscle, and elastin. Microscopic studies suggest that this fascia may be histologically indistinct from the deep vaginal wall, and not a separate "fascia."

The pelvic fascia consists of two leaves—the endopelvic fascia (abdominal side) and the perivesical fascia (vaginal side). The urethra, bladder, vagina, and uterus are all contained within these two layers of fascia. The two leaves fuse laterally to insert along the arcus tendineus.

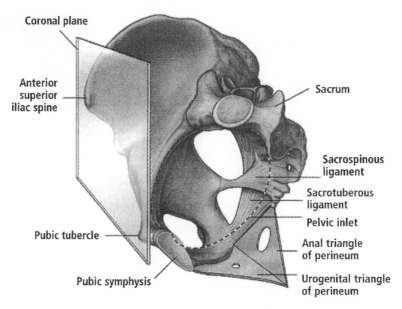

▲ **Figure 40–1.** Orientation of the bony pelvis in an upright woman. (Reproduced, with permission, from Drake RL et al (eds): Gray's Anatomy for Students. Churchill Livingston, Philadelphia, 2005.)

There are three important components of the pelvic fasciae. Anteriorly, the pubourethral ligaments attach to the lower portion of the pubis and insert on the proximal third of the urethra. Laterally, the arcus tendineus fascia pelvis extends from the pubourethral ligament (inferior portion of pubic symphysis) to the ischial spine. The arcus tendineus fascia pelvis is a thickening of the fascia overlying the iliococcygeus muscle. It corresponds to the lateral attachment of the anterior bladder wall to the pelvic sidewall (Figure 40–3). Fascia extending medially from this arc carries a variety of names (pubourethral, pubocervical, urethropelvic, vesicopelvic) and provides important support to the urethra and anterior vaginal wall. Posterior to the ischial spine, the fascia fans out to either side of the rectum and attaches to the pelvic sidewall as the strong cardinal and uterosacral ligaments (Figure 40–4). The cardinal and uterosacral ligaments hold the uterus and upper vagina in their proper place over the levator plate.

▶ **Innervation**

Many anatomic and surgical texts suggest that the levator ani muscles are dually innervated from the pudendal nerve on the perineal surface and direct branches of the sacral nerves on the pelvic surface. However, recent anatomic, neurophysiologic, and experimental evidence indicates that the levator ani muscles are innervated solely by a nerve traveling on the intrapelvic surface of the muscles without contribution of the pudendal nerve. This nerve originates from S3, S4, and/or S5 and innervates both the coccygeus and the levator ani muscle complex. After exiting the sacral foramina, it travels 2–3 cm medial to the ischial spine and ATLA across the coccygeus, iliococcygeus, pubococcygeus, and puborectalis. Given its location, the levator ani nerve is susceptible to injury during parturition and pelvic surgery.

The pudendal nerve innervates the striated urethral and anal sphincters as well as the deep and superficial perineal muscles and provides sensory innervation to the external genitalia. This nerve follows a complex course that originates from S2–S4 and travels behind the sacrospinous ligament just medial to the ischial spine, exiting the pelvis through the greater sciatic foramen. It then enters the ischiorectal fossa through the lesser sciatic foramen and travels through the pudendal canal (Alcock's canal) on the medial aspect of the obturator internus muscles before separating into several terminal branches that terminate within the muscles and skin of the perineum.

PATHOPHYSIOLOGY

Pelvic prolapse is prevented by several mechanisms. The most important support is from the continuous contraction of the levator ani pelvic muscles. The activity of skeletal muscle is a combination of basic tone, reflex contraction or relaxation, and voluntary contraction or relaxation. In patients with multiple deliveries, there is widening and descent of the levator plate. Therefore, the musculature becomes less important, and the "fascial" structures become the more important elements of support as the organs cross the pelvic floor.

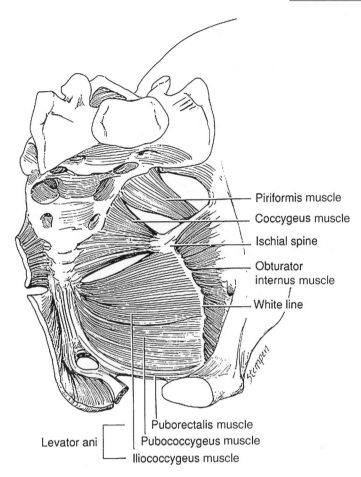

Piriformis muscle

Coccygeus muscle

Ischial spine

Obturator internus muscle

White line

Puborectalis muscle

Levator ani   Pubococcygeus muscle

Iliococcygeus muscle

▲ **Figure 40–2.** Muscular support of the pelvis. The pubococcygeus, the puborectalis, and the iliococcygeus comprise the levator ani muscles. (Reproduced, with permission, from Walsh PC et al (eds): Campbell's Urology, 8th edn. WB Saunders, Philadelphia, 2002, p. 49.)

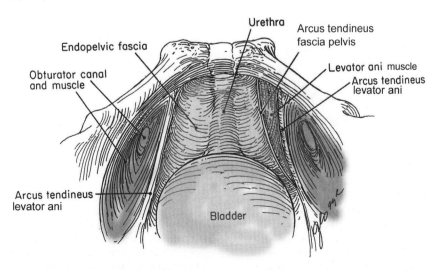

Urethra

Arcus tendineus fascia pelvis

Endopelvic fascia

Levator ani muscle

Arcus tendineus levator ani

Obturator canal and muscle

Arcus tendineus levator ani

Bladder

▲ **Figure 40–3.** Diagram of the arcus tendineus levator ani and arcus tendineus fascia pelvis.

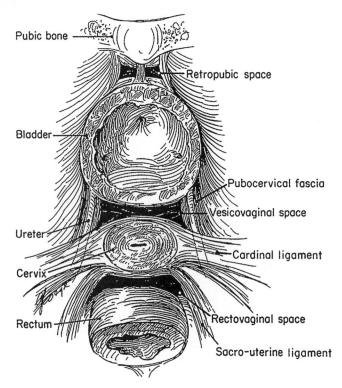

▲ Figure 40–4. Fascial support of the urethra and vagina. (Reproduced, with permission, from Walsh PC et al (eds): Campbell's Urology, 8th edn. WB Saunders, Philadelphia, 2002, p. 1103.)

Because of the complexity of pelvic organ support, vaginal prolapse is likely multifactorial: myopathic or neuropathic disorders, aging, atrophy, chronic increase in abdominal pressures, multiple deliveries, hysterectomy, and hormonal changes. However, intrinsic collagen abnormalities and other individual predisposing factors, such as genetics, differences in pelvic architecture, inherent quality of the pelvic musculature, and tissue response to injury, might explain why patients with known risk factors do not develop prolapse and many patients without risk factors do.

CLASSIFICATION

A number of classification systems have been published to facilitate standardization of clinical findings and enable communication about patients. Until recently, none of the systems have been validated. In 1996, the International Continence Society accepted standardization of the terminology for prolapse, known as the POPQ system for pelvic organ prolapse quantification. Although most clinicians still use the Baden-Walker system (Grades 1–4), the POPQ system is the accepted standard for clinical studies and published data on prolapse (Figure 40–5).

The POPQ system is a site-specific quantitative description of support that locates six defined points around the vagina (two anterior, two posterior, and two apical) with respect to their relationship to the hymenal ring. Negative numbers (in centimeters) are assigned to structures that have not prolapsed and positive numbers to those that protrude, with the plane of the hymen defined as zero. Points Aa and Ap are 3 cm above the hymenal ring. Points Ba and Bp are defined as the lowest points of the prolapse. The apex anteriorly is C (cervix), and posteriorly is D (pouch of Douglas). When the uterus is absent, point C is the vaginal cuff and D is omitted. TVL is total vaginal length at rest. GH is the genital hiatus measured from the middle of the urethral meatus to the posterior hymenal ring. PB is the perineal body measured from the posterior aspect of GH to the midanal opening (Figures 40–6 and 40–7).

The terminology avoids assigning a specific label, such as cystocele or rectocele, to the prolapsing part of the vagina, acknowledging that the actual organ(s) frequently cannot be determined on physical examination. Although it is more difficult to learn than traditional systems, reproducibility studies document interobserver and intraobserver reliability.

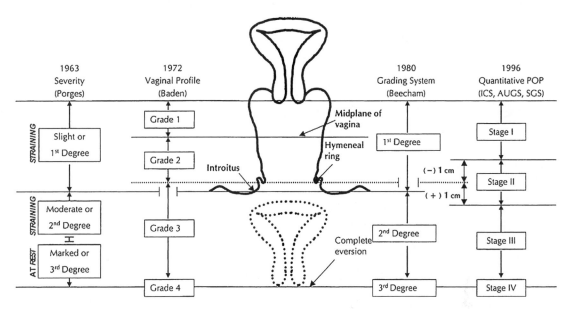

▲ **Figure 40–5.** Comparison of various classification systems of pelvic organ prolapse. (Reproduced, with permission, from Theofrastous JP, Swift SE: The clinical evaluation of pelvic floor dysfunction. Obstet Gynecol Clin North Am 1998;25:783.)

DIAGNOSIS

▶ Symptoms

Pelvic organ prolapse is often asymptomatic until it is severe. Many women present with symptoms in addition to the vaginal bulge, as a result of the associated organ dysfunction.

The most common complaint due to anterior compartment prolapse (cystocele) is vaginal bulging, with or without suprapubic pressure and pain. Other symptoms include urgency, frequency, urge incontinence, and recurrent urinary tract infections. Obstructive voiding symptoms are due to urethral kinking when the bladder descends beyond the pubic ramus, but the urethra remains fixed. This is commonly seen in the setting with previous surgery (eg, bladder neck suspension, urethropexy, sling). Patients may describe using unusual positions to void, such as pelvic tilting, squatting, or standing. Acute urinary retention and hydronephrosis are rare in patients with pelvic prolapse.

Many women with severe prolapse report that their stress incontinence improved as the prolapse worsened. Reduction of the prolapse during examination can produce stress incontinence in more than 50% of clinically continent patients. This unmasking of occult stress incontinence warrants attention when considering surgical therapy.

Constipation and difficult defecation with distal stool trapping or excessive straining are symptoms commonly attributed to posterior compartment prolapse (rectocele). The patient may report having to manually splint the perineum or vagina to assist evacuation.

▶ Physical Examination

A thorough physical examination should be done with a comfortably full bladder, at rest and with straining, in the supine (lithotomy) position. Depending on the patient's ability to strain, examination in the upright position may be performed to accentuate the degree of prolapse to match that reported by the patient. The goal of examination is to determine the degree of prolapse, the specific anatomic defects, and the presence of concomitant organ prolapse in other compartments or incontinence. In the supine position, the origin of prolapse should be determined. Using a half-speculum blade, the posterior vaginal wall is retracted; the patient is asked to strain while the anterior defect is evaluated. After characterizing the anatomic defects, an attempt can be made to reduce the cystocele in order to elicit occult stress urinary incontinence and hypermobility. Similarly, the anterior vaginal wall is retracted to determine the presence of any posterior defect. A digital rectal exam assesses rectal tone, the presence of impacted stool, attenuation of the pre-rectal fascia, and perineal laxity. Using both blades of speculum, the vaginal vault or cervix can be examined for uterine descent, vault prolapse, and enterocele.

EVALUATION

The basic evaluation for prolapse includes a history, physical examination, measurement of postvoid residual volume, and urinalysis. Additional testing may be needed in the setting of a large introital bulge where it may be difficult to differentiate between a severe cystocele, an enterocele, or

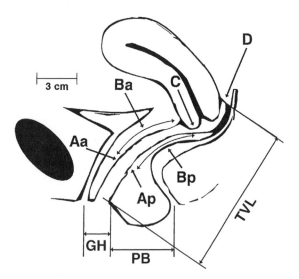

▲ **Figure 40–6.** The pelvic organ prolapse quantification system. Aa, anterior vaginal wall 3 cm from hymen; Ba, lowest point of anterior vaginal wall prolapse; C, distance from hymen to cervix; D, distance from hymen to posterior fornix (pouch of Douglas); Ap, posterior vaginal wall 3 cm from hymen. Bp, lowest point of posterior vaginal wall prolapse; TVL, total vaginal length; GH, genital hiatus measured from midurethral meatus to posterior hymen; PB, perineal body measured from posterior hymen to midanus. (Reproduced, with permission, from Bump RC et al: The standardization of terminology of female pelvic organ prolapse and pelvic floor dysfunction. Am J Obstet Gynecol 1996;175:10.)

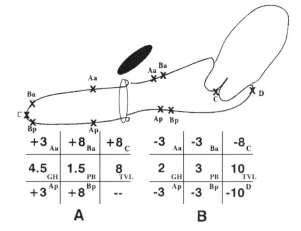

+3 Aa	+8 Ba	+8 C	-3 Aa	-3 Ba	-8 C
4.5 GH	1.5 PB	8 TVL	2 GH	3 PB	10 TVL
+3 Ap	+8 Bp	--	-3 Ap	-3 Bp	-10 D
A			**B**		

▲ **Figure 40–7.** ***A:*** Example of complete vaginal prolapse (eversion) using POPQ classification. This occurs after a hysterectomy; therefore, there is no point D. Points Aa and Ap are maximally distal. Points Ba, C, and Bp are maximally everted. ***B:*** Normal support with no vaginal wall descent. (Reproduced, with permission, from Bump RC et al: The standardization of terminology of female pelvic organ prolapse and pelvic floor dysfunction. Am J Obstet Gynecol 1996;175:10.)

high rectocele by physical examination only. Imaging studies can be performed to identify which organs are prolapsing. An ideal study should provide precise information about which structures are prolapsed, the presence of urinary retention and obstruction, urethral hypermobility, and urinary incontinence.

▶ Cystourethrography

The patient is upright with a full bladder. Films are taken in a lateral position during both rest and strain. This exam provides information about bladder position, bladder neck funneling, urethral mobility, stress incontinence, and postvoid residual. The normal position of the base of the bladder should be above the pubococcygeal line (Figure 40–8). The presence of a rectocele can also be inferred when bowel gas is identified below the pubic symphysis. This exam is static and does not provide information about other pelvic organs or soft tissues of the pelvic floor.

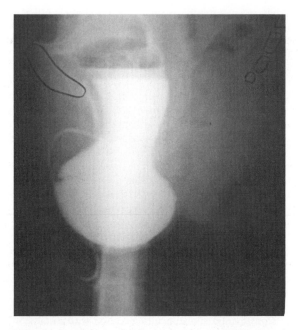

▲ **Figure 40–8.** Example of a cystocele. Lateral image of contrast-filled bladder extending well past the pubococcygeal line (line drawn from inferior edge of pubis to coccyx).

► Ultrasonography

Ultrasound is an attractive imaging modality because it is easy to perform, minimally invasive, and avoids radiation exposure. Tubo-ovarian and renal disease can also be assessed during examination. There is evidence that ultrasound is useful in evaluating bladder neck hypermobility; however, transvaginal imaging for pelvic prolapse does not provide adequate visualization of the soft tissues. Translabial ultrasound can be used to quantify prolapse, although it appears to be better for the anterior compartment and uterine descent than for the posterior compartment.

► Dynamic Magnetic Resonance Imaging

Recently, magnetic resonance imaging (MRI) has been used to evaluate pelvic prolapse. It is performed quickly, without contrast or ionizing radiation, and permits visualization of the soft tissues as well as the upper urinary tract. Gousse and colleagues (2000) have shown that in comparison with findings at surgery, MRI has a 100% sensitivity, 83% specificity, and a positive predictive value of 97% when assessing cystoceles. MRI does not require intravesical catheterization, does not require contrast, is fast, and is noninvasive. The drawback is that it may underestimate the extent of cystocele and enterocele because the exam must be performed in the supine position, which diminishes the downward forces that can be generated with abdominal straining. Standing MRIs will be the ultimate modality in obtaining an even more precise study for prolapse. Cost is the main reason that prohibits the wide use of MRIs currently (Figures 40–9A and B).

► Video Urodynamic Study

A urodynamic study can be done with or without video assistance. Both methods provide information about bladder compliance, capacity, sensation of filling, detrusor overactivity, and contractility. An advantage in performing videourodynamics is the capability to watch the position and funneling of the bladder neck during filling and straining. This combines cystourethrography with the urodynamic study. Choosing to use fluoroscopy should be based on cost, availability, and familiarity with this method.

The importance of documenting the presence of urinary incontinence in patients with large cystoceles is controversial. The incidence of occult stress urinary incontinence is felt to be as high as 22–80% among patients with high-stage vaginal prolapse. Due to the known masked urinary incontinence, and the high incidence of postoperative "de novo" stress incontinence, many pelvic reconstruction surgeons routinely perform a concomitant anti-incontinence surgery in all anterior vaginal reconstruction, independent of the continence status. This, however, remains a point of debate.

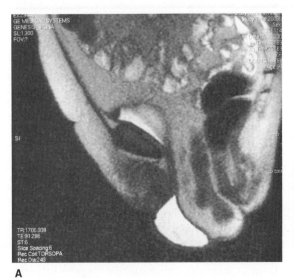

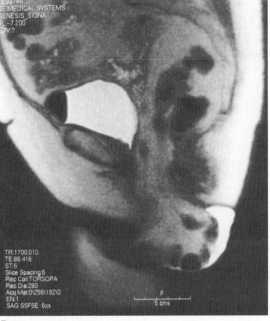

A   B

▲ **Figure 40–9.** **A:** Sagittal MRI image of cystocele and enterocele. Small intestine protrudes posterior to the prolapsed bladder (*white*). **B:** Sagittal MRI image of an enterocele only. Bladder does not prolapse past the pubococcygeal line.

Determining the presence of bladder overactivity is important in preoperative counseling because it can affect the postoperative result. In the majority of cases (60–80%), urgency may resolve after surgery. However, some patients may have no change in urgency or a worsening of their urgency with sling placement and/or bladder neck elevation. Urodynamic study may also suggest urinary obstruction with elevated voiding pressure, low urinary flow, or radiographic evidence of urethral kinking.

▶ Cystourethroscopy

This exam is performed to rule out concurrent pathology in the bladder and urethra, such as bladder carcinoma, urethral diverticulum, stones, or foreign bodies (ie, suture material) from previous surgery. Cystoscopic illumination can also be used to differentiate an enterocele from a cystocele. A pelvic exam is performed with the cystoscope in the bladder. The bladder transilluminates through the anterior vaginal wall so that the extent of the bladder prolapse is demarcated. It can also be used as a bedside urodynamic exam, assessing filling sensation, postvoid residual, and visual cystometrics for bladder contractions. With a full bladder, a supine Valsalva stress test can be performed, looking for urethral leakage.

▶ Upper Urinary Tract Evaluation

Patients with a high-stage cystocele should have upper-tract imaging because there is a 4–7% incidence of moderate hydroureteronephrosis amongst patients with severe vaginal prolapse. This risk is greater in patients with procidentia, compared with vault prolapse. Ultrasound, excretory urography, computed tomography, or MRI can be used. An advantage of MRI is the ability to simultaneously evaluate the upper urinary tract, tubo-ovarian disease, and pelvic organ prolapse simultaneously.

▶ Laboratory Evaluations

Patients must have sterile urine prior to proceeding with an operative procedure. In preparation for surgery, a complete blood count, basic metabolic panel, coagulation profile, and urine culture should be obtained.

TREATMENT

▶ Nonsurgical Therapy

When surgery is contraindicated or must be deferred, a patient can be made comfortable with a vaginal pessary. They are of primarily two types, ring and support. Pessaries should be used with care. Without close monitoring of the patient and frequent examinations, ulcerations of the vaginal mucosa and fistula formation to the bladder can occur. Proper sizing, care, cleansing, and estrogen replacement can minimize complications. Vaginal estrogen cream has been shown to have beneficial effects on vaginal epithelium by improving vascu-

larity and total skin collagen content, especially in preparation for surgical correction.

Other nonsurgical treatments include pelvic floor muscle exercises as well as measures to improve the associated factors such as chronic cough, obesity, and constipation. These may help alleviate symptoms and prevent worsening of the prolapse, but the actual prolapse usually will not spontaneously disappear.

▶ Surgical Repairs

The goal of repair is to restore pelvic anatomical support. This is rarely an independent surgery. Often, surgery entails addressing incontinence as well as prolapse of the other compartments. The end result must restore anatomy and function by restoring normal vaginal axis and depth while preserving urinary, bowel, and sexual function. Because the various forms of organ prolapse are interrelated owing to shared support mechanisms, some recommend that all defects be repaired at the same time because occult weaknesses in other sites may be acquired.

▶ Anterior Compartment

Anterior colporrhaphy was initially introduced in 1914. It is a transvaginal approach that reduces the herniation of the bladder by plicating the redundant tissue, imbricating the detrusor, and approximating the tissue in the midline (Figure 40–10). The long-term results have been disappointing. There have been numerous modifications to the anterior colporrhaphy, including the use of synthetic or allograft materials, variations in suture placement, and anchoring techniques. One method places a piece of mesh into the fold of the imbricated bladder wall. Another places the prosthetic layer over the plication sutures and anchors it in place laterally in the arcus tendineus fasciae pelvis or obturator fascia bilaterally. These repairs supported by a piece of biomaterial appear to be more durable than a simple anterior colporrhaphy.

The vaginal paravaginal repair is another technique with various modifications. It involves reapproximation of the weakened lateral vaginal attachments to the arcus tendineus. Two to three interrupted permanent sutures are placed on each side between the arcus tendineus laterally and the pubocervical fascia medially from the back of the pubis to the ischial spine.

Cystoceles can also be repaired abdominally by suturing the endopelvic fascia and lateral vaginal sulcus to the arcus tendineus with interrupted permanent sutures. As a result of multiple modifications to these techniques and the addition of anti-incontinence procedures that are performed concomitantly, the durability of each procedure is uncertain. However, many pelvic reconstruction surgeons have evolved to repairing anterior compartment defects with a graft material to support the bladder with or without anterior colporrhaphy.

as 11%. Therefore, cystoscopy after intravenous indigo carmine is essential.

The vaginal vault can also be elevated to the sacrospinous ligament that extends from the ischial spine to the sacrum. Transvaginal placement of sutures needs to be performed with care as the pudendal nerve, artery, and vein are located immediately deep to the sacrospinous ligament, and damage to these structures can cause significant morbidity.

Fixation of the vaginal apex to the iliococcygeus fascia and/or muscle is another method to resuspend the vaginal vault. One or two sutures are placed into the iliococcygeus just anterior to the ischial spine. If the patient is not sexually active, this can be performed without a vaginal incision by placing a monofilament permanent suture at full thickness through the vaginal wall into the muscle either unilaterally or bilaterally. A potential benefit is the absence of critical structures in the area. Very recently, the use of polypropylene mesh to support vaginal vault suspensions has been reported with good success.

Abdominal sacrocolpopexy is considered by most surgeons to be the gold-standard procedure for vaginal vault prolapse. The procedure entails suspension of the vaginal apex to the sacral promontory with or without using a graft bridge. Autologous, allogenic, and synthetic materials have all been described (Figure 40–11). Although this procedure

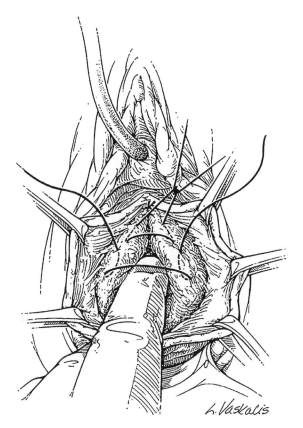

▲ **Figure 40–10.** Anterior colporrhaphy. (Reproduced, with permission, from Nichols DH, Clarke-Pearson DL (ed.): Gynecologic, Obstetric, and Related Surgery. 2nd edn. Mosby, St. Louis, MOP, 2000.)

More recent innovative approaches for anterior vaginal wall repair anchor an allograft, xenograft, or polypropylene mesh without tension via strips placed through the obturator foramen with a special device (Perigee, American Medical Systems; Anterior Prolift, Gynecare). These techniques await safety and efficacy studies but are increasing in use.

▶ Apical Compartment

An enterocele has a hernia sac behind vaginal epithelium that lacks musculofascial support of the vaginal vault. Repair involves transvaginal dissection of the peritoneal sac from the vaginal wall laterally, the bladder anteriorly, and the rectum posteriorly. Obliteration and ligation of the sac is performed by the use of purse string sutures. Because an enterocele presents due to weakened vault support, the vaginal vault must also be resuspended.

Vaginal vault suspension can be performed by transvaginal reattachment of the uterosacral ligaments to the vaginal apex. Excellent anatomic outcomes have been described, but ureteral injury is a possible complication, with rates as high

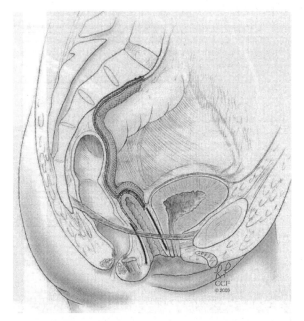

▲ **Figure 40–11.** Abdominal sacrocolpopexy using a polypropylene bridge from the sacral promontory to the vaginal apex. (Reproduced, with permission, from Biller DH, Davila GW: Vaginal vault prolapse: Identification and surgical options. Cleve Clin J Med 2005;72(Suppl 4):S12.)

requires an abdominal incision and there is the risk of bleeding from the sacral promontory and postoperative ileus, the resultant anatomy carries the greatest longevity and least risk of sexual dysfunction and dyspareunia. The laparoscopic approach appears to be just as successful in experienced hands. In addition, abdominal sacrocolpopexy also has the potential to resuspend the bladder in cases of concomitant cystocele.

▶ Posterior Compartment

The aims of posterior colporrhaphy for the repair of rectocele are to plicate the prerectal and pararectal fascia in the midline, narrow the posterior aspect of the levator hiatus, and repair the perineal body. Rectocele repair is indicated only if the patient is symptomatic because increased dyspareunia as well as worsening defecatory symptoms occurs in some patients. There is some evidence and opinion that asymptomatic rectoceles should be repaired at the time of repair of other defects because new defects may be acquired if a weakness exists. Until there is compelling evidence of benefit, the decision to repair asymptomatic rectoceles is left to the surgeon's clinical judgment. There is some clinical support to perform the posterior colporrhaphy using mesh or fascia for augmentation. However, there are no definitive recommendations for the exact procedure to be utilized.

CONCLUSION

Proper treatment of pelvic organ prolapse entails a thoughtful preoperative evaluation, strong knowledge of pelvic floor anatomy, and restoration of the vagina to its normal position and axis while maintaining normal physiologic and sexual function.

FEMALE SEXUAL DYSFUNCTION

INTRODUCTION

Sexual dysfunction is a perturbation of normal sexual function that interferes with an individual's ability to engage in satisfactory sexual activity. Sexual dysfunctions are largely defined and described as disruptions of particular parts of the sexual response cycle.

The traditional view of a sexual response is an orderly progression through discrete phases in sequence (desire, arousal, orgasm, and resolution). This linear model, advocated by Masters and Johnson and later by Kaplan, has recently been challenged principally by Basson, who has advocated a circular model that emphasizes the interrelationships between the psychoemotional aspects of sexuality in women (Figure 40–12). In this model, innate sexual desire may play a variable role in an individual woman's sexual response, influencing a woman's sexual incentives, receptiveness, and response to stimuli. There is continuing con-

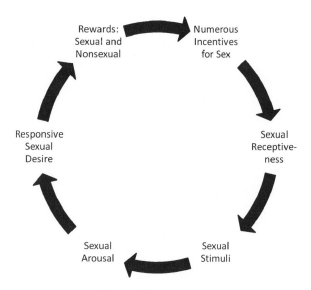

▲ **Figure 40–12.** Circular female sexual response cycle of Basson. (Adapted from Basson R et al: Summary of the recommendations on sexual dysfunction in women. J Sex Med 2004;1(1):24–34.)

troversy regarding the accuracy of these competing models, although data are emerging that the circular model of Basson may be more frequently endorsed by women with sexual dysfunction. This is parsimonious as women who have difficulties with, or reduced interest in, sex may be primarily motivated to engage in sex for emotional and psychosocial reasons.

Disorders of female sexual function are summarized in Table 40–1. Many existing definitions of female sexual dysfunction are based on scant empiric evidence, although distress regarding the situation is an important component of most modern definitions. Traditionally, sexual desire disorders have been diagnosed in the setting of infrequent sexual thoughts and fantasies. However, sexual thoughts are infrequent in many women without apparent sexual dissatisfaction and the frequency of sexual fantasies or sexual thoughts has shown little correlation with sexual satisfaction in women. Most contemporary definitions incorporate an absence of receptive desire, that is, interest in sex initiated by a partner's initiation of a sexual encounter. Arousal disorders may be subdivided into subjective arousal disorders, genital arousal disorders, and combined (mixed) arousal disorder. Of note, the Diagnostic and Statistical Manual of Mental Disorders Volume IV Text Revision (DSM-IV-TR) focuses specifically on lubrication in their definition of sexual arousal disorder, whereas the American Urological Association (AUA) definitions do make a distinction between subjective and genital arousal response. There are no defined cut-off scores (objective or subjective) to establish the diagnosis of

Table 40–1. Definitions of sexual dysfunction.

APA Definition[a]	AUA Definition[b]
Hypoactive sexual desire disorder Persistent or recurrent deficiency or absence of sexual fantasies and desire for sexual activity. Judgment of deficiency is made by the clinician, taking into account factors that affect sexual functioning	Sexual desire/interest disorder Absent or diminished feelings of sexual interest or desire, absent sexual thoughts or fantasies, and a lack of responsive desire. Motivations for attempting to become sexually aroused are scarce or absent. Lack of interest goes beyond a normal lessening with increasing age and relationship duration Combined arousal disorder Absent or markedly reduced feelings of sexual arousal (sexual excitement and sexual pleasure) from any type of stimulation, and absent or impaired genital sexual arousal (vulvar swelling and lubrication) Subjective arousal disorder Absent or markedly reduced feelings of sexual arousal (sexual excitement and sexual pleasure) from any type of stimulation. Vaginal lubrication and other signs of physical response still occur
Female sexual arousal disorder Persistent or recurrent inability to attain, or to maintain until completion of sexual activity, adequate lubrication, and swelling response of sexual excitement	Genital arousal disorder Absent or impaired genital sexual arousal (minimal vulvar swelling or vaginal lubrication from any type of sexual stimulation, and reduced sexual sensations when genitalia are caressed). Subjective sexual excitement still occurs from nongenital sexual stimuli (eg, erotica, breast stimulation, kissing)
Female orgasmic disorder Persistent or recurrent delay or absence of orgasm after a normal sexual excitement phase	Orgasmic disorder Lack of orgasm, markedly diminished intensity of orgasmic sensations, or marked delay of orgasm from any kind of stimulation, despite self-reported high sexual arousal or excitement
Dyspareunia Recurrent or persistent genital pain associated with intercourse	Dyspareunia Persistent or recurrent pain with attempted or complete vaginal entry and/or vaginal intercourse
Vaginismus Recurrent or persistent involuntary spasm of the musculature of the outer third of the vagina that interferes with sexual intercourse	Vaginismus Persistent difficulties to allow vaginal entry of a penis, a finger, and/or any object, despite the woman's expressed wish to do so. Structural or other physical abnormalities must be ruled out/addressed Sexual aversion disorder Extreme anxiety and/or disgust at the anticipation of/or attempt to have any sexual activity Persistent genital arousal disorder Spontaneous, intrusive, and unwanted genital arousal (eg, tingling, throbbing, pulsating) in the absence of sexual interest and desire. Any awareness of subjective arousal is typically but not invariably unpleasant.

[a]Data from the American Psychiatric Association (APA) Diagnostic and Statistical Manual Mental Disorders Volume IV Text Revision (DSM-IV-TR).
[b]Data from the 2003 Second International Consultation on Sexual Medicine sponsored by the American Urological Association (AUA).

arousal disorder and therefore the diagnosis is based purely on patient report for both subjective and genital arousal disorders. At the time of this writing, there is controversy over whether there will be a distinction between sexual desire and sexual arousal disorders in the upcoming DSM-V; currently, there is an impetus to combine these disorders into a unifying diagnosis that incorporates both disorders, consistent with the model of Basson.

The diagnosis of an orgasmic disorder per both American Psychiatric Association (APA) and AUA guidelines necessitates that an acceptable and preferred form of sexual stimulation

has occurred and orgasm has not resulted. A substantial proportion of the female population does not climax from coital intercourse and absence of climax from coitus should not be diagnosed as a sexual dysfunction unless it represents a distressing change from a woman's prior state of affairs.

PHYSIOLOGY

The basis of desire and perceived arousal in women is poorly understood, but it involves complex interactions among the central nervous system, sex hormones, and psychoemotional factors. The sexual response cycle incorporates numerous changes throughout the body as well; for the purpose of brevity in this chapter, we will focus on genital responses.

The genital arousal response in women is mediated in large part by activity of the parasympathetic and sympathetic nervous system as well as the vascular endothelium. These systems release nitric oxide and vasointestinal polypeptide. These messengers promote vasodilatation, which in turn leads to genital vasocongestion. In the clitoris, this causes engorgement of the corporal bodies and clitoral erection. In the vagina, increased oncotic pressure leads to production of a transudate fluid that is expressed through the vaginal epithelium, producing lubrication. It is important to note that there is no evidence for a glandular component to vaginal lubrication; vaginal wetness is derived entirely from this transudate.

Genital vasocongestive responses occur in women within seconds after erotic stimulation. Interestingly, the genital arousal response appears to be an automated response to sexual stimulation; indeed, it has been shown in many studies that women may exhibit an arousal response to stimuli that are not of subjective interest. For instance, it has been shown that women often exhibit a genital arousal response (increased blood flow) in response to viewing of erotic videos, irrespective of the subject matter, sexual orientation, and personal interest in the sexual activities depicted. Genital arousal response may also occur in response to depictions of nonpreferred activities, such as threat. The reason for this automatic "priming" of genital response is unclear but may be an evolutionarily protective mechanism to ensure adequate genital lubrication for possible sexual activity.

The effect of estrogen levels on sexual function is complex. Although low estrogen levels and vaginal atrophy are associated with reduced measures of vaginal congestion when the woman is not receiving sexual stimulation, the percent increase in congestion in response to erotic stimuli is similar in the presence of low and high estrogen levels (ie, pre- and postmenopausal women). Similarly, changes in the volume of the vaginal wall and clitoris and the relative volume of regional blood in response to sexual stimulation are similar before and after menopause. Estrogen deficiency does not necessarily preclude adequate lubrication, provided that stimulation is sufficient. It is important to note that a woman who is postmenopausal will generally have less baseline lubrication and therefore the necessity of adequate stimulation to prevent painful intercourse is often more apparent in women who are postmenopausal.

Indirect evidence suggests that testosterone and dopamine play a role in modulating sexual response, since testosterone supplementation or treatment with a dopaminergic agonist can augment sexual response. However, large population studies have failed to find the expected positive correlations between sexual function and baseline serum testosterone levels. One possible explanation is that serum levels do not reflect the intracellular production of testosterone from adrenal and ovarian precursors.

Numerous psychosocial factors have been associated with reduced subjective arousal. These include distractions from other life stressors, expectations of a negative experience (eg, as a result of dyspareunia, the partner's sexual dysfunction, or negative experiences in the past), sexual anxiety, fatigue, and depression. Medications including selective serotonin-reuptake inhibitors and oral contraceptives have also been implicated in decreased sexual arousal. Oral contraceptives increase levels of sex hormone–binding globulin, which in turn reduces free testosterone levels; it is hypothesized that some women are particularly sensitive to these effects and may exhibit symptoms, whereas others would not.

On the basis of survey data, several factors have been closely linked to women's sexual satisfaction and desire. These include stable past and current mental health, positive emotional well-being and self-image, rewarding past sexual experiences, positive feelings for the partner, and positive expectations for the relationship. Certain diseases such as multiple sclerosis, renal failure, and premature menopause induced by chemotherapy are also associated with a high incidence of sexual dysfunction. In women, unlike men, vascular diseases associated with age (diabetes, metabolic syndrome, atherosclerosis) have not been clearly correlated with sexual dissatisfaction and problems in women.

EVALUATION

A detailed history is the main tool in the assessment and diagnosis of sexual dysfunction and is best obtained from both partners. Important aspects of the history include the quality of the couple's relationship, the woman's mental and emotional health, the quality of past sexual experiences, specific concerns related to sexual activity (such as insufficient nongenital and nonpenetrative genital stimulation), and the woman's thoughts and emotions during sexual activity. A description of a recent sexual encounter may be instructive as it may reveal details that are not immediately disclosed in the history.

A physical examination, including a pelvic examination, is part of routine care. It is of primary usefulness in cases of dyspareunia to rule out superficial conditions (such as candidiasis, vestibulitis) and pelvic conditions (uterine leiomyomas, ovarian pathology) that may be associated with pain during sexual activity. Table 40–2 details features that are potentially relevant to sexual dysfunction that need to be assessed during an examination.

The possibility that laboratory testing will identify causes of sexual dysfunction is low. Estrogen deficiency, for example, can typically be detected by history and physical examination alone. In addition, serum testosterone has not been shown to clearly correlate with sexual function. Measurement of these hormones is of course warranted if supplementation of some

Table 40–2. Physical examination findings potentially relevant to sexual dysfunction.

External genitalia	Sparsity of pubic hair, suggestive of low adrenal androgen levels Vulvar skin disorders (eg, lichen sclerosus) Cracks or fissures in interlabial folds suggestive of candidiasis Labial abnormalities that may cause embarrassment
Introitus	Vulvar atrophy Lichen sclerosus Splitting of posterior fourchette Abnormalities of the hymen Labial adhesions Swelling of vestibular glands Vestibulitis Pelvic organ prolapse Abnormal vaginal discharge
Internal	Hypertonicity of pelvic muscles Presence of tender "trigger points" on palpation of levator ani muscles Fixed retroversion of uterus, tenderness of vaginal fornix on bimanual exam causing deep dyspareunia Endometriosis Uterine leiomyoma Ovarian cysts

kind is contemplated. Measurement of prolactin or thyrotropin is warranted if other symptoms or signs suggest the presence of abnormal levels.

TREATMENT

The management of sexual dysfunction in women is guided by the history. Data from randomized trials that support the use of any particular intervention are limited.

▶ Psychological

Cognitive behavioral therapy focuses on identifying and modifying factors that contribute to sexual dysfunction, such as maladaptive thoughts, unreasonable expectations, behaviors that reduce the partner's interest or trust, insufficient erotic stimuli, and insufficient nongenital physical stimulation. Strategies are suggested to improve the couple's emotional closeness and communication and to enhance erotic stimulation. Sex therapy for couples is focused on similar issues but also includes sensate focus techniques, consisting initially of nonsexual physical touch, with gradual progression toward sexual touch; partners are encouraged to alternately touch each other and to provide feedback about what touches are pleasurable. These techniques may help to reduce performance pressure in situations where a "goal-oriented" approach toward sexual activity detracts from sexual enjoy-

ment. Attention should also be directed to life stressors and relationship stress, as these factors are likely to exert an influence on a woman's sexual enjoyment.

▶ Pharmacologic

Other than estrogen therapy for dyspareunia related to genitourinary atrophy, no medications are currently approved by the US Food and Drug Administration (FDA) for the treatment of sexual dysfunction in women. However, a testosterone patch for management of hypoactive sexual desire disorder has been approved for use in several European countries. In the United States, off-label use of several drugs has been reported, although data about effectiveness are sparse.

▶ Nonhormonal

The involvement of nitric oxide in neurogenic vasodilatation suggests that phosphodiesterase type 5 inhibitors (PDE5I, used most commonly for erectile dysfunction in men) may ameliorate genital arousal disorder. In a small, laboratory-based, randomized trial, a single 50-mg dose of sildenafil (Viagra, Pfizer) increased subjective arousal, genital sensations, and ease of orgasm in some women with genital arousal disorder. The benefit was observed only among women who had a marked reduction in the normal vasocongestive response to subjectively arousing visual erotic stimulation. Sildenafil has also been shown to enhance orgasmic response in women with sexual dysfunction related to selective serotonin reuptake inhibitors (SSRIs). However, most large-scale studies of women with sexual dysfunction have not demonstrated meaningful improvements in sexual satisfaction amongst women treated with PDE5I. It is logical to speculate that PDE5I may be useful in women with a physical condition that tends to retard genital response with no or limited subjective component to the arousal disturbance; however, evidence to support this hypothesis is generally scant. Future studies are warranted to determine the potential role of PDE5I in this subset of women.

The prevalence of sexual disorders that are associated with the use of antidepressants in women is estimated at 22–58%, with higher rates reported for selective SSRIs and lower rates reported for bupropion. A recent meta-analysis of strategies to ameliorate dysfunction associated with antidepressants did not recommend any particular drug, although the potential advantages of adding bupropion were noted.

Flibanserin is a centrally acting agent with complex actions (both agonist and antagonist) on serotonergic and dopaminergic receptors. Flibanserin has reported efficacy in the treatment of hypoactive sexual desires disorder in women based on a series of phase III clinical trials in women. Approval for flibanserin was not granted by the FDA and its current status as a potential treatment for sexual problems in women is unclear.

▶ Hormonal

Supraphysiologic androgen therapy has been prescribed for sexual dysfunction since the 1930s. More recently, testosterone at lower doses has been studied in randomized trials. The results of four recent randomized trials of testosterone in women have generally shown increases in sexually satisfying events, sexual desire, and response. Important limitations of these studies include their brevity (which is of particular importance, given the expected long-term use of the drug) and that their results are generalizable only to women in whom menopause was surgically induced and who also receive estrogen therapy. In some women who have undergone natural menopause, the ovaries continue to be an important source of androgens, and thus, the effects of androgen supplementation may differ from those whose ovaries have been surgically removed.

There are ongoing health concerns about the long-term supplementation of either androgens or estrogens. There are scant safety or efficacy data of testosterone supplementation for estrogen-deficient women. A chief concern with long-term androgen use is a potential increase in insulin resistance, which could predispose a woman to the metabolic syndrome or exacerbate the syndrome if it is already present. This is in addition to concerns regarding cosmetic side effects including hirsutism and acne.

The role of systemic estrogen in increasing desire and subjective arousal remains unclear. In the Women's Health Initiative trial, no significant differences were found between the estrogen and placebo groups in reported satisfaction after sexual activity. However, sexual dysfunction was not a primary focus of the trial, and the assessment tool was inadequate.

RECOMMENDATIONS AND CONCLUSIONS

Recommendation guidelines for the evaluation and management of sexual dysfunction in women advocate attention to mental and physical health. Careful attention must also be directed toward both interpersonal and personal psychological issues. Local estrogen therapy is recommended for dyspareunia that is associated with vulvar atrophy that results in reduced sexual motivation. Testosterone therapy and PDE5I should be viewed as investigational and should be prescribed only by clinicians who are knowledgeable about sexual dysfunction in women.

A better understanding is needed of the endogenous and environmental factors that mediate sexual desire and arousal. Randomized clinical trials are also needed to assess the effects of psychological and pharmacologic therapies alone and in combination. The risks and benefits of long-term testosterone therapy require further study. The search for a nonhormonal medical treatment for female sexual dysfunction continues, although recent setbacks may lessen interest in this line of inquiry.

BIBLIOGRAPHY

Introduction

Bump RC, Norton PA: Epidemiology and natural history of pelvic floor dysfunction. Obstet Gynecol Clin North Am 1998;25:723.

Popovic JR, Kozac LJ: National hospital discharge survey: Annual summary, 1998. National Center for Health Statistics. Vital Health Stat 2000;13(148):1–194.

Anatomy

Barber MD et al: Innervation of the female levator ani muscles. Am J Obstet Gynecol 2002;187:64.

Bremer RE et al: Innervation of the levator ani and coccygeus muscles of the female rat. Anat Rec 2003;275:1031.

DeLancey JOL: Anatomic aspects of vaginal eversion after hysterectomy. Am J Obstet Gynecol 1992;166:17.

Farrell SA et al: Histologic examination of "fascia" used in colporrhaphy. Obstet Gynecol 2001;98(5):794.

Percy JP et al: Electrophysiological study of motor nerve supply of pelvic floor. Lancet 1981;1:16.

Vanderhorst VG, Holstege G: Organization of lumbosacral motoneuronal cell groups innervating hindlimb, pelvic floor, and axial muscles in the cat. J Comp Neurol 1997;382:46.

Pathophysiology

Bump RC, Norton PA: Epidemiology and natural history of pelvic floor dysfunction. Obstet Gynecol Clin North Am 1998;25:723.

Mant J et al: Epidemiology of genital prolapse: Observations from the Oxford Family Planning Association study. Br J Obstet Gynaecol 1997;104:579.

Classification

Baden WF, Walker TA: Genesis of the vaginal profile: A correlated classification of vaginal relaxation. Clin Obstet Gynecol 1972;15:1048.

Bump RC et al: The standardization of terminology of female pelvic organ prolapse and pelvic floor dysfunction. Am J Obstet Gynecol 1996;175:10.

Hall AF et al: Inter- and intra-observer reliability of the proposed International Continence Society, Society of Gynecologic Surgeons, and American Urogynecologic Society pelvic organ prolapse classification system. Am J Obstet Gynecol 1996;175:1467.

Diagnosis

Romanzi LJ et al: The effect of genital prolapse on voiding. J Urol 1999;161(2):581.

Theofrastous JP, Swift SE: The clinical evaluation of pelvic floor dysfunction. Obstet Gynecol Clin North Am 1998;25:783.

Evaluation

Barbaric ZL et al: Magnetic resonance imaging of the perineum and pelvic floor. Top Magn Reson Imaging 2001;12(2):83.

Beverly CM et al: Prevalence of hydronephrosis in patients undergoing surgery for pelvic organ prolapse. Obstet Gynecol 1997;90:37.

Comiter CV et al: Grading pelvic prolapse and pelvic floor relaxation using dynamic magnetic resonance imaging. Urology 1999;54(3):454.

Dietz HP et al: Ultrasound in the quantification of female pelvic organ prolapse. Ultrasound Obstet Gynecol 2001;18(5):511.

Gallentine ML, Cespedes RD: Occult stress urinary incontinence and the effect of vaginal vault prolapse on abdominal leak point pressures. Urology 2001;57(1):40.

Gousse AE et al: Dynamic half Fourier acquisition, single shot turbo spin-echo magnetic resonance imaging for evaluating the female pelvis. J Urol 2000;164(5):1606.

Kelvin FM et al: Female pelvic organ pro-lapse: A comparison of triphasic dynamic MR imaging and triphasic fluoroscopic cysto-colpoproctography. Am J Roentgenol 2000;174(1):81.

Vandbeckevoort D et al: Comparative study of colpocystodefography and dynamic fast MR imaging. J Magn Reson Imaging 1999;9:373.

Vasavada SP et al: Cystoscopic light test to aid in the differentiation of high-grade pelvic organ prolapse. Urology 1999;54(4):1085.

Treatment

Biller DH, Davila GW: Vaginal vault prolapse: Identification and surgical options. Cleve Clin J Med 2005;72(Suppl 4):S12.

Goldberg RP et al: Protective effect of suburethral slings on postoperative cystocele recurrence after reconstructive pelvic operation. Am J Obstet Gynecol 2001;185:1307.

Kelly HA, Dumm WM: Urinary incontinence in women without manifest injury to the bladder. Surg Gynecol Obstet 1914;18:444.

Kobashi KC, Leach GE: Pelvic prolapse. J Urol 2000;164:1879.

Rutman MP et al: Repair of vaginal vault prolapse and pelvic floor relaxation using polypropylene mesh. Neurourol Urodyn 2005; 24(7):654.

Shull BL et al: A transvaginal approach to repair of apical and other associated sites of pelvic organ prolapse with uterosacral ligaments. Am J Obstet Gynecol 2000;183:1365.

Weber AM et al: Anterior colporrhaphy: A randomized trial of three surgical techniques. Am J Obstet Gynecol 2001;185:1299.

Sexual Dysfunction

Avis NE et al: Correlates of sexual function among multi-ethnic middle-aged women: Results from the Study of Women's Health Across the Nation (SWAN). Menopause 2005;12:385.

Bancroft J et al: Distress about sex: A national survey of women in heterosexual relationships. Arch Sex Behav 2003;32:193.

Basson R et al: Definitions of women's sexual dysfunction reconsidered: advocating expansion and revision. J Psychosom Obstet Gynaecol 2003;24:221.

Physiology

Braunstein G et al: Safety and efficacy of a testosterone patch for the treatment of hypoactive sexual desire disorder in surgically menopausal women: A randomized, placebo-controlled trial. Arch Intern Med 2005;165:1582.

Buster JE et al: Testosterone patch for low sexual desire in surgically menopausal women: A randomized trial. Obstet Gynecol 2005; 105:944.

Clayton AH et al: Prevalence of sexual dysfunction among newer antidepressants. J Clin Psychiatry 2002;63:357.

Davis SR et al: Circulating androgen levels in self-reported sexual function in women. JAMA 2005;294:91.

Davis SR et al: The efficacy and safety of a testosterone patch for the treatment of hypoactive sexual desire disorder in surgically menopausal women: A randomized, placebo controlled-trial. Menopause 2006;13(3):387.

Dennerstein L, Lehert P: Modeling mid-aged women's sexual functioning: A prospective, population-based study. J Sex Marital Ther 2005;30:173.

Ganz PA et al: Quality of life in long-term, disease-free survivors of breast cancer: A follow-up study. J Natl Cancer Inst 2002;94:39.

Labrie F et al: Is dehydroepiandrosterone a hormone? J Endocrinol 2005;187:169.

Laumann EO et al: Sexual problems among women and men aged 40–80 y: Prevalence and correlates identified in the Global Study of Sexual Attitudes and Behaviors. Int J Impot Res 2005;17:39.

Maravilla KR et al: Dynamic MR imaging of the sexual arousal response in women. J Sex Marital Ther 2003;29(Suppl 1):71.

Palmer BF: Sexual dysfunction in men and women with chronic kidney disease and end-stage kidney disease. Adv Ren Replace Ther 2003;10:48.

Panzer C et al: Impact of oral contraceptives on sex hormone-binding globulin and androgen levels: A retrospective study in women with sexual dysfunction. J Sex Med 2006;3:104.

Sanders SA et al: A prospective study of the effects of oral contraceptives on sexuality and well-being and their relationship to discontinuation. Contraception 2001;64:51.

Santoro A et al: Correlates of circulating androgens in mid-life women: The Study of Women's Health Across the Nation. J Clin Endocrinol Metab 2005;90:4836.

Segraves RT et al: Bupropion sustained release for the treatment of hypoactive sexual desire disorder in premenopausal women. J Clin Psychopharmacol 2004;24:3390.

Simon J et al: Testosterone patch increases sexual activity and desire in surgically menopausal women with hypoactive sexual desire disorder. J Clin Endocrinol Metab 2005;90:5226.

van Lunsen RHW, Laan E: Genital vascular responsiveness in sexual feelings in midlife women: Psychophysiologic, brain, and genital imaging studies. Menopause 2004;11:741.

Evaluation

Davis SR et al: Circulating androgen levels in self-reported sexual function in women. JAMA 2005;294:91.

Santoro A et al: Correlates of circulating androgens in mid-life women: The Study of Women's Health Across the Nation. J Clin Endocrinol Metab 2005;90:4836.

Management

Basson R et al: Efficacy and safety of sildenafil citrate in women with sexual dysfunction associated with female sexual arousal. J Womens Health Gend Based Med 2002;11:367.

Basson R, Brotto LA: Sexual psychophysiology and effects of sildenafil citrate in oestrogenised women with acquired genital arousal disorder and impaired orgasm: A randomised controlled trial. BJOG 2003;110:1014.

Braunstein G et al: Safety and efficacy of a testosterone patch for the treatment of hypoactive sexual desire disorder in surgically menopausal women: A randomized, placebo-controlled trial. Arch Intern Med 2005;165:1582.

Buster JE et al: Testosterone patch for low sexual desire in surgically menopausal women: A randomized trial. Obstet Gynecol 2005; 105:944.

Davis SR et al: The efficacy and safety of a testosterone patch for the treatment of hypoactive sexual desire disorder in surgically menopausal women: A randomized, placebo controlled-trial. Menopause 2006;13(3):387.

Hays J et al: Effects of estrogen plus progestin on health-related quality of life. N Engl J Med 2003;348:1839.

Labrie F et al: Is dehydroepiandrosterone a hormone? J Endocrinol 2005;187:169.

Nurnberg HG et al: Sildenafil treatment of women with antidepressant-associated sexual dysfunction: a randomized controlled trial. JAMA 2008;300:395.

Simon J et al: Testosterone patch increases sexual activity and desire in surgically menopausal women with hypoactive sexual desire disorder. J Clin Endocrinol Metab 2005;90:5226.

Stahl SM et al: Multifunctional pharmacology of flibanserin: Possible mechanism of therapeutic action in hypoactive sexual desire disorder. J Sex Med 2011;8:15.

Taylor MJ et al: Strategies for managing antidepressant-induced sexual dysfunction: Systematic review of randomised controlled trials. J Affect Disord 2005;88:241.

Trudel G et al: The effect of a cognitive-behavioral group treatment program on hypoactive sexual desire in women. Sex Relat Ther 2001;16:145.

Disorders of the Penis & Male Urethra

41

Jack W. McAninch, MD, FACS, FRCS(E)(Hon)

CONGENITAL ANOMALIES OF THE PENIS

APENIA

Congenital absence of the penis (apenia) is extremely rare. In this condition, the urethra generally opens on the perineum or inside the rectum.

Patients with apenia should be considered for assignment to the female gender. Castration and vaginoplasty should be considered in combination with estrogen treatment as the child develops.

MEGALOPENIS

The penis enlarges rapidly in childhood (megalopenis) in boys with abnormalities that increases the production of testosterone, for example, interstitial cell tumors of the testicle, hyperplasia, or tumors of the adrenal cortex. Management is by correction of the underlying endocrine problem.

MICROPENIS

Micropenis is a more common anomaly and has been attributed to a testosterone deficiency that results in poor growth of organs that are targets of this hormone. A penis smaller than 2 standard deviations from the norm is considered a micropenis (see Table 41–1). The testicles are small and frequently undescended. Other organs, including the scrotum, may be involved. Early evidence suggests that the ability of the hypothalamus to secrete luteinizing hormone-releasing hormone (LHRH) is decreased. The pituitary–gonadal axis appears to be intact, since the organs respond to testosterone, although this response may be sluggish at times. Studies have shown that topical application of 5% testosterone cream causes increased penile growth, but its effect is due to absorption of the hormone, which systemically stimulates genital growth. Patients with micropenis must be carefully evaluated for other endocrine and central nervous system anomalies.

Retarded bone growth, anosmia, learning disabilities, and deficiencies of adrenocorticotropic hormone and thyrotropin have been associated with micropenis. In addition, the possibility of intersex problems must be carefully investigated before therapy is begun.

The approach to management of micropenis has undergone gradual change in recent years, but androgen replacement is the basic requirement. The objective is to provide sufficient testosterone to stimulate penile growth without altering growth and closure of the epiphyses. A regimen of 25 mg orally every 3 weeks for no more than four doses has been recommended. Penile growth is assessed by measuring the length of the stretched penis (pubis to glans) before and after treatment. Therapy should be started by age 1 year and aimed at maintaining genital growth commensurate with general body growth. Repeat courses of therapy may be required if the size of the penis falls behind as the child grows. For undescended testicles, orchiopexy should be done before the child is 2 years old. In the future, treatment with LHRH may correct micropenis as well as cause descent of the testicles, but at present, LHRH is not approved for such use.

ADULT PENILE SIZE

In recent years, penile augmentation and enhancement procedures have been done with increasing frequency, although no validation of success has been documented. Suspensory ligament release with pubic fat pad advancement, fat injections, and dermal fat grafts have been used in attempts to enhance penile size. Many consider that these procedures have not been proved safe or efficacious in normal men. Wessells et al (1996) evaluated penile size in the flaccid and erect state in otherwise normal adult men and found very good correlation between stretched and erect length ($R^2 = 0.793$; Table 41–2). This information can provide a guideline for physicians whose patients are concerned with their penile dimensions.

Table 41–1. Size of unstretched penis and testis from infancy to adulthood.

Age (years)	Length of penis (cm ± SD)	Diameter of testis (cm ± SD)
0.2–2	2.7 ± 0.5	1.4 ± 0.4
2.1–4	3.3 ± 0.4	1.2 ± 0.4
4.1–6	3.9 ± 0.9	1.5 ± 0.6
6.1–8	4.2 ± 0.8	1.8 ± 0.3
8.1–10	4.9 ± 1	2 ± 0.5
10.1–12	5.2 ± 1.3	2.7 ± 0.7
12.1–14	6.2 ± 2	3.4 ± 0.8
14.1–16	8.6 ± 2.4	4.1 ± 1
16.1–18	9.9 ± 1.7	5 ± 0.5
18.1–20	11 ± 1.1	5 ± 0.3
20.1–25	12.4 ± 1.6	5.2 ± 0.6

Source: Reproduced, with permission, from Winter JSD, Faiman C: Pituitary-gonadal relations in male children and adolescents. Pediatr Res 1972;6:126.

CONGENITAL ANOMALIES OF THE URETHRA

DUPLICATION OF THE URETHRA

Duplication of the urethra is rare. The structures may be complete or incomplete. Resection of all but one complete urethra is recommended.

URETHRAL STRICTURE

Congenital urethral stricture is uncommon in infant boys. The fossa navicularis and membranous urethra are the two most common sites. Severe strictures may cause bladder damage and hydronephrosis (see Chapter 11), with symptoms of obstruction (urinary frequency and urgency) or uri-

Table 41–2. Adult penile size: relationships among flaccid, stretched, and erect measurements.[a]

Penile state	Length (cm)	Circumference (cm)
Flaccid	8.8	9.7
Stretched	12.4	—
Erect	12.9	12.3

[a]Data represent the mean of measurements in 80 men and are drawn from Wessells H, Lue TF, McAninch JW: Penile length in the flaccid and erect states: Guidelines for penile augmentation. J Urol 1996;156:995.

nary infection. A careful history and physical examination are indicated in patients with these complaints. Excretory urography and excretory voiding urethrography often define the lesion and the extent of obstruction. Retrograde urethrography (Figure 41–1) may also be helpful. Cystoscopy and urethroscopy should be performed in all patients in whom urethral stricture is suspected.

Strictures can be treated at the time of endoscopy. Diaphragmatic strictures may respond to dilation or visual urethrotomy. Other strictures should be treated under direct vision by internal urethrotomy with the currently available pediatric urethrotome. It may be necessary to repeat these procedures in order to stabilize the stricture. Single-stage open surgical repair by anastomotic urethroplasty, buccal mucosa graft, or penile flap is desirable if the obstruction recurs.

POSTERIOR URETHRAL VALVES

Posterior urethral valves, the most common obstructive urethral lesions in infants and newborns, occur only in males and are found at the distal prostatic urethra. The valves are mucosal folds that look like thin membranes; they may cause varying degrees of obstruction when the child attempts to void (Figure 41–2).

▶ Clinical Findings

A. Symptoms and Signs

Children with posterior urethral valves may present with mild, moderate, or severe symptoms of obstruction. They often have a poor, intermittent, dribbling urinary stream. Urinary infection and sepsis occur frequently. Severe obstruction may cause hydronephrosis (see Chapter 11), which is apparent as a palpable abdominal mass. A palpable midline mass in the lower abdomen is typical of a distended bladder. Occasionally, palpable flank masses indicate hydronephrotic kidneys. In many patients, failure to thrive may be the only significant symptom, and examination may reveal nothing more than evidence of chronic illness.

B. Laboratory Findings

Azotemia and poor concentrating ability of the kidney are common findings. The urine is often infected, and anemia may be found if infection is chronic. Serum creatinine and blood urea nitrogen levels and creatinine clearance are the best indicators of the extent of renal failure.

C. X-Ray Findings

Voiding cystourethrography is the best radiographic study available to establish the diagnosis of posterior urethral valves. The presence of large amounts of residual urine is apparent on initial catheterization done in conjunction with radiographic studies, and an uncontaminated urine

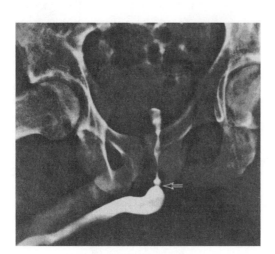

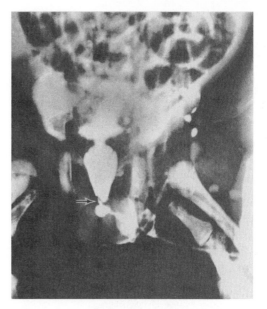

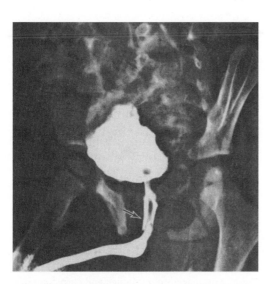

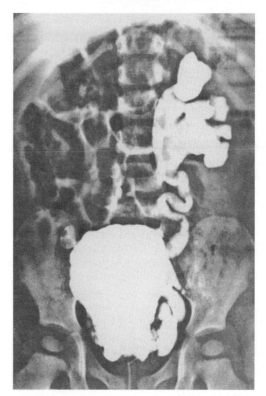

▲ **Figure 41–1.** ***Upper left:*** Retrograde urethrogram showing congenital diaphragmatic stricture. ***Upper right:*** Posterior urethral valves revealed on voiding cystourethrography. *Arrow* points to area of severe stenosis at distal end of prostatic urethra. ***Lower left:*** Posterior urethral valves. Patient would not void with cystography. Retrograde urethrogram showing valves (*arrow*). ***Lower right:*** Cystogram, same patient. Free vesicoureteral reflux and vesical trabeculation with diverticula.

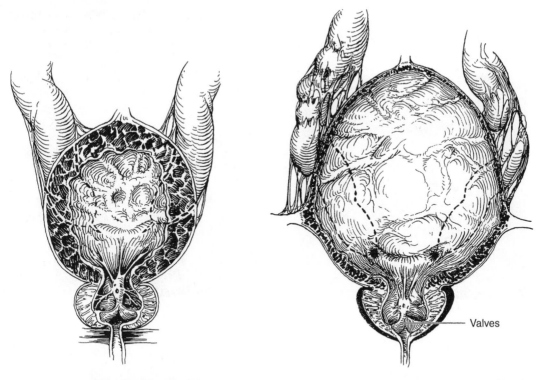

▲ **Figure 41–2.** Posterior urethral valves. **Left:** Dilatation of the prostatic urethra, hypertrophy of vesical wall and trigone in stage of compensation; bilateral hydroureters secondary to trigonal hypertrophy. **Right:** Attenuation of bladder musculature in stage of decompensation; advanced ureteral dilatation and tortuosity, usually secondary to vesicoureteral reflux.

specimen should be obtained via the catheter and sent for culture. The cystogram may show vesicoureteral reflux and the severe trabeculations of long-standing obstruction, and the voiding cystourethrogram often demonstrates elongation and dilatation of the posterior urethra, with a prominent bladder neck (Figure 41–1). Excretory urograms may reveal hydroureter and hydronephrosis when obstruction is severe and long standing.

D. Ultrasonography

Ultrasonography can be used to detect hydronephrosis, hydroureter, and bladder distention in children with severe azotemia. It can also detect fetal hydronephrosis, which is typical of urethral valves, as early as 28 weeks of gestation; when the obstruction is from valves, an enlarged bladder with bilateral hydroureteronephrosis is usually present.

E. Instrumental Examination

Urethroscopy and cystoscopy, performed with the patient under general anesthesia, show vesical trabeculation and cellules and, occasionally, vesical diverticula. The bladder neck

and trigone may be hypertrophied. The diagnosis is confirmed by visual identification of the valves at the distal prostatic urethra. Supravesical compression shows that the valves cause obstruction.

▶ Treatment

Treatment consists of destruction of the valves, but the approach depends on the degree of obstruction and the general health of the child. In children with mild to moderate obstruction and minimal azotemia, transurethral fulguration of the valves is usually successful. Occasionally, catheterization, cystoscopy, or urethral dilation by perineal urethrostomy destroys the valves.

The more severe degrees of obstruction create varying grades of hydronephrosis requiring individualized management. Treatment of children with urosepsis and azotemia associated with hydronephrosis includes use of antibiotics, catheter drainage of the bladder, and correction of the fluid and electrolyte imbalance. Vesicostomy may be of benefit in patients with reflux and renal dysplasia.

In the most severe cases of hydronephrosis, vesicostomy or removal of the valves may not be sufficient, because of ureteral atony, obstruction of the ureterovesical junction from trigonal hypertrophy, or both. In such cases, percutaneous loop ureterostomies may be done to preserve renal function and allow resolution of the hydronephrosis. After renal function is stabilized, valve ablation and reconstruction of the urinary tract can be done.

The period of proximal diversion should be as short as possible, since vesical contracture can be permanent after prolonged supravesical diversion.

It has been noted that approximately 50% of children with urethral valves have vesicoureteral reflux and that the prognosis is worse if the reflux is bilateral. After removal of the obstruction, reflux ceases spontaneously in about one-third of patients. In the remaining two-thirds of patients, the reflux should be corrected surgically.

Long-term use of antimicrobial drugs is often required to prevent recurrent urosepsis and urinary tract infection even though the obstruction has been relieved.

▶ Prognosis

Early detection is the best way to preserve kidney and bladder function. This can be accomplished by ultrasonography in utero, by careful physical examination and observation of voiding in the newborn, and by thorough evaluation of children who have urinary tract infections. Children in whom azotemia and infection persist after relief of obstruction have a poor prognosis.

ANTERIOR URETHRAL VALVES

Signs of anterior urethral valves, a rare congenital anomaly, are urethral dilatation or diverticula proximal to the valve, bladder outlet obstruction, postvoiding incontinence, and infection. Enuresis may be present. Urethroscopy and voiding cystourethrography will demonstrate the lesion, and endoscopic electrofulguration will effectively correct the obstruction.

URETHRORECTAL AND VESICORECTAL FISTULAS

Urethrorectal and vesicorectal fistulas are rare and are almost always associated with imperforate anus. Failure of the urorectal septum to develop completely and separate the rectum from the urogenital tract permits communication between the two systems (see Chapter 2). The child with such a fistula passes fecal material and gas through the urethra. If the anus has developed normally (ie, if it opens externally), urine may pass through the rectum.

Cystoscopy and panendoscopy usually show the fistulous opening. Radiographic contrast material given by mouth will reach the blind rectal pouch, and the distance between the end of the rectum and the perineum can be seen on appropriate radiograms.

Imperforate anus must be opened immediately and the fistula closed, or if the rectum lies quite high, temporary sigmoid colostomy should be performed. Definitive surgery, with repair of the urethral fistula, can be done later.

HYPOSPADIAS

In hypospadias, the urethral meatus opens on the ventral side of the penis proximal to the tip of the glans penis (Figure 41–3).

Sexual differentiation and urethral development begin in utero at approximately 8 weeks and are complete by 15 weeks. The urethra is formed by the fusion of the urethral folds along the ventral surface of the penis, which extends to the corona on the distal shaft. The glandular urethra is formed by canalization of an ectodermal cord that has grown through the glans to communicate with the fused urethral folds (see Chapter 2). Hypospadias results when fusion of the urethral folds is incomplete.

Hypospadias occurs in 1 in every 300 male children. Estrogens and progestins given during pregnancy are known to increase the incidence. Although a familial pattern of hypospadias has been recognized, no specific genetic traits have been established.

▶ Classification

There are several forms of hypospadias classified according to location: (1) glandular, that is, opening on the proximal glans penis; (2) coronal, that is, opening at the coronal sulcus; (3) penile shaft; (4) penoscrotal; and (5) perineal. About 70% of all cases of hypospadias are distal penile or coronal.

Hypospadias in the male is evidence of feminization. Patients with penoscrotal and perineal openings should be considered to have potential intersex problems requiring appropriate evaluation. Hypospadiac newborns should not be circumcised, because the preputial skin may be useful for future reconstruction.

▶ Clinical Findings

A. Symptoms and Signs

Although newborns and young children seldom have symptoms related to hypospadias, older children and adults may complain of difficulty directing the urinary stream and stream spraying. Chordee (curvature of the penis) causes ventral bending and bowing of the penile shaft, which can prevent sexual intercourse. Perineal or penoscrotal hypospadias necessitates voiding in the sitting position, and these proximal forms of hypospadias in adults can be the cause of infertility. An additional complaint of almost all patients is the abnormal (hooded) appearance of the penis, caused by deficient or absent ventral foreskin. The hypospadiac meatus may be stenotic and should be carefully examined and calibrated. (A meatotomy should be done when stenosis exists.) There is an increased incidence of undescended testicles in children with hypospadias; scrotal examination is necessary to establish the position of the testicles.

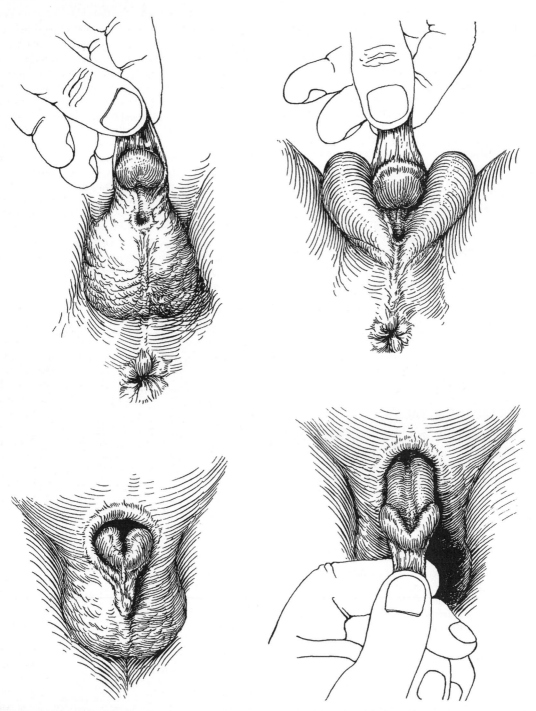

▲ **Figure 41–3.** Hypospadias and epispadias. **Upper left:** Hypospadias, penoscrotal type. Redundant dorsal foreskin that is deficient ventrally; ventral chordee. **Upper right:** Hypospadias, midscrotal type. Chordee more marked. Penis often small. **Lower left:** Epispadias. Redundant ventral foreskin that is absent dorsally; severe dorsal chordee. **Lower right:** Traction on foreskin reveals dorsal defect.

B. Laboratory, X-Ray, and Endoscopic Findings

Since children with penoscrotal and perineal hypospadias often have a bifid scrotum and ambiguous genitalia, a buccal smear and karyotyping are indicated to help establish the genetic sex. Urethroscopy and cystoscopy are of value to determine whether internal male sexual organs are normally developed. Excretory urography is also indicated in these patients to detect additional congenital anomalies of the kidneys and ureters.

Some authors recommend routine use of excretory urography for all patients with hypospadias; however, this seems to be of little value in the more distal types of the disorder, because there appears to be no increased incidence of upper urinary tract anomalies.

▶ Differential Diagnosis

Any degree of hypospadias is an expression of feminization. Perineal and scrotal urethral openings should be carefully evaluated to ascertain that the patient is not a female with androgenized adrenogenital syndrome. Urethroscopy and cystoscopy will aid in evaluating the development of internal reproductive organs.

▶ Treatment

For psychological reasons, hypospadias should be repaired before the patient reaches school age; in most cases, this can be done before age 2.

More than 150 methods of corrective surgery for hypospadias have been described. Currently, one-stage repairs with foreskin island flaps and incised urethral plate are performed by many urologists. It now appears that buccal mucosa grafts are more advantageous than others and should be considered the primary grafting technique when indicated. Fistulas occur in 15–30% of patients, but the fistula repair is considered a small, second-stage reconstruction.

All types of repair involve straightening the penis by removal of the chordee. The chordee removal can be confirmed by producing an artificial erection in the operating room following urethral reconstruction and advancement. Most successful techniques for repair of hypospadias use local skin and foreskin in developing the neourethra. In recent years, advancement of the urethra to the glans penis has become technically feasible and cosmetically acceptable.

▶ Prognosis

After corrective surgery, most patients are able to void in the standing position as well as to deposit semen into the vagina. The overall cosmetic appearance and the prevention of fistula formation remain the greatest challenges in these repairs.

CHORDEE WITHOUT HYPOSPADIAS

Congenital ventral chordee without hypospadias is seen occasionally and is caused by a short urethra, fibrous tissues surrounding the corpus spongiosum, or both. The urethral opening is in the normal position on the glans penis; only with erection does the penis bow, thus preventing satisfactory vaginal penetration. During examination, if the patient cannot achieve an erection naturally, erection can be induced by injecting saline solution into the corpus cavernosum after placing a tourniquet at the base of the penis. This technique should also be used during corrective surgery to be certain that the penis will be straight after the operation.

If the penis is adequate in length, the dorsal surface can be shortened (1) by excising elliptic portions of the tunica albuginea on the dorsum of the penis on either side of the midline or (2) by making transverse cuts in a similar position and then closing them longitudinally, thus shortening the dorsum. Fibrous tissue found in association with the urethra and corpus spongiosum should be totally excised.

EPISPADIAS

The incidence of complete epispadias is approximately 1 in 120,000 males and 1 in 450,000 females. The urethra is displaced dorsally, and classification is based on its position in males. In glandular epispadias, the urethra opens on the dorsal aspect of the glans, which is broad and flattened. In the penile type, the urethral meatus, which is often broad and gaping, is located between the pubic symphysis and the coronal sulcus. A distal groove usually extends from the meatus through the splayed glans. The penopubic type has the urethral opening at the penopubic junction, and the entire penis has a distal dorsal groove extending through the glans.

Patients with glandular epispadias seldom have urinary incontinence. However, with penopubic and penile epispadias, incontinence is present in 95% and 75% of cases, respectively.

Females with epispadias have a bifid clitoris and separation of the labia. Most are incontinent.

Urinary incontinence is a common problem because of maldevelopment of the urinary sphincters. Dorsal curvature of the penis (dorsal chordee) is also present (Figure 41–3). The pubic bones are separated as in exstrophy of the bladder. Epispadias is a mild form of bladder exstrophy, and in severe cases, exstrophy and epispadias coexist.

Surgery is required to correct the incontinence, remove the chordee to straighten the penis, and extend the urethra out onto the glans penis. Repair of the urinary sphincter has not been very successful. Chordee excision and urethroplasty with advancement of the meatus have been successful in achieving acceptable cosmetic and functional results. Bladder augmentation combined with the artificial sphincter may be required in patients in whom incontinence cannot be corrected.

ACQUIRED DISEASES AND DISORDERS OF THE PENIS AND MALE URETHRA

PRIAPISM

Priapism is an uncommon condition of prolonged erection. It is usually painful for the patient, and no sexual excitement or desire is present. The disorder is idiopathic in 60% of cases, while the remaining 40% of cases are associated with diseases (eg, leukemia, sickle cell disease, pelvic tumors, pelvic infections), penile trauma, spinal cord trauma, or use of medications (trazodone). Currently, intracavernous injection therapy for impotence may be the most common cause. Although the idiopathic type often is initially associated with prolonged sexual stimulation, cases of priapism due to the other causes are unrelated to psychic sexual excitement.

Priapism may be classified into high- and low-flow types. High-flow priapism (nonischemic) usually occurs secondary to perineal trauma, which injures the central penile arteries and results in loss of penile blood-flow regulation. Aneurysms of one or both central arteries have been observed. Aspiration of penile blood for blood–gas determination demonstrates high oxygen and normal carbon dioxide levels. Arteriography is useful to demonstrate aneurysms that will respond to embolization; erectile function is usually preserved.

The patient with low-flow priapism (ischemic) usually presents with a history of several hours of painful erection. The glans penis and corpus spongiosum are soft and uninvolved in the process. The corpora cavernosa are tense with congested blood and tender to palpation. The current theories regarding the mechanism of priapism remain in debate, but most authorities believe the major abnormality to be physiologic obstruction of the venous drainage. This obstruction causes buildup of highly viscous, poorly oxygenated blood (low O_2, high CO_2) within the corpora cavernosa. If the process continues for several days, interstitial edema and fibrosis of the corpora cavernosa will develop, causing impotence.

Ischemic priapism must be considered a urologic emergency. Epidural or spinal anesthesia can be used. The sludged blood can then be evacuated from the corpora cavernosa through a large needle placed through the glans. The addition of adrenergic agents administered via intracavernous irrigation has proved helpful. Monitoring intracavernous pressure ensures that recurrence is not imminent. Multiple wedges of tissue can be removed with a biopsy needle to create a shunting fistula between the glans penis and corpora cavernosa. This technique, which has been very successful, provides an internal fistula to keep the corpora cavernosa decompressed. To maintain continuous fistula drainage, pressure should be exerted intermittently (every 15 minutes) on the body of the penis. The patient can do this manually after he has recovered from anesthesia.

If the shunt described fails, another shunting technique may be used by anastomosing the superficial dorsal vein to the corpora cavernosa. Other effective shunting methods are corpora cavernosa to corpus spongiosum shunt by perineal anastomosis; saphenous vein to corpora cavernosa shunt; and pump decompression.

Patients with sickle cell disease have benefited from massive blood transfusions, exchange transfusions, or both. Hyperbaric oxygen also has been suggested for these patients. Patients with leukemia should receive prompt chemotherapy. Appropriate management of any underlying cause should be instituted without delay. Such treatment should not prevent aggressive management of the priapism if the erection persists for several hours.

Impotence is the worst sequel of priapism. It is more common after prolonged priapism (several days). Early recognition (within hours) and prompt treatment of priapism offer the best opportunity to avoid this major problem.

PEYRONIE'S DISEASE

Peyronie's disease (plastic induration of the penis) was first described in 1742 and is a well-recognized clinical problem affecting middle-aged and older men. Patients present with complaints of painful erection, curvature of the penis, and poor erection distal to the involved area. The penile deformity may be so severe that it prevents satisfactory vaginal penetration. The patient has no pain when the penis is in the nonerect state.

Examination of the penile shaft reveals a palpable dense, fibrous plaque of varying size involving the tunica albuginea. The plaque is usually near the dorsal midline of the shaft. Multiple plaques are sometimes seen. In severe cases, calcification and ossification are noted and confirmed by radiography. Although the cause of Peyronie's disease remains obscure, the dense fibrous plaque is microscopically consistent with findings in severe vasculitis. The condition has been noted in association with Dupuytren's contracture of the tendons of the hand, in which the fibrosis resembles that of Peyronie's disease when examined microscopically.

Spontaneous remission occurs in about 50% of cases. Initially, observation and emotional support are advised. If remission does not occur, p-aminobenzoic acid powder or tablets or vitamin E tablets may be tried for several months. However, these medications have limited success. In recent years, a number of operative procedures have been used in refractory cases. Excision of the plaque with replacement with a dermal or vein graft has been successful, as has the use of tunica vaginalis grafts after plaque incision. Other authors have incised the plaque and inserted penile prostheses in the corpora cavernosa. Additional methods include radiation therapy and injection of steroids, dimethyl sulfoxide, or parathyroid hormone into the plaque. The success of such treatments is poorly documented.

PHIMOSIS

Phimosis is a condition in which the contracted foreskin cannot be retracted over the glans. Chronic infection from poor local hygiene is its most common cause. Most cases occur in uncircumcised males, although excessive skin left after circumcision can become stenotic and cause phimosis. Calculi and squamous cell carcinoma may develop under the foreskin. Phimosis can occur at any age. In diabetic older men, chronic balanoposthitis may lead to phimosis and may be the initial presenting complaint. Children younger than 2 years seldom have true phimosis; their relatively narrow preputial opening gradually widens and allows for normal retraction of foreskin over the glans. Circumcision for phimosis should be avoided in children requiring general anesthesia; except in cases with recurrent infections, the procedure should be postponed until the child reaches an age when local anesthesia can be used.

Edema, erythema, and tenderness of the prepuce and the presence of purulent discharge usually cause the patient to seek medical attention. Inability to retract the foreskin is a less common complaint.

The initial infection should be treated with broad-spectrum antimicrobial drugs. The dorsal foreskin can be slit if improved drainage is necessary. Circumcision, if indicated, should be done after the infection is controlled.

PARAPHIMOSIS

Paraphimosis is the condition in which the foreskin, once retracted over the glans, cannot be replaced in its normal position. This is due to chronic inflammation under the redundant foreskin, which leads to contracture of the preputial opening (phimosis) and formation of a tight ring of skin when the foreskin is retracted behind the glans. The skin ring causes venous congestion leading to edema and enlargement of the glans, which make the condition worse. As the condition progresses, arterial occlusion and necrosis of the glans may occur.

Paraphimosis usually can be treated by firmly squeezing the glans for 5 minutes to reduce the tissue edema and decrease the size of the glans. The skin can then be drawn forward over the glans. Occasionally, the constricting ring requires incision under local anesthesia. Antibiotics should be administered and circumcision should be done after inflammation has subsided.

CIRCUMCISION

Although circumcision is routinely performed in some countries for religious or cultural reasons, it is usually not necessary if adequate penile cleanliness and good hygiene can be maintained. There is a higher incidence of penile carcinoma in uncircumcised males, but chronic infection and poor hygiene are usually underlying factors in such instances. Circumcision is indicated in patients with infection, phimosis, or paraphimosis (see preceding sections).

URETHRAL STRICTURE

Acquired urethral stricture is common in men but rare in women. (Congenital urethral stricture is discussed earlier in the chapter.) Most acquired strictures are due to infection or trauma. Although gonococcal urethritis is seldom a cause of stricture today, infection remains a major cause—particularly infection from long-term use of indwelling urethral catheters. Large catheters and instruments are more likely than small ones to cause ischemia and internal trauma. External trauma, for example, pelvic fractures (see Chapter 17), can partially or completely sever the membranous urethra and cause severe and complex strictures. Straddle injuries can produce bulbar strictures.

Urethral strictures are fibrotic narrowings composed of dense collagen and fibroblasts. Fibrosis usually extends into the surrounding corpus spongiosum, causing spongiofibrosis. These narrowings restrict urine flow and cause dilation of the proximal urethra and prostatic ducts. Prostatitis is a common complication of urethral stricture. The bladder muscle may become hypertrophic, and increased residual urine may be noted. Severe, prolonged obstruction can result in decompensation of the ureterovesical junction, reflux, hydronephrosis, and renal failure. Chronic urinary stasis makes infection likely. Urethral fistulas and periurethral abscesses commonly develop in association with chronic, severe strictures.

▶ Clinical Findings

A. Symptoms and Signs

A decrease in urinary stream is the most common complaint. Spraying or double stream is often noted, as is postvoiding dribbling. Chronic urethral discharge, occasionally a major complaint, is likely to be associated with chronic prostatitis. Acute cystitis or symptoms of infection are seen at times. Acute urinary retention seldom occurs unless infection or prostatic obstruction develops. Urinary frequency and mild dysuria may also be initial complaints.

Induration in the area of the stricture may be palpable. Tender enlarged masses along the urethra usually represent periurethral abscesses. Urethrocutaneous fistulas may be present. The bladder may be palpable if there is chronic retention of urine.

B. Laboratory Findings

If urethral stricture is suspected, urinary flow rates should be determined. The patient is instructed to accumulate urine until the bladder is full and then begin voiding; a 5-second collection of urine should be obtained during midstream maximal flow and its volume recorded. After the patient repeats this procedure eight to ten times over several days in a relaxed atmosphere, the mean peak flow can be calculated. With strictures creating significant problems, the flow rate will be <10 mL/s (normal 20 mL/s).

Urine culture may be indicated. The midstream specimen is usually bacteria free, with some pyuria (eight to ten white blood cells [leukocytes] per high-power field) in a carefully obtained first aliquot of urine. If the prostate is infected, bacteria will be present in a specimen obtained after prostatic massage. In the presence of cystitis, the urine will be grossly infected.

C. X-Ray Findings

A urethrogram or voiding cystourethrogram (or both) will demonstrate the location and extent of the stricture. Sonography has also been a useful method of evaluating the urethral stricture. Urethral fistulas and diverticula are sometimes noted. Vesical stones, trabeculations, or diverticula may also be seen.

D. Instrumental Examination

Urethroscopy allows visualization of the stricture. Small-caliber strictures prevent passage of the instrument through the area. Direct visualization and sonourethrography aid in determining the extent, location, and degree of scarring. Additional areas of scar formation adjacent to the stricture may be detected by urethroscopy.

The stricture can be calibrated by passage of bougies à boule.

▷ Differential Diagnosis

Benign or malignant prostatic obstruction can cause symptoms similar to those of stricture. After prostatic surgery, bladder neck contracture can develop and induce stricture-like symptoms. Rectal examination and panendoscopy adequately define such abnormalities of the prostate. Urethral carcinoma is often associated with stricture; urethroscopy demonstrates a definite irregular lesion, and biopsy establishes the diagnosis of carcinoma.

▷ Complications

Complications include chronic prostatitis, cystitis, chronic urinary infection, diverticula, urethrocutaneous fistulas, periurethral abscesses, and urethral carcinoma. Vesical calculi may develop from chronic urinary stasis and infection.

▷ Treatment

A. Specific Measures

1. Dilation—Dilation of urethral strictures is not usually curative, but it fractures the scar tissue of the stricture and temporarily enlarges the lumen. As healing occurs, the scar tissue reforms.

Dilation may initially be required because of severe symptoms of chronic retention of urine. The urethra should be liberally lubricated with a water-soluble medium before instrumentation. A filiform is passed down the urethra and gently manipulated through the narrow area into the bladder. A follower can then be attached (see Chapter 10) and the area gradually dilated (with successively larger sizes) to approximately 22F. A 16F silicone catheter can then be inserted. If difficulty arises in passing the filiform through the stricture,

urethroscopy should be used to guide the filiform under direct vision.

An alternative method of urethral dilation employs Van Buren sounds. These instruments are best used by an experienced urologist familiar with the size and extent of the stricture involved. First, a 22F sound should be passed down to the stricture site and gentle pressure applied. If this fails, a 20F sound should be used. Smaller sounds should be used with care, because they can easily perforate the urethral wall and produce false passages. Bleeding and pain are major problems caused by dilation.

2. Urethrotomy under endoscopic direct vision—Lysis of urethral strictures can be accomplished using a sharp knife attached to an endoscope. The endoscope provides direct vision of the stricture during cutting. A filiform should be passed through the stricture and used as a guide during lysis. The stricture is usually incised circumferentially with multiple incisions. A 22F instrument should pass with ease. A catheter is left in place for a short time to prevent bleeding and pain. Results of this procedure have been satisfactory in short-term follow-up in 70–80% of patients, but long-term success rates are much lower. The procedure has several advantages: (1) minimal anesthesia is required—in some cases, only topical anesthesia combined with sedation; (2) it is easily repeated if the stricture recurs; and (3) it is very safe, with few complications.

3. Surgical reconstruction—If urethrotomy under direct vision fails, open surgical repair should be performed. Short strictures (≤2 cm) of the anterior urethra should be completely excised and primary anastomosis done. If possible, the segment to be excised should extend 1 cm beyond each end of the stricture to allow for removal of any existing spongiofibrosis and improve postoperative healing.

Strictures >2 cm in length can be managed by patch graft urethroplasty. The urethra is incised in the midline for the full length of the stricture plus an additional 0.5 cm proximal and distal to its ends. A full-thickness skin graft is obtained—preferably from the penile skin or buccal mucosa—and all subcutaneous tissues are carefully removed. The graft is then tailored to cover the defect and meticulously sutured into place (Figure 41–4).

In very long, densely fibrotic strictures, the distal penile fasciocutaneous flap technique has been successful in >80% cases. This single-stage procedure can be combined with buccal mucosa grafting in panurethral strictures. In adults, grafts from buccal mucosa or penile skin should be applied with an onlay technique in the bulbar region of the urethra to maximize graft vascularization from the corpus spongiosum.

Strictures involving the membranous urethra ordinarily result from external trauma (see Chapter 17) and present problems in reconstruction. Most can be corrected by a perineal approach with excision of the urethral rupture defect and direct anastomosis of the bulbar urethra to the prostatic

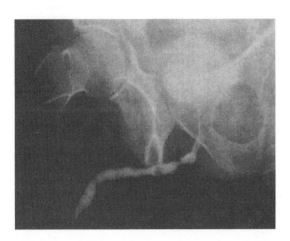

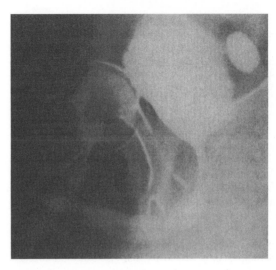

▲ **Figure 41–4.** ***Left:*** Urethrogram demonstrating multiple anterior urethral strictures. ***Right:*** Voiding cystourethrogram following a patch skin graft of 14 cm in the same patient. There are no residual strictures.

urethra (Figure 41–5). At times, partial pubectomy from the perineal approach can be done to improve urethral approximation without tension on the anastomosis. Rarely, total pubectomy combined with the perineal approach is required to accomplish the direct end-to-end anastomosis.

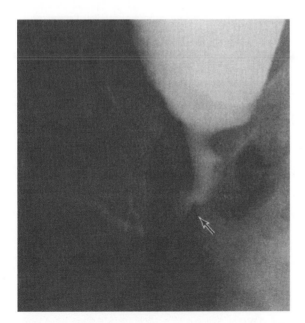

▲ **Figure 41–5.** Voiding urethrogram following repair of traumatic posterior urethral stricture. *Arrow* indicates that area of repair is stricture free.

These single-stage procedures have a high success rate and create a urethra free of hair—a major problem seen with two-stage procedures. Although seldom required, two-stage procedures are important reconstructive techniques to be considered in complex urethral strictures.

B. Treatment of Complications

Urinary tract infection in patients with strictures requires specific antimicrobial therapy, followed by long-term prophylactic therapy until the stricture has been corrected. Periurethral abscesses require drainage and use of antimicrobial drugs. Urethral fistulas usually require surgical repair.

▶ Prognosis

A stricture should not be considered "cured" until it has been observed for at least 1 year after therapy, since it may recur at any time during that period. Urinary flow rate measurements and urethrograms are helpful to determine the extent of residual obstruction.

URETHRAL CONDYLOMATA ACUMINATA (URETHRAL WARTS)

Condylomata acuminata are uncommon in the urethra and are almost always preceded by lesions on the skin. They are wart-like papillomas caused by a papilloma virus and are usually transmitted by direct sexual contact but may be transmitted nonsexually.

Patients commonly complain of bloody spotting from the urethra and occasionally have dysuria and urethral discharge. Examination of the urethral meatus often reveals a small, protruding papilloma. If a lesion is not found in this location, the meatus should be separated with the examining fingers so that the distal urethra can be inspected. About 90% of such lesions are situated in the distal urethra. Complete urethroscopy must be done to be certain other lesions do not exist.

Lesions of the meatus can be treated by local excision. A local anesthetic is applied to the area at the base of the lesions, and the pedunculated lesions are sharply incised with small scissors. The area is then fulgurated by electrocautery. Meatotomy may be indicated for excision of lesions in the fossa navicularis and glandular urethra.

Deeper lesions may be fulgurated transurethrally with a resectoscope or Bugby electrode. Recently, lesions have been successfully destroyed using a carbon dioxide or holmium laser. Laser therapy does minimal damage to the urethral mucosa, and stricture formation seems less likely with its use.

Multiple lesions have also been treated with fluorouracil, 5% solution or cream. The drug is instilled in the urethra for 20 minutes twice a week for 5 weeks. Care must be taken to protect the penile skin and scrotum from coming in contact with the medication, since it may produce severe irritation.

Lesions may become infected and ulcerated. This suggests carcinoma, and histopathologic confirmation of the diagnosis should be obtained. Rarely, giant condylomata (Buschke-Löwenstein tumors) involving the glans penis and often the urethra may be seen. Such lesions suggest carcinoma and a biopsy must be done. Surgical excision is the treatment of choice.

To prevent recurrence of condylomata acuminata, the sexual partner must also be examined and treated if necessary.

STENOSIS OF THE URETHRAL MEATUS

Newborns are often suspected of having meatal stenosis of some degree. This condition is thought to be secondary to ammonia dermatitis following circumcision and resulting in prolonged irritative meatitis.

Calibration is important, since the visual appearance of the meatus does not correlate well with its actual size. The urethra should easily accept the tip of an 8F pediatric feeding tube. The significance of metal stenosis is debated, but a meatal caliber <5F in children <10 years of age is an indication for meatotomy.

PENILE PHLEBOTHROMBOSIS AND LYMPHATIC OCCLUSION

Superficial veins and lymphatic vessels of the dorsal penile shaft just proximal to the corona may become irritated and inflamed. A careful history usually indicates that minor trauma to the area (eg, from prolonged sexual intercourse) has occurred. Examination reveals a tender, indurated, cord-like structure on the distal penile shaft. Slight erythema may be present.

For clinical purposes, there is no need to distinguish lymphatic and venous causes, since both penile phlebothrombosis and lymphatic occlusion will resolve spontaneously. The patient must be reassured.

BIBLIOGRAPHY

Congenital Anomalies
Penis and Urethra

Akman Y et al: Penile anatomy under the pubic arch: Reconstructive implications. J Urol 2001;166:225.

Barbagli G: Editorial comment on: Surgical treatment of 31 complex traumatic posterior urethral strictures associated with urethrorectal fistulas. Eur Urol 2010;57(3):520–521.

Confer SD et al: Megacystis with an anterior urethral valve: Case report and review of literature. J Pediatr Urol 2010;6(5):459–462.

de Oliveira MC et al: Surgical treatment of penile duplication. J Pediatr Urol 2010;6(3):257.e1–257.e3.

Fine MS et al: Posterior urethral valve treatments and outcomes in children receiving kidney transplants. J Urol 2011;185(6, Suppl): 2507–2511.

Gad YZ et al: 5 alpha-reductase deficiency in patients with micropenis. J Inherit Metab Dis 1997;20:95.

Ishii T et al: The effect of intramuscular testosterone enanthate treatment on stretched penile length in prepubertal boys with hypospadias. Urology 2010;76(1):97–100.

Sarhan OM et al: Posterior urethral valves: Multivariate analysis of factors affecting the final renal outcome. J Urol 2011;185(6, Suppl): 2491–2495.

Tsang S: When size matters: A clinical review of pathological micropenis. J Pediatr Health Care 2010;24(4):231–240. Review.

Wan J, Rew KT: Common penile problems. Prim Care 2010;37(3): 627–642, x. Review.

Wessells H et al: Penile length in the flaccid and erect states: Guidelines for penile augmentation. J Urol 1996;156:995.

Yanai T et al: Minimally invasive repair of hypospadiac urethral duplication. Pediatr Surg Int 2011;27(1):115–118.

Hypospadias

Acimi S: Comparative study of two techniques used in distal hypospadias repair: Tubularized incised plate (Snodgrass) and tubularized urethral plate (Duplay). Scand J Urol Nephrol 2011;45(1):68–71.

Barbagli G et al: Retrospective descriptive analysis of 1,176 patients with failed hypospadias repair. J Urol 2010;183(1):207–211.

Baskin LS: Hypospadias and urethral development. J Urol 2000; 163:951.

Bhangoo A et al: Isolated micropenis reveals partial androgen insensitivity syndrome confirmed by molecular analysis. Asian J Androl 2010;12(4):561–566.

Castagnetti M, El-Ghoneimi A: Surgical management of primary severe hypospadias in children: Systematic 20-year review. J Urol 2010;184(4):1469–1474.

Hensle TW et al: Hypospadias repair in adults: Adventures and misadventures. J Urol 2001;165:77.

Powell CR et al: Comparison of flaps versus grafts in proximal hypospadias surgery. J Urol 2000;163:1286.

Roberts J: Hypospadias surgery past, present and future. Curr Opin Urol 2010;20(6):483–489.

Snodgrass W: Hypospadias reporting—How good is the literature? J Urol 2010;184(4):1255–1256.

Thorup J et al: What is new in cryptorchidism and hypospadias—A critical review on the testicular dysgenesis hypothesis. J Pediatr Surg 2010;45(10):2074–2086.

Wan J, Rew KT: Common penile problems. Prim Care 2010;37(3):627–642.

Ziada A et al: Outcomes of hypospadias repair in older children: A prospective study. J Urol 2011;185(6, Suppl):2483–2485.

Epispadias

Baird AD et al: Reconstructive lower urinary tract surgery in incontinent adolescents with exstrophy/epispadias complex. Urology 2005;66:636.

Ben-Chaim J, Gearhart JP: Current management of bladder exstrophy. Scand J Urol Nephrol 1997;31:103.

Gearhart JP: Re: Results of complete penile disassembly for epispadias repair in 42 patients. J Urol 2004;171:2386.

Grady RW, Mitchell ME: Management of epispadias. Urol Clin North Am 2002;29:349.

Hammouda HM: Results of complete penile disassembly for epispadias repair in 42 patients. J Urol 2003;170:1963.

Acquired Diseases and Disorders of the Penis and Male Urethra

Park S et al: Extramammary Paget's disease of the penis and scrotum: Excision, reconstruction and evaluation of occult malignancy. J Urol 2001;166:2112.

Rosenstein D, McAninch JW: Urologic emergencies. Med Clin North Am 2004;88:495.

Priapism

Chinegwundoh F, Anie KA: Treatments for priapism in boys and men with sickle cell disease. Cochrane Database Syst Rev 2004;18(4): CD004198.

Costa WS et al: Structural analysis of the corpora cavernosa in patients with ischaemic priapism. BJU Int 2010;105(6):838–841; discussion 841.

Montague DK et al: American Urological Association guideline on the management of priapism. J Urol 2003;170:1318.

Montague DK: Sexual dysfunction: Immediate penile prosthesis for acute ischemic priapism. Nat Rev Urol 2010;7(4):187–188.

Shrewsberry A et al: Recent advances in the medical and surgical treatment of priapism. Curr Urol Rep 2010;11(6):405–413. Review.

Stember DS, Mulhall JP: Ischemic priapism and implant surgery with sharp corporal fibrosis excision. J Sex Med 2010;7(6):1987–1990; quiz 1991.

Tabibi A et al: Erectile function and dysfunction following low flow priapism: A comparison of distal and proximal shunts. Urol J 2010;7(3):174–177.

Volkmer BG et al: Prepubertal high flow priapism: Incidence, diagnosis and treatment. J Urol 2001;166:1018.

Peyronie's Disease

Breyer BN et al: Are sonographic characteristics associated with progression to surgery in men with Peyronie's disease? J Urol 2010; 183(4):1484–1488.

Chung E et al: Five-year follow-up of Peyronie's graft surgery: Outcomes and patient satisfaction. J Sex Med 2011;8(2):594–600.

Eisenberg ML et al: Tunica-sparing ossified Peyronie's plaque excision. BJU Int 2011;107(4):622–625.

Heidari M et al: Evaluation of intralesional injection of verapamil in treatment of Peyronie's disease. J Pak Med Assoc 2010;60(4):291–293.

Hellstrom WJ: Medical management of Peyronie's disease. J Androl 2009;30(4):397–405.

Mulhall JP et al: Basic fibroblast growth factor expression in Peyronie's disease. J Urol 2001;165:419.

Seftel AD: Incidentally diagnosed Peyronie's disease in men presenting with erectile dysfunction. J Urol 2005;173:2076.

Simonato A et al: Penile dermal flap in patients with Peyronie's disease: Long-term results. J Urol 2010;183(3):1065–1068.

Tal R et al: Peyronie's disease following radical prostatectomy: Incidence and predictors. J Sex Med 2010;7(3):1254–1261.

Wilson SK et al: Long-term followup of treatment for Peyronie's disease: Modeling the penis over an inflatable penile prosthesis. J Urol 2001;165:825.

Phimosis

Hayashi Y et al: Prepuce: Phimosis, paraphimosis, and circumcision. ScientificWorldJournal 2011;11:289–301.

Minhas S et al: Penile cancer—Prevention and premalignant conditions. Urology 2010;76(2, Suppl 1):S24–S35.

Nobre YD et al: To circ or not to circ: Clinical and pharmacoeconomic outcomes of a prospective trial of topical steroid versus primary circumcision. Int Braz J Urol 2010;36(1):75–85.

Pieretti RV et al: Late complications of newborn circumcision: A common and avoidable problem. Pediatr Surg Int 2010; 26(5):515–518.

Paraphimosis

Olson C: Emergency treatment of paraphimosis. Can Fam Physician 1998;44:1253.

Circumcision

Fitzgerald DW et al: An Ad5-vectored HIV-1 vaccine elicits cell-mediated immunity but does not affect disease progression in HIV-1-infected male subjects: Results from a randomized placebo-controlled trial (the Step study). J Infect Dis 2011;203(6):765–772.

Mahanta J et al: Circumcision and herpes simplex virus-2 infection among spouses. Sex Transm Infect 2010;86(7):487.

Mokhless IA et al: Penile advancement and lengthening for the management of post-circumcision traumatic short penis in adolescents. Urology 2010;76(6):1483–1487.

Wawer MJ et al: Effect of circumcision of HIV-negative men on transmission of human papillomavirus to HIV-negative women: A randomised trial in Rakai, Uganda. Lancet 2011;377(9761):209–218.

Urethral Stricture

Anger JT et al: Trends in stricture management among male Medicare beneficiaries: Underuse of urethroplasty? Urology 2011; 77(2):481–485.

Breyer BN et al: Multivariate analysis of risk factors for long-term urethroplasty outcome. J Urol 2010;183(2):613–617.

Burks FN, Santucci RA: Complicated urethroplasty: A guide for surgeons. Nat Rev Urol 2010;7(9):521–528.

Chapple C: Anterior urethral surgery: Current concepts and future directions. Eur Urol 2010;58(1):42–45.

Ching CB et al: The Cleveland Clinic experience with adult hypospadias patients undergoing repair: Their presentation and a new classification system. BJU Int 2011;107(7):1142–1146.

Erickson BA et al: The use of uroflowmetry to diagnose recurrent stricture after urethral reconstructive surgery. J Urol 2010; 184(4):1386–1390.

Lumen N et al: Ventral longitudinal stricturotomy and transversal closure: The Heineke-Mikulicz principle in urethroplasty. Urology 2010;76(6):1478–1482.

Mundy AR, Andrich DE: Urethral strictures. BJU Int 2011;107(1): 6–26.

Myers JB, McAninch JW: Perineal urethrostomy. BJU Int 2011;107(5):856–865.

Myers JB, McAninch JW: Surgery illustrated—Surgical atlas perineal urethrostomy. BJU Int 2011;107(5):856–857.

Santucci R, Eisenberg L: Urethrotomy has a much lower success rate than previously reported. J Urol 2010;183(5):1859–1862.

Schwentner C et al: Anterior urethral reconstruction using the circular fasciocutaneous flap technique: Long-term follow-up. World J Urol 2011;29(1):115–120.

Whitson JM et al: Long-term efficacy of distal penile circular fasciocutaneous flaps for single stage reconstruction of complex anterior urethral stricture disease. J Urol 2008;179(6):2259–2264.

Urethral Condylomata Acuminata (Urethral Warts)

Stefanaki C et al: Prognostic factors for the response to treatment in males with genital warts. J Eur Acad Dermatol Venereol 2009;23(10): 1156–1160.

Penile Phlebothrombosis and Lymphatic Occlusion

Conkbayir I et al: Superficial dorsal penile vein thrombosis (Mondor disease of the penis) involving the superficial external pudendal vein: Color Doppler sonographic findings. J Ultrasound Med 2010;29(8):1243–1245.

Disorders of the Female Urethra

42

Donna Y. Deng, MD, MS, & Emil A. Tanagho, MD

CONGENITAL ANOMALIES OF THE FEMALE URETHRA

DISTAL URETHRAL STENOSIS IN INFANCY AND CHILDHOOD (SPASM OF THE EXTERNAL URINARY SPHINCTER) AND DYSFUNCTIONAL VOIDING

There has been considerable confusion about the site of lower tract obstruction in young girls who have enuresis, a slow and interrupted urinary stream, recurrent cystitis, and pyelonephritis and who, on thorough examination, often exhibit vesicoureteral reflux. Treatment has been directed largely to the bladder neck on rather empiric grounds. Most of these children, however, have congenital distal urethral stenosis with secondary spasm of the striated external sphincter rather than bladder neck obstruction.

Lyon and Tanagho (1965) found that the distal urethral ring calibrates at 14F at age 2 and at 16F between the ages of 4 and 10. Even though from the hydrodynamic standpoint, such a stenotic area should not be obstructive, almost all observers agree that dilatation of the ring does relieve symptoms in these children and that it results in cure or amelioration of persistent infection or vesical dysfunction in 80% of cases (Kondo et al, 1994). Tanagho et al (1971) measured pressures in the bladder and in the proximal and mid urethra simultaneously in symptomatic girls and found high resting pressures, some as high as 200 cm of water (normal, 100 cm of water) in the midurethral segment. Attempts at voiding caused intravesical pressures as high as 225 cm of water (normal, 30–40 cm of water) to develop. Under curare, the urethral closing pressures dropped to normal (40–50 cm of water), proving that these obstructing pressures were caused by spasm of the striated sphincter muscle. If the distal urethral ring was treated and symptoms abated, repeat pressure studies showed normal midurethral and intravesical voiding pressures. It seems clear, therefore, that the likely cause of urinary problems in young girls is spasm of the external sphincter and not vesical neck stenosis (Smith, 1969).

In addition to recurrent urinary tract infections, these patients have hesitancy in initiating micturition and a slow, hesitant, or interrupted urinary stream. Enuresis and involuntary loss of urine during the day are common complaints. Abdominal straining may be required in order to void. Small amounts of residual urine are found, which impair the vesical defense mechanism. A voiding cystourethrogram may reveal an open bladder neck and ballooning of the proximal urethra secondary to spasm of the external sphincter (Figure 42–1).

The voiding cystourethrogram may reveal evidence of the distal ring, but typical findings are not always seen, particularly if the flow rate is slow. Definitive diagnosis is made by bougienage.

Historically, the simplest and least harmful treatment is overdilatation with sounds up to 32–36F). The ring "cracks" anteriorly, with some bleeding. Recurrence of the ring is rare. The results of internal urethrotomy were poor, since incising the urethra along its entire length does not cut the external sphincter (Kaplan et al, 1973).

In the past two decades, it has been recognized that many of these symptoms are due to functional, rather than neurologic or anatomic causes of obstruction. Children must achieve adult patterns of urinary control and disturbances, especially around the time of toilet training. This may cause a variety of symptoms that result from voiding against a voluntarily closed urethral sphincter (dysfunctional voiding). These range from severe functional obstruction with urinary retention, altered bladder anatomy, and vesicoureteral reflux (known as Hinman's syndrome) to less severe incomplete control of urination. They are often accompanied by bowel symptoms, such as constipation or encopresis. Treatment requires bladder retraining, including psychologic help and biofeedback, as well as restoration of normal bowel habits, including dietary changes and laxatives.

LABIAL FUSION (SYNECHIA VULVAE)

Some children with recurring urinary infection are found to have fused labia minora, which are apt to obstruct the flow of

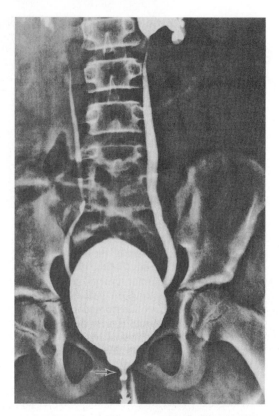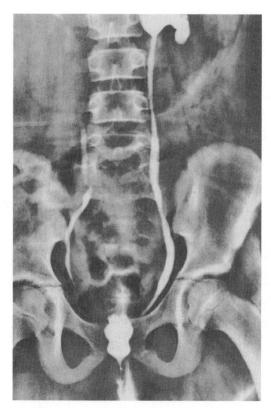

▲ **Figure 42–1.** Distal urethral stenosis with reflux spasm of voluntary urethral sphincter. **Left:** Voiding cystourethrogram showing bilateral vesicoureteral reflux, a wide-open vesical neck, and severe spasm of the striated urethral sphincter in the mid portion of the urethra (*arrow*) secondary to distal urethral stenosis. **Right:** Postvoiding film. The bladder is empty and the vesical neck open, but the dilated urethra contains radiopaque fluid proximal to the stenotic zone. Bacteria in the urethra thus can flow back into the bladder. (Courtesy of AD Amar.)

urine, causing it to pool in the vagina. Local application of estrogen cream twice daily for 2–4 weeks usually causes spontaneous separation, with minimal side effects (Aribag, 1975; Leung et al, 2005). Forceful separation or dissection has its advocates (Christensen and Oster, 1971).

It is uncommonly seen as an acquired disease after puberty, caused by genital trauma (sexual abuse, vaginal delivery, surgery, etc) (Kumar et al, 2006). In cultures where "female circumcision" is performed, this may be a relatively common complication (Adekunle et al, 1999).

ACQUIRED DISEASES OF THE FEMALE URETHRA

ACUTE URETHRITIS

Acute urethritis frequently occurs with gonorrheal (*Neisseria gonorrhoeae*) or trichomoniasis (*Trichomonas vaginalis*) infection in women, and it may less commonly occur with infection by *Chlamydia trachomatis* (approximately 25% of cases are symptomatic). Urinary symptoms are often present at the onset of the disease. Cultures and smears establish the diagnosis. Prompt cure can be achieved with antimicrobial drugs, usually to cover both gonorrhea and chlamydia, such as a combination of intramuscular ceftriaxone and oral azithromycin or doxycycline. Treatment is important, as 40% of women with untreated chlamydia infections will have pelvic inflammatory disease, which may lead to ectopic pregnancy, pelvic pain, and infertility (Simms and Stephenson, 2000).

The detergents in bubble bath and some spermicidal jellies may cause vaginitis and urethritis. Symptoms of vesical irritability may occur (Bass, 1968; Marshall, 1965).

CHRONIC URETHRITIS

Chronic urethritis is one of the most common urologic problems of females. The distal urethra normally harbors pathogens, and the risk of infection may be increased by wearing contaminated diapers, by insertion of an indwelling catheter, by spread from cervical or vaginal infections, or by intercourse with an infected partner. Urethral inflammation may also occur from the trauma of intercourse or childbirth, particularly if urethral stenosis, either congenital or following childbirth, is present.

▶ Clinical Findings

The urethral mucosa is reddened, quite sensitive, and often stenotic. Granular areas are often seen, and polypoid masses may be noted just distal to the bladder neck.

A. Symptoms

The symptoms resemble those of cystitis, although the urine may be clear. Complaints include burning on urination, frequency, and nocturia. Discomfort in the urethra may be felt, particularly when walking.

B. Signs

Examination may disclose redness of the meatus, hypersensitivity of the meatus and of the urethra on vaginal palpation, and evidence of cervicitis or vaginitis. There is no urethral discharge.

C. Laboratory Findings

When the initial and midstream urine are collected in separate containers, the first glass contains pus and the second does not (Marshall et al, 1970). *Ureaplasma urealyticum* (formerly called T strains of mycoplasmas) is often identifiable in the first glass. These findings are similar to those of nongonococcal (chlamydial) urethritis in males. Clinically, the presence of white blood cells (leukocytes) in the absence of bacteria on a routine stain or culture suggests nongonococcal urethritis. In other cases, various bacteria (eg, *Streptococcus faecalis, Escherichia coli*) may be cultured from both the urethral washings and a specimen taken from the introitus.

D. Instrumental Examination

A catheter, bougie à boule, or sound may meet resistance because of urethral stenosis. Panendoscopy reveals redness and a granular appearance of the mucosa (Krieger, 1988). Inflammatory polyps may be seen in the proximal portion of the urethra. Cystoscopy may show increased injection of the trigone (trigonitis), which often accompanies urethritis.

▶ Differential Diagnosis

Differentiation of urethritis from cystitis depends on bacteriologic study of the urine; panendoscopy demonstrates the urethral lesion. Both urethritis and cystitis may be present. Chronic noninflammatory urethritis may be a manifestation of psychic stressors. Patients with anxiety or other temporary or chronic psychologic disorders may present with symptoms

that are very suggestive of urethritis. Alternatively, women with long-standing symptoms may have these symptoms as an adult version of childhood voiding dysfunction (see earlier discussion). It is important to understand that chronic dysuria in the absence of a real bacteriologic source is often a manifestation of chronic pelvic pain syndrome (ie, interstitial cystitis, painful bladder syndrome).

▶ Treatment and Prognosis

Gradual urethral dilatations (up to 36F in adults) are indicated for urethral stenosis; this allows for some inevitable contracture. However, true urethral stenosis is not common in women, and diagnosis should be confirmed by cystoscopy and urethral calibration. If pelvic dysfunction is the underlying issue, calibration under anesthesia will show normal caliber urethra. Immergut and Gilbert (1973) prefer internal urethrotomy (Farrar, 1980). *U. urealyticum* and chlamydial urethritis usually respond to doxycycline or azithromycin.

ATROPHIC URETHRITIS

After physiologic (or surgical) menopause, hypoestrogenism occurs and atrophic changes take place in the vaginal mucosa, so it becomes dry and pale (Smith, 1972); atrophic vaginitis affects 20–30% of postmenopausal women. This is likely a significant underestimation because women are unwilling to report symptoms due to either embarrassment or lack of knowledge that there are treatments available (Johnston, 2004). Similar changes develop in the lower urinary tract, which arises from the same embryologic tissues as the female reproductive organs. Some eversion of the mucosa about the urethral orifice, from atrophy of the vaginal wall, is usually seen. This is commonly misdiagnosed as caruncle.

▶ Clinical Findings

A. Symptoms

Many postmenopausal women have symptoms of vesical irritability (burning, frequency, urgency) and stress incontinence. Dysuria may occur due to urine contact with the inflamed atrophic tissues themselves or because of the increased incidence of urinary tract infections in these women. They may complain of vaginal and vulval itching or tightness, discharge, dyspareunia, and may have bloody vaginal spotting, especially after intercourse.

B. Signs

The vaginal epithelium is dry and pale, with a decrease in the rugae. The mucosa at the urethral orifice is often reddened and hypersensitive; eversion of its posterior lip from atrophy of the urethrovaginal wall is common. Atrophic vaginitis also increases the risk for urinary tract infections, and approximately 10–15% of women older than 60 years have frequent urinary tract infections.

C. Laboratory Findings

The urine is usually free of microorganisms. The diagnosis can be made by the following procedure: A dry smear of vaginal epithelial cells is stained with Lugol's solution. The slide is then washed with water and immediately examined microscopically while wet. In hypoestrogenism, the cells take up the iodine poorly and are therefore yellow. When the mucosa is normal, these cells stain a deep brown because of their glycogen content. The diagnosis may also be confirmed by a Papanicolaou smear. Postmenopausal status is associated with a higher vaginal pH, a decrease in vaginal lactobacillus colonization, and increased colonization with *E. coli*.

D. Instrumental Examination

Cystourethroscopy may demonstrate a reddened and granular urethral mucosa. Some urethral stenosis may be noted. More commonly, the mucosa at the meatus is reddened, but the remainder of the urethra is quite normal.

▶ Differential Diagnosis

Atrophic urethritis is often mistaken for urethral caruncle. Eversion of the posterior lip of the urinary meatus is evident in both conditions; however, a hypersensitive vascular mass is not present in atrophic urethritis.

▶ Treatment

Atrophic urethritis responds well to local estrogen treatment to the vagina (Sturdee, 2010). There are several formulations available: conjugated equine estrogen cream, a sustained-release intravaginal estradiol ring which delivers low level of estradiol over a 3-month period, or a low-dose estradiol tablet. Local application has the advantage of minimal change of systemic blood level and thus avoids the side effects associated with systemic hormone therapy. There is insufficient data to recommend annual endometrial surveillance in asymptomatic women using local estrogens. However, for those who have had breast or gynecologic cancers, consultation with their oncologist is important.

▶ Prognosis

Topical estrogen vaginal cream is an effective treatment in postmenopausal women with recurrent infections (Quinlivan, 1965). In one study, patients treated with the estrogen cream averaged 0.5 infections per year, compared with about 6.0 infections per year in women who were not treated (Raz and Stamm, 1993).

URETHRAL CARUNCLE

Urethral caruncle is a benign, red, raspberry-like, friable vascular tumor involving the posterior lip of the external urinary meatus. It is rare before menopause. Microscopically, it

consists of connective tissue containing many inflammatory cells and blood vessels and is covered by an epithelial layer (Lee, 1995).

▶ Clinical Findings

Symptoms include pain on urination, pain with intercourse, and bloody spotting from even mild trauma. A sessile or pedunculated red, friable, tender mass is seen at the posterior lip of the meatus.

▶ Differential Diagnosis

Carcinoma of the urethra may involve the urethral meatus. Palpation reveals definite induration. Biopsy establishes the true diagnosis. Atrophic urethritis is often associated with a polypoid reaction of the urinary meatus and in fact is the most common cause of masses in this region. The diagnosis can be made by verifying the patient's hypoestrogenic status and by demonstrating a favorable response to estrogen replacement therapy. Biopsy should be done if doubt exists (Neilson, 1989; Young, 1996).

Thrombosis of the urethral vein presents as a bluish, swollen, tender lesion involving the posterior lip of the urinary meatus. It has the appearance of the thrombosed hemorrhoid. It usually subsides without treatment; however, persistence or pain will require excision to control symptoms.

▶ Treatment

Local excision is indicated only if symptoms are troublesome.

▶ Prognosis

True caruncle is usually cured by excision, but in a few instances, it does recur.

▶ Prolapse of the Urethra

Prolapse of the female urethra is not common. It usually occurs only in children or in paraplegics suffering from a lower motor neuron lesion. The protruding urethral mucosa presents as an angry red mass that may become gangrenous if it is not reduced promptly (Kleinjan, 1996). When a young girl has a protruding mass, urethral prolapse must be differentiated from prolapse of a ureterocele (Fernandes et al, 1993; Valerie et al, 1999).

After reduction, cystoscopy should be done to rule out ureterocele. Recurrences are rare following reduction; the accompanying inflammation probably "fixes" the tissue in place as healing progresses. If the prolapsed urethra cannot be reduced or if it recurs, an indwelling catheter should be inserted, traction placed on it, and a heavy piece of suture material tightly tied over the tissue and catheter just proximal to the mass. The tissue later sloughs off. Using this same technique, the tissue can be resected, preferably with an electrosurgical cautery (Devine, 1980).

URETHROVAGINAL FISTULA

Urethrovaginal fistulas may follow local injury secondary to fracture of the pelvis or obstetric or surgical injury. A common cause in the industrial world is accidental trauma to the urethra or its blood supply in the course of surgical repair of a cystocele or excision of urethral diverticula. In the developing world, obstructed and prolonged labor is the most common cause (Elkins, 1994). Other causes may include radiation therapy for pelvic malignancy, trauma/pelvic fracture, and vaginal neoplasms. Diagnosis can usually be made on physical examination and urethroscopy. Vaginal urethroplasty is indicated, and these surgeries may be very challenging due to poor quality local tissue; often, two or more procedures may be necessary (Webster et al, 1984). A Martius labial fat flap can be used as interposition layer to augment repair and prevent recurrence of fistula.

URETHRAL DIVERTICULUM

The incidence of diverticulation of the urethral wall is between 0.6% and 5% (Andersen, 1967; Davis and Robinson, 1970). Diverticula are at times multiple or lobulated. Most cases are probably secondary to obstetric urethral trauma or severe urethral infection. A few cases of carcinoma in such diverticula have been reported (Kato, 1998; Marshall, 1977; Nakamura et al, 1995). Urethral diverticula are usually associated with recurrent attacks of cystitis, irritative voiding symptoms, and urethral pain. A mnemonic is the three Ds: dribbling, dyspareunia, and dysuria. Purulent urethral discharge is sometimes noted as the infected diverticulum empties. On occasion, the diverticulum may be large enough to be discovered by the patient.

The diagnosis is usually made on feeling a rounded cystic mass in the anterior wall of the vagina that leaks pus from the urethral orifice when pressure is applied. Urethroscopy may reveal the urethral opening, although the openings are often very difficult to locate. The postvoiding film of an excretory urographic series may demonstrate the lesion. It may be possible to introduce a small catheter through which radiopaque fluid can be instilled. Appropriate x-ray films are then exposed (Figure 42–2). The plain film may show a stone in the diverticulum (Presman, 1964). If these methods fail, the following procedures can be used:

1. Empty the diverticulum manually. Via a catheter, instill 5 mL of indigo carmine and 60 mL of contrast medium into the bladder. Remove the catheter and have the patient begin to void. Occlude the meatus with a finger. This maneuver usually causes the diverticulum to fill with the test solution. Take appropriate x-rays, and perform urethroscopy to look for leakage of blue dye from the mouth of the diverticulum.

2. Insert a Davis-TeLinde catheter (aka double balloon catheter). This looks like a Foley catheter but is surrounded by a second movable balloon. Pass the catheter to the bladder and inflate the proximal balloon. While exerting tension on the catheter, slide the second balloon against the urinary meatus and inflate it. Then inject contrast medium into the catheter. The radiopaque fluid will exit from the catheter through a hole between the balloons and will fill the urethra and diverticulum, after which x-rays can be exposed. Occasionally, urethral diverticulum is elusive and difficult to visualize. Transvaginal ultrasonography (Baert, 1992; Mouritsent, 1996; Siegel et al, 1998; Vargas-Serrano et al, 1997) or pelvic magnetic resonance imaging

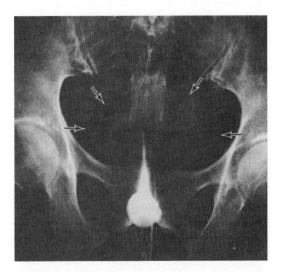 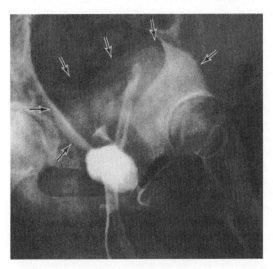

▲ **Figure 42–2.** Urethral diverticulum containing stone. **Left:** Plain film showing stone. *Arrows* outline bladder. **Right:** Diverticulum filled with radiopaque fluid instilled through ureteral catheter. Bladder outlined by *arrows*.

(MRI) (Chaudhari, 2010; Debaere et al, 1995; Kim, 1993) can be helpful in diagnosis; MRI is reported to be much more sensitive in detecting diverticulae than double-balloon urethrography (Neitlich et al, 1998), especially when an endoluminal coil is placed in the vagina to enhance the periurethral imaging (Dwarkasing, 2011). MRI is useful to assess urethral diverticula but there are limitations. A study by Chung et al (2010) revealed 24% discrepancy between MRI and surgical findings. Examples include misdiagnosis of the diverticulum as Bartholin's cyst, a sterile abscess incorrectly diagnosed as a diverticulum, and missed detection of cancer within the diverticulum.

Treatment consists of removal of the sac through an incision in the anterior vaginal wall and care being taken not to injure the urethral sphincteric musculature. Incision is carried down to the diverticular mucosa, and the plane of cleavage is followed all around to the neck of the diverticulum. The diverticular sac is completely excised and the defect in the urethra repaired. A suprapubic cystostomy or urethral catheter should be left in place for 2–3 weeks following surgical excision of the diverticulum.

The outcome is usually good unless the diverticulum is so situated that its excision injures the external urinary sphincter mechanism. In a few cases, urethrovaginal fistula may develop. If the fistula does not close with adequate drainage, surgical repair will be necessary 2–3 months later.

URETHRAL STRICTURE

True organic stricture of the adult female urethra is not common. (Functional urethral obstruction is more common, due to pelvic floor dysfunction.) It may be congenital or acquired. The trauma of intercourse and especially of childbirth may lead to periurethral fibrosis with contracture, or the stricture may be caused by the surgeon during vaginal repair. It may develop secondary to acute or chronic urethritis.

Persistent hesitancy in initiating urination and a slow urinary stream are the principal symptoms of stricture. Burning, frequency, nocturia, and urethral pain may occur from secondary urethritis or cystitis. If secondary infection of the bladder is present, pus and bacteria will be found in the urine. A fairly large catheter (22F) may pass to the bladder only with difficulty. Urethroscopy may demonstrate the point of narrowness and disclose evidence of urethritis. Cystoscopy often reveals trabeculation (hypertrophy) of the bladder wall.

Chronic cystitis may cause similar symptoms, but urinalysis reveals evidence of infection. Cancer of the urethra causes progressive narrowing of the urethra, but induration and infiltration of the urethra are found on vaginal examination. Panendoscopy with biopsy establishes the diagnosis. Bladder tumor involving the bladder neck causes hesitancy and impairment of the urinary stream. Cystoscopy and biopsy is definitive. Chronic urethritis commonly accompanies urethral stenosis; either may be primary. Recurrent or chronic cystitis is often secondary to stenosis.

Treatment consists of gradual urethral dilatation (up to 36F) at weekly intervals. Slight overstretching is necessary, since some contracture will occur after therapy is discontinued. Measures to combat urethritis and cystitis also must be employed. Internal urethrotomy has its proponents (Essenhigh, 1968). With proper overdilatation of the urethra and specific therapy of the urethritis that is usually present, the prognosis is good. Formal urethroplasty can be performed with high success rates in cases that do not respond to urethral dilations (Onol, 2011).

BIBLIOGRAPHY

Distal Urethral Stenosis

Immergut MA, Gilbert EC: Internal urethrotomy in recurring urinary infections in girls. J Urol 1973;109:126.

Kaplan GW et al: A blind comparison of dilatation, urethrotomy and medication alone in the treatment of urinary tract infection in girls. J Urol 1973;109:917.

Kondo A et al: Functional obstruction of the female urethra: Relevance to refractory bed wetting and recurrent urinary tract infection. Neurourol Urodyn 1994;13(5):541–546.

Lyon RP, Marshall S: Urinary tract infections and difficult urination in girls: Long-term follow-up. J Urol 1971;105:314.

Smith DR: Critique on the concept of vesical neck obstruction in children. JAMA 1969;207:1686.

Tanagho EA et al: Spastic external sphincter and urinary tract infection in girls. Br J Urol 1971;43:69.

Labial Fusion (Synechia Vulvae)

Adekunle AO et al: Female genital mutilation—Postcircumcision vulval complications in Nigerians. J Obstet Gynaecol 1999;19:632.

Aribarg A: Topical oestrogen therapy for labial adhesions in children. Br J Obstet Gynaecol 1975;82:424.

Christensen EH, Oster J: Adhesions of labia minora (synechia vulvae) in childhood: A review and report of fourteen cases. Acta Paediatr Scand 1971;60:709.

Kumar RK et al: Labial adhesions in pubertal girls. Arch Gynecol Obstet 2006;273:243.

Leung AK et al: Treatment of labial fusion with topical estrogen therapy. Clin Pediatr (Phila) 2005;44:245.

Acute Urethritis

Bass HN: "Bubble bath" as an irritant to the urinary tract of children. Clin Pediatr 1968;7:174.

Marshall S: The effect of bubble bath on the urinary tract. J Urol 1965; 93:112.

Simms I, Stephenson JM: Pelvic inflammatory disease epidemiology: What do we know and what do we need to know? Sex Transm Infect 2000;76:80.

Chronic Urethritis

Bruce AW et al: Recurrent urethritis in women. Can Med Assoc J 1973;108:973.

Farrar DJ et al: An evaluation of Otis urethrotomy in female patients with recurrent urinary tract infections: A review after 6 years. Br J Urol 1980;52:68.

Krieger JN et al: Evaluation of chronic urethritis: Defining the role for endoscopic procedures. Arch Intern Med 1988;148:703.

Marshall S et al: Nonspecific urethritis in females. Calif Med 1970; 112:9.

Simpson T et al: Vaginal douching among adolescent and young women: More challenges than progress. J Pediatr Adolesc Gynecol 2004;17:249.

Atrophic Urethritis

Johnston SL et al: The detection and management of vaginal atrophy. J Obstet Gynaecol Can 2004;26:503.

Quinlivan LG: The treatment of senile vaginitis with low doses of synthetic estrogens. Am J Obstet Gynecol 1965;92:172.

Raz R, Stamm WE: A controlled trial of intravaginal estriol in post-menopausal women with recurrent urinary tract infections. N Engl J Med 1993;329:753.

Smith P: Age changes in the female urethra. Br J Urol 1972;44:667.

Sturdee DW, Panay N: Recommendations for the management of postmenopausal vaginal atrophy. Climacteric 2010;13:509.

Urethral Caruncle

Lee WH et al: The aetiology of postmenopausal bleeding—A study of 163 consecutive cases in Singapore. Singapore Med J 1995;36:164.

Neilson D et al: Squamous intra-epithelial neoplasia presenting as a urethral caruncle. Br J Urol 1989;64:200.

Young RH et al: Urethral caruncle with atypical stromal cells simulating lymphoma or sarcoma—A distinctive pseudoneoplastic lesion of females. A report of six cases. Am J Surg Pathol 1996;20:1190.

Prolapse of the Urethra

Devine PC, Kessel HC: Surgical correction of urethral prolapse. J Urol 1980;123:856.

Fernandes ET et al: Urethral prolapse in children. Urology 1993; 41:240.

Kleinjan JH, Vos P: Strangulated urethral prolapse. Urology 1996; 47:599.

Valerie E et al: Diagnosis and treatment of urethral prolapse in children. Urology 1999;54:1082.

Urethrovaginal Fistula

Creatsas G et al: Reconstruction of urethrovaginal fistula and vaginal atresia in an adolescent girl after an abdominoperineal-vaginal pull-through procedure. Fertil Steril 1997;68:556.

Elkins TE: Surgery for the obstetric vesicovaginal fistula: A review of 100 operations in 82 patients. Am J Obstet Gynecol 1994;170:1108.

Webster GD et al: Urethrovaginal fistula: A review of the surgical management. J Urol 1984;132:460.

Urethral Diverticulum

Andersen MJ: The incidence of diverticula in the female urethra. J Urol 1967;98:96.

Baert L et al: Endovaginal sonography: New diagnostic approach for urethral diverticula. J Urol 1992;147:464.

Chaudhari VV et al: MR imaging and US of female urethral and peri-urethral disease. Radiographics 2010;30:1857.

Chung DE et al: Urethral diverticula in women: Discrepancies between magnetic resonance imaging and surgical findings. J Urol 2010;183:2265.

Davis BL, Robinson DG: Diverticula of the female urethra: Assay of 120 cases. J Urol 1970;104:850.

Debaere C et al: MR imaging of a diverticulum in a female urethra. J Belge Radiol 1995;78:345.

Dwarkasing RS et al: MRI evaluation of urethral diverticula and differential diagnosis in symptomatic women. AJR Am J Roentgenol 2011;197:676.

Elik M: Diverticulum of the female urethra: A new method of ablation. J Urol 1957;77:243.

Kato H et al: Carcinoembryonic antigen positive adenocarcinoma of a female urethral diverticulum: Case report and review of the literature. Int J Urol 1998;5:291.

Kim B et al: Diagnosis of urethral diverticula in women: Value of MR imaging. AJR Am J Roentgenol 1993;161:809.

Marshall S, Hirsch K: Carcinoma within urethral diverticula. Urology 1977;10:161.

Mouritsen L, Bernstein I: Vaginal ultrasonography: A diagnostic tool for urethral diverticulum. Acta Obstet Gynecol Scand 1996;75:188.

Nakamura Y et al: A case of adenocarcinoma arising within a urethral diverticulum diagnosed only by the surgical specimen. Gynecol Obstet Invest 1995;40:69.

Neitlich JD et al: Detection of urethral diverticula in women: Comparison of a high resolution fast spin echo technique with double balloon urethrography. J Urol 1998;159:408.

Presman D et al: Calculus formation within a diverticulum of the female urethra. J Urol 1964;91:376.

Siegel CL et al: Sonography of the female urethra. AJR Am J Roentgenol 1998;170:1269.

Vargas-Serrano B et al: Transrectal ultrasonography in the diagnosis of urethral diverticula in women. J Clin Ultrasound 1997;25:21.

Urethral Stricture

Essenhigh DM et al: A study of the bladder outlet in lower urinary tract infections in women. Br J Urol 1968;40:268.

Onol FF et al: Techniques and results of urethroplasty for female urethral strictures: Our experience with 17 patients. Urology 2011;77:1318.

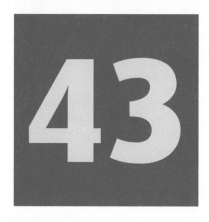

43

Disorders of Sex Development

Laurence S. Baskin, MD

What defines our sexuality is a complex interaction between our genetic makeup, environmental stimulus, and cultural influences. The origins of our sexuality occur at the time of conception when the genetic material from two sources of the opposite sex coalesces into a new individual. From that moment, sexual differentiation occurs by a highly organized process. Sex chromosomes and autosomes dictate the development of gonads; the gonads in turn produce hormones, which then direct the development of the internal and external genitalia. Disorders of sex development (DSD) or differentiation arise from abnormalities in chromosomes, gonadal development, or hormonal production/activity.

Patients with DSD become apparent (1) during the newborn period as having ambiguous genitalia or a discordant phenotypic from the genotype found at the time of amniocentesis, (2) as having inappropriate pubertal development, (3) as having delayed pubertal development, or (4) later in life as having infertility.

NORMAL SEXUAL DIFFERENTIATION

▶ Chromosomal Sex

The genetic material necessary for the development of the male phenotype is normally located on the short arm of the Y chromosome (Wilson et al, 1981). The critical gene or sex-determining region on the Y chromosome is known as the SRY region. The gene products of the SRY genetic cascade direct the development of the testis by interacting with multiple other genes such as *SOX-9* (Conte and Grumbach, 2007). Genetic information that is known to be necessary for male and female development beyond gonadal differentiation is located on the X chromosome and on the autosomes.

▶ Gonadal Differentiation

The gonads develop from the urogenital ridges (Figure 43–1), which are formed during the 4th week of gestation by the

proliferation of the coelomic epithelium and condensation of the underlying mesenchyme along the mesonephros. The germ cells, located in the endoderm of the yolk sac, migrate to the genital ridges. At the early stage of development, the gonad is bipotential, capable of forming into either a testis or an ovary. During the 6th–7th week of gestation, at least four different genes, Wilms' tumor suppressor gene (*WT-1*), Fushi-Tarza Factor-1 (*FTZ-F1*), steroidogenic Factor-1 (*SF-1*), and *LIM-1*, induce the development of the testis. The primordial germ cells differentiate into the Sertoli cells and associated Leydig cells, which aggregate into spermatogenic cords. Loose mesenchymal tissue condenses into a thick layer, the tunica albuginea, which surrounds the testis and separates its connection with the coelomic epithelium, thereby preventing further migration of mesonephric cells into the testis.

Classic teaching is that the female phenotype is the default developmental pathway in the absence of the SRY cascade. It is now known that at least one gene, dosage-sensitive sex reversal (*DAX-1*), is essential for ovarian development. *DAX-1* is located on the short arm of the X chromosome. The gene products of SRY and *DAX-1* compete to stimulate the steroidogenic acute regulatory protein (StAR). The StAR protein is the first step in steroidogenesis, facilitating the conversion of cholesterol to pregnenolone. In the normal XY male, SRY overwhelms the one functional *DAX-1* gene, stimulating testicular development and subsequent testosterone production. In the normal XX female, two *DAX-1* genes are present without the competitive SRY, downregulating StAR, hence inhibiting testicular development, which results in ovarian development. In the fetal ovaries, the germ cells differentiate and are arrested in the last phase of meiotic prophase, forming the oocytes. The cells in the genital ridges develop into granulosa cells, which surround the oocytes and complete the formation of the ovaries.

▶ Hormones

At 3.5 weeks' gestation, the Wolffian system appears as two longitudinal ducts connecting cranially to the mesonephros

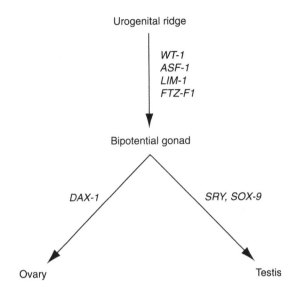

Urogenital ridge

WT-1
ASF-1
LIM-1
FTZ-F1

Bipotential gonad

DAX-1   SRY, SOX-9

Ovary   Testis

▲ **Figure 43–1.** Sex-determining genes involved in testes and ovarian development.

and caudally draining into the urogenital sinus (Figure 43–2). At approximately the 6th week of gestation, the Müllerian duct develops as an evagination in the coelomic epithelium just lateral to the Wolffian duct.

During the 8th–9th week of gestation, Sertoli cells of the fetal testis secrete a glycoprotein, Müllerian-inhibiting substance (MIS), or anti-Müllerian hormone. This protein induces the regression of the Müllerian ducts through the dissolution of the basement membrane and condensation of mesenchymal cells around the Müllerian duct. Because MIS acts locally, Müllerian duct regression occurs only on the ipsilateral side of the fetal testis producing this hormone. MIS also induces the formation of seminiferous tubules and further differentiation of the testis. At the 9th or 10th week of gestation, the Leydig cells appear in the testis and begin to synthesize testosterone. This hormone transforms the Wolffian duct into the male genital tract, which is completed by the end of the 11th week of gestation.

Beginning in the 9th week of gestation, testosterone also induces the development of the external genitalia (Figure 43–3) from the genital tubercle, urogenital sinus, and genital swellings (Jirasek et al, 1968). At the molecular level, testosterone is converted to 5α-dihydrotestosterone (DHT) by the microsomal enzyme, type 2 5α-reductase, for complete differentiation of the penis with a male-type urethra and glans (Wilson et al, 1993). Testosterone dissociates from its carrier proteins in the plasma and enters cells via passive diffusion. Once in the cell, testosterone binds to the androgen receptor (AR) and induces changes in conformation, protecting it from degradation by proteolytic enzymes. This conformational change is also required for AR dimerization, DNA binding, and transcriptional activation, all necessary for testosterone to be expressed. Androgen binding also displaces heat shock proteins, possibly relieving constraints on receptor dimerization or DNA binding. After entering the nucleus, the AR complex then binds androgen response element DNA regulatory sequences within the androgen responsive genes and activates them. DHT also binds the AR, with enhanced androgenic activity, in part because of its slow dissociation rate from the AR.

DHT then binds to nuclear receptors, forming a complex that regulates the transformation of these tissues into the glans penis, penile and cavernous urethra, Cowper's glands, prostate, and scrotum. Between the 28th and 37th week of gestation, testicular descent into the scrotum begins. While the mechanism of this process is not completely understood, it is clearly androgen dependent.

▶ Development of the Female Genitalia

The female internal genitalia develop from the Müllerian ducts. Without the hormones produced by the testis, the Wolffian ducts regress at the 9th week of gestation. At the same time, the Müllerian ducts begin to differentiate; the cranial portions form the fallopian tubes, while the caudal portions fuse to form the uterus, cervix, and the upper portion of the vagina. Concurrently, the external genitalia defined as the lower portion of the vagina, the vestibule, Bartholin and Skene glands, the clitoris, and labia minora and majora develop from the urogenital sinus and genital tubercles. Like the testis, the ovary undergoes a partial transabdominal descent. However, transinguinal descent of the ovary does not occur, leaving the ovaries just below the rim of the true pelvis. The role of estrogen in the differentiation of the female phenotype is unclear.

▶ Development of the Male External Genitalia

Formation of the external male genitalia is a complex developmental process involving the SRY genetic programming, cell differentiation, hormonal signaling, enzyme activity, and tissue remodeling. By the end of the 1st month of gestation, the hindgut and future urogenital system reach the ventral surface of the embryo at the cloacal membrane. The urorectal septum divides the cloacal membrane into a posterior, or anal, half and an anterior half, the urogenital membrane. Three protuberances appear around the latter. The most cephalad is the genital tubercle. The other two, the genital swellings, flank the urogenital membrane on each side. Up to this point, the male and female genitalia are essentially indistinguishable. Under the influence of testosterone in response to a surge of luteinizing hormone from

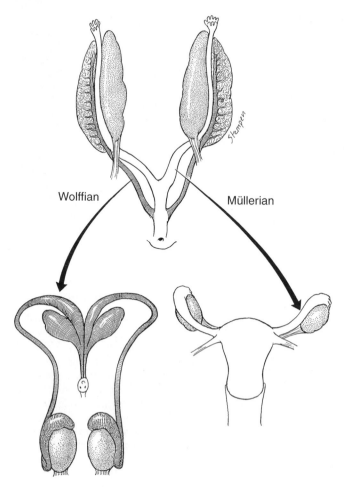

▲ **Figure 43–2.** Schematic of male (Wolffian) and female (Müllerian) internal and external genital development from common origin.

the pituitary, masculinization of the external genitalia takes place. One of the first signs of masculinization is an increase in the distance between the anus and the genital structures, followed by elongation of the phallus, formation of the penile urethra from the urethral groove, and development of the prepuce.

At 8 weeks' gestation, the external genitalia remain in the indifferent stage. The urethral groove on the ventral surface of the phallus is between the paired urethral folds. The penile urethra forms as a result of fusion of the medial edges of the endodermal urethral folds. As development progresses, the ectodermal edges of the urethral groove begin to fuse to form the median raphe (Figure 43–4A). By 11–12 weeks, the coronal sulcus separates the glans from the shaft of the penis. By 16 weeks' gestation, the urethral folds have completely fused in the midline on the ventrum of the penile shaft (Figure

43–4B). Note the normal ventral penile curvature, or chordee, that occurs during development and resolves by the 20th week (Figure 43–4C).

The glandular urethra, which consists of a squamous epithelial-lined tube different from the urothelial-lined anterior urethra, also completes its formation during this period. The mechanism of the glandular urethral formation remains controversial. Evidence suggests two possible explanations (Figure 43–5): (1) endodermal cellular differentiation where the glandular urethra forms by an extension of urogenital sinus epithelium that undergoes transdifferentiation versus (Kurzrock et al, 1999) (2) primary intrusion of the ectodermal tissue from the skin of the glans penis. Cross-sectional histologic analysis at 24 weeks' gestation reveals complete penile development (Figures 43–6A–H). Note the extensive neuronal innervation just above the tunica of the

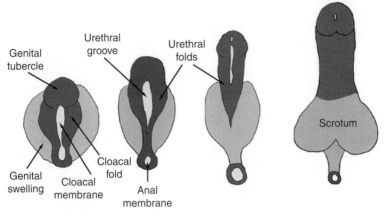

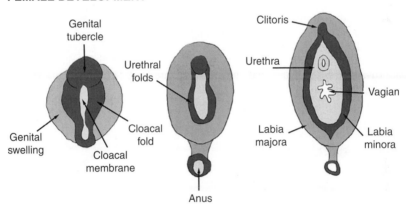

▲ **Figure 43–3.** Differentiation of the male and female external genitalia from the indifferent stage to full differentiation (8–16 weeks). (Illustrations by Dr Hiep Nguyen.)

corporeal bodies. Three-dimensional reconstruction of the fetal male penis illustrates the extensive neuronal distribution (Figure 43–7). Note the nerve density in the glans (Figures 43–7E and F).

Anatomical and immunohistochemical studies advocate the new theory of endodermal differentiation, which shows that epithelium of the entire urethra is of urogenital sinus origin. The entire male urethra, including the glandular urethra, is formed by dorsal growth of the urethral plate into the genital tubercle and ventral growth and fusion of the urethral folds. Under proper mesenchymal induction, urothelium has the ability to differentiate into a stratified squamous phenotype with characteristic keratin staining, thereby explaining the cell type of the glans penis.

The future prepuce is forming at the same time as the urethra and is dependent on normal urethral development. At about 8 weeks' gestation, low preputial folds appear on both sides of the penile shaft, which join dorsally to form a flat ridge at the proximal edge of the corona. The ridge does not entirely encircle the glans because it is blocked on the ventrum by incomplete development of the glandular urethra. Thus, the preputial fold is transported distally by active growth of the mesenchyme between it and the glandular lamella. The process continues until the preputial fold (foreskin), covers all of the glans, forming a midline seam (Figure 43–4D). The fusion is usually present at birth, but subsequent desquamation of the epithelial fusion allows the prepuce to retract. If the genital folds fail to fuse, the preputial tissues do not form ventrally; consequently, in

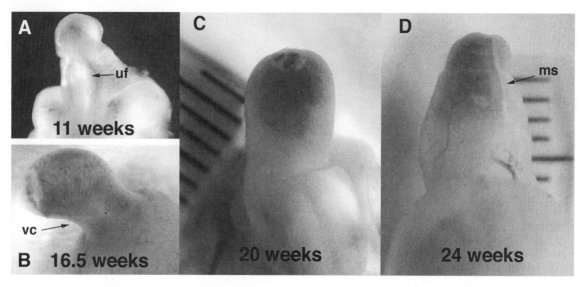

▲ **Figure 43–4.** Male human fetal external genitalia during gestation. **A:** 11 weeks. Note the urethra is open and urethral fold (uf) and groove are prominent in the transillumination view of the phallus. **B:** 16.5 weeks. Note the normal ventral curvature (vc) as well as the foreskin, which is almost completely formed. **C:** At 20 weeks' gestation, penile and urethral development looks complete, with the prepuce covering the glans and the penile curvature resolving. **D:** At 24 weeks, the prepuce covers the whole glans. Note the midline seam (ms). Note the progression of natural curvature to a straight phallus during development.

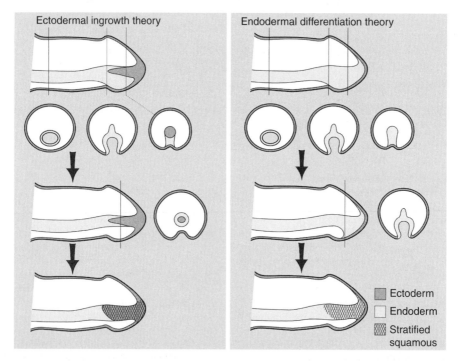

▲ **Figure 43–5.** Theories of human penile urethral development. The ectodermal ingrowth theory as described in most textbooks of embryology postulates that the glanular urethra is formed by ingrowth of epidermis. More recent data support the formation of the entire urethra via endodermal differentiation alone.

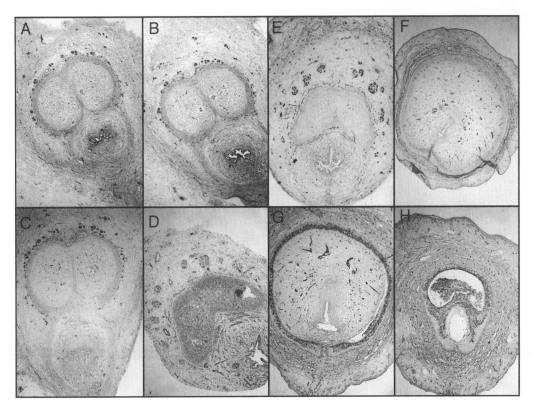

▲ **Figure 43–6.** Normal human fetal penis, 24 weeks **(A–H)**. Transverse histologic sections show immunohistochemical localization with the neuronal marker S-100 (25×). Note localization of S-100 nerve marker (dark staining) completely surrounding the cavernous bodies up to the junction with the urethral spongiosum along the penile shaft except at the 12 o'clock position **(A–D)**. On the proximal penis at the point where the corporeal bodies split into two **(E)** and continue in a lateral fashion inferior and adjacent to the pubic rami, the nerves localize to an imaginary triangular area at the 11 o'clock and 1 o'clock positions. At this point **(E)**, the nerves reach their furthest vertical distance from the corporeal body (approximately one-half the diameter of the corporeal body) and continue **(F–G)** in a tighter formation at the 11 o'clock and 1 o'clock positions well away from the urethra.

hypospadias, preputial tissue is absent on the ventrum, and excessive dorsally.

▷ Disorders of Sexual Differentiation

Disorders of abnormal sexual differentiation may be divided into the following three categories.

A. Disorders of Chromosomal Sex

These result from abnormalities in the number or structure of the sex chromosomes. These abnormalities may arise from nondisjunction, deletion, breakage, rearrangement, or translocation of genetic material on these chromosomes. These disorders are summarized in Table 43–1.

B. Disorders of Gonadal Sex

These result from abnormalities in gonadal development. In these disorders, the karyotype is normal (ie, 46,XX or 46,XY). However, mutations in the sex chromosomes or autosomes, teratogens, or trauma to the gonads interfere with their normal development. These disorders are summarized in Table 43–2.

C. Disorders of Phenotypic Sex

These result from abnormalities in hormonal production or activity. The etiologies include defective synthesis by the gonads, abnormal production by the adrenal glands, the presence of exogenous sources, or abnormalities in receptor activity. These disorders are summarized in Table 43–3.

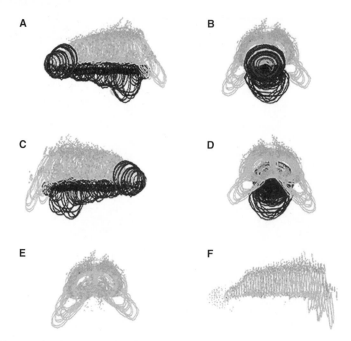

▲ **Figure 43–7.** Normal human fetal penis, 45 weeks' gestation. Four views of a computer-generated three-dimensional reconstruction (**A**, side; **B**, front; **C**, side; **D**, back, **E**, front [without urethra]; **F**, side [without urethra]). Note the nerves along the outside of the tunica of the corporeal bodies and their absence at the 12 o'clock position. Note the impressive glandular innervation in **E** and **F**.

CLINICAL EVALUATION OF PATIENTS WITH AMBIGUOUS GENITALIA

The accurate diagnosis of a patient with ambiguous genitalia is a challenging process. Based on the diagnosis, decisions will be made for gender assignment, which will have a great impact not only on the patient but also on the patient's family (Daaboul and Frader, 2001; Morland, 2001; Conte and Grumbach, 2007). In most societies, the accepted norm is two sexes, either male or female. When a new baby arrives and the proclamation as to whether it is a boy or a girl cannot be made immediately, an anticipated celebration turns into a stressful family dilemma. With prenatal amniocentesis and routine ultrasound, sex determination is often known well before birth. This can compound the emotional trauma when the known and anticipated genotype does not match the newborn's phenotype. Furthermore, in cases such as severe salt-wasting congenital adrenal hyperplasia (CAH), accurate diagnosis is lifesaving.

▶ History

A detailed history is of great importance. Since many of the disorders such as XX male syndrome and true hermaphrodites are hereditary, a family history should carefully be examined for similarly affected individuals, unexplained death during infancy, infertility, amenorrhea, and hirsutism. Furthermore, drugs ingested during pregnancy (such as progesterone) and virilizing signs in the mother during pregnancy should be ascertained.

▶ Physical Examination

The abdomen and rectum should be carefully palpated for midline structures such as a uterus. These examinations will provide information regarding the presence of Müllerian duct derivatives. Other helpful physical findings include dehydration, failure to thrive, pigmentation (in patients with salt-wasting CAH), and the presence of other associated anomalies such as cardiac murmurs or web neck (in patients with Turner's or Klinefelter syndrome).

It is important to palpate for gonads in the labioscrotal fold or the scrotum. Since ovaries do not descend, it is likely to be a testis and hence unlikely to represent a case of 46,XX DSD (female pseudohermaphroditism). Based on the presence or absence of gonads, an algorithm can be followed to determine the differential diagnosis of patients with ambiguous genitalia (Figure 43–8). It is important to look at the

Table 43–1. Disorders of chromosomal sex.

Disorder	Pathology	Chromosomes	Incidence	Gonads	Internal genitalia	External genitalia	Other features	Risk of cancer	Treatment
47,XXY (Klinefelter syndrome)	Extra X chromosome	47,XXY 46,XY/47,XXY	1 in 500	Hyalinized testis No spermatogenesis	Wolffian	Male	Gynecomastia Tall stature Mild mental retardation Elevated FSH/LH Low testosterone Elevated estradiol Infertility	Breast Extragonadal germ cell	Supplemental androgens Surgery for severe gynecomastia
XX male (XX sex reversal)	No Y chromosome Usually TDF (+)	46,XX	1 in 20,000–24,000	Hyalinized testis No spermatogenesis	Wolffian	Male	Gynecomastia Short stature Inc. incidence of hypospadias Normal mental status May be familial	Rare germ cell	Same as Klinefelter
45,X (Turner's syndrome)	Absence of X chromosome	45,X 46,XX/45,X Some contain Y chrom. elements	1 in 2700	Streak gonads No germ cells	Müllerian	Immature female	Short stature Little breast development Web neck and other somatic abn. Cardiovascular abn. (ie, coarctation) Renal abn. (Horseshoe or malrotation) Autoimmune dz. (hypothyroid, diabetes) Infertility Amenorrhea	Germ cell Y-chrom mosaic	Supplemental estrogen Removal of streak gonads in Y-chrom. mosaic
45,X/46,XY DSD (Mixed gonadal dysgenesis)	Incompl. virilization & Müllerian regression	45,X/46,XY (70%) Undetected mosaic		One testis (usually undescended) and streak gonad	Wolffian and Müllerian	Usually ambiguous 60% reared as female	Somatic features like 45,X	Germ cell	Female —Prophylactic gonadectomy Male —Streak gonads removed —Intra-abd. testis excised unless can be relocated and no ipsilateral Müllerian structure present
Ovotesticular DSD (True hermaphrodite)	Unknown	46,XX (70%) 46,XY (10%) Mosaic	Unknown	Bilateral ovotestis Ovotestis & ovary or testis (40%) One ovary & testis (40%)	Wolffian and Müllerian	Usually ambiguous 70% reared as male	Gynecomastia at puberty Menstruation at puberty May be familial	Rare germ cell	Reconstructive surgery Poss. remove gonads

Table 43–2. Disorders of gonadal sex.

Disorder	Pathology	Chromosomes	Incidence	Gonads	Internal genitalia	External genitalia	Other features	Risk of cancer	Treatment
Complete gonadal dysgenesis (Swyer Syndrome)	Unknown mutation prevents nl. differentiation of gonads	46,XX 46,XY	1 in 8000	Bilateral streak gonads	Müllerian	Immature female	Normal to tall stature Minimal somatic abn. Female: estrogen def. Male: testosterone def. May be familial	Germ cell in 46,XY	Estrogen supplement Remove gonads in 46,XY
Absent testes syndrome	Mutation, teratogen or trauma to testis	46,XY	Unknown	Absent/ rudiment testis No streak gonads	Wolffian	Var. virilization	Normal	Usually none	Female —Estrogen supplement —Reconstructive surgery Male —Androgen supplement

size of phallus (Table 43–4) and the location of the urethral meatus (Camurdan et al, 2007). Any patients with bilateral cryptorchidism or with unilateral cryptorchidism with hypospadias should be suspected of having abnormalities in sexual differentiation. As noted, other helpful physical findings include hyperpigmentation of the areola and labioscrotal fold, common in patients with CAH.

Chromosomal Evaluation

Examination of buccal mucosal cells for Barr body (inactivated second X chromosome) cannot be relied on to make an accurate diagnosis in patients with ambiguous genitalia.

A more accurate but more time-consuming method (2–3 days) is the direct assessment of chromosomes from cultured peripheral blood leukocytes. This method provides the exact chromosomal complements, the presence of mosaicism, and structural features of the chromosomes.

In the case of mosaicism, several different tissue samples may be required to accurately confirm the genotype.

Biochemical Evaluation

In the case of CAH, the specific enzyme defect can be determined based on the presence or absence and the type of steroid excreted in the urine. Figure 43–9 depicts the steroid synthesis pathway from cholesterol to aldosterone, steroids, or DHT. Note the enzymes necessary for conversion from precursors to products (also see Table 43–3).

In other disorders caused by hormonal abnormalities (such as 5α-reductase deficiency and androgen resistance), direct measurement of plasma testosterone is often not helpful, since abnormalities in testosterone levels in these pathologic states have not been consistently characterized. A more useful test is the testosterone response following stimulation by human chorionic gonadotropin (hCG) (2000 IU/day for 4 days). If plasma testosterone levels rise >2 ng/mL from baseline, the abnormality is consistent with androgen resistance rather than a defect in testosterone synthesis. In addition, this test is also used to diagnose 5α-reductase type 2 deficiency. A post-hCG stimulation ratio of testosterone to DHT >30 establishes this diagnosis.

Radiographic Evaluation

In patients with intersex disorders, ultrasonography provides the least invasive and safest means of imaging the abdomen and pelvis. Identification of Müllerian-derived structures such as the uterus and fallopian tubes will be important in determining the diagnosis (Figure 43–10A). The adrenal glands can also be examined for enlargement. While this finding is not diagnostic for CAH, it is suggestive and can direct further evaluation. Magnetic resonance imaging can provide a more detailed examination of the abdomen for internal genital structures. However, in most cases, anesthesia is needed for a good-quality magnetic resonance imaging examination. Injecting radiographic contrast material through the opening in the urogenital sinus is helpful in delineating the internal duct structures. It is most useful in assessing the presence of vagina, cervix, fallopian tube, utricle, and the connection with the urethra (Figures 43–10B and C). Genitography will also provide needed anatomical information for future reconstructive surgery.

Diagnostic Laparotomy or Laparoscopy

Occasionally, surgery is needed to delineate the internal genitalia and obtain a biopsy specimen of the gonads. It is indicated in patients in whom the biopsy result will influence sex assignment. In addition, surgery may be needed to remove streak or dysgenetic gonads in patients who are at risk for cancer (incomplete testicular feminization, Turner's

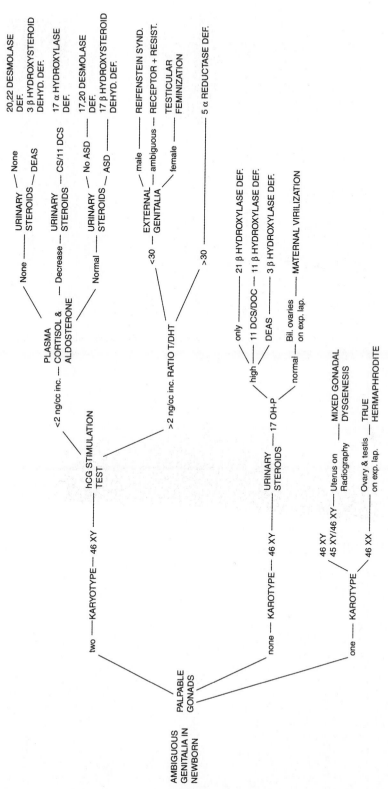

▲ **Figure 43–8.** Clinical approach to intersex. Algorithm based on palpating gonads. Bil., bilateral; CS/11 DCS, corticosterone/deoxycortisol; DEAS, 1,3-bis[4-(diethylamino)-2-hydroxy phenyl]-2,4-dihydroxycyclobutenediylium dihydroxide, bis(inner salt); DCS/DOC, deoxycortisol costerone; def., deficiency; dehyd., dehydration; 17 OH-P, 17 hydroxy progesterone; exp. lap., exploratory laparoscopy; resist., resistance; synd., syndrome; T/DHT, testosterone/dihydrotestosterone.

Table 43–3. Disorders of phenotypic sex.

Disorder	Pathology	Chromosomes	Incidence	Gonads	Internal genitalia	External genitalia	Other features	Urinary steroids	Risk of cancer	Treatment
46,XX DSD (Female Pseudohermaphrodite)										
3 β-Hydroxysteroid dehydrogenase def.	Excess androgens	46,XX	Second most common of CAH	Ovary	Müllerian	Mild ambiguous	Severe salt wasting, No cortisol, No aldosterone	DEAS	None	Replacement mineralocorticoids and glucocorticoids, Reconstruction as needed
11 β-Hydroxy lase def.	Excess androgens	46,XX	Rare	Ovary	Müllerian	Ambiguous	Hypertension, Dec. cortisol, Dec. aldosterone	11 DCS, 11 DOC	None	Replacement glucocorticoids
21 α-Hydroxylase def. —Partial	Excess androgens	46,XX	1 in 5000–15,000	Ovary	Müllerian	Ambiguous	Normal cortisol, Inc. aldoster one	17 OH-P	None	Reconstruction as needed
—Severe	Excess androgens	46,XX		Ovary	Müllerian	Ambiguous	Severe salt wasting, Dec. cortisol, Dec. aldosterone	17 OH-P	None	Replacement mineralocorticoids and glucocorticoids, Reconstruction as needed
Excess maternal androgens	Excess androgens	46,XX		Ovary	Müllerian	Ambiguous	Drugs such as progestational agents, Virilizing ovarian, Adrenal tumors	None	None	None
46,XY DSD (Male Pseudohermaphrodite)										
20,22 Desmolase def.	Defect in testosterone synthesis	46,XY		Testis	Wolffian	Ambiguous	Severe salt wasting, No cortisol, No aldosterone	None	None	Replacement mineralocorticoids and glucocorticoids
3 β-Hydroxy steroid dehydrogenase def.	Defect in testosterone synthesis	46,XY	Second most common in CAH	Testis	Wolffian	Ambiguous	Severe salt wasting, No cortisol, No aldosterone	DEAS	None	Replacement mineralocorticoids and glucocorticoids, Reconstruction as needed

Disorder	Defect	Karyotype/Inheritance	Frequency	Gonad	Internal ducts	External genitalia	Clinical features	Associated		Treatment
17 α-Hydroxylase def.	Defect in testosterone synthesis	46,XY		Testis	Wolffian	Ambiguous	Hypokalemic alkalosis Hypertension Dec. cortisol Dec. aldosterone Gynecomastia	CS 11 DCS	None	Replacement glucocorticoids
17,20 Desmolase def.	Defect in testosterone synthesis	46,XY	Rare	Testis	Wolffian	Ambiguous	Normal cortisol and aldosterone		None	Supplemental testosterone
17 β-Hydroxysteroid dehydrogenase def.	Defect in testosterone synthesis	46,XY	Most common	Testis	Wolffian	Ambiguous	Virilization and puberty	ASD	None	Decision reared as female or male
5 α-Reductase def.	Defect in androgen action	46,XY —Autosomal rec.		Testis with spermatogenesis	Wolffian	Female	No gynecomastia Nl. testosterone Nl. virilization	None	None	None
Complete androgen Insensitivity syndrome	Androgen receptor defect	46,XY —X linked	1 in 20,000–64,000	Testis not fertile	Absent	Female reared as female	Inc. testosterone Inc. estrogen	None	Germ cells	Remove gonads after puberty Estrogen replacement
Partial androgen Insensitivity syndrome	Androgen receptor defect	46,XY —X linked rec.	1/10th of complete	Testis not fertile	Wolffian	Female Versus severe hypospadias	Inc. testosterone Inc. estrogen	None	Germ cells	Depends on sex of rearing
Infertile male syndrome	Androgen receptor defect	46,XY —? X linked rec.		Testis not fertile	Wolffian	Male	Infertility Nl. or inc. testosterone Nl. or inc. estrogen	None	None	None
Persistent Müllerian duct syndrome	Persistent Müllerian ducts	Unknown		Testis	Wolffian with rudimentary uterus and tubes	Male usually cryptorchid	Nl. testosterone Nl. estrogen	None	None	Orchiopexy Leave uterus and tubes

Table 43–4. Normal values for stretched penile length.

Age	Length (cm) (Mean ± SD)
Premature 30 wk	2.5 ± 0.4
Full-term newborn	3.5 ± 0.4
0–5 months	3.9 ± 0.8
6–12 months	4.3 ± 0.8
1–2 y	4.7 ± 0.8
2–3 y	5.1 ± 0.9
3–4 y	5.5 ± 0.9
5–6 y	6.0 ± 0.9
10–11 y	6.4 ± 1.1
Adult	12.4 ± 2.7

Y variant, and mixed gonadal dysgenesis). Laparoscopic surgery has provided an alternative to open surgery in patients with intersex disorders. It can be performed safely in newborns and only requires 1–3 3-mm incisions for placement of the laparoscopic ports. Simple surgical procedures such as hernia repair, orchidopexy, and resection of discordant organs can be readily performed laparoscopically. More complex procedures may require 5-mm ports and larger instruments.

▶ Sex Assignment

In the past, the baby born with ambiguous genitalia was considered incomplete until either a male or female sex was assigned. Unfortunately, a prompt but inappropriate assignment, although timely and comforting for family, physicians, nurses, and staff, can lead to more complex problems in the future. The issue of sexual determination remains complex. We reaffirm the teaching of our mentors by advocating an immediate and thorough attempt to make a definitive and accurate diagnosis. Fortunately, for most patients with ambiguous genitalia (ie, CAH), this can be accomplished. In patients where ambiguity remains after initial testing and the diagnosis cannot be made, or when the diagnosis is clear but sex assignment remains difficult, we would now advocate for a more cautious approach. Foremost, this would include a reversible or nonbinding sex assignment. Experience has shown that patients themselves may reassign their sex. For example, in cases of cloacal exstrophy or iatrogenic penile injuries, past treatment was based on the absence of an "adequate" phallic structure. These patients were converted from genetic males to females with surgical orchiectomy, removal of any excess male genitalia, vaginoplasty, and future hormonal treatment for breast development. Although surgical results can be anatomically successful, these women will not menstruate or have fertility potential, and their sexual function is not known. A number of these patients went through adolescence, have identified as females, and have not had major issues with their assigned discordant, genetic sexual

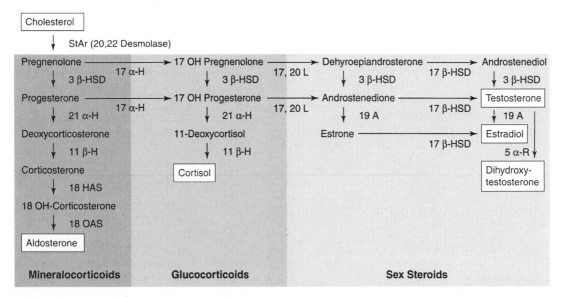

▲ **Figure 43–9.** Pathway of steroid hormone biosynthesis and possible enzyme deficiencies. 3β-HSD, 3β-hydroxysteroid dehydrogenase; 21α-H, 21α-hydroxylase; 11β-H, 11β hydroxylase; 17β-HSD, 17β-hydroxysteroid dehydrogenase; 18 HAS, 18 hydroxy-aldosterone synthetase; 18 OAS, 18 oxidase-aldosterone synthetase; 5α-R, 5α reductase; 19A, 19 aromatase; StAR, steroidogenic acute regulatory protein.

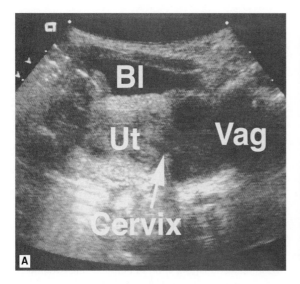

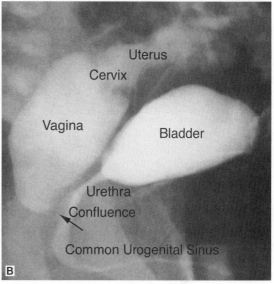

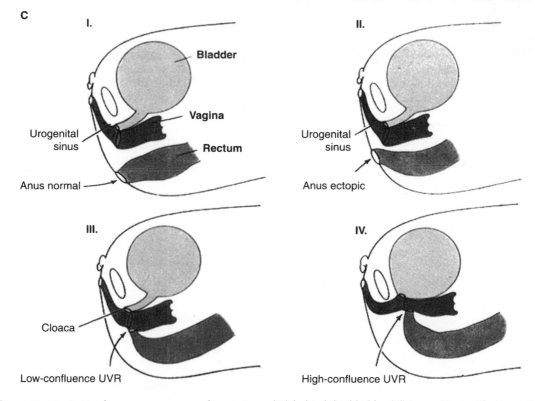

▲ **Figure 43-10.** **A:** Newborn sonogram revealing a uterus (Ut) behind the bladder (Bl) in a patient with congenital adrenal hyperplasia. Note the dilated vagina (Vag), the cervix (*arrow*), and the bladder. **B:** Genitogram showing a high confluence (*arrow*) of the urethra and vagina with a long common urogenital sinus in a patient with congenital adrenal hyperplasia. **C:** Schematic of possible genitogram findings: I. and II. Urogenital sinus anomalies with two openings on the perineum (common urogenital sinus and rectum). III. and IV. Cloacal anomalies with 1 perineal opening. Note the low and high confluence of the urethra, vagina, and rectum (UVR). (Modified with permission from Dr Hardy Hendron.) Genitogram showing the common urogenital sinus.

identity. In contrast, some of these patients have subsequently identified with their genetic sex and demanded or reassigned their sex from female to male. In cases where the genotype does not match the phenotype, it is clear that surgical reconstruction from male to female does not guarantee a successful sexual identity.

The clinical experience exemplifies the complexity of sexual determination. It is clear that social factors, or the "nurturing" hypothesis, and biologic factors, or the "genetic" hypothesis, both play a role in determining our sexual identity. The nurturing hypothesis is based on the parent's perception of their child's genitalia. This perception will influence interactions such as naming, clothes, play orientation, and social organization. Clearly, how a parent perceives his or her child and the type of environment used to raise the baby is critical to the child's identity.

In contrast, the genetic hypothesis states that sexual identity is predetermined by the genetic makeup. Increasing laboratory evidence is accumulating to support the genetic hypothesis. For example, animal experimentation supports the concept of steroid or androgen imprinting of the brain. The human evidence supporting masculinization of the brain is supported by (1) women with virilizing CAH, (2) iatrogenic penile ablation in males raised as females, and (3) males with 5α-reductase deficiency who were raised as females. The common theme in these patients is the high level of in utero exposure to androgens theoretically masculinizing the brain and conferring a male identity. Another example of hormonal influence on sexual orientation can be found in women exposed to diethylstilbestrol. Human retrospective studies looking at these women reveal an increase in bisexual and homosexual orientation.

The process of sexual identity in both humans and experimental animals is not an all-or-none process, meaning that male and female characteristics exist as a continuum. For example, although the "garbage removal, plumbing, and TV-channel-flipping gene" seems to exist almost exclusively on the Y chromosome, these traits may also be found in the female sex.

Two issues must be separated when evaluating patients with intersex or ambiguous genitalia: (1) gender identity (Is the person's sense of identity male or a female?) and (2) sexual orientation. The incidence of discordant gender identity is approximately 1 in 30,000 males and 1 in 100,000 females. The incidence of same-sex orientation in both males and females is estimated to be approximately 5–10% of the population consistent with normal variation.

▶ Practical Approach to the Diagnosis of Intersex

In the newborn period, patients with ambiguous genitalia can be approached in a logical fashion (Figure 43–11) (Lee et al, 2006). As noted earlier, history, physical examination, laboratory evaluation, and radiographic and in some cases surgical exploration are necessary to make an accurate diagnosis. Once the karyotype is known, along with the gonadal status, an appropriate test can lead to a diagnosis (Figure 43–11 and Table 43–5). Patients may also present at puberty (inappropriate or delayed development) with sexual differentiation abnormalities or later in life with infertility. The differential diagnosis for these disorders is diagrammed in Figure 43–12.

TREATMENT OF SPECIFIC DISORDERS

▶ 46,XX DSD (Female Pseudohermaphrodites)

46,XX disorders of sex development (DSD) are characterized by a 46,XX genotype, nonpalpable gonads or normal ovaries, and variable degrees of virilization of the external genitalia.

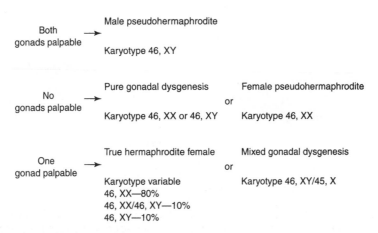

▲ **Figure 43–11.** Algorithm for initial workup of intersex based on physical examination and karyotype.

Table 43–5. Differential diagnosis for a newborn with ambiguous genitalia.

	Common karyotype	Gonad status	Genitalia	Uterus	Urinary/ Serum steroids
46,XX DSD (Female pseudohermaphrodite) (CAH)	XX	Ovary	Hypospadias	Present	Elevated
46,XY DSD (Male pseudohermaphrodite)	XY	Testes	Hypospadias/ micropenis	Absent	Normal
45,X/46,XY DSD (Mixed gonadal dysgenesis	XY/XO	Streak dysgenetic	Hypospadias	Variable/ rudimentary	Normal
Ovotesticular DSD (True hermaphrodite)	XX/mosaic	Ovotestis or ovary and testes	Hypospadias	Variable/ rudimentary	Normal

A. Congenital Adrenal Hyperplasia

CAH is the most common cause of female ambiguous genitalia or pseudohermaphroditism and accounts for approximately 70% of all patients with ambiguous genitalia. CAH accounts for >95% of the cases of female pseudohermaphroditism, with exposure to maternal androgens accounting for the remaining 5%. Mutations in one of five genes result in impaired cortisol secretion, which in turn causes excess secretion of adrenocorticotropic hormone (ACTH) and consequently adrenal hyperplasia (Speiser, 2007). Four of the five genes code for enzymes necessary for steroid hormone synthesis, and the fifth encodes for an intracellular cholesterol transport protein (StAR) (Figure 43–9). Deficiencies in 21α-hydroxylase and 11β-hydroxylase result in masculinization of the female fetus, while they have no effects on the genitalia of the male fetuses. In contrast, infants with deficiencies in 3β-hydroxysteroid dehydrogenase, 17α-hydroxylase,

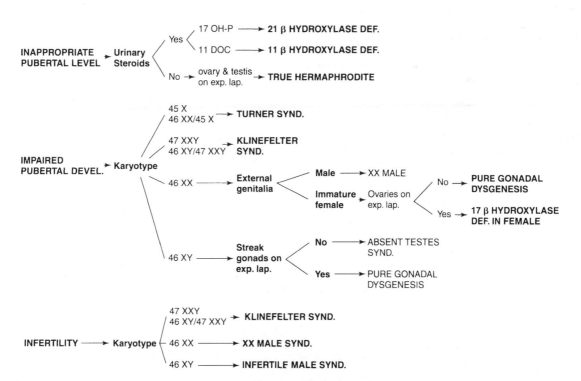

▲ **Figure 43–12.** Differential diagnosis of patients with inappropriate pubertal development, impaired pubertal development, and infertility. Def., deficiency; devel., development; DOC, 11-deoxycorticosterone; exp. lap., exploratory laparoscopy; 17 OH-P, 17 hydroxy progesterone; synd., syndrome.

and StAR have defects in both the synthesis of cortisol and steroid hormones. Affected males have varying degree of ambiguous genitalia due to deficiency in testosterone synthesis, while affected females may or may not be virilized.

21α-Hydroxylase deficiency is the most common cause of CAH, accounting for 90% of cases. The metabolites 17-hydroxyprogesterone and 17-hydroxypregnelone, which build up above the 21α-hydroxylase deficiency, are metabolized to androgens, resulting in virilization of the female external genitalia. Three forms of 21α-hydroxylase deficiency exist: classic, simple virilizing, and nonclassic. Each of these disorders is characterized by the activity level of the gene. Patients with the classic disease have both virilization and salt wasting, those with simple virilizing have masculinization without salt losing, and the nonclassic patients present after puberty with virilization.

In general, the classic form of 21α-hydroxylase deficiency exhibits the more severe forms of virilization (Figure 43–13). Impaired cortisol and aldosterone secretion leads to electrolytes and fluid losses, producing hyponatremia, hyperkalemia, acidosis, increased plasma renin, dehydration, and eventual vascular collapse unless recognized and treated. In affected males, deficiency in 21α-hydroxylase does not result in abnormal genitalia, and consequently, salt loss may occur unnoticed. Aggressive fluid resuscitation with normal saline should be instituted immediately and repeat serum electrolyte measurement should be obtained to monitor the progress of the resuscitation. Diagnosis is based on an elevated level of 17-hydroxyprogesterone in the urine and blood. After diagnosis and stabilization, replacement therapy should be instituted with glucocorticoids, mineralocorticoids, and salt. Regular measurement of serum electrolytes, renin, and ACTH helps to monitor the adequacy of hormonal replacement. Untreated patients with 21α-hydroxylase deficiency exhibit excessive growth, virilization, advanced bone age, and early closure of epiphyseal growth plates (Hughes, 2007).

11β-Hydroxylase deficiency accounts for most of the remaining cases of CAH (approximately 9%). Patients with 11β-hydroxylase accumulate 17-hydroxyprogesterone as well as DOC and 11-deoxycortisol, which results in salt accumulation leading to hypertension. Patients with 11β-hydroxylase deficiency are more likely to present with hypertension secondary to the salt-retaining metabolites DOC and 11-deoxycortisol, in contrast to the hypovolemic shock associated with 21α-hydroxylase deficiency. Hypokalemia is also common secondary to an increase in mineralocorticoid activity.

Since CAH is hereditary, it is possible to counsel and offer treatment to families wishing further children. Maternal treatment with dexamethasone prior to the 10th week of gestation can significantly reduce the risk of masculinization of the female fetus (Miller, 1998). Standard prenatal treatment is 20 mg/kg two times daily beginning as soon as the pregnancy is confirmed (5th week of gestation) in a family with a positive history of CAH. At 9–10 weeks' gestation, chorionic villus sampling can confirm karyotype and test for the presence of the gene *CYP 21*, which is present in 21α-hydroxylase deficiency (90% of CAH cases). If the karyotype is XY or the CAH gene *CYP 21* is not present, the maternal dexamethasone treatment is stopped. Statistically, 50% of the fetuses will be male, and of the females, only 25% will be

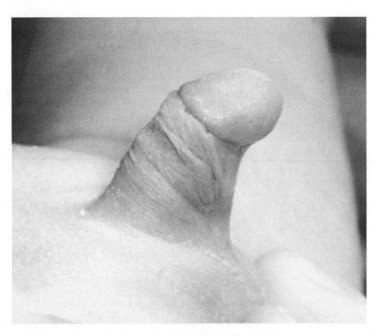

▲ **Figure 43–13.** Patient with severe masculinization from congenital adrenal hyperplasia.

Table 43–6. Drugs that may induce disorder of sex development if taken during pregnancy.

C21-steroid medroxyprogesterone acetate (progesterone)
Finasteride (Proscar)
Leuprolide acetate (Lupron)
Stilbestrol
Danazol
Norethynodrel
Ethisterone
Norethindrone

affected secondary to the recessive inheritance pattern of 21α-hydroxylase deficiency. Unfortunately, this will result in unnecessary prenatal steroid exposure in seven of eight fetuses with unknown long-term health consequences, such as hypertension. Although the short-term success of decreasing female virilization has been documented, long-term follow-up of fetuses exposed to steroids needs to be documented.

B. Maternal Hormonal Sources of Virilization

Maternal tumors are a rare cause of virilization of the female fetus. The most common type are luteomas of the ovary, which also virilize the mother. Diagnosis can be made by maternal blood samples and imaging studies (sonogram and magnetic resonance imaging). Maternal ingestion of medication is another rare cause of abnormalities in genital development (Table 43–6). Progesterone is a common agent being used early in pregnancy to prevent abortions as well as during in vitro fertilization treatments.

The female fetus that is exposed to high concentrations of progesterone can virilize secondary to direct action of progesterone on the AR. In the male fetus, hypospadias can develop by progesterone-inhibiting testosterone synthesis and downregulating the AR. A prenatal history of progesterone exposure should be elicited in the differential diagnosis of patients with abnormalities of the external genitalia.

▶ 46,XY DSD (Male Pseudohermaphrodites)

46,XY DSD are characterized by a 46,XY genotype, normal testes (usual palpable), and partial or complete masculinization of the external genitalia. The differential diagnosis is outlined in Figure 43–14.

Two forms of androgen resistance related to male pseudohermaphrodites are complete androgen insensitivity and partial androgen insensitivity.

A. Complete Androgen Insensitivity

Androgen resistance ranges from partial to complete due to a defect in the AR. Patients with complete androgen resistance or androgen insensitivity syndrome (AIS) (previously called testicular feminization) have a 46,XY karyotype but have unambiguous female external genitalia, hypoplastic labia majora, a blind vaginal pouch, and an absent uterus (Wisniewski et al, 2000). Since a functional AR is necessary for the development of axillary and pubic hair, complete AIS patients have sparse to nonexistent hair growth in these areas. Complete AIS patients either inherit the disease by an X-linked recessive pattern or develop a spontaneous mutation that renders the AR nonfunctional. Patients with complete AIS appear to identify as females. Presumably, the functional defect in the AR also exists in the brain, preventing "masculinization." There is not enough long-term follow-up to assess issues with sexual identity in these patients.

Complete androgen resistance should be suspected in phenotypic females who present with an inguinal hernia that contains a testis (approximately 1% of all prepubertal females undergoing hernia repair) (Oakes et al, 2008). The most common presentation for complete AIS is amenorrhea in adolescent females. Breast development occurs in AIS patients secondary to the peripheral conversion of testosterone to estradiol from aromatase enzyme. After puberty, the testes have approximately a 10% risk of developing cancer, the most common tumor being a seminomatous germ cell. Because of the significantly increased cancer risk, removal of the gonads is recommended after postpubertal breast development. Alternatively, the gonads can be removed at the time of diagnosis, with estrogen replacement therapy initiated in the pubertal time period. Since the vagina may be inadequate in length, some patients may need augmentation procedures. Self-vaginal dilation is the most common technique, followed by vaginal augmentation procedures using skin grafts or bowel.

B. Partial Androgen Insensitivity

In contrast to complete AIS, patients with partial androgen resistance may have external genitalia ranging from mild to severe hypospadias (with or without cryptorchidism) to micropenis or clitorimegaly with partial labial fusion (Figure 43–15) (Griffin et al, 1995). The testes may be located in the labia, inguinal canal, or abdomen. The testes are histologically normal before puberty. However, after puberty, spermatogenesis is usually absent and there is Leydig cell hyperplasia. The testes are predisposed to malignant transformation in 4–9% of the patients (Fallat and Donahoe, 2006).

The defect in partial androgen resistance is typically due to a single base pair mutation in the AR. Inheritance may be X-linked, autosomal recessive, or from a spontaneous mutation. Interestingly, the same genetic defect within a family may have a different phenotypic expression. The variability of phenotypic expression makes counseling difficult in affected families.

In patients with partial androgen resistance, the sex of rearing depends on the degree of androgen resistance and the degree of genital ambiguity. In patients who respond to high-dose androgen therapy (2 mg/kg initially followed by 4 mg/kg) with phallic growth, the sex of rearing as male has been

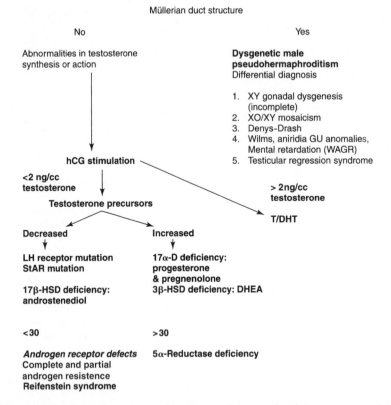

Müllerian duct structure

No   Yes

Abnormalities in testosterone
synthesis or action

**Dysgenetic male
pseudohermaphroditism**
Differential diagnosis

1. XY gonadal dysgenesis
   (incomplete)
2. XO/XY mosaicism
3. Denys-Drash
4. Wilms, aniridia GU anomalies,
   Mental retardation (WAGR)
5. Testicular regression syndrome

hCG stimulation

<2 ng/cc
testosterone

> 2ng/cc
testosterone

Testosterone precursors

T/DHT

Decreased

Increased

**LH receptor mutation
StAR mutation**

**17α-D deficiency:
progesterone
& pregnenolone**
3β-HSD deficiency: DHEA

**17β-HSD deficiency:
androstenediol**

<30

>30

Androgen receptor defects
**Complete and partial
androgen resistence
Reifenstein syndrome**

5α-Reductase deficiency

▲ **Figure 43–14.** Differential diagnosis of patients with male pseudohermaphroditism. 17α-D, 17(α)-hydroxylase; DHEA, dehydroepiandrosterone; GU, genitourinary; hCG, human chorionic gonadotropin; HSD, hydroxy-steroid dehydrogenase; LH, luteinizing hormone; StAR, steroidogenic acute regulatory protein; T/DHT, testosterone/dihydrotestosterone.

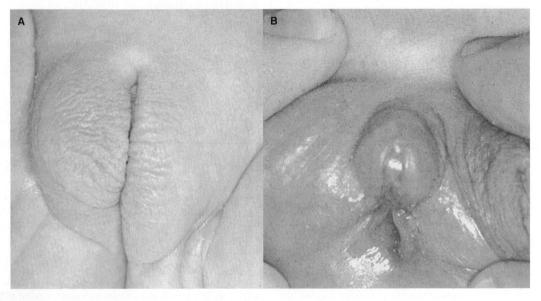

▲ **Figure 43–15.** Partial androgen receptor defect resulting in severe hypospadias with curvature *(A)* and a small phallus *(B)*.

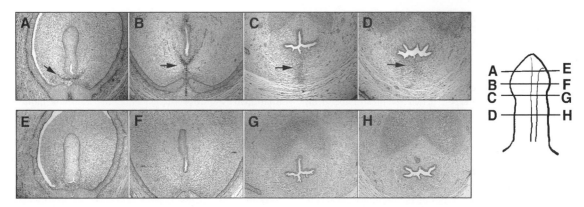

▲ **Figure 43-16.** Immunohistochemical localization of 5α-reductase type 2 *(A–D)* and the androgen receptor (AR) *(E–H)* in the same human fetal penis at 16.5 weeks of gestation (reduced from 25×). Note the strong expression of 5α-reductase type 2 along the urethral seam area (*arrows*).

successful. Genital reconstruction repairing the hypospadias and undescended testes is performed at an early age. Patients who have a poor response to androgen stimulation fall into a difficult category of intersex. In the past, patients who were raised as females had feminizing genital surgery and gonadectomy typically in the first year of life. At the time of puberty, estrogen replacement is instituted. Presumably in partial androgen insensitivity, sexual identity is influenced by the effects of androgens on central imprinting. A discord may exist between the external genitalia that partially responds to androgen stimulation and the effects of androgens on determining sexual identity in the brain (Zucker, 2003). The fact that some patients with severe hypospadias and a small phallus have had difficulty with sexual identity in adulthood makes sex assignment difficult. Presently, it seems reasonable to delay irreversible surgery until after the patient has developed a sexual identity and can drive the decision for reconstructive surgery.

▶ 5α-Reductase Type 2 Deficiency

5α-Reductase type 2 deficiency is an autosomal recessive transmitted disorder affecting the formation of the male genitalia (Wilson et al, 1993). 5α-Reductase is responsible for the conversion of the less potent testosterone to the five to ten times more potent DHT. Type 2 5α-reductase predominates in the tissue of the external genitalia and the prostate, whereas type 1 5α-reductase localizes to the skin and nongenital tissues. Numerous mutations have been described in the 5α-reductase type 2 gene consistent with the variation in clinical spectrum seen in patients with this defect. Immunohistochemical localization of 5α-reductase type 2 reveals that the enzyme is located in the midline urethral seam (Figure 43–16) (Kim et al, 2002). The midline seam localization is consistent with the formation of hypospadias in patients with 5a-reductase type 2 gene defects in that the epithelial

edges of the urethral seam would fail to fuse, resulting in hypospadias.

Clinically, patients with 5α-reductase type 2 present with a small phallus, severe hypospadias, bifid scrotum, and a residual prostatic utricle or blind-ending vaginal pouch (Figure 43–17). The testes are often undescended in the inguinal

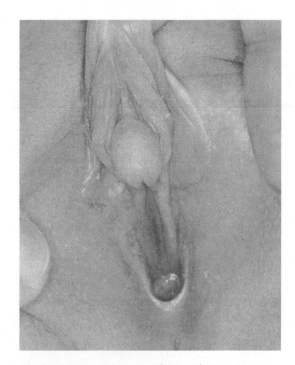

▲ **Figure 43–17.** A patient with 5α-reductase type 2 deficiency. Note severe hypospadias with a small phallus, bifid scrotum, and visible prostatic utricle or blind-ending vaginal pouch.

canal. Untreated patients will typically virilize during puberty when elevated levels of the less potent testosterone either overwhelm the functioning androgen gene or the functioning 5α-reductase type 1 enzyme cross-reacts with the excess testosterone, converting it to DHT.

Sexual identity appears to be intact for karyotype XY males with 5α-reductase type 2 deficiency, presumably from an intact masculinization of the brain. In specific geographic areas such as the Dominican Republic, where the incidence of 5α-reductase type 2 deficiency is relatively high, it is generally accepted that these children will change from an initial "in-between" sex to a male sexual identity at the time of puberty.

The diagnosis of 5α-reductase type 2 deficiency should be considered in severe phenotypes of hypospadias, especially with associated scrotal anomalies and undescended testes. Diagnosis is based on an increase in ratio of testosterone to DHT. Since these patients have a small phallus, attempts at enlargement with DHT cream are reasonable, although DHT is difficult to obtain in the United States. Reconstructive surgery for the hypospadias and undescended testes is indicated. Fertility has not been reported in patients with 5α-reductase type 2, although sperm production has been documented.

▶ Persistent Müllerian Duct Syndrome

Müllerian-inhibiting substance or factor (anti-Müllerian duct hormone) causes regression of the structures that would have formed the uterus, fallopian tube, and upper part of the vagina. Defects in the MIS gene or MIS receptor result in retained Müllerian structures typically inherited as an autosomal recessive defect. Male siblings of affected patients, especially with cryptorchidism, should undergo screening; they have a 25% chance of being affected (Rey et al, 1999).

Clinically, patients with persistent Müllerian duct syndrome present, unexpectedly, at the time of surgery for cryptorchidism (Figure 43–18). Hence, the alternate name for persistent Müllerian duct syndrome is hernia uterine inguinale. Within the hernia sac, a fallopian tube, uterus, or both are found attached to the testicular cord structures. What makes the treatment difficult is that these structures and hence the diagnosis are found unexpectedly at the time of surgery for cryptorchidism. If persistent Müllerian duct structures are found during orchiopexy, it is reasonable to abort the procedure until a correct diagnosis can be determined. At the initial exploration, a clear description of gonad and surrounding Müllerian structures should be documented, with a biopsy specimen of the gonad taken and a karyotype obtained.

Once a definitive diagnosis is made, reconstructive surgery can then be performed. Separation of inappropriate Müllerian structures from the cord without disturbing the vas deferens, the testicular artery, or both is the goal; however, this may be impossible if the vas runs through the Müllerian structures, which is a common outcome. Fertility is usually impaired in patients with persistent Müllerian duct syndrome even though testosterone levels may be normal. Whether this is a consequence of primary gonadal dysfunction or secondary to the cryptorchid testes is controversial. Efforts should be made to remove the Müllerian structures

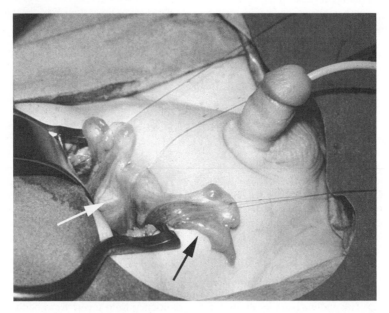

▲ **Figure 43–18.** Hernia uterine inguinale or persistent Müllerian duct syndrome. Note the presence of a fallopian tube (*black arrow*) and uterus attached (*white arrow*) to the testicular cord structures.

and deliver the testes into the scrotum or at least a palpable position in the groin for subsequent cancer surveillance. Testes cancer has been reported in 2–10% of patients. In patients where the testes remains in the abdomen or cannot be separated from the Müllerian structures, orchiectomy is indicated.

▶ Abnormal Gonadal Function Syndromes

A. 45,X DSD (Turner's Syndrome)

Turner's syndrome is relatively common, occurring in 1 in every 2000 female births. The genotype in patients with Turner's syndrome is a complete or mosaic X monosomy, 45,X, or 45,X/46,XX) (Loscalzo, 2008). Turner stigmata consist of a web neck, shield chest, aortic valve defects, coarctation of the aorta, horseshoe kidney, short stature, and absent puberty. During fetal development in patients with Turner's syndrome, the ovaries develop but subsequently degenerate to streak gonads. The streak gonads are not at risk for cancer (unless Y chromatin material is present) and therefore do not need to be removed. Therapy is directed toward growth augmentation with growth hormone therapy in childhood. Subsequently, estrogen replacement is begun in late adolescence so as not to interfere with maximum growth.

B. 46,XX DSD Complete Gonadal Dysgenesis

Patients with 46,XX complete gonadal dysgenesis are typically diagnosed following a workup for delayed puberty or primary amenorrhea. Patients have a normal female phenotype without the stigmata of Turner's syndrome, normal external and internal Müllerian structures, and bilateral streak gonads. Sexual identity is female. Unlike patients with 46,XY gonadal dysgenesis, risk of tumor formation is rare and treatment is directed at hormonal replacement, with removal of the streaks gonads unnecessary.

C. 46,XY DSD Gonadal Dysgenesis (Swyer's Syndrome)

Patients with 46,XY gonadal dysgenesis are characterized by absent testicular function in the presence of a Y chromosome. Classically, patients with 46,XY gonadal dysgenesis have a female phenotype. Patients come to medical attention if the prenatal karyotype (XY) is discordant with the child's phenotype (female), delayed puberty, amenorrhea, or precocious puberty from a hormonally functional gonadal tumor. The incidence of gonadal tumors is as high as 60%, with gonadoblastoma being the most common, although dysgerminomas, seminomas, and nonseminomatous germ cell tumors have also been reported.

In pure XY gonadal dysgenesis, Müllerian duct structures usually are present secondary to failure of MIS secretion, and Wolffian duct structures are vestigial or absent secondary to lack of testosterone secretion. Laboratory analysis reveals female levels of baseline testosterone with no increase in response to hCG stimulation. Surgical exploration reveals streak gonads, fallopian tubes, and a uterus. With a 60% chance of tumor, the gonads need to be removed once the diagnosis is confirmed. These patients should be raised as females with estrogen replacement at the time of puberty.

D. 45,X/46,XY DSD (Mixed Gonadal Dysgenesis)

Patients with mixed gonadal dysgenesis usually have a 45,X/46,XY, 46,XY, or other mosaic karyotype. They typically have one streak and one dysgenetic testis. Most children with mixed gonadal dysgenesis have incomplete virilization resulting in ambiguous genitalia or hypospadias with cryptorchidism. The other classic presentation is a mosaic genotype diagnosed on prenatal amniocentesis (Chang et al, 1990). Interestingly, the subsequent phenotype of patients with a prenatal karyotype of 45,X/46,XY is 90% normal male external genitalia. However, with a prenatal genotype of 45,X/46,XY, the patient is at risk for progressive gonadal changes leading to fibrosis and decreased fertility and low testosterone levels. The incidence of gonadal tumors does not seem to be increased. Most notably, 20% of these children have mental retardation or autism.

In patients who present with ambiguous genitalia, one gonad is typically palpable in the scrotum or inguinal canal and the other gonad (streak) is nonpalpable. The phallus size is typically small with a proximal or more severe hypospadias (Figure 43–19). Testosterone levels are normal with an appropriate response to hCG. MIS levels are usually normal. At surgery, the dysgenetic gonad (streak) may grossly appear normal but have microscopic abnormalities such as hypoplastic tubules surrounded by ovarian or fibrotic stroma. Variable Müllerian duct structures, such as fallopian tubes and uterus, are present depending on the degree of gonadal dysgenesis. On biopsy, the contralateral gonad in the scrotum or inguinal canal is either a normal or dysgenetic testis. In patients with mixed gonadal dysgenesis, the risk of gonadoblastoma is 15–30% (Levin, 2000). Gonadoblastoma is a steroid hormone–secreting gonadal tumor composed of large germ cells, Sertoli cells, and stromal derivatives. The incidence of gonadoblastoma appears to be higher in more undervirilized patients and the most common associated karyotype is 46,XY. Sixty percent of gonadoblastomas arise in an indeterminate gonad, 22% in streak gonads, and 18% in dysgenetic cryptorchid testis. Two cases occurring in a testis located in the scrotum have been reported. One-third of the patients have bilateral disease. Sixty percent of gonadoblastomas are associated with subsequent malignant germ cell tumor (germinoma, seminoma, and dysgerminoma but also embryonal teratoma, embryonal carcinoma, endodermal sinus tumor, or choriocarcinoma). Metastases develop in 10% of patients with germinomas arising within the gonadoblastoma.

In children who are undervirilized, female sex assignment is an option, and the streak and dysgenetic gonads should be removed at the time of diagnosis due to increased risk of malignancy. Hormonal replacement with estrogen will be

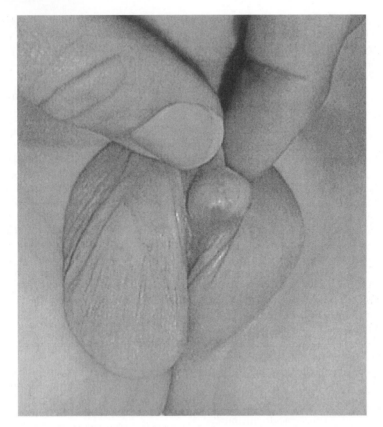

▲ **Figure 43–19.** Presentation of mixed gonadal dysgenesis with ambiguous genitalia and a unilateral palpable gonad on the right side.

necessary during adolescence. If male gender is assigned, management of the scrotal testis is controversial, ranging from serial observation to surveillance biopsy. In the virilized patients who are raised as males, the testis will inevitably reveal poor hormonal and fertility potential (Woodhouse, 2001). These patients will require testosterone supplementation in adulthood (Birnbacher et al, 1999).

In 5% of patients, mixed gonadal dysgenesis is associated with Wilms' tumor, ambiguous genitalia, and progressive glomerulopathy known as the Denys-Drash syndrome. Wilms' tumor occurs in the first 2 years of life and is often bilateral. Classic presentation is an infant with ambiguous genitalia, hypertension, and nephrotic syndrome.

E. 17β-Hydroxysteroid Dehydrogenase Deficiency

Patients with a defect in the enzyme 17β-hydroxysteroid dehydrogenase do not efficiently convert androstenedione to testosterone. 17β-Hydroxysteroid dehydrogenase is predominantly located in the testes. The rare disorder of 17β-hydroxysteroid dehydrogenase deficiency is inherited via an autosomal recessive pattern. This disorder is indigenous to the Arab population of the Gaza strip in the Middle East. Clinical presentation in a patient with XY genotype is mild virilization of the external genitalia, with clitoral hypertrophy, and a blind-ending utricle (vagina). The testes are undescended in the abdomen or inguinal canal or descended into the labioscrotal folds. If the virilization is mild, the diagnosis becomes apparent at puberty, with penile growth and male secondary sexual characteristics. At puberty, the increased levels of androstenedione are converted by nongenital, nonmutant 17α-hydroxysteroid dehydrogenase to testosterone. These patients may also present with gynecomastia at puberty by the peripheral conversion of androstenedione to estradiol by aromatase. Diagnosis is based on an increased ratio of androstenedione to testosterone postpubertal or in the prepubertal state in response to an hCG-stimulation test.

If the diagnosis is suspected in infancy, treatment with testosterone, reconstruction of the hypospadias, and male sex assignment are indicated. At puberty in the Gaza strip, gender conversion from female to male is common practice. Long-term outcomes of patients raised as females initially and reassigned to males at puberty await documentation.

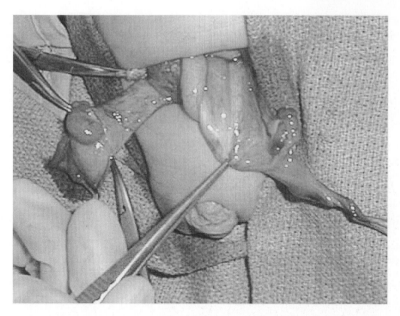

▲ **Figure 43–20.** Finding at the time of surgical exploration in a true hermaphrodite. On the patient's right side, note the testes, and on the left, note the fallopian tube, uterus, and biopsy-proven ovary.

▶ Ovotesticular DSD (True Hermaphroditism)

True hermaphroditism is defined as the presence of both ovarian and testicular tissue within the same individual (Figure 43–20). The most common karyotype in patients with true hermaphroditism is 46,XX (predominately in African Americans), followed by 46,XY/46,XX mosaicism. The latter karyotype in a patient with ambiguous genitalia strongly suggests the diagnosis of true hermaphroditism. Only 7% of patients with this disorder have a 46,XY karyotype. Interestingly, not all true hermaphrodites express the SRY gene, suggesting that non-SRY genes play a role in the development of the testes in these patients.

In patients with true hermaphroditism, the gonads are a combination of ovotestis, ovaries, or testis. The most common configuration is ovotestis/ovary in 35%, followed by bilateral ovotestis in 25%, ovary/testes in 25%, and ovotestis/testes in the remaining 15%. One or both gonads are palpable in at least 60% of the patients. For unexplained reasons, the testis is more likely to be found on the right side. The testis and ovaries are located in their respective normal position, and the level of descent of the ovotestis is dependent on the amount of testicular tissue. While ovarian histology and function may be normal, testicular histology and function is usually abnormal. Ovotestis can be bilobar in configuration, with the ovarian and testicular tissue relatively separate, or the ovarian and testicular tissue may be intermingled and difficult to surgically separate. At the time of diagnosis, deep biopsies are necessary to determine the histologic status of the gonad. The internal structures tend to correlate with the type of gonad. Approximately 80% of true hermaphrodites will have a functional or rudimentary uterus. The uterus may be found in the abdomen or associated with an inguinal hernia. In patients with normal uterine structures and ovarian histology, fertility and normal pregnancies have been reported.

The external genitalia are usually ambiguous, although 60% of patients are masculinized, with a well-developed hypospadiac phallus. The hypospadias can be severe perineal or penile scrotal with incomplete fusion of the labioscrotal folds. The degree of masculinization is dependent on the amount of functional testicular tissue present. In childhood, testicular tissue has been documented to have normal spermatogonia. With maturation, however, testicular fibrosis occurs, with fertility in males a rare event. Testicular tumor is uncommon, occurring only in 1–2% of the patients.

The diagnosis of true hermaphroditism should be suspected in patients with virilized ambiguous genitalia who have a 46,XX (African American) or mosaic genotype 46,XX/46,XY associated with the finding of Müllerian structures. Diagnosis is confirmed by gonadal biopsy confirming the presence of both ovarian and testicular tissue. After a decision regarding sex gender assignment has been made, gonadal tissue inappropriate for sex gender assignment should be removed. In patients who are raised as females, removal of all functioning testicular tissue is critical to prevent virilization at puberty. Surgical correction of the urogenital sinus to expose the vagina is necessary. In patients raised as males—who account for approximately 30% of all true hermaphrodites—the hypospadias and undescended testes should be reconstructed. In males, since testicular failure is common at puberty, testosterone supplementation may be required.

▶ Unclassified Forms of Abnormal Sexual Development

A. Hypospadias

Hypospadias except in the most severe situation is not a form of DSD (intersex) (Figure 43–21) (Baskin and Ebbers, 2006). The etiology can be defined in less than 5% of patients. This leaves most cases without a defined etiology. The variable expression of the AR in the ventral versus the dorsal urethra may play a role in the etiology of hypospadias (Figure 43–22) (Baskin et al, 1998; Kim et al, 2002). Recent theories suggest an abnormality in closure of the midline urethral seam. Another possible etiology explaining the increase in incidence of hypospadias in western countries over the last 25 years is an increase in exposure to environmental endocrine disruptors (Baskin et al, 2001).

In controlled studies, most patients with hypospadias undergo successful surgical reconstruction and have acceptable long-term outcomes. Patients with hypospadias have an unambiguous male sexual identity. In severe forms of hypospadias with perineal or scrotal urethral openings, severe curvature and the phallus buried within the scrotum are the critical issues confirming the correct diagnosis. This is also the case for patients with hypospadias and a nonpalpable or undescended testis. If any doubt exists, patients with severe hypospadias, hypospadias in association with an undescended testis, or both, a karyotype should be checked to document genotype (McAleer and Kaplan, 2001). In severe cases of hypospadias where penile size is difficult to assess secondary to severe chordee, an hCG stimulation will assess the gonadal axis and confirm an intact AR by eliciting penile growth.

B. Micropenis

A penis less than 2.5 cm in stretched penile length without hypospadias in a full-term male is defined as micropenis

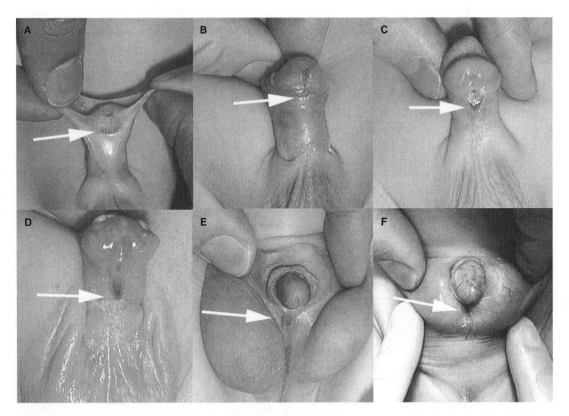

▲ **Figure 43–21.** The spectrum of hypospadias, which is not an ambiguous or intersex condition. **A:** Anterior, where the meatus is on the inferior surface of the glans penis. **B:** Coronal, where the meatus is in the balanopenile furrow. **C:** Distal, on the distal third of the shaft. **D:** Penoscrotal, at the base of the shaft in front of the scrotum. **E:** Scrotal, on the scrotum or between the genital swellings. **F:** Perineal, where the meatus is behind the scrotum or genital swellings.

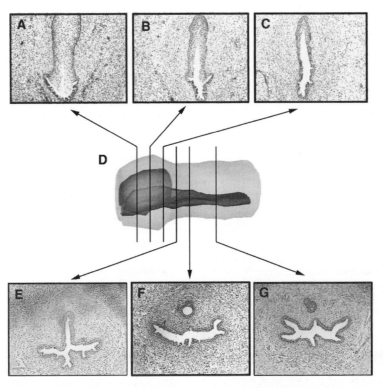

▲ **Figure 43–22.** Androgen receptor (AR) expression in the human fetal penis at 16.5 weeks. A greater density of AR-positive cells is seen in the ventral portion of the urethral epithelium in the distal glans *(A)*, midglans *(B)*, and proximal glans *(C)*. In the distal *(E)*, mid *(F)*, and proximal *(G)* shaft of the penis, all portions of the urethral epithelium show the same density of expression. Three-dimensional reconstruction was performed to demonstrate the urethral AR expression pattern *(D)*. Note the weaker density of AR in the dorsal aspect of the glanular urethra.

(Figure 43–23 and Table 43–4). Micropenis can be caused by multiple etiologies, the most common being fetal testosterone deficiency followed by partial defects in the AR or 5α-reductase enzyme (Table 43–7). Fetal testosterone synthesis can be divided into two categories: (1) primary testicular failure (Leydig cell) and (2) central failure. Central failure can be from congenital hypopituitarism or isolated gonadotropin deficiency. Patients with decreased fetal testosterone production either from (Fallat and Donahoe, 2006) Leydig cell failure or lack of Leydig cell stimulation from gonadotropin deficiency respond to treatment with supplementary testosterone enanthate intramuscular injections 25–50 mg each month for 3 consecutive months.

Long-term outcomes of patients with micropenis have documented that final adult penile length is normal for >90% of patients treated with multiple short courses of testosterone enanthate. In addition, patients with micropenis identified with the male gender had normal erections, ejaculation, and orgasm. In rare patient who does not respond to testosterone stimulation, gender conversion to female had been advocated in the past. Presently, gender conversion would not be considered based solely on the small phallus size.

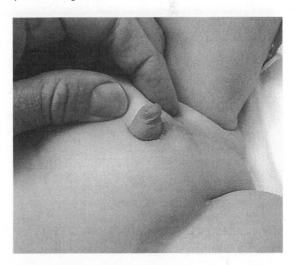

▲ **Figure 43–23.** Micropenis. Normal corporeal bodies are palpable within the foreskin. The urethral meatus is at a terminal position within the glans. Stretched penile length is <2.5 cm in this full-term infant.

Table 43–7. Etiologies of micropenis.

I. Deficient testosterone secretion
  A. Hypogonadotrophic hypogonadism
    1. Kallmann syndrome
    2. Prader-Willi syndrome
    3. Laurence-Moon syndrome
    4. Bardet-Biedl syndrome
    5. Rudd syndrome
  B. Primary hypogonadism ("Bum Gonads")
    1. Anorchia
    2. Klinefelter syndrome
    3. Gonadal dysgenesis (partial)
    4. LH receptor defects (partial)
    5. Noonan syndrome
    6. Trisomy 21
    7. Robinow syndrome
    8. Bardet-Biedl syndrome
    9. Laurence-Moon syndrome
    10. Testosterone synthesis defects (partial)

II. Defects in testosterone action
  A. Androgen receptor defects (partial)
  B. 5α-Reductase deficiency
  C. Growth hormone/insulin growth factor-1 deficiency
  D. Fetal hydantoin syndrome

III. Developmental anomalies
  A. Aphallia
  B. Cloacal exstrophy
  C. Iatrogenic injuries
    1. Circumcision
    2. Trauma

Reassignment to the female gender with removal of the gonads and feminizing genitoplasty in patients with penile agenesis, iatrogenic penile amputation, or circumcision injury had been standard treatment. In complete penile agenesis, the testicles are normal, corporeal bodies are absent, and the urethra opens into the anterior rectum or perineum. These patients have normal prenatal androgen levels, and hence, the brain has received signals for male gender identity (Wisniewski et al, 2001). The same is true for the rare patient who has a severe penile injury during circumcision. As in micropenis, gender conversion would now not be considered based solely on the absence or small size of the phallus. Penile reconstruction, although not technically ideal, may provide the best overall outcome.

C. Cloacal and Exstrophy Anomalies

In the past, patients with the most severe and rare form of lower abdominal congenital malformation, cloacal exstrophy (incidence of 1 in 200,000 live births), were usually left to die. Significant problems associated with surgical reconstruction of cloacal exstrophy include omphalocele; numerous gastrointestinal anomalies such as short gut, malrotation, duplication, duodenal atresia, and Meckel's diverticulum; and significant genitourinary anomalies such as separate bladder halves, upper-tract renal anomalies, and bifid genitalia. Patients with cloacal exstrophy can also have neurologic and orthopedic anomalies such as tethered cord, myelomeningocele, lower extremity paralysis, club-foot, and hip dislocation.

Historically, newborn males with cloacal exstrophy (Figure 43–24) were often gender converted to female as a result of

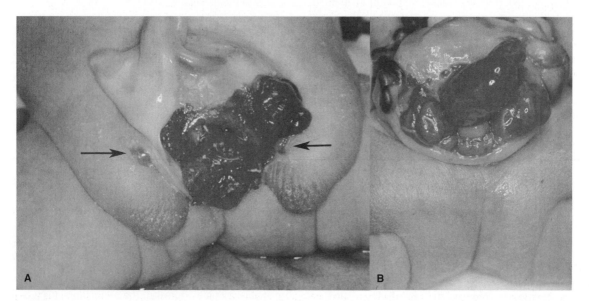

▲ **Figure 43–24. A:** Male with cloacal exstrophy. **B:** Female with cloacal exstrophy. In the male, note the split scrotal appearance and the small hemiphallus (*arrow*). In the female, the clitoral bodies/genitalia are not visible.

inadequate genital development and the poor prognosis for surgically developing a normal male phenotype. In rearing genetic males as females, although the surgical reconstruction can match the assigned female phenotype, a new set of issues was created, such as the need for hormonal replacement with estrogen during adolescence and the issue of a nonmenstruating infertile female. In addition, the fetal and neonatal androgen imprinting on the brain does not seem to be reversible.

Because some of these XY, gender-converted females have self-reassigned their sex during adolescence to coincide with their genetic karyotype, there has been reevaluation of the practice of rearing genetic males as females. With the exact determinates of sexual identity not completely defined, a pragmatic approach is to delay any irreversible surgery such as orchiectomy or phallic removal/reduction in these patients. With modern surgical techniques and a multidisciplinary approach to their care, children with this complex disorder can have a normal *sexual* identity.

SURGICAL MANAGEMENT OF DSD

The surgical management of patients with intersex is undergoing a reevaluation. The determination of a patient's *sexual* identity is strongly influenced by the genetic karyotype and steroid/androgen action on the developing brain.

The environmental and social impacts are certainly important but presently seem to have a less dominating influence.

We would advocate surgical management of patients with intersex when the diagnosis is clearly established and the long-term outcome for the diagnosis is favorable. Surgery falls into five categories: (1) diagnostic/biopsy, (2) gonadectomy and removal of inappropriate Müllerian structures, (3) clitoral reduction, (4) vaginoplasty, and (5) phallic reconstruction.

Diagnostic techniques have improved with the widespread use of laparoscopy to assess the morphology of the internal genital structures. Laparoscopic techniques allow the gonads and associated structures to be visualized and in some cases have a biopsy specimen taken without the need for a open incision. Once the diagnosis is established, it is possible to remove an inappropriate gonad, Müllerian remnant, or both via laparoscopic techniques.

CLITOROPLASTY

Clitoroplasty is presently a controversial topic. No studies exist to clearly document whether androgen stimulation resulting in a large clitoris requires reduction or can be left intact. Clearly, surgery on the clitoral structures can result in nerve damage and removal of erectile tissue.

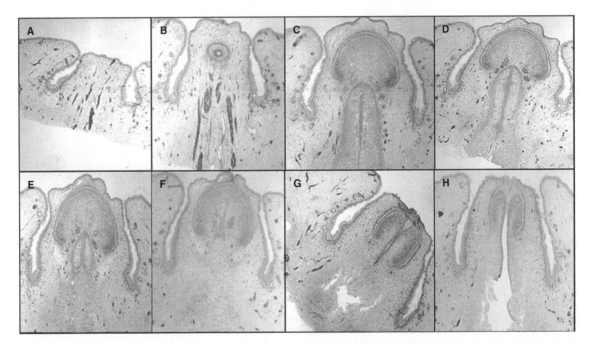

▲ **Figure 43–25.** Normal human fetal clitoris at 24 weeks' gestation (40×) immunostained with the neuronal marker S-100 (dark stain). ***A:*** Clitoral hood, labia minora, and majora. ***B:*** Nerves on top of the erectile body and top of glans clitoris. ***C–E:*** Glans clitoris and erectile bodies. ***F–G:*** Lower part of glans clitoris with midline cleft. ***H:*** End of glans clitoris and vaginal introitus.

Historically, the enlarged clitoris/phallic structure has been dealt with by amputation (Gross and Crigler, 1966). Subsequently, more refined techniques such as recession clitoroplasty were developed where the entire clitoral organ is preserved by imbricating and burying the proximal corporeal shaft and excess glans clitoris. The disadvantage of the clitoral recession procedures may not become apparent until puberty, when the recessed corporeal bodies become enlarged and painful during sexual stimulation. This leads to the need for a procedure involving subtotal resection of the shaft of the clitoris with preservation of the glans.

In cases where clitoroplasty is performed, the goal is to recreate the normal female anatomy. Presently, more conservative procedures have been employed to preserve both the sensory and cosmetic aspects of the clitoris. An understanding of normal female anatomy has benefited the design of reconstructive surgery in patients with CAH (Figures 43–25 and 43–26) (Baskin et al, 1999). A contemporary reduction

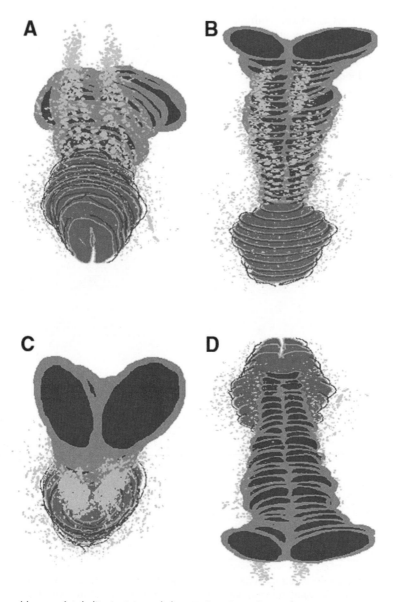

▲ **Figure 43–26.** Normal human fetal clitoris, 24 weeks' gestation. Four views of a computer-generated three-dimensional reconstruction (*A:* top; *B:* bottom; *C:* back/top; *D:* bottom). Note the pathway of the nerves (light gray) with a paucity of nerves on the bottom of the clitoris as well as in the top midline.

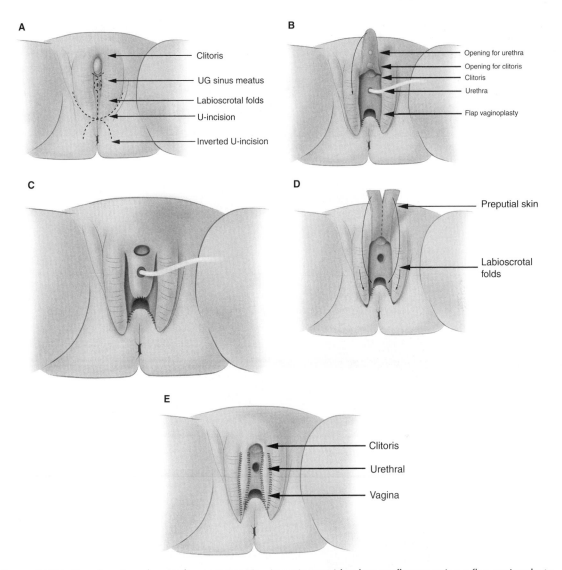

A

- Clitoris
- UG sinus meatus
- Labioscrotal folds
- U-incision
- Inverted U-incision

B

- Opening for urethra
- Opening for clitoris
- Clitoris
- Urethra
- Flap vaginoplasty

C

D

- Preputial skin
- Labioscrotal folds

E

- Clitoris
- Urethral
- Vagina

▲ **Figure 43–27.** Female external genitalia reconstruction in patients with a low confluence using a flap vaginoplasty. **A:** Surgical schematic of the perineum in patients with common urogenital sinus. **B:** The anterior flap for the vagina can be created using the phallic skin or the distal portion of the urogenital sinus. Two openings are created in the midline of the preputial skin flap to accommodate the clitoris and urethra. The preputial skin flap is then brought down and sutured to the anterior wall of the vagina. **C:** The completed repair. **D:** Alternatively, the preputial skin can be split in the midline and used for reconstruction of the vaginal introitus and the anterior vaginal wall. **E:** The completed repair. (Used with permission from Nguyen HT, Baskin LS: A Child with Ambiguous Genitalia. American Urological Association Patient Management Problems, Vol. 6. Decker Electronic Publishing Inc, 2002, p. 2.)

clitoroplasty is based on anatomical observations from fetal anatomical dissections. Presently, the tunica of the corporeal body can be preserved to spare as much of the dorsal nerve as possible. The concept of lifting the dorsal nerve off the tunica at the 11 and 1 o'clock positions seems inconsistent with the fact that the nerves fan out extensively around the dorsal and lateral aspects of the clitoral body.

A second issue is the removal of erectile tissue. In severe cases of masculinization of the genitalia (Prader V), consideration may be given to reduce the amount of erectile tissue.

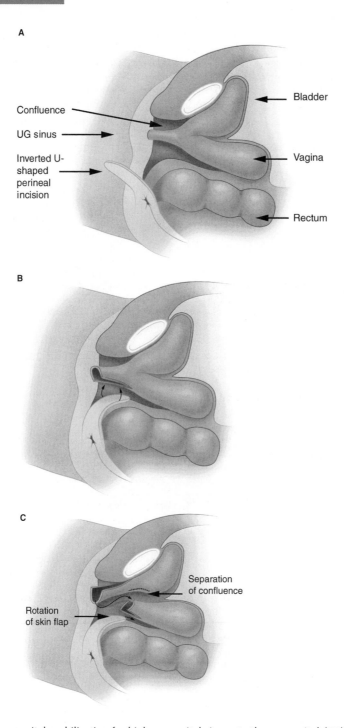

A

Confluence

UG sinus

Inverted U-shaped perineal incision

Bladder

Vagina

Rectum

B

C

Separation of confluence

Rotation of skin flap

▲ **Figure 43–28.** Partial urogenital mobilization for high urogenital sinus. **A:** The urogenital (UG) sinus is separated from the rectum posteriorly and the pubic bone anteriorly. **B:** The posterior skin flap (*arrows*) is assessed for length to reach the vagina. **C:** The confluence of the vagina and urethra (*arrow*) is separated. (Used with permission from Nguyen HT, Baskin LS: A Child with Ambiguous Genitalia. American Urological Association Patient Management Problems, Vol. 6. Decker Electronic Publishing Inc, 2002, p. 2.)

Standard treatment was to amputate the erectile body of the clitoris at the pubic arch, leaving each crural body and the neurovascular bundle with a strip of dorsal tunica. The long-term effects of removing this erectile tissue on sexual function are unknown. In contrast, leaving too much erectile tissue has been reported to cause pain in patients at the time of puberty. This, however, may be from fixing the corporeal tissue to the pubic bone, a practice that is no longer advocated. A compromise is to incise the erectile body on the ventral surface at the 6 o'clock position away from the nerves and remove erectile tissue within the tunica to reduce the size of the erectile body, thereby preserving some erectile tissue and the nerves of the clitoris.

▶ Vaginoplasty

The timing of vaginoplasty is also a controversial issue in genital reconstruction. The presence of a vagina is not necessary until puberty and initially only to allow the passage of menstrual fluids. Later the vagina is necessary for vaginal penetration, fertility, and, in most females, a healthy female *sexual* identity. This may not be the case for all females, for example, a woman with a small vagina and a female *sexual* identity with a female sexual preference may not desire a larger vagina. In patients with absent Müllerian structures (specifically a functional uterus) who have a female *sexual* identity, menstruation is not an issue and timing of vaginoplasty can be driven by the patient's wishes and motivation. In patients with a common urogenital sinus and hidden vagina, there are advantages and disadvantages of early surgery in the first year of life versus late surgery prior to puberty (Farkas et al, 2001). The advantage of early vaginoplasty is the closeness of the vagina to the perineum and the reported decreased bleeding in the early years of life. The major disadvantages are the smallness of the structures and that secondary surgery at the time of puberty may be necessary to correct vaginal stenosis. In contrast, delaying surgery has the advantages of operating on larger structures and the possibility that the patient can perform postoperative vaginal dilation to prevent stenosis (Hensle et al, 2006).

The type of vaginoplasty depends on the level of masculinization. For low urogenital sinus anomalies, a flap vaginoplasty will usually allow for an adequate introitus with separation of the urethra and vagina (Figure 43–27). For high urogenital sinus anomalies, partial urogenital mobilization and use of the elongated common urogenital sinus as an anterior vaginal flap may be necessary (Figure 43–28) (Rink and Cain, 2008). In the case of an absent vagina or a very short vagina, substitution vaginoplasty with bowel or skin grafting maybe required (Thomas and Brock, 2007). More recently autologous buccal mucosa has been successfully for used vaginal reconstruction (Samuelson and Baker, 2006).

▶ Phallic Reconstruction

Phallic reconstruction is a formidable task. Nevertheless, it is critical that reconstructive efforts continue in this area, especially for patients with penile agenesis or iatrogenic injuries and a XY genotype and functional AR. Several techniques have been devised, such as free microanastomosis, innervated radial forearm flaps, tubed abdominal flaps with a penile prosthesis, and rectus abdominus myocutaneous flaps. In the free radial forearm flap, the pudendal nerve is anastomosed to the lateral cutaneous nerve of the forearm. The radial artery and vein are anastomosed to the inferior epigastrics, the internal pudendals, or the femoral vessels. The major complications with these procedures are fistula, prosthesis erosion, and poor sensation. The technical nuances of microvascular anastomosis require that these procedures be performed in adolescents and adulthood. The psychological implications of relatively late reconstruction have not been determined. More recently, a technique to create a neonatal phallus from abdominal wall tissue has been described by De Castro et al (2007). Early results are encouraging but longer follow-up and the need for revision at the time of puberty will need to be determined. With newer tissue engineering techniques, better phallic reconstruction procedures may be on the horizon.

BIBLIOGRAPHY

Baskin LS et al: Anatomical studies of hypospadias. J Urol 1998;160(3, Pt 2):1108–1115; discussion 1137.

Baskin LS et al: Anatomical studies of the human clitoris. J Urol 1999;162(3, Pt 2):1015–1020.

Baskin LS et al: Hypospadias and endocrine disruption: Is there a connection? Environ Health Perspect 2001;109(11):1175–1183.

Baskin LS, Ebbers MB: Hypospadias: Anatomy, etiology, and technique. J Pediatr Surg 2006;41(3):463–472.

Birnbacher R et al: Gender identity reversal in an adolescent with mixed gonadal dysgenesis. J Pediatr Endocrinol Metab 1999; 12(5):687–690.

Camurdan AD et al: Current stretched penile length: Cross-sectional study of 1040 healthy Turkish children aged 0 to 5 years. Urology 2007;70(3):572–575.

Chang HJ et al: The phenotype of 45,X/46,XY mosaicism: An analysis of 92 prenatally diagnosed cases. Am J Hum Genet 1990;46(1):156–167.

Conte FA, Grumbach MM: Disorders of sexual determination and differentiation, Chapter 15. In: DG Gardner, D Shoback (eds.). Greenspan's Basic and Clinical Endocrinology, 8th ed. McGraw-Hill, New York, 2007, pp. 562–610.

Daaboul J, Frader J: Ethics and the management of the patient with intersex: A middle way. J Pediatr Endocrinol Metab 2001; 14(9):1575–1583.

De Castro R et al: Phalloplasty and urethroplasty in children with penile agenesis: Preliminary report. J Urol 2007;177(3):1112–1116; discussion 1117.

Fallat ME, Donahoe PK: Intersex genetic anomalies with malignant potential. Curr Opin Pediatr 2006;18(3):305–311.

Farkas A et al: 1-Stage feminizing genitoplasty: 8 years of experience with 49 cases. J Urol 2001;165(6, Pt 2):2341–2346.

Griffin J et al: The androgen resistance syndromes: Steroid 5 alpha-reductase deficiency, testicular feminization and related disorders.

In: Scriver C (ed.) The Metabolic and Molecular Bases of Inherited Disease, Vol. 3. McGraw-Hill, Philadelphia, PA, 1995, pp. 2967–2998.

Gross R, Crigler R: Clitorectomy for sexual abnormalities, indications and techniques. J Surg 1966;59:300–308.

Hensle TW et al: Sexual function following bowel vaginoplasty. J Urol 2006;175(6):2283–2286.

Hughes IA: Congenital adrenal hyperplasia: A lifelong disorder. Horm Res 2007;68(Suppl 5):84–89.

Jirasek J et al: The relationship between the development of gonads and external genitals in human fetuses. Am J Obstet Gynecol 1968;101:830.

Kim KS et al: Expression of the androgen receptor and 5 alpha-reductase type 2 in the developing human fetal penis and urethra. Cell Tissue Res 2002;307(2):145–153.

Kurzrock E et al: Ontogeny of the male urethra: Theory of endodermal differentiation. Differentiation 1999;64:115–122.

Lee PA et al: Consensus statement on management of intersex disorders. International Consensus Conference on Intersex. Pediatrics 2006;118(2):e488–e500.

Levin HS: Tumors of the testis in intersex syndromes. Urol Clin North Am 2000;27(3):543–551, x.

Loscalzo ML: Turner syndrome. Pediatr Rev 2008;29(7):219–227.

McAleer IM, Kaplan GW: Is routine karyotyping necessary in the evaluation of hypospadias and cryptorchidism? J Urol 2001;165 (6, Pt 1):2029–2031; discussion 2031–2032.

Miller W: Prenatal treatment of congenital adrenal hyperplasia—A promising experimental therapy of unproven safety. Trends Endocrinol Metab 1998;9:290–293.

Morland I: Management of intersex. Lancet 2001;358(9298):2085–2086.

Oakes MB et al: Complete androgen insensitivity syndrome—A review. J Pediatr Adolesc Gynecol 2008;21(6):305–310.

Rey RA et al: Evaluation of gonadal function in 107 intersex patients by means of serum antimullerian hormone measurement. J Clin Endocrinol Metab 1999;84(2):627–631.

Rink RC, Cain MP: Urogenital mobilization for urogenital sinus repair. BJU Int 2008;102(9):1182–1197.

Samuelson ML, Baker LA: Autologous buccal mucosa vulvovaginoplasty for high urogenital sinus. J Pediatr Urol 2006;2(5):486–488.

Speiser PW: Prenatal and neonatal diagnosis and treatment of congenital adrenal hyperplasia. Horm Res 2007;68(Suppl 5): 90–92.

Thomas JC, Brock JW III: Vaginal substitution: Attempts to create the ideal replacement. J Urol 2007;178(5):1855–1859.

Wilson JD et al: The hormonal control of sexual development. Science 1981;211(4488):1278–1284.

Wilson JD et al: Steroid 5 alpha-reductase 2 deficiency. Endocr Rev 1993;14(5):577–593.

Wisniewski AB et al: Complete androgen insensitivity syndrome: Long-term medical, surgical, and psychosexual outcome. J Clin Endocrinol Metab 2000;85(8):2664–2669.

Wisniewski AB et al: Congenital micropenis: Long-term medical, surgical and psychosexual follow-up of individuals raised male or female. Horm Res 2001;56(1–2):3–11.

Woodhouse CR: Prospects for fertility in patients born with genitourinary anomalies. J Urol 2001;165(6, Pt 2):2354–2360.

Zucker KJ: Re: Androgen imprinting of the brain in animal models and humans with intersex disorders: Review and recommendations. J Urol 2003;169(6):2306; author reply 2306.

Male Infertility

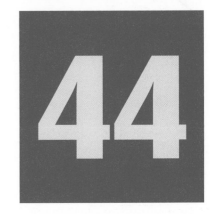

Thomas J. Walsh, MD, MS, & James F. Smith, MD, MS

Infertility is defined as the failure to conceive despite 1 year of regular unprotected intercourse. Approximately 15% of couples will experience infertility, and of these, 20% will have a male factor that is solely responsible; male factors will contribute in an additional 30% of cases. In general, male infertility is identified by abnormalities on a semen analysis; however, other issues can contribute to infertility despite normal semen.

The causes of male infertility are widely varied and are best evaluated by a urologist. Some causes of male infertility can be identified and reversed (or improved) with *specific* surgery or medication while other causes can be identified but not reversed. Occasionally, the underlying cause of infertility or an abnormal semen analysis cannot be identified, in which case it is termed idiopathic. These cases may be amenable to *empiric* treatment to improve the chances of conception. Before discussing the diagnosis and treatment of male infertility, a review of basic reproductive endocrinology, physiology, and anatomy is in order.

MALE REPRODUCTIVE PHYSIOLOGY

▶ The Hypothalamic–Pituitary–Gonadal Axis

The hypothalamic–pituitary–gonadal (HPG) axis plays a critical role in both the endocrine (testosterone production) and exocrine (sperm maturation) functions of the testes. Several endocrine concepts must be reviewed.

A. Hormone Classification (Figure 44–1)

Both peptide and steroid hormones are required for communication in the reproductive axis. Peptide hormones are small secretory proteins that bind receptors on the cell surface membrane and induce a series of intracellular events. Hormone signals are transduced by second-messenger pathways whose actions culminate in the phosphorylation of

various proteins that alter cell function. The key peptide hormones of the HPG axis are luteinizing hormone (LH) and follicle-stimulating hormone (FSH).

Steroid hormones are derived from cholesterol and, unlike peptide hormones, are not stored in secretory granules. As a result, steroid secretion is limited by the rate of production. Since they are lipophilic, steroid hormones are generally cell membrane permeable. In plasma, steroid hormones are largely bound to serum proteins, with only a small "free" component available to diffuse into the intracellular space and bind receptors. Once bound to an intracellular receptor, steroids are translocated to deoxyribonucleic acid (DNA) recognition sites within the nucleus where they act by regulating the transcription of target genes. The key steroid hormones of the HPG axis are testosterone (T) and estradiol (E2).

B. Feedback Loops

Normal endocrine and exocrine function of the testes depends on the orchestrated action of numerous hormones. Positive and negative feedback is the principal mechanism through which hormonal regulation occurs. By this mechanism, a hormone can regulate the synthesis and action of itself or of another hormone. Further coordination is provided by hormone action at multiple sites and through multiple responses. In the HPG axis, negative feedback is responsible for minimizing hormonal perturbations and maintaining homeostasis.

▶ Anatomy of the Hypothalamic–Pituitary–Gonadal Axis (Figure 44–2)

A. Hypothalamus

The hypothalamus receives and integrates neuronal input from the amygdala, thalamus, pons, retina, and cortex. The pulsatile secretion of gonadotropin-releasing hormone (GnRH) from the hypothalamus causes the cyclical secretion

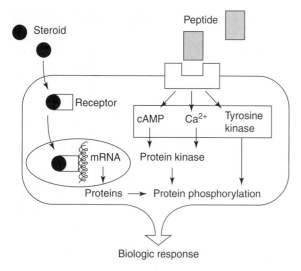

▲ Figure 44–1. Two kinds of hormone classes mediate intercellular communication in the reproductive hormone axis: peptide and steroid.

Table 44–1. Substances that modulate GnRH secretion.

GnRH modulator	Type of feedback	Examples
Opioids	Negative/inhibitory	β-Endorphin
Catecholamines	Variable	Dopamine
Peptide hormones	Negative/inhibitory	FSH, LH
Sex steroids	Negative/inhibitory	Testosterone
Prostaglandins	Positive/stimulatory	PGE$_2$

FSH, follicle-stimulating hormone; LH, luteinizing hormone; PGE$_2$, prostaglandin E$_2$.

of pituitary and gonadal hormones. It is anatomically linked to the pituitary gland by both a portal vascular system and neuronal pathways, thus avoiding the systemic circulation. GnRH is a 10-amino acid peptide secreted from neurons in the preoptic and arcuate nuclei of the hypothalamus. Once secreted into the pituitary portal circulation, GnRH has a half-life of approximately 5–7 minutes, almost entirely removed on the first pass through the pituitary where it stimulates the secretion of FSH and LH.

GnRH secretion is highly responsive to a variety of hormonal and pharmacologic inputs (Table 44–1) and may also be impacted by stress, exercise, and diet. The pulse frequency of GnRH secretion varies from once or twice in 24 hours to every hour and can be abolished by the administration of GnRH agonists.

B. Anterior Pituitary

The anterior pituitary gland is located within the sella turcica of skull and secretes a series of peptide hormones, including the gonadotropins. GnRH stimulates both production and release of FSH and LH by a calcium flux-dependent mechanism. The sensitivity of the pituitary gonadotrophs for GnRH varies with patient age and hormonal status.

LH and FSH are both glycoproteins composed of alpha and beta subunits, each coded by a separate gene. The alpha subunits of each hormone are identical and are similar to that of all other pituitary hormones; thus, their unique biologic activities are conferred by the beta subunits. Pulsatile secretion of LH varies from 8 to 16 pulses per day with variation in amplitude by one- to threefold. The pulse patterns reflect GnRH release and are regulated by androgens and estrogens through negative feedback. Pulsatile secretion of FSH occurs approximately every 1.5 hours and also demonstrates amplitude variation. Because FSH secretion is smaller in amplitude and has a longer serum half-life, its responsiveness to GnRH is more difficult to measure. In addition to its regulation by serum steroid hormones, FSH appears to have unique and independent responsiveness to the gonadal proteins inhibin and activin.

In the testis, LH stimulates steroidogenesis within Leydig cells by inducing the mitochondrial conversion of cholesterol to pregnenolone and testosterone. FSH binds to Sertoli cells and spermatogonial membranes within the testis and is the major stimulator of seminiferous tubule growth during

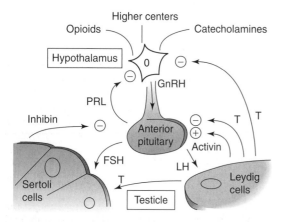

▲ Figure 44–2. Major components of the HPG axis and recognized hormone feedback pathways. HPG, hypothalamic–pituitary–gonadal; GnRH, gonadotropin-releasing hormone; PRL, prolactin; T, testosterone; FSH, follicle-stimulating hormone; LH, luteinizing hormone; +, positive feedback; –, negative feedback.

development and initiates spermatogenesis at puberty. In adults, the major physiologic role of FSH is to maintain quantitatively normal spermatogenesis. Both FSH and LH bind cell surface receptors that activate adenylate cyclase and cause increases in intracellular cyclic adenosine monophosphate (cAMP).

Prolactin is also produced and secreted by the anterior pituitary and can impact both the HPG axis and fertility. Prolactin is a large (23 kDa), globular protein that potentiates milk production and lactation during pregnancy. The role of prolactin in men is poorly understood, but it may increase the concentration of LH receptors on the Leydig cell and may help sustain high intratesticular testosterone levels. It may also potentiate the effects of androgens on the growth and secretions of male accessory sex glands. Normal prolactin levels may be important in the maintenance of libido. Elevated prolactin appears to abolish gonadotropin pulsatility by interfering with episodic GnRH release. Importantly, a markedly elevated prolactin may be evidence of a prolactin-secreting adenoma of the pituitary (prolactinoma) that requires further evaluation.

C. The Testis

Normal male reproduction requires that the testes have both endocrine (steroid production) and exocrine (sperm maturation and excretion) function. Both of these functions are under the control of the HPG axis. Steroidogenesis occurs in the interstitial compartment, where Leydig cells reside. Spermatogenesis occurs in the seminiferous tubules with the support of Sertoli cells.

1. Endocrine testis—Men normally produce approximately 5 g/day. Approximately 2% of testosterone circulates "free" in the serum and is considered the biologically active fraction. The remaining testosterone is bound to sex hormone–binding globulin (SHBG) and, to a slightly lesser extent, albumin within the blood. Several conditions can alter SHBG levels within the blood and thus changing the amount of free or bioavailable testosterone available for tissues. Elevated estrogens and thyroid hormone decrease plasma SHBG and increase the free testosterone fraction, whereas androgens, growth hormone, and obesity increase SHBG levels and decrease the active androgen fraction. Further, as men age, SHBG levels rise. Testosterone is a primary regulator of its own production through negative feedback on the HPG axis.

Testosterone is metabolized into two primary metabolites in target tissues: (1) dihydrotestosterone (DHT) by the enzyme 5-alpha-reductase and (2) estradiol by the enzyme aromatase. DHT is a more potent androgen than testosterone, and in many tissues, the conversion of testosterone to DHT is required for androgen action. While aromatase is present in many tissues, adipocytes play a significant role in the aromatization of testosterone to estradiol. While the mechanisms are still being elucidated, estradiol appears to have a pivotal role in the regulation of the HPG axis.

2. Exocrine testis—FSH acts primarily on Sertoli cells within the seminiferous tubules to induce the production of a number of proteins necessary for spermatogenesis, including androgen-binding protein, transferrin, lactate, ceruloplasmin, clusterin, plasminogen activator, prostaglandins, and several growth factors. Through these actions, seminiferous tubule growth is stimulated during development, and sperm production is initiated during puberty and maintained in adulthood.

3. Inhibin and activin—Inhibin is a 32-kDa protein derived from Sertoli cells that inhibits FSH release from the anterior pituitary. Inhibin production is stimulated by FSH and acts by negative feedback at the pituitary and hypothalamus. Activin, a peptide hormone with structural homology to transforming growth factor-beta, appears to stimulate FSH secretion through its action on the hypothalamus and pituitary. Activin receptors are found in a host of extragonadal tissues, suggesting that this hormone may have a variety of growth factor or regulatory roles in the body.

SPERMATOGENESIS

Spermatogenesis is a complex process during which primitive, multipotent stem cells divide to either renew themselves or produce daughter cells (mitosis) that further divide (meiosis) to become spermatozoa. These processes occur within the seminiferous tubules of the testis and 80–90% of testis volume is made up of the seminiferous tubules and germ cells at various developmental stages. Thus, it is not surprising that testicular hypotrophy and atrophy are strongly correlated to semen parameters.

▶ Sertoli Cells

Sertoli cells line the seminiferous tubules and are linked by tight junctions. These junctional complexes divide the seminiferous tubule space into basal (basement membrane) and adluminal (lumen) compartments and form the basis for the blood–testis barrier. As a result of this tight junction barrier, spermatogenesis occurs in an immunologically privileged site. Sanctuary from the immune system is critical given that spermatozoa are produced at puberty and therefore contain foreign antigens; immune recognition develops during the first year of life.

Sertoli cells foster spermatogenesis and participate in germ cell phagocytosis. FSH binding to high-affinity FSH receptors on Sertoli cells induces production and secretion of androgen-binding protein. Within the luminal fluid, this protein binds testosterone leading to levels 20–50 times that found in serum. Other regulatory effects of Sertoli cells include the production of inhibin and ligand-receptor complexes, such as c-*kit* and kit ligand.

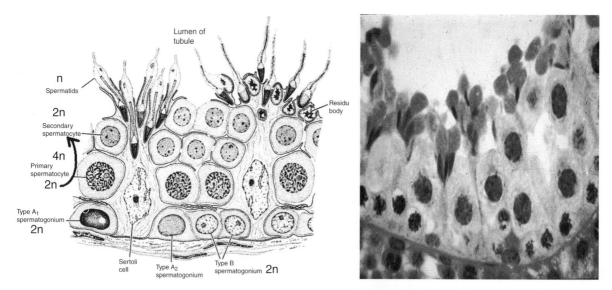

▲ Figure 44–3. Testicular germ cell maturation from spermatogonium to spermatid.

▶ Germ Cells

Germ cells are highly ordered within the cross section of the seminiferous tubules. Spermatogonia sit directly on the basement membrane and are followed by primary spermatocytes, secondary spermatocytes, and finally spermatids within the tubular lumen. Thirteen stages of germ cell differentiation have been identified in humans. The tight junctions of Sertoli cells support spermatogonia and early spermatocytes within the basal compartment while all subsequent stages of germ cell development occur within the adluminal compartment. Germ cells are staged by their histologic morphology; there are dark type A (Ad) and pale type A (Ap) and type B spermatogonia and preleptotene, leptotene, zygotene, and pachytene primary spermatocytes, secondary spermatocytes, and Sa, Sb, Sc, Sd_1, and Sd_2 spermatids (Figure 44–3).

Spermatogenesis is a cyclic process that involves the division of spermatogonial stem cells into elongated spermatids. Several individual cycles of spermatogenesis coexist within the germinal epithelium at a given time. In humans, an entire spermatogenic cycle requires approximately 60–80 days. Cohorts of developmentally similar germ cells are linked by cytoplasmic bridges and mature in unison. This cytoplasmic linkage of cells is organized in a spiral pattern along the seminiferous tubule and results in consistent and stable production of mature sperm.

▶ Genetics of Spermatogenesis

Mitosis is the process by which somatic cells are replicated to form genetically identical daughter cells. Meiosis is the process by which germ cells replicate. As the result of meiosis, daughter cells called *gametes* are formed which contain one half the genetic material of the parent cell and thus allow for reproduction. This fundamental difference in cell replication generates genetic diversity through natural selection.

A cell's life is divided into cycles that are each associated with different DNA replication activities. Only 5–10% of the cell cycle is spent in the mitotic phase (M), during which time genetic (DNA) and cellular division occur. Mitosis is a precise series of events that requires complete duplication of the genetic material (chromosomes), degeneration of the nuclear envelope, and equal division of chromosomes and cytoplasm into two daughter cells (Table 44–2). The difference between mitotic and meiotic replication is that in mitosis, a single DNA duplication is followed by one cell division; however, in meiosis, two-cell divisions take place to create

Table 44–2. Phases of the cell cycle and mitosis.

Mitotic phase	Cell cycle	Description of events
Interphase	G_1, S, G_2	DNA doubling occurs
Prophase	M	Nuclear envelope degenerates; spindle forms
Metaphase	M	Chromosomes align at cell equator
Anaphase	M	Duplicated chromosomes separate
Telophase	M	Chromosomes to poles, cytoplasm divides

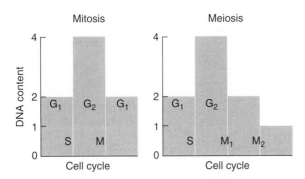

▲ **Figure 44–4.** Changes in nuclear DNA content with mitosis and meiosis. G, growth phase; S, DNA synthesis phase; M, mitotic phase.

four daughter cells (Figure 44–4). As a consequence, following meiosis, daughter cells (gametes) contain only half of the chromosome content of the parent cell and are said to be haploid (n) as opposed to diploid (2n). Other major differences between mitosis and meiosis are outlined in Table 44–3.

Stages of Spermatogenesis

From puberty onward, the process of spermatogenesis requires rapid and organized cell division, the likes of which are not seen in other cell lines of the human body. As a result, these highly specialized cells are produced in large quantities; up to 300 sperm per gram of testis tissue per second. Type B spermatogonia undergo mitosis to produce diploid primary spermatocytes (2n), which then duplicate their DNA during interphase. After the first meiotic division, each daughter cell contains a single partner of the homologous chromosome pair and are termed secondary spermatocytes (2n). During the second meiotic division, the chromatids separate at the centromere, yielding haploid spermatids (n).

Table 44–3. Essential differences between mitosis and meiosis.

Mitosis	Meiosis
Occurs in somatic cells	Occurs in sexual cycle cells
One cell division, two daughter cells	Two cell divisions, four daughter cells
Chromosome number maintained	Chromosome number halved
No pairing, chromosome homologs	Synapse of homologs, prophase I
No crossovers	>1 crossover per homolog pair
Centromeres divide, anaphase	Centromeres divide, anaphase II
Identical daughter genotype	Genetic variation in daughter cells

Spermiogenesis

Spermiogenesis is the process by which spermatids mature to become elongated spermatozoa within the basilar compartment of the seminiferous tubules. This process requires several weeks, and requires the following: (1) formation of the acrosome from the Golgi body, (2) formation of the flagellum from the centriole, (3) reorganization of the mitochondria around the midpiece, (4) extensive compaction of nuclear material, and (5) elimination of residual cytoplasm.

Many cellular elements contribute to the cellular morphologic changes during spermiogenesis, including chromosome structure, associated chromosomal proteins, the perinuclear cytoskeletal theca layer, the microtubules in the nucleus, subacrosomal actin, and Sertoli cell interactions. With completion of spermatid elongation, the Sertoli cell cytoplasm retracts around the developing sperm, stripping it of all unnecessary cytoplasm and extruding it into the tubule lumen. The mature sperm has remarkably little cytoplasm.

Sperm Maturation

Testicular spermatozoa have limited or no motility and are therefore incapable of naturally fertilizing an egg (which has significant clinical implications). They become functional only after traversing the epididymis and where further maturation occurs. Anatomically, the epididymis is divided into three regions: caput or head, corpus or body, and cauda or tail. While the process of epididymal sperm maturation is still being elucidated, it is clear that several changes occur in sperm as they transit through the epididymis. These changes include alterations in cell membrane polarity, membrane protein composition, immunoreactivity, phospholipid and fatty acid content, and adenylate cyclase activity. A sperm's transit time through the epididymis is approximately 10–15 days.

FERTILIZATION

During natural conception, fertilization generally occurs within the ampullary portion of the fallopian tubes. Ovulation typically occurs during the middle of the female menstrual cycle and can be predicted by timing, change in body temperature, chemical detection of the luteinizing hormone surge, or by changes in cervical mucus. This mucus becomes more abundant and watery, thereby facilitating the entry of sperm into the uterus and protecting it from the acidic vaginal environment. Once within the female reproductive tract, sperm undergo physiologic changes referred to as capacitation.

Upon making contact with the egg, sperm undergo hyperactivation, characterized by profound changes in motility (large, lashing motions of the sperm tail). Lytic enzymes are released from the acrosome to allow penetration of the outer surface of the egg. Upon completion of the acrosome reaction, contact between sperm and egg is mediated by specific ligands and receptors on the surface of each gamete.

Once a single sperm enters the zona pellucida of the ovum, it becomes impenetrable to additional sperm. Upon fertilization, the egg resumes meiosis and forms a metaphase II spindle. The sperm centriole, contained within the midpiece, is crucial for early spindle formation and ongoing embryogenesis.

DIAGNOSIS OF MALE INFERTILITY

The purpose of the male infertility evaluation is to (1) identify and correct the reversible causes of male infertility with the goal of allowing a couple to conceive through intercourse, or with the least amount of technology; (2) identify irreversible conditions that may be amenable to treatment with assisted reproductive technology (ART) using the male partner's sperm; (3) identify irreversible conditions in which the man's sperm are not obtainable, in which case the couple may consider donated sperm or adoption; (4) identify medical diseases that may be associated with infertility and require treatment; and (5) identify specific genetic causes of infertility that may be transmitted to and impact offspring. Given that a male factor can be the cause of infertility in 30–40% of couples and is a contributing factor in 50% of cases, it is important to evaluate both partners in parallel. A complete urologic evaluation is important because male infertility may be the presenting symptom of otherwise occult but significant systemic disease. A complete evaluation must be comprehensive.

HISTORY

A man's evaluation begins with a thorough reproductive, medical, and surgical history (Table 44–4). Important components of this history include (1) duration of infertility, coital timing and frequency, and sexual health; (2) prior paternity or fertility treatments; (3) childhood illnesses and development; (4) medical illnesses, prior infections, and medications; (5) prior surgeries or traumas; and (6) exposure to potential gonadal toxins, such as heat, radiation, chemical solvents, or pesticides.

A sexual history is important as many couples do not know how to precisely time intercourse to achieve a pregnancy. Following intercourse, sperm reside within the cervical mucus and crypts for 1–2 days and can survive longer; thus, an appropriate frequency of intercourse is every 2 days. Water-based lubricants such as K-Y Jelly, most skin lotions, and saliva can reduce sperm motility in vitro and should be avoided. If needed, acceptable lubricants include vegetable, safflower, and peanut oils as well as egg whites.

A general medical and surgical history is also important. Fever or acute infection can decrease testis function and semen quality. Given that spermatogenesis generally requires

Table 44–4. Components of the infertility history.

Fertility history
  Previous pregnancies (all partners)
  Duration of infertility
  Previous infertility treatments
  Female evaluation

Sexual history
  Erections
  Timing and frequency
  Lubricants

Developmental history
  Cryptorchidism
  Childhood cancer/treatment
  Mumps orchitis
  Pubertal development

Medical history
  Fevers
  Systemic illness—diabetes, cancer, infection
  Genetic diseases—cystic fibrosis, Klinefelter syndrome

Surgical history
  Orchidopexy, cryptorchidism
  Herniorrhaphy
  Trauma, torsion
  Pelvic, bladder, or retroperitoneal surgery
  Transurethral resection for benign prostatic hyperplasia
  Pubertal onset

Family history
  Cryptorchidism
  Midline defects (Kartagener syndrome)
  Hypospadias
  Exposure to diethylstilbestrol
  Other rare syndromes—prune belly, etc.

Medications
  Testosterone
  Nitrofurantoin
  Cimetidine
  Sulfasalazine
  Spironolactone
  Alpha-blockers

Social history
  Ethanol
  Smoking/tobacco
  Cocaine
  Anabolic steroids

Occupational history
  Exposure to ionizing radiation
  Chronic heat exposure (saunas)
  Aniline dyes
  Pesticides
  Heavy metals (lead)

at least 60 days to complete, the impact of such insults may not be observable in the semen until 2 months after the event. Surgical procedures on the bladder, retroperitoneum, or pelvis can lead to infertility by causing ejaculatory dysfunction due to damage to the bladder neck, sympathetic nerves, or pelvic nerve plexus, respectively. Hernia surgery can result in obstruction of the vas deferens in 1% of cases; this incidence may be rising because of the recent increased use of highly inflammatory mesh patches.

Childhood diseases can have a significant impact on fertility. Severe unilateral orchitis occurs in approximately one-third of postpubertal mumps infections and bilateral orchitis in 10%. Mumps orchitis likely causes pressure necrosis of testis tissue due to severe edema with the later development of testis atrophy. Cryptorchidism is associated with decreased sperm production. This is true for both unilateral and bilateral cases. Longitudinal studies of affected boys have shown that abnormally low sperm counts can be found in 30% of men with unilateral cryptorchidism and 50% of men with bilateral undescended testes. While difficult to study from an epidemiologic standpoint, cryptorchidism appears to result in a higher risk of infertility. Similar to testicular cancer risk, early orchidopexy may reduce the risk of spermatogenic failure.

Exposure and medication histories are very relevant to fertility. Decreased sperm counts have been demonstrated in workers exposed to specific pesticides, which may alter normal testosterone/estrogen hormonal balance. Exposure to ionizing radiation can cause temporary reductions in sperm production with as little as 10 cGy and more permanent or severe reductions with higher doses. Several medications (Table 44–5) and ingestants such as tobacco, cocaine, and marijuana have all been implicated as gonadotoxins. The effects of these agents may be reversible on withdrawal. Anabolic steroids, often taken to increase muscle mass and development, act as contraceptives by inhibiting the pituitary–gonadal axis. Routine exposure to moist heat by use of hot tubs or saunas should be discouraged, as these activities can elevate intratesticular temperature and impair

Table 44–5. Medications associated with impaired ejaculation.

| Antihypertensive agents (Thiazides) |
| Alpha-adrenergic blockers (Prazosin, Phentolamine) |
| Antipsychotic agents |
| Mellaril (thioridazine) |
| Haldol (haloperidol) |
| Librium |
| Antidepressants |
| Imipramine |
| Amitriptyline |

sperm production. Other characteristics associated with impaired fertility include obesity, electromagnetic radiation exposure (eg, significant exposure to high-voltage power lines, cell phones in the "on" position), occupational status (eg, dry cleaners, painters, farm workers), and job-related or other psychological stress.

The family and developmental histories may also provide clues to the infertility etiology. A family history of cystic fibrosis (CF), a condition associated with congenital absence of the vas deferens (CAVD), or intersex conditions is important. The existence of siblings with fertility problems may suggest that a Y chromosome microdeletion or a cytogenetic (karyotype) abnormality is present in the family. A history of delayed onset of puberty could suggest Kallmann or Klinefelter syndrome. A history of recurrent respiratory tract infections may suggest a ciliary defect characteristic of the immotile cilia syndromes. It is important to remember that reproductive technologies enable most men afflicted with such conditions to become fathers and therefore allow for the perpetuation of genetic abnormalities that may not be normally sustained.

PHYSICAL EXAMINATION

A complete examination of the infertile male is important to identify general health issues associated with infertility. For example, the patient should be adequately virilized; signs of decreased body hair or gynecomastia may suggest androgen deficiency.

The scrotal contents should be carefully palpated with the patient standing. As it is often psychologically uncomfortable for young men to be examined, one helpful hint is to make the examination as efficient and matter of fact as possible. Two features should be noted about the testis: size and consistency. Size is assessed by measuring the long axis and width; as an alternative, an orchidometer can be placed next to the testis for volume determination (Figure 44–5). Standard values of testis size have been reported for normal men and include a mean testis length of 4.6 cm (range, 3.6–5.5 cm), a mean width of 2.6 cm (range, 2.1–3.2 cm), and a mean volume of 18.6 mL (± 4.6 mL) (Figure 44–6). Consistency is more difficult to assess but can be described as firm (normal) or soft (abnormal). Testes that are smaller than normal volume are termed hypotrophic, whereas those that are softer than normal are termed atrophic. Both conditions suggest impaired spermatogenesis.

The peritesticular area should also be examined. Irregularities of the epididymis, located posterior-lateral to the testis, include induration, tenderness, or cysts. The presence or absence of the scrotal vas deferens is critical to observe, as 2% of infertile men may present with CAVD.

Engorgement of the pampiniform plexus of veins in the scrotum is indicative of a varicocele. Asymmetry of the spermatic cords is the usual initial observation, followed by the feeling of a "bag of worms" when retrograde blood flow

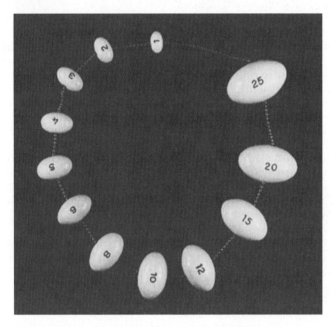

▲ **Figure 44–5.** Prader orchidometer for measuring testicular volume. (Reproduced, with permission, from McClure RD: Endocrine investigation and therapy. Urol Clin North Am 1987;14:471.)

through the pampiniform veins occurs with a Valsalva maneuver. Varicoceles are usually found on the left side (90%) and are commonly associated with atrophy of the left testis. A discrepancy in testis size between the right and left sides should alert the clinician to this possibility.

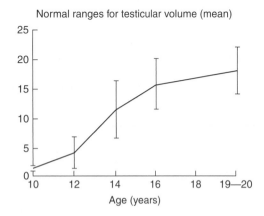

▲ **Figure 44–6.** Normal values for testicular volume in relation to age. (Redrawn and reproduced, with permission, from Zachman M et al: Testicular volume during adolescence: Cross-sectional and longitudinal studies. Helv Paediatr Acta 1974;29:61; and McClure RD: Endocrine investigation and therapy. Urol Clin North Am 1987;14:471.)

Prostate or penile abnormalities should also be noted. Penile abnormalities such as hypospadias, abnormal curvature, or phimosis could result in inadequate delivery of semen to the upper vaginal vault during intercourse. Prostatic infection may be detected by the finding of a boggy, tender prostate on rectal examination. Prostate cancer, often suspected with unusual firmness or a nodule within the prostate, can occasionally be diagnosed in infertile men. Enlarged seminal vesicles, indicative of ejaculatory duct obstruction (EDO), may also be palpable on rectal examination.

LABORATORY TESTING

Laboratory testing is an important part of the male infertility evaluation.

▶ Semen Analysis

A carefully performed semen analysis is the primary source of information on sperm production and reproductive tract patency. However, it is not a measure of fertility. An abnormal semen analysis simply suggests the likelihood of decreased fertility. Studies have established that there are certain limits of adequacy below which it may be difficult to initiate a pregnancy. These semen analysis values were identified by the World Health Organization (2009) and are considered the minimum criteria for "normal" semen quality (Table 44–6). It is statistically more difficult to achieve a pregnancy if a

Table 44–6. Semen analysis—minimal standards of adequacy.

Ejaculate volume	>1.5 mL
Sperm concentration	$>215 \times 10^6$ sperm/mL
Motility	≥40%
Progressive motility	≥30%
Morphology	>4% morphologically normal forms

Note: No agglutination (clumping), white cells, or increased viscosity.

semen parameter falls below any of those listed. Of these semen variables, the count and motility appear to correlate best with fertility.

A. Semen Collection

Semen quality can vary widely in a normal individual from day to day, and semen analysis results are dependent on collection technique. For example, the period of sexual abstinence before sample collection is a large source of variability. With each day of abstinence (up to 1 week), semen volume can rise by up to 0.4 mL, and sperm concentration can increase by 10–15 million/mL. Sperm motility tends to fall when the abstinence period is longer than 5 days. For this reason, it is recommended that semen be collected after 48–72 hours of sexual abstinence.

To establish a baseline of semen quality, at least two semen samples are needed. Semen should be collected by self-stimulation; by coitus interruptus (less ideal); or with a special, nonspermicidal condom into a clean glass or plastic container. Because sperm motility decreases after ejaculation, the specimen should be analyzed within 1 hour of procurement. During transit, the specimen should be kept at body temperature.

B. Physical Characteristics and Measured Variables

Fresh semen is a coagulum that liquefies 15–30 minutes after ejaculation. Ejaculate volume should be at least 1.5 mL, as smaller volumes may not sufficiently buffer against vaginal acidity. Low ejaculate volume may indicate retrograde ejaculation, EDO, incomplete collection, or androgen deficiency. Sperm concentration should be >20 million sperm/mL. Sperm motility is assessed in two ways: the fraction of sperm that are moving and the quality of sperm movement (how fast, how straight they swim).

Sperm cytology or morphology is another measure of semen quality. By assessing the exact dimensions and shape characteristics of the sperm head, midpiece, and tail, sperm can be classified as "normal" or not. In the strictest classification system (Kruger morphology), only 14% of sperm in the

ejaculate are normal looking. In fact, this number correlates with the success of egg fertilization in vitro and thus is ascribed real clinical significance. In addition, sperm morphology is a sensitive indicator of overall testicular health, because these characteristics are determined during spermatogenesis. The role of sperm morphology in the male infertility evaluation is to complement other information and to better estimate the chances of fertility.

C. Computer-Assisted Semen Analysis

In an effort to remove the subjective variables inherent in the manually performed semen analysis, computer-aided semen analyses (CASAs) couple video technology with digitalization and microchip processing to categorize sperm features by algorithms. Although the technology is promising, when manual semen analyses are compared with CASA on identical specimens, CASA can overestimate sperm counts by 30% with high levels of contaminating cells such as immature sperm or leukocytes. In addition, at high sperm concentrations, motility can be underestimated with CASA. CASA has accepted value in the research setting and in some clinical laboratories.

D. Semen Leukocyte Analysis

White blood cells (leukocytes) are present in all ejaculates and play important roles in immune surveillance and clearance of abnormal sperm. Leukocytospermia or pyospermia, an increase in leukocytes in the ejaculate, is defined as $>1 \times 10^6$ leukocytes/mL semen but is not a significant cause of male subfertility and its treatment is debated. The prevalence of leukocytospermia ranges from 2.8% to 23% of infertile men. In general, neutrophils predominate among inflammatory cells (Table 44–7). This condition is detected by a variety of diagnostic assays, including differential stains (eg, Papanicolaou), peroxidase stain that detects the peroxidase enzyme in neutrophils, and immunocytology.

Antisperm antibodies (ASAs) can be found in three locations: serum, seminal plasma, and sperm bound. Among these, sperm-bound antibodies are the most relevant. The antibody classes that appear to be clinically relevant include

Table 44–7. Cells involved in leukocytospermia.

Cell type	Relative abundance
Neutrophils	++++
Monocyte/macrophage	+
T-helper lymphocytes	+
T-suppressor lymphocytes	++
B lymphocytes	+

Table 44–8. Frequency of semen analysis findings in infertile men.

	Percent
All normal	55
Isolated abnormal	37
Low motility	26
Low count	8
Volume	2
Morphology	1
No sperm	8

immunoglobulin G (IgG) and IgA. IgG antibody is derived from local production and from transudation from the bloodstream (1%). IgA is thought to be purely locally derived.

▶ Adjunctive Semen Tests: Seminal Fructose and Postejaculate Urinalysis

Fructose is a carbohydrate that is secreted in high concentration from the seminal vesicles and is normally present in the ejaculate. When absent, seminal vesicle agenesis or obstruction may exist. Seminal fructose testing is indicated in men with low ejaculate volumes and no sperm. A postejaculate urinalysis inspects the first voided urine after ejaculation for the presence of sperm. If sperm is identified in the urine, a diagnosis of retrograde ejaculation is made. This test is indicated when the ejaculate volume is below normal (Table 44–8).

▶ Antisperm Antibody Test

The testis is an immunologically privileged site due to the blood–testis barrier formed by the sertoli cell tight junctions. Autoimmune infertility may result when the blood–testis barrier is broken and the body is exposed to sperm antigens. Trauma to the testis and vasectomy are two common ways in which this occurs, giving rise to ASAs. ASA may be associated with impaired sperm transport through the reproductive tract or impairment in egg fertilization. An assay for ASA should be considered when (1) semen analyses show persistent sperm agglutination or clumping; (2) low sperm motility with history of testis injury or surgery; (3) idiopathic leukocytospermia; or (4) unexplained infertility.

▶ Hypoosmotic Swelling Test

Motility is the most commonly used measure of a sperm's viability. Studies have suggested, however, that some nonmotile sperm may still be viable. Indeed, there are clinical conditions, such as immotile-cilia syndrome or testicular sperm, in which there may be immotile but otherwise healthy, viable sperm. Given that these sperm may be used in conjunction with intracytoplasmic sperm injection (ICSI) to form healthy embryos, it is clinically important that they are identifiable. Cell viability can be evaluated noninvasively by using the physiologic principle of hypoosmotic swelling. Viable cells with functional membranes swell when placed in a hypoosmotic environment. This response is easily observed in sperm as tail coiling generally accompanies head swelling. This sperm test is indicated in cases of complete absence of sperm motility.

▶ Sperm Penetration Assay

It is possible to measure the ability of human sperm to penetrate a specially prepared hamster egg in the laboratory setting. The hamster egg allows interspecies fertilization but no further development. This form of bioassay can give important information about the ability of sperm to undergo the capacitation process as well as penetrate and fertilize the egg. Infertile sperm would be expected to penetrate and fertilize a lower fraction of eggs than normal sperm. The indications for the diagnostic sperm penetration assay (SPA) are limited to situations in which functional information about sperm is needed, that is, to further evaluate couples with unexplained infertility and to help couples decide whether intrauterine insemination (IUI) (good SPA result) or in vitro fertilization (IVF) and micromanipulation (poor SPA result) is the appropriate next treatment.

▶ Sperm DNA Fragmentation Assay

There is growing evidence that the integrity of sperm DNA is important for male fertility. Double- and single-stranded breaks in sperm DNA can be measured by several methods, including the COMET and TUNEL assays with or without the use of flow cytometry. These tests assess the degree of DNA fragmentation that occurs after chemically stressing the sperm DNA–chromatin complex, and can indirectly reflect the quality of sperm DNA–chromatin complex and can indirectly reflect the quality of sperm DNA integrity. Abnormally fragmented sperm DNA rarely occurs in fertile men, but can be found in a larger percentage of infertile men with otherwise normal semen analyses. This test can detect infertility that is missed on a conventional semen analysis. Often reversible, causes of DNA fragmentation include tobacco use, medical disease, hyperthermia, air pollution, infections, and varicocele.

▶ Hormone Assessment

Evaluation of the pituitary–gonadal axis provides valuable information on the state of sperm production. Furthermore,

Table 44-9. Characteristic endocrine profiles in infertile men.

Condition	T	FSH	LH	PRL
Normal	NL	NL	NL	NL
Primary testis failure	Low	High	NL/High	NL
Hypogonadotropic hypogonadism	Low	Low	Low	NL
Hyperprolactinemia	Low	Low/NL	Low	High
Androgen resistance	High	High	High	NL

T, testosterone; FSH, follicle-stimulating hormone; LH, luteinizing hormone; PRL, prolactin; NL, normal.

abnormal function of the HPG axis can be an underlying cause of poor sperm production and infertility (hyperprolactinemia, gonadotropin deficiency, congenital adrenal hyperplasia). In general, FSH and testosterone should be measured in infertile men with sperm concentrations of $<10 \times 10^6$ sperm/mL. Testosterone is a measure of overall endocrine balance and likely plays a critical role in spermatogenesis. In most cases, FSH reflects the state of sperm production: when spermatogenesis is impaired at the testicular level, FSH should be elevated. This combination of tests will detect most (99%) endocrine abnormalities. Serum LH and prolactin levels may be obtained if testosterone and FSH are abnormal. In the setting of low testosterone, free testosterone should be assessed. Given the role of estradiol in regulating the HPG axis, it too should be assessed if there is evidence of poor virilization or obesity. Thyroid hormone, liver function, and other organ-specific tests should be obtained if there is clinical evidence of active disease, as uncontrolled systemic illness can affect sperm production. The common patterns of hormonal disorders observed in infertility are given in Table 44-9.

With relatively normal spermatogenesis, low levels of plasma LH and FSH have no clinical meaning; likewise, an isolated low LH with normal testosterone is not significant. Additional indications for hormone evaluation of infertile men include impaired sexual function (low libido, erectile dysfunction) and findings suggestive of a specific endocrinopathy (eg, thyroid). On initial testing, approximately 10% of infertile men will have an abnormal hormone level, with clinically significant endocrinopathies occurring in 2% of men.

GENETIC TESTS

▶ Chromosomal Studies

Subtle genetic abnormalities can present as male infertility. It is estimated that between 2% and 15% of infertile men with azoospermia (no sperm count) or severe oligospermia

(low sperm counts) will harbor a chromosomal abnormality on either the sex chromosomes or autosomes. A blood test for cytogenetic analysis (karyotype) can determine if such a genetic anomaly is present. Patients at risk for abnormal cytogenetic findings include men with small, atrophic testes; elevated FSH values; and azoospermia. Klinefelter syndrome (XXY) is the most frequently detected sex chromosomal abnormality among infertile men (Figure 44-7).

▶ Cystic Fibrosis Mutation Testing

A blood test is indicated for infertile men who present with CF or the much more subtle condition, CAVD. Similar genetic mutations are found in both patients, although the latter group is generally considered to have an atypical form of CF, in which the scrotal vas deferens is nonpalpable. Approximately 80% of men without palpable vasa will harbor a CF gene mutation. Recent data also indicate that azoospermic men with idiopathic obstruction and men with a clinical triad of chronic sinusitis, bronchiectasis, and obstructive azoospermia (OA) (Young syndrome) may be at higher risk for CF gene mutations.

▶ Y Chromosome Microdeletion Analysis

As many as 7% of men with oligospermia and 15% of men with azoospermia have small, underlying deletions in one or more gene regions on the long arm of the Y chromosome (Yq). Several regions of the Y chromosome have been implicated in spermatogenic failure, identified as *AZFa, b,* and *c* (Figure 44-8). Deletion of the *DAZ* (deleted in azoospermia) gene in the *AZFc* region is the most commonly observed microdeletion in infertile men. Fertility is possible in most men with these deletions with IVF and micromanipulation of sperm. A polymerase chain reaction–based blood test can examine the Y chromosome from peripheral leukocytes for these gene deletions and is recommended for men with low or no sperm counts and small, atrophic testes.

ADJUNCTIVE TESTS

▶ Urinalysis

A urinalysis is a simple test that can be performed during the initial office visit. It may indicate the presence of infection, hematuria, glucosuria, or renal disease, and as such may suggest anatomic or medical problems within the urinary tract.

▶ Semen Culture

Seminal fluid that passes through the urethra is routinely contaminated with bacteria. This can make the interpretation of semen culture difficult. Semen cultures should only be obtained in selected situations and approximately 13% of

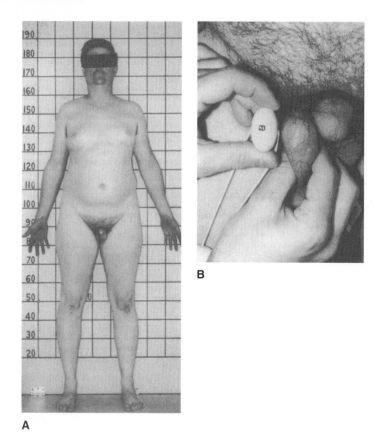

▲ **Figure 44–7.** Klinefelter syndrome. **A:** Note the eunuchoid habitus, female escutcheon, gynecomastia, and lack of temporal balding. **B:** Characteristic firm, small testes. (Reproduced, with permission, from McClure RD: Endocrine investigation and therapy. Urol Clin North Am 1987;14:471.)

infertile men will have positive semen cultures; the relationship between bacterial cultures and infertility is controversial. Semen cultures should be considered when there is evidence of infection, including (1) a history of genital tract infection, (2) abnormal expressed prostatic secretion, (3) the presence of >1000 pathogenic bacteria per milliliter of semen, and (4) the presence of $>1 \times 10^6$ leukocytes/mL of semen (pyospermia).

The agents most commonly responsible for male genital tract infections are listed in Table 44–10. Gonorrhea is the most common infection. About 10–25% of chlamydial infections may be asymptomatic. *Trichomonas vaginalis* is a protozoan parasite responsible for 1–5% of nongonococcal infections; it is usually symptomatic. *Ureaplasma urealyticum* is a common inhabitant of the urethra in sexually active men (30–50% of normal men) and is responsible for one-fourth of all cases of nongonococcal infections. *Escherichia coli* infections are relatively uncommon in young men and are usually symptomatic. Mycoplasmas are aerobic bacteria that

are known to colonize the male reproductive tract. Rarer but possible causes of infection include anaerobic bacteria and tuberculosis.

▶ Radiologic Testing

A. Scrotal Ultrasound

High-frequency ultrasound of the scrotum is commonly performed for the evaluation of testicular, paratesticular, and scrotal lesions that cannot be completely evaluated on physical examination. Scrotal ultrasound is indicated in men who have a hydrocele, whereby the testis is nonpalpable. Any abnormality of the peritesticular region should also undergo a scrotal ultrasound to determine its characteristics or origin.

Scrotal color Doppler ultrasonography has been used to investigate varicoceles (Figure 44–9). By combining measurements of blood-flow patterns (the presence of retrograde venous flow) and vein size, both physiologic and anatomic information can be obtained to confirm the diagnosis.

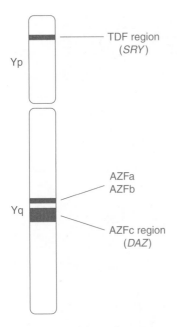

▲ **Figure 44–8.** Regions of the Y chromosome that have been associated with male infertility include azoospermia factor (AZF) regions *a, b,* and *c.* The *AZFc* region contains the *DAZ* gene, one of the few true infertility genes isolated to date. TDF, testis-determining factor.

Although diagnostic criteria that define a varicocele vary widely, a pampiniform venous diameter of >3 mm is considered abnormal. Retrograde blood flow through the veins with a Valsalva maneuver is a key radiologic feature of a varicocele.

B. Venography

Historically, venography has been described as the most sensitive way to diagnose varicoceles. Although found by palpation in approximately 30–40% of subfertile men, varicoceles can be detected by venography in 70% of patients. This test is

Table 44–10. Most common organisms in male genital infection.

Neisseria gonorrhoeae	Cytomegalovirus
Chlamydia trachomatis	Herpes simplex II
Trichomonas vaginalis	Human papilloma virus
Ureaplasma urealyticum	Epstein–Barr virus
Escherichia coli (other gram-negative bacilli)	Hepatitis B virus
Mycoplasma hominis	Human immunodeficiency virus

invasive, expensive, and technician dependent; at present, its main indications are to guide simultaneous percutaneous varicocele embolization and it is virtually never utilized as a stand-alone diagnostic test. The test is performed through percutaneous canalization of the internal jugular vein or common femoral vein. Venographically, a varicocele is defined by a Valsalva-induced retrograde flow, of contrast material from the renal vein into the scrotal pampiniform plexus.

C. Transrectal Ultrasound

High-frequency (5–7 mHz) transrectal ultrasound (TRUS) can provide good anatomic detail of the prostate, seminal vesicles, and ejaculatory ducts. Dilation of the seminal vesicles (>1.5 cm in width) or ejaculatory ducts (>2.3 mm) in association with a cyst, calcification, or stones along the duct is highly suggestive of obstruction (Figure 44–10). Among infertile men, TRUS is indicated in cases of low ejaculate volume (<1.5 mL) not explained by retrograde ejaculation or abnormal hormones.

D. Computed Tomography Scan or Magnetic Resonance Imaging of the Pelvis

The imaging techniques of computed tomography (CT) and magnetic resonance imaging (MRI) can further define reproductive tract anatomy. However, since the advent of TRUS, these studies have relatively few indications. They include evaluation of a patient with a solitary right varicocele, which may be associated with retroperitoneal pathology, and evaluation of the nonpalpable testis.

▶ Testis Biopsy and Vasography

The diagnostic testis biopsy is an important adjunct to the infertility evaluation as it provides direct information regarding the state of spermatogenesis. Most commonly, the technique involves a small, open incision in the scrotal wall and testis tunica albuginea under local or general anesthesia. A small sample of testis tissue is removed, fixed in formalin or Bouin's solution, and examined histologically. Abnormalities of seminiferous tubule architecture and cellular composition are then categorized into several patterns. This procedure is generally reserved for azoospermic men, in whom it may be difficult to distinguish between a failure of sperm production (nonobstructive azoospermia [NOA]) and obstruction within the reproductive tract ducts (OA). A testis biopsy allows delineation between these conditions and can guide further treatment options in azoospermic men (Figure 44–11).

In azoospermic men with normal ejaculate volume and evidence of normal spermatogenesis by testis biopsy, formal investigation of the reproductive tract to identify the site of obstruction is warranted. A vasogram involves the injection of contrast media into the vas deferens toward

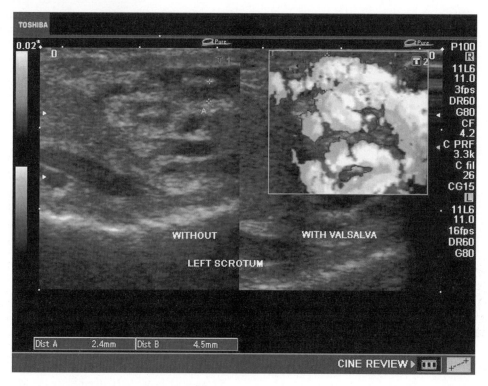

▲ **Figure 44–9.** Scrotal ultrasound. Varicoceles are imaged as tubular echo-free structures. (Reproduced, with permission, from McClure RD, Hricak H: Scrotal ultrasound in the infertile male. Detection of subclinical unilateral and bilateral varicoceles. J Urol 1986;135:711.)

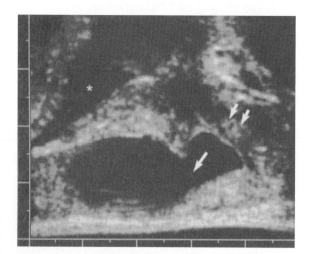

▲ **Figure 44–10.** Transrectal ultrasonography (sagittal view) in a man with low ejaculate volume and low sperm counts and motility. Ejaculatory duct cyst (*white arrow*); urethra (*double white arrows*); bladder (*asterisk*).

the bladder from the scrotum. In plain film radiographs or fluoroscopy, contrast material can delineate the proximal vas deferens, seminal vesicle, and ejaculatory duct anatomy and determine whether obstruction is present. Similar information, albeit without anatomic detail, can be obtained with chromotubation, whereby dye (indigo carmine, methylene blue) is injected while the ejaculatory ducts are visualized by cystourethroscopy. Sampling of vasal fluid during the same procedure can also determine whether sperm exist within the testicular end of the vas deferens. Vasal sperm presence implies that there is no obstruction in the testis or epididymis. With this information, the site of obstruction can be accurately determined and potentially surgically corrected.

Biopsy is generally not indicated for oligospermia unless it is severe or alternates with azoospermia (cryptozoospermia). While a unilateral testis biopsy is usually sufficient, the finding of asymmetric testes warrants bilateral biopsies. This situation may reflect a unilateral unobstructed failing testis paired with a normal obstructed testis. Historically, testis biopsy has been proposed to identify patients at high risk for intratubular germ cell neoplasia. This premalignant

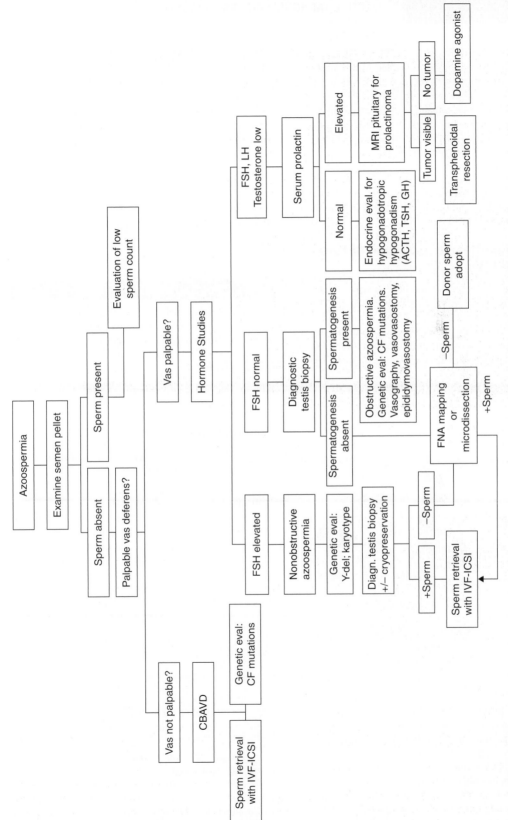

▲ **Figure 44–11.** Algorithm for evaluation of azoospermia or no sperm in the ejaculate. CBAVD, congenital bilateral absence of the vas deferens; FSH, follicle-stimulating hormone; LH, luteinizing hormone; MRI, magnetic resonance imaging; CF, cystic fibrosis; ACTH, adrenocorticotrophic hormone; TSH, thyroid-stimulating hormone; GH, growth hormone; FNA, fine-needle aspiration. (Adapted with permission from Turek PJ. Practical approach to the diagnosis and management of male infertility. Nat Clin Pract Urol 2005;2:1.)

condition exists in 5% of men with a contralateral germ cell tumor of the testis and is more prevalent in infertile men than in fertile men. Importantly, while there is strong evidence that infertile men have higher risk for testicular cancer, their absolute risk for cancer remains low and most cancers will present with a painless testicular mass. In general, the purpose of biopsy is for identifying the presence or absence of sperm, and not for cancer diagnosis.

Testis biopsy may also be performed to obtain sperm for use with ART. Testicular sperm that are harvested by biopsy are now routinely used to help men with severe male-factor infertility to achieve fatherhood. Sperm retrieval techniques are discussed in subsequent sections.

▶ Multisite Fine-Needle Aspiration of Testes (Figure 44–12)

Testicular sperm is used with IVF and ICSI to achieve pregnancies; however, there is a failure to obtain sperm in 25–50% of men with spermatogenic failure. When testis biopsies fail to retrieve sperm, IVF cycles are canceled at great emotional and financial cost. To minimize the chance of failed sperm retrieval, percutaneous fine-needle aspiration (FNA) of the testis has

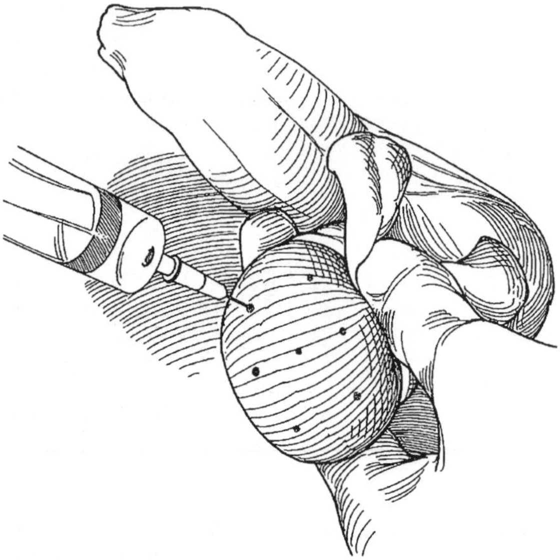

▲ **Figure 44–12.** Technique of percutaneous fine-needle aspiration "mapping" for sperm in the testis. Cytologic samples are taken from various systematically sampled areas of the testis, guided by marks on the scrotum. (Reproduced, with permission, from Turek PJ, Cha I, Ljung BM: Systematic fine needle aspiration of the testis: Correlation to biopsy and the results of organ "mapping" for mature sperm in azoospermic men. Urology 1997;49:743.)

been described. This technique can accurately diagnose and classify the severity of disease in men with azoospermia or severe oligospermia. Cytological analysis with FNA has a high correlation with histological specimens from open testicular biopsies. In some men, FNA may be more sensitive at detecting a heterogenous pattern of intratesticular spermatogenesis.

Similar to a testis biopsy, FNA is performed under local anesthesia. Percutaneously aspirated (with a 23G needle) seminiferous tubules from various locations in the testis are smeared on a slide, fixed, stained, and read by an experienced andrologist or cytopathologist for the presence of sperm. The information gained from this technique can fully inform patients of their chances of subsequent sperm retrieval for IVF and ICSI.

CAUSES OF MALE INFERTILITY

The causes underlying male infertility are numerous and best categorized by effects at one or more of the following levels: pretesticular, testicular, and posttesticular.

PRETESTICULAR

Conditions that cause infertility that act at the pretesticular level tend to be hormonal in nature (Table 44–11).

▶ Hypothalamic Disease

A. Gonadotropin Deficiency (Kallmann Syndrome)

Kallmann syndrome (1:30,000) is characterized by central hypogonadism, delayed in puberty, and infertility. Other clinical features include anosmia, small testes and occasionally renal agenesis, bimanual synkinesia, cleft lip, and dental agenesis. When anosmia is not present, the condition is termed

Table 44–11. Pretesticular causes of infertility.

Hypothalamic disease
  Gonadotropin deficiency (Kallmann syndrome)
  Isolated LH deficiency ("fertile eunuch")
  Isolated FSH deficiency
  Congenital hypogonadotrophic syndromes
Pituitary disease
  Pituitary insufficiency (tumors, infiltrative processes, operation, radiation, deposits)
  Hyperprolactinemia
  Exogenous hormones (estrogen-androgen excess, glucocorticoid excess, hyper- and hypothyroidism)
  Growth horm one deficiency

Note: Virilization and fertility can be achieved when FSH and LH are given to stimulate testis function.

idiopathic hypogonadotrophic hypogonadism (IHH). The clinical diagnosis of Kallmann syndrome is confirmed by hormonal assessment revealing low testosterone, low LH, low FSH, and normal prolactin levels. Infertility is treatable with gonadotropin (LH and FSH) replacement over 12–18 months, which induces sperm in the ejaculate in 80% of men. The condition is inherited as a familial disorder in one-third of cases and both X-linked and autosomal inheritance patterns have been described. In the X-linked recessive form, deletions of the *KAL1* gene prevent migration of GnRH neurons to the preoptic area of the hypothalamus during embryologic development.

B. Isolated Gonadotropin Deficiencies

These deficiencies are rare. As the result of a partial LH deficit, there is enough LH to stimulate intratesticular testosterone production and spermatogenesis but insufficient testosterone to promote virilization. The results are a eunuchoid body habitus, variable virilization, and gynecomastia. These men usually have normal size testes, but sperm concentration is low. Plasma FSH levels are normal, but serum LH and testosterone levels are low normal.

With insufficient FSH production by the pituitary, patients are normally virilized, testicular size is normal, and LH and testosterone levels are normal. FSH levels are uniformly low and do not respond to stimulation with GnRH. Sperm counts range from azoospermia to severely low numbers (oligospermia).

C. Congenital Hypogonadotrophic Syndromes

Several syndromes may be associated with secondary hypogonadism. Prader–Willi syndrome (1:20,000) is characterized by obesity, mental retardation, small extremities, and hypogonadism and is caused by a deficiency of hypothalamic GnRH. The cause of this condition appears to be a single gene deletion on chromosome 15. Similar to Kallmann syndrome, spermatogenesis can be induced by treatment with FSH and LH. Bardet–Biedl syndrome is an autosomal recessive form of hypogonadotrophic hypogonadism that also results from GnRH deficiency. It is characterized by mental retardation, retinitis pigmentosa, polydactyly, and hypogonadism. The presentation is similar to Kallmann syndrome but includes obesity and may also be treated with gonadotropin administration. Cerebellar ataxia can be associated with hypogonadotrophic hypogonadism. Cerebellar involvement includes abnormalities of speech and gait and these patients can have a eunuchoid appearance with atrophic testes. Hypothalamic–pituitary dysfunction due to pathologic changes in cerebral white matter is thought to underlie infertility.

▶ Pituitary Disease
A. Pituitary Insufficiency

Pituitary insufficiency may result from tumors, infarcts, surgery, radiation, or infiltrative and granulomatous processes.

In sickle cell anemia, pituitary and testicular microinfarcts result from sickling of red blood cells potentially leading to both hypogonadism and spermatogenic failure. Men with sickle cell anemia have decreased testosterone and variable LH and FSH levels. Beta-thalassemia occurs primarily in patients of Mediterranean or African origin and is caused by mutations in the beta-globulin that leads to abnormal hemoglobin composition and subsequent red cell lysis. Infertility results from the deposition of hemosiderin in the pituitary gland and testes. Similarly, hemochromatosis results in iron deposition within the liver, testis, and pituitary and is associated with testicular dysfunction in 80% of cases.

B. Hyperprolactinemia

Elevations of circulating prolactin can cause hypogonadotropic hypogonadism. If hyperprolactinemia is identified, secondary causes such as stress during the blood draw, systemic illness, or medications should be ruled out. With these causes excluded, the most common and important cause of hyperprolactinemia is a prolactin-secreting pituitary adenoma, or prolactinoma. MRI of the sella turcica has classically been used to distinguish between microadenoma (<10 mm) and macroadenoma (>10 mm) forms of tumor.

Stratification of disease based on radiologic diagnosis alone is misleading, as surgery for hyperprolactinemia almost always reveals a pituitary tumor. Elevated prolactin typically results in suppression of gonadotropin production, with subsequent declines in testosterone levels and spermatogenesis. Symptoms of hyperprolactinemia may include loss of libido, erectile dysfunction, gynecomastia, and galactorrhea. Signs and symptoms of other pituitary hormone derangements (adrenocorticotropic hormone, thyroid-stimulating hormone) should also be investigated.

C. Exogenous or Endogenous Hormones

1. Estrogens—An excess of sex steroids, either estrogens or androgens, may cause infertility due to an imbalance of the testosterone estrogen ratio, which is normally 10:1. Liver cirrhosis increases endogenous estrogens due to augmented aromatase activity within the diseased liver. Likewise, obesity may be associated with testosterone and estrogen imbalance owing to increased peripheral aromatase activity in adipocytes. Less commonly, adrenocortical tumors, Sertoli cell tumors, and interstitial testis tumors may produce estrogens. Excess estrogens cause spermatogenic failure by decreasing pituitary gonadotropin secretion, thus inducing secondary testis failure.

2. Androgens—An excess of androgens can suppress pituitary gonadotropin secretion and lead to secondary testis failure. The use of exogenous androgenic steroids (anabolic steroids) by as many as 15% of high school athletes, 30% of college athletes, and 70% of professional athletes may result in temporary sterility due to suppression of the normal HPG axis. Treatment includes immediate discontinuation of steroids and reevaluation of semen quality every 3–6 months until spermatogenesis returns. The most common reason for excess endogenous androgens is congenital adrenal hyperplasia caused by 21-hydroxylase deficiency. The resultant absence of cortisol synthesis and excessive adrenocorticotropic hormone production leads to elevated androgenic steroids by the adrenal cortex. High androgen levels in prepubertal boys result in precocious puberty, with premature development of secondary sex characteristics and abnormal enlargement of the phallus. The testes are characteristically small because of central gonadotropin inhibition by androgens. In young girls, virilization occurs with clitoral enlargement. In cases of classic congenital adrenal hyperplasia that presents in childhood, normal sperm counts and fertility have been reported, even without glucocorticoid treatment. This disorder is one of the few intersex conditions associated with potentially normal fertility. Other sources of endogenous androgens include hormonally active adrenocortical tumors or Leydig cell tumors of the testis.

3. Hyper- and hypothyroidism—Thyroid abnormalities are a rare cause (0.5%) of male infertility. Abnormally high or low levels of serum thyroid hormone impact spermatogenesis at the level of both the pituitary and testis. Euthyroidism is important for normal hypothalamic hormone secretion and for normal sex hormone–binding protein levels that govern the testosterone–estrogen ratio.

TESTICULAR

Many conditions that cause infertility act at the testicular level (Table 44–12.) Unlike many pretesticular conditions, which are treatable with hormonal manipulation, testicular defects are mostly irreversible.

Table 44–12. Testicular causes of infertility.

Chromosomal (Klinefelter syndrome [XXY], XX sex reversal, XYY syndrome)

Noonan syndrome (male Turner syndrome)

Myotonic dystrophy

Vanishing testis syndrome (bilateral anorchia)

Sertoli-cell-only syndrome (germ cell aplasia)

Y chromosome microdeletions (*DAZ*)

Gonadotoxins (radiation, drugs)

Systemic disease (renal failure, liver failure, sickle cell anemia)

Defective androgen activity

Testis injury (orchitis, torsion, trauma)

Cryptorchidism

Varicocele

Idiopathic

▶ Common Genetic Causes

A. Y Chromosome Microdeletions

Approximately 7% of men with low sperm counts and 13% of men with azoospermia have a structural alteration in the long arm of the Y chromosome (Yq). The testis-determining region genes that control testis differentiation are intact, but there may be gross deletions in other regions that may lead to defective spermatogenesis. The recent explosion in molecular genetics has allowed for sophisticated analysis of the Y chromosome. At present, three gene sites are being investigated as putative AZF (azoospermia factor) candidates: *AZFa, b,* and *c.* The most promising site is *AZFc,* which contains the *DAZ* gene region. The gene, of which there are at least six copies in this region, appears to encode a ribonucleic acid (RNA)-binding protein that regulate the meiotic pathway during germ cell production. Homologs of the *DAZ* gene are found in many other animals, including mouse and *Drosophila.* A quantitative polymerase chain reaction–based assay is used to test blood for these deletions. In the future, sperm DNA may also be tested as part of a semen analysis. Since men with these microdeletions can have sperm in the ejaculate, they are likely to pass them on to offspring if ART is used.

B. Klinefelter Syndrome

Abnormalities in chromosomal constitution are well-recognized causes of male infertility. In a study of 1263 infertile couples, a 6.2% overall prevalence of chromosomal abnormalities was detected. Among men whose sperm count was <10 million/mL, the prevalence was 11%. In azoospermic men, 21% had significant chromosomal abnormalities. For this reason, cytogenetic analysis (karyotype) of autosomal and sex chromosomal anomalies should be considered in men with severe oligospermia and azoospermia.

Klinefelter syndrome is the most common chromosomal aneuploidy and a common genetic cause of azoospermia, accounting for up to 14% of cases in some series (overall incidence 1:500 males). The classic triad of findings is small, firm testes; gynecomastia; and azoospermia. Some men may present with delayed sexual maturation, increased height, decreased intelligence, varicosities, obesity, diabetes, leukemia, increased likelihood of extragonadal germ cell tumors, and breast cancer (20-fold higher than in normal men). Among men with Klinefelter syndrome, 90% have an extra X chromosome (47,XXY) and 10% are mosaic, with a combination of XXY/XY chromosomes. The testes are usually <2 cm in length and always <3.5 cm; biopsies show sclerosis and hyalinization of the seminiferous tubules with normal numbers of Leydig cells. Hormones usually demonstrate decreased testosterone and frankly elevated LH and FSH levels. Serum estradiol levels may also be elevated. With age, testosterone levels decline, and most men will require androgen replacement therapy both for virilization and for normal sexual function. Paternity with this syndrome is rare but more likely in the mosaic or milder form of the disease. Some men will have limited spermatogenesis, whereby sperm may be retrieved from the testicles and used with ICSI to cause pregnancy.

▶ Other Genetic Causes and Syndromes

A. XX Male Syndrome

XX male syndrome is a structural and numerical chromosomal condition, a variant of Klinefelter syndrome that presents as gynecomastia at puberty or as azoospermia in adults. Average height is below normal, and hypospadias is common. Male external and internal genitalia are otherwise normal. The prevalence of mental deficiency is not increased. Hormone evaluation shows elevated FSH and LH and low or normal testosterone levels. Testis biopsy reveals absent spermatogenesis with fibrosis and Leydig cell clumping. The most obvious explanation is that sex-determining ratio (SRY), or the testis-determining region, is translocated from the Y to the X chromosome. Thus, testis differentiation is present; however, the genes that control spermatogenesis on the Y chromosome are not similarly translocated, resulting in azoospermia.

B. XYY Syndrome

The prevalence of XYY syndrome is similar to that of Klinefelter, but the clinical presentation is more variable. Typically, men with 47,XYY are tall, and 2% exhibit aggressive or antisocial behavior. Hormone evaluation reveals elevated FSH and normal testosterone and LH levels. Semen analyses show either oligospermia or azoospermia. Testis biopsies vary but usually demonstrate arrest of maturation or Sertoli-cell-only syndrome.

C. Noonan Syndrome

Also called male Turner syndrome, Noonan syndrome is associated with clinical features similar to Turner syndrome (45,X). However, the karyotype is either normal (46,XY) or mosaic (X/XY). Typically, patients have dysmorphic features like webbed neck, short stature, low-set ears, wide-set eyes, and cardiovascular abnormalities. At birth, 75% have cryptorchidism that limits fertility in adulthood. If testes are fully descended, then fertility is possible and likely. Associated FSH and LH levels depend on the degree of testicular function.

D. Myotonic Dystrophy

Myotonic dystrophy is the most common reason for adult-onset muscular dystrophy. In addition to having myotonia, or delayed relaxation after muscle contraction, patients usually present with cataracts, muscle atrophy, and various endocrinopathies. Most men have testis atrophy, but fertility has been reported. Infertile men may have elevated FSH and LH with low or normal testosterone, and testis biopsies show seminiferous tubule damage in 75% of cases. Pubertal development is normal; testis damage seems to occur later in life.

E. Vanishing Testis Syndrome

Also called bilateral anorchia, vanishing testis syndrome is rare, occurring in 1:20,000 males. Patients present with bilateral nonpalpable testes and sexual immaturity due to the lack of testicular androgens. The testes are lost due to fetal torsion, trauma, vascular injury, or infection. In general, functioning testis tissue must have been present during weeks 14–16 of fetal life, since Wolffian duct growth and Müllerian duct inhibition occur along with appropriate growth of male external genitalia. Patients have eunuchoid body proportions but no gynecomastia. The karyotype is normal. Serum LH and FSH levels are elevated, and serum testosterone levels are extremely low. There is no treatment for this form of infertility; patients receive lifelong testosterone for normal virilization and sexual function.

F. Sertoli-Cell-Only Syndrome

Sertoli-cell-only syndrome is characterized by the complete absence of germinal cells on histologic examination of testes biopsies from an azoospermic man. Several causes have been proposed, including genetic defects, congenital absence of normal germ cell migration during embryogenesis, and androgen resistance. Clinically, men are normally virilized with smaller than normal testes with normal consistency. Endocrine function of the testes is preserved and testosterone and LH levels are normal; however, FSH levels are usually (90%) elevated. The use of the word "syndrome" implies that no recognized insult has occurred, since gonadotoxins such as ionizing radiation, chemotherapy, and mumps orchitis can also render the testes aplastic of germ cells. There is no known treatment for this condition. In some patients, extensive testis sampling with FNA mapping or multiple biopsies can reveal sperm that can be used for pregnancy with ARTs.

G. Defective DNA Mismatch Repair

Defective DNA repair has been suspected to play an etiologic role in certain cancers. Data from mice suggest that mutations in genes needed for DNA repair (PMS2, Mlh1) also lead to infertility characterized by meiotic arrest with a pattern of maturation arrest seen in testis pathology. Male infertility characterized by azoospermia and both germ cell maturation arrest and Sertoli-cell-only syndrome has also been described in association with abnormalities in DNA mismatch repair. This provides evidence that certain forms of male infertility could involve the inability to properly repair germline DNA. The relationship between defective DNA repair in infertile men and their risk of cancer as well as the risk of cancer among their biological offspring certainly merits further research.

Gonadotoxins

A. Radiation

The effects of radiotherapy on sperm production have been well described. Clifton and Bremner (1983) examined the effects of ionizing irradiation on semen quality and spermatogenesis among a population of healthy prisoners in the 1960s. Before a vasectomy, each of the volunteers was exposed to various levels of radiation and found a distinct dose-dependent, inverse relationship between irradiation and sperm count. Sperm count was significantly reduced at 15 cGy, and azoospermia was temporarily induced at 50 cGy. Persistent azoospermia was induced at 400 cGy, without evidence of recovery for a minimum of 40 weeks. In most subjects, sperm counts rebounded to preirradiation levels with cessation of exposure.

Histologic examination of testis tissue after irradiation has shown that spermatogonia are most sensitive to irradiation while Leydig cell mass is relatively preserved. Given the sensitivity of germ cells to irradiation, some studies have focused on the testicular radiation exposure that occurs during radiation therapy for cancer. During abdominal radiation with gonadal shielding, the estimated mean unintended gonadal exposure is approximately 75 cGy. There does not appear to be an increase in congenital birth defects in offspring of irradiated men. Importantly, recent data have suggested that environmental or occupational exposure to electromagnetic radiation may also reduce semen quality.

B. Drugs

A list of gonadotoxic medications can be found in Table 44–13. These can result in infertility by various mechanisms. Ketoconazole, spironolactone, and alcohol inhibit testosterone synthesis, whereas cimetidine is an androgen antagonist. Recreational drugs such as marijuana, heroin, and methadone are associated with lower testosterone levels. Certain pesticides, like dibromochloropropane, are likely to have estrogen-like activity. Importantly, the gonadotoxic potential of many pharmaceutical and over-the-counter medications is unknown. Therefore, couples should consider discontinuing

Table 44–13. Medications associated with infertility.

Calcium channel blockers	Allopurinol
Cimetidine	Alpha-blockers
Sulfasalazine	Nitrofurantoin
Valproic acid	Lithium
Spironolactone	Tricyclic antidepressants
Colchicine	Antipsychotics

and unnecessary medication or supplements prior to their attempt to conceive.

Chemotherapies intended for their cytotoxic effects on rapidly dividing cancer cells also have a profound impact on germ cells that are normally dividing at a rapid rate. Spermatogonia are the germ cells most sensitive to cytotoxic chemotherapy. Alkylating agents such as cyclophosphamide, chlorambucil, and nitrogen mustard are the most toxic agents. The effects of chemotherapeutic drugs vary according to dose and duration of treatment, type and stage of disease, age and health of the patient, and baseline testis function. Despite this toxicity, the mutagenic effects of chemotherapy agents do not appear to be significant enough to increase the chance of birth defects or genetic diseases among offspring of treated men. Patients should wait at least 6 months after chemotherapy ends before attempting to conceive.

Systemic Disease

A. Renal Failure

Uremia is associated with infertility, decreased libido, erectile dysfunction, and gynecomastia. The cause of hypogonadism is controversial and probably multifactorial. Testosterone levels are decreased, and FSH and LH levels can be elevated. Serum prolactin levels are elevated in 25% of patients. Hyperestrogenemia may play a role in hormone axis derangements and impaired spermatogenesis. Medications and uremic neuropathy may cause uremic-related impotence and a decline in libido. Renal transplantation can result in improvement in hypogonadism.

B. Liver Cirrhosis

Hypogonadism related to liver failure may have various contributing factors. The reason for organ failure is important. Hepatitis is associated with viremia, and associated fevers can affect spermatogenesis. Excessive alcohol intake inhibits testicular testosterone synthesis, independent of its liver effects. Liver failure and cirrhosis are associated with testicular atrophy, impotence, and gynecomastia. Levels of testosterone and its metabolic clearance are decreased; estrogen levels are increased owing to augmented conversion of androgens to estrogens by aromatase. Decreased testosterone levels are not accompanied by proportionate elevations in LH and FSH levels, suggesting that a central inhibition of the HPG axis may accompany liver failure.

C. Sickle Cell Disease

As mentioned earlier, sickle cell disease can cause pituitary dysfunction, likely due to the sludging of erythrocytes and associated microinfarcts. This same mechanism may also occur in testis tissue and contribute to primary hypogonadism. As a result, spermatogenesis is decreased, accompanied by lower serum testosterone levels.

D. Diabetes Mellitus

Prolonged diabetes can result in significant cardiovascular disease, as well as peripheral neuropathy. The impact of such disease on erectile and ejaculatory function has been well described. In addition to poor sexual function, neuropathy involving the parasympathetic and sympathetic pelvic plexus can lead to poor contractility of the bladder neck and ejaculatory organs resulting in retrograde or anejaculation.

▶ Defective Androgen Activity

Peripheral resistance to androgens occurs with two basic defects: (1) a deficiency of androgen production through the absence of 5-alpha-reductase and (2) a deficiency in the androgen receptor. In general, these conditions are a consequence of single gene deletions.

A. 5-Alpha-Reductase Deficiency

5-Alpha-reductase deficiency results in normal development of the testes and Wolffian duct structures (internal genitalia) but ambiguous external genitalia. The ambiguity results from an inborn deficiency of the 5-alpha-reductase enzyme that converts testosterone to DHT in androgen-sensitive tissues like the prostate, seminal vesicle, and external genitalia. Thus far, 29 mutations have been described in the culprit enzyme. The diagnosis is made by measuring the ratio of testosterone metabolites in urine and confirmed by finding decreased 5-alpha-reductase in genital skin fibroblasts. Spermatogenesis has been described in descended testes; however, fertility has not been reported in these patients. The lack of fertility may be due largely to functional abnormalities of the external genitalia.

B. Androgen Receptor Deficiency

Androgen receptor deficiency is an X-linked genetic condition marked by resistance to androgens. The androgen receptor, a nuclear protein, is absent or functionally altered such that testosterone or DHT cannot bind to it and activate target cell genes. Since androgens have no effect on tissues, both internal and external genitalia are affected. Fertility effects depend on the specific receptor abnormality. Some patients are 46,XY males with complete end-organ resistance to androgens. They have female external genitalia with intra-abdominal testes. Testes show immature tubules and the risk of testis cancer is elevated: Tumors will develop in 10–30% of patients without orchiectomy. Fertility is absent. Patients with mild receptor defects may present as normal-appearing infertile men. Spermatogenesis may be present, although impaired. It is unclear exactly how common this occurs in infertile men.

▶ Testis Injury

A. Orchitis

Inflammation of testis tissue is most commonly due to bacterial infection, termed epididymo-orchitis. Viral infections also occur in the testis in the form of mumps orchitis. Orchitis is observed in approximately 30% of postpubertal males who develop mumps parotitis. Testis atrophy is a significant and frequent result of viral orchitis but is less common with bacterial infections.

B. Torsion

Ischemic injury to the testis secondary to twisting of the testis on the spermatic cord pedicle is common in prepubertal and early postpubertal boys. When diagnosed and corrected surgically within 6 hours of occurrence, the testis can usually be saved. Torsion may result in inoculation of the immune system with testis antigens that may predispose to later immunological infertility. It recognized that the "normal" contralateral mate of a torsed testis could also exhibit histologic abnormalities. It has not been clearly demonstrated whether this is related to the actual torsion or to an underlying abnormality in testes predisposed to torsion.

C. Trauma

Trauma to the testis can result in infertility. Because of the unique immunologic status of the testis in the body (ie, it is an immunologically privileged site), trauma to the testis can invoke an abnormal immune response in addition to atrophy resulting from injury. Both may contribute to infertility. Trauma to the testis that results in fracture of the testis tunica albuginea should be surgically explored and repaired to minimize exposure of testis tissue to the body.

▶ Cryptorchidism

Undescended testis is a common urologic problem, observed in 0.8% of boys at 1 year of age. It is considered a developmental defect and places the affected testis at higher risk of developing testicular germ cell cancer. Although the newborn undescended testis is morphologically normal, deterioration in germ cell numbers is often seen by 2 years of age. The contralateral, normally descended testis is also at increased risk of harboring germ cell abnormalities. Thus, males with either unilaterally or bilaterally undescended testes are at risk for infertility later in life. Historically, orchidopexy was performed solely for the purpose of testicle palpation to allow for cancer detection. However, more recent data have shown that when performed prior to puberty, orchidopexy reduces the risk of cancer development. Other data have suggested that early orchidopexy can improve spermatogenesis in cryptorchid boys.

▶ Varicocele

Varicocele is defined as dilated and incompetent veins within the pampiniform plexus of spermatic cord. Varicocele has been described as the most common surgically correctable cause of male subfertility. This is a disease that develops during puberty when both endocrine and exocrine function of the testicle dramatically increases, along with testicular blood flow. Varicocele is only rarely detected in boys <10 years of age. A left-sided varicocele is found in 15% of healthy young men. In contrast, the incidence of a left varicocele in subfertile men approaches 40%. Bilateral varicoceles are uncommon in healthy men (<10%) but are palpated in up to 20% of subfertile men. In general, varicoceles do not spontaneously regress. An accurate physical examination remains the cornerstone of varicocele diagnosis.

Several anatomic features contribute to the predominance of left-sided varicoceles. The left internal spermatic vein is longer than the right and it typically joins the left renal vein at a right angle compared with the oblique insertion of the right spermatic vein into the inferior vena cava. As a result of these characteristics, higher venous pressures fare transmitted to the left spermatic cord veins and result in retrograde reflux of blood.

Varicoceles are associated with testicular atrophy and varicocele correction can reverse atrophy in adolescents. There is strong evidence that the varicocele affects semen quality. Varicocele can cause abnormalities in concentration, motility, and morphology; however, deficits in motility can be the most profound. The finding of semen abnormalities constitutes the most common indication for varicocele surgery in infertile men.

The mechanism by which varicocele exerts an effect on the testicle remains unclear. Several theories have been postulated and it is likely that a combination of effects results in infertility. Pituitary–gonadal hormonal dysfunction, internal spermatic vein reflux of renal or adrenal metabolites, and an increase in hydrostatic pressure associated with venous reflux are also postulated effects of a varicocele. The most intriguing theory of how varicoceles affect testis function invokes an inhibition of spermatogenesis through the reflux of warm corporeal blood around the testis, with disruption of the normal countercurrent heat exchange balance and elevation of intratesticular temperature.

▶ Idiopathic

It has been estimated that nearly half of male infertility has no readily identifiable cause. The etiology of male infertility is likely multifactorial, encompassing genetic, endocrine, and environmental factors. In addition, modifiable lifestyle characteristics may make a significant contribution to the disease. The effects of physical activity, obesity, alcohol and tobacco use, psychological stress, and cell phone usage on male infertility have been examined in a few observational studies, yet results are inconclusive due to limitations in study design.

POSTTESTICULAR (TABLE 44–14)

▶ Reproductive Tract Obstruction

The posttesticular portion of the reproductive tract includes the epididymis, vas deferens, seminal vesicles, and associated ejaculatory apparatus.

Table 44–14. Posttesticular causes of infertility.

Reproductive tract obstruction
  Congenital blockages
  Congenital absence of the vas deferens (CAVD)
  Young syndrome
  Idiopathic epididymal obstruction
  Polycystic kidney disease
  Ejaculatory duct obstruction
  Acquired blockages
  Vasectomy
  Groin surgery
  Infection
  Functional blockages
  Sympathetic nerve injury
  Pharmacologic
Disorders of sperm function or motility
  Immotile cilia syndromes
  Maturation defects
  Immunologic infertility
  Infection
Disorders of coitus
  Impotence
  Hypospadias
  Timing and frequency

A. Congenital Blockages

1. Cystic fibrosis—CF is the most common autosomal recessive genetic disorder in the United States with a carrier frequency of 1:20 among Caucasians. The disease is caused by defective chloride ion transport across cell membranes resulting in fluid and electrolyte abnormalities (abnormal chloride–sweat test). CF typically presents with chronic lung obstruction and pulmonary infections, pancreatic insufficiency, and infertility. More than 95% of men with CF also have congenital bilateral absence of the vas deferens (CBAVD). In addition to the vas, parts of the epididymis, seminal vesicles, and ejaculatory ducts may be atrophic or absent, causing obstruction. Although spermatogenesis is quantitatively normal, recent data suggest that sperm from men with CF may lack the normal capacity to fertilize an egg. Furthermore, some carriers of abnormal CF genes may also have functional sperm defects. CBAVD accounts for 1–2% of infertility cases. On physical examination, no palpable vas deferens is observed on one or both sides. As in CF, the rest of the reproductive tract ducts may also be abnormal and unreconstructable. This disease is related to CF. Even though most of these men demonstrate no symptoms of CF, up to 80% of patients will harbor a detectable CF mutation. In addition, 15% of these men will have renal malformations, most commonly unilateral agenesis.

2. Young syndrome—Young syndrome presents with a triad of chronic sinusitis, bronchiectasis, and OA. The obstruction is in the epididymis. The pathophysiology of the condition is unclear but may involve abnormal ciliary function or abnormal mucus quality. Reconstructive surgery is associated with lower success rates than that observed with other obstructed conditions.

3. Idiopathic epididymal obstruction—Idiopathic epididymal obstruction is a relatively uncommon condition found in otherwise healthy men. There is recent evidence linking this condition to CF in that one-third of men so obstructed may harbor CF gene mutations.

4. Adult polycystic kidney disease—Adult polycystic kidney disease is an autosomal dominant disorder associated with numerous cysts of the kidney, liver, spleen, pancreas, epididymis, seminal vesicle, and testis. Disease onset usually occurs in the twenties or thirties with symptoms of abdominal pain, hypertension, and renal failure. Infertility with this disease is usually secondary to obstructing cysts in the epididymis or seminal vesicle.

5. Blockage of the ejaculatory ducts—Blockage of the ejaculatory ducts, the delicate, paired, collagenous tubes that connect the vas deferens and seminal vesicles to the urethra, is termed EDO. It is the cause of infertility in 5% of azoospermic men. Obstruction can be congenital and result from Müllerian duct (utricular) cysts, Wolffian duct (diverticular) cysts, or congenital atresia or is acquired from seminal vesicle calculi or postsurgical or inflammatory scar tissue. It presents as hematospermia, painful ejaculation, or infertility. The diagnosis is confirmed by finding a low-volume ejaculate and TRUS showing dilated seminal vesicles or dilated ejaculatory ducts.

B. Acquired Blockages

1. Vasectomy—Vasectomy is performed on more than ½ million men per year in the United States for contraception. Subsequently, 6% of these men have the vasectomy reversed, most commonly because of remarriage.

2. Groin and hernia surgery—Groin and hernia surgery can result in inguinal vas deferens obstruction in 1% of cases. There has been concern that Marlex mesh used for hernia repairs may add to perivasal inflammation and increase the likelihood of vassal obstruction.

3. Bacterial infections—Bacterial infections (*E. coli* in men age >35 or *Chlamydia trachomatis* in young men) may involve the epididymis, with scarring and obstruction.

C. Functional Blockages

Besides physical obstruction, functional obstruction of the seminal vesicles may exist. Functional blockages may result from nerve injury or medications that impair the contractility of seminal vesicle or vasal musculature. A classic example of nerve injury affecting ejaculation is after retroperitoneal lymph node dissection for testis cancer. This can cause either retrograde ejaculation or complete anejaculation, depending on the degree of injury to postganglionic sympathetic fibers arising from the thoracolumbar spinal cord. These autonomic nerves overlie the inferior aorta and coalesce as the hypogastric plexus within the pelvis and control seminal emission. Multiple sclerosis and diabetes are other conditions that result in disordered ejaculation.

Evidence from animal models indicates that the seminal vesicles possess contractile properties similar to those of the urinary bladder, suggesting that seminal vesicle organ dysfunction may underlie some cases of ejaculatory duct "obstruction." Medications implicated in this functional problem are those classically associated with ejaculatory impairment. Table 44–5 lists these medications.

▶ Disorders of Sperm Function or Motility

A. Immotile Cilia Syndromes

Immotile cilia syndromes are a heterogeneous group of disorders (1:20,000 males) in which sperm motility is reduced or absent. The sperm defects are due to abnormalities in the motor apparatus or axoneme of sperm and other ciliated cells. Normally, nine pairs of microtubules are organized around a central microtubule pair within the sperm tail and are connected by dynein arms (ATPase) that regulate microtubule and therefore sperm tail motion. Various defects in the dynein arms cause deficits in ciliary and sperm activity. Kartagener syndrome is a subset of this disorder (1:40,000 males) that presents with the triad of chronic sinusitis, bronchiectasis, and situs inversus. Most immotile cilia cases are diagnosed in childhood with respiratory and sinus difficulties. Cilia present in the retina and ear may also be defective and lead to retinitis pigmentosa and deafness in Usher's syndrome. Men with immotile cilia characteristically have nonmotile but viable sperm in normal numbers. The diagnosis can only be confirmed with electron microscopy of sperm.

B. Immunologic Infertility

Autoimmune infertility has been implicated as a cause of infertility in 10% of infertile couples. The testis is an immunologically privileged site, probably owing to the blood–testis barrier, which consists of Sertoli cell tight junctions and locally downregulated cellular immunity. Autoimmune infertility may result from an abnormal exposure to sperm antigens as the result of vasectomy, testis torsion, or biopsy, which then incites a pathologic immune response. Antibodies may disturb sperm transport or disrupt sperm–egg interaction. Many assays are available to detect ASAs, but assays that detect sperm-bound, and not serum, antibodies are the most clinically relevant.

C. Infection

The agents most commonly responsible for male genital tract infections are listed in Table 44–10. Various products of activated leukocytes can exist in infected semen. A correlation exists between leukocytes in semen and the generation of superoxide anions, hydrogen peroxide, and hydroxyl radicals (reactive oxygen species), all of which can damage sperm membranes. Sperm are highly susceptible to the effects of oxidative stress because they possess little cytoplasm and therefore little antioxidant activity. Damage to sperm from oxidative stress has been correlated to loss of function and damaged DNA. Although genital tract infection has been linked to infertility in epidemiologic studies, the correlation between individual organisms and infertility is unclear. Uncontrolled studies suggest that pregnancy rates may improve after treatment, but controlled studies do not confirm these findings.

Disorders of Coitus

A. Impotence

Sexual dysfunction stemming from low libido or impotence is a frequent cause of infertility. The male hormonal evaluation can detect organic reasons for such problems. Most cases of situational impotence, in which the stress of attempting to conceive results in poor erections, are treated with sexual counseling and oral phosphodiesterase inhibitors.

B. Hypospadias

Anatomic problems like hypospadias can cause inappropriate placement of the seminal coagulum too distant from the cervix and result in infertility.

C. Timing and Frequency

Simple problems of coital timing and frequency can be corrected by a review of the couple's sexual habits. An appropriate frequency of intercourse is every two days, performed within the periovulatory period, the window of time surrounding ovulation when egg fertilization is possible. Charting of basal body temperature by the female partner allows for the calculation of that period for the next ovulatory cycle. Home kits that detect the LH surge in the urine before ovulation are also helpful. Couples should be counseled to avoid lubricants if at all possible. It is also wise to discontinue any unnecessary medications during attempts to conceive. Other coital toxins include heat exposure from regular saunas, hot saunas, hot tubs, or Jacuzzis and the use of cigarettes, cocaine, marijuana, and excessive alcohol.

TREATMENT OF MALE INFERTILITY

SURGICAL TREATMENTS

The role of surgery in the treatment of certain causes of male infertility is well established and cost-effective when compared with high-technology approaches. Surgeries that attempt to reverse specific anatomic or pathophysiologic defects may result in normalization or improvement in semen quality, thus allowing a couple to conceive naturally rather than the use of ART. Other surgeries are for the purpose of obtaining sperm directly from the testis or epididymis and are intended to be used in conjunction with ART.

Varicocele

The association of varicoceles with male infertility is well established. Several treatment modalities, both surgical and nonsurgical, are available for varicoceles. These include ligation of the veins through the retroperitoneal, inguinal, or subinguinal approaches; percutaneous embolization; and laparoscopy. The common goal of all treatments is to stop the retrograde flow of venous blood through the internal spermatic veins. Treatments can be compared in terms of expected success rates (semen improvement and pregnancy), cost, and outcomes (pain pills, return to work or other activity), and their relative merits can be analyzed. A basic comparison of three treatment options is outlined in Table 44–15. Remember that if watchful waiting is chosen, a pregnancy rate of 16% can be expected. If IVF is chosen, a pregnancy rate of 35% can be expected. An overall complication rate of 1% is associated with the incisional approach, compared with a 4% complication rate for laparoscopy and 10–15% for radiologic occlusion. A significant problem with the radiologic approach is technical failure, meaning the inability to access and occlude the spermatic vein.

Vasectomy Reversal

More than 500,000 men per year undergo vasectomy in the United States, and nearly 6% will eventually wish to have their vasectomy reversed. The most common reasons relate to changes in a man's social circumstances and include remarriage and the loss of a child. Causes of vasal obstruction other than vasectomy include infection, congenital, trauma, and previous surgery and are less frequent indications for

Table 44–15. Varicocele treatments: comparison of outcomes.

Outcome parameter	Treatment		
	Incisional	Laparoscopic	Radiologic
Semen improvement	66%	50–70%	60%
Pregnancy rate	35%	12–32%	10–50%
Recurrence	0–15%	5–25%	0–10%
Technical failure	Negligible	Small	10–15%
Pain pills	9.4	11	Minimal
Days to work	5.0	5.3	1

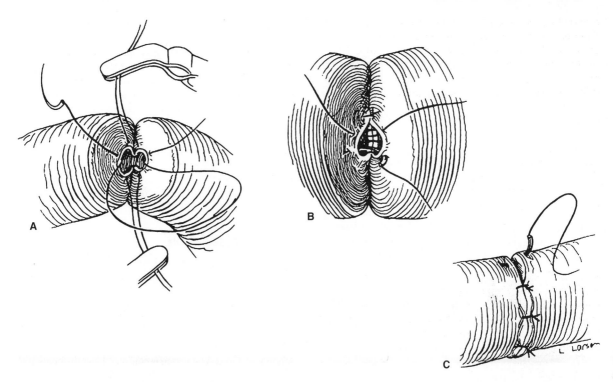

▲ **Figure 44–13.** Two-layer microsurgical vasovasostomy. **A:** Mucosal stitches of 10–0 nylon are placed in the "back wall" of the vas lumen, incorporating mucosa and a small amount of submucosal tissue. **B:** The "front wall" mucosal sutures are then placed. **C:** Finally, serosal sutures of 9–0 nylon are placed in the outside wall of the vas deferens to complete the anastomosis. (Reproduced, with permission, from McClure RD: Microsurgery of the male reproductive system. World J Urol 1986;4:105.)

vasovasostomy or epididymovasostomy. A problem with duct obstruction should be suspected in men with normal testis size, normal hormones, and azoospermia.

Several methods have been described for vasovasostomy. None has been proved superior to any other, except that magnification with an operating microscope results in better success rates. In general, either a single-layer anastomosis or a double-layer anastomosis is performed (Figure 44–13). Although these procedures are technically different, the experience of the surgeon is the most important factor for success. Depending on these factors, 95% or more of patients may have a return of sperm after a vasovasostomy. If vasal fluid below the level of the vasectomy does not contain sperm, there may be a secondary obstruction in the epididymis. Such obstruction may result from rupture of the epididymal tubules in response to increased luminal pressure. A prolonged period of vasectomy or a vasectomy close to the epididymis increases the risk of an epididymal blockage. In this case, the vas must be connected to the epididymis above the area of rupture in an operation called an epididymovasostomy. Although this is a technically challenging operation,

given improvements in surgical techniques and instrumentation, approximately 60–65% of men will have sperm in the ejaculate following epididymovasostomy.

The achievement of sperm in the ejaculate after vasovasostomy depends largely on surgical technique, but pregnancy after surgery is dependent upon the fertility potential of the couple. Therefore, it is critical to understand the reproductive health of the female partner before embarking on the procedure. Other reasons that reproductive tract microsurgery fails are (1) the quality of preblockage semen may not have been normal; (2) ASAs develop in roughly 30% of men who have had vasectomies (high antibody levels may impair fertility); (3) postsurgical scar tissue can develop at the anastomotic site, causing another blockage; (4) when the vas deferens has been blocked for a long time, the epididymis is adversely affected and sperm maturation may be compromised.

▶ Ejaculatory Duct Obstruction

EDO should be suspected when the ejaculate volume is <1.5 mL and no retrograde ejaculation or hormonal deficit

Table 44–16. Classification of ejaculatory duct obstruction by semen analysis parameters.

	Incomplete or partial	Complete	Functional
Ejaculate volume	Low or low-normal	Low	Low
Sperm count	Low	Absent	Absent or low
Sperm motility	Low	Absent	Absent or low
Ejaculate fructose	Present	Absent	Absent or low

has been identified. EDO can take several forms (Table 44–16). *Complete or classic* EDO is the physical blockage of both ejaculatory ducts and presents with low-volume azo-ospermia. *Incomplete or "partial"* EDO is the unilateral, physical blockage of one of the paired ducts or the partial blockage of both ducts. This condition is generally associated with low ejaculate volume and low sperm concentrations and severely impaired motility. *Functional* EDO is a form of ejaculatory dysfunction that presents as classic EDO but without anatomical evidence of physical blockage. Clinical suspicion can be confirmed by TRUS demonstration of dilated seminal vesicles or dilated ejaculatory ducts. Patients with EDO sufficient to cause coital discomfort, recurrent hematospermia, or infertility should be considered for treatment.

Transurethral resection of the ejaculatory ducts (TURED) is performed cystoscopically (Figure 44–14). A small

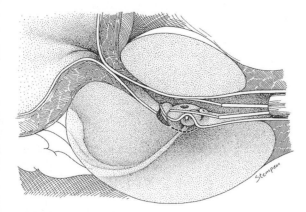

▲ **Figure 44–14.** Transurethral resection of the ejaculatory ducts. A cystoscope with a resecting loop is used to remove the verumontanum and unroof, an associated obstructing cyst that has compressed and obstructed the ejaculatory ducts. (Reproduced, with permission, from Turek PJ: Seminal vesicle and ejaculatory duct surgery. In: Graham SD (ed.): Glenn's Urologic Surgery, 5th edn. Lippincott, Philadelphia, 1998.)

resectoscope is inserted, and the verumontanum is resected in the midline until the ducts are visualized. The concomitant use of real-time TRUS may increase the accuracy of resection. Since the area of resection is at the prostatic apex, near the external urethral sphincter and the rectum, careful positioning of the resectoscope is essential. Sixty-five to seventy percent of men show significant improvement in semen quality after TURED and a 30% pregnancy rate can be expected. The complication rate from TURED is approximately 20%. Most complications are self-limited and include hematospermia, hematuria, urinary tract infection, epididymitis, and a watery ejaculate. Rarely reported complications include retrograde ejaculation, rectal perforation, and urinary incontinence.

▶ Electroejaculation

A complete failure of emission and ejaculation occurs most commonly from spinal cord injury (10,000 cases/year in the United States) and as a result of deep pelvic or retroperitoneal surgery that injured the pelvic sympathetic nerves. With rectal probe electroejaculation, the pelvic sympathetic nerves undergo controlled stimulation, with contraction of the vas deferens, seminal vesicle, and prostate, such that a reflex ejaculation is induced. The semen is collected from the penis and the bladder as retrograde ejaculation is often associated with electroejaculation. Semen acquired in this way at minimum requires the use of IUI to allow for pregnancy.

In men with anejaculation after retroperitoneal surgery or spinal trauma, successful recovery of sperm with electroejaculation is possible in the majority of patients. Sperm motility tends to be lower than normal when obtained in this way, an effect independent of electrical or heat effects inherent to the procedure. In men with spinal cord injuries above the T5 level, it is often possible to induce a reflex ejaculation with high-frequency penile vibration, termed vibratory stimulation. With the use of handheld vibrators set to a frequency of 110 cycles/s at an amplitude of 3 mm, patients may be taught to perform the procedure and attempt to conceive at home with cervical insemination.

▶ Sperm Retrieval

Sperm retrieval techniques are indicated for men in whom ejaculation of sperm is not possible because the ductal system is absent, surgically unreconstructable, or because the couple has elected to use ART rather than vasectomy reversal. Testicular sperm retrieval is also indicated in men with NOA who may harbor areas of reduced spermatogenesis within the testes. Given these widely varied indications, retrieval techniques have evolved to include minimally invasive aspiration procedures and more invasive dissections of the testis with the aid of an operating microscope. Sperm are routinely aspirated from the vas deferens, epididymis, or testicle. It is important to realize that IVF is required to achieve

Table 44–17. Sources of retrieved sperm and associated reproductive technologies.

Procedure	Source	IVF	Micromanipulation
Vasal aspiration	Vas deferens	Usually	No
Epididymal aspiration	Epididymis	Yes	Yes
Testis biopsy	Testicle	Yes	Yes

IVF, in vitro fertilization.

a pregnancy with these procedures. Thus, success rates are intimately tied to a complex program of assisted reproduction for both partners (Table 44–17). In cases of sperm aspiration from the testicle and epididymis, IVF along with ICSI is required. An obvious prerequisite for these procedures is sperm production. Although evaluated indirectly by hormone levels and testis volume, the most direct way to verify sperm production is with a testis biopsy.

A. Vasal Aspiration

After a scrotal incision and with an operating microscope, a hemivasotomy is made, and leaking sperm are aspirated into culture medium. Once enough sperm are obtained (>10–20 million), the vasotomy is closed with microscopic sutures. Vasal aspiration provides the most mature sperm.

B. Epididymal Sperm Aspiration

Epididymal sperm aspiration may be performed by two distinct techniques. With microscopic epididymal sperm aspiration (MESA), sperm are directly collected from a single, isolated epididymal tubule (Figure 44–15). After sperm are obtained, the epididymal tubule is closed with fine, microscopic suture, and the sperm are processed. When the epididymis is palpable, sperm may also be obtained with percutaneous epididymal sperm aspiration (PESA). Although this technique is a less invasive, the blind insertion of a needle into the epididymis may be more likely to result in tubule injury, thus reducing the chances for successful subsequent vasectomy reversal. Epididymal sperm are not as mature as vasal sperm; as a consequence, epididymal sperm require ICSI to fertilize the egg. Egg fertilization rates of 65% and pregnancy rates of 50% are possible with epididymal sperm, but results vary among individuals because of differences in sperm and egg quality.

C. Testis Sperm Retrieval

Testicular sperm extraction (TESE) is indicated for patients in whom there is an unreconstructable blockage in the epididymis, or in cases of severe testis failure, in which so few sperm are produced that they cannot reach the ejaculate. Testicular sperm retrieval procedures are highly variable in

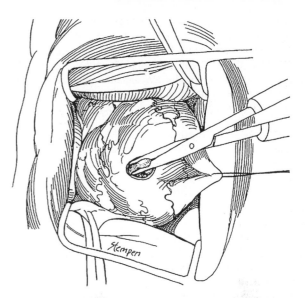

▲ **Figure 44–15.** Microscopic epididymal sperm aspiration. A small "window" incision is made in the scrotum and held open with a small retractor. Under 20× magnification, the epididymis is dissected, and a single epididymal tubule is incised with microscissors. Fluid containing sperm is aspirated for use with in vitro fertilization.

terms of their surgical invasiveness. Whenever possible, the least invasive approach necessary to acquire adequate sperm should be used. In traditional TESE, a small piece of testis tissue is taken in a manner similar to that of a regular testis biopsy. When spermatogenesis is known or suspected to be normal, or is reduced but uniformly distributed throughout the testicle, then testicular sperm aspiration (TESA) should be considered. In distinction to this, if spermatogenesis is markedly reduced, as in many cases of NOA, the greatest changes for successful sperm retrieval will achieved by meticulously dissecting all testicular tissue with the aid of a surgical microscope (micro-TESE). The testis tissue is specially treated in the laboratory to separate sperm from other cells. High egg fertilization rates (60–75%) and pregnancy rates (40–50%) are possible with testis sperm despite the fact that normal motility is usually lacking.

▶ Orchidopexy

An undescended testis occurs in 0.8% of male infants at 1 year of age and the incidence may be increasing. Historically, orchidopexy was done to allow for palpation of a testis that was at increased risk for cancer. More recent evidence suggests that early orchidopexy reduces cancer risk and may improve spermatogenesis later in life. Histologic studies of undescended testis show that significant decreases in spermatogonial numbers occur between birth and 2 years of age. Orchidopexy has been recommended within 2 years of age to potentially prevent this germ cell degeneration. Given that sperm can be retrieved from very atrophic testes and used with assisted reproduction, orchidopexy and not orchiectomy should be the primary goal in these cases.

Torsion of the testis is a urologic emergency. Data from animal studies suggest that the unaffected, contralateral testis may also develop impaired spermatogenesis termed sympathetic orchidopathia. This phenomenon may be immunologic in nature and is the basis for the recommendation that a nonviable torsed testicle be removed at diagnosis. However, given the advances in ARTs, such recommendations should be reconsidered.

▶ Pituitary Ablation

Hyperprolactinemia from a pituitary adenoma can be treated medically and surgically. If the adenoma is radiologically visible (macroadenoma), then transsphenoidal surgical ablation of the lesion is possible. If the adenoma is not visible (microadenoma), then medical therapy with the dopamine agonist bromocriptine or a derivative is more appropriate. Studies have suggested that hyperprolactinemia alone independent of gonadotropin deficiencies can suppress normal testicular function.

NONSURGICAL TREATMENTS

▶ Specific Therapy

Specific therapy refers to treatments aimed at reversing known pathophysiology in an effort to improve spermatogenesis and fertility. These therapies should be contrasted to empiric therapies that aim to overcome a pathologic condition. Whenever possible, specific therapies should be elected over empiric therapies.

A. Leukocytospermia

Elevated leukocytes in semen is termed leukocytospermia and has been associated with (1) subclinical genital tract infection, (2) elevated reactive oxygen species, and (3) poor sperm function and infertility. The treatment of leukocytospermia is controversial in the absence of overt bacteriologic infection. It is important to evaluate the patient for sexually transmitted diseases, penile discharge, prostatitis, or epididymitis. An expressed prostatic secretion is examined for leukocytes; urine can be assayed for chlamydial, gonococcal, and mycoplasma infections. The use of broad-spectrum antibiotics such as doxycycline and trimethoprim–sulfamethoxazole may reduce seminal leukocyte concentrations or improve sperm function; however, this remains a debated topic. In general, the female partner is also treated. Importantly, the histologic appearance of immature germ cells can be confused with leukocytes in a semen sample. Therefore, is critical

to avoid treating leukocytospermia purely on the basis of elevated "round cells." Specific staining for leukocyte esterase with a concentration of cells greater than one million per milliliter confirms the diagnosis.

In cases of confirmed leukocytospermia, frequent ejaculation (more than every 3 days) and doxycycline may result in a more durable resolution than antibiotic treatment alone. There is increasing evidence that the antioxidant vitamins (A, C, and E) as well as glutathione and Omega-3 fatty acids (fish oil) may help scavenge reactive oxygen species within semen and improve sperm motility in cases of leukocytospermia.

B. Coital Therapy

Simple counseling on issues of coital timing, frequency, and gonadotoxin avoidance can improve fertility. It is important to review the essentials of basal body temperature charting or home kits that detect the LH surge in the urine immediately (<24 hours) before ovulation. Since sperm reside in the cervical mucus for 48 hours and are released continuously, it is not necessary that coitus and ovulation occur at the exact same time. In general, coitus every other day around ovulation is an appropriate recommendation. Coital lubricants should be avoided if possible, as many commercially available products are toxic to sperm. If necessary, vegetable oils, olive oil, and egg whites are the safest.

Retrograde ejaculation results from a failure of the bladder neck to close during ejaculation. Diagnosed by the finding of sperm within the postejaculate bladder urine, it can be treated with sympathomimetic medications. Approximately 30% of men will respond to treatment with some degree of antegrade ejaculation. Begun several days before ejaculation, imipramine (25–50 mg twice a day), or Sudafed Plus (60 mg three times a day), has been used with success. For medication failure, sperm harvesting techniques can be used with IUI to achieve a pregnancy. Premature ejaculation occurs when men ejaculate before the partner is ready. Sexual counseling combined with tricyclic antidepressants or serotoninergic uptake inhibitors can be effective.

C. Immunologic Infertility

ASAs are a complex problem underlying male infertility. Available treatment options include corticosteroid immune suppression, sperm washing, IUI, IVF, and ICSI. Steroid suppression is based on the concept that the immune system can be weakened to reduce antibodies on sperm; however, this modality is rarely used given the potential for significant side effects. IUI places more sperm nearer the ovulated egg to optimize the sperm–egg environment. Pregnancy rates with this technique generally fall in the 10–15%/cycle range. ART with IVF and ICSI is very effective in this scenario. In general, if >50% of sperm are bound with antibodies, then treatment should be offered. In addition, head-directed or midpiece-directed sperm antibodies appear more relevant than tail-directed antibodies.

D. Medical Therapies

Hormone therapy is effective when it is used as specific and not empiric treatment. Specific replacement therapy seeks to reverse well-established, pathophysiologic states. Empiric treatments attempt to overcome pathologic conditions that are ill defined or have no proven treatment.

1. Hyperprolactinemia—Normal levels of prolactin in men help sustain high intratesticular testosterone levels and affect the growth and secretions of the accessory sex glands. Hyperprolactinemia abolishes gonadotropin pulsatility by interfering with episodic GnRH release. Visible lesions are generally treated with transsphenoidal surgery, and nonvisible lesions are treated with bromocriptine, 5–10 mg daily, to restore normal pituitary balance.

2. Hypothyroidism—Both elevated and depressed levels of thyroid hormone can impair spermatogenesis. Replacement or removal of low or excessive thyroid hormone is effective treatment for infertility. As these diseases are clinically evident, routine thyroid screening is not recommended for infertility patients.

3. Congenital adrenal hyperplasia—Most commonly, the 21-hydroxylase enzyme is deficient resulting in cortisol deficiency and excess androgen production. The testes fail to mature because of gonadotropin inhibition due to excessive androgens. The diagnosis is rare and classically presents as precocious puberty; careful laboratory evaluation is essential. In both sexes, the condition and the infertility associated with it are treated with corticosteroids.

4. Testosterone excess/deficiency—Patients with Kallmann syndrome lack GnRH that stimulates normal pituitary function. Infertility associated with this condition can be very effectively treated with hCG, 1000–2000 U three times weekly, and recombinant FSH 75 IU twice weekly, to replace LH and FSH. It is also possible to give GnRH replacement in a pulsatile manner, 25–50 ng/kg every 2 hours, by a portable infusion pump. Individuals with fertile eunuch syndrome or isolated LH deficiency respond well to hCG therapy alone. One can expect to find sperm in the ejaculate beginning 9–12 months after therapy is started. Since injectable drug regimens are long, complex, and costly, it is good practice for men to cryopreserve motile sperm once achieved in the ejaculate. Anabolic steroids are a common and underdiagnosed reason for testicular failure in which excess exogenous testosterone and metabolites depress the pituitary–gonadal axis and spermatogenesis. Initially, the patient should discontinue the offending hormones to allow the return of normal homeostatic balance. Second-line therapy generally consists pituitary stimulation with clomiphene citrate (see later) or with testis stimulation with hCG and FSH as with Kallmann syndrome.

▶ Empiric Medical Therapy

Nearly a quarter of men evaluated for infertility will not have an identifiable cause. Because the pathophysiology is ill defined, this is termed idiopathic infertility. Additionally, other men in whom an abnormality is identified on semen analysis may have no specific target for therapy. Both groups of men are candidates for empiric medical therapy. This form of therapy seeks to overcome pathologic conditions that are ill defined or have no proven treatment. As a rule, it is important to establish a timeline of therapy and decide with the patient when empiric treatment is to be discontinued and other avenues pursued.

A. Clomiphene Citrate

Clomiphene citrate is a synthetic, nonsteroidal antiestrogen that blocks the action of the normally low levels of estrogen on the male hormone axis resulting in increased secretion of GnRH, FSH, and LH. The enhanced output of these hormones generally increases testosterone production and may improve spermatogenesis. Its use in male infertility treatment is "off-label," as it is FDA approved only for the treatment of female infertility. Clomiphene therapy is given for idiopathic low sperm count in the setting of low-normal LH, FSH, and testosterone levels. The dose is 12.5–50 mg/day either continuously or with a 5-day rest period each month. Serum gonadotropins and testosterone should be monitored at 3 weeks and the dose adjusted to keep the testosterone level within the normal range. Higher than normal testosterone levels may result in hyperestrogenemia and decreased semen quality. Therapy should be discontinued if no semen quality response is observed in 6 months. Although there have been more than 30 published trials on clomiphene since 1964, only a few include control arms. In general, the results of these studies have been equivocal with regard to the effectiveness of clomiphene citrate as an empiric therapy. Recent data have suggested that treatment of nonobstructive azoospermic men with clomiphene citrate may improve the odds of successful surgical sperm retrieval.

B. Antioxidant Therapy

There is evidence that up to 40% of infertile men have increased levels of reactive oxygen species in the reproductive tract. These species (OH, O_2 radicals, and hydrogen peroxide) can cause lipid peroxidation damage to sperm membranes that leads to deficits in sperm motility and overall function. Treatment with scavengers of these radicals may protect sperm from oxidative damage. Proposed agents have included glutathione, vitamin E, and fish oil. These agents may be useful in a subgroup of infertile men with elevated levels of seminal reactive oxygen species. Unfortunately, well-controlled studies demonstrating the effectiveness of these supplements are small or not available.

ASSISTED REPRODUCTIVE TECHNOLOGIES

If neither surgery nor medical therapy is appropriate for male infertility treatment, assisted reproductive techniques can be used to achieve a pregnancy. Generally speaking, ARTs represents the most profound implementation of empiric therapies.

▶ Intrauterine Insemination

IUI represents the least technological of all ARTs and is generally classified separately from *in vitro* fertilization. IUI involves the placement of a washed pellet of ejaculated sperm beyond the cervix, within the female uterus. The specific indication for IUI is for a cervical factor; if the cervix is bypassed, then pregnancies may ensue. IUI is also used for low sperm quality, for immunologic infertility, and in men with mechanical problems of sperm delivery (eg, hypospadias). IUI is commonly used for idiopathic infertility. There should be at least 5–40 million motile sperm in the ejaculate (volume × concentration × motility) to make this procedure worthwhile. Success rates vary widely and are directly related to female reproductive potential; given this, pregnancy rates of 8–16% per cycle have been reported with IUI as a treatment for male infertility. Success rates are improved if the female partner is treated with medication to stimulate ovulation.

▶ In Vitro Fertilization and ICSI (Figure 44–16)

In vitro fertilization involves controlled ovarian stimulation and ultrasound-guided transvaginal egg retrieval from the ovaries before normal ovulation occurs. Eggs are then combined with washed sperm in petri dishes to allow fertilization to occur. Importantly, significant numbers of postwash, motile sperm (500,000 to 5 million) are necessary for traditional IVF to be successful. In 1992, microscopic injection of a single sperm into the subzonal space of an egg to cause a pregnancy was described. This technology, termed ICSI, has revolutionized the treatment of severe male factor infertility. The sperm requirement for egg fertilization has dropped from hundreds of thousands for IVF to 1 viable sperm for ICSI. This has led to the development of aggressive new surgical techniques to provide sperm for egg fertilization from men with azoospermia. The availability of these techniques has pushed urologists to look beyond the ejaculate and into the male reproductive tract to find sperm for biologic pregnancies. At present, sources of sperm include the vas deferens, epididymis, and testicle. Since IVF and ICSI eliminate many natural selection barriers that exist during natural fertilization, genetic defects that caused the infertility are expected to be passed on to offspring. Because ICSI is a relatively new technique, long-term data concerning future health and fertility of children

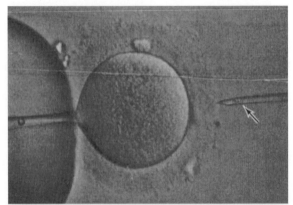
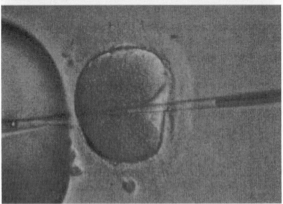

▲ **Figure 44–16.** The intracytoplasmic sperm injection procedure. (**Top**) A mature oocyte (left) is readied for injection with a sperm (**arrow**) in a micropipet under the microscope. (**Bottom**) The micropipet is placed directly into the oocyte, and the sperm is deposited into the cytoplasm.

conceived with ICSI is not yet available. Some studies have reported the increased incidence of hypospadias in babies conceived through ICSI. Furthermore, because some causes of male infertility are familial and related to genetic problems (Y microdeletions), male offspring may also suffer from impairments in spermatogenesis, inherited from their fathers.

▶ Preimplantation Genetic Diagnosis

Preimplantation genetic diagnosis is a specialized technique that enables the laboratory to precisely define the genetic normality of embryos. In patients with heritable, possibly life-threatening, diseases, it is possible that offspring conceived with IVF and ICSI may have these diseases transmitted to them. This complex technique involves the removal of single cells from the early embryo while it is grown in petri dishes before transfer to the uterus. The genetic material from these "biopsied" cells can then be examined to determine whether the embryo carries an abnormal chromosome or gene. Through preimplantation genetic diagnosis, early human embryos that result from IVF and ICSI can be individually examined as they develop for the presence or absence of suspected genetic traits. Because of the real-time nature of the technique, decisions regarding embryo transfer are made within 24 hours and help ensure that lethal diseases are not transmitted to offspring. Remarkably, the removal of a few cells from the embryo is not detrimental to the survival and normal development of most embryos.

▶ Nonreproductive Implications of Male Infertility

Beyond the significant psychosocial and marital stress, which is associated with male infertility, several epidemiologic studies have suggested that male infertility may be a marker for overall health. A large, longitudinal Danish study suggested that male fertility may be associated with overall longevity, whereby men with better semen quality may have lower age-adjusted mortality than men with worse semen quality. Other studies have demonstrated that male infertility is a strong risk factor for the development of testicular germ cell cancer later in life. A large US cohort study found that infertile men were nearly three times more likely to develop testis cancer, and on average, men presented with infertility more than a decade prior to developing cancer. Other studies have suggested that male subfertility may be risk factor for prostate cancer; however, these studies have yet to be confirmed and further investigation is warranted. While male infertility and its treatments are unlikely to be causative with regard to cancer, it is highly likely that these diseases share a common underlying etiology. Given that men present with reproductive failure relatively early in life, the epidemiologic study of infertile men may provide the opportunity to identify and remove exposure to carcinogenic agents.

BIBLIOGRAPHY

Male Reproductive Physiology

Aitken RJ et al: Leukocytic infiltration into the human ejaculate and its association with semen quality, oxidative stress, and sperm function. J Androl 1994;15:343. [PMID: 7982803]

Gui YL et al: Male hormonal contraception: Suppression of spermatogenesis by injectable testosterone undecanoate alone or with levonorgestrel implants in Chinese men. J Androl 2004;25:720. [PMID: 15292101]

Hess RA et al: A role for estrogens in the male reproductive system. Nature 1997;390:509. [PMID: 9393999]

Von Eckardstein S et al: Serum inhibin B in combination with FSH is a more sensitive marker than FSH alone for impaired spermatogenesis in men, but cannot predict the presence of sperm in testicular tissue samples. J Clin Endocrinol Metab 1999;84(7): 2496. [PMID: 10404826]

Diagnosis of Male Infertility

Agarwal A et al: Clinical relevance of oxidative stress in male factor infertility: An update. Am J Reprod Immunol 2008;59:2. [PMID: 18154591]

Carlsen E et al: Evidence for decreasing quality of semen during the past 50 years. Br Med J 1992;105:609. [PMID: 1393072]

Carlsen E et al: History of febrile illness and variation in semen quality. Hum Reprod 2003;18:2089. [PMID: 14507826]

Chemes HE: Phenotypes of sperm pathology: Genetic and acquired forms in infertile men. J Androl 2000;21:799. [PMID: 11105905]

Clifton DK, Bremner WJ: The effect of testicular X-irradiation on spermatogenesis in man: A comparison with the mouse. J Androl 1983;4:387. [PMID: 6654753]

Gandini L et al: Effect of chemo- or radiotherapy on sperm parameters of testicular cancer patients. Hum Reprod 2006;21:2882. [PMID: 16997940]

Guzick DS et al: Sperm morphology, motility and concentration in fertile and infertile men. N Engl J Med 2001;345:1388. [PMID: 11794171]

Hammoud AO et al: Impact of male obesity on fertility: A critical review of the current literature. Fertil Steril 2008;90:897. [PMID: 18929048]

Jarow JP et al: Male Infertility Best Practice Policy Committee of the American Urological Association Inc. J Urol 2002;167:2138. [PMID: 11956464]

Kruger TF et al: Predictive value of abnormal sperm morphology in in vitro fertilization. Fertil Steril 1988;49:112. [PMID: 3335257]

Meinertz H et al: Antisperm antibodies and fertility after vasovasostomy: A follow-up study of 216 men. Fertil Steril 1990;54:315. [PMID: 2379630]

Sallmen M et al: Reduced fertility among overweight and obese men. Epidemiology 2006;17:520. [PMID: 16837825]

Sigman M, Jarow JP: Medical evaluation of infertile men. Urology 1997;50:659. [PMID: 9372871]

Smith JF et al: Ejaculatory duct obstruction. Urol Clin North Am 2008;35(2):221 [PMID: 18423242]

Turek PJ et al: Diagnostic findings from testis fine needle aspiration mapping in obstructed and non-obstructed azoospermic men. J Urol 2000;163:1709. [PMID: 10799166]

Turek PJ: Practical approach to the diagnosis and management of male infertility. Nat Clin Pract Urol 2005;2:1.

Urban MD et al: Adult height and fertility in men with congenital virilizing adrenal hyperplasia. N Engl J Med 1978;299:1392. [PMID: 152409]

Walsh TJ et al: Increased risk of testicular germ cell cancer among infertile men. Arch Intern Med 2009;169(4):351. [PMID: 19237718]

World Health Organization: WHO Laboratory Manual for the Examination of Human Semen and Sperm-Cervical Mucus Interaction, 4th edn. Cambridge University Press, Cambridge, 2009, pp. 60–61.

Xu WM et al: Cystic fibrosis transmembrane conductance regulator is vital to sperm fertilizing capacity and male fertility. Proc Natl Acad Sci U S A 2007;104(23):9816. [PMID: 17873061]

Zini A et al: Prevalence of abnormal sperm DNA denaturation in fertile and infertile men. Urology 2002;60:1069. [PMID: 12475672]

Causes of Male Infertility—Pretesticular

Aiman J et al: Androgen insensitivity as a cause of infertility in otherwise normal men. N Engl J Med 1979;300:223. [PMID: 7598691]

Carter JN et al: Prolactin-secreting tumors and hypogonadism in 22 men. N Engl J Med 1978;299:847. [PMID: 211411]

Fujisawa M et al: Growth hormone releasing hormone test for infertile men with spermatogenetic maturation arrest. J Urol 2002;168:2083. [PMID: 12394714]

Goffin V et al: Prolactin: The new biology of an old hormone. Annu Rev Physiol 2002;64:47. [PMID: 11826263]

Griffin JE: Androgen resistance: The clinical and molecular spectrum. N Engl J Med 1992;326:611. [PMID: 1734252]

Oliveira LMB et al: The importance of autosomal genes in Kallmann syndrome: Genotype-phenotype correlations and neuroendocrine characteristics. J Clin Endocrinol Metab 2001;86:1532. [PMID: 11297579]

Wu SM, Chan WY: Male pseudohermaphroditism due to inactivating luteinizing hormone receptor mutations. Arch Med Res 1999;30:495. [PMID: 10714363]

Causes of Male Infertility—Testicular

Aiman J, Griffin JE: The frequency of androgen receptor deficiency in infertile men. J Clin Endocrinol Metab 1982;54:725. [PMID: 6801070]

Hopps CV et al: Detection of sperm in men with Y chromosome microdeletions of the AZFa, AZFb and AZFc regions. Hum Reprod 2003;18:1660. [PMID: 12871878]

Kostiner DR et al: Male infertility: Analysis of the markers and genes on the human Y chromosome. Hum Reprod 1998;13:3032. [PMID: 9853850]

Lipshultz LI et al: Testicular function after orchiopexy for unilaterally undescended testis. N Engl J Med 1976;295:15. [PMID: 5671]

Nagler HM et al: Testicular torsion: Temporal considerations. Fertil Steril 1984;42:257. [PMID: 6745459]

Richardson I et al: Outcomes of varicocele treatment: An updated critical analysis. Urol Clin North Am 2008;35:191. [PMID: 18423240]

Walsh TJ et al: Prepubertal orchidopexy for cryptorchidism may be associated with lower risk of testicular cancer. J Urol 2007;178:1440. [PMID: 17706709]

Walsh TJ et al: Differences in the clinical characteristics of primarily and secondarily infertile men with varicocele. Fertil Steril 2009;91:826 [PMID: 18314114]

World Health Organization: The influence of varicocele on parameters of fertility in a large group of men presenting to infertility clinics. Fertil Steril 1992;57:1289. [PMID: 1601152]

Causes of Male Infertility—Posttesticular

Chillon M et al: Mutations in the cystic fibrosis gene in patients with congenital absence of the vas deferens. N Engl J Med 1995;332:1475. [PMID: 7739684]

Handelsman DJ et al: Young's syndrome: Obstructive azoospermia and chronic sinopulmonary infections. N Engl J Med 1984;310:3. [PMID: 6689737]

Matsuda T et al: Obstructive azoospermia of unknown origin: Sites of obstruction and surgical outcomes. J Urol 1994;151:1543. [PMID: 8189567]

Genetic Causes of Male Infertility

Anguiano A et al: Congenital bilateral absence of the vas deferens: A primarily genital form of cystic fibrosis. JAMA 1992;267:1794. [PMID: 1545465]

Kenti-First MG et al: Infertility in intracytoplasmic-sperm-injection-derived sons. Lancet 1996;348:332. [PMID: 8709700]

Kurda-Kawaguchi T et al: The AZFc region of the Y chromosome features massive palindromes and uniform recurrent deletions in infertile men. Nat Genet 2001;29:279. [PMID: 11687796]

Prycr JL et al: Microdeletions in the Y chromosome of infertile men. N Engl J Med 1997;336:534. [PMID: 9023089]

Reijo R et al: Diverse spermatogenic defects in humans caused by Y chromosome deletions encompassing a novel RNA-binding protein gene. Nat Genet 1995;10:383. [PMID: 7670487]

Walsh TJ et al: The genetics of male infertility. Semin Reprod Med 2009;27(2):124 [PMID: 19247914]

Xu EY et al: A gene family required for human germ cell development evolved from an ancient meiotic gene conserved in metazoans. Proc Natl Acad Sci U S A 2001;98:7414. [PMID: 11390979]

Treatment of Male Infertility

Baker WHG et al: Protective effect of antioxidants on the impairment of semen motility by activated polymorphonuclear leukocytes. Fertil Steril 1996;65:411. [PMID: 8566272]

Belker AM et al: Results of 1,469 microsurgical vasectomy reversals by the vasovasostomy study group. J Urol 1991;145:505. [PMID: 1997700]

Bennett CJ et al: Sexual dysfunction and electroejaculation in men with spinal cord injury: Review. J Urol 1988;139:453. [PMID: 3278126]

Branigan EF, Muller CH: Efficacy of treatment and recurrence rate of leukocytospermia in infertile men with prostatitis. Fertil Steril 1994;62:580. [PMID: 7520396]

Cayan S et al: Response to varicocelectomy in oligospermic men with and without defined genetic infertility. Urology 2001;57:530. [PMID: 11248633]

Cayan S et al: Can varicocelectomy significantly change the way couples use assisted reproductive technologies? J Urol 2002;167:1749. [PMID: 11912402]

Cox G et al: Intracytoplasmic sperm injection may increase the risk of imprinting defects. Am J Hum Genet 2002;71:162. [PMID: 12016591]

Damani MN et al: Post-chemotherapy ejaculatory azoospermia: Fatherhood with sperm from testis tissue using intracytoplasmic sperm injection. J Clin Oncol 2002;20:930. [PMID: 11844813]

DeBaun M et al: Association of in vitro fertilization with Beckwith-Wiedemann syndrome and epigenetic alterations of LIT1 and H19. Am J Hum Genet 2003;72:156. [PMID: 12439823]

Eisenberg ML et al: Ejaculatory duct manometry in normal men and in patients with ejaculatory duct obstruction. J Urol 2008;180:255. [PMID: 18499178]

Eisenberg ML et al: Racial differences in vasectomy utilization in the United States: Data from the national survey of family growth. Urology 2009;74:1020. [PMID 19773036]

Evers JLH, Collins JA: Assessment of efficacy of varicocele repair for male subfertility: A systematic review. Lancet 2003;361:1849. [PMID: 12788571]

Fuchs EF, Burt RA: Vasectomy reversal performed 15 years or more after vasectomy: Correlation of pregnancy outcome with partner age and with pregnancy results of in vitro fertilization with intracytoplasmic sperm injection. Fertil Steril 2002;77:516. [PMID: 11872205]

Guzick DS et al: Efficacy of superovulation and intrauterine insemination in the treatment of infertility. National Cooperative Reproductive Medicine Network. N Engl J Med 1999;340:177. [PMID: 9895397]

Haas GG Jr, Manganiello P: A double-blind, placebo-controlled study of the use of methylprednisolone in infertile men with sperm-associated immunoglobulins. Fertil Steril 1987;47:295. [PMID: 3545909]

Hendry WF et al: Comparison of prednisolone and placebo in subfer-tile men with antibodies to spermatozoa. Lancet 1990;335:85. [PMID: 1967425]

Kadioglu A et al: Does response to treatment of ejaculatory duct obstruction in infertile men vary with pathology? Fertil Steril 2001;76:138. [PMID: 11438332]

Madgar I et al: Controlled trial of high spermatic vein ligation for varicocele in infertile men. Fertil Steril 1995;63:120. [PMID: 7805900]

Matthews GJ et al: Patency following microsurgical vasoepididymostomy and vasovasostomy: Temporal considerations. J Urol 1993;154:2070. [PMID: 7500460]

Meng M et al: Surgery or assisted reproduction? A decision analysis of treatment costs in male infertility. J Urol 2005;174:1926. [PMID: 16217347]

Ovesen P et al: Growth hormone treatment of subfertile males. Fertil Steril 1996;66:292. [PMID: 8690119]:2272. [PMID: 17509339].

Yang G et al: The kinetics of the return of motile sperm to the ejaculate after vasectomy reversal. J Urol 2007;177(6):2272–2276.

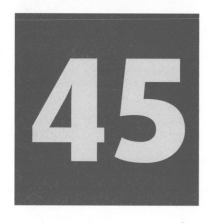

The Aging Male

James F. Smith, MD, MS, & Thomas J. Walsh, MD, MS

INTRODUCTION

The proportion of individuals older than 65 years will rise significantly over the next 25 years. According to US census data, the number of Americans older than 65 years will rise from approximately 35 million today (12.4% of all Americans) to nearly 55 million in 2020 (16.3% of total), and nearly 87 million in 2050 (20.7% of total). As a consequence, the health care system will likely experience a dramatic increase in age-related health problems, such as cancer, cerebrovascular and ischemic heart disease, and hormone deficiency. A substantial body of literature supports the assertion that hormonal changes in the aging male can be associated with significant health problems. This chapter reviews the epidemiology of testosterone deficiency in older men; alterations in testis biology that occur with age; and the effects that these changes may have on semen quality, fertility, birth defects in offspring, and on the overall health of older men.

EPIDEMIOLOGY

Hypogonadism may affect up to 4 million Americans, with a minority receiving treatment. From a population standpoint, the effect of aging on circulating testosterone levels is highly significant. The Baltimore Longitudinal Study of Aging (BLSA) found that 12%, 20%, 30%, and 50%, respectively, of men in their 50s, 60s, 70s, and 80s were hypogonadal using a total serum testosterone threshold of 325 ng/dL. Age has been shown to be an independent risk factor for hypogonadism even after adjustment for chronic medical conditions, such as obesity, diabetes mellitus, and hyperthyroidism.

CHANGES IN TESTIS BIOLOGY WITH AGE

▶ The Endocrine Testis

A. Leydig Cells

The quest to understand the underlying mechanism behind the epidemiological and clinical observations that aging men experience a gradual decline in testosterone levels led to the analysis of Leydig cell populations in human testes. Leydig cells produce 95% of adult male testosterone and are found in the interstitial space between seminiferous tubules. Kaler and Neaves (1978), in a study of testes retrieved at autopsy after sudden death among men aged 18–87, noted that total Leydig cell volume declines significantly with age and that decline is directly proportional to a fall in the total number of Leydig cells. From such studies, it is estimated that a pair of young testes (20-year-old) contains 700 million Leydig cells and undergoes an attrition of about 80 million cells per decade of life. Other studies have also shown that serum luteinizing hormone (LH) levels are significantly higher in older men compared with younger men, providing physiologic corroboration of the Leydig cell studies.

B. Testosterone

Although the decline of testosterone levels in older males has been described by the terms andropause, male climacteric, male menopause, late onset hypogonadism (LOH), and partial androgen deficiency in the aging male (PADAM), only LOH and PADAM accurately reflect these changes. Serum testosterone levels in men fall progressively from the third decade to the end of life, primarily due to the decline in testicular Leydig cell mass. This decline may be associated with changes in the circadian rhythm and hypothalamic–pituitary homeostatic control of LH secretion, which regulates testosterone production. Thus, mechanisms exist both at the testicular and hypothalamic–pituitary levels that may result in decreased testosterone with age.

Testosterone exists in several different forms in plasma, with each having different bioactivity (Figure 45–1). Free or unbound testosterone is fully bioavailable, but protein-bound testosterone is only partly bioavailable. Among protein-bound forms, albumin-bound testosterone is more freely bioavailable than sex hormone-binding globulin (SHBG)-bound testosterone, which is considered an inactive form of testosterone (Figure 45–2). Population-based studies have demonstrated that aging and several medical comorbidities are

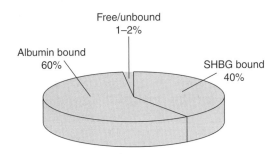

▲ **Figure 45–1.** Relative amounts of various forms of testosterone in the blood. Albumin-bound testosterone is considered "bioavailable" and has physiologic activity, but the SHBG-bound testosterone is chemically unavailable. SHBG, sex hormone-binding globulin.

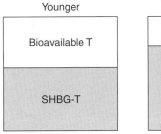
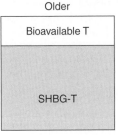

▲ **Figure 45–3.** Changes in sex hormone-binding globulin (SHBG) with age. Although total testosterone levels may be similar in younger and older men, there is less "available" testosterone due to an increase in SHBG with age. T, testosterone.

associated with an increase in SHBG. This increase in SHBG leads to increased binding to and inactivation of testosterone, lowering the levels of bioavailable androgens (Figure 45–3). Fifty percent of men older than 60 years have below normal levels of non–SHBG-bound testosterone. The age-related onset, rate, and degree of change in testosterone production are all variable; however, a general rule of thumb is that mean testosterone levels decrease approximately 1% annually after the age of 50. Indeed, the concentration of bioavailable testosterone in men decreases by as much as 50% between the ages of 25 and 75 years. In contrast, dihydrotestosterone (DHT) and estradiol levels (a primary metabolite of testosterone and potent androgen) show minimal and mild declines, respectively, as men age.

▶ The Exocrine Testis

A. Sertoli Cells

Age-related declines in Sertoli cells have been observed in anatomical studies. These studies revealed that Sertoli cell

populations in the young adult male testis have approximately 500 million Sertoli cells compared with 300 million for older men (Table 45–1). Concurrent declines in testicular mass and the numbers of round spermatids have also been observed.

SPERMATOGENESIS

▶ Production

The changes that occur in the seminiferous tubules with age include a decrease in total volume of the testis occupied by seminiferous tubules and a decrease in actual tubule length. Calculations of mature sperm production in testis tissue homogenates also suggest that daily sperm production decreases significantly with age (Table 45–2). The age-related decrease in sperm production in older testes appears to result from a decrease in primary spermatocytes or a decrease in spermatogonial proliferation rather than cellular degeneration. Correspondingly, follicle-stimulating hormone (FSH) levels increase significantly with age, with mean values threefold higher in older men than in younger men.

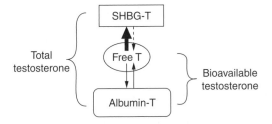

▲ **Figure 45–2.** Diagram outlining the various forms of testosterone in the blood. Total testosterone includes all forms of the hormone, both free and bound. The affinity of sex hormone-binding globulin (SHBG) for testosterone is much higher (*thick arrow*) than that of albumin. Available forms of testosterone that exert physiologic activity include free and albumin-bound fractions. T, testosterone.

Table 45–1. Comparison of Sertoli cells and germ cells in younger and older men.

Testis parameter	Age range	
	20–48 years	50–85 years
Average testis weight	19 g	16 g
No. of Sertoli cells/testis	503 million	312 million
No. of round spermatids	55 million/g testis	41 million/g testis
No. of spermatids/Sertoli cell	4.0	4.3

Data from Johnson L et al: Quantification of human Sertoli cell population: Its distribution, relation to germ cell numbers and age-related decline. Biol Reprod 1984;31:785.

Table 45–2. Age-related changes in seminiferous tubules and sperm production.

Testis parameter	Age range	
	20–48 years	50–90 years
Paired testis weight	41 g	31 g
Seminiferous tubule volume	24 mL/person	18 mL/person
Daily sperm production	250 million	121 million

Data from Johnson L et al: Age-related variations in seminiferous tubules in men. A stereologic evaluation. J Androl 1986;7:316.

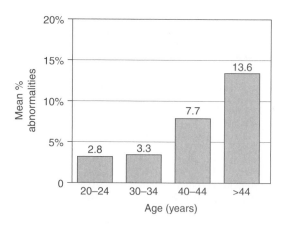

▲ **Figure 45–4.** Incidence of sperm chromosomal structural anomalies by paternal age. (Data from Martin RH, Rademaker AW: The effect of age on the frequency of sperm chromosomal abnormalities in normal men. Am J Hum Genet 1987;41:484.)

Semen Quality

Although an age-related decrease in semen quality might be expected from calculated changes in testis biology with age, this has not been obvious to demonstrate clinically. Cross-sectional studies have observed both decreased and unchanged ejaculated sperm concentrations in older versus younger men. However, most studies show that sperm motility is consistently lower in older men compared with younger men, with a decrease of approximately 0.7% motility per year after the third decade. These declines can be difficult to attribute to age, given the wide variability in semen analysis results between repeated samples from the same individual and the lack of prospective, population-based studies to confirm the findings found in cross-sectional analyses.

Fertility

The effect of paternal age on fertility is controversial. Studies that address this issue are confounded by the variables of the aging female partner and decreased coital frequency that occurs with age. Despite these limitations, several studies have demonstrated delays in the time to achieve a pregnancy in men older than 35 compared with men younger than 30, even after controlling for maternal age. Advancing paternal age has also been implicated as a risk factor for developmental and chromosomal abnormalities in their offspring. The mechanism of these declines is not yet clear; however, researchers have demonstrated that increased levels of reactive oxygen species are found in the semen of older men in addition to higher levels of genetic abnormalities.

Genetics

A. Sperm Chromosomal Anomalies

Early sperm cytogenetic studies in fertile men stratified by age showed a 10% overall incidence of sperm chromosomal abnormalities, but no relationship between paternal age and the frequency of numerical abnormalities (aneuploidy) in sperm chromosomes. Recent studies using more sensitive fluorescence in situ hybridization (FISH) technology have

shown more subtle paternal age effects on sperm aneuploidy. Interestingly, paternal age appears to increase the fraction of sperm with sex chromosomal aneuploidies. Even more pronounced is the highly significant positive, linear relationship demonstrated between paternal age and the frequency of structural anomalies in sperm ($r = 0.63$, Figure 45–4).

It is possible that continued cell divisions that characterize spermatogenesis place the germ cells at risk for chromosomal injury, especially given the extended exposure to clastogens, such as reactive oxygen species, that occur with age. However, it is important to realize that studies of live newborns or prenatally diagnosed fetuses do not support the assertion that de novo structural chromosomal anomalies, with the exception of inherited reciprocal translocations, are found more commonly in the offspring of older men.

B. Sperm Genetic Mutations

Single gene defects in sperm can result from errors in the DNA replication process. Numerous studies have cataloged the association between advanced paternal age and new cases of conditions associated with single gene deletions (Table 45–3). One mechanism for the development of new single gene mutations with advanced paternal age implicates the characteristic and continuous process of spermatogonial cell division in spermatogenesis. By puberty, 30 cell divisions of spermatogonia have occurred, resulting in a large pool of undifferentiated cells. After puberty, 23 divisions per year occur; in a 35-year-old man, these cells will have undergone 540 divisions. The simple fact that the spermatogonial stem cells of older men having undergone numerous cell divisions may make them more likely to contain errors in DNA transcription, the source of single gene defects.

Table 45–3. Selected genetic disorders associated with advanced paternal age.

Achondroplasias	Aniridia
Apert syndrome	Bilateral retinoblastoma
Crouzon syndrome	Fibrodysplasia ossificans
Hemophilia A	Lesch-Nyhan syndrome
Marfan syndrome	Neurofibromatosis
Oculodentodigital syndrome	Polycystic kidney disease
Polyposis coli	Progeria
Treacher-Collins syndrome	Tuberous sclerosis
Waardenburg syndrome	

Table 45–4. Testosterone effects in the normal male.

Target organ	Effects
Male sex organs	Growth, development, maintenance of secondary sex characteristics, sperm production, erections, and prostatic function
Behavior	Improved libido, mood, memory, and energy
Bone	Linear growth, closure of the epiphyses, and increased bone mineral density
Fat tissue	Body and visceral fat reduction
Muscle	Anabolic; increases muscle mass and possibly strength
Liver	Stimulates production of serum proteins
Kidney	Stimulates erythropoietin production
Heart	Causes coronary vasodilation
Blood	Suppression of clotting factors (II, V, VII), low HDL-cholesterol
Bone marrow	Stimulates stem cell production
Hair	Influences body hair growth, especially facial hair

C. Paternal Age and Birth Defects and Disease in Offspring

There is little doubt of the association between advanced paternal age and an increased probability of autosomal-dominant diseases in offspring (Table 45–3). This risk of autosomal mutations due to advanced paternal age has been quantified by investigators who demonstrated that for men aged 40–44, the risk of a mutation occurring in offspring was 4.5 per 1000 births compared with 0.22 per 1000 births among men younger than 29. Analogously, aneuploid conceptions associated with female age demonstrate a similar pattern. It has been suggested that this underlying genetic mechanism may explain the consistent association between paternal age and schizophrenia found among offspring from a range of countries around the world.

Paternal age has been the source of several studies of anatomic birth defects. One demonstrated that paternal age older than 40 was associated with a 20% increase in the incidence of having offspring with a serious birth defect, such as situs inversus, atrial septal defects, or ventricular septal defects. Because of these relationships, guidelines for sperm donors recommend that donors be younger than 50 years.

THE DIAGNOSIS OF ANDROGEN DEFICIENCY

▶ Organ System Effects of Testosterone

Testosterone affects an impressively varied number of target organs. In the brain, it may modulate or influence aspects of cognition, mood, sexual interest (ie, libido), and male aggression. Cognitively, verbal memory, visual-spatial skills, and memory have been improved in older men taking testosterone replacement therapy. Testosterone stimulates production of erythropoietin and stem cells in the kidney and bone marrow, while in bone, testosterone causes accelerated linear growth and closure of epiphyses for prepubertal

males. Testosterone is responsible for an increase in muscle strength and growth. Among young males, testosterone allows for maturation of sexual organs and penile growth. In postpubertal males, endogenous testosterone enhances spermatogenesis and supports prostatic growth and function. The male external appearance is influenced by testosterone as it induces specific body hair growth patterns, temporal balding, and other secondary characteristics. Consequently, normal male growth, maturation, and reproductive and sexual function are strongly influenced by testosterone levels (Table 45–4).

In 2002, the National Institute on Aging and the United States National Cancer Institute charged the Institute of Medicine (IOM) with conducting an analysis of the effects of testosterone replacement in aging men. This report summarized many of the effects testosterone treatment has on a wide range of organ systems. They found that significant declines in testosterone (and estradiol) are associated with bone loss in men. Despite this, the IOM report found insufficient evidence to conclude that fracture risk was higher among hypogonadal aging men. Consistent studies have demonstrated increased lean muscle mass in men receiving testosterone supplementation; however, these studies have not always demonstrated subsequent improvements in muscle strength. Although some evidence exists to support a link between cognitive improvements after testosterone replacement, clinical trials have not consistently demonstrated a benefit. This pattern was also seen for the relationship between mood, depression, and testosterone levels. Some studies have demonstrated benefit, while others have been equivocal. Studies suggest that currently depressed men were more likely to benefit from testosterone replacement. By stimulating erythropoietin production, testosterone replacement increases the red blood cell production (hematocrit) in aging men. Low testosterone levels are significantly associated with hypertension, atherogenic lipid profiles, prothrombotic factors, and type 2 diabetes, all important cardiovascular risk factors. Despite this association with cardiovascular risk factors, no studies have conclusively demonstrated that testosterone replacement alters cardiovascular morbidity or mortality.

Specific aspects of sexual function can improve with testosterone replacement. Most studies support the relationship between libido and testosterone levels. Testosterone replacement has more consistent effects on improving libido than on erectile function. Erectile dysfunction in older men can result from endothelial dysfunction, decreased penile vascular supply (eg, atherosclerotic changes in penile arteries), neurological abnormality (eg, diabetes, surgery for pelvic cancer), or psychological or relationship difficulties. Although testosterone can occasionally be an effective treatment for erectile dysfunction in the hypogonadal men, specific treatments for erectile dysfunction are available. More recent data suggest that androgen replacement therapy and type 5 selective phosphodiesterase inhibitors (PDEI-5s) may work synergistically to improve erectile function, or that a threshold testosterone level must be achieved for PDEI-5s to work effectively.

► Patient History and Examination

Given the wide range of organs affected by testosterone levels, it is no surprise that the PADAM syndrome is characterized by a variety of nonspecific physical and intellectual alterations. Because of this complexity, most clinicians agree that symptoms or physical findings need to accompany the laboratory demonstration of low testosterone to consider treatment for PADAM.

A. Symptoms

Adult onset of hypogonadism can result in loss of or a decrease in libido, loss of nocturnal erections, loss of body hair, and reduced muscle strength. A decrease in sexual frequency can often accompany the decrease in sexual desire. Flushes and/or sweating, breast discomfort or gynecomastia, and infertility are also more specific symptoms of testosterone deficiency. Symptoms that are less specific to hypoandrogenism include fatigue, depression, declines in memory or other cognitive function, increased body fat, diminished work performance, and sleep disturbances.

B. Signs

Examination of the man with suspected hypogonadism may reveal breast tenderness or gynecomastia, a decline in lean body mass with associated reduced muscle volume and strength and increases in visceral fat (abdominal girth). Decreased or thinning facial and chest hair and skin alterations such as increases in facial wrinkling and pale-appearing skin suggestive of anemia may also be noted. Anemia tends to be mild and of a normochromic, normocytic type. Low bone mineral density with osteopenia or osteoporosis can also be associated with low circulating testosterone levels. Examination of the genitalia may reveal testicular atrophy with either reduced testis volume or soft consistency may exist.

The diagnosis of PADAM does not require all of these symptoms and signs to be present. However, for many men, the natural process of aging, underlying depression or other mood disorders, or other medical comorbidities can be associated with many of these characteristics. For example, studies have demonstrated that frailty with aging is a major socioeconomic and health care problem that can reduce independent living. Symptoms typical of testosterone deficiency such as decreased mood, impaired cognition, loss of muscle strength, and bone fractures can all be found in older men despite normal testosterone levels. Despite these observations, the association of such symptoms with documentation of testosterone deficiency implicates PADAM as a possible underlying etiology.

► Laboratory Findings

There is considerable debate as to what laboratory test should be ordered to diagnose androgen deficiency in aging men. For most men, a total serum testosterone obtained between 7 and 11 AM along with a serum SHBG are the two initial tests. A recently published consensus statement supported the diagnosis of testosterone deficiency for serum testosterone values lower than 230 ng/dL (8 nmol/L). For serum testosterone levels less than 150 ng/dL (5.2 nmol/L), serum prolactin should be obtained to evaluate the possibility of a prolactinoma. Values between 230 and 350 ng/dL (8–12 nmol/L) should be confirmed with additional testing with a repeat serum total testosterone, bioavailable testosterone, free testosterone, or calculated free testosterone (using SHBG, serum albumin, and total testosterone; www.issam.ch/freetesto.htm). These confirmatory tests are important to quantify all of the non–SHBG-bound testosterone. Although reference ranges for bioavailable and free testosterone have been published, these have not been rigorously validated. Reference ranges are not age dependent, as testosterone effects on end organs are the same regardless of a man's age. Free testosterone levels measured by equilibrium dialysis are generally reliable but less available than the analog displacement assay. This assay, though widely available, is not a reliable measure of free testosterone. If the measured or calculated active or bioavailable testosterone levels are normal in this situation, then androgen deficiency is unlikely. A working management algorithm for the laboratory diagnosis of androgen deficiency is outlined in Figure 45–5. Currently, the assessment

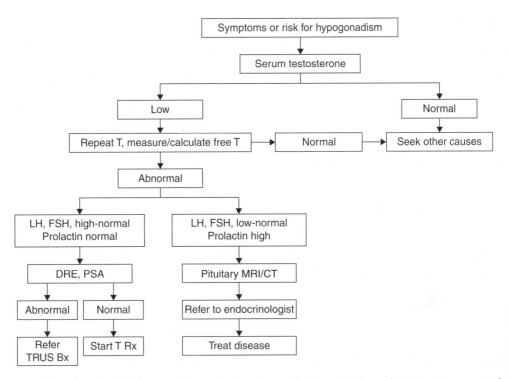

▲ **Figure 45–5.** Algorithm for the laboratory diagnosis of androgen deficiency in the male. T, testosterone; LH, luteinizing hormone; FSH, follicle-stimulating hormone; TRUS Bx, transrectal ultrasound and prostate biopsy; MRI, magnetic resonance imaging; CT, computed tomography scan.

of levels of testosterone metabolites (eg, DHT, estradiol, and dihydroandrosteindione [DHEA]) is not recommended or helpful in the diagnosis of androgen deficiency. An assessment of red blood cell mass with a hemoglobin or hematocrit may be helpful to confirm hypogonadal anemia and is important to establish a baseline prior to the initiation of treatment.

▶ Radiological Testing

As hypogonadism is frequently associated with low bone mineral density and a higher fracture risk, baseline hip and spine bone densitometry should be obtained. Although plain-films x-rays have been used in the past to assess bone mineral density, the DEXA scan is currently the most accurate method. This is an enhanced form of x-ray technology, termed dual-energy x-ray absorptiometry (DXA or DEXA) that is a quick and noninvasive procedure for measuring bone loss. The DEXA machine sends low-dose x-rays with two distinct energy peaks through the body. One peak is absorbed mainly by soft tissue and the other by bone. Soft tissue absorption is subtracted from the total absorption, resulting in calculated levels of bone absorption that are converted into bone density equivalents. The amount of

radiation used is extremely small—less than one-tenth the dose of a standard chest x-ray. Portable devices are also available that measure the wrist, fingers, or heel and are sometimes used for screening. The test is scored in two ways: (1) the T score is the amount of bone present compared with a young adult of the same gender with normal bone mass. A score above −1 is considered normal. A score between −1 and −2.5 is classified as osteopenia, the first stage of bone loss. A score below −2.5 is defined as osteoporosis and can be used to estimate the risk of developing a fracture; (2) the Z score reflects the amount of bone present compared with others of similar age, size, and gender. Regardless of treatment chosen, bone density assessments should be repeated in 1–2 years to determine whether adequate bone mass is maintained.

TREATMENT OF ANDROGEN DEFICIENCY

▶ Formulations

The primary aims of testosterone replacement treatment for PADAM is to restore eugonadal levels of testosterone and ameliorate symptoms and signs of low testosterone, while minimizing the potential for side effects of these treatments.

Table 45–5. Types of testosterone replacement therapy available in the United States.

Available preparation	Formula	Dose	Specific risk	Retail cost
Parenteral	Testosterone cypionate Testosterone enanthate	100–400 mg IM every 2–3 weeks	Deep IM injection. Gives supraphysiologic peaks and low trough hormone levels; mood fluctuations	Cypionate: $112/10 cc (200 mg/cc) Enanthate: $100/5 cc (200 mg/cc)
Transdermal patch	Testoderm (scrotal) Testoderm TTS Androderm	4–6 mg/day 5 mg/day	Scrotal patch: requires daily shaving, variable absorption Nonscrotal patch: high incidence of skin welts at placement site	Androderm 2.5 g, 60 patches $320 5 g, 30 patches $340
Testosterone pellet	Testopel (pellets inserted subQ through 5 mm incision in abdomen with local anesthesia)	(Available as 75 mg/pellet; initial placement is 8–10 pellets q 3–4 months)	Local site infections, extravasation, mood swings, elevated hematocrit	$60/ pellet
Transdermal gel	AndroGel, Testim (applied to clean, dry skin of arm, back, thigh)	2.5–5 mg/day 5 mg/day	Transference of hormone to partner or children. Musky odor (Testim)	Testim 1%, 30 tubes (5 g/tube) $330 Androgel, 30 tubes (5 g/tube) $325 Androgel pump, 120 pumps (1.25 g/pump) $325

IM, intramuscular.

Four major types of hormone replacement are available in the United States: oral, injectable, transdermal, and buccal mucosal systems (Table 45–5). The most popular formulations are the transdermal gels, injectables, and transdermal patches, in that order. Oral testosterone replacement is associated with an unacceptably high rate of liver toxicity and should no longer be used. More than 95% of prescribed testosterone medication is administered through a transdermal or injectable route. Risks of specific testosterone formulations are summarized in Table 45–5, while general risks are summarized in the next section.

▶ **Risks**

Cardiovascular disease: A relationship between cardiovascular disease (CAD) and elevated testosterone levels was proposed on the basis of a higher incidence of cardiovascular events among men compared with women; however, several studies have demonstrated that this relationship is not causal. In fact, several studies have demonstrated that higher testosterone levels may decrease the risk of CAD. Furthermore, studies of testosterone replacement for hypogonadal men have not revealed an increased risk of CAD. Despite these reassuring findings, the long-term effects of testosterone replacement on cardiovascular functioning are yet to be determined.

Lipid profiles: Although supraphysiologic doses of testosterone, particularly oral nonaromatizable androgenic steroids, appear to lower HDL levels, numerous studies have demonstrated that physiologic doses of testosterone do not have a significant effect on HDL, total cholesterol, and LDL levels. Testosterone formulation does not appear to alter these relationships.

Polycythemia: Evidence suggests that testosterone levels are associated with erythropoiesis. Pubertal boys experience a 15–20% increase in hemoglobin levels in conjunction with increasing testosterone levels. Hypogonadal men often have mild anemia that is improved with testosterone therapy, and testosterone replacement therapy in men with normal hemoglobin levels can result in supraphysiologic hemoglobin levels. The utilization of testosterone injections is most often associated with this side effect.

Spermatogenesis and infertility: Exogenous testosterone of any type generally leads to spermatogenic arrest through negative feedback inhibition of both pituitary LH and FSH secretion. Azoospermia occurs in >90% of patients within 10 weeks. With cessation, sperm levels rebound usually within 18 months, but some patients may remain azoospermic. Patients receiving hormone replacement therapy should be informed that fertility will be impaired on this treatment.

Hepatotoxicity: Liver toxicity has been reported with oral administration of methyl testosterone and fluoxymesterone; however, it is only rarely observed with parenteral, transdermal, and transbuccal formulations. Testosterone undecanoate is an oral testosterone formulation that does not appear to increase hepatic toxicity, but it is not available in the United States.

Prostate cancer: Since Huggins first described the relationship between suppression of testosterone levels and regression of prostate cancers in the 1940s, treatments designed to reduce testosterone levels have been used to treat advanced prostate cancer. For many years, the question of increasing the risk of prostate cancer with testosterone supplementation has been unanswered. Early case reports suggested that testosterone therapy unmasked occult prostate cancers. Larger, prospective studies, however, have failed to confirm these anecdotal observations. In fact, the preponderance of evidence would suggest that testosterone replacement therapy is not associated with an increased risk of prostate cancer. Despite these reassuring data, proper monitoring with digital rectal examinations and serum prostate specific antigen (PSA) levels are important to diagnose any occult prostate cancers that may occur after initiating testosterone replacement therapy.

Benign prostatic hyperplasia: It is known that prostatic enlargement is an androgen-dependent process. Chemical or surgical castration causes a clear decrease in the volume of prostate tissue. Testosterone replacement therapy has been associated with an increase in prostate volume to a level similar to that of eugonadal men. Despite these findings, no changes in urinary flow rate, lower urinary tract symptoms, or postvoid residuals have been noted with testosterone treatment. Furthermore, a higher rate of urinary retention has not been noted with this treatment. However, it is prudent to monitor voiding symptoms as a standard part of routine monitoring.

Exacerbation of sleep apnea: Testosterone therapy can worsen preexisting sleep apnea. Although not a cause of sleep apnea, testosterone can exacerbate the problem in patients predisposed to the condition (ie, elderly men, obese men, and patients with chronic obstructive pulmonary disease). All potential patients should be questioned for sleep-related breathing disorders before androgen replacement is considered. This side effect appears to be dose related. A centrally mediated mechanism has been postulated, as no upper airway changes have been noted in men taking testosterone therapy who develop worsening sleep apnea.

Fluid and electrolyte disturbances: Water retention is known to occur with androgen therapy. In aging men, it can lead to hypertension, peripheral edema, or exacerbation of congestive heart failure. Moreover, retention of sodium, chloride, potassium, calcium, and inorganic phosphates can occur. Weight and blood pressure monitoring are important for at-risk patients.

Gynecomastia or breast tenderness: Painful breast enlargement due to elevated levels of estrogen (a metabolite of testosterone) frequently develops, and may occasionally persist, in patients on testosterone therapy. Estrogen receptor blockers can be used to treat this side effect.

Miscellaneous: Local skin irritation is commonly reported with the use of the testosterone patch. Acne, headaches, emotional lability, insomnia, and hot flushes have been reported with testosterone therapy. The transfer of testosterone to significant others after gel application is minimized by washing the skin site 10 minutes after application. A component of Testim gel, pentadecalactone, has a musky odor that some men find unappealing. Transbuccal formulations (Striant) may cause gingivitis, stinging of the lips, toothache, and has a bitter taste. Despite these side effects, 60% of men when given the option preferred to continue with a transbuccal treatment approach.

▶ Contraindications and Precautions

Testosterone replacement therapy should not be given to men with prostate cancer, breast cancer, and/or untreated melanoma, as this treatment may increase the growth of these tumors. For men with bladder outlet obstruction related to severe benign prostatic hypertrophy and severe sleep apnea, testosterone replacement therapy should be administered with caution as these symptoms may be exacerbated with this treatment.

At present, there is insufficient evidence to justify the use of testosterone supplementation (not replacement) in men of any age with low-normal but not truly "androgen-deficient" testosterone levels. The IOM consensus statement from 2003 concluded that there was insufficient evidence to justify the use of testosterone therapy for widespread, generalized use for preventing age-related disease or to enhance strength or mood in otherwise healthy older men.

▶ Monitoring Treatment

Testosterone replacement for PADAM is normally a lifelong treatment. Monitoring of the patient with PADAM should be performed at baseline, at 1–2 months after initiating treatment, at intervals of 3–6 months during the first year, and annually thereafter. A digital rectal examination, serum PSA and hematocrit/hemoglobin determination, assessment of voiding function, and sleep apnea are mandatory at the baseline evaluation (Table 45–6). Within a month or two after treatment is started, the efficacy of treatment and serum testosterone levels should be assessed. As testosterone levels can fluctuate, particularly after intramuscular (IM) administration, clinical indicators may be a better guide for adjusting the dose of testosterone. During the first year of therapy, patients should be followed every 3–6 months to assess clinical and biochemical response, with serial digital rectal examinations and PSA levels if they are older than 40 years. The history and physical examination at these time points should evaluate the presence of gynecomastia, urinary side effects, and changes in degree of sleep apnea. After the first year, patients who remain stable may subsequently be followed annually. Annual evaluations should include testosterone, hemoglobin, liver function tests, lipid profile, and PSA measurements. Bone density and psychological evaluations should be performed depending on the initial indications for androgen supplementation.

Table 45–6. Patient monitoring before and during testosterone treatment.

Time period	Indicated assessment
Baseline (pretreatment)	Hgb, HCT, and PSA level Digital rectal exam Ascertain symptoms of voiding dysfunction and sleep apnea Consider DEXA scan for bone mineral density
1-2 months of treatment	Assess treatment efficacy: testosterone level and symptom relief. Consider adjusting dose for either variable
3-6 month intervals during first year	Assess symptomatic response to treatment, voiding symptoms and sleep apnea Perform physical exam with DRE and obtain testosterone, LFTs, lipid profile, PSA, and Hgb levels
Annually after first year	Assess symptomatic response to treatment, voiding symptoms, and sleep apnea Perform physical exam with DRE and obtain testosterone, LFTs, lipid profile, PSA, and Hgb levels

DEXA, dual-energy x-ray absorptiometry. DRE, digital rectal exam; Hgb, hemoglobin; HCT, hematocrit; LFTs, liver function tests; PSA, prostate specific antigen.

FUTURE TREATMENTS FOR ANDROGEN DEFICIENCY

▶ 5α-Dihydrotestosterone

The natural androgen 5α-DHT is a metabolite of testosterone, resulting from the conversion of testosterone to 5α-DHT by 5-alpha reductase in the scrotum and skin. One of its primary benefits is that it is a very potent androgen, binding to androgen receptors more tightly than testosterone, but is not converted to estrogen. It is currently available in Europe as a gel application and creates a steady state within 2–3 days of application. Trials have demonstrated improvements in sexual function and lean muscle mass with its use; paradoxically, a decline in prostate volume has been observed after this therapy. This may be due to the fact that estrogens may work synergistically with androgens to cause prostatic growth with age and DHT, as a selective androgen, may result in lower estrogen levels during treatment.

▶ Selective Androgen Receptor Modulators

Selective androgen receptor modulators (SARMs) offer a theoretical advantage of tissue specificity. Animal models have demonstrated promising results and early clinical trials in humans are underway.

▶ Selective Estrogen Receptor Modulators

Treatment with selective estrogen receptor modulators (SERMs), such as clomiphene citrate (Clomid™), has demonstrated significant improvements in hypogonadal symptoms in men with secondary hypogonadism. In one recent randomized trial, the majority of men treated with clomiphene reported improvements in sexual function and gonadotropin levels. A second study demonstrated improvements in serum testosterone levels. This treatment can be an effective treatment for hypogonadism in men who desire to preserve fertility. Importantly, since SERMs act by stimulating the hypothalamic–pituitary–gonadal axis, this form of therapy will only be effective among men with sufficient Leydig cell mass to respond to increased secretion of gonadotropins.

▶ Human Chorionic Gonadotropin

Human chorionic gonadotropin (hCG) can increase the production of testosterone by binding to Leydig cells and stimulating the release of testosterone. Injections with 1000–2000 IU two to three times per week can result in significant increases in serum testosterone levels. For some men, this treatment can also improve spermatogenesis and, as noted for clomiphene citrate, is a good choice for hypogonadal men wishing to preserve fertility.

▶ 7α-methyl-19-nortestosterone

This medication, also known as MENT, is ten times more potent than testosterone, is not bound to SHBG, and is aromatized to estradiol, but does not undergo 5α-reduction to DHT. It has been shown to enhance sexual function with minimal prostatic effect. Lean muscle mass paradoxically declined at high doses with associated increases in prostatic volume.

▶ Dehydroepiandrosterone

DHEA is available in over-the-counter formulations in the United States. DHEA is a steroid hormone made by the adrenal gland and exhibits a progressive decline in serum levels beginning the third decade of life and beyond. As a consequence of this decline, studies have attempted to correlate levels of DHEA and DHEA sulfate with a myriad of health conditions. Clinical trials that have investigated the DHEA for multiple conditions have shown largely inconsistent findings. Placebo-controlled studies suggest that doses of 30–50 mg of oral DHEA may produce physiologic androgen levels.

Clinical trials suggest that 50 mg of oral DHEA, but not <30 mg, can increase serum androgen levels to within the physiologic range for young adults with primary and secondary adrenal insufficiency, and improve sexual function, mood and self-esteem, and decrease fatigue/exhaustion. Although DHEA replacement therapy may be effective in patients with adrenal insufficiency, its efficacy in aging males is not well established.

BIBLIOGRAPHY

Changes in Testis Biology with Age

Eskenazi B et al: The association of age and semen quality in healthy men. Hum Reprod 2003;18:447. [PMID: 12571189]

Ford WCL et al: Increasing paternal age is associated with delayed conception in a large population of fertile couples: Evidence for declining fecundity in older men. Hum Reprod 2000;15:1703. [PMID: 10920089]

Johnson L et al: Quantification of human Sertoli cell population: Its distribution, relation to germ cell numbers and age-related decline. Biol Reprod 1984;31:785. [PMID: 6509142]

Johnson L et al: Age-related variations in seminiferous tubules in men. A stereologic evaluation. J Androl 1986;7:316. [PMID 3771369]

Kaler LW, Neaves WB: Attrition of the human Leydig cell population with advancing age. Anat Rec 1978;92:513. [PMID: 736271]

Malaspina D et al: Advancing paternal age and the risk of schizophrenia. Arch Gen Psychiatry 2001;58:361. [PMID:11296097]

Martin RH, Rademaker AW: The effect of age on the frequency of sperm chromosomal abnormalities in normal men. Am J Hum Genet 1987;41:484. [PMID: 3631081]

The Diagnosis of Androgen Deficiency

AACE Hypogondadism Task Force. American Association of Clinical Endocrinologists Medical Guidelines for Clinical Practice for the Evaluation and Treatment of Hypogonadism in Adult Male Patients-2002 Update. 2002. Available at: http://www.aace.com/pub/pdf/guidelines/hypogonadism.pdf, 2009.

Arver S, Lehtihet M: Current guidelines for the diagnosis of testosterone deficiency. Front Horm Res 2009;37:5–20.

Calof OM et al: Adverse events associated with testosterone replacement in middle-aged and older men: A meta-analysis of randomized, placebo-controlled trials. J Gerontol A Biol Sci Med Sci 2005;60:1451. [PMID: 16339333]

Center JR et al: Mortality after all major types of osteoporotic fracture in men and women: An observational study. Lancet 1999;353;878. [PMID: 10093980]

Cherrier MM et al: Cognitive changes associated with supplementation of testosterone or dihydrotestosterone in mildly hypogonadal men: A preliminary report. J Androl 2003;24:568. [PMID: 12826696]

Fisch H: Older men are having children, but the reality of a male biological clock makes this trend worrisome. Geriatrics 2009;64(1):14–17.

Harman SM et al: Longitudinal effects of aging on serum total and free testosterone levels in healthy men. Baltimore Longitudinal Study of Aging. J Clin Endocrinol Metab 2001;86:724. [PMID: 11158037]

Harman SM et al: Longitudinal effects of aging on serum total and free testosterone levels in healthy men. Baltimore Longitudinal Study of Aging. J Clin Endocrinol Metab 2001;86(2):724–731.

Kouri EM et al: Changes in lipoprotein-lipid levels in normal men following administration of increasing doses of testosterone cypionate. Clin J Sport Med 1996;6:152. [PMID: 8792045]

Pfeil E, Dobs AS: Current and future testosterone delivery systems for treatment of the hypogonadal male. Expert Opin Drug Deliv 2008;5(4):471–481.

Rhoden EL, Morgantaler A: Risks of testosterone-replacement therapy and recommendations for monitoring. N Engl J Med 2004;350:482. [PMID: 14749457]

Seftel AD: Male hypogonadism. Part I: Epidemiology of hypogonadism. Int J Impot Res 2006;18(2):115–120.

Seftel A: Male hypogonadism. Part II: Etiology, pathophysiology, and diagnosis. Int J Impot Res 2006;18(3):223–228.

Snyder PJ et al: Effect of testosterone treatment on bone mineral density in men over 65 years of age. J Clin Endocrinol Metab 1999;84:1966. [PMID: 10372695]

Wang C et al: Testosterone replacement therapy improves mood in hypogonadal men—A clinical research center study. J Clin Endocrinol Metab 1996;8:3578. [PMID: 8855804]

Wang C et al: Investigation, treatment and monitoring of late-onset hypogonadism in males: ISA, ISSAM, EAU, EAA and ASA recommendations. Eur J Endocrinol 2008;159(5):507–514.

Whitsel EA et al: Intramuscular testosterone esters and plasma lipids in hypogonadal men: A meta-analysis. Am J Med 2001;111:261. [PMID: 11566455]

Normal Laboratory Values*

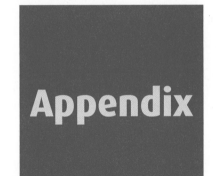

Appendix

Jack W. McAninch, MD, FACS, FRCS(E)(Hon)

Values may vary with method of measurement and population.

HEMATOLOGY

Antithrombin III: [P] 86–120%

Bleeding time: Template method, 3–9 minutes (180–540 seconds)

Cellular measurements of red blood cells (erythrocytes):

Average diameter = 7.3 μm (5.5–8.8 μm)

Mean corpuscular volume (MCV): Men, 80–94 fL; women, 81–99 fL (by Coulter counter)

Mean corpuscular hemoglobin (MCH): 27–32 pg

Mean corpuscular hemoglobin concentration (MCHC): 32–36 g/dL; erythrocytes (32–36%)

Color, saturation, and volume indices: 1 (0.9–1.1)

Clot retraction: Begins in 1–3 hours; complete in 6–24 hours. No clot lysis in 24 hours.

Fibrin D-dimer: [P] 0–250 ng/mL

Fibrinogen split products: <10 μg

Fragility of erythrocytes: Begins at 0.45–0.38% NaCl; complete at 0.36–0.3% NaCl

Glucose-6-phosphate dehydrogenase (G6PD): [B] 4–8 μg/g Hb

Hematocrit (PCV): Men, 40–52%; women, 37–47%

Hemoglobin: [B] Men, 14–18 g/dL (2.09–2.79 mmol/L as Hb tetramer); women, 12–16 g/dL (1.86–2.48 mmol/L). [S] 2–3 mg/dL

Partial thromboplastin time: Activated, 25–37 seconds

Platelets: 150,000–400,000/mL (0.15–0.4 × 10^{12}/L)

Prothrombin: International normalized ratio (INR), 1–1.4

Erythrocyte count: Men, 4.5–6.2 million/μL (4.5–6.2 × 10^{12}/L); women, 4–5.5 million/μL (4–5.5 × 10^{12}/L)

Reticulocytes: 0.6–1.8% of erythrocytes

Sedimentation rate: <20 mm/h (Westergren)

White blood count (leukocytes) and differential: 5,000–10,000/μL (5–10 × 10^{9}/L)

Segmented neutrophils	40–70%
Myelocytes	0%
Juvenile neutrophils	0%
Band neutrophils	0–15%
Lymphocytes	15–45%
Eosinophils	1–3%
Basophils	0–5%
Monocytes	0–7%

Lymphocytes: Total, 1500–4000/μL	
B cell	5–25%
T cell	60–88%
Suppressor	10–43%
Helper	32–66%
H:S	>1

BLOOD, PLASMA, OR SERUM CHEMICAL CONSTITUENTS (Values vary with method used)

Acetone and acetoacetate: [S] 0.3–2 mg/dL (3–20 mg/L)

Aldolase: [S] Values vary with method used.

α-Amino acid nitrogen: [S, fasting] 3–5.5 mg/dL (2.2–3.9 mmol/L)

Aminotransferases:

Aspartate aminotransferase (AST; SGOT): [S] 15–55 IU/L

Alanine aminotransferase (ALT; SGPT): [S] 10–70 IU/L. Values vary with method used.

---

*Blood [B], Plasma [P], Serum [S], Urine [U].

Ammonia: [B] 9–33 µmol/L

Amylase: [S] 80–180 units/dL (Somogyi). Values vary with method used.

α₁-Antitrypsin: [S] >180 mg/dL

Ascorbic acid: [P] 0.4–1.5 mg/dL (23–85 33 µmol/L)

Base, total serum: [S] 145–160 mEq/L (145–160 mmol/L)

Bicarbonate: [S] 24–28 mEq/L (24–28 mmol/L)

Bilirubin: [S] Total, 0.2–1.2 mg/dL (3.5–20.5 µmol/L). Direct conjugated, 0.1–0.4 mg/dL (<7 µmol/L). Indirect, 0.2–0.7 mg/dL (<12 µmol/L).

Calcium: [S] 8.5–10.3 mg/dL (2.1–2.6 mmol/L). Values vary with albumin concentration.

Calcium, ionized: [S] 4.25–5.25 mg/dL; 2.1–2.6 mEq/L (1.05–1.3 mmol/L)

β-Carotene: [S, fasting] 50–300 µg/dL (0.9–5.58 µmol/L)

Ceruloplasmin: [S] 25–43 mg/dL (1.7–2.9 µmol/L)

Chloride: [S or P] 96–106 mEq/L (96–106 mmol/L)

Cholesterol: [S or P] 150–240 mg/dL (3.9–6.2 mmol/L). (See Lipid fractions.) Values vary with age.

Cholesteryl esters: [S] 65–75% of total cholesterol

CO_2 content: [S or P] 24–29 mEq/L (24–29 mmol/L)

Complement: [S] C3 (b1C), 90–250 mg/dL. C4 (β₁E), 10–60 mg/dL. Total (CH_{50}), 75–160 mg/dL

Copper: [S or P] 100–200 µg/dL (16–31 µmol/L)

Cortisol: [P] 8:00 AM, 5–25 µg/dL (138–690 nmol/L); 8:00 PM, <14 µg/dL (385 nmol/L)

Creatine kinase (CK): [S] 10–50 IU/L at 30°C. Values vary with method used.

Creatine kinase MB fraction: [S] <4% total CK

Creatinine: [S or P] 0.7–1.5 mg/dL (62–132 µmol/L)

Cyanocobalamin: [S] 200 pg/mL (148 pmol/L)

Epinephrine: [P] Supine, <0.1 µg/L (<0.55 nmol/L)

Erythropoietin: [S] 5–20% IU/L

Ferritin: [S] Adult women, 20–120 ng/mL; men, 30–300 ng/mL. Child to 15 years, 7–140 ng/mL.

α-Fetoprotein: [S] 0–8.5 ng/mL

Folic acid: [S] 2–20 ng/mL (4.5–45 nmol/L). [Erythrocytes] >100 ng/mL (>318 nmol/L)

Glucose: [S or P] 65–110 mg/dL (3.6–6.1 mmol/L)

α-Glutamyl transpeptidase: [S] 8–78 IU/L

Glycosylated hemoglobin (HbA_{10}): [B] 4–7%

Haptoglobin: [S] 40–200 mg of hemoglobin-binding capacity

Iron: [S] 40–175 µg/dL (9–31.3 µmol/dL)

Iron-binding capacity: [S] Total, 250–410 µg/dL (44.7–73.4 µmol/L). Percent saturation, 20–55%.

Lactate: [B, special handling] Venous, 4–16 mg/dL (0.44–1.8 mmol/L)

Lactate dehydrogenase (LDH): [S] 55–140 IU/L. Values vary with method used.

Lipase: [S] 0.2–1.5 U

Lipid fractions: [S or P] Desirable levels: High-density lipoprotein (HDL) cholesterol, >40 mg/dL; low-density lipoprotein (LDL) cholesterol, <150 mg/dL; VLDL cholesterol, <40 mg/dL. (To convert to mmol/L, multiply by 0.026.)

Lipids, total: [S] 450–1000 mg/dL (4.5–10 g/L)

Magnesium: [S or P] 1.8–3 mg/dL (0.75–1.25 mmol/L)

Myoglobin: [P] 15–100 ng/mL

Norepinephrine: [P] Supine, <0.5 µg/L (<3 nmol/L)

Osmolality: [S] 280–296 mOsm/kg water

Oxygen:

    Capacity: [B] 16–24 vol%. Values vary with hemoglobin concentration.

    Arterial content: [B] 15–23 vol%. Values vary with hemoglobin concentration.

    Arterial % saturation: 94–100% of capacity

    Arterial P_{O_2} (Pa_{O_2}): 80–100 mm Hg (10.67–13.33 kPa) (sea level). Values vary with age.

Pa_{CO_2}: [B, arterial] 35–45 mm Hg (4.7–6 kPa)

pH (reaction): [B, arterial] 7.35–7.45 (H^+ 44.7–45.5 nmol/L)

Phosphatase, acid: [S] 1–5 U (King-Armstrong), 0.1–0.63 U (Bessey-Lowry)

Phosphatase, alkaline: [S] 38–126 IU/L

Phospholipid: [S] 145–200 mg/dL (1.45–2 g/L)

Phosphorus, inorganic: [S, fasting] 3–4.5 mg/dL (1–1.5 mmol/L)

Potassium: [S or P] 3.5–5 mEq/L (3.5–5 mmol/L)

Prostate-specific antigen (PSA): [S] 0–4 ng/mL

Protein:

    Total: [S] 6–8 g/dL (60–80 g/L)

    Albumin: [S] 3.5–5.5 g/dL (35–55 g/L)

    Globulin: [S] 2–3.6 g/dL (20–36 g/L)

    Immunoglobulin: [S] IgA 78–400 mg/dL. IgG 690–1400 mg/dL. IgM 35–240 mg/dL

    Fibrinogen: [P] 0.2–0.6 g/dL (2–6 g/L)

Prothrombin clotting time: [P] By control. INR, 1–1.4.

Pyruvate: [B] 0.6–1 mg/dL (70–114 mmol/L)

Serotonin: [B] 0.05–0.2 µg/mL (0.28–1.14 µmol/L)

Sodium: [S or P] 136–145 mEq/L (136–145 mmol/L)

Specific gravity: [B] 1.056 (varies with hemoglobin and protein concentration). [S] 1.0254–1.0288 (varies with protein concentration).

Sulfate: [S or P] As sulfur, 0.5–1.5 mg/dL (156–468 µmol/L)

Transferrin: [S] 200–400 mg/dL (23–45 µmol/L)

Triglycerides: [S] <165 mg/dL (1.9 mmol/L). (See Lipid fractions.)

Troponin: [S] <0.5 ng/mL

Urea nitrogen: [S or P] 8–25 mg/dL (2.9–8.9 mmol/L). Do not use anticoagulant-containing ammonium oxalate.

Uric acid: [S or P] Men, 3–9 mg/dL (0.18–0.54 mmol/L); women, 2.5–7.5 mg/dL (0.15–0.45 mmol/L)

Vitamin A: [S] 15–60 µg/dL (0.53–2.1 µmol/L)

Vitamin B$_{12}$: [S] >200 pg/mL (>148 pmol/L)

Vitamin D: [S] Cholecalciferol (D$_3$): 25-hydroxycholecalciferol, 8–55 ng/mL (19.4–137 nmol/L); 1,25-dihydroxycholecalciferol, 26–65 pg/mL (62–155 pmol/L); 24,25-dihydroxycholecalciferol, 1–5 ng/mL (2.4–12 nmol/L)

Volume, blood (Evans blue dye method): Adults, 2990–6980 mL. Women, 46.3–85.5 mL/kg; men, 66.2–97.7 mL/kg.

Zinc: [S] 50–150 µg/dL (7.65–22.95 µmol/L)

HORMONES, SERUM, OR PLASMA

Adrenal:

Aldosterone: [P] Supine, normal salt intake, 2–9 ng/dL (56–250 pmol/L); increased when upright.

Cortisol: [S] 8:00 AM, <5–20 µg/dL (0.14–0.55 µmol/L); 8:00 PM, <10 µg/dL (0.28 µmol/L)

Deoxycortisol: [S] After metyrapone, >7 µg/dL (>0.2 µmol/L)

Dopamine: [P] <135 pg/mL

Epinephrine: [P] <0.1 ng/mL (<0.55 nmol/L)

Norepinephrine: [P] <0.5 µg/L (<3 nmol/L). See also Miscellaneous Normal Values.

Gonad:

Testosterone, free: [S] Men, 10–30 ng/dL; women, 0.3–2 ng/dL. (1 ng/dL = 0.035 nmol/L)

Testosterone, total: [S] Prepubertal, <100 ng/dL; adult men, 300–1000 ng/dL; adult women, 20–80 ng/dL; luteal phase, up to 120 ng/dL

Estradiol (E$_2$): [S, special handling] Men, 12–34 pg/mL; women, menstrual cycle 1–10 days, 24–68 pg/mL; 11–20 days, 50–300 pg/mL; 21–30 days, 73–149 pg/mL (by radioimmunoassay [RIA]). (1 pg/mL = 3.6 pmol/L)

Progesterone: [S] Follicular phase, 0.2–1.5 ng/mL; luteal phase, 6–32 ng/mL; pregnancy, >24 ng/mL; men, <1 ng/mL (by RIA). (1 ng/mL = 3.2 nmol/L)

Islets:

Insulin: [S] 4–25 µU/mL (29–181 pmol/L)

C-peptide: [S] 0.9–4.2 ng/mL

Glucagon: [S, fasting] 20–100 pg/mL

Kidney:

Renin activity: [P, special handling] Normal sodium intake: Supine, 1–3 ng/mL/h; standing, 3–6 ng/mL/h. Sodium depleted: Supine, 2–6 ng/mL/h; standing, 3–20 ng/mL/h

Parathyroid: Parathyroid hormone levels vary with method and antibody. Correlate with serum calcium.

Pituitary:

Growth hormone (GH): [S] Adults, 1–10 ng/mL (46–465 pmol/L) (by RIA)

Thyroid-stimulating hormone (TSH): [S] <10 µU/mL

Follicle-stimulating hormone (FSH): [S] Prepubertal, 2–12 mIU/mL; adult men, 1–15 mIU/mL; adult women, 1–30 mIU/mL; castrate or postmenopausal, 30–200 mIU/mL (by RIA)

Luteinizing hormone (LH): [S] Prepubertal, 2–12 mIU/mL; adult men, 1–15 mIU/mL; adult women, <30 mIU/mL; castrate or postmenopausal, >30 mIU/mL

Corticotropin (ACTH): [P] 8:00–10:00 AM, up to 100 pg/mL (22 pmol/L)

Prolactin: [S] 1–25 ng/mL (0.4–10 nmol/L)

Somatomedin C: [P] 0.4–2 U/mL

Antidiuretic hormone (ADH; vasopressin): [P] Serum osmolality 285 mOsm/kg, 0–2 pg/mL; >290 mOsm/kg, 2–12+ pg/mL

Placenta:

Estriol (E$_3$): [S] Men and nonpregnant women, <0.2 µg/dL (<7 nmol/L) (by RIA)

Chorionic gonadotropin: [S] β-Subunit: Men, <9 mIU/mL; pregnant women after implantation, >10 mIU/mL

Stomach:

Gastrin: [S, special handling] Up to 100 pg/mL (47 pmol/L). Elevated, >200 pg/mL

Pepsinogen I: [S] 25–100 ng/mL

Thyroid:

Thyroxine, free (FT$_4$): [S] 0.8–2.4 ng/dL (10–30 pmol/L)

Thyroxine, total (TT$_4$): [S] 5–12 µg/dL (65–156 nmol/L) (by RIA)

Thyroxine-binding globulin capacity (T$_4$): [S] 12–28 µg/dL (150–360 nmol/L)

Triiodothyronine (T$_3$): [S] 80–220 ng/dL (1.2–3.3 nmol/L). Reverse triiodothyronine (rT$_3$): [S] 30–80 ng/dL (0.45–1.2 nmol/L).

Triiodothyronine uptake (rT$_3$U): [S] 25–36%; as TBG assessment (rT$_3$U ratio), 0.85–1.15.

Calcitonin: [S] <100 pg/mL (<29.2 pmol/L)

NORMAL CEREBROSPINAL FLUID VALUES

Appearance: Clear and colorless.

Cells: Adults, 0–5 mononuclear cells/µL; infants, 0–20 mononuclear cells/µL

Glucose: 50–85 mg/dL (2.8–4.7 mmol/L). (Draw serum glucose at same time.)

Pressure (reclining): Newborns, 30–88 mm water; children, 50–100 mm water; adults, 70–200 mm water (avg = 125)

Proteins: Total, 20–45 mg/dL (200–450 mg/L) in lumbar cerebrospinal fluid. IgG, 2–4 mg/dL (0.02–0.04 g/L)

Specific gravity: 1.003–1.008

RENAL FUNCTION TESTS

ρ-Aminohippurate (PAH) clearance (RPF): Men, 560–830 mL/min; women, 490–700 mL/min

Creatinine clearance: Calculation from serum creatinine:

Men: $\dfrac{(140 - age) \times (wt\ in\ kg)}{72 \times serum\ creatinine\ mg/dL}$ = creatinine clearance mL/min

Women: calculated mg/dL × 0.85

Creatinine clearance, endogenous (GFR): Approximates inulin clearance (see below).

Inulin clearance (GFR): Men, 110–150 mL/min; women, 105–132 mL/min (corrected to 1.73 m^2 surface area)

Maximal glucose reabsorptive capacity (Tm_G): Men, 300–450 mg/min; women, 250–350 mg/min

Maximal PAH excretory capacity (Tm_{PAH}): 80–90 mg/min

Osmolality: On normal diet and fluid intake: Range 500–850 mOsm/kg water. Achievable range, normal kidney: Dilution 40–80 mOsm; concentration (dehydration) up to 1400 mOsm/kg water (at least three to four times plasma osmolality).

Specific gravity of urine: 1.003–1.030

MISCELLANEOUS NORMAL VALUES

Adrenal hormones and metabolites:

Aldosterone: [U] 2–26 μg/24 h (5.5–72 nmol). Values vary with sodium and potassium intake.

Catecholamines: [U] Total, <100 μg/24 h. Epinephrine, <10 μg/24 h (<55 nmol); norepinephrine, <100 μg/24 h (<591 nmol). Values vary with method used.

Cortisol, free: [U] 20–100 μg/24 h (0.55–2.76 mmol)

11,17-Hydroxycorticoids: [U] Men, 4–12 mg/24 h; women, 4–8 mg/24 h. Values vary with method used.

17-Ketosteroids: [U] <8 years, 0–2 mg/24 h; adolescents, 2–20 mg/24 h. Men, 10–20 mg/24 h; women, 5–15 mg/24 h. Values vary with method used. (1 mg = 3.5 mmol)

Metanephrine: [U] <1.3 mg/24 h (<6.6 μmol) or <2.2 μg/mg creatinine. Values vary with method used.

Vanillylmandelic acid (VMA): [U] Up to 7 mg/24 h (<35 μmol).

Fecal fat: <30% dry weight

Lead: [U] <80 μg/24 h (<0.4 μmol/d)

Porphyrins:

δ-Aminolevulinic acid: [U] 1.5–7.5 mg/24 h (11.4–57.2 μmol)

Coproporphyrin: [U] <230 μg/24 h (<345 nmol)

Uroporphyrin: [U] <50 μg/24 h (<60 nmol)

Porphobilinogen: [U] <2 mg/24 h (<8.8 μmol)

Urobilinogen: [U] 0–2.5 mg/24 h (<4.23 μmol)

Urobilinogen, fecal: 40–280 mg/24 h (68–474 μmol)

Index

Note: Page numbers followed by f and t denotes figure and table repectively.